GUIDE TO PSYCHIATRY

GUIDE TO PSYCHIATRY

MYRE SIM
M.D. (Edin.), F.R.C.P.E., F.R.C. Psych., D.P.M.
Consultant Psychiatrist, United Birmingham Hospitals
and Midland Centre for Neurosurgery and Neurology.
Lecturer in Psychiatry, University of Birmingham

Third Edition

with a chapter on
LEGAL ASPECTS OF PSYCHIATRY
in the United States of America
by JOHN DONNELLY
M.D., F.R.C. Psych. (G.B.), F.A.C.P., F.A.P.A.
Psychiatrist-in-Chief, Institute of Living, Hartford, Conn., U.S.A.

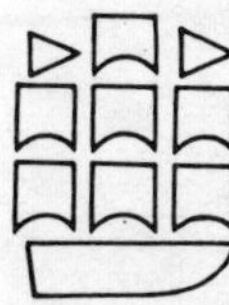

CHURCHILL LIVINGSTONE
Edinburgh and London 1974

CHURCHILL LIVINGSTONE
Medical Division of Longman Group Limited

Distributed in the United States of America by Longman Inc., New York, and by associated companies, branches and representatives throughout the world.

First Edition 1963
Second Edition 1968
Reprint 1969
Third Edition 1974

ISBN 0 443 01161 3

Library of Congress Catalog Card Number 73-94257

PRINTED IN GREAT BRITAIN BY
T.&A. CONSTABLE, LTD., EDINBURGH

COMPUTER TYPESETTING BY PRINT ORIGINATION
BOOTLE, LANCS, L20 6NS

Preface to the Third Edition

The favourable reception of the Second Edition, which was reprinted, would suggest that the format and style of the 'Guide' is acceptable and that it would be unwise to make radical changes. I have had several requests to alter chapter headings such as 'Mental Deficiency' and 'Psychopathic Personality', to bring them into line with the latest 'classification'. If these changes were really based on scientific advances, there would be good reason to comply, but they are merely changes in words in deference to an unduly sensitive attitude to the previous terms by a few psychiatrists and some members of the public. I can see no real advantage in substituting 'Subnormality' or 'Retardation' for 'Deficiency', or 'Personality Disorder' for 'Psychopathic Personality', or 'Sexual Deviation' for 'Psychopathia Sexualis'.

The old legal maxim: 'When it is not necessary to change, it is necessary not to change', is more commendable than being a slave to fashion. Changes in names do not change a condition. If the condition is debased in the public mind, the change in words merely debases more words and does little, if anything, to improve the social situation; it may even retard progress.

Developments in psychiatry continue, so that the whole text has had to be revised and updated and in certain chapters this has also meant considerable additions with a regrettable but necessary increase in size. Another area of growth is the section dealing with references. Many readers have told me how useful they find them, so there should be no complaint about that. I have also rewritten the entire index, for it had many glaring omissions and I, like some critics, have frequently been exasperated, knowing that an item was in the text but failing to find it in the index. This, too, has added to the size of the 'Guide', but is, I consider, fully justified.

Overall, the third edition is a considerable improvement on its predecessors, and this is due, in no small part, to the many helpful suggestions and criticisms I have had from students, colleagues and reviewers.

MYRE SIM

BIRMINGHAM, 1974

Preface to the First Edition

Not only is psychiatry a rapidly expanding subject, but its role in the teaching and practice of medicine is rapidly changing. Medical students, who at one time received only a few demonstrations of the grosser psychotic states, are now given a comprehensive course in psychiatry which extends from the pre-clinical to the final and even pre-registration years. In many medical schools there is more formal instruction in psychiatry for undergraduates than used to be provided in post-graduate courses for the diploma in psychological medicine.

Textbooks of psychiatry tended to fall into two groups: small ones for the medical student and general practitioner, and large ones for the would-be specialist. But psychiatry is no longer the isolated speciality it once was, and general practitioners, physicians, surgeons and paediatricians have need of a guide which not only gives them access to psychiatric literature, but which also provides a frank appraisal of current theory and practice. There are others, for example, in social science and psychology, whose work demands of them more than a superficial knowledge of certain aspects of psychiatry, and while there are many excellent monographs and works of reference, a reasonably small and comprehensive guide should meet their needs for a handy 'bench book'. Library facilities for the undergraduate have improved considerably, and medical students are encouraged to refer to original papers, and critically assess them. They, too, should be offered a guide to psychiatry which is in keeping with the present accent on medical education.

In the wide field that is now covered by psychiatry, it is difficult to know what and how much to include. If one were to be partisan in the traditional sense, this 'Guide' would point to either dynamic or organic psychiatry, but the needs of the patient frequently demand a practitioner with a knowledge of both. With the increasing integration of the psychiatrist in the work of the general hospital, he should be familiar with the organic problems his colleagues will refer to him. He should also be able to provide an expert dynamic outlook in assessment and treatment, for in that field lies his unique contribution to medical practice. Due emphasis has therefore been given to both sides.

To those who use this 'Guide' to study for examinations, either undergraduate or post-graduate, I make a special plea. Do not confine your reading to the text, but extend it also to the references. One can acquire a superficial knowledge of a place by reading about it in a guide-book, but to practise psychiatry effectively and enjoy it, the habit of reading the literature should be cultivated from one's first introduction to the subject.

I beg the reader's pardon for the above exhortation, and if I appear, at times, in the text to be over-critical or even dogmatic, it is because I am conscious of the fact that as well as writing a Guide to Psychiatry, I am writing a Guide for the Perplexed.

MYRE SIM

BIRMINGHAM, 1963.

Acknowledgement

The preparation of this third edition could never have been completed without the unstinting help of my wife. Her continued support throughout all three editions has stimulated me to persevere with a task which, at times, appeared too formidable.

Contents

CHAPTER 1

Psychology

Psychology has been defined as the science which studies the behaviour of man and other animals. This short definition includes a whole range of subdivisions each of which constitutes a subject in itself, such as educational, industrial, experimental, social, statistical, comparative and medical. As this chapter is primarily concerned with the basic requirements of the doctor-in-training, only those aspects which have a direct bearing on medical practice are included and it is not intended to be even the briefest introduction to general psychology.

As psychology is a young science, it has tended to make ready use of the instruments of measurement developed by the senior sciences of astronomy, physics and physical chemistry. But the use of instruments, no matter how precise, does not confer exactness and psychology had for some time in this century been too preoccupied with the means of measuring, rather than with what should be measured. The situation has been stated by Hogben (1961) thus:

> . . . It is more true to say that no branch of science attains to the status of being as exact as it might be until it has undertaken the preliminary taxonomical task of sorting out what facts are relevant and what are not relevant to the end in view. If we assume that our own species, by which I mean inter-fertile local varieties of *Homo sapiens,* made its appearance about 30,000 years ago, we may be sure that twenty thousand years of patient observation of the night sky by hunting and food-gathering nomads elapsed before a more settled way of life made it possible to construct a calendar based on the solar year and equipped with numerical symbols for the task. In my view, the neglect of this elementary consideration during the past four decades has forced social sciences in general, and psychology in particular, to follow a futile trail of gamesmanship in the illusion that measurement is intrinsically elevating regardless of the fruitfulness of what one is measuring. A single irresponsible and somewhat silly aphorism of the late Lord Kelvin has made measurement intrinsically respectable regardless of relevance, the more so if upholstered with an elegant sufficiency of irrelevant algebra.

The history of psychology has not been entirely confined to irrelevant measurement. Weber (1795–1878) used the laboratory and produced a generalization from his observations, called *Weber's Law,* which stated: *A difference that is just perceptible bears a constant ratio to the size of the standard stimulus.* This is regarded as the first quantitative law in psychology and was based on observations of weights and lines and the recognition of differences. More weight had to be added to a heavier weight for the difference to be perceived, than would be necessary for a lighter weight, and similarly for length of line. Fechner (1801–87) was impressed with Weber's findings and considered that he was able to relate mental processes to physical processes and that this relationship could be expressed symbolically as:

$$S = K \log R,$$

where S = sensation, K = constant, R = stimulus (German, *Reiz*) and that in this way sensation could be measured.

The founder of modern experimental psychology was Wilhelm Wundt (1832–1920) and much of his work was with the special senses, especially vision. From his laboratory, workers went forth to universities all over the world and experimental psychology had arrived as an independent subject with its own problems. Some of these were related to instincts, affects, conation, intelligence, learning and personality.

Instincts

Instinct is usually defined as unlearned, patterned, goal-directed behaviour, which is species-specific, as illustrated by nest building in birds or by the migration of salmon.

There has been much controversy over the presence or absence of instincts in man, particularly as some regarded them as inborn or hereditary. The long period of infantile dependence gives the child ample opportunity to acquire a variety of behaviour patterns which could be regarded as inborn. Support for the rejection of the term 'instinct' has come from those who have made a special study of what used to be called instinctive behaviour but is now referred to as 'species-specific behaviour'. A new specialty has been created called Ethology, by Tinbergen (1951), Hinde (1959), and Lorenz (1937). They were zoologists who confined their observations to animals and birds, but the challenge of human behaviour has encouraged a number of ethologists to transfer their observations from the mating habits of birds and monkeys to the social organization of man, whether it be in the acute psychotic ward of a mental hospital or the highly stylized behaviour at a 'teenage' dance. This activity used to be the province of the social anthropologist but the urge to relate human to animal behaviour even when inappropriate, is strong.

There are various ways of regarding an instinct. For example, the term is used for forms of behaviour which approximate to reflex activity in lower organisms, and in humans for that powerful energy and drive which is evident in the furtherance of aims. In animals, instincts are regarded as genetically transmitted, unlearned and stereotyped patterns of behaviour which are of biological value to the organism, while as humans they are capable of development, arrest, elaboration and even perversion. These differences in definition depend on methods of study as well as essential differences in the organism, for the biologist can accurately observe insects, birds and other animals in a relatively uncomplicated and generally recurring setting, but in humans the picture is much more complex. In general the unimpeded expression of an instinct is alleged to give pleasure, and its denial is followed by feelings of frustration.

Affect

This is the feeling tone associated with emotion and it may also influence instinctive behaviour. It is not the same as *emotion* which is primarily the pattern of behaviour which gives somatic expression to affect and is dependent on autonomic and cerebral factors. The term 'affective' is used for those psychiatric disorders where feeling tone is disturbed.

Lists of emotions were as long as those of instincts and at one time enjoyed a similar popularity. Interest is now being directed to the bodily changes accompanying such emotions as fear, anger, pleasure and anxiety. Hilgard (1962), describes ten somatic fields which are affected by the emotions, but these are so well-known to medical students and others that any elaboration here is unnecessary. It is sufficient to list them: (1) galvanic skin response, (2) blood distribution, (3) heart rate, (4) respiration, (5) pupillary responses, (6) salivary secretion, (7) pilomotor response, (8) gastro-intestinal motility, (9) muscle tension and tremor, (10) blood composition. There definition and quantitative estimation are constantly being revised and improved and new fields are being defined. Though emotion and affect as words are regarded as the province of the psychologist, the major experimental work designed to elucidate their mode and sites of action comes from clinical departments of cardio-respiratory diseases, neuro-surgery, endocrinology, psychiatry and gastro-enterology.

This association with psychosomatic disorders must already be apparent and a more detailed account of this relationship will be found in the appropriate chapter.

Conation

This is a term which stems from the old 'Faculty Psychology' where different mental activities were regarded as independent faculties. It is the urge of striving of the personality and is therefore the essence of the instinctive drive as defined (see p.2). It is basic to the concept of a dynamic psychiatry where behaviour is motivated and instincts conflict with each other and give rise to neurotic illness or are sublimated in socially acceptable behaviour.

Intelligence

An adequate definition does not exist though it has been loosely defined as the capacity to adjust to or change environment. It is impossible to measure such a capacity with any precision, but there are tests which in spite of their impractical nature and theoretical shortcomings, do provide a very useful measure of many aspects of human ability.

Binet and Simon are credited with the design of the first standardized tests for school children. Performance scores were converted to Mental Age and Terman developed from the Intelligence Quotient (or I.Q.) which is:

$$\frac{\text{Mental Age} \times 100}{\text{Chronological Age}}$$

The concept of the I.Q. has been greatly criticized and it has been said: 'Give a child a high I.Q. and he will spend the rest of his life trying to live up to it; give him a low I.Q. and he will spend the rest of his life trying to live it down.' It is not a constant measurement for it is easily influenced by emotional and environmental factors and experienced testers are prepared to accept an error of five points on either side of the score. Tests have to be standardized on well-defined populations, for the subjects are just as important as the problems put to them. Tests are therefore 'tailored' to the subject. In infancy and early childhood the I.Q. is not nearly as helpful as the D.Q. (Developmental Quotient) which is based on the child's age and 'milestones', among which are, following an object with the eyes, grasping an object, smiling, sitting up, walking and talking. Most tests in general use have been designed for school children, but there are also tests for adults, and special ones for mechanical aptitudes, intellectual deterioration and brain damage. They are of proved value in the selection of children for grammar and technical schools or in their modern counterpart within the 'Comprehensive' educational system, in placing dull children in their proper educational milieu and in the selection of servicemen, officer cadets, university entrants and junior executives.

As psychology has occupied itself mainly with the subject of intelligence and its measurement since the beginning of the century, there is a wealth, if not a surfeit of data on its relationship to educational attainments, ethnic groups, hereditary factors, occupational requirements, and social influences as well as on the many attempts to define its essential composition. Further details will be given later in the section on 'Psychological Tests', where the more common intelligence tests are described. The clinical application of relevant data will be found in Chapters 16 and 17 on Mental Deficiency and Child Psychiatry respectively.

LEARNING

Definition

This has been defined by Hilgard (1962) as the process by which an activity originates or is changed through responding to a situation.

As learning is common to all living objects, lower and higher forms of animal life have been studied and it is important to know whence the conclusions are drawn so that analogies are not confused with experimental proof.

Lower Forms of Learning include:

Habituation. This is the gradual suppression of an inborn impulse to a repeated stimulus and is a very early form of adjustment or learning. It is generally temporary, as exhibited in the *knee jerk* where repeated taps result in a lessened response and in the *eye blink,* though in this, habituation is speedier, due presumably to cortical interference. It is a negative form of learning.

The Conditioned Reflex. This was originally a physiological study reported in a series of papers by Pavlov (1927) and full details can be found in a text book of physiology. *Classical conditioning* as seen in the salivating dog, depends on a conditioned stimulus, such as a light or bell, an unconditioned stimulus, food, eventually giving rise to a conditioned response, namely salivating to the sound of the bell. These responses can be reinforced, extinguished and recover spontaneously after extinction. The conditioned stimulus which may be a specific tone can be generalized to a range of tones or restricted to a more discriminatory stimulus.

Operant Conditioning. This occurs when the stimulus is not directly concerned with the response, such as food with salivation. An example is when a rat gets food by pressing a bar in its cage. If food is obtained when the bar is pressed and a light appears, the rat may regard the light as part of the reinforcement. Such conditioning can be defined as the strengthening of a stimulus-response association by following the response with a reinforcing stimulus, usually one which can satisfy a drive. The elaboration of experiments in operant conditioning including secondary reinforcement, where poker chips could be used to obtain food for a chimpanzee from a vending machine (the Chimp-o-mat), has inevitably brought the concept of operant conditioning into explanations of human learning and treatment of mental illness.

A secondary reinforcer has a wide application and once established it can strengthen responses other than that used in its original establishment, and with motives other than the prevailing motives during original training. The deductive use of conditioning principles in learning was emphasized by Hull (1951) who applied the following mathematical model.

Two aspects were considered to be present in any learned performance:

1. Habit strength, to which the symbol $g^H R$ is applied. This was said to be the result of association learning under reinforcement as one finds in operant conditioning.

2. Drive, to which the symbol D is applied and which is a non-associative component.

The fundamental formula is:

$$g^E R \text{ (excitatory potential)} = D \text{ (drive)} \times g^H R \text{ (habit strength)}$$

D (drive) can be influenced by hunger, so a hungry rat would presumably learn its way through a maze to a food goal more quickly than a well-fed rat which was equally experienced with the maze. A *law of habit formation* was then expressed by the formula $g^H R = 1 - 10^{-aN}$ where N is the number of evenly distributed reinforced trials and a is a constant.

The law states that other things being equal, habit strength increases regularly with reinforcement to a maximum of strength 1.00 (in arbitrary units). The resulting error is one of decreasing gains. As the theory was further developed by Hull's collaborator, Spence, it is referred to as the Hull-Spence theory (Logan, 1959). Other mathematical models for learning have been devised, a more commonly quoted one being that of Estes (1959) who in addition attempts to explain time-dependent phenomena such as spontaneous recovery and forgetting.

B.F. Skinner (1904–) published his first major work (Skinner, 1938) in which he argued that the simple reflex open to Pavlovian conditioning plays little part in ordinary behaviour. He placed the major stress on *'operants'*, *i.e.* motor responses that are emitted spontaneously rather than elicited by particular external stimuli. Like reflexes, or in Skinner's term, *'respondents'*, operants may likewise be conditioned, and for their study he devised the 'Skinner Box', in which the animal learns to press a bar for food reward, which is delivered automatically according to a pre-arranged schedule. Since he held that most human behaviour was operant rather than respondent, he considered that work on operant conditioning in animals might throw more light on human behaviour than Pavlovian conditioning.

He laid greater stress than Pavlov on *reinforcement*, which is the increase in strength or frequency of a response resulting from reward contingent upon its execution. He demonstrated that reinforcement and performance were more complicated than Pavlov had supposed and that they depended greatly on the particular 'schedule' of reinforcement adopted. For instance, animals continue to press a bar much more frequently and for longer periods if the reward is delivered periodically, say after every eight responses, than if it is given after every single response.

Unlike some of his contemporary neo-behaviourists such as Clark L. Hull, he never professed great interest in learning *per se* and his work has been styled 'descriptive behaviourism', its object being to explore the relations between performance and contingencies of reinforcement and thereby to provide the outline of a technology of education. Apart from the laboratory experiments, the principles he evolves embody little more than is common knowledge to parents, teachers or trainers of performing animals. He suffers from what has been called a well-known occupational disease of psychologists, namely, premature generalization from limited evidence.

Operant Conditioning of Autonomic Responses

This technique was developed in rats where heart rate could be controlled to a certain extent when rewarded and similarly for intestinal contractions and that these changes could operate independently (Miller & Banuazizi, 1968). These experiments indicate that visceral learning can be specific to an organ system and is not the result of some general factor such as an overall level of activation. Similar work with human subjects has had similar results.

It is difficult at this stage to see what bearing these models have on the practice of psychiatry, for as Hull himself pointed out, they are valid in the animal experiments, other things being equal, and initial inequality is the most certain statistical fact in human behaviour. These theories are, however, being increasingly invoked in the recent enthusiasm for behaviour therapy and the doctor should know on what theoretical construct others would treat patients. The elaboration of these models proceeds apace, and while a doctor need not be familiar with the host of symbols and equations that now proliferate, he should know what is now a main preoccupation with many psychologists and be in a position to critically evaluate their efforts in applying these theories to the treatment of illness. One major criticism which has already been made is that in the healer-patient relationship there are factors operating which hardly influenced the rats of Hull, Spence or even Estes. This aspect will be discussed more fully under Behaviour Therapy (Chapter 19).

Peters (1957) disapproves of the uncritical transfer of information derived from animal experiment to human situations and states:

> We know so much about human beings and our knowledge is incorporated in our language. Making it explicit could be a more fruitful preliminary to developing a theory than gaping at rats or grey geese.

Vickers (1965) commented thus on the above statement:

> None the less, the rat in the maze and the judge on the bench display differences (as well as similarities) of behaviour which cannot at present be contained within a single conceptual framework. No doubt even judges might sometimes behave in every respect like rats; but rats never behave in every respect like judges.

Trial and Error Learning. This was first systematically studied by Thorndike in his experiments on problem-solving in cats. The animal after several attempts was able to get at food placed outside its cage and the theory was put forward that learning could be accelerated by satisfaction in one situation and by frustration or pain in another. These hypotheses are included in the *Law of Effect* which states that the greater the satisfaction or discomfort consequent on an act, the greater the strengthening or weakening of its bond with the prevailing situation. Similar conclusions have been drawn from studies on maze-solving in rats.

Stimulus Equivalence. This is seen even in conditioned reflexes where there is a degree of generalization and what is 'learnt' can be transferred to other situations. This process is more applicable in higher forms of learning where one learned pattern can be applied to many new situations.

Higher Forms of Learning include:

Combination and Insight. These are the capacity to combine simple habits which had been acquired at different times, and use them to solve new problems. The classical studies of Kohler on the mentality of apes showed that the animal could not only use a tool directly to reach fruit outside its cage, but could also join two sticks together to give it the requisite length to reach the fruit and this latter conduct could be regarded as insightful or intelligent.

Development of Skill. This illustrates certain aspects of learning and has been intensively studied by Bartlett who claimed that the best single measure of skill in any field is its degree of resistance to disintegrating conditions. Skills are retained under a wide variety of conditions. The loss of skill under stress is associated with emotional changes such as irritability and dissatisfaction and even a tendency not to bother to correct errors. The growth of skill also has its emotional aspect and depends on information reaching the subject about his progress and thus providing satisfaction and incentive. Formal examinations make use of these principles.

Reasoning and Problem-solving in Man. The average person does not use logic in solving practical problems but rather a variety of methods from trial and error to careful reasoning. It is suggested that the following three factors are involved: *(a)* a tendency to set up and test hypotheses; *(b)* the emergence of a solution after some delay and resembling the 'insightful' behaviour of some animals; and *(c)* the operation of a form of thinking which is not conscious. This last factor has been stressed by many who claim that the surest way to solve a problem is to sleep on it.

Engram. Penfield (1968) defined an engram as: 'The writing left behind in the brain after conscious experience'. He based this on the twin responses to stimulation of the interpretative cortex: (*a*) sudden signal of interpretation accompanied by feelings of familiarity and strangeness; (*b*) activation of past experience.

He was unable to reactivate silent thought, physical exercise, sleeping, eating or sexual activity. Auditory and visual components were always prominent.

Bilateral removal of the hippocampus and hippocampal gyrus in man produces loss of recent memory. As soon as he has turned his attention to something else, the patient is unable to remember what was happening a moment earlier. It is as though he made no record of present experience *or* having made the record as usual, he has lost the mechanism that enabled him to reactivate the record by voluntary initiation. He defines memory as the power or the process of responding or recalling what has been learned.

PERSONALITY

This is a most complex aspect of psychology and the following definition from Hilgard (1962) indicates some of the complexities:

> . . . the configuration of individual characteristics and ways of behaving which determines an individual's unique adjustments to his environment. We stress particularly those personal traits that affect the individual's getting along with other people and with himself. Hence personality includes any characteristics that are important in the individual's personal adjustment, in his maintenance of self-respect. Any description of the individual personality must take into account appearance, abilities, motives, emotional reactivity and the residues from experiences that have shaped the person as we find him.

Factors which contribute to personality structure are: maturation, training in infancy, social motives, intelligence (*e.g.* a gifted child will have an entirely different experience of life compared with a subnormal one), culture, physique, temperament and heredity.

Allport (1961) elaborated a theory of personal dispositions which runs counter to the belief that all traits are shared by all. He believed in individual patterns of traits with a hierarchical structure for *cardinal* through *central* to *secondary*. Cardinal traits dominate an individual and may even typify him, so that one may label a person a Casanova or Don Juan or a James Bond. Usually it requires a short list of central traits to label a person, and Allport quotes a description of the psychologist William James, as having the traits of 'sensibility, vivacity, humanity and socialibity'.

Cattell (1946) arrived at uniqueness in the individual by varying combinations of common traits which are present in different strengths. He describes *surface traits* grouped together through cluster analysis which is arrived at by collecting all traits that intercorrelate ·60 or higher. The other group consists of source traits which are divined by factor analysis. Tests have been designed to measure them (Cattell, 1957), and 16 in all have been assessed.

Psychoanalytical theories on personality development are dealt with in Chapter 2 (Psychopathology).

There are numerous definitions of personality or what it should embrace but none is sufficiently comprehensive, for there are still large gaps in our knowledge. There are, however, a number of facets of the problem which are recognized and are being actively studied. Among these are the following.

1. **Temperament.** This is considered to be inherited and to influence our moods and emotional reactions. It is also said to be affected by body build, and both Kretschmer and Sheldon have described body types and their relationship to temperament. The former used the terms schizoid and cycloid, while the latter talked of endo-, meso- and ecto-morphic somato-types with their associated temperaments of viscero-tonic (greedy), somato-tonic (athletic) and cerebro-tonic (intellectual). There have been many other classifications of temperament, all having some validity, but also deficiencies.

2. **Character.** This has a variety of definitions in ordinary English usage. In psychiatry it has come to mean traits acquired in childhood which persist into adult life and manifest as personality disturbances or *character disorders*. Much of the theoretical basis for the foregoing statement is based on Adlerian and Freudian psychology (see Chapter 2).

3. **Cerebral Influences.** A number of organic brain diseases, injuries or operations like pre-frontal leucotomy can produce personality changes leading to disorders of social conduct. The neurophysiological basis of these influences is dealt with in Chapter 5.

Memory

This implies previous learning with retention and is dependent on *attention* at the time of the initial and/or subsequent experiences. The following aspects of memory have been studied and defined.

Recall. This is the most easily tested by giving the subject a series of numbers to repeat forward or backward, either immediately or after an interval. The *'memory-drum'* is an instrument which permits syllables, words or symbols to appear one at a time. The subject after one run through is asked to state in advance the next item that will appear.

Recognition. This plays some part in recall and many laboratory tests for memory are really designed to define faulty recognition, for the subject is presented with items which approximate to the one he had been shown.

Forgetting. To the student who has to amass facts, this can be a tragic experience, but in emotional life it can play a vital part in relieving anxiety and is closely linked with the dynamic concept of repression (see below). Theories of forgetting other than the dynamic are:

(a) *Passive Decay through Disuse.* Objections to this theory are based on the ability of senile patients to remember events of long ago, though forgetting recent ones..

(b) *Systematic Distortion of the Memory Trace.* This is attributed to changes in the brain and is based on some early experimental evidence by Wulf, who defined three patterns:

(i) *levelling,* where the figures moved towards greater regularity and symmetry;
(ii) *sharpening,* where the irregularity was the most prominent feature but in subsequent reproductions becomes caricaturized; and
(iii) *assimilating,* where the figure approximates to something it resembles. The 'memory-trace' has not yet been established experimentally and is assumed.

(c) *Retroactive Inhibition.* This is based on the theory that retention of the old is impaired by acquisition of new information and *pro-active inhibition* means that prior learning can interfere with retention of subsequent learning.

There is some experimental evidence to support all these theories and though it is still not possible to say what part each plays in the process of forgetting, it is likely that the dynamic or *motivated forgetting* is the most important in human experience.

Redintegration. This is a technical term and means remembering the whole of an earlier experience on the basis of partial cues and is usually concerned with events in the personal history of the subject with the attendant circumstances. It is an aspect of memory which is rarely tackled by experimental psychologists, but is frequently used by psychotherapists and hypnotherapists in their efforts to reactivate early experiences which may have a bearing on the patient's problems.

PSYCHOLOGICAL TESTS

Historical

Though tests of personal attributes must have been in use for centuries, an early example being that used by Gideon before his battle with the Midianites (Judges vii. 7), it was not until the nineteenth century that any systematic approach to the problem was made. With the renewed interest during that period in the mentally abnormal, classification became important and Esquirol (1838) devoted a considerable amount of his work to the grading of mental defectives. At about the same time Séguin (1866), who had been a pioneer in the training of the feeble-minded, had devised apparatus with which the subject was asked to fit assorted shapes into matching recesses as quickly as possible. What was originally designed as an exercise in sensory discrimination and motor control became a 'performance' test—the *Séguin Form Board.*

Psychological testing was formally launched by Sir Francis Galton, who in 1882 established a laboratory in London and charged a fee for measuring individual differences in visual and auditory acuity, reaction time and other attributes, and collected a large amount of data (Galton, 1883). He devised his own tests, defined sensory parameters, used rating scales and questionnaires and introduced mathematical techniques in the form of statistical procedures for the analysis of test data. His influence in this respect has not been an unmixed blessing, for a pre-occupation with *averages* tends to dissolve the essential biological features and one may be left with only meaningless numbers.

Cattell (1890) was the first to use the term 'mental test' in psychological literature, when he described tests to determine the intellectual levels of college students. Since then, the development of mental tests has been prolific, and there is hardly a human attribute, real or imagined, which has not got at least one 'standardized' test. It was, however, Binet and Simon (1905) who made the greatest impact on the measurement of human intelligence in response to the establishment of a commission to study the education of subnormal children in Paris schools. They elaborated tests and defined the *mental age* which was a comparison between the chronological age of the child and the age level of the tests he could do. Terman (1916) revised their test for American children and produced what is called the Stanford-Binet test and defined the Intelligence Quotient or I.Q.

Perhaps the greatest stimulus to mental testing was General Pershing's telegram to the Secretary of State in the First World War asking him to arrange for better material to be sent out to France for the American Expeditionary Force. The American Psychological Association appointed a committee and they produced the Army Alpha and Beta tests. These became a model for group intelligence tests which spread to schools, colleges, hospitals, prisons and other institutional groups. To these tests were added those for special aptitudes and for personality and attitudes, and there was also considerable pre-occupation with what was being tested. Spearman (1927) defined a general '*g*' factor and special '*s*' factors, and Thurstone (1935) elaborated techniques of factor analysis in their application to the problem. An extension of this development has been the designing of *differential aptitude batteries* which in place of a score or I.Q. provided a separate score for each aptitude, thus making the test more comprehensive and in certain circumstances, such as the selection of candidates for special branches of Service training, more meaningful.

Criteria of Tests

Anastasi (1954), who has written a comprehensive textbook on the subject, gives the following definition: 'A psychological test is essentially an objective and standardized measure of a sample of behaviour'.

Standardization. This implies a uniformity of procedure in the administration and scoring of the test and is really an effort to control as many variables as possible, the one variable which cannot be controlled being the subject.

Norms. These are average performances for the individual's age, social or cultural background, the emphasis varying according to the test employed, and it is with these norms that the individual's performance is compared.

Reliability. This is assessed by objective evaluation and if the test *constantly* measures what it set out to measure it is reliable.

Validity. This is the degree to which the test actually measures what it purports to measure (Anastasi, 1954). It is not the same as reliability which is concerned with consistency of performance rather than the conclusions that can be drawn from the performance. The purpose of the test is usually a practical one, such as success of candidates for medical school or an army signals course, and if this is high after using the test for selection purposes it therefore has a high *validity co-efficient.*

Most reliable and valid tests (as well as a number that are not) are copyright, so it is not possible to reproduce these tests. All one can do in the available space is to give a short description of the commoner ones and the reader should make himself familiar with the test materials which can be obtained through scientific suppliers. There is no alternative to using a test in order to gauge its relevance to the task in hand. Descriptions of the tests can only act as signposts.

The Stanford-Binet Scale

This is used primarily for children and has two forms (L and M) consisting of 129 items or tests, grouped into 20 age levels ranging from 2 years to 'superior adult' which comes after average adult, which in turn comes after the tests for the 14-year age group. Test materials include toy objects for the younger age levels (2–6 years), a record form and a test manual giving the instructions on how to administer and score the test. Manipulative tests at the earliest ages measure eye-hand coordination and use a form board like that of Séguin, block-building and stringing beads. Drawing and copying and perceptual tests such as discrimination and recognition, picture completion, similarities and differences between objects, are all included as well as ordinary arithmetic. In the higher age levels verbal answers are more prominent and scores would tend to favour children with a high verbal facility.

The test is valuable not only because of the wide variety of items it measures, but because it is extensively used and a large body of information about is has accumulated. Anastasi (1954) writes: 'For many clinicians, educators and others concerned with the evaluation of general ability level, the Stanford-Binet I.Q. has become almost synonymous with intelligence'. Burt has standardized a similar test for London school children.

Group Intelligence Tests

The Army Alpha and Beta were earliest in the field and there have been numerous developments since for use in schools, universities, industry and the services, some making free use of multiple choice answers, in which the correct answer is given among others and the candidate has to indicate which is the correct one. Most group tests can also be given individually, and a well-known example in Britain is:

Raven's Progressive Matrices. This test was designed to measure Spearman's '*g*' factor and is non-verbal. It consists of 60 matrices of abstract designs grouped in five sets of 12. From each design a part is missing and the candidate selects what he considers is the missing part from the group of six or eight which are illustrated below the test piece. The test becomes more difficult with each succeeding group and no time limit is set. Scores are converted into percentiles according to norms devised by Raven who standardized the test on a large British army population during the Second World War. There is a simpler coloured version for children and it has also been used for deteriorated adults. The standard tests gained a high reputation for efficiency in the selection of recruits and other grades of military personnel.

Non-verbal tests are of particular importance in deaf and dumb subjects and where language barriers exist. Unfortunately cultural barriers are not entirely overcome by such tests which are standardized on literate communities, though some have devised allegedly 'culture-free' tests.

Percentile or Centile Scale

If ranks in the scores of a test are converted to positions between 0 and 100, then such ranks may be given a percentile rating. If a person were placed in 90th percentile of a large group it would mean that only 10 per cent of the group scored higher. Similarly, somebody in the 50th percentile would be halfway between the top and bottom of his group.

The percentiles are computed thus: Scores are placed in order, the highest score receiving the rank 1, but in centile language this would be equivalent to near 100, for the lowest score would be equivalent to zero. The centile position is derived from the following formula.

$$\text{Centile position} = 100 - \frac{100\,(\mathrm{R} - 0{\cdot}5)}{N}$$

when R = rank (with 1 high), and N = No. of cases ranked.
Example: A student is ranked 10th in a class of 50 students

$$\text{Centile position} = 100 - \frac{100\,(10 - 0{\cdot}5)}{50}$$

$$= 100 - 19 = 81.$$

Ordinary reasoning would have given the student a centile position of 80 in that there are 40 scores below him representing 80 per cent of the sample. In the middle scores the formula is more helpful. For example, ranks of 25 and 26 lie on either side of the middle and the formula clearly separates them by giving them centiles of 51 and 49 respectively.

Performance Tests

These depend on the manipulation of material and are particularly useful where language is a barrier as they are non-verbal and do not depend on educational attainment.

Pintner-Paterson Performance Scale. This was described in 1917 and it included 15 tests, though 10 are more commonly used. Form boards (including Séguin), picture completion and manikin assembly are some of the subjects used. As a time limit is set, speed of response is important and this would tend to handicap some children with physical defects.

Porteous Maze. A number of mazes are used and there is no time limit. It is regarded as a measure of foresight and planning capacity.

Kohs Block Design (1923). The patient is asked to arrange a number of identical one-inch cube blocks which have red, white, yellow, blue, red and white, and yellow and blue sides to match coloured designs on cards, of which there are 17. The number of moves and the time taken to solve each card is scored and an intelligence rating is obtained by reference to tables. In clinical practice, the test is of value in recognizing patients with spatial disorientation, particularly, in the author's experience, those with Alzheimer's disease, where the parietal lobes are usually involved.

Goodenough Draw-a-Man Test. This is frequently used for children and in the setting of a child guidance clinic is a useful test for the psychiatrist. It helps to establish rapport, while at the same time offering an opportunity to gauge the child's motor skills and whether there is any apraxia present. The mental age achieved depends on the completeness of the drawing; the top score will require the man to have arms, feet, hands, fingers, eyes, ears and clothes, including shoes.

Wechsler Adult Intelligence Scale

This test, which is the most commonly used for assessing adult intelligence, was first presented by Wechsler (1939) as the Wechsler-Bellevue scale. There are now two scales, I and II, so that retesting is possible, though some have found the two scales not entirely interchangeable. It is divided into two, a verbal section and a performance section, which in turn are subdivided as follows:

Verbal Scale. This consists of the following subtests: *information, e.g.* 'How many weeks are there in a year?'; *comprehension,* this tests logical thinking, *e.g.* 'Why are laws necessary?'; *arithmetic; similarities,* naming a common factor in a pair, *e.g.* dog and lion;

digit span, a test of immediate recall of numbers forward and backward; and *vocabulary.*

Performance Scale. This consists of the following subtests: *digit symbol,* symbols are linked with numerals and in a given time the subject copies the symbols into blank spaces with the numerals as a guide; *picture completion,* part of the picture is missing and the subject has to identify the missing part; *block design,* the subject has to arrange coloured blocks to represent a design on a card; *picture arrangement,* pictures have to be arranged in a logical sequence to tell a story; *object assembly,* pieces of cardboard are arranged to make an object such as a face or hand.

It is the nearest approach in the measurement of adult intelligence to the Stanford-Binet and gives a high degree of reliability and validity. It has also been used for testing intellectual deterioration (see below). A Wechsler scale for children has also been designed and some regard it as being as well standardized as the Stanford-Binet.

Tests for Intellectual Deterioration

Babcock Test (1930). This was one of the first to be standardized. The subject's Stanford-Binet vocabulary score is used to estimate his expected performance on a series of tests of memory, learning and motor speed, and the difference between the actual and estimated score is computed as an 'Efficiency Index'.

Shipley-Hartford. This is based on the Babcock scale but is much simpler to administer and score. It consists of a 40 item vocabulary scale and an 'abstraction' scale, the latter having 20 items of the series-completion type. The difference between these two scales is referred to a table which provides the Conceptual Quotient or C.Q. If the C.Q. is below 70 (normal is 100) organic mental deterioration can be suspected; if below. 60 it is likely, and so on. One of the disadvantages of the test is that in affective disorders in the elderly, the C.Q. may be very low due to a lack of interest or application and in the very instance where one would like to rule out cerebral deterioration the test result may simulate it where it does not exist.

Wechsler Adult Intelligence Scale. Just as it is probably the best test of adult intelligence, it is also the most useful for measuring intellectual deterioration. The scatter of the score in the various subgroups may often be diagnostic. High scores on vocabulary and information with low scores on block design, object assembly, similarities and arithmetic may be very suggestive. The shape of the 'profile'—that is the linking up of the various scores by a continuous line—will reveal 'troughs' of low performance and indicate the organic nature of the patient's difficulties. Though there are many valid criticisms by psychologists of its limitations, it is a very useful test for the psychiatrist and the author has made a practice of ensuring that his registrars become thoroughly familiar with its use, as it stands them in good stead, especially when asked to see these difficult border-line problems.

Memory Tests. Although clinically, the inability of a patient to remember the names of a number of given objects is considered a useful pointer to organic intellectual impairment, formal memory tests such as those included in the Wechsler are not nearly as helpful as one would have thought. The repeating of digits forwards is particularly unhelpful and digits backwards involves factors other than memory, so that it is difficult to decide what one is measuring.

Tests for Conceptual Thought. Some of these have already been mentioned, *e.g.* in the Wechsler and Kohs Blocks, but the series devised by Goldstein, who elaborated the principle of categorical and conceptual thinking (p. 107) is widely used.

Goldstein-Scheerer Cube. This is similar to Kohs Blocks and in fact uses mainly the same blocks. If the subject is unable to do the test certain aids are supplied which lower the conceptual or abstract quality of the test and make it more concrete. It is then possible to see if the patient has 'learned' to transfer what he gained from the concrete to the abstract situation.

Weigl-Goldstein-Scheerer Colour-Form Sorting. Twelve objects consisting of four circles, four squares and four triangles in colours red, green and yellow and on the reverse white, are used. The objects are mixed together and the patient is asked to arrange them in the way he thinks they are connected (form or colour). Again aids can be given to make the situation more concrete. It is obviously a test to be used in the grossly deteriorated or in those patients who have localized dominant parietal lobe damage.

Goldstein-Scheerer Stick. Thirty sticks of four lengths are used and the subject is asked to copy simple geometric designs with them. He is then asked to produce the design with the sticks from memory. The patient's verbal facility in explaining his efforts is also assessed.

Gelb-Goldstein Sorting. Woollen skeins of different colours and brightness are sorted according to these qualities. A more concrete situation is structured by asking the patient to do simple matching.

Goldstein-Scheerer Object Sorting. A variety of objects like plates, cigars, knives, forks, spoons, nails, screwdrivers are used. The examiner hands the patient an article and asks him to pick out those others which belong with it. He may also be asked to group articles according to his own inclination.

Variations of the above tests are included in the Vigotsky which is a sorting test using coloured wooden blocks of different shapes and though introduced as a diagnostic aid in schizophrenia, has its uses in the brain-damaged. Hanfmann and Kasanin (1942) introduced it from Russia to the U.S.A.

Perceptual Tests. Some of the preceding tests involve the ability to perceive spatial relations but the *Bender-Gestalt* (1938) test is based on Gestalt psychology and is in fact selected from a larger series of designs used by Wertheimer who was one of the founders of that school. Gestalt psychology depends on certain mechanisms used in perception such as gap-filling and bump-erasing, so that irregularities in objects are smoothed out to create the harmonious shapes the mind prefers to see. Nine simple designs on cards are presented singly to the patient who is asked to copy them. It has been standardized on normal subjects, and it was found that scores were independent of drawing ability. It has been regarded as a useful rapid screening test in psychotic disturbance, though one would expect it also to be of value in the study of the brain-damaged.

Aptitude Tests. These are designed to see whether a person has a special skill, potential or character trait, and have been used extensively in personnel selection. In the British Army, in addition to the non-verbal Progressive Matrices which is regarded as the main indication of intelligence, there are tests for mechanical aptitude (practical and comprehension), instruction and arithmetic. These tests and others are usually presented in battery form and the subject can then be placed in what is presumably the job which would use his latent and actual talents to the full. It does not always work out that way, though these batteries were very useful during the Second World War in selecting personnel for courses, with good prospects that they would absorb the necessary training in the allotted time. This is of course a very different situation to peace-time placement which should permit an individual to realize his full potential. Application, interest and ambition may count for more than the results of an aptitude test and there should always be flexibility in its use to ensure that some who may be very successful are not excluded, or what may be even more harmful to society, that somebody is not selected for a task which he can do and is thereby prevented from doing something which provides for him a greater challenge and which might call out from him reserves of strength of which neither he nor his testers were aware.

Special Aptitude Tests. These are more restricted in their aim and may be used for specific qualities such as reaction time, visual acuity, hearing acuity, manual dexterity.

Achievement or Attainment Tests. An educational system should take stock of its handiwork and measure the success or otherwise of its efforts. There are therefore tests for reading, spelling, arithmetic, general knowledge and other subjects which have been standardized for school children. Remedial training is given for the backward and the success of this training is measured by these tests. In a society where literacy is standard, failure to read can prove a greater handicap than a physical disability and there is therefore likely to be an increasing accent on such attainment tests.

Personality Tests

It has always been popular to categorize people according to certain traits they are considered to possess. These may be physical or mental and the one would frequently be regarded as intimately connected with the other. The splenic, choleric and phlegmatic, the fat and the lean, the tough and the tender, the extravert and the introvert are examples which were popular in their day. It soon became apparent that a couple or several traits could not classify the whole range of human personality and therefore these tests became more and more detailed in their attempt to plumb the foundations of an individual's personality. Personality profiles were designed, multiple choice inventories were drawn up and the following are some of the more commonly used tests.

The Minnesota Multiphasic Personality Inventory (MMPI). This is a very comprehensive test which was introduced in 1940 and in the Manual (Hathaway & McKinley, 1951) it states that the inventory sets out 'to assay those traits that are commonly characteristic of disabling psychological abnormality'. There are 550 affirmative statements on cards which the patient is asked to place in three stacks—True, False and Cannot Say. It has also been designed as a group test. The range of statements is wide and includes among others religion, politics, sex, family, neurotic and psychotic symptoms, ideas of reference, sadistic and masochistic drives. A number of scales have been prepared for Hypochondriasis (HS), Depression (D), Hysteria (Hy), Psychopathic deviation (Pd), Masculinity or femininity of interest pattern (Mf), Paranoia (Pa), Psychasthenia (P), Schizophrenia (Sc) and Hypomania (Ha).

The test includes in itself four 'validity' scales which are inserted to check carelessness or the frank malingerer. Anastasi (1954) is critical of its value and while admitting that as a screening test for disturbed people it may be useful, adds that there are shorter and simpler tests which are equally reliable. When used as a diagnostic test, it has been shown that schizophrenics do not score higher on the Sc scale than on other scales. She states: '. . . the construction and use of personality inventories are beset with special difficulties over and above the common problems encountered in all psychological testing'. A recent stimulus to its use has been the programming of a computer to facilitate scoring. This does not make the test more valid, but more popular.

Projective Techniques

These depend on setting the patient an 'unstructured' task, thus permitting a wide variety of responses which is limited only by the individual's ability to interpret.

Rorschach Test. This is an ink-blot test which was designed by Rorschach in 1921 and translated into English in 1942. The ink blots are on 10 cards, five with colours and five in black and grey, and are presented one at a time to the patient who is asked to comment on them. After he has seen them all, he is asked systematically about those parts of the ink blot he had previously mentioned or described. Scoring is elaborate and depends on the number of responses, whether whole or part, the reaction time, failure to answer or rejection of a card, form, movement and colour, animal or human. These are further subdivided and D, which stands for 'detail', can be reduced to Dd, meaning smaller detail and so on. It has a large following as a test, particularly among clinical psychologists, yet efforts to evaluate and define the factors on which it is alleged to be based have not been successful and there has been serious and well-substantiated criticism. One wonders whether Rorschach's death in 1922, one year after he completed his work, inspired some of the reverence with which the test has been regarded. Rorschach himself was more modest than many of his followers and in his preface stated: 'The conclusions drawn, therefore, are to be regarded more as observations than as theoretical deductions'. The theoretical foundation for the experiment is, for the most part, still quite incomplete. The clinical material he used totalled 405 patients of whom 117 were 'normals', 188 schizophrenics, 20 psychopaths, 20 epileptics, 10 senile dements and 12 mental defectives.

Psychiatrists may find the test useful as a talking point with inhibited patients or with those who are not very communicative and their responses may betray obsessional or schizophrenic features. It is not as reliable as a well-trained clinical opinion, and seems to engender among psychiatrists either enthusiasm for its use or a complete aversion, but it is still popular with non-medical workers.

Murray's Thematic Apperception Test (TAT). Murray (1943) devised this test, using 19 cards with black and white pictures and one blank card. The pictures are capable of a variety of interpretations and the patient is asked to make up a story to fit each picture, the events before and after the incident portrayed, and his interpretation of the picture itself. With the blank card, he is asked to imagine a picture on it and tell a story about it. Although formal scoring is difficult, the responses can be helpful to the psychiatrist in that they may declare the patient's phantasy life. As with the Rorschach, it has also been used as a group test by making lantern slides of the pictures.

Rosenzweig Picture-Frustration Study. This test was described by Rosenzweig *et al.* (1947) and there are adult and child forms. These consist of 24 cartoons of two principal characters, one of whom is involved in a common and mildly frustrating situation, while the other is saying something which either contributes to it or points it out. The patient is asked to write in the blank space what the frustrated person would answer, giving the first reply that comes to mind. There are two kinds of frustrating experience depicted: (1) 'ego-blocking', where the individual is directly frustrated; and (2) 'super-ego blocking', where the individual is insulted or accused. It is based on the patient identifying with the frustrated character in the picture and reactions are classified as: *(a)* 'obstacle-dominance', *(b)* 'ego-defence' and (*c*) 'need-persistence'. Aggression is described as 'extrapunitive', 'intropunitive' or 'impunitive'. Modifications of the test have been used to study the attitudes of minority groups.

Szondi Test. Pictures are again used here and the patient is shown 48 photographs of psychiatric patients of both sexes, in sets of eight, each containing a homosexual, a sadistic murderer, an epileptic, a hysteric, a catatonic schizophrenic, a paranoid schizophrenic, a depressive and a manic. The patient is asked to select two which he likes most and two which he dislikes most in each set. The test has been described by Deri (1949) and there is some system of scoring which is very complex. Anastasi (1954) regards it as 'one of the least acceptable of the currently popular projection techniques. Its theoretical orientation . . . is particularly weak and fallacious'. This last remark may well be applied to most projection tests, but they all have their enthusiasts.

Word Association Tests. Though introduced originally by Galton, it was Jung (1910) who made the most striking contributions. He used stimulus words with emotional significance and analysed reaction time and content of the responses. The patient's attitude was also noted and the test in certain instances gave dramatic results. It can be structured to suit a particular problem, and since Jung there have been many developments of the test, such as *Sentence Completion, Storytelling* and *Argument Completion.*

Other projection techniques are drawing, painting, the use of toys and puppets, drama and creating a world (Lowenfeld, 1939), in which the child is given a number of models of houses, people, animals, fences, trees, cars, etc., and is asked to create anything he wishes. Interpretation is used, sometimes freely, and it has been used for therapy as well as in diagnosis.

Anastasi (1954) lists the following advantages of projection techniques: Malingering and dissimulation is more difficult, rapport can more readily be established, and they are useful in young children, illiterates, and persons with language handicaps and speech defects. As one would expect, *disadvantages* are the difficulties of standardization, the definition of norms, as well as their general unreliability and lack of validity in both the technical and ordinary senses.

Concept

Definition. A learned response to a class of events or a grouping of things into a single category on the basis of one or more features which they share. Concept formation requires abstraction, which defines what several objects have in common, and generalization, which defines other objects which share this attribute. It is usually dependent on language but can precede language as in the newborn child in the human race, and of course, in the animal kingdom.

Functions: *(a)* to reduce the complexity of the environment; *(b)* to identify objects and their properties; (*c*) to predict the nature of objects.

Concepts and Reasoning. (*a*) Concept formation (see Piaget in Chapter 17), *(b)* concept attainments. Bruner *et al.* (1956) analysed the four systematic strategies in problem-solving and their application according to the type of concept and its nature.

Concept and Personality. Environmental and social variables will influence concepts as will the unique experience of the individual. For example, those that have proved successful in prediction will be retained while those that were unsuccessful will be discarded.

The specific meaning attached to a concept will vary from person to person, for each concept has a public (extensional) meaning which is general and a private (intensional) meaning which is unique for that individual. Study of the concepts used by individuals has been used to elaborate theories of personality.

Kelly's Personal Construct Theory

Man in his efforts to understand, predict and control his world elaborates a unique system of concepts or a personal construct system through which he perceives his world. Constructs differ from Concepts in being bipolar (kind-cruel; black-white) but are otherwise similar. The theory of personal constructs is concerned with its relationship to behaviour, particularly interpersonal relationships. Thus, *emotion* is awareness of a state of change or transition in one's construct system; *anxiety* is awareness that events lie mostly outside its range of convenient function; *hostility* is the continued effort to obtain evidence in support of an already failed social prediction.

Kelly's Repertory Grid

This is a technique to enable the above construct systems of individuals to be analysed and described quantitatively. It is not standardized but is flexible so that the person being tested rates people and objects. It has become popular as a personality test in clinical assessment (Slater, 1969).

Semantic Differential

This is a method of measuring connotative meanings more precisely (Snider & Osgood, 1969). The subject is asked to rate the word according to a number of bipolar adjective pairs, e.g. 'strong-weak'. One member of the pair is placed at one end of a seven-point scale, the other member at the opposite end. The subject indicates the direction and intensity of his judgment by rating the word under study at some point along the scale. For example, the word 'polite' can be rated along a scale with polar opposites such as 'angular-rounded'; 'weak-strong'; 'rough-smooth'; 'active-passive'; 'small-large'; 'cold-hot'; 'good-bad'; 'tense-relaxed'; 'wet-dry'; 'fresh-stale'. When two groups are presented with the scale, their interpretations of the meaning of the word 'polite' can approximate very closely even though the adjectives bear little relation to the quality 'politeness'.

After considerable experiment it was found that the connotative meaning of most words could be expressed in three basic dimensions:

1. *Evaluative* (good-bad; clean-dirty).
2. *Potency* (strong-weak; light-heavy).
3. *Activity* (fast-slow; sharp-dull).

These dimensions apply to connotative meaning in a wide variety of languages and the semantic differential has been used to distinguish and reveal similarities in cultural groups.

Disordered Use of Concept

1. *Concreteness.* (See under Goldstein's Theory in Chapter 5).
2. *Overinclusiveness.* An inability to preserve the boundaries of concept results in their becoming vague and ill-defined and possessing features which are only remotely related to the concept.
3. *Personal Constructs.* Schizophrenic patients have loose and inconsistent construct systems and it has been suggested that these result from repeated invalidation of their concepts, but they may be the result rather than the cause.

Relevance of Personal Construct Theory to Psychiatry

It is difficult to see what it has contributed except to provide another area of measurement. 'Man Must Measure' but this obsession which has accurately charted the movements of the planets has also given us the pseudo-sciences of astrology and numerology. The evidence to date has not yet placed it in the first category. It could well be another form of 'scientism' which was defined by Hayek (1970) thus:

> The characteristic feature of scientism now seems to me to be that it insists on applying the techniques that were developed for the explanation of essentially simple phenomena to the explanation of essentially complex phenomena. There are wide fields in which explanation cannot successfully be accomplished by relying on 'laws' which represent a magnitude as a function of at most two or three others as physics has so successfully done for many phenomena which for this reason are regarded as 'physical' or 'mechanical'. There exist in the world essentially complex phenomena in the sense that they occur only when a great multiplicity of different events interact—events which are not yet numerous enough to make them accessible to statistical treatment. It is in the scientific treatment of these 'problems of organized complexity' as Dr. Warren Weaver has called them that the prejudice of scientism has done so much harm.

He recalls his earlier contribution in 1942 when he coined the term 'scientism'. 'The scientistic as distinguished from the scientific view is not an unprejudiced but a very prejudiced approach which before it has considered its subject claims to know what is the most appropriate way of investigating it'.

HUMAN TERRITORIALITY

Ethologists have testified to the territorial instinct in animals and birds. They have noted that behaviour and motor patterns are clearly linked with the need for self-preservation which makes domination and control of territory essential for hunting and mating. Lorenz had described the phenomenon of human territoriality and Bowlby (1959) had identified similarities in the psychoanalytic concepts of instinct, its developmental manifestations and discharge patterns with those of the comparative ethologists.

Sarwer-Foner (1972) noted during psychoanalytic treatment of patients, specific human psychic and behavioural expressions of territoriality. He states that man needs personal living space, but he also cathects his areas of interest. He can symbolize functions and occupations in reference to his social position relative to his fellows in much the same way as lower animals treat essential geographic territory. The affective responses seen demonstrate the strength of the neurophysiological mechanism triggered to express this cathexis.

The author claims that there is clear evidence that the affective components and their motor manifestations are triggered and mediated largely through the visceral brain and that the 'symbolized territories' are treated by the CNS as though they were hunting, mating and living territories which should be experienced through the senses. The adequate connections with the hypothalamic motor centres permit efficient, affective integrated motor responses, while the poorer synaptic connections with the neocortex lend a strong instinctive (biological) colour to such reactions, which impair cerebral reasoning and therefore efficient ego control and reality testing. He suggests that it is this neurophysiological stimulation of the 'old brain' which reinforces, mediates or even initiates the cathexis of the id and ego drives, but gives them a primitive urgency characteristic of primary process phenomena and thus weakens the ego's capacity to integrate, synthesize and test reality.

Comment: The neurophysiological analogy is of interest and appears valid but it is dependent on a certain stage of our appreciation of these mechanisms. The 'telephone exchange' model is rapidly giving way to the biochemical one, especially as far as effective responses are concerned and a new explanation would then be needed.

CHAPTER 2

Psychopathology

Humoral, demonic, astrological and physical theories have been used to explain the morbid mental states of man, but it is mainly in the present century that a number of theories have been elaborated which purport to explain psychiatric disorders in a 'logical' manner and which have been based on an intensive study of these disorders.

FREUDIAN THEORY

This theory, though given the name of the founder of the psychoanalytic movement, owes much to the efforts of a whole school of thought. Sigmund Freud himself was born in 1856 in Freiberg, Moravia (now Czechoslovakia), went with his parents to Vienna at an early age and studied medicine there. His main post-graduate interests were initially neurology and neuropharmacology; he had made a serious contribution to the study of spastic diplegia in children, and was co-discoverer with Karl Koller of the local anaesthetic effects of cocaine. His personal history is admirably presented by his biographer Ernest Jones (1953–7). In 1885, he went to Paris for post-graduate studies in neurology under Charcot, who at that time was experimenting with the use of hypnosis in cases of hysteria, and Freud developed a keen interest in this work. (For an excellent description of Charcot's work with his hysterics at the Salpêtrière in Paris, see Axel Munthe's *Story of San Michele*). At about this time Pierre Janet (1893), a pupil of Charcot, in his efforts to explain the phenomena of hysteria, introduced the concepts of *dissociation,* the *subconscious* and *psychological tension.* Weakness of the psychic tension or energy could be caused by emotional shocks and traumatic memories, and as a result certain mental processes could be dissociated from the main stream of consciousness, leaving the individual, on the surface, calm and apparently unperturbed, a state which Janet referred to as '*la belle indifférence*'.

This was the age of Bergson (1859–1941) who had put forward his views on the '*élan vital*' and had given a dynamic interpretation to human conduct. He considered that the cerebral mechanism was so arranged as to push back into the unconscious almost the whole of our past and to allow beyond the threshold only that which will further the action in hand. It was also the age of William James (1890) who described the case of the Reverend Ansell Bourne who disappeared and two months later a man woke up in a fright saying his name was Bourne, but in the intervening time he had moved from Rhode Island to Pennsylvania and had rented a confectioner's shop in the name of a Mr A. J. Brown. These vagaries of the mind were becoming of increasing interest to investigators and probably the most celebrated was that of Miss Beauchamp decribed by Morton Prince (1906). She exhibited multiple personalities (triple to be exact) and significantly he gave his book the title *The Dissociation of a Personality*. Robert Louis Stevenson, who as the supreme story-teller had earlier noticed the potential these characters had for the novelist, described one in his book *Dr Jekyll and Mr Hyde* (Stevenson, 1886).

Freud returned to Vienna and published his *Studies in Hysteria* (Breuer & Freud, 1895). This was the start of a long and productive journey into the unconscious of man. Even the concept of the unconscious was vigorously challenged by philosophers of that time and he had to prove its presence, which he did through the phenomena of hypnosis, the signs of hysteria, slips of the tongue, motivated forgetting and above all, the mental activity during dreams. By many he has been accredited the role of the infallible and the discoverer of all psychological truth including the discovery of the unconscious. A healthy corrective to this uncritical adoration is provided by Brown (1961):

In fact he originated neither the term nor the concept but learned them in the sixth form in his school in Vienna, where he was taught the psychology of Herbart at about the same time that William James in America was popularizing the word 'subconscious' and showing the importance of this type of motivation in mental life. Freud was a very great man, but it is preposterous to assume with the uncritical that all his basic concepts were entirely original or with the very erudite that they originated from such exalted sources as Plato, Spinoza, Nietzsche and Schopenhauer. On the contrary, they were based on ideas which in one form or another happened to be in the air at the time he was developing his theories and amongst psychiatrists, psychologists and physicians rather than amongst philosophers, whose work he is unlikely to have studied during those early years. Certainly he was not acquainted with the works of either Nietzsche or Schopenhauer until quite late in life, and all that need be assumed in the way of influences is that Freud, like most scientists of his time, was a rationalist and materialist with a great admiration for Darwin, whence came his evolutionary and biological approach; that he learned the Herbartian doctrine of the unconscious at school and later became a physician specializing in neurology but, finding that many of his patients were suffering from psychological rather than organic complaints, went to Paris, where he saw that hypnosis could both produce and remove hysterical symptoms and was told by Charcot that 'sex is always at the bottom of the trouble'; that, finally, on his return to Vienna he found Breuer using hypnosis in a new way but, not being a particularly good hypnotist himself, was driven to achieve the same results by other means. As a result of these experiences Freud's picture of the unconscious differed considerably from that of his predecessors in that he pictured it as a dynamic force rather than as a mere waste-paper basket of ideas and memories which had fallen below the threshold of awareness because they were relatively unimportant and lacked the mental energy to force their way into consciousness. He was able to show that precisely the opposite was the case, that the unconscious plays a predominant part in mental life, since it takes its energy from the instinctual drives, and its contents are kept out of awareness not because they lack significance but because they may be so significant as to constitute what is felt as a threat to the ego . . .

Freud may not have been the first to postulate the 'unconscious', but no man has had to defend the concept more vigorously and no man has done it so well.

He was bitterly attacked because of his theories of infantile sexuality; he was accused of translating findings from a few abnormal people to the 'normal'. He was attacked for his rationalism and atheism and at the same time for being a Jew, but he persevered in his studies and elaborated a theory of the unconscious and psycho-sexual development, which even if not universally valid made a tremendous contribution to the understanding and treatment of mental illness. His four postulates—psychic determinism, the role of the unconscious, the goal-directed nature of behaviour, and the developmental or historical approach—are now generally accepted by all schools of dynamic psychiatry and much of his work which used to shock and anger is now invested with an air of respectability. At one time 'orthodox' psychiatrists would joke about Freudian theory and practice, but now that the alienist has emerged from behind the walls of the mental hospital, he has had to face up to a variety of clinical problems which could not be dealt with by an institutional regime and where powers of understanding were more important than powers of description. The author, who sits on selection committees for psychiatric appointments, has been struck in recent years by the tendency for candidates to claim even more experience of Freudian psychopathology than they actually possessed, whereas previously it was considered a doubtful move to admit any experience whatever. Freud escaped from Vienna in 1938 at the time of the *Anschluss* when Hitler invaded Austria, and he and his family were given refuge in London, where he died in 1939.

Freud described the three main components of the mind thus:

1. **The Id.** The term is a latinized derivation from Groddeck's (1928) *das Es*. The new-born child is regarded as being completely 'Id-ridden', that is, it is a mass of instinctive drives and impulses each seeking gratification. The id is responsible for our basic drives such as food, sex and aggressive impulses, and demands immediate satisfaction. It is amoral and egocentric; ruled by the pleasure-pain principle; is without a sense of time; completely illogical; primarily sexual; infantile in its emotional development; will not take 'no' for an answer; is without verbal representation and therefore does not enter consciousness. It is regarded as the reservoir of the libido or 'love-energy'. The portrayal of the new-born child as the prime example of the id-ridden individual has been underlined by the following humorous definition of the new-born child—'an alimentary tract with no sense of responsibility at either end'.

2. **The Ego.** The ego is largely conscious; uses logic; deals with the outer world; is usually influenced by the super-ego; has moral standards; has time perception; is verbalized; and sleeps but has a dream censorship. It makes contact with the environment through the sensory processes and is able to evaluate the information received and effect compromises. It therefore has to modify the impulses of the id and the demands of the super-ego, and is or should be concerned with the reality-principle. It is involved in a variety of forms of behaviour, which are called ego-defences which may be responsible for symptom-formation. One speaks of a 'weak' ego when it is unable to effect the necessary compromises with life and instinctive drives, without falling back on neurotic or psychotic patterns of behaviour, while a 'strong' ego is one where the instinctive drives are healthily channelled and the stresses of life are adequately contained.

3. **The Super-ego.** This is the differentiated part of the ego which arises out of the need to face society's moral prohibitions. It is primarily unconscious and therefore inaccessible to the ego; exercises some control over the ego; though a neighbour of the id in the unconscious, it is frequently disapproving; is the moral critic responsible for the sense of guilt borne by the ego; though regarded as the voice of conscience is much more rigid. It contains the 'Oedipus complex' and the emotional complications derived from it.

It is claimed that a super-ego which is developed from fear and punishment makes for a more brittle ego structure than one based on identification with the standards of one's parents and teachers and the introjection of these standards. There are however other factors which may cause the super-ego to 'hypertrophy' and lead to psychotic breakdown or crippling obsessive-compulsive behaviour.

The Permissive Society and the Super-ego

Lowenfeld and Lowenfeld (1970) explain that Freud's concept of civilization grew out of his clinical work and that the development of civilization required drive restrictions. He then saw both the dangers of the suppression and liberation of instinctual drives. For many, suppression was not possible without neurosis, but on the other hand drive liberation threatens civilization. Freud recognized that environmental changes could resolve neurotic illness but did not share the optimism of those who claimed that liberation from sexual prohibitions would eliminate neurosis and make for a healthier society, and indeed they have been proved wrong.

Freud advocated a rational education which would lead to the control of drives and the preservation of civilization. The rapid growth of science and technology, the decline of religious belief and the rationally-orientated drive liberation in education have all contributed to cultural changes which deny the power of the basic drives and have led to the formation of a weak ego and an incompletely developed super-ego with consequent regression and aggression manifesting strongly in individual development.

The core of the super-ego is determined by the earliest parental images. Lack of effective discipline over the pregenital, oral and aggressive drives of children, a less marked latency period, the indulgent education and general social climate of permissiveness have all contributed to a weakened image of the parental figures and to the formation of a poorly functioning super-ego which cannot solve the task of control and sublimation, but still maintains its powers of punishment and self-destruction.

As parental authority and the influence of monotheism decline, the influence of the group becomes increasingly powerful and encompasses younger ages. Disappointment in the parents leads to youth's contempt of the cultural traditions of civilization which they represent and neurotic manifestations and their analyses reflect this. The authors illustrate their thesis with three case histories where complaints of dissatisfaction, self-hate, no motivation, inability to love and poor control of the drives are manifest. They point out that analysis is increasingly difficult in a social climate where the super-ego is thought of as a superfluous appendix.

They conclude that sexual freedom has not produced greater mental health but only new neurotic constellations. Culture is based on a balance of psychological forces and is threatened if this balance is impaired by losing one of its supports. The decline of the super-ego disturbs the equilibrium to a dangerous degree.

The Psychopathology of Shame

Levin (1971) lists as the most significant external factors in the arousal of shame: criticism; ridicule; scorn; and abandonment by others. The ego, in accordance with the pleasure principle, attempts to avoid such feelings which in the process of development call on the following defences: (*a*) the limiting of self-exposure; (*b*) repression of certain internalized thoughts, feelings and impulses which evoke shame in the absence of self-exposure; (*c*) the development of the ego-ideal, *i.e.* the wish to perform in such a manner as to protect oneself from being shamed by others; (*d*) the limiting of libidinal investment; and (*e*) the discharge of aggression, *e.g.* the blaming of others for one's own failures.

Shame begins to appear in early childhood and may undergo major reinforcement during the oedipal or latency phases. It later concentrates on aspects of the self which are exposed to others and may therefore be manifest through obsessive concern with parts of thc body, *e.g.* size or shape of nose, and this can be displaced to external objects such as parents or friends. Those with strong shame reactions are highly sensitive and may develop a secondary shame for reacting so strongly and attempt to counter these feelings by denying their sensitivity or inhibitions. The author stresses the importance of the analysis of shame since it represents one of the major motives for defence.

THE LIBIDO THEORY

This deals with that energy which is attached to the sexual instinct. Originally Freud regarded the sex instinct as it is understood in the everyday sense, but he later applied it to any pleasurable sensation relating to the bodily function, and also, through the process of sublimation, to socially approved forms of behaviour such as fellow-feeling and enjoyment of work and social responsibilities. Brown (1961) explains:

> . . . he used the word to refer to what would ordinarily be described as 'desire'.

The reason Freud gave for defining sex in this unusual way was the obvious fact that adult sex strivings are not necessarily exclusively directed towards persons of the opposite sex; in the perversions they may be directed towards persons of the same sex, towards the individual himself, towards animals, or even towards inanimate objects. Nor, for that matter, is genital union necessarily the object of sexual behaviour; for the mouth and anus may also be involved. Lastly, in the behaviour of infants, actions are observable which resemble those of adult perverts (*e.g.* interest in urination and defaecation, thumb-sucking, or showing the naked body and taking pleasure in observing others naked).

The libido can therefore be attached to a variety of objects and Freud pointed out the chronological sequence that such attachments follow and defined three phases:

1. The Oral Phase

This starts at birth and continues for approximately 18 months. It has been suggested that oral eroticism stems from the pleasure derived by the infant from breast feeding, but sucking movements have been described prior to sucking. The importance of the breast as a source of nourishment is obvious and when it is withdrawn, alternatives which give erotic 'nourishment' are sought and in infancy these include thumb-sucking or putting other objects in the mouth. This oral eroticism persists into adult life and is seen in kissing, smoking and eating as well as in overt sexual perversions (p. 407). Although the libido is primarily fixated at an oral level, it is, in earliest infancy, diffusely spread all over the body and auto-eroticism is paramount; this narcissism may persist into adult life. In early infancy the ego is undifferentiated, *i.e.* it has not yet reached the stage when it can distinguish 'self' from 'not self', and the first love-object, the breast, may be regarded by the infant as an extension of itself and it is only when it is withdrawn that this universality of self is broken and that external love-objects are identified. The early oral phase is a passive one, but when the child acquires teeth it assumes a more aggressive role. Brown (1961) points out that this later oral phase was described by Karl Abraham, who contributed greatly to the libido theory.

Abraham had been an embryologist before taking up psychoanalytic work, and it was natural for him to think in terms of maturational processes which caused libidinal development to take place in an orderly sequence of stages each with its typical zone and aim.

2. The Anal Phase

This overlaps the oral one and is said to continue till 3 years. Erogenic zones are anus, rectum and bladder, and pleasure is derived from excretion and later retention of urine and faeces. It is then that an ambivalent attitude develops towards adults who both thwart and gratify the child's desires, and characteristics such as cleanliness, neatness and punctuality are also established.

3. The Phallic Phase

This overlaps the anal one and continues to develop till the child is about 7 years old. There are naturally differences between the sexes.

(a) *In boys,* awareness of penis sensitivity may lead to masturbation at an early age and associated phantasies are usually those of the mother. The father is seen as a rival for the mother's love and the boy develops hostile thoughts towards him. This situation is referred to as the *Oedipus complex,* after the main character in Sophocles' tragedy *Oedipus Rex,* who killed his father and married his mother, without knowing the identity of either. The gods were angry, for incest was denied to mortals and a plague was visited on Thebes and Oedipus suffered symbolic castration by having his eyes put out. The working through of the Oedipus situation is a very important part of psycho-sexual development and the individual usually works through it by the fourth to fifth year. At about the same time the boy becomes aware of the female lack of a penis, which in association with his guilt over the Oedipus situation creates a fear of punishment and what is known as '*castration anxiety*'.

(b) *In girls* the situation is more complex. The discovery of a penis in the male creates what is called '*penis envy*' and this is associated with a tendency to blame the mother for depriving her of this object. It is then that she turns from her mother to her father and has phantasies of getting from him either a penis or a baby and the mother becomes her rival from the father's love. This has been called the Electra complex, again from a Greek myth in which Electra connives at the death of her mother Clytemnestra who had murdered her father Agamemnon. It is said to occur when the girl has renounced the hope of masculinity and reconciled herself to castration as an accepted fact.

There are therefore fundamental differences between these two processes. The boy fears he will be castrated or punished, while the girl feels that she has already been castrated or punished. The working through of the Oedipus situation marks the termination of infantile sexuality, while an unconscious tendency to perpetuate Oedipal strivings forms the basis for many neurotic processes.

Following these three phases, there is a fourth stage, which is called the *Latency Period,* and is said to exist between 7 and 12 years, or the onset of puberty. During it the Oedipus situation is resolved and a stronger super-ego developed, with increased moral responsibility. Curiosity is directed into non-sexual channels and the child makes rapid progress in scholastic and physical activities. It is during this period that group loyalties such as gang-membership and hero-worship outside the family circle (usually from someone of the same sex) occur. After the latency period there is *adolescence* when the sex interest is strongly re-awakened, with consequent masturbation and interest in the opposite or same sex, depending on the degree of resolution of the Oedipal situation. Much of this increased sexual activity is of course due to hormonal changes.

During all these phases the libido is supplying and directing the love-energy but the above descriptions do not convey the economic and environmental factors which are also associated with it. The following is a masterly summary by Brown (1961):

(1) Libido is best conceived as drive energy, the principal components of which are sexual (in the broad sense defined above), but Freud never subscribed to the view that no other instincts existed or that 'everything is sex'. Component instincts such as scoptophilia, the desire to look, and motility are described, and it was made quite clear that the sexual instinct was singled out because it was regarded as the most important one and, subject to repression, 'the one we know most about'. The term 'life force' is too metaphysical to apply to a concept which is a purely biological one.

(2) In its economic aspects, libido in an individual is regarded as a closed energy system regulated by the physical law of conservation of energy, so that libido withdrawn from one area must inevitably produce effects elsewhere. Hence the psychoanalyst's conviction that any symptom removed by suggestion (*i.e.* without release of the energy maintaining it) will make its appearance in some other form, *e.g.* cessation of smoking may be replaced by over-eating, cessation of habitual masturbation or intercourse by anxiety. In his theory of wit Freud saw laughter as an explosion of energy previously employed to repress antisocial feelings which for the moment society is prepared to permit in partially disguised form. Jokes about God or mothers-in-law under the disguise of 'just for fun' lift the repression from sadistic feelings embodying real hate or irreverence which are temporarily permitted expression in an implied playful contest. This realization is embodied in G. K. Chesterton's insight that we only laugh at serious things which would ordinarily produce sympathy, grief, fear, or awe, although obviously this applies to only one form of humour.

(3) Libido passes through the stages of maturation already described, each of which is biologically determined, is centred on a specific erotogenic zone (mouth, anus, penis), and has a specific aim of gratification (sucking, incorporating, and biting, retention and aggressive expulsion, penetration). Adult genital sexuality represents a fusion of pregenital with genital drives, and a sexual perversion is said to be present only when pregenital drives in the adult become primary and supersede the genital one as goal. But although the stages of libido development are biologically determined, it is recognized that their development is influenced by the reaction of significant figures to the child's behaviour while it is passing through them; the effects of upbringing, the parental attitudes to early bowel training and masturbation or prohibitions

generally, have an immediate influence upon the relative emphasis or frustration of the particular zones and their aims, as also does the early or later timing of their application. The immediate effect, however, is of less significance than the delayed results of maturation and learning on the adult personality in terms of fixation, regression, object relationships, symptom formation, and character. The timing of maturation and learning is important because the same act on the part of the mother will produce different effects at different times in the child's life (phase specificity), and the interaction between events experienced at various stages of development must also be taken into account. Naturally, quantitative variations in the constitutional strength of a drive or in the strength of stimulation and the length of time it is applied have an important influence on the final result.

Libido-direction. This not only varies in its localization such as anal, oral and genital, but also in its object choice and here too it goes through stages. The first is *auto-erotic,* where the child is both lover and loved one and this is entirely an *id* activity. The second is *narcissistic* which occurs where the ego is differentiated from external reality; self-awareness results and libidinal impulses are self-directed. The child may seek satisfaction from himself in the face of reality, and this process may persist into adult life. These two stages, both meaning self-love, are not identical. The former is independent of the concept of a personality and is really a form of animal self-stimulation. Narcissism, though mediating through auto-eroticism, is a sequel of ego-differentiation. A third stage is allo-eroticism, which is the seeking of a love-object outside oneself and is at the core of the Oedipus situation.

The fate of the libido can therefore be allo-erotic or narcissistic. The latter can be primary as described already, or secondary where the libido is frustrated and is turned inwards to the ego which now becomes identified as a love-object. This can be a normal phase but it can be evidence of severe mental breakdown.

The libido can also be *fixated.* Normally there is a progression of love-objects from mother to mate, but arrest can occur at any time at the mother or mother-substitute level. It can also *regress,* which implies previous maturity, but in the face of a traumatic situation the libido has returned to an earlier love-object from which it had derived greater security. Libido may be *repressed,* which is a defensive mechanism to prevent the flooding of consciousness with painful or distasteful material. It can be used to keep the normal quota of homosexuality under control, so that the average person who is neither a latent nor overt homosexual can be said to be an effectively repressed one. Lastly the libido may be *sublimated* or expressed in a socially approved form where the energy of the sex desire is directed into non-sexual channels. Great social contributions such as the creative activity of artists have been attributed to sublimation.

MENTAL MECHANISMS

If there is any contribution from psychoanalysis which has given us greater understanding of mental illness and which has had almost universal acceptance, it is that relating to mental or adaptive mechanisms. The key to all these mechanisms is *repression* which has two functions, (1) to exclude material from rising into consciousness or *primal* function, and (2) to expel material from consciousness, or *after-expulsion* function. The problem of the ego is to come to terms with reality, the super-ego and the id, and therefore ideas are excluded which may lead to tension or anxiety. Repression is therefore a means of avoiding conflict and on occasions super-ego impulses as well as those of the id may be repressed.

Displacement

This is said to occur when an undesirable idea which might provoke anxiety does not reach consciousness in its original form, but is transferred to another object, person or situation, so that it is more acceptable to the ego. An emotional attitude such as love or hate is usually involved and the displaced object is not nearly so disturbing to the ego. This mechanism can be recognized in paranoid states, where the object of the hostility is a substitute, or in obsessional neurosis when the purification rites are a displacement of earlier guilt feelings.

Dissociation

This occurs when a painful experience may be incapable of displacement because of its extensive associations, and as a result a large part of the ego-content is split off, resulting in gross amnesia or some other hysterical reaction. Effective repression is obtained at the price of functional incapacity but the ego is freed of conflict for it can no longer morally recognize or be responsible for that which is now unconscious. This mechanism has already been mentioned as that responsible for multiple personality and massive amnesia, but it need not always be so gross and there is a more localized form called *conversion* which is the somatization of a psychological conflict which is the basis of hysterical symptomatology of a motor or sensory nature, *e.g.* paralysis and anaesthesias. An interesting prediction of a conversion process is the Psalmist's plea—'If I forget thee, O Jerusalem, may my right hand forget its cunning' (Psalm 137 v.5).

Reaction-formation

This is the process whereby the repressed object produces an attitude in consciousness which is the reverse of the disapproved one. Over-solicitousness for the health of a parent may be an attempt to deny hostile impulses while at the same time satisfying the dictates of the super-ego. Extreme personality traits, such as over-aggressiveness, over-submissiveness or over-politeness may be the results of unconscious efforts to conceal their opposites.

Projection

This is the externalization of personal insecurities. At a simple level, the man who has dishonest intentions (albeit unconscious) may be preoccupied with frustrating the dishonesty of others. It is the basis of the paranoid reaction in which the patient accuses others of acts or intentions to which he himself unconsciously subscribes. It is seen in young children who have great difficulty in assuming personal responsibility for naughtiness and are prone to believe that others are to blame. It is a very common mechanism in the mentally ill and also in everyday life where it is seen most clearly in certain 'fringe' individuals or groups who have a pathological hatred and are constantly attributing to their enemies their own unconscious hostilities. It is more comforting for the ego to feel that the hostile impulses have found what it considers a legitimate object rather than an illicit one, or more reassuring still, have not been directed against itself. The ego thus protected can function more efficiently, but there is always the threat of ego-disintegration, which may be manifest by the appearance of delusions and even hallucinations. In order to counter disintegration, the individual may strive to convert others to his way of thinking in the hope that if other people share his ideas he may not feel so abnormal. The mechanism carries within itself many of the features of displacement, but has a much more sinister clinical significance.

Identification

This occurs when the person patterns himself on another individual or on a group, and is found in the Oedipus situation where the boy identifies with his father, and at a more pathological level, where a person living with another of unsound mind accepts and identifies with the delusional system expressed (*folie à deux* or communicable insanity). It can play an important part in the healthy development of the ego, or be evidence of gross mental disorder. It can also account for the sympathy law-abiding citizens frequently show for the criminal, even to the extent of attacking the policeman who is trying to make an arrest. Unconsciously the person is saying 'There, but for the grace of God . . .' It is also seen in the champion of lost causes and in members of hospital staff who pattern themselves on their chiefs. The slightest idiosyncrasy is seized on and may unconsciously be caricaturized. Christmas concerts in hospital afford an excellent opportunity for identification, and of course for other less flattering mechanisms.

Rationalization

This is an attempt by the ego to make an emotionally toned and irrational attitude appear logical. It is seen in delusional states, but is very common in everyday life where the ego is under attack or where it is necessary to boost it by depreciating the efforts of others. But to see all criticism of oneself or one's friends as rationalizations by the offending party is more likely to be an example of the mechanism than evidence of insight into the motives of others.

Introversion

This has a highly specialized meaning in psychoanalysis. Freud used it for phantasy-cathexis, which means that the libido achieves gratification from phantasies of objects and situations as in day-dreaming, which is prefixed with the word 'compensatory' when the phantasies form a substitute or retreat from painful experiences.

Polarities

These are opposite pairs which are frequently invoked in psychoanalytic theory. Examples are love-hate, pleasure-pain, life-death and sado-masochism. One pole may represent the other in consciousness as in reaction-formation.

Restitution

This is the lightening of a load of guilt by some form of expiation.

It is seen in the normal in the 'day's good deed', but can become pathological in the person who is obsessed with his benevolent drives and who may react catastrophically when the channels for expression are blocked.

FREUD'S THEORY OF DREAMS

Freud regarded dreams as 'the royal road to the unconscious' and his researches raised their interpretation from the darkened tents of the soothsayers to the consulting room of the physician and the hospital clinic. He said that dreams were the mode of reaction of the mind to stimuli acting upon it during sleep, though these stimuli need not be exclusively psychological, and laid down the following three basic principles in dream interpretation: (1) The function of the dream is to preserve sleep; (2) there is a latent as well as a manifest content and it is frequently the former which is the more significant; and (3) it represents the gratification of an unfulfilled wish which is usually infantile. Dream analysis therefore gives clues to repressed urges which were disguised by the manifest content. In the waking state censorship or repression is more effective, but in sleep it is alleged to be relaxed and an impasse in therapy can often be resolved by dream analysis.

Efforts to disguise the dream are called *the dream-work* and Freud described four mechanisms whereby it operates. Three of these are regressive with archaic forms of expression showing conspicuous absence of abstract thinking. They are: (1) *dramatization* where abstract ideas are given solid or concrete shape with the free use of symbols representing the repressed activities or experiences; (2) *condensation* which is a form of abbreviation or shorthand which conceals from the dreamer some of the latent content by omission, or by using a part, sometimes a very small part, to represent a whole, or by the fusing of a variety of latent elements sharing a common feature into one piece; (3) *displacement* which is the replacement of the latent content by a remotely associated element which is no more than an allusion or oblique reference, or shifting the accent so that the latent content is barely recognizable; (4) *secondary elaboration* which occurs just as full consciousness is regained and continues for a time during the waking state, thus making the dream appear more rational. As secondary elaboration is ego-inspired, it is advisable to get the patient to write down his dreams immediately on waking before this distortion begins to operate.

Dream Interpretation

This is practised by using free-association to convert the manifest content to latent, and the material produced is handled as neurotic symptoms, on the assumption that each dream represents a wish, probably infantile, which the patient cannot tolerate in the waking state, but in its disguised form can achieve gratification and sleep. A familiarity with dream symbols is essential for the therapist and the following are a selected sample: exalted persons such as kings and queens for parents; reference to water for birth; going on a journey for dying; clothes or uniform for nakedness or shame; the number three for male genitalia; long, straight objects like poles, trees, sticks or sharp objects like daggers or guns and revolvers for the penis; serpent, balloons, fast racing cars, flying in aircraft for erection; a variety of receptacles, such as caves, jars, pockets or a jewel case for the female genitalia.

ANALYTICAL PSYCHOLOGY

This was founded by C. G. Jung (1875–1961) who was an early associate of Freud but after a few years broke with the psychoanalytic movement as he had ascribed to the unconscious functions which were considered beyond those necessary for orthodox psychoanalytic theory. He was keenly interested in symbols and found during analysis that some recurred more frequently than others and were common to a variety of cultures, particularly in myths and legends. Jung considered that these were not part of the individual's personal experience but were, like his body, made up of his racial past and profoundly influenced behaviour, forming part of the racial or collective unconscious as opposed to the personal one. This accent on race has been misconstrued by those obsessed with racial theory and particularly supremacy, but it is unlikely that Jung subscribed to this view and he would appear rather to be pleading for the appreciation of a number of 'experiences' in our unconscious which could not have got there post-natally. These he called *archetypes*, which, though showing some cultural differences, had universal application. Examples are gods, witches, demons and spirits which are punitive and devouring; the eternal compassionate mother; and magic numbers of geometrical designs such as the mandala, a four-sided figure with a central circle. Personality he regarded as the *persona* or mask worn by Roman actors and was therefore that part of consciousness exposed to the gaze of the world. Those aspects of mental life which are denied in consciousness develop in the unconscious and form the personal unconscious or 'shadow', which plays an important part in dreams and is explained in terms of Jungian typology.

PSYCHOLOGICAL TYPES

These, which form one of Jung's major studies, were based on two attitudes, extraversion and introversion, and originally to each he ascribed a fundamental function, to the former, feeling and to the latter, thought. This does not mean that the introvert is incapable of feeling or the extravert of thought, but that these functions are unconscious. When the introvert is faced with a situation demanding feeling rather than thought, a conflict arises because of tension between these opposing faculties. Jung later modified this relatively simple plan by ascribing the four functions, thinking, feeling, intuition and sensation to each individual, and qualifying them as 'superior' and 'inferior', with thought and feeling, intuition and sensation as paired opposites. Diagrammatically (Fig. 1), if thought were 'superior', feeling was 'inferior', with sensation and intuition coming in between. The scheme was further complicated by introducing empirical thinking between thinking and sensation, emotional feeling between sensation and feeling, intuitive feeling between feeling and intuition, and speculative thinking between intuition and thinking. Add to these the attitudes extraversion and introversion, and the mariner's compass loses on points!

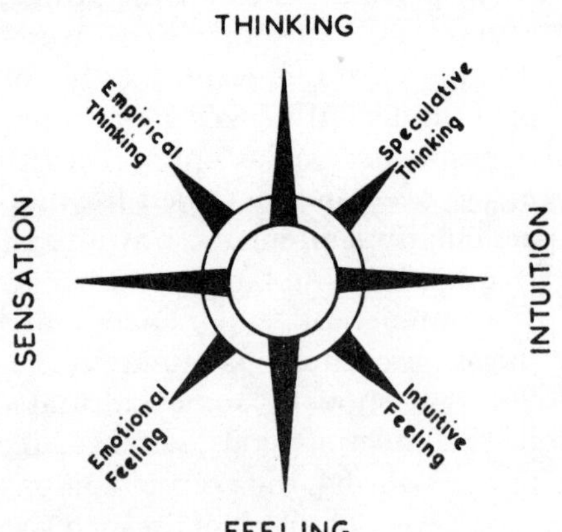

Figure 1. Psychological types.

Jung laid great stress on dream analysis, but his interpretations, while in some respects similar to those of Freud, took into account the archetypes and he dismissed the idea of a censorship preventing the emergence of unconscious material into consciousness. He regarded a symbol as not only evidence of repression, but an attempt to point out the way to the dreamer. The Jungian analyst is expected to use his knowledge of anthropology and world classical literature to interpret dreams and is not restricted by the dreamer's personal inexperience of these data, for, he argues, they are part of his collective or racial unconscious. Analysis of the personal unconscious is therefore only the first part of the treatment; the second and more difficult is that of the racial unconscious. The libido is seen differently too, as a primal and universal force corresponding to Bergson's *élan vital*.

The psyche is said to have an unconscious presentation which is the sexual counterpart of the true sexual expression of the individual and either sex may project its opposition. The feminine unconscious persona is called the *anima* and the male the *animus*. Because Jung considered the woman to be monogamous, her animus is multiform and George Eliot, the authoress, is quoted as an example of an active and multiform animus which is projected into her writings.

Jungian analysis, if properly conducted, calls for great scholarship and training and it may be that this has deterred recruitment. It has, however, made serious contributions, particularly to our understanding of some schizophrenic processes, and its founder has earned his place in psychology and psychiatry, not only for his early work on schizophrenia, his Word-Association test and his elaboration of the archetypes, but for many other contributions. Brown (1961) quotes Murphy's (1947) comments on Jung:

> Jung's method—it is no more than a friendly exaggeration to say this—is to argue that because A is somewhat like B and B can, under certain circumstances, share something with C, and C has been known on occasions to have been suspected of being related to D, the conclusion in full-fledged logical form is that A = D. As the language of *science* this is meaningless.

Brown's own comments are worth quoting:

> . . . the present writer . . . gets much the same impression from reading Jung as might be obtained from reading the scriptures of the Hindus, Taoists or Confucius; although well aware that many wise and true things are being said, he feels that they could have been said just as well without involving us in the psychological theories upon which they are supposedly based.

Although Jung has not had anything like the impact on medical psychology as Freud, he has a fascination for theologians and a number have adopted Jung's theories in their 'pastoral psychology' or more generally in their mission of healing.

INDIVIDUAL PSYCHOLOGY

This is the name given to the system of psychology devised by Alfred Adler (1870–1937). He was the first of Freud's associates to break away and establish his own theory which he regarded as a key to the understanding of the whole of mental life. He expressed his basic tenet thus (Adler, 1938): 'To be a human being means the possession of a feeling of inferiority that is constantly pressing on towards its own conquest.' His writings are strongly influenced by Nietzschean philosophy, and terms such as 'organ inferiority' with strivings to over-compensate for this inferiority, and the 'will to power' are frequently referred to. He considered that man has to make major adjustments to society, vocation and love, and his capacity to make these would depend on childhood experiences and the 'life-style' patterned on them. He explained that the helplessness of the child gives it an 'inferiority complex' which can be accentuated by an organ inferiority or unsuitable early handling such as spoiling, sarcasm or snubbing. Inferiority is dealt with by the individual in three ways: (1) by successful compensation, as, for example, Beethoven with his deafness and Demosthenes with his stammer; (2) defeat is followed by retreat, which is regarded as the normal pattern in some cultures; (3) compromise or over-compensation, the former being a tendency to attribute the failure to the physical inferiority, while the latter is a ridiculous protest against it. Examples of the latter are the little man who is always aggressive and challenging, and the dull man who affects an intellectual pose. Over-compensation can result in decompensation and neurosis.

Adler used the term 'neurosis' in an all-embracing sense and paid no heed to differences in diagnosis. He made sweeping generalizations, such as 'every neurosis can be understood as an attempt to free oneself from a feeling of inferiority in order to gain a feeling of superiority'. His concept of aetiology was not localized in the unconscious but in the child's environment and family style. The inferior organ he regarded as occasionally conditioned by psychological factors and serving as a defence mechanism and in practically all illness he defined three factors: the structural, the functional, and the psychic, the last being the major one in neurotic illness. This concept has found a place in the field of psychosomatic medicine, but as with many speculations, adequate proof is elusive. The idea of 'organ jargon', where the inferior or affected part is in fact communicating its psychological stress, is an Adlerian concept. Neurotic or delinquent behaviour may stem from the child's erroneous solution to its problems. Over-compensation may result in a phantasy goal which is virtually unattainable and give rise to abnormal behaviour patterns, or to much compensatory day-dreaming and withdrawal from reality.

Treatment is largely a matter of imparting insight and depends on a painstaking analysis of the early childhood experiences and life and family 'styles', paying particular attention to birth rank, sibling rivalry, family careers and adverse environmental factors. An appreciation of the patient's strivings or 'masculine protest' would then emerge and repetition of behaviour patterns become evident. Efforts to overcome the handicap include advice and even practical help, for the Adlerian does not adhere to the detached 'scientific' attitude of the psychoanalyst. It is not surprising, therefore, that social rehabilitation units, out-patient social clubs and day hospitals have been largely inspired by Adlerian theory, though it could be argued that such expedients would have evolved in any case. It is essentially a system of psychology for the teacher and the 'practical' doctor who have a high regard for the role of environment in the production and removal of neurotic illness. Like other analytical therapies, it requires knowledge and experience, though as it does not involve 'depth' processes, personal analysis is not essential.

Although Adler has formally had nothing like the influence on psychotherapy as Freud, much of his teaching has been incorporated by others and even Freudian analysts now pay more attention to the ego and non-sexual factors in the causation of neurosis. His methods appeal to those searching for shorter techniques in psychotherapy and Stekel (1868–1940), who elaborated his own methods, incorporated much of Adler's teaching. He interpreted the life-style or life-line of the patient as the 'life-lie', for he regarded the patient as pursuing a series of fictive goals.

BRITISH CONTRIBUTIONS TO PSYCHOTHERAPY

These enjoyed their own vintage years, starting with the First World War and petering out after the Second. Although Ernest Jones (1879–1958) was one of the leaders of the psychoanalytical movement and authoritatively introduced Freud's work into this country, there were less orthodox psychotherapists who elaborated their own forms of treatment. They were prepared to adopt what they considered best in any school and adapt it to the culture in which they lived. They styled themselves 'Eclectics', and though that label in orthodox analytic circles has now an unsavoury reputation, it was borne and still is borne by psychotherapists of great distinction. W. H. R. Rivers, in association with the eminent neurologist, Head

(Head & Rivers, 1920), experimented with sensory receptors in the skin and described the *protopathic* or crude and gross reaction, and the *epicritic* or fine and more localized reaction. By generalizing on this distinction, he concluded there was a protopathic life in lower organisms which precedes in development the epicritic life in higher organisms and that the distinction between these two functions permeated the whole nervous system. Young children show an 'all or none' reaction which in the course of development becomes more graduated and Rivers, who practised psychiatry with Service patients during the First World War, regarded the reactions he treated as evidence of the primitive, protopathic factor. He defined five types of reaction: aggression, flight, manipulative activity, immobility and collapse, the term 'manipulative activity' being used to define a vacillating state between aggression and flight, with the carrying out of purposeless actions in a state of apparent mental confusion. It is not difficult to see the resemblance between this condition and some aspects of the 'catastrophic reaction' as defined by Goldstein (p. 107). His theory was certainly applicable to the gross hysterical reactions that abounded during the First World War, and though they were largely confined to other ranks and were not nearly so much in evidence during the Second World War, they were observable phenomena for which treatment was necessary and they do in fact still occur. Rivers (1920) also appreciated there were unconscious factors in neurotic illness and described cases where early traumatic experiences led to phobias in later life.

Suttie's Modifications of Freudian Theory (Suttie, 1935)

This is in accord with the orthodox Freudian's accent on separation anxiety, but while Freud considered that culture developed from the thwarting of the sex-impulse, Suttie maintained that it derived from the activity of play which gives the individual that reassuring contact with his fellows which he lost when the mother's nurtural services were no longer required or offered. Anger is aimed not at the direct removal of frustration or attainment of the goal of the moment still less at (the mother's) destruction, but *at inducing the mother to accomplish these wishes for the ehild.* Brown (1961) in a review of Suttie's psychopathic theory describes the striving of the neurotic as an insistent demand for the help of others. The infant who has a strong need for love and security may be deprived by the mother's neurotic inability to give affection, a new baby, cultural factors such as bowel training, or economic factors such as the mother's need to return to work. The child tries to remove the cause of his anxiety and thereby change his feelings of anxiety and hate into love and security. The mechanism used is similar to the 'life-style' described by Adler and it may influence personality development. Four attitudes are described:

1. 'Mother is always good—if she does not love me it is because I am bad'. This could later lead to depressive states or an 'inferiority complex'.
2. 'Mother is bad for not loving me—I will not trust her'. This could lead to a persecutory attitude.
3. 'If I become a baby again, mother will be good to me as she was before'. This predisposes to hysterical and regressive behaviour.
4. 'You must love me or I will bite you—I *will* get attention somehow'. Delinquency may arise from such an attitude.

Though Suttie accepted Freud's general observations on sexual development in the child he paid great importance to cultural factors. The anal stage derives its accent from the cultural attitude to physical cleanliness; the Oedipus complex is not necessarily universal but derives from certain aspects in the mother's character and her relationship with her husband and son. Some see Suttie's views as being similar to those of Adler but here too he denied the universality of Adler's power drive and described it as 'an anxiety-reaction to a particular mode of upbringing and hence contingent upon certain cultural influences'.

He commented on the modern 'taboo on tenderness' and interpreted epithets such as 'mummy's boy', 'milk-sop', 'soppy' and 'cry-baby' as anti-feminist in contrast with the idealization of toughness, aggressiveness and hardness. He considered these values as a reaction against early weaning and a revenge upon and repudiation of the weaning mother. He opposed Freud's views on 'penis envy' in the female as patriarchal and antifeminist bias and pointed out other forms of envy in the male, such as his jealousy of the female's ability to produce children or 'Zeus jealousy'. This attitude is found in all cultures from the primitive Aranda tribe of Australian aborigines who believe that man can bear children, to the modern equivalent of the 'Couvade'*. Suttie did not share Freud's atheism and could not subscribe to the view that religion was a 'universal obsessional neurosis' but regarded it as a form of psycho-social therapy which like psychotherapy operated by restoring mental health through love.

Crichton-Miller (1945) was the epitome of the British Eclectics and in his little book, *Psychoanalysis and its Derivatives,* he gives a lucid appraisal of the major divisions, enlightened by his own penetrating criticism. He founded the Tavistock Clinic in 1920 and

* In Western society this refers to psychosomatic complaints from a husband which are related to his wife's pregnancy.

from humble beginnings developed it into a major psychotherapeutic centre whose pioneer work on Human Relations and Group Therapy has been widely recognized. Balint (1957) initiated at the Tavistock Clinic courses in psychotherapy for general practitioners, thus filling a great need. The doctors attend regularly as a group and discuss their own patients' problems and at the same time gain insight into their own resistances and emotional difficulties which are raised in their dealings with these patients. The popularity of these courses and the demand that they be duplicated in other parts of the country, has been regarded by some as a temporary feature which will end when the medical schools impart adequate psychiatric training to their students. This is speculative, for it presumes that undergraduates who are still not legally responsible for their patients' treatment can be given that responsibility in the psychiatric field which they have not in the medical or surgical fields. That they will be under supervision does not produce a parallel situation, for Balint's pupils are mature doctors with complete responsibility for their patients in all departments. It is doubtful even if such experience can be imparted at the house physician or intern level, though a considerable amount of training for psychotherapy can be absorbed during that period.

T. A. Ross, though not noted as an original contributor to the theory and practice of psychotherapy (he was rather a British advocate of du Bois and Déjerine or the persuasive schools, where the patient was given heavy suggestion as to his capacity to overcome his handicap), nevertheless has a special place. His prestige was such that at a time when many doubted, he made psychotherapy a respectable pursuit for the physician and he was the first director of the Cassel Hospital which was founded specifically for the treatment of the neuroses. His book (Ross, 1937) *The Common Neuroses,* though by present standards rather superficial, was a landmark in that it brought a practical and easily understood system of psychotherapy within reach of all medical practitioners.

Halliday has made a major contribution to the definition and limitations of psychosomatic medicine. His 'psychosomatic formula' (Halliday, 1943) helped to bridge the gap between the theoretical psychologist and the clinician and provided a formula which both could accept and thus paved the way for fruitful cooperation.

Foulkes has not only made pioneer contributions to group therapy, but by introducing his methods to a military neurosis centre during the Second World War, brought the technique within range of a great number of psychiatrists. It is largely due to his influence that these group techniques have been so freely adopted in mental hospitals and have given to psychiatrists in training, not only in the analytically orientated centres, but in mental hospitals all over the country, an insight into dynamic psychiatry, which they might otherwise not have received. In a recent paper (Foulkes, 1961) he pointed out the limitations of psychotherapy and illustrated the change in thinking which has taken place in the last half-century. While to Freud the limitations were biological, they are now being increasingly recognized as cultural, the neurotic being the weakest link in the chain of what is, in fact, a family neurosis and that when a patient improves, some other member of the family may go under.

Millais Culpin brought a critical psychiatric appraisal to the problems of occupational diseases (Smith *et al.*, 1927; Culpin, 1929) and disability associated with telegraphist's cramp and miner's nystagmus were shown to be primarily of neurotic origin. These studies set the pattern for the estimation of neurosis in industry and its influence on morbidity rates.

Maxwell Jones undertook what was probably the most difficult of tasks in psychiatry, namely, the treatment of the psychopath *en masse*. Individually the problem is a formidable one, but when it is concentrated, it is well nigh impossible. Yet for years he directed (if that is the word for it) his Social Rehabilitation Centre at Belmont and introduced analytical concepts to the group situation. Though the percentage of therapeutic successes may not have been particularly high, it was a prolonged experiment which very few could have carried out, and the lessons gained from it have had more than local significance. Joshua Bierer introduced the Day Hospital to Britain and by adapting Adlerian methods, provided a theoretical basis for what might have become haphazard improvization (Bierer, 1951). Out-patient social clubs, too, owe much to his influence and the impulse to get and keep people out of the mental hospital could not have been maintained at its present strength if these essential ancillary services were not available. The impact of the Day Hospital is spreading beyond the borders of the psychiatric clinic and is already being seriously considered by other branches of medicine.

There are many other workers who by their researches have made valuable contributions to British psychiatry in its academic, educational and therapeutic aspects, and the above examples have been selected mainly because of their social impact.

The object of listing these names is to show that major contributions to psychotherapy are not exclusively a psychoanalytic monopoly and that British eclecticism has played an important part in initiating and coordinating theories and techniques of psychotherapy. As will be seen later, there are still more schools of psychotherapy, and if history is a guide it is unlikely that their adherents will be capable of presenting an unbiased account of their advantages and limitations. It is therefore very important that eclecticism should be maintained, not as the last refuge of the unbeliever, but for well-informed psychiatrists who have no special interest in propagating the *Weltanschauung* of the individual schools but desire to increase man's understanding of man and place the benefits at the service of patients. Rivalry between schools may lead to, and in fact has led to, victory of one over the others with initial rejection of the others' achievements. The much ridiculed Adler who lost to the Freudians was not so far out with his emphasis on the ego, the 'here and now' situation had his failure to give pride of place to the id, and we are now seeing the incorporation of some of his views by his previous opponents.

POST-FREUDIAN SCHOOLS OF PSYCHOTHERAPY

H. S. Sullivan (1892–1949). He was an American-born psychiatrist who had a unique understanding of schizophrenia and made important contributions to its psychotherapy. His views are presented in his book (Sullivan, 1948) but although they have been widely appreciated in the United States, they have not been popular in Britain. He itemized personality development in the following way:

Personality Development

1. *Infancy.* Empathy is the important influence; an increasing awareness of self; realization of one's capacities.
2. *Childhood.* Follows infancy and is distinguished by the acquiring of language; cultural indoctrination begins and thought processes are evident; clashes occur between the parent and child.
3. *Juvenile.* Co-operation with compeers; group solidarity; competition and the desire to belong.
4. *Pre-adolescence.* From 8½ years to 12 years (or early puberty). Egocentricity gives way to social responsibility and personal friends are regarded as important as oneself.
5. *Adolescence.* Subdivided into (*a*) Early (*b*) Mid (onset of genital behaviour) (*c*) Late (establishment of durable intimate relationships).
6. *Maturity.*

In his approach to personality he was much influenced by the philosopher J. G. Fichte's dictum: 'the "I" is not a fact but an act'. He held that the Ego is the only ultimate reality and that it exists because it posits itself. This extreme subjectivism was a departure from previous attitudes which held that the self could be detached and observe the world from its own fastness. Previous claims by philosophers and psychologists that we are as if in an ivory tower leaving it periodically to satisfy our physical and mental needs to return basically unaffected are denied by Sullivan. He claimed that we do not merely *have* experiences—we *are* our experiences.

He divided human performances into two categories:

1. Pursuit of satisfactions such as drive or physical needs for sleep, food, drink and sex.
2. Pursuit of securities. These are mainly cultural and include . . . all those movements, actions, speech, thoughts, reveries and so on which pertain more to the culture which has been embedded in a particular individual than to the organization of his tissues and glands.

The child learns to absorb the standards of its culture and to accept the cultural attitude to 'good' and 'bad' under threat of punishment or withdrawal of approval. Feeling 'good' is identified with achievement of satisfaction and security, derived from approved behaviour, while feeling 'bad' is associated with biological urges which cannot be satisfied through approved cultural attitudes. Feeling 'bad' is therefore equated with 'anxiety'. These two categories are generally intermingled producing a complex picture with components of both feelings. A third category which is intermediate between pursuit of satisfaction and security is that of loneliness which results from a need to be physically close to another member of society.

Sullivan used 'anxiety' in a psychosomatic sense, pointing out that satisfaction of drives decreases tension particularly in voluntary and involuntary muscles and that it is related to autonomic (parasympathetic) activity.

Insecurity or frustration would produce the opposite effect and was associated with autonomic (sympathetic) activity leading to heightened tone in involuntary and voluntary muscles. The natural cycle in the infant is: sleep—hunger (pangs)—crying—satisfaction—sleep. Skeletal muscles are not utilized in this stage, for crying in itself may evoke a maternal reponse. This phase Sullivan called 'oral dynamism', which includes the respiratory and food-taking apparatus. Later, oral dynamism is less effective in securing satisfaction and skeletal muscles are used, though the muscles associated with crying may still show in increase in tone and give rise to the feeling associated with crying.

Empathy. This term is used by Sullivan to describe the 'emotional contagion or communion' which the child has for its mother or nurse and is particularly evident between the sixth and twenty-seventh months. It may give rise to feeding difficulties which are engendered by the mother's emotional distress and is said to occur also in animals and to be independent of the ordinary sensory channels. C. G. Jung (1909) held similar views. He said:

> It is not the good and pious precepts, nor is it any other inculcation of pedagogic truths that have a moulding influence upon the character of the developing child, but what most influences him is the peculiarly affective state which is totally unknown to his parents and educators. The concealed discord between the parents, the secret worry, the repressed hidden wishes, all these produce in the individual a certain affective state with its objective signs which slowly but surely, though unconsciously, works its way into the child's mind, producing therein the same conditions and hence the same reactions to external stimuli . . . The father and mother impress deeply into the child's mind the seal of their personality; the more sensitive the child, the deeper is the impression. Thus even things that are never spoken about are reflected in the child. The child imitates the gesture, and just as the gesture of the parent is the expression of an emotional state, so in turn the gesture gradually produces in the child a similar feeling, as it feels itself, so to speak, into the gesture.

Empathy, by making the child aware of its mother's emotional states, is subjected to her reaction to the child's failure to control micturition and defaecation and this may play an important part in habit training. Similarly her approval for good performance will be reflected in the communicative release of her tension.

Sullivan, as one would expect from his adherence to Fichte, regarded the individual's capacity to avoid anxiety as his 'power motive'. This gives him a feeling of ability in the handling of interpersonal relationships leading to respect of self and others. Self-respect which arises in childhood from the attitudes of others is later determined by the individual's attitude to himself. Empathy is said to be responsible for engendering opposite states in the child, anxiety or euphoria, tension or relaxation, comfort or discomfort and the chronically hostile, anxious parent will therefore produce resentment or anxiety in the child.

The Self. Once this has developed, it tends to maintain its own form and direction as a system whose basic function is to avoid anxiety. Earliest experiences are most deep-seated and pervasive and though at a later stage the individual may question and compare his experiences he never escapes those early influences. This 'homeostasis' of the 'self' is due to the production of anxiety by experiences which threaten to disrupt or come into conflict with its organization and the institution of behaviour designed to nullify this anxiety. In Freudian terms this is equivalent to a mobilization of the ego-defences, but Sullivan uses the analogy of the amoeba which digests meat and rejects glass, even when the glass is coated with meat extract. The self-structure is built up during the formative years and thereafter is determined to maintain its integrity, even should it be a poor one.

Even when the self is a derogatory and hateful system it will inhibit and misinterpret any disassociated feeling or experience of friendliness towards others; and it will misinterpret any gestures of friendliness from others. The direction and characteristics given to the self in infancy and childhood are maintained year after year at an extraordinary cost, so that most people in this culture, and presumably in any other, because of inadequate and unfortunate experience in early life, become 'inferior caricatures of what they might have been'.

It is not difficult to see how such a development could lead to a paranoid type of personality. In Sullivan's system, the individual seeks freedom from anxiety, the achievement of security and the release from tension *under all circumstances.* A hateful self no less than a pleasing one is motivated by the need to avoid anxiety and arises when the child's need for tenderness is rebuffed by the parent. When tenderness is shown he may feel he is showing the 'bad me' and his behaviour is thus 'malevolently transformed'.

Other ways of dealing with experiences which threaten self-esteem are by sublimation in which the forbidden impulse is combined with socially approved patterns, and by anger, which can temporarily neutralize anxiety.

The Self-System. This is the part of the personality which can be observed. True-self is the core of potential which may or may not have been developed and is influenced by cultural factors, since man is moulded by his culture and attempts to break with it produce anxiety. Modifications in later life are possible by people with whom the individual identifies such as parents, teachers and friends and as the self is the sum of 'reflected appraisals' what we think of ourselves may depend on what others have thought of us.

Parataxic Distortion. This is the mechanism whereby one may attribute to others traits taken from significant people in one's past. This goes on in most inter-personal relationships so that what is overt does not incorporate all that really goes on between them. The interpretation and removal of these distortions is one of the main purposes of Sullivan's psychotherapy. The patient's evaluations may be compared with those of the psychotherapist on the principle that if one's views differ from those of a person one esteems, these views may be changed. These changes are unlikely to occur in frankly delusional situations but can be effected where neurotic interpretations exist and when insight is possible such as in parataxic distortion.

Even though Sullivan's theories have a limited appeal, he was essentially a clinician and the practising psychiatrist will derive much useful information from his writings, particularly in his work *The Psychiatric Interview* (Sullivan, 1954). Here he lays down a pattern for initial history-taking, emphasizing that it is the onset of therapy.

Karen Horney (1885–1952)

For a number of years she practised as an orthodox Freudian at the Berlin Psychoanalytic Institute, but when she came to America her views changed and she became a prolific writer of serious and semi-popular works which were very much at variance with orthodox Freudian theory. Brown (1961) writes:

> The direct influences upon Horney herself are not far to seek. There was firstly her long-standing distaste for Freud's antifeminist bias, as revealed in almost all her early papers: 'On the Genesis of the Castration Complex in Women', 'The Flight from Womanhood', 'The Dread of Women', 'The Denial of the Vagina' (*International Journal of Psycho-Analysis,* v. 1924; vii, 1926; xiii, 1932; xiv, 1933) are typical titles of papers attributing sexual differences to social rather than biological factors. Secondly, although unadmitted, must have been the Marxism which during the 1920's she shared with Fromm, Reich, and of course the vast majority of Socialists and progressive thinkers in Central Europe throughout that decade, even if it did not survive the end of the Popular Front. Thirdly, there was the debt to Adler . . . Lastly, and most emphasized by Horney herself, was the influence of America, where, as she describes in *New Ways in Psychoanalysis,* she found following her arrival in the early 1930's that '. . . the greater freedom from dogmatic beliefs . . . alleviated the obligation of taking psychoanalytical theories for granted, and gave me the courage to proceed along the lines which I considered right. Furthermore, acquaintance with a culture which in many ways is different from the European taught me that many neurotic conflicts are ultimately determined by cultural conditions'.

She puts forward her main criticism of Freud in her book, *New Ways in Psychoanalysis* (Horney, 1939), in which she states that Freud's main contribution to modern psychology was the fundamental triad of concepts: (1) that psychic processes are strictly determined, (2) that actions and feelings may be unconsciously motivated and (3) that the motivations are emotional in nature. She then proceeds to comment on these three principles. Psychic determinism she accepts, but she differs in her concept of unconscious motivation for she regards the Freudian sense too formalistic and adds:

> Awareness of an attitude comprises not only the knowledge of its existence but also the knowledge of its forcefulness and influence and the knowledge of its consequences and the function which it serves. If this is missing it means that the attitude was unconscious, even though at times glimpses of knowledge may have reached awareness.

This is a much wider interpretation than that of Freud, and as Brown (1961) points out, it would include Stekel's concept of scotomatization and Adler's fictive goals as 'she would label any mental process "unconscious" if the individual were unaware of its full implications, power and results'.

She pointed out that many of Freud's basic assumptions were determined by the prevailing philosophical beliefs of the nineteenth century. These were:

1. *Biological orientation.* This is seen in his instinct theories and his emphasis on heredity and constitution and his efforts to explain psychological sexual differences on an anatomical basis. This gave rise to his emphasis of 'penis envy' and 'castration anxiety'.

2. *Ignorance of modern anthropology and sociology.* The 'culture concept' that human societies can differ from each other radically is of relatively recent origin. In Freud's time it was agreed that one's own culture had universal application and he therefore considered cultural phenomena to be derived from biological and instinctual factors.

3. *Tendency to dualistic thinking.* Opposite pairs of polarities are a feature of Freudian psychopathology. Ego and Id, Life and Death instincts, Love and Hate are not only paired but rigidly contrasted opposites. His theoretical models are mechanistic and based on physical systems such as energy which is expended in one area is lost to another, *e.g.* giving love impairs self-love and *vice versa.*

4. *Deliberate abstention from moral judgments.* This is the attitude of the detached scientist and may be exercised when recording and interpreting in the physical sciences. Horney points out that the psychologist cannot and should not be neutral.

5. *Mechanistic-evolutionistic thinking.* This derives from Darwinian theory for which Freud had a great admiration. It implies that not only are present manifestations conditioned by the past (which is reasonable) but they contain nothing but the past. Hence adult attitudes are nothing but a repetition of the same attitudes in the child and nothing much happens in development after the age of five and as birth is the first manifestation of anxiety, later forms of anxiety are repetitions of this. Horney argues that it is wrong to suppose that later anxiety is *exactly the same.*

She interprets Freud's libido theory on the basis of these criticisms and then exposes its inadequacies:

> . . . not only the striving for power, but every kind of self-assertion is (to be) interpreted as an aim-inhibited expression of sadism. Any kind of affection becomes an aim-inhibited expression of libidinal desires. Any kind of submissive attitude towards others becomes suspect of being an expression of a latent passive homosexuality.

The theory of the Death Instinct which asserts that we have to destroy others in order not to destroy ourselves runs counter to the whole process of natural selection which eliminates traits which are harmful to survival. Brown (1961) comments:

> . . . it seems strange that innate human aggression should be so strong that the only solution is universal analysis.

The sceptic might add that even universal analysis is unlikely to be effective. If man is naturally self-centred and aggressive and his sociability an expression of aim-inhibited sex, one might legitimately ask why he ever came to form social groups. Similarly, in cultural anthropology there are examples where aggression is lacking as in the Arapesh of New Guinea (Mead 1931). Horney comments:

> That over-kindliness may be a reaction-formation against sadistic trends does not preclude the possibility of a genuine kindliness which arises out of basically good relations with others. That generosity may be a reaction-formation against greediness does not disprove the existence of genuine generosity.

She regards Freud's libido theory as inadequate. As an instinct theory it does help one to see how a single trend affects a personality, but it also assumes that the libido is the source of all trends. That the only deep analytical interpretations are those connected with infantile drives is a dangerous illusion for the following reasons:

1. It gives a false impression of human relationships, the nature of neurotic conflicts and the role of cultural factors.
2. It pretends that a machine can be understood out of one wheel instead of by a study of the interrelation of all parts.
3. It leads the therapist to assume final limitations to therapy (based on biological factors) when they do not exist.

Her views on the Oedipus complex are close to those of Ian Suttie and Alfred Adler. She does not accept it as universal or arising from innate factors, but that it is derived from the possible environmental situations (1) the witting or unwitting sexual stimulation of the child by the frustrated father or mother; (2) the child's anxiety to compensate for hostile tendencies or a frustrating home situation. In order to allay anxiety it may cling to a parent to receive reassuring affection. This may look like the complex described by Freud as there will be a passionate clinging to and monopolizing of one parent with resentment at the other's interference, but it arises from neurotic conflict and is not biologically determined.

Self-aggrandisement which Freud regarded as self-love or narcissism and Adler as power over others is considered by Horney in much the same light as Suttie (see above). If others do not love and respect him for what he is they should at least pay attention to him and admire him. This aim is substituted for love, and thus self-aggrandisement is a result of the failure to obtain love rather than self-love. This attitude is supported by Erich Fromm (1944) who said 'It is true that selfish persons are incapable of loving others, but they are not capable of loving themselves either'.

In her criticism of Freud's view that women wish they were men because of their biological inferiority she states:

It is necessary not to take at face value a woman's tendency in one way or another to base her inferiority feelings on the fact that she is a woman; rather it must be pointed out to her that every person belonging to a minority group or to a less privileged group tends to use that status as a cover for inferiority feelings of various sources, and that the important thing is to try to find out these sources.

Brown (1961) remarks that this view is in strong opposition to those of such Freudian writers as Helene Deutsch who has supposed that women are basically masochistic wishing to be violated and raped in intercourse, and humiliated in mental life. She rejects the concept of a universal normal psychology, for behaviour which is regarded as neurotic in one culture may be regarded as normal elsewhere, but she accepts two traits which are present in all neurotics.

1. *Rigidity in reaction.* While normal people have a flexibility suited to their environment, the neurotic tends to react in predetermined ways, *e.g.* suspicion in the normal is engendered by the environment, while the neurotic brings his suspiciousness with him.

2. *Discrepancy between potentialities and accomplishments.* The individual may be frustrated by harsh realities which cause him to fail in spite of himself, but the neurotic brings about his own failure.

Her definition of neurosis (Horney 1945) is, of course, a necessary ingredient for understanding her views. It is: 'a psychic disturbance brought about by fears and defences against these fears, and by attempts to find compromise solutions for conflicting tendencies'.

For her, neurosis is 'basic anxiety' which she describes as feeling small, insignificant, helpless, and endangered in a world that is out to abuse, cheat, attack, humiliate, betray and envy. Such feelings are present in children whose parents are incapable of genuine warmth and affection and have therefore never experienced 'the blissful certainty of being wanted'. Because of this the environment is:

. . . felt to be unreliable, mendacious, unappreciative, unfair, unjust, begrudging, and merciless. According to this concept the child not only fears punishment or desertion because of forbidden drives, but he feels the environment as a menace to his entire development and to his most legitimate wishes and strivings. He feels in danger of his individuality being obliterated, his freedom taken away, his happiness prevented. In contrast to the fears of castration this fear is not fantasy, but is well founded on reality. In any environment in which the basic anxiety develops, the child's free use of energies is thwarted, his self-esteem and self-reliance are undermined, fear is instilled by intimidation and isolation, his expansiveness is warped through brutality or over-protective 'love'.

New Ways in Psychoanalysis

In the child's efforts to escape from this anxiety, the following neurotic personality trends are developed:

1. *Neurotic striving for affection.* In normal love the primary need is for affection, but in the neurotic, it is based on the need for reassurance. This leads to approval-hunger which can never be satisfied. Sex becomes a means of buying affection or reassurance. Because of his childhood experiences he cannot really trust people and is unable to return love for fear of emotional dependence. He cannot therefore establish a mature relationship but becomes promiscuous, demanding from others unconditional love regardless of his own shortcomings.

2. *Neurotic striving for power.* Though this trait was regarded as fundamental by Adler, it is considered by Horney to be one of several. In the neurotic it arises out of fear, anxiety and feelings of inferiority and consequently he wishes to be superior in everything; he is hostile to others and will try to disparage and defeat them and as he fears retaliation he builds up his strength so that he cannot be harmed. These measures can of course only be considered neurotic if there is no factual basis for the person's fear and anxiety and it would be wrong to suggest that the world is yet free from hostility.

3. *Neurotic withdrawal.* Self-sufficiency is equated with safety and the formula 'If I avoid people, they cannot harm me' is applied.

4. *Neurotic submissiveness.* Because he feels helpless he readily accepts the views of the traditional, the powerful and the influential and represses his own, the formula being: 'If I submit to the will of others or help them, I shall avoid being hurt'.

These neurotic attitudes could if persistently practised yield a character who could lead a reasonably effective life, but the neurotic frequently exploits all four and often inappropriately and then gets into serious trouble. Horney considers that conflict over helplessness, hostility and isolation form the core of a neurosis and she calls it the 'basic conflict'. She presents the following allegory to describe her theory of neurosis:

> Let us assume that a man with a shady past has found his way into a community by false pretence. He will, of course, live in dread of his former

status being disclosed. In the course of time his situation advances; he makes friends, secures a job, founds a family. Cherishing his new position, he is beset with a new fear, the fear of losing these goods. His pride in his respectability alienates him from his unsavoury past. He gives large sums to charity and even to his old associates in order to wipe out his old life. Meanwhile the changes that have been taking place in his personality proceed to involve him in new conflicts, with the result that in the end his having commenced his present life on false premises becomes merely an undercurrent in his disturbance.

Defence mechanisms which are used to solve the basic conflict are:

1. Eclipse of part of the conflict with prominence given to the opposite trend. This is equivalent to *reaction-formation.*
2. *Isolation* from people.
3. *Idealized image* of himself. He asks society to look at his high ideals—generous, independent, honest and pure. Genuine ideals however make for humility; these make for arrogance.
4. *Externalize.* This can take the form of identifying with the oppressed or expressing anger with those who exhibit his own shortcomings. The latter is very similar to Freud's 'projection'.

Horney considers neurosis to be a social manifestation which may not be abnormal in certain cultures, but if it is used to solve intrapsychic conflicts then, even though it may be normal behaviour in other cultures, it is neurotic for that individual. This definition does, of course, also apply to delusional states, which must also be seen within the context of the individual's culture.

Erich Fromm (1900–)

Like Karen Horney, he practised as an analyst in Berlin before going to America. He was also a sociologist, his main interest being the relationship of the individual to his society and the psychology of authoritarianism, which he elaborated in his book, *The Fear of Freedom* (Fromm, 1942). In his political thinking he was profoundly influenced by Karl Marx and analysed Freudian theory in Marxian terms.

(Human) relations as Freud sees them are similar to the economic relations to others which are characteristic of the individual in capitalist society. Each person works for himself, individualistically, at his own risk, and not primarily in cooperation with others. But he is not a Robinson Crusoe; he needs others, as customers, as employees, or as employers. He must buy and sell, give and take. The market, whether it is the commodity or the labour market, regulates these relations. Thus the individual, primarily alone and self-sufficient enters into economic relation with others as means to one end: to sell and to buy. Freud's concept of human relations is essentially the same: the individual appears fully equipped with biologically given drives which need to be satisfied. In order to satisfy them, the individual enters into relations with other 'objects'. Other individuals are always a means to one's end, the satisfaction of strivings which in themselves originate in the individual before he enters into contact with others. The field of human relations in Freud's sense is similar to the market—it is an exchange of satisfaction of biologically given needs, in which the relationship to the other individual is always a means to an end, but never an end in itself.

Fromm did not accept these implications of Freudian theory and put forward his own assumptions:

1. The satisfaction or frustration of an instinct is not in itself the fundamental problem of psychology, which is more dependent on the relationship of the individual to his world.

2. This relationship is not, as Freud suggested, a static one, but is constantly changing. Though organic drives such as hunger, thirst, sex are common to all men, the *differences* between people (sensuality, puritanism, love, hate, desire for power etc.) are produced by the social process. Society can create as well as suppress and human nature is a cultural product limited by, but not entirely dependent on biological factors.

He gives historical examples of how man and his nature varied as between the Middle Ages and the Renaissance, but does not accept that man is entirely moulded by his environment and challenges those like Marx who would 'reduce the psychological facts to a shadow of culture patterns'. His aim is to show:

> . . . not only how passions, desires, anxieties, change and develop as a *result* of the social process, but also how man's energies thus shaped into specific forms, in their turn become *productive forces, moulding the social process.* 'Man is not only made by history—history is made by man'.

Fromm considered that Freud's concept of '*instinct*' contained two distinct components:

1. A specific action pattern determined by the physical structure of the nervous system. A variety of activities such as the migrating cycle of the salmon, the social behaviour of ants and other complex behaviour of bees and birds come within this group.

2. Biological needs and drives such as sex, hunger and thirst. Although man shares these with other animals, the manner in which they are satisfied is culturally or socially determined. These cultural influences may negative the essential biological function, for men may give away their last piece of bread, sacrifice their lives for their convictions and frequently exasperate politicians by acting contrary to their real interests.

Evolution in man has produced entirely new qualities which have separated him even more from other animals. He has this awareness of being a separate being, can store the knowledge of the past, visualize the future and through his imagination he reaches far beyond the range of his senses. Fromm regarded him as a freak of nature:

> . . . a part of nature, subject to her physical laws and unable to change them, yet he transcends the rest of nature. He is set apart while being apart; he is homeless, yet chained to the home he shares with all creatures. Cast into this world at an accidental place and time, he is forced out of it, again accidentally. Being aware of himself, he realizes his powerlessness, and the limitations of his existence. He visualizes his own end: death. Never is he free from the dichotomy of his existence: he cannot rid himself of his mind, even if he should want to; he cannot rid himself of his body as long as he is alive—and his body makes him want to be alive.

He described two dichotomies 'existential' and 'historical'. The former depends on the relatively short span of man's life in the historical process and the limits set by the existing level of culture; the latter includes the problems of war, hunger in the midst of plenty, disease, etc., which can be solved given the time and the will. In his Marxist way he points out that those who benefit from historical dichotomies attempt to convince others that they are inevitable like existential dichotomies. Contradictions and anomalies in social life he states would normally produce the desire to solve them, so those with a vested interest in preserving the *status quo* deny their existence. Ideologies serve for the masses the same purpose as rationalization does for the individual. The common examples are presented. In the Middle Ages, it was the doctrine of the static society ordained by God; in early capitalist society it was the free market as the guarantee that the best man would rise to the top and therefore the poor were poor, because they did not deserve better. Ideologies serve man to give him a feeling of equilibrium and mental comfort and therefore religion is not as Freud would have it a universal neurosis for it comforts man and fulfils some of his basic needs. Neurosis (presumably an obsessional one) is however a private religion, and has no general acceptance by the culture but is needed by the individual to help him to come to terms (unsuccessfully) with himself.

Fromm continues with his Marxist analogy:

> . . . the mode of life, as it is determined for the individual by the peculiarity of an economic system, becomes the primary factor in determining his whole character structure, because the imperative need for self-preservation forces him to accept the conditions under which he has to live. This does not mean that he cannot try, together with others, to effect certain economic and political changes; but primarily his personality is moulded by the particular mode of life, as he has already been confronted with it as a child through the medium of the family, which represents all the features that are typical of a particular society or class.

He traces the history of man from his emergence from a state of oneness with nature which has protected him from loneliness, though he is blocked as a free self-determining productive individual. By the Middle Ages he had lost his feelings of unity with nature though he still had social solidarity. The free market did not operate and personal, economic and social life was governed by rules laid down by the Church. With the Renaissance individualism emerged in all classes and pervaded all forms of activity and with this new-found freedom, emotional security was lost. This was accentuated with the growth of Protestantism which became closely identified with the new Capitalism. Man constantly longs for the Golden Age when he was at one with the world and did not have to bear the heavy burden of individual freedom. Modern totalitarianism has tried to woo man from his freedom by offering him membership of a uniform (literally) group. Industrial society with its mergers and other arrangements makes it more and more difficult for the individual to impose any rational order on things or even to identify with a group. In the face of these problems, the individual elaborates the following psychic mechanisms which are analogous to the 'neurotic character traits' described by Horney:

1. *Moral Masochism.* This corresponds to Horney's 'neurotic need for affection' and may be expressed in feelings of inferiority and inadequacy, which Fromm sees as a need for dependence. These masochistic feelings may be disguised by the individual as those of 'love', 'devotion' or 'loyalty' but they are really based on a neurotic compulsion.
2. *Sadism.* This corresponds to Horney's 'neurotic striving for power' and can manifest by making others dependent on oneself, exploiting them or making them suffer.
3. *Destructiveness.* Though related to the sado-masochistic complex it has different origins. The individual has unbearable feelings of powerlessness and isolation and says 'I can only escape the feelings of my own powerlessness in comparison with the world outside of myself by destroying it'.
4. *Automation Conformity.* This corresponds to Horney's 'neurotic submissiveness' and is an attempt to eliminate the differences between himself and others and reach identity with them. He therefore substitutes a pseudo-self for the real self.

Gardner Murphy (1947) summarizes Fromm's views on the human story thus:

> Fromm and Horney make the point that with the loss of security in the medieval system, the primary problem has become the struggle for status, the struggle to be somebody . . . (They) both suggest that we have paid a terrific price for freedom to come and go, to rise and fall. Not that we would wish to give it up. But we live competitively only at great cost; and in times of grave stress many of us strive to 'escape from freedom' through recourse to a pattern of authority.

Fromm's Classification of Character

He considers that man relates to the world in two ways, (a) by acquiring and assimilating things; (b) by relating to other people and to himself:

> Man can acquire things by receiving or taking them from an outside source or by producing them through his own effort. But he must acquire and assimilate them in some fashion in order to satisfy his needs . . . Man can relate himself to others in various ways: he can love or hate, he can compete or cooperate; he can build a social system based on equality or authority, liberty or oppression; but he must be related in some fashion and the particular form of relatedness is expressive of his character.

To the four methods of relating to others (masochism, sadism, destructiveness, automaton conformity), he adds a fifth, the normal approach, which is love. The methods of assimilation which correspond to these methods of socialization form the basic character types. *Character* he defines as the relatively permanent form in which human energy is canalized in the process of assimilation and socialization. The types are not found in pure form but frequently predominate, giving a recognizable character type. Character itself is influenced by inherited temperament which he classifies in the Hippocratic manner as choleric, sanguine, phlegmatic and melancholic. The family, which he describes as the 'psychic agency of society', moulds the character, producing patterns according to society's specification. For a society to function well its members '. . . have to *desire* what objectively is necessary for them to do. *Outer force* is replaced by *inner compulsion,* and by the particular kind of human energy which is channelled into character traits'. (Fromm, 1944). The five characters are:

1. *The Receptive.* He believes that everything he wishes, whether goods, knowledge, pleasure or love, must come from outside. He is dependent on a protector and relates to others in terms of 'moral masochism' like Horney's 'neurotic need for affection' and Freud's 'oral-receptive character'.
2. *The Exploitative.* He satisfies his desires by force or cunning and is aggressive, preferring to take or steal rather than produce by his own efforts. He resembles Horney's 'neurotic need for power' and Freud's 'oral-aggressive' character.
3. *The Hoarding.* His security is based on saving and keeping what he has gathered and he has little interest in what he has not produced for himself. He is orderly, punctual and pedantic and tends to insulate himself from the outside world. He resembles Horney's 'neurotic withdrawal' and Freud's 'anal-erotic' character.

4. *The Marketing.* His approach to socialization is equivalent to 'automaton conformity' and he adapts and sells himself to others as if his personality were a commodity which can be bought and sold. This has been compared to Horney's 'neurotic submissiveness' and Freud's 'phallic' character.

5. *The Productive.* He is considered normal and capable of genuine love relationships and corresponds with Freud's 'genital' character.

Fromm does not regard self love and love for others in the Freudian sense as polar opposites but as associated. He does not see it in terms of energy economics where if some is directed outwards, less is directed inwards.

He differs from Freud in his interpretation of the Oedipus complex, adopting a position nearer to that of Otto Rank (see below). He emphasizes that the Freudian interpretation is only valid in a patriarchal society, but in matriarchal societies infantile sexuality is not directed towards the mother but is auto-erotic or directed towards other children. He is aware of the frustration and anxiety which arises from social organization of which the Oedipal situation is only one. The resultant anxiety and uncertainty need not lead to neurosis but can be

> . . . a necessary condition to compel man towards further development, and . . . if he faces the truth without panic he will recognize that there is no meaning to life except the meaning man gives his life by the unfolding of his powers. (Fromm, 1947.)

While Marxist theory may no longer be applicable to the economic problems of our time, Fromm has introduced a freshness of outlook into psychopathology which not only takes into account cultural factors, but provides a contemporary analogy which is recognizable. It is not particularly helpful in the understanding of the severer forms of mental illness, but is useful in providing a framework for character types and assessing the 'life-style'.

Otto Rank (1884–1939)

He was impressed by the similarities of the physiological concomitants of anxiety and those accompanying birth, and because of this denied that the Oedipus complex occupied the central position in the aetiology of neurosis but considered that all neurosis originated in the birth trauma, which in essence is separation from the mother. Further separation experiences such as weaning (separation from the breast) and symbolic castration (separation from the penis) or separation from a loved object or person could reactivate this anxiety. He divided this anxiety into two forms:

1. *The Life Fear.* This occurs when the individual becomes aware of creative capacities within himself which if asserted would threaten him with independence and therefore the separation from existing relationships.
2. *The Death Fear.* This is the fear of losing one's individuality and being swallowed up in the whole.

Throughout life each person is spurred forward by the need to express his individuality yet is restrained by the fear that by doing so he may cut himself off from society. Two solutions are possible: (1) *normal* or the wholehearted acceptance of society's standards as one's own, and (2) *creative* or standing alone and producing one's own standards. The neurotic can accept neither.

Like Fromm, he saw society as both patriarchal and matriarchal, and religion in terms of sublimation of the fears of the primal birth trauma. Resurrection is therefore a conquering of the birth trauma and Paradise is a return to the mother and her protecting womb. He has his followers who practise psychotherapy according to his principles, but he has a limited appeal. His main book *The Trauma of Birth* (Rank, 1952*a*) gives an account of his psychoanalytic theory and practice while *The Myth of the Birth of the Hero* (Rank, 1952*b*) is his major anthropological study.

Karl Jaspers

With the recent translation into English of Jasper's large text which is entitled *General Psychopathology* (Jaspers, 1963) there has been an increasing awareness of his contributions among English-speaking psychiatrists. The book has not changed materially from its first German edition in 1913, which would appear to make Jaspers as inflexible as the earlier theorists, Kraepelin, Kretschmer and Freud whom he severely criticizes. He saw psychopathology as being chiefly concerned with conscious psychic events though he appreciates that extraconscious mechanisms and unconscious mental processes also play a part. He therefore limits it to the study of the psychic state as experienced by patients and the 'meaningful connexions' within the psyche and the 'causal connexions' between psychic and extrapsychic events. These causal factors he regards as always extrapsychic while abnormal mental phenomena are based on personality development or on an intercurrent illness.

He argues his case with considerable logic and it is understandable that Jaspers has a greater reputation among European (including British) schools of philosophy than with British psychiatrists. It is all over-simplified and though the phenomenology of psychiatric illness is described with great accuracy and detail, Jaspers fails to see that much of it is dependent on the institutional milieu in which the patients then lived. He therefore is unaware of some of the meaningful links, and 'real causes' like genetics which were considered proven at the time the first edition appeared are no longer tenable. This work has however greatly influenced German psychiatric thinking and some who are unhappy over the logical inconsistencies of Freudian psychopathology or who would wish to subscribe to anything but Freud will find in Jaspers an adequate intellectual exercise. It will not help towards an understanding of the apparent illogicalities and contradictions of emotionally toned behaviour and is therefore very dated and out of touch with modern advances in psychiatry.

The Psychopathology of Research

There is an increasing tendency to transfer the interpretations of psychopathology from the field of clinical psychiatry to social situations such as the political field or to interpersonal relationships. While this may prove a satisfying exercise for the practitioner and permit him to score against his adversary, it can have overtones which are not only undesirable for the field in which they are used, but can contribute to undesirable changes in society itself.

Wilkinson (1973) uses as his model the psychopathology of research, but it need not be so restricted. He points out that the use of terms like 'ethnocentrism', 'achievement orientation', 'Protestant ethic' and the 'authoritarian personality' are part of an armoury of descriptive and quasi-descriptive concepts which provide a mode of denigration and covert moral criticism.

He states: 'The older rhetoric praised a man for controlling himself: the newer rhetoric denigrates a man for not letting himself go. Its archetype of psychological disease is an examplar of the Protestant ethic, who controls his impulses exercises responsibility and authority without too much self-doubt, achieves success or distinction, attempts difficult tasks, feels uneasiness over his failure, moral and otherwise, works within a framework of routine and agreed conventions, feels loyalty to his country and religion, and likes to be clean and tidy'.

He attacks many psychoanalysts, who, by using an aggressive system of 'insight', can discount what a person says or believes and avoid any direct confrontation with him. They can claim to know the 'real' person and thereby commandeer his identity. This is a power exercised behind the guise of autonomy. Prejudice shifts from

Jews and Blacks to the 'not very bright', 'polyannas', police, races, *e.g.* Luther, Germans and Japanese.

This needed saying, for pscyhoanalysts and others are prone to use their jargon for personal or political advantage.

Z. J. Lipowski

In a thoughtful paper (Lipowski, 1966) he takes up a position intermediate between the phenomenological approach of Jaspers and the dynamic approach of the Freudian schools. He points out that a scientific evaluation of psychopathology is long overdue and lays down the following main tasks:

1. Observation, description, classification.
2. Study of methods of making and recording observations.
3. Formulation and testing of explanatory hypotheses.
4. Critical scrutiny and clearer definition of our linguistic apparatus, i.e. the descriptive and theoretical terms used by psychopathologists.
5. Analysis of our theoretical conceptions and systems for their logical consistence.

The value of Lipowski's statement is the lack of prejudice built into it and its intellectually honest approach. Each point is in itself a monstrous task, but the 'manifesto' does provide a yardstick by which information and theories derived from them can be assessed.

Whom to Believe?

Those with little experience in the clinical problems of psychiatry may well quail before the welter of psychopathological theories, of which the foregoing is only a selection. For those who seek a cult, there are plenty within and without orthodox psychiatry which can provide a rigid framework of reference and appear to be superficially all-embracing. For those who are strictly scientific and would not consider the application of any theory unless it has satisfied all the criteria put forward by Lipowski (see above), the application of psychopathology to their clinical practice will have to wait—perhaps for ever. To those who are neither fanatical devotees nor sceptics, there is much in existing theories which has clinical validity and can be very helpful in the understanding and treatment of mental illness. Eclecticism based on what is most useful in any theory is the best that can be offered at present to the very wide range of mental illness it is our privilege and responsibility to treat. The author's predilections will be readily recognizable as the 'Guide' progresses and there is no need to declare them at this stage.

CHAPTER 3

Genetics

'Like father, like son' in terms of likeness may have a certain degree of validity but the resemblance may well stop at that. Yet for centuries it has been claimed that most mental diseases are inherited and it is only in recent times that serious efforts have been made to test the hypothesis. A few rare disorders which are associated with mental symptoms have an indisputable genetic factor, dominant or recessive, but in the vast majority of psychiatric disturbances, particularly those where no organic disease has yet been demonstrated, clear-cut evidence of genetic transmission is still elusive.

Studies of uniovular twins are alleged to prove the hereditary aspect of some forms of mental illness, yet temperament in identical twins can vary at least as much as their proneness to infection or other environmental hazards and this has been noted in pairs who have been reared together. A notorious example is that of Chang and Eng, the original 'Siamese' (they were really Chinese) twins. Penrose (1959) writes:

> What Chang liked to eat, Eng detested; Eng was very good-natured, Chang cross and irritable. He drank heavily and, though at times he got drunk, Eng never felt any influence from the debauch of his brother. The twins often quarrelled; they sometimes came to blows, and on one occasion they were summoned to court for this.

The subject is very controversial and it is still a matter of patiently accumulating evidence in what is a most difficult field. In the second part of this chapter a critical attitude is adopted towards existing claims, but this does not in any way detract from the valuable work of some devoted investigators. Their assembly of facts has given rise in some instances to criticism of methodology and of criteria of twinning, but their efforts are the essential first steps. There are still large gaps in our knowledge and it is only by the dedication of these workers that methods will be refined and these gaps filled.

To a few the issue of genetic transmission of the common forms of mental illness is no longer in doubt and they would urge counselling on marriage and procreation on existing evidence and even initiate eugenic programmes. They point out the dangers of modern medicine interfering with natural selection, which they declare will result in a gradual increase of poorly adapted carriers with a chance of reproduction. It can all sound so plausible, the unintelligent breed more rapidly and the level of national intelligence is bound to go down (Cattell, 1937); the neurotic is protected in a welfare state and will reproduce his kind; the psychotics are no longer segregated in institutions, but are released to the community in varying degrees of remission, and they, too, will perpetuate their kind. If we are to believe all this, we are rapidly heading for a moronic society with an ever-increasing yield of neurotics, psychotics and other less common disorders. The prophecy can, however, be projected, so that society will eventually lack the capacity to salvage the weak and the tainted and natural selection will again operate. However we still know so little about human genetics compared even with animal genetics which is to date best understood in the fruit fly, and it is a far cry from those established human genetic conditions like Huntington's chorea and tuberous sclerosis to hysteria and schizophrenia. There is the old adage: 'a stock can mend as well as end'. It remains now to review the available evidence.

THE LANGUAGE OF GENETICS

Though there are great differences in our knowledge between human and animal and plant genetics, the language on the subject is a common one. The advantages are great in that it makes it easier to introduce the advances from the non-human to the human study, but at the same time it does not sufficiently emphasize some essential differences. These are mainly in research techniques for, unlike animals, human beings cannot be studied in isolation and animals do not have nearly the same impact on the environment which in turn can materially influence human behaviour.

The following are some terms and definitions which are in common use:

Alleles are the family of elements which are always found at the same locus, the adjective being *allelic*.

Aneuploidy. An irregular number of chromosomes (*e.g.* 45, 47 or 48 in man) caused by the addition or loss of one or more or part of a chromosome.

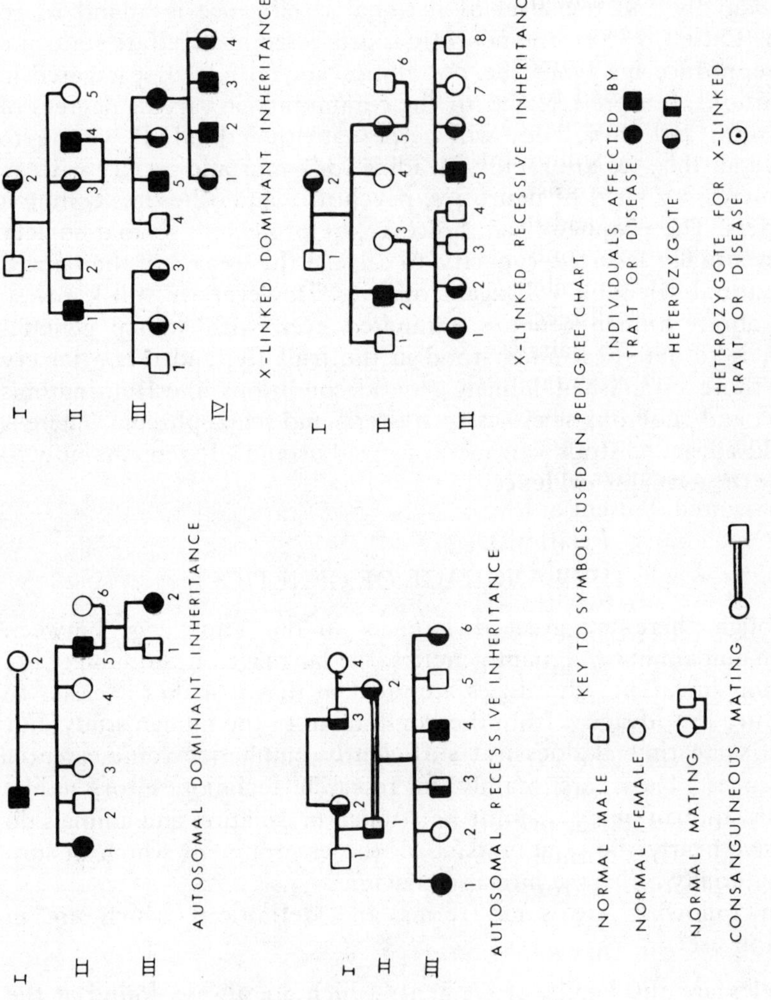

Figure 2. Pedigree charts.

Autosomes are those 22 pairs of chromosomes other than the pair carrying the sexual characters which are two X-chromosomes in the female and XY-chromosomes in the male. Distribution of autosomal genes (dominant or recessive) is usually equal between the sexes.

Barr Body. The sex chromatin mass in somatic cells of the female.

Carrier. An individual who carries a recessive gene, either autosomal or sex-linked, together with its normal allele, but who does not himself show the full effects of the gene; *i.e.* a heterozygote for a recessive gene.

Chromatid. A chromosome at prophase or metaphase consists of two strands attached to the centromere. Each strand is a chromatid.

Chromosomes are parallel strands or filaments of a material which can be stained by aniline dyes and are contained in the cell nucleus. They are said to consist of desoxyribose-nucleic acid or DNA and grow like crystals, and in humans each individual carries in his cells two complete sets, one from each parent; these are called *homologous* pairs. The number of pairs varies in different animals and in humans this was till recently accepted as 24 pairs, but with improved techniques only 23 pairs (46 chromosomes) can be identified. They are seen in cells from rapidly growing tissues such as bone marrow or the embryo and in cultured cells. This chromosome apparatus acts as a storehouse of information for the organism and this information is located in a number of *loci* in the chromosome.

Congenital. Present at birth. Not synonymous with genetic.

Consanguinity. Relationship by descent from a common ancestor.

Coupling and Repulsion. In lower organisms it has been shown that if genes for two traits are close together on the chromosome, they are likely to appear together in the pedigree, and if they are far apart they rarely appear together. In man, the search for coupling and repulsion has not been fruitful largely because of the small size of families and random mating.

Crossing-over. The exchange of corresponding segments between maternal and paternal homologous chromosomes occurring when these are paired during prophase of the first meiotic division.

Diploid. The normal complement of chromosomes (22 pairs of homologous chromosomes and the sex chromosomes in humans).

Dizygotic (or Dizygous) twins. Twins resulting from the simultaneous fertilization of two ova by two spermatozoa. Recurrence in families is common.

Dominant is applied to the genes of a heterozygous pair which produce the trait in the offspring. It is frequently preceded by the name 'Mendelian' after its originator, Gregor Mendel (1865).

Empiric Risk. The prediction of probability that a genetic or congenital abnormality will occur in a family.

Expressivity. The extent to which a dominant trait is manifested. The phenotypic expression may be slight or pronounced.

Gamete. A male or female reproductive cell; a spermatozoon or ovum.

Gene Frequency. The relative proportion of each of two or more alleles of a particular gene in a given population. It is expressed as a percentage or as a probability (0 to 1).

Genes are segments of DNA consisting of large numbers of nucleotides and replication may be achieved by separation of complementary nucleotide chains with the formation of new daughter chains. At one time it was thought that one gene unit occupied one locus on the chromosome, but it is realized that numerous genes can be located in these stations and each gene itself may be a complex of genes.

Genetic Code. The sequential order of the bases of DNA which carry the genetic information.

Genome. All the genes found in a diploid set of chromosomes.

Genotype is the fundamental gene formula of an individual. It need not present in the phenotype as in heterozygosity when the gene is carried by the individual but is not expressed by him.

Haploid. The number of chromosomes in a normal gamete which contains only one member of each chromosome pair. In man the haploid number is 23.

Hemizygous. Since males have only one X chromosome they are said to be hemizygous with respect to X-linked genes.

Hermaphrodite. An individual with both male and female gonadal tissue, not necessarily functioning.

Heterologous. Chromosomes or chromosomal segments which are non-homologous or non-identical.

Heterozygous is when the person receives the gene from only one parent and at the corresponding locus of the chromosome there is a different gene from the other parent.

Homologous. Chromosomes or chromosomal segments which are identical with respect to genetic loci and visible structure, *e.g.* two normal chromosomes 15's.

Homozygous is the term used for a person or animal who carries an identical pair of single genes derived from each parent and under environmental conditions will exhibit the characteristic associated with that gene.

Incidence. Number of infants born with a condition per number of live births in a given population.

Isochromosome. One in which the arms on either side of the centromere are identical.

Karyotype. The full complement of chromosomes, including numbers, relative sizes and morphology.

Linkage. Genes are said to be *linked* if they have their loci on the same chromosome. Also used to describe traits transmitted by a gene of known locus on a specific chromosome.

Locus. The precise location of a gene on a chromosome. Different forms of the gene (alleles) are always found at the same locus.

Meiosis. Nuclear division during formation of gametes. Two consecutive meiotic divisions occur but only one division of the chromosomes. Thus the number of chromosomes is reduced from diploid (46) to haploid (23). During meiosis pairing of homologous chromosomes occurs followed by chromosomal breakage and crossing-over. The end result is four cells each with one half the number of chromosomes possessed by the original cells.

Metaphase. That stage of cell division (mitosis or meiosis) during which the chromosomes line up on the spindle equatorial plate.

Mitosis. Nuclear division in which each chromosome splits lengthwise by replication, one chromatid of each chromosome passing to one daughter cell and the other to the second daughter cell. Thus each daughter cell receives the full complement of 46 chromosomes. Mitosis is characteristic of somatic cells and of germ cells before meiosis.

Modifier Genes are those subsidiary genes which cause quantitative changes in the expression of a major gene which normally bred true (mutation).

Mosaic. An individual with two or more cell lines differing in genotype.

Mutation is that variability in the gene structure which is either spontaneous or induced (*e.g.* by irradiation). There are two kinds recognized: (1) those which consist of rearrangement, breakage and junction of chromosomes, and (2) those which affect single loci by producing new allelic genes or point *mutations*. Mutations can account for the spontaneous emergence in several generations of a dominant characteristic which is biologically unfavourable and its subsequent disappearance. Examples are achondroplasia, tuberous sclerosis and retinoblastoma.

Mutation Rate. Frequency of detectable mutations per genic locus per generation.

Penetrance is that capacity for the gene to express itself, and this can be influenced by a variety of factors which usually operate by reducing penetrance. In genetic arguments in psychiatry this phenomenon is freely produced to explain the lack of consistency of expression of a gene which is alleged to be homozygous.

Other explanations are incomplete dominance and recessiveness, that the phenotypic expression of a gene is not a fixed entity but that it merely sets in train a series of events which can be modified by environmental factors as well as by other genes.

Phenocopy. An individual with all the hallmarks of a particular genetic disorder but with no hereditary evidence.

Phenotype is the visible expression of characters in a group of individuals whose heredity is different. A recessive trait should be homozygous before it can be expressed in the phenotype.

Polygenic or Multifactorial Inheritance. Inheritance of a trait governed by many genes. Each gene may act independently with cumulative total effect. Examples are height, weight and other body dimensions.

Population Genetics. The study of mutant genes in populations rather than in individuals.

Prevalence. The number of individuals with a specific condition in a given population.

Proband. The abnormal individual whose relatives are studied to determine the hereditary or genetic aspects of the trait.

Prophase. The first stage of cell division during which the chromosomes can be visually identified.

Recessive is applied to the gene of a heterozygous pair which does not express itself in the offspring.

Ring Chromosome. A circular chromosome resulting from breakage in both arms of a chromatid followed by fusion of the broken ends to form a ring. Varying amounts of chromosomal material are lost or deleted from both arms.

Segregation. The separation of the two alleles of a pair during meiosis so that they pass to different gametes.

Sex Chromatin (Synonym: Barr body). A chromatin mass in the nucleus of the interphase cells of females. It represents a single X chromosome which is inactive in the metabolism of the cell. Normal females are therefore *chromatin-positive;* normal males are *chromatin-negative*.

Sex chromosomes. These are responsible for sex determination. (XX in females: XY in males).

Sex-limited. Affecting one sex.

Sex-linkage occurs when traits are caused by genes located on that pair of chromosomes which determines sex. It is almost exclusively concerned with the X-chromosome though it should be theoretically possible for gene interchange to occur between the X-

and Y-chromosomes. Those genes on the Y-chromosome would determine those characters transmitted exclusively from affected father to sons. Classical examples of sex linkage are colour blindness and haemophilia, and as one sex (usually the female) carries the gene as a recessive and is unaffected, propagation of the condition demands that the gene is present in both partners and is therefore more likely to occur in consanguineous marriages.

Sex may influence autosomal hereditary characters without sex linkage. This is seen in baldness where the endocrine structure of the female protects her from the condition.

Sib, Sibling. Brother or sister.

Translocation. A change in location of genetic material either within a chromosome or from one chromosome to another.

Trisomy. The presence of 3 rather than 2 chromosomes in a particular set, *e.g.* XXX, XXY or XYY are trisomic for sex chromosomes.

X-Chromosome. A sex chromosome which occurs singly in the normal male and in duplicate in the normal female.

Y-Chromosome. A sex chromosome which occurs singly in the normal male but is absent in the normal female.

METHODS OF STUDY

Family Histories

These constitute probably the earliest studies and while they have produced some classical findings like that of Scott (1778) who described an authentic and genetically understandable family history of colour blindness which has stood the test of time, they have also contributed a mythology which has retarded progress. It is natural to expect that desirable and undesirable qualities in the parents will appear in the children. This belief is especially held in regard to socially disapproved diseases and characteristics. The example of syphilis was seen by some early observers as a genetic tainting rather than the transmission of infection, and alcoholism was also regarded as an heredo-degenerative phenomenon. The reason may be rooted in the Decalogue where it is stated: '. . . for I the Lord thy God am a jealous God, visiting the iniquity of the fathers upon the children unto the third and fourth generation of them that hate me, . . .' (Deut. v.9). This may well have inspired the studies of the Kallikak and Jukes families and the results, which showed an overwhelming degree of crime, alcoholism, prostitution and vagrancy.

Galton (1869) attempted a study of hereditary genius and was able to cite families, like Bernoulli, in mathematics, Bach in music, and Bellini in painting. He realized the difficulties of trying to establish a scientific basis for hereditary traits on reputation and hearsay evidence and introduced measurements by using the **correlation co-efficient.** A co-efficient approximating to unity would indicate a strong resemblance in the trait and one approximating to zero would indicate practically no resemblance. This demonstration of the presence of a factor has, by some, been too readily accepted as evidence of a genetic factor and the cult of factor analysis has produced a number of results which though statistically valid, are remote from clinical experience and suggest that some of the premises are false.

Census

Some circumscribed communities may yield valuable information by this method, but it can be used only when the data are of an unequivocal nature and diagnostic criteria are not in doubt. These reservations almost exclude it in psychiatric studies and apart from some rare biochemical abnormalities which are easily detected such as phenylketonuria, it is not reliable.

Twin Studies

Galton (1875) postulated that since identical twins have the same genetic structure, any differences they may exhibit are due to their environment. Non-identical twins of the same sex provide a convenient group for comparison, for their gene structure is no closer than ordinary brothers and sisters, but they have the advantage that like identical twins they are of the same age.

In European communities, twins occur about once in every 88 confinements, but as a number do not survive because of their high infant mortality, the chances of an adult having a twin, instead of being 1 in 44, is 1 in 60. The ratio of identical to fraternal twins is 1 : 2½, and Penrose (1959) suggests that the incidence of identical twinning is about 1 in 300 confinements. Identical twins are called *monozygotic*, while fraternal twins are called *dizygotic*.

Though identical twins are regarded as ideal subjects for study, there are occasionally minor differences even in the finger-prints. In rare instances where identical twins have been reared apart, some investigators have assumed that similarities could not be attributed to environmental factors, but Penrose points out that the very important period before birth is not controlled. He also stresses the fallacy of assuming that because identical twins have the same trait, this proves the trait is hereditary and exposes it by the following imaginary example:

> . . . Suppose that a student of heredity should hail from another planet and that he should be required to use the twin method to find out whether or not people's clothes were a direct consequence of heredity. He would find that identical twins were very often dressed alike, down to quite small details, and that this was uncommon with fraternal twins. He would confidently conclude that the choice of clothes was almost an exclusively hereditary trait and might even suppose them to be a part of the natural skin of the human animal by the exercise of superificial reasoning.

Certain facts have emerged from twin studies. A recessive trait always appears in both members of an identical pair. Identical twins who may suffer from the same disease do not disclose to us the mode of inheritance but merely indicate the possibility that the disease in question has a genetic factor. This is particularly so in organic diseases like tuberculosis where the predisposition may be inherited though there is no doubt that the disease is due to infection by the tubercle bacillus. Penrose sums up the situation thus: '. . . Indeed, the study of twins, from being regarded as one of the easiest and most reliable kinds of researches in human genetics, must now be considered as one of the most treacherous'.

Morbidity-risk Data. This implies considerable statistical expertize and a knowledge of a variety of procedures to define the expectancy rates of certain traits. The frequency of a gene in a population can be assessed and it has been applied with great accuracy to blood groups by Bernstein (1924); there is as yet however no reliable information that the common psychiatric diseases are genetically determined and in fact it is difficult to see how even the most sophisticated of statistical methods can be profitably used in such a complex field. Still less is it possible to make genetical predictions in psychiatric disease. It is almost an axiom that the commoner a condition is the more difficult it is to predict. For genetic purposes a common condition is one with an incidence of 1 in 1000 and common genes are liable to modification by 'modifier genes' or by environment. If a single gene is responsible for the condition and the exact mode of transmission is known it should be possible to make a valid prediction, but even then only in terms of probability. Absolute certainty does not exist and a wrong prediction is for the unfortunate parent a 100 per cent error. Even with an established recessive trait the probability of a subsequent child being affected where one already exists is one in four. In the common mental disorders there is no real point in trying to predict; we just do not know.

BIOCHEMICAL ASPECTS OF GENETICS

In addition to the biochemical nature of gene influence, there are specific biochemical defects which have a genetic aspect and some of these have cerebral effects. These are recessive and are divided into four categories:

Lipids

The cerebral lipoidoses, consisting of Tay-Sachs disease (amaurotic family idiocy) and gargoylism, have a common neuro-histology (pp. 728-729).

Amino Acids

(a) Phenylpyruvic amentia is alleged to be due to a deficiency of phenylalanine hydroxylase which interferes with the metabolism of phenylalanine and causes excessive urinary excretion of phenylpyruvic acid (p. 723).

(*b*) Wilson's disease (hepatolenticular degeneration) is associated with a generally determined deficiency of ceruloplasmin, a plasma copper protein which as an oxidase regulates the absorption of ingested copper (p. 729).

Carbohydrates

(*a*) Galactosaemia is caused by a failure to metabolize galactose because of an absence of phospho-galactose-uridyl transferase (p. 726).

(*b*) Glycogenosis (von Gierke's disease) is due to a failure in the breakdown of glycogen with resultant accumulation of the carbohydrate in various organs. The deficiency of the enzyme, glucose-6-phosphatase is alleged to be responsible.

Pigments

In Hallevorden-Spatz disease there is an accumulation of pigment in the globus pallidus and substantia nigra.

There are other less well defined biochemical abnormalities of genetic origin some with demonstrable brain lesions, and a formidable list has been prepared for the biochemist to unravel. These include Huntington's chorea, Pick's disease, Alzheimer's disease, retinoblastoma, hereditary ataxias and tuberous sclerosis, which are regarded by some as being transmitted by a dominant gene as well as a number of diseases considered to be transmitted by recessive genes. Such is the present fascination with biochemistry, that a number of mental disorders with no cerebral organic lesion or for that matter with no definite biochemical lesion, are being regarded as of genetic (biochemical) origin. These include manic-depressive psychosis, schizophrenia, and even homosexuality and alcoholism, and so the pendulum within the space of a century has swung right back.

CHROMOSOMES

Prior to 1956 the human chromosome count was regarded as 48 but since then, by a new technique it has been shown to be 46. Behind this bald statement lies a romance of improved techniques of staining, the 'squash' technique of making preparations, the use of hypotonic saline or citrate to expand the cell and separate the chromosomes, and the use of colchicine on mitoses which halts them in a half-complete state. Colchicine also inhibits spindle formation and prevents crowding of chromosomes on the spindle, making counting much easier.

A colchicine preparation of chromosomes shows them to be nearly split into *chromatids*, adherent at the *centromere*. The limbs of the chromatids bend away from the centromere, so that if this is central (metacentric) the structure is X-shaped, and if near the end (acrocentric) it is V-shaped. Each structure is a partly split chromosome and the other member of the chromosome pair is elsewhere in the preparation. The centromere does not stain with the usual stain and therefore presents as a gap. As each chromosome pair has identical length and division of arms, this permits identification.

Lennox (1961) in his most lucid paper 'Chromosomes for Beginners', describes the various techniques used both in the preparation and counting of the specimens and summarizes what one can and cannot tell from a chromosome count:

1. The total number of chromosomes can be accurately counted and if the number is abnormal, one can say which is missing or in excess.
2. If a structural abnormality is substantial, it can be recognized, *e.g.* the loss of half a micron from a chromosome 22, because this amounts to nearly half its long arm, but a much larger loss from a chromosome 1 would be unnoticed.
3. The genetic lesion of traditional Mendel-inherited disorders like haemophilia or phenylketonuria cannot be detected by this method. '. . . These depend on a disorder of the desoxyribonucleic acid chain—perhaps the misplacement of a single base in the chain, one dash written for a dot in an enormously long Morse code message. It is like hoping to detect a single false note in a recording of a symphony speeded up so fast that we hear the whole in a second. The most

we can manage at present is to identify the symphony from its length and the position of its main interval.'

4. Loss of one whole chromosome (*monosomy*) from a pair is nearly always fatal, but gain of a chromosome (*trisomy*) is damaging but not fatal.

5. Loss or gain of the sex chromosomes is well tolerated and sex chromosome monosomy (a single X or XO) is the only form of monosomy yet recognized which is compatible with life.

Clinical Syndromes Associated with Chromosomal Abnormalities

1. **Trisomy-21.** (*Down's syndrome.*) An extra chromosome 21 is generally associated with this condition while a few cases of Down's syndrome have the normal 46 chromosomes, but these are the 'translocation' cases in which the bulk of the extra 21 is still present but attached to another chromosome.

2. **Trisomy-X.** (*The XXX syndrome.*) This is found in about 1 per cent of female subnormals who may be fertile with normal offspring and is diagnosed mainly by buccal smear which shows the duplicated sex-chromatin bodies in the nuclei. Cases with four or more X-chromosomes occur but three are by far the commonest.

3. **Trisomy-XY.** (*XXY Klinefelter's syndrome.*) This is found in males who in addition to having small testicles and being infertile may exhibit eunuchoidism, gynaecomastia and mental defect. The presence of sex chromatin in the buccal smear is diagnostic and the condition accounts for over 1 per cent of all male defectives and for 3 per cent of men who are infertile.

Nielson (1971) reported 198 men referred for observation to a forensic psychiatric clinic and found that 2·4 per cent had a sex chromosome abnormality (expected frequency 0·36 per cent). Klinefelter's syndrome was found in 0·5 per cent; XYY in 1·9 per cent; large Y in 8·1 per cent. The mean Y/F index for the total tested population was 0·91 which was significantly higher than the mean Y/F index of 0·83 in a random sample of 1400 newborn boys. Four patients had XYY syndrome and they were impulsive and hot-tempered but with average intelligence.

The author concludes that not only is the risk of criminality affected by the length of the Y chromosome, but also the type of criminality, with more violence associated with the larger Y.

4. **Monosomy-X.** (*XO Turner's syndrome.*) This is found in females who are usually dwarfed with gonadal hypoplasia, webbed neck, irregular ears and hairline, cubito valgus, shield-shaped chest with

wide-spaced nipples, cardiovascular defects (coarctation) and generally average intelligence.

Christodorescu *et al.* (1970) report 3 cases of Turner's syndrome with psychiatric disturbances. They rightly point out that there are complex factors at work, *e.g.* (1) gonosomal anomaly with possible direct effect on the CNS; (2) endocrine insufficiency; and (3) patient's psychogenic reaction to her sexual and statural deficiency. Unlike Klinefelter's syndrome, and the XYY patient, Turner's syndrome does not manifest with severely antisocial behaviour, probably because they are both women and dwarfs.

Their psychosexual orientation is feminine, their fantasies in childhood and adolescence being typical for girls of their age, although genitopelvic eroticism is low. Despite their low sexual impulse, they are preoccupied with sexuality and aware of their deficient femininity, often causing them to mask it by exaggerated feminine attitudes and dress. The authors suggest that because of the relative frequency of EEG anomalies along with space-form dysgnosia and sometimes mental retardation or neurological signs, it may be an organic brain syndrome determined by the chromosomal abnormality. The dysgnosia is not constant and its severity and expression are variable.

5. **The XYY Syndrome.** Out of 315 men in a State Psychiatric Criminal Institution (Carstairs, Scotland) Price and Whatmore (1967) found 9 with XYY chromosomes. Their personalities showed extreme instability and irresponsibility and an incapacity to tolerate the mildest frustration though they adjusted well to the hospital and rarely became violent. In their criminal behaviour they were less violent than control patients.

Nielsen *et al.* (1968) found 42 out of 155 patients in Herstedvester with XYY chromosomes and found that 'a significant number' (2 out of a total of 3) were involved in arson. It would be unwise to generalize from this apparently 'significant' finding.

The 47 XYY Male and Behaviour. Price and Jacobs (1970) discuss three chromosome surveys at maximum security hospitals in which a relatively large number of men with a 47 XYY karyotype were found. They were significantly taller, tended to be immature and exhibited inadequate control. It is still not possible to say how representative these XYY males are of those who are non-institutionalized. Estimates of incidence in the general population indicate fairly clearly that those identified in institutions are only a small minority of the total. While the authors lean to a causal relationship between the genetic abnormality and the behaviour disorder, this has to be seen against the even greater number of XYY in the community who do not exhibit behaviour disorders. Environmental factors could well be relevant, and Daly (1969) showed that his 10 patients with XYY in a maximum security hospital were reared in environments which would ordinarily be considered far less than optimal for the development of normal personality and character.

Legal Implications of the XYY Syndrome. Although the extra Y chromosome is not necessarily associated with violence, this has not deterred the XYY argument being introduced as an excuse for criminal acts by giving the accused an 'elevated aggressiveness potential' or causing him to be 'unrestrainedly aggressive'. Russell and Bender (1970) review a number of criminal trials where this argument was introduced. It was generally offered as part of a 'not guilty by reason of insanity' plea, though the authors suggest that were the syndrome to become medically substantiated the 'irresistible impulse' might be more appropriate.

The XYY syndrome as presented in court is very similar to arguments on behalf of the classical psychopathic personality whose criminal responsibility, although a subject of medical controversy, has always been rigidly upheld by the courts. Furthermore, if the court accepted the plea, it would have to assume that the accused would commit aggressive, antisocial acts in future and be detained indefinitely. In any case, the general opinion is that the current knowledge of the relationship between genetics, criminality and mental illness does not meet 'reasonable medical certainty' standards for admission into evidence.

6. **Other Abnormalities**. These are being increasingly recognized and trisomics have been described for other pairs. In the main they are found in mentally defective children with multiple congenital defects and multiple trisomics like a Down-Klinefelter combination occur.

CHROMOSOMAL MOSAICISM

This denotes the presence in one individual of cells which differ in their complement of chromosomes.

The Lyon Hypothesis

Lyon (1961) put forward the theory that normal women are in fact mosaics with regard to their two X chromosomes. Though microscopically the cells all look alike and there is no abnormal nuclear division, she postulates that about the twelfth day after fertilization one of the X chromosomes in each cell of the female foetus becomes inactive in a random manner. The net result is that in about half the cells of the body the maternal X chromosome will be inactivated and the paternal one active, whereas the reverse will hold in the other half. Since the maternal and paternal X chromosomes may be carrying different sets of X-linked genes, the results in a visible character such as coat colour in an animal might be patchiness. It was this phenomenon which she noticed in the mouse. The 'non-working' X chromosome is only genetically inactive for it can and does replicate, and once the 'working' and 'non-working' X has been decided for each cell all descendants will follow the same pattern. As men have only one X chromosome this 'works' in every cell. The hypothesis helps to explain several phenomena. It is known that an extra autosome always leads to mental deficiency and the lack of one is always lethal. Yet this is not so with the X chromosome. XO in the mouse is normally fertile and in humans Turner's syndrome is associated with normal intelligence. Again, though XXX is found in the mentally subnormal this is not invariable.

In the cells of normal females there is a dark-staining mass which is absent in the cells of normal males and is called the *Barr body*. There is always one less present than the number of X chromosomes and it is therefore regarded as the inactive X chromosome. Its DNA is tightly coiled and stains more deeply than all the other chromosomes and it has been shown that it replicates later. The tight coiling has been used as the explanation of the impairment in production and release of R.N.A. which is said to bear chemical 'instructions' from the genes and why the chromosome is genetically inactive. Lyon's hypothesis suggests why the sexes are not more different from one another than they are. If both X chromosomes were active women would have nearly twice as many 'working' sex-linked genes as men. That this is not so has been shown by studies showing that normal women do not make twice as much glucose-6-phosphate-dehydrogenase (G.-6-P.D.) as normal men. Furthermore, women known to be heterozygous for G.-6-P.D. deficiency can be shown to have two races of red cells, one producing the enzyme and the other not, according to whether the normal or the abnormal X was the 'working' one in the nucleated-precursor.

It remains to be seen what influence the Lyon hypothesis will have on genetic studies and if it will have any relevance at all to the genetics of psychiatry. That it may help to explain some problems associated with mental deficiency and with body habitus in the sexes is sufficient grounds for its inclusion in this chapter.

Origin of the Anomalies

During meiosis in the phase of preparation for reduction division, the two chromosomes of each pair come briefly together (for the only time) before parting to each daughter cell (haploid with 23 chromosomes). If this process fails either in pairing off or in separation when formed, both members of one pair may find themselves in one gamete. For example, if Down's syndrome is associated with non-disjunction in the mother, faulty division of the oocyte can result in a cell with two 21's, and another with none at all. As each normal spermatozoon brings its single 21, if it fertilizes an ovum with two 21's, the result is a zygote with three 21's which is associated with Down's syndrome. If it fertilizes an ovum with no 21's, the final zygote has only one 21 and this dies at an early stage in the pregnancy.

As non-disjunction increases with maternal age, the mothers of patients with Down's syndrome and the XXX syndrome tend to be older.

Translocation

This is an exchange of material between two chromosomes of different pairs (exchange with the other member of the same pair is a normal part of meiosis). This exchange does not have an immediate effect, but as the chromosomes affected are now different from their original partners they cannot pair off properly during meiosis and as a result there are irregularities in the offspring. For example a translocation may exist which results in the bulk of one 21 chromosome being attached to a larger one. This in itself does not matter and it may continue for several generations, but it affects meiosis so that occasional members of the family acquire an extra dose of 21 and so present Down's syndrome and provide a familial example of the condition. Familial cases of Down's syndrome form the only example of chromosomal anomaly which has to date been recognized as transmissible. All other anomalies cease with the appearance of the case.

Deletion or loss of part of a chromosome has also been regarded as responsible for disease in man.

Acquired Chromosome Anomalies

The conditions described above are congenital, the lesion being present in the fertilized ovum or (for mosaics) its immediate successors. Acquired lesions do occur, for example in most cases of chronic myeloid leukaemia there is a deletion of part of one of the smallest autosomes—a 21 or a 22. Another example is the effect of a single dose of 250 rad of deep X-rays to the spine or 100 mC of radio-iodine which can produce a temporary but abundant crop of chromasomal anomalies.

The Genetics of Dermal Ridges

Holt (1969) summarizes the characteristic changes in children with chromosome abnormalities. These are: (1) Down's syndrome (G-trisomy) where the distal position of the palmar or T-triradius is the most useful single feature; (2) Edward's syndrome (E-trisomy) with a high proportion of arches on the fingers; (3) Patan's syndrome (D-trisomy) where the T-triradius is even more distal than in Down's syndrome.

Behavioural Genetics

Money (1970) defines behavioural genetics as the science of ascertaining: (a) the environmental limits within which the genetic code can operate and unfold itself into a normal phenotype; (b) the limits which environmental extremes may impose on the genetic code without destroying it, but obligating it to unfold into a defective or abnormal but viable phenotype. He cites Turner's and Klinefelter's syndromes and XYY as illustrative examples. While it is unlikely that any dramatic discovery will result, the concept is an extension of previous approaches to the problem and this in itself is welcome.

GENES AND ENVIRONMENT

While some cautionary remarks have been made about environmental influences, one must repeat that no characteristic is inherited—either normal or abnormal, but only genetic material. This material sets the individual's reaction pattern, physical and psychological, to environmental experiences. These experiences include nutrition, exposure to infection, prenatal influences, traumatic events and age and, of course, the psychological impact of life in all its variety. If one could classify traits into those which are hereditary and those which are environmental, the issue would be much simpler, but most, if not all traits are a mixture of both.

There is an essential difference between human and animal and plant genetics apart from the complexity of man. The medical application of genetics in the human is (and should be) guided by the principle that in man one looks for ways to manipulate the environment and not to manipulate the genetic structure of the human population. Some would argue against this principle and point to the example of malarial resistance in people with a sickle-cell gene which results in abnormal haemoglobin, but most would question whether the deliberate fostering of sickle-cell anaemia was justified as an antimalarial measure, especially as there are effective means of controlling the parasite and protecting the patient from the disease. The chairman of a recent conference on genetics made this statement:

> . . . The spiritual, artistic and emotional qualities in man will long seem far more important than disease resistance. There is even a bare possibility that disease susceptibility will conduce to these high qualities. Our greatest human beings have not always been perfect physical specimens. We must not forget the divine spark that characterizes man at his highest, if not always his healthiest.

CHAPTER 4

Cybernetics

The word 'cybernetics' was introduced by Wiener (1948) from the Greek *κυβερνητης* = steersman, and has been defined as 'the branch of science which studies, in complex mechanisms, **the lines of communication**, which may be established between part and part, the **information** which may be transmitted along them, the **control** which each part thereby establishes over the other, and the coordination which is thereby achieved' (Ashby, 1950). The latinized version of cybernetics is 'governor' which was the name given to Watt's self-correcting device for his steam engine and one of the earliest examples of regulation in mechanical invention. Prior to this application, machines were controlled by the human brain through a system of levers; later, energy was stored in the machine as in the clock-spring; later still, as in Watt's steam engine, the machine became capable of transforming energy and to a certain extent controlling the output.

Military technology provided a great stimulus to the production of target-seeking guns and missiles which depended on information which could constantly be fed back to the control mechanism. Servo-mechanisms kept the machine informed as to its relationship with the outside as well as the situation within itself and its 'behaviour' would be modified accordingly. Wiener (1948) was struck by the resemblance between the faults these machines developed and disorders of the nervous system such as tremor, nystagmus, ataxia and clonus, and he elaborated hypotheses based on servo-mechanistic analogies to explain these phenomena. Analogies for central nervous activity are not new and have been borrowed from earlier mechanical devices, particularly that of the clockwork, and have found their way into every day speech. We therefore still speak of being 'run down', 'wound up' and 'ticking over'. It may be that when the analogies were introduced people really believed that the structure of the brain was similar to these mechanisms though the machines themselves were limited in their function and did not exhibit the 'intelligence' of the modern computer. It is claimed that these new machines not only operate in some ways like the central nervous system (CNS) but that by a careful study of their mode of action, one can learn more about the CNS itself. It is also claimed that even though all activity cannot yet be explained by cybernetics, it has provided a language which in itself gives us a much clearer insight, and permits the design of experiments and the production of models to test brain function. A new language which is based largely on telecommunication theory has arisen to describe CNS activity and some familiarity with it is now required by the student of psychiatry.

Control

The behaviour of a machine depends on the action of one part on another, and in simpler machines control belonged to that part which supplied the energy to the others. In the newer machines energy need not be a factor in control and control can flow towards energy as well as from it and this degree of control can be measured quantitatively. Furthermore the amount of control which say A can exert over B depends on the number of values which A can take as a variable. Ashby (1950) gives the following biological example from Beach (1948):

> An immature female rat responds to a single sex hormone, oestrogen, in two ways. When approached by an adult male rat she exhibits the avoiding reaction but if the oestrogen level is artificially raised above the ordinary threshold a characteristic mating reaction replaces it. The reaction to oestrogen is therefore either present or absent, and the control which A (oestrogen) exerts on B (the immature female rat) depends not on its complexity as a molecule, nor on its strength but on the number of values which B can take as a variable—in this case, two—avoidance or mating.

Information

This depends primarily not on *what is said*, but on *what could have been said*, so that the information carried by a message is obtainable only by comparing the actual message with the possible number of averages or their respective probabilities. The telegraph operator is not concerned with the content of his messages, but the sequence of signals, and the 'capacity' of the channel he is using determines how much he can transmit. Ashby states: 'We must consider not the message but the statistical ensemble'. Machines which transmit information develop a basic random activity called 'noise' (it is heard on the radio), and Ashby considers that this may well be a factor in CNS activity and that cybernetic techniques will prove essential to its study. Information can be stored (see below) but when lost or destroyed it can never be recovered.

Storage of Information

In a complex machine certain information may have to wait before it can be correlated and this holding of information for subsequent use is called 'memory' which is, of course, an over-simplification of the psychological counterpart. There are two methods used for longer term storage:

1. **Static.** Localized structural changes which persist. *Example:* events are punched automatically on cards and the perforations are later used to determine future action.
2. **Dynamic.** Events may be kept going for hours by transforming them into wave patterns through a column of mercury. At the other end the wave pattern regenerates.

If, as Ashby suggests, these two are the only processes possible, they may well represent the mechanisms responsible for an equivalent aspect of memory, and in that case the latter would depend on reverberating neuronic circuits (see below).

Control by Pattern

Response to a pattern of events in spite of changes in position is a fundamental aspect of Gestalt psychology. This is now a property of some complex machines. This recognition of patterns can be achieved by a variety of mechanisms one of which is *group scanning.* The mechanism is presented a pattern and generates from it all the other equivalents to make a complete set to which it will alone react. It can then be said to react to a *type of pattern* belonging to the set and not to a specific pattern. Ashby suggests that this method may be used in the visual and auditory cortex for pattern recognition with the alpha rhythm functioning as the scanner.

Feedback is present if the controls of part on part form a re-entrant circuit (Ashby, 1950). This is seen in Watt's governor:

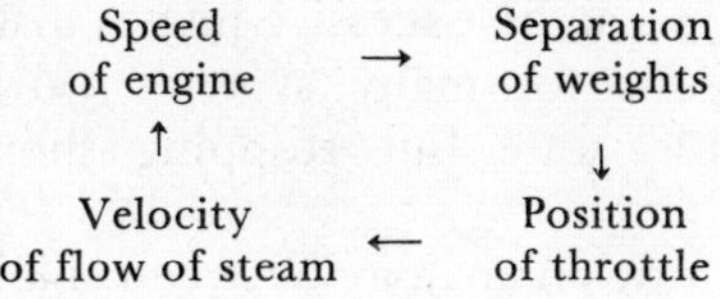

Machines with feedback can correct their own errors and can therefore be said to be goal-seeking. Circuits with feedbacks have been demonstrated in the CNS by Lorente de Nó (1933) who defined his Law of Reciprocity of Connexions thus: 'If a cell-complex A sends fibres to cell or cell-complex B, then B also sends fibres to A, either direct or by means of one internuncial neuron'. In a body, **homeostatic mechanisms** depend on feedback, *e.g.* the pH of the blood influences the respiratory centre, which controls the rate of CO_2 elimination from the blood, which controls the pH of the blood–a re-entrant circuit. In walking, an intact reflex arc is essential to give sensory information but when this is lost as in tabes dorsalis, ataxia results. Feedback of this nature is **negative** and the restoring force is opposite to the deviation, and equilibrium results. In **positive** feedback, the error is self-augmenting and gross instability of the mechanism can result.

Goal-seeking Behaviour

Watt's governor automatically keeps to a set speed independent of the degree of displacement. The goal here is the *set* speed. In the more complex systems, an anti-aircraft gun can react to pulses from the target aircraft and its own shells, and will correct its aim and is only limited by the nature of the target, *e.g.* a heavy gun could not adequately track a swallow. To the observer, the gun would appear to be following the target on its own account '. . . Goal-seeking behaviour, then, is the prerogative, not of the living system, but of the system with feedback' (Ashby, 1950).

Stability

In addition to the advantages of feedback, there is the disadvantage of **instability**, for the error may not be self-correcting. '*A system is stable if to a bounded disturbance it produces a bounded response.*' The more complex the feedback the more difficult it is to achieve stability and 'all large systems with much feedback should be regarded as unstable unless there is evidence to the contrary'. Stability in a machine is capable of mathematical study and when this is applied to input and output the system's **transfer function** can be calculated. Stability can be excessive just as instability may not be entirely disadvantageous for many systems work best when they approach the unstable state but stopping short of a **'run-away'** reaction.

It is tempting to draw an analogy between stability and instability in machines and the human organism. Melancholia and catatonic stupor have been cited as examples of excessive stability as they are alleged to respond only to very strong stimuli though this assumption may be queried. Mania and catatonic excitement have also been put forward as examples of extreme instability for a slight stimulus can provoke a major response which can resemble a 'run-away' state and be self-generating.

Circulating Processes

In the most complex machines there are a number of subsystems which are given work to do by other parts of the machine and a certain amount of 'freedom of action' and 'memory' are built in to give greater versality if not virtuosity. This, however, increases the possibility of disorder and the machine may develop an error which is regenerative and a **circular** process results which is self-perpetuating. Special corrective devices are introduced to avoid these processes, and the cyberneticist considers they are present in the human brain though they have not yet been demonstrated. The part these processes may play in human instability becomes evident when one considers their effects on the machine, as stated by Ashby:

1. The parts used by the process are no longer available for normal use.
2. Other parts in contact with the affected part will receive distorted messages and have their function upset.
3. The spread of these distorted messages makes new circulating disorders more likely for as they are not static they will either disappear or bring the rest of the mechanism into their orbit.
4. These processes can occur in a machine which when examined part by part, may show no mechanical fault.

'Treatment'

The following instructions are laid down for machines that develop faults:

1. Switch off the whole machine and start again, for then some components may start from different positions and the coincidence which led to the original fault will have disappeared.
2. Switch off or remove suspect part of the machine, which may permit efficient function, though at the cost of speed.
3. If the exact error can be located, a special signal can be sent to the abnormal circuit and disrupt it so that it can again be linked with normal activity.
4. Apply to the machine a brief but maximal electric impulse. The effect of the shock soon disappears because of the machine's self-correcting devices but the abnormal process may also disappear. This sudden and general increase in

activity tends to disrupt the abnormal ones which are already maximal.

This last method has been compared to the use of electroplexy in psychiatric disorders.

Learning and Adaptation

Feedback depends on certain constants which are built into the machine. If these constants can respond to the behaviour of the machine, a second order **feedback** results and the machine appears 'intelligent' and can 'learn'. The second order feedback depends on **step-functions** which differ from the constants determining the first order feedback. These step-functions can change value at the moment of change in behaviour. Under certain conditions, second order feedback has as its goal, not a particular state, but a stable, goal-seeking behaviour.

Ashby (1948) built a machine which he called the **homeostat** which illustrates this principle. In addition to primary feedback it has a second order feedback which is goal-seeking and self-correcting and will bring back the primary feedbacks to their normal pattern if they are disturbed. He compares this behaviour and learning of living organisms with second order feedback and claims that the latter is goal-seeking for stable arrangements and may use the method of trial and error. Other experimental models have been constructed which appear to behave like an animal. One such is the 'turtle' of Grey Walter (1953) which followed white lines on the floor and would run to electrical outlets to recharge its batteries when low and would behave differently when 'spanked'.

Further studies of the CNS as a telecommunication device with the aim of constructing theories of nervous function have been and are being pursued. In an important paper Mackay and McCullough (1952) discuss two types of coding in telecommunication (1) **amplitude modulation** and (2) **frequency modulation**, and they consider that there is evidence that both are used in synaptic transmission in the nervous system. They found frequency modulation was several times more efficient in information transmission and therefore assume, that as the optimum method it is predominantly used in the CNS.

BRAIN FUNCTIONS AND THE MACHINE

Ashby (1963) examines some of the brain's functions in terms of the cybernetic analogy. He directs his attention to what could be regarded as a selected sample of the brain's 'human' qualities and which would be lacking in a conventional machine, namely, induction, deduction, prediction, decision-making and selection. The cyberneticist questions the basic philosophical assumptions on which these qualities are based and insists that cybernetics and information theory are practical, pragmatic and empirical, winning knowledge piece by piece. Statements are neither true nor false but are probabilities ranging from one to zero and these extremes are rarely achieved. The Greeks and their logic are seen only in terms of their scientific contributions and their capacity to wrest information from nature. Ashby defines these 'human' qualities as follows:

Induction

This is simply the collecting of information and what can be said at any moment is absolutely bounded by the quantity of information that has been taken in. There is no magic theorem or algorithm which enables us to say much after receiving little information. A minimum amount of information is necessary before induction comes into existence, *e.g.* two points of a curve are essential before the 'tangent' becomes definable; three, before we can speak of curvature; and four, before torsion becomes meaningful. Induction is therefore the taking in of information.

Deduction

This is the carrying through of some *well-defined* and consistently reproducible process. A digital computer deduces the numerical form of a Bessel function; an analogue computer deduces the flow past an aerofoil; and a network of relays deduces the consequences of a set of propositions. Whether one can reduce the roots of an equation depends on whether one can carry through a well-defined process. The usefulness of a deduction rests on totally independent criteria and has nothing to do with the process itself. There is no essential mystery about deduction; a complex deduction system is only a matter of time and labour.

Prediction

Wiener said that to predict the future is to perform an operation on the past. The agent in the act of prediction depends wholly on the actual past and not in the least on the actual future. When one says of a trained rat that it will not jump through a hole because it *will* receive a shock on the other side, one is guilty of confused thinking. One can in fact demonstrate that the actual future does not influence the situation by arranging for the rat *not* to receive a shock. Cybernetics sees nothing peculiar about prediction: it is simply an organism (or anti-aircraft gun) reacting to an immediate and remote past in the way every system does. The fact that the gun crew make it point ahead of the plane is a consequence of its design (several years ago) and its input (in the last few seconds). Prediction is meaningful only when the past shows some constraint and some redundancy and the organism makes use of this constraint. It ensures that present action shall have a better chance than probability of combining with the events in the real world to achieve the desired goal.

Decision-making

Machines have no trouble decision-making; they just act. Even if a car engine refuses to start, the refusal is as much its decision as starting up. One may however classify according to good or successful decisions.

Selection

Any system which achieves appropriate selection to a degree better than chance does so as a consequence of information received. Violation of this law arouses suspicion as with the examination candidate who gives the correct answer before the question has been put. The rules for decision will always take the same form. The possible outcomes are initially many, mixed, good and bad. The set has to be cut down and the amount of cutting down is absolutely bounded by the amount of information. When the information by its finite quantity has been used up, no further selection can be justified. The process has reached its 'field of ignorance' and there is no justification for further selection.

Trial and Error

The philosopher has often dismissed this process as trivial. As a mere grab at success which fails it is valueless, but as a means of obtaining new information, it reduces the field of ignorance. It is an essential feature in solving a maze. When discussing the merits of brain and computer, the latter is often criticized for using the method of trial and error, while the brain is regarded as using a superior method. When similarly situated, such as in maze-solving they may both use the same method.

MAN AND MACHINE

Is man then a machine? Cybernetics does not accept that this is a proper question as it denies that one can classify the world's systems into mechanical and non-mechanical. *Every system* has mechanistic aspects as far as it is law-abiding and orderly in its behaviour. The human brain also shows a good deal of orderliness in its methods, including induction. Is man therefore more than a machine? This will depend on one's definition of a machine. It is only when the idea of a machine is pushed to its limits that one can decide the answer and the cyberneticist says with some justification that he with his greater knowledge of the limits of the machine is most able to answer that question.

Comment

The above are some of the arguments in favour of the cybernetic analogy. The main question the psychiatrist would ask is, how far has it contributed to one's understanding of mental illness? While cybernetics has concentrated on learning and the intellectual functions of the brain, with some success, it has, as yet, made no significant contribution to the emotional aspects of mental life. Joy, anger, grief, depression, anxiety, interest, apathy, jealousy, shame, guilt and love are still absent from machines, yet these factors play an important part in mental function. Only a most rigid subscriber to 'Faculty' psychology would submit that intellectual function is divorced from the affective state.

This has not deterred cyberneticists from speculating freely on mental disturbance. They have been guilty of the error of assuming that a word has the same meaning in their own field as it has in everyday use. For example, instability is regarded as of cybernetic validity and conditions like melancholia and stupor are described as being due to extreme degrees of stability, no doubt because the overt physical features are associated with relative immobility, while mania and catatonic excitement are regarded as the reverse. Obsessional preoccupation is compared with circuit activity and phobic states with avoidance reactions. One cannot say that cybernetics will not make great contributions to our understanding of mental illness, but, to date, it lacks much of the basic knowledge which is more likely to come from the neurophysiologist. Untutored comment on mental illness even if dressed in cybernetic analogy will not substitute for true knowledge of clinical facts.

Analogies are not new and all-embracing ones are suspect. Cybernetics does convey an air of precision which because of its veneer of mathematical certainty will find adherents and even fanatical devotees. The models used are physical and while illustrating possible methods of storing information in the brain and of learning, they are seriously deficient in other biological and human functions. The human brain is not nearly as sensitive as the machine to trauma and has considerable compensatory powers when deprived of large areas either through disease or surgery. It also has emotional functions which are lacking in the machine. It is possible to say that the machine looks 'puzzled' or 'angry' but these are illusions, for feeling has not yet reached the machine.

Rapoport's (1959) cautionary remark is pertinent. 'Behavioural scientists who feel that cybernetics and allied subjects have something of value to contribute to their area of investigation will do well to draw from those fields of knowledge some of their disciplines as well as their inspirations.'

Computers

The increasing sophistication of computers has led some to believe that all previous objections to regarding them as facsimiles of the human brain are no longer valid. Pfalzner (1970) puts the matter into a more up-to-date perspective. He stresses that:

> ... computers are not retarded juveniles who by education, training and experience may improve their judgment and intellect. A computer is an electro-mechanical tool devised by human intelligence and like other tools, is an extension of a human hand and brain. It was grossly misleading to speak of computers in anthropomorphic terms. No-one teaches a computer anything—a computer is programmed by a human programmer to carry out certain specific and circumscribed processes intended by the programmer.
>
> A computer, no matter how sophisticatedly programmed, will always be a 'linear thinker', i.e. can only carry out logical (rote), 'programmable' tasks, and so cannot be 'taught' much less 'taught to teach itself'. Paradox, intuition, emotion, humour, ethics, aesthetics, everything creative and idiosyncratic are human faculties only. Computers can be programmed to imitate certain human thought processes. Some people think that in this way they may be able to learn about the human brain—but it seems unlikely that this is so. At least, not until I find a computer that is able to make jokes!

Dreaming and the Machine

Evans (1966) uses the cybernetic analogy to explain the dreaming process. He bases his theory on the work of Dement (1960) who demonstrated rapid eye movement (R.E.M.) as a feature of dreaming. The act of going to sleep he regards as equivalent to taking the computer off-line. A dream is the actual running through and modification of the existing programmes in the light of the previous day's experiences and events. When the individual is disturbed in the course of the clearing process, modified programmes are caught in the act, as it were, by the conscious mind and a dream is experienced. A dream, according to the above analogy is therefore an *interrupted* dream, for dreams which achieve their purpose are never interrupted and are not consciously experienced or remembered.

The resemblance between this last statement and the Freudian postulate that the purpose of the dream is to preserve sleep is striking. It would carry more conviction if the cybernetic theory were based on stronger experimental evidence.

CHAPTER 5

Organic Psychiatry

Organic disease does not confer immunity to psychiatric illness and *vice versa.* Behind this short statement lies a multiplicity of facts and theories which range over many aspects of medicine and even surgery, and the information, while available in textbooks on these subjects does demand a psychiatric inflection which is not usually available other than in a textbook of psychiatry. At its most general interpretation, all physical illness has its mental accompaniment, if only in the personality of the patient. In addition many diseases have specific mental features which form an essential part of the clinical picture and which may, because of behaviour disturbances require treatment in a unit where such behaviour can be properly evaluated and controlled. This, by tradition, has been the mental hospital, and although there have been developments in the general hospital to cater for the needs of these patients, it is usually the psychiatrist who is responsible for, or advises on their treatment.

Examples that instantly spring to mind are cerebral diseases, such as tumours, degenerative changes, vascular disease and trauma but the list is a long one and as many of these conditions may present *initially* with psychiatric symptoms, like severe depression, it behoves the psychiatrist to be thoroughly familiar with their differential diagnosis. This will entail not only a knowledge of cerebral localization, but some acquaintance with modern neurophysiology, psychological testing, biochemical aspects of disease, toxicology, and even genetics.

It used to be popular for psychiatrists to demonstrate to their colleagues, patients who had been regarded as organic but who were really suffering from 'functional' disease, but there has always been the other side of the coin. Physicians are not at a loss to find patients who have been regarded as 'functional', who were really suffering from organic disease. As there is a tendency for the two groups of specialists to work in isolation, the one group may consider the other to be the main offender, but whoever is most guilty, the psychiatrist has least cause to be. While the physician may diagnose the functional by excluding the organic, the psychiatrist has a similar responsibility in excluding the organic, but should not diagnose the functional on this criterion alone, but on finding positive evidence of functional disturbance.

The problem can be made to appear much greater than it is, for the missed diagnosis is a constant reproach, but Jacobs and Russell (1961) who followed up after five years a series of 100 out-patients from the 5 per cent who had been labelled 'functional', found that 78 were in good health and of the remainder only six patients developed disease which may have accounted for the original symptoms. Of these six, one had disseminated sclerosis and another myxoedema and the other four may well have developed their trouble in the course of the five years. This could, of course, be regarded as a tribute to a thorough clinical appraisal at the initial out-patient examination, but it does suggest that not more than 2 per cent out of 5 per cent (or 1 in 1000) of a series are likely to be misdiagnosed and this in the highly complex borderlands of neurology.

Herridge (1960) who studied 209 consecutive admissions to a psychiatric unit found that 5 per cent had a major physical disease as the principal diagnosis, yet these had been referred as 'functional', so that standards do vary. Comparing these two papers does, however, illustrate that the problem need not be a serious one, provided sufficient care is taken with the organic assessment.

Evidence that organic disease can masquerade as functional illness has led many to consider that all functional illness is organically determined and there are a number of theories to account for it all. While appreciating the vast amount of work that has been undertaken to provide 'proof' and the ingenious explanations, a scrupulous concern for factual evidence is still essential, for historically, clinical judgment has frequently been sacrificed for spurious theory.

General Medicine and Psychiatry

From the author's experience over many years in the practice of psychiatry in a general hospital, the well-trained psychiatrist is more able to exclude the functional than his medical and surgical colleagues are to exclude the organic. This is no reflection on the expertise of the latter but a clinical reality. For example, is a patient with multiple sclerosis whose plantars become extensor on one day, free of organic disease the day before? The chances are high that the disease process has been active for some time but present methods of physical examination are unable to detect this. The same could be said of diseases in other systems. The psychiatrist's role in the general hospital is to tell his colleagues that he can detect no functional disease and that further observation and investigation may well reveal a physical cause for the patient's complaints. The good physician will respect this opinion, and indeed this may prove to be the most valuable contribution the psychiatrist can make to hospital medical practice. The day when the psychiatrist in the general hospital passively accepted all patients referred to him as functional because the organic had been 'excluded' has gone. It also provides a greater challenge to the psychiatrist's diagnostic expertise, and one which he should be able to meet.

A less controversial field, but an important one, is that of general medical problems occurring in a psychiatric hospital. It has for long been recognized that mentally ill patients have more than their share of physical illness and Davies (1964) has reported his unique experiences. His appointment is that of a general physician (internist) to a mental hospital of 700 beds which has a higher quota of elderly patients than other mental hospitals in the area. In a six-month period he had 34 in-patients referred with intercurrent physical disease. Examples: Chronic paranoid state with backache—secondary deposits in spine from malignant reticulosis; chronic hypochondriasis—acoustic neuroma; chronic schizophrenia with hypotension—reactivated pulmonary tuberculosis with a positive sputum. In addition there were 11 patients admitted with a psychiatric diagnosis and *unsuspected* physical disease yet the degree of physical morbidity was no less than that described above.

That the situation is not all that bad and may even be improving is suggested in the report by Eastwood *et al.* (1970) who investigated the frequency of physical disorder among 100 consecutive new referrals to the Maudsley Hospital Emergency Clinic. Only 16 patients had a physical condition which had not been previously diagnosed and 10 of these had hypertension. Only one patient was found to be suffering from a purely physical disease. The authors suggest that all could have been detected by a small number of screening tests which they recommend as a routine.

Every psychiatrist is aware of these diagnostic pitfalls but it is just as well to be reminded of them, so that their importance is re-emphasized in our practice and teaching.

The complexity of the neurological borderlands has already been mentioned and Symonds (1960) quotes a case of a young man, labelled hysterical, who, when he approached a corner, walked hesitatingly with outstretched arms and would not turn till he felt he was at the corner, yet he could estimate with some accuracy the length of the ward but not the examination room. This patient explained that he arrived at the first estimate by multiplying the width of a bed (which he guessed) by the number of beds in the ward. It was evident that he had local brain damage (a fact which was supported by a recent penetrating gunshot wound in the occipital region). He had lost the perception of distance.

This is a unique example, but such rare instances have persuaded many that all mental abnormality is due to disordered brain function. This attitude may have been influenced by Jackson (1894) who in his essay on 'The Factors of Insanities', stated:

> In every insanity more or less of the highest cerebral centres is out of function, temporarily or permanently, from some pathological process; for my present limited purpose it matters little what that process may be. It only matters as the pathological processes produce loss of function, that is dissolution, of more or less of the highest centres. I do not use the term function in the sense often given to it in clinical accounts of nervous maladies, as, for example, when it is said of a patient that 'his case is entirely functional'. I do not believe there is such a thing as loss or defect of function of any nervous elements without a proportionate material alteration of their structure and nutrition. Of course, the separation into structure, nutrition and function of the nervous system is artificial; it is merely a convenient device, just as the separation into the surface, weight and mass of a body is.

He firmly believed that different regions of the highest cerebral centres could undergo dissolution in different kinds of insanity and he quoted melancholia and general paralysis as two examples.

Jackson's theory goes much further than the legitimate conclusions derived from clinical observations, which are, that apparent functional states may have an organic basis. He in fact stated that all functional states have an organic basis. There is powerful support for this theory in that post-encephalitic states can produce psychiatric illness which is almost indistinguishable from that with no history of encephalitis; epileptic psychoses, particularly with schizophrenic features, can closely resemble the 'functional' variety, and hallucinogenic drugs can create mental changes which have some of the features of a 'functional psychosis'. If with all this evidence, one denies the existence of the unconscious and of psychopathology because of lack of 'proof', then the stage is set for an organic explanation for every psychiatric symptom.

Bleuler (1951) did not take such an extreme view. He stated: '. . . I approve, of course, of the modern concept of psychosomatic medicine, which considers both—structure and function, body and mind—as equivalent and inseparable expressions of life itself'. He considered that it was possible through psychopathological studies to differentiate between mental derangement with and without brain pathology, but his use of the term 'psychopathology' was rather different to that of 'dynamic' psychiatry and was really another word for psychiatric symptoms; his criteria will be described in greater detail (see below).

Organic disease associated with mental changes is not confined to structural changes in the brain, but includes endocrine disease and biochemical abnormalities. Some have tried to explain the major psychoses on an endocrine and biochemical basis, but, significantly, established workers in the field are more cautious in their claims. Simpson (1957) summarizes the position thus:

> . . . In so far as major endocrine disorders, with a preponderant excess or gross deficiency of one or more hormones, are frequently associated with characteristic behaviour patterns, as well as with psychoneuroses and psychoses, it seems reasonable to conclude that the excess or deficiency of hormones is causative or influential, and not merely coincidental—a view which is further supported by successful organic treatment, but which does not necessarily exclude the existence of non-endocrine genetic factors modifying the response of individuals to hormonal stimuli, excessive or deficient . . . I qualify my conclusions by an unqualified admission of the importance of non-endocrine factors in determining behaviour patterns, and even more so in the case of the psychoneuroses and psychoses, the majority of the latter of which are not due to endocrine factors.

It is not possible to classify 'organic syndromes' with complete logicality, as the essential mechanisms by which the symptoms are produced are still very imperfectly understood, but there is already a 'traditional' approach. There are those disorders which are in part or wholly associated with brain involvement which may be the result of structural change or less well defined insults. Others are associated with general systemic disturbances which are primarily rooted in other organs but which have cerebral overtones, though the features of both these groups may overlap. Generally the physical signs and symptoms of the underlying disease are discernible and lead to an accurate diagnosis, but occasionally and particularly in the prodromal stage, mental symptoms alone may present and it is by studying their nature that the organic nature of the condition may be defined. Some have labelled these conditions with a primary organic basis other than cerebral as the *Symptomatic Psychoses*, and naturally are identified by their somatic symptomatology.

Frequently one finds a psychotic picture which, though obviously related to an organic disease, is almost indistinguishable from a true functional psychosis. Bleuler (1951) considered that when this occurs in association with cerebral disease, such as brain tumour, it is not due to the lesion itself, but to the uncovering of a constitutional predisposition. He found that among the relatives of patients with brain tumours associated with schizophrenic and manic-depressive disorders, there was a higher incidence of these psychoses than among the relatives of patients who had no psychotic features complicating their brain tumours. He concluded that constitutional factors may determine some of the differences in symptomatology that frequently occur with brain tumour.

Classification

This should not be an end in itself, for if imperfectly based, it may conceal more valid associations. As the site, nature, rate of development, previous personality and environmental demands all influence the mental picture, it is not proposed to present a 'systematic' classification of these disorders, but merely to state the facts as they are known, yet at the same time to attempt some grouping which it is hoped will make their study less irksome. It is a complex field which borders on general medicine and neurology, and it is difficult to steer a course which is primarily psychiatric, for a textbook of psychiatry which encroaches on these subjects not only treats them inexpertly, but diminishes itself in its prime object; yet the effort should be made.

ORGANIC BRAIN SYNDROMES

These include all cerebral pathology which may lead to mental changes, such as infection, tumour, and other space-occupying lesions, vascular abnormalities, trauma, degenerative changes, toxic reactions, and encephalopathic states based on biochemical disturbances. They are frequently classified under acute and chronic reactions in addition to their specific aetiology, and it would be opportune here to state the essential features of these two reactions to avoid subsequent repetition.

Acute Reaction

This term has not necessarily been confined to conditions of sudden onset, but rather to the reversible process, and this would appear to be an unsatisfactory definition for there are chronic conditions such as pellagra and dementia paralytica which are reversible. It is also true that there are conditions of sudden onset which can deteriorate rapidly and if reversibility were the sole criterion, then such conditions should be labelled chronic. It is a pity that psychiatric nomenclature should spread its confusion to organic diseases which can be classified in a more orderly and comprehensible manner. The label should therefore be reserved for conditions of acute onset, whether reversible or not. If recovery does not take place then, as in other medical conditions, it can be said to become chronic.

The clinical picture is that of clouding of consciousness which can range from mild confusion to delirium and coma. Memory may be impaired with lack of concentration and at times distractibility, and in some instances a true dysmnesic syndrome.

Chronic Reaction

This has been defined as irreversible but there are objections to this definition which have already been stated. It too may become manifest with impairment of consciousness, but not to the degree of the acute stage, although there can be acute exacerbations with delirium superimposed on the chronic state. There is usually memory impairment though this is variable and may depend on the site of the lesion and it can take the form of a general loss, or present as the dysmnesic syndrome. Dementia in all its grades is a dominant feature and this has been classified by Mayer-Gross and Guttmann (1937) under the following headings:

1. A difficulty in retention (the amnesic syndrome).
2. Disturbance of attention, and more particularly, difficulty in focusing attention.
3. Lack of spontaneity, though occasionally there is an excess of spontaneity.
4. Poverty of ideas.
5. Forced responsiveness to stimuli; or perhaps an extreme selectiveness for stimuli.
6. Some degree of disturbed consciousness.
7. Undue tidiness; or on the other hand, slovenliness.
8. Affective disorders.
9. Proclivity to various catastrophic reactions.

The author has felt that present 'classification' is not only unsatisfactory in that it is illogical, but that it fails to recognize some of the more readily definable features of the chronic brain syndromes. Too much attention has been focused on the intellectual aspects of deterioration and the term dementia has been largely concerned with these aspects. Not only are there marked qualitative differences at the cognitive level but there are other aspects of mental deterioration which may be more important in determining the patient's capacity to live in the community.

In mental deficiency it has long been recognized that intellectual defect is a poor index of this capacity; social behaviour was far more important. So with dementia; social, emotional and behavioural deficits are of greater importance. A patient may have lost very little in intellectual functioning, but because of disturbing behaviour, depraved social habits or emotional immaturity his work and home may reject him. One should consider dementia in a 'global' sense and then one may be able to identify the dementia 'differentials'. A whole new field of classification is opening up and it is the clinician rather than the psychologist who should provide the structure on which it will be based.

GOLDSTEIN'S CONTRIBUTION TO THE ORGANIC CEREBRAL REACTION

Perhaps the most original contributions in recent years to the study of the brain-damaged patient are those of Goldstein (1939). In his challenging book *The Organism*, he combines a careful clinical approach with a capacity to see relationships and formulate theory.

He bases his conclusions on 'three methodological postulates' which are:

1. All the phenomena presented by the patient should be considered without giving preference in description to any one, *i.e.* no symptom is greater or lesser in importance than another. He cites the example of amnesic aphasia or difficulty in finding words, which was considered to be the main disability, because it was the one which presented most strikingly and in turn, gave rise to a false theory about the reduced capacity to evoke speech images. He found that these patients had not lost this capacity, but were unable to use words as the bearers of *meaning* and when this aspect was not involved and words were used in a concrete situation the words were available, and he concludes: 'The inability to find and use words voluntarily is not due to the primary defect of the speech mechanism, but to a change in their total personality which bars them from the situation where meaning is required.'

2. There must be accurate description of the observable phenomena, and not merely a description of their effects, for the effect may

not be expressive of the underlying function and in some instances give unreliable information. The 'plus or minus method' of recording can be erroneous, for the result may be achieved by a roundabout way which unless carefully analysed is ignored in the final reading. He cites the example of the patient with loss of 'categorical behaviour' who may have difficulty in naming a colour according to a category such as redness or greenness. Yet when this patient is asked to select the red group of the Holmgren wool samples, he may place them serially from light to dark red. One might assume that the patient had the concept of brightness in mind and placed the wools accordingly, but Goldstein points out that this would be an error of observation which overlooked the differences between this behaviour and one based on categorical thought. In fact the patient cannot proceed categorically and does not arrange things in order of brightness when asked to do so. What he does is to place one shade after another in pairs, the second pair being related to the one immediately before it and so on, and the procedure is one of sorting by successive pairs rather than by a concept of the order of brightness. This can be shown by removing the skein last placed in position, which will render the patient incapable of completing the series. Similarly a wrong response should not be marked down as a simple failure, for it may help us to understand the patient's mental functions. It may be that normal response was not practicable for that patient and that his failure represents a local rather than a general defect.

3. 'No phenomenon should be considered without reference to the organism concerned, and to the situation in which it appears'. This principle is of course taken from Hughlings Jackson but Goldstein has revitalized it. His approach demands the greatest patience and capacity to see relationships where previously none had been suspected and he emphasizes that: '. . . One single extensive analysis of this sort is much more valuable than many examinations involving many patients, but yielding only imperfect conclusions'.

He defines the performance of an organism as '. . . any kind of behaviour, activity, or operation—whole or in part—which expresses itself overtly and bears reference to the environment'. He has a remarkable faculty for enumerating laws which have the ring of universal truth and the following are a few examples:

1. A single performance field will never drop out *alone* for invariably *all* performance fields are affected although the degree to which the individual field is involved varies.

2. A single performance field will never drop out *completely*.

Some individual performances are always preserved.

3. Although a patient may present different symptoms in different fields, these symptoms are expressions of the same basic disturbance.

4. The basic disturbance can be regarded as a change of behaviour or as an impairment of brain function and the behaviour change is usually a failure to handle the abstract and a retention of the capacity to manipulate concrete situations. This principle pervades a variety of responses such as action, perception, thinking and volition.

> The patient acts, perceives, thinks, has the right impulses of will, feels like others, calculates, pays attention, retains, etc., as long as he is provided with the opportunity to handle objects concretely and directly. He fails when this is possible. This is the reason why he does not succeed in intelligence tests. This is also the reason why he can grasp a little story as long as it concerns a familiar situation in which he, himself, has participated. But he will not understand a story—certainly no more difficult for the average person—requiring him to place himself, in imagination, in the position of someone else. He does not comprehend metaphors or puzzles. He can manipulate numbers in a practical manner, but has no concept of their value. He can talk if there is some concrete subject matter present for him to depend upon, but he cannot recount material unrelated to him, or report it purely conceptually. He is incapable of representation of direction and localities in objective space, nor can he estimate distances; but he can find his way about very well, and can execute actions which are dependent upon perception of distance and size.

He calls this **disturbance of categorical behaviour.**

Disruption of function first attacks the most highly organized and later the more basic functions are impaired. Consequent on this, there is a gradual loss of the faculties which are most characteristic of the individual, till he is left with those of the gross dement. The highest form he calls 'ordered' and the other he calls 'disordered or catastrophic'. In the 'ordered' responses appear constant, correct and adequate for the respective organism as well as to the respective circumstances. This is not synonymous with normal behaviour. 'Catastrophic' reactions are inadequate, disordered, inconstant and inconsistent and the patient exhibits anxiety. It is therefore a function of the organism to move towards ordered behaviour which is free of anxiety and to try and avoid the catastrophic reaction, which he does by 'substitute performances'. These consist of efforts to hold to the preserved performance level and not undertaking tasks which will extend the patient. They may result in action which in itself is meaningless, but in the context of a threatened catastrophic reaction the meaning is clear. Conduct may be stereotyped or maintain a uniform and undisturbed condition, thus giving rise to descriptions such as apathy and lack of volition, again illustrating how fallacious it is to draw conclusions from a final behavioural act without taking into account its purpose. There may be a **'tendency to orderliness'** which has by some been labelled obsessional behaviour but it is really designed to help the patient to find his articles with the least possible distress. Other features mentioned by Goldstein are:

Avoidance of 'Emptiness'. This can be seen when the patient is given a sheet of blank paper. The patient will very rarely use the middle of the sheet, but will write at the top edge and crowd the writing very closely. One of his patients would only write on a blank sheet if allowed to draw a line parallel to the upper margin.

Relative Maintenance of Ordered Behaviour by Shrinkage of Milieu according to Defect. From this Goldstein enunciated the law: 'A defective oganism achieves ordered behaviour only by a shrinkage of its environment in proportion to the defect'.

Tendency to Optimal Performance. This he illustrates by an example from hemianopic patients with total destruction of the calcarine cortex of one hemisphere (the central termination of the optic tract). These patients are totally blind in the corresponding halves of the visual field of both eyes but in everyday life they fail to indicate that they see nothing in one-half of the visual field and they can recognize objects within an area, where stimulation, during perimetrical examination, is ineffective. Subjectively they are aware only of impaired vision, but they are not aware of the rigidly defined hemianopia of perimetry or even that they see less distinctly on one side. These patients have their vision arranged round the centre as in the normal; this is the area of sharpest vision and they are therefore able to preserve this organization in spite of the defect, thus demonstrating the above tendency.

Goldstein, while fully cognizant of localization in the cerebral cortex, has re-emphasized Lashley's theory of Mass Action—that impaired function of the brain depends to a considerable extent on the quantity of brain tissue involved, and has applied a corrective to those who would represent mental function by a topographical map of the brain.

PERSEVERATION

This is a feature found in a variety of organic states. In the clinical sense, perseveration implies the continuation or repetition of a purposeful response which is entirely appropriate to the first of two stimuli but is inappropriate to the second one, though it is provoked by it. Allison (1966 *a & b*) in his Croonian lectures emphasizes that it is not specific to any one disease of the central nervous system either focal or diffuse but is also found in schizophrenia. In organic states it is generally associated with a variety of other symptoms such as clouding of consciousness, impairment of recent memory, inability to learn, disorientation in time and place, and altered mood.

It can be difficult to distinguish perseveration associated with organic disease from that associated with schizophrenia. Freeman and Gathercole (1966) who contrasted its occurrence in schizophrenic patients and organic dementias distinguished 3 types:

1. The act is frequently repeated, *e.g.* when the patient is asked to put out his tongue he continues to put it out and in for several minutes. This they equate with Luria's (1965) *efferent motor perseveration* or *compulsive repetition.*
2. That seen in alternation tests involving 'switching', *i.e.* where one object is substituted for another and the patient reports it to be the former object.
3. Ideational perseveration, *i.e.* where the same concepts which were originally arrived at by a process of deduction are offered inappropriately in response to different questions.

They found that although more organic dementing patients gave evidence of impairment of switching, and schizophrenics showed compulsive repetition, there was no significant overall difference. The dementing patients showed perseveration on an average of 5·8 tests and the schizophrenics averaged 5·4 tests.

INFECTIONS OF BRAIN AND MENINGES ASSOCIATED WITH MENTAL ILLNESS

1. DEMENTIA PARALYTICA (General Paralysis of the Insane)

This disease occupies a special place in psychiatric history. The first description is usually accredited to Haslam (1798) who was an apothecary at Bethlem Hospital. His report, which was one in a series of 29 cases which came to autopsy, reads as follows:

Case XV. J.A., a man, forty-two years of age, was first admitted into the house on June 27, 1795. His disease came on suddenly whilst working in a garden, on a very hot day, without any covering to his head. He had some years before travelled with a gentleman over a great part of Europe; his ideas ran particularly on what he had seen abroad; sometimes he conceived himself the king of Denmark, at other times the king of France. Although naturally dull and wanting common education, he professed himself a master of all the dead and living languages; but his most intimate acquaintance was with the old French: and he was persuaded he had some faint recollection of coming over to this country with William the Conqueror. His temper was irritable, and he was disposed to quarrel with everybody about him. After he had continued ten months in the hospital, he became tranquil, relinquished his absurdities, and was discharged well in June 1796. He went into the country with his wife to settle some domestic affairs, and in about six weeks afterwards relapsed. He was re-admitted into hospital August 13th.

He now evidently had a paralytic affection; his speech was inarticulate, and his mouth drawn aside. He shortly became stupid, his legs swelled, and afterwards ulcerated: at length his appetite failed him; he became emaciated, and died December 27th of the same year.

It was the French physician Bayle (1822) who for his M.D. thesis made a systematic study of a number of cases who had presumably acquired their infection as a result of the increased incidence of syphilis in the Napoleonic Wars, and in France the condition is still referred to as Bayle's disease. The label 'general paralysis of the insane' also stems from France, where Calmeil (1826) referred to the disease as *paralysie générale des aliénés,* which is now familiarly called 'G.P.I.' .

It is sometimes difficult to appreciate that a disease which at one time accounted for nearly 20 per cent of mental hospital admissions, did not have its aetiology defined till Noguchi and Moore (1913) demonstrated the *Treponema pallidum* in the brain in cases of general paralysis. Yet Esmarch and Jessen (1857) had over 50 years earlier published a paper on the relation between syphilis and insanity. There were however many medical 'personalities' who at that time pontificated against its syphilitic origin and exercised considerable influence, and as long as 'proof' was confined to clinical appraisal alone, their views prevailed, but laboratory methods were steadily gaining ground. Schaudinn (1905) had identified the causative organism, Wassermann (1906) had devised a test which gave a positive reaction in the blood and spinal fluid, and it only needed Noguchi and Moore to complete the chain of evidence and refute the opinions of such giants in medicine as Henry Maudsley and Virchow, both of whom had denied its syphilitic origin. G.P.I. has an additional interest for psychiatrists, for it was the first major disease in the asylum hitherto regarded as incurable to respond to medical treatment, and thus the status of the asylum was raised almost overnight. Its doctors had now developed skills in treating a disease which by its nature was not admitted to general hospitals, and the asylum became the mental hosptial.

INCIDENCE

This is difficult to assess, for once the Wassermann reaction was used as an index of diagnosis, any condition which remotely resembled G.P.I. was so labelled, if the W.R. was positive. False positives were initially imperfectly understood and even now they can cause considerable doubt, and it is only by the Treponema immobilization test (T.P.I.) that the diagnosis can be made with certainty and this procedure, for very good reasons, is not generally employed. Yet there has been a marked downward trend in incidence, which could only in part be due to better diagnosis and one must assume that the reduction is real. One can only speculate as to the reasons, but propaganda with emphasis on prophylaxis has probably had some effect, while antibiotics have also played their part and the incidence in mental hospital populations has dropped from 20 per cent to 2 per cent. But there are fallacies in trying to assess incidence, for many cases are now admitted and treated in general hospitals and in the Queen Elizabeth Hospital, Birmingham, England, out of 15 cases admitted between 1953–62, only two were initially seen in the psychiatric department. The recent downwards trend in Britain is in danger of being reversed, for we are now approaching the end of the incubation period for infections acquired in the Second World War. Teenagers are at present very prone to venereal infection because of a loosening of moral values (Schofield, 1965) and the prevalence of modern contraceptive clinics, which are not 'preventative' against venereal disease. Adults are no less at risk. While many will be treated and cured, a number may not be initially recognized and will eventually add to the total.

PATHOLOGY

Most of the evidence is from advanced cases. The meninges are thickened, cloudy and adherent. The brain is shrunken with atrophy of the cerebral convolutions, particularly in the frontal and parietal regions. The ventricles are usually enlarged with a granular ependymitis, and the brain weight may be considerably reduced.

Microscopically

1. There is cellular infiltration of small vessels and capillaries particularly in the cortex and corpus striatum. The cells are mainly plasma cells and lymphocytes, the former being identified by pinkish protoplasm (with Nissl stain), a clock-face arrangement of the

chromatin in the nucleus, and a clear area immediately round the nucleus. Their shape is also said to be characteristic and they may appear square, irregular or fit together like paving stones and are present in the adventitial spaces and at times in the tissue, while a degenerative form, called the 'mulberry' cell, may also be found in the tissue.

2. Endarteritis of small cortical vessels.

3. Glial changes. These consist of: (*a*) proliferation of large astrocytes; (*b*) proliferation under the ependyma of the ventricles; (*c*) proliferation of Hortega cells which in the cortex and striatum show as *rod cells*. These are elongated microglia arranged in parallel, and perpendicular to the surface of the cortex. Although seen with Nissl stain, their real extent can only be gauged by a special glial stain for Hortega cells.

4. Intra-adventitial iron deposits, which appear yellowish-green with Nissl stain, but can be demonstrated in fresh material with Spatz stain and in alcohol fixed material with Turnbull blue. They occur mainly in adventitial cells and may lie free in the adventitial spaces and occasionally in Hortega cells. They are diffusely spread over cortex and striatum.

5. Cell changes in the parenchyma are varied and include: (*a*) 'dropping out' of nerve cells over wide or circumscribed areas; (*b*) disturbance of the cytoarchitectonics of the cortex, with nerve cells and their processes running parallel instead of perpendicular to the cortex; (*c*) circulatory determined cell changes, such as is seen in the Sommer section of the *cornu Ammonis*.

6. Distribution of lesions is diffuse, but they tend to concentrate in the anterior part of the brain and decrease toward the posterior pole, with the *cornu Ammonis* being particularly involved. The cerebellum may be affected and generally grey matter is more vulnerable than white matter. Nerve cell destruction is also more marked in the front of the brain.

Wertham and Wertham (1934) state:

> Despite the great variety of histopathological findings in dementia paralytica, it is possible to single out a few *cardinal histological signs* which characterize the process. These are the plasma cell infiltrations of small vessels, the Hortega cell proliferation and the iron deposits occurring in the intra-adventitial spaces and in Hortega cells.

Spirochaetes are present in large numbers in the brains of untreated patients, but they tend to disappear in treated subjects. This also applies to the other histological evidence of the disease.

CLINICAL PICTURE

In an organically determined disease, much of the symptomatology is organic and though the mental symptoms have an organic flavour, it is convenient to describe them separately.

Physical Signs

In the early stage these may be entirely absent but the disease may be diagnosed by blood Wassermann or by a lumbar puncture performed for some unrelated purpose. Physical signs such as convulsions, transient hemiplegia or aphasia may, however, precede the mental changes by several months. Others have characteristics which have been traditionally associated with the disease and are as follows:

1. *Speech disorders,* consisting of difficulty in articulation, hesitation and slurring. In the early stages, test phrases such as 'Methodist Episcopal Church', 'Royal Irish Constabulary', 'The Leith police dismisseth us' and 'Biblical Criticism' are put to the patient who is unable to pronounce them correctly. These are only a sample of a number of 'tongue twisters' which are favoured, but all generally depend on variations of vowel and consonant, which demand a high degree of articulation, and similar tests have been used in assessing drunkenness and in experiments in sedation threshold. The speech disorder eventually deteriorates to complete incoherence.

2. *Pupillary changes* of varying nature are in the early stages present in not more than 90 per cent of cases, but with deterioration they become one of the most constant findings, Argyll Robertson (1869 *a & b*) described a pupil which is regarded as diagnostic and is found in over 50 per cent of paretics. It is miotic or excessively contracted, and though reacting to accommodation effort, does not react to light. It should not be confused with the Holmes-Adie myotonic pupil which, as in tabo-paresis, may also be associated with absent knee jerks. In the Holmes-Adie syndrome the pupil is not contracted; it may even be dilated and if exposed to light after a long spell in the dark, may slowly contract.

3. *Optic atrophy* may occur in varying degrees in 50 per cent of cases and may progress to complete blindness. The discs are pale and there are visual defects either in the field or of colour sensitivity.

4. *Handwriting* is frequently involved and shows considerable deterioration with misspelling, omissions and repetitions as well as disorganization in the formation of the letters themselves. Though it may be due partly to tremor, it may also be due to difficulty in

arranging things in space and the patient usually shows little insight into his writing mistakes.

5. *Tremor* is usually coarse and is seen particularly in the fingers, lips and tongue which when protruded shows the 'trombone' effect.

6. *Facial appearance* tends to be mask-like with flattening and smoothing of the nasio-labial folds and the faculty of expression and mobility is deficient.

7. *Convulsions* are common and when the disease was more prevalent they were regarded as an important early indication, if occurring for the first time in a patient over the age of 35 years. With the reduction in incidence of the disease and the more accurate diagnosis of cerebral tumours and aneurysms, the presence of convulsions does not carry the specific import it did; yet from 60 to 70 per cent of patients do have convulsions at some time during the illness.

8. *Muscular incoordination* is manifest by difficulty in buttoning clothing or in dressing, though this may be partly due to the tremor. If tabetic features are also present, there will be gross ataxia with the high 'steppage' gait.

9. *Sphincter* disturbances are more common in the terminal stages, though urinary incontinence can occur earlier.

10. *Knee jerks* are usually exaggerated, with ankle clonus and spasticity, but if a tabetic process co-exists, they are absent.

11. *Apoplectic attacks* are similar to convulsions but are followed by hemiplegia or more localized lesions. The prognosis is usually more favourable than in the arteriosclerotic type and recovery is the rule.

12. *Aortitis and aneurysm* are frequently associated, but these are usually found at autopsy, for in life they are commonly asymptomatic.

13. *Special Investigations*

(a) *C.S.F.*

(i) W.R. and Khan tests are positive in about 100 per cent of untreated cases. Other conditions which give a positive W.R. such as disseminated lupus erythematosus should be borne in mind and in a few instances, a Treponema immobilization test (T.P.I.) is justified. A fluorescent antibody technique using conjugated syphilitic serum has been used in the diagnosis of syphilis in exudate from lesions and in tissues where the *Treponema pallidum* is present. It is not as specific as the T.P.I. for false positives still result, and the T.P.I. is still the final court of appeal.

(ii) Cells are increased (10–50) per ml.).

(iii) Increased protein, particularly the globulin fraction.

(iv) Paretic Lange (colloidal gold) curve, *e.g.* 5555444322, though it may be tabo-paretic, *e.g.* 1122345432.

If the patient has had an antibiotic such as penicillin, these features may be masked.

(b) *EEG*. Abnormal tracings in the untreated will depend on the severity of the disease, but may be present in 80 per cent. The tracings are not characteristic but if convulsions have occurred there will probably be evidence to support them. Disturbances will be more likely localized to the frontal region indicating frontal lobe damage. As with the C.S.F., previous therapy tends to mask EEG abnormalities.

Mental Symptoms

Information about early psychiatric disturbance is usually obtained from relatives for the patient may be unable to remember or even comprehend. The first symptom is frequently alleged to be a dramatic one, but this may be because it was so dramatic that it registered, while earlier and less obvious aspects went unrecognized. This could account for those tales of respectable lawyers singing bawdy songs instead of proposing toasts—the surgeon making an autopsy incision instead of that for appendicectomy, and the politician at the party convention sitting on the platform and picking his nose (Mayer-Gross *et al.,* 1960). Occasionally one does get a history of gradual deterioration with repeated mislaying of articles and other memory disturbances.

1. *Memory disturbance*. Some have tried to distinguish this in the patient with G.P.I. from the senile dement, saying that the latter lives in the past while the former lives apathetically in the present (Noyes & Kolb, 1958). It does have certain features in common with senile dementia, for recent events are forgotten while remote events are accurately retained. Confusion frequently accompanies the memory defect and the patient may behave erratically because of it, forgetting the time of day or what he has just done, while other incidents are unaffected.

2. *Mood* has traditionally been described as grandiose and expansive, with optimism and euphoria, but in fact apathy and dullness are also common and there is a shallow affectivity, the patient being relatively unmoved by events which in the normal would evoke a marked emotional response. The euphoria is therefore not quite as intense as in true mania, and there is a lack of brightness and intelligence behind it, the whole appearance being rather facile such as one sees in a Korsakoff psychosis. Occasionally the patient is depressed and tearful.

3. *Delusions* are traditionally described as grandiose, the patient claiming to have done the most fantastic things which would make even the celebrated Baron Munchausen blush. They own everything, can do or have done everything, and occupy the most exalted positions. In their delusions they lack all judgment, contradicting one system with another and showing no embarrassment. One patient claimed he was an Admiral of the Fleet, an Air Marshal and a Field Marshal as well as owning all the castles and palaces in the land and was a millionaire many times over. The facility with which some of these delusions are produced is very reminiscent of the confabulation one meets in Korsakoff psychosis. There is an element of fashion associated with these grandiose delusions, the patient believing he is the Prince of Wales or General Montgomery, Mr Churchill or Stalin. Delusions of grandeur occur in not more than 50 per cent of patients with G.P.I. but because of their high anecdotal value, they are usually reported at length while the more pedestrian mental disturbances go unrecorded. Delusions of persecution and bizarre nihilistic ones have also been described.

4. *Mental deterioration,* in the early stages, is manifest as tactlessness such as is found after leucotomy and later it extends to impaired judgment with deterioration in behaviour which extends into the emotional field, the patient being no longer able to make full rapport with those around him and exhibiting conduct lacking the usual aesthetic and moral qualities he once possessed. As dementia progresses it may be associated with violent and destructive outbursts, and with the concomitant march of the general paralysis, the terminal picture is one of complete dementia with complete paralysis. This state is now rarely seen for antibiotics, if not able to control the dementia, can arrest the paralytic process.

5. *Delirium* is seen in rapidly developing states and may well be associated with an acute meningitic reaction.

A variety of psychiatric syndromes have been described which tend to cover the full scale of psychotic illness. The incidence of each type varies and Dewhurst (1969) described the types and their percentage incidence in the table on p. 121.

While these figures may not be universally applicable, they do show that the majority of cases are neither expansive nor euphoric. One might expect that in those countries where certain functional psychoses predominate, they will colour the picture of G.P.I. and this is borne out by Borges Fortes (1956) who reported a higher rate of schizophrenic syndromes from South America. These types are of course not discrete and there is usually considerable overlap but they do tend to group together selected members of a bewildering variety of symptoms and have the additional merit of clinical validity.

Simple Dementing Type

The dementia is insidious and progressive with no delusions or excitement. There is a falling off in interest with impairment of judgment, memory defect, and a general apathy which is seen initially as a lack of ambition and drive. A benign euphoria may be present and the patient puts on weight which together with the facial appearance described above completes a picture which has for long been recognized as characteristic. Remissions are rare and the condition if untreated slowly deteriorates.

Expansive Type

This is the variety which is frequently reported because of the drama surrounding the patient's delusions. Initially the patient may be good-humoured and apparently enjoy what he believes to be the admiration of all, but he may later become very irritable and aggressive, though he can be humoured, and this is one of the very few instances where it is justifiable to accept the patient's delusions without question and not betray one's judgment. This attitude can, however, be carried too far by inexperienced staff who may take an unhealthy delight in stimulating the patient to relate his grandiose delusions. Occasionally the psychomotor activity is increased to the point of mania, and exhaustion may supervene.

Depressed Type

Though not generally reported, this variety is not uncommon and may present with classical features of melancholia such as nihilistic and hypochondriacal delusions. The mood is never as intense as in the unadulterated melancholic for there is an associated emotional deterioration with a shallow affectivity. Nevertheless a number do express delusions of unworthiness and suicidal attempts have been reported. Dementia though not an obvious feature in the early stages is usually present and can be demonstrated.

Circular Type

Here there are the usual swings of mood seen in cyclothymia and some psychiatrists have (probably correctly) postulated an underlying cyclothymic personality. Just as alternating types are uncommon in the manic-depressive psychoses, so in G.P.I. this type tends to be rare. It is mentioned here because it can very closely simulate its functional counterpart and the diagnosis may be missed.

Schizophrenic Type

As with the other varieties, this closely resembles the functional picture with feelings of influence and passivity freely expressed and there may also be auditory hallucinations and paranoid features. There was the classical patient of Bumke (1948) who had been regarded for some time as a catatonic schizophrenic till he died of paralysis.

Lissauer's Type

This variety was first described by Lissauer and Storch (1901) who indicated that there are atypical forms of G.P.I. It is characterized by unilateral atrophy of either a whole cerebral region or a group of convolutions, the areas affected being primarily the pre-central and post-central gyri and less frequently the occipital and rolandic areas. It is a gross form of parenchymatous brain damage and the resulting specimen looks rather moth-eaten and it is not difficult to appreciate the clinical findings of epileptic and apoplectic attacks. Unilateral lesions may be gross and cause hemiparesis but they may also be localized and cause aphasia, apraxia, and other examples of selective cortical involvement.

Tabo-paretic Type

As one would expect from the name, this type presents features of both tabes and G.P.I. The absent tendon reflexes, sensory involvement, root pains, ataxic gait and classical C.S.F. changes (see above) in the presence of a clinical picture of G.P.I. should establish the diagnosis.

Juvenile G.P.I.

Clouston (1877) is given the credit of first describing this condition in an adolescent aged 16 years. It is a very rare form of the disease and even among congenital syphilitics, it does not account for more than 1 per cent of the total. The infection is transmitted to the child via the placenta and the incubation period before the diease is manifest corresponds to that of the adult, namely 5–20 years. A number become feeble-minded in childhood, but some can go on to adolescence before the disease makes any impact. One such patient served in the army as a gunner in North Africa during the Second World War before the disease impaired his efficiency. The clinical picture is generally one of simple dementia and the usual pupillary and C.S.F. changes are present. Expansive and grandiose types are rarely described. The development of the Maternity and Child Welfare Services with the wide recognition of congenital syphilis and the efficient methods of treating the affected mother have made juvenile G.P.I. a very rare phenomenon indeed.

Present-day Features of Neurosyphilis

Dewhurst (1969) tried to determine the incidence of neurosyphilitic psychotic illness of sufficient severity to be admitted to a mental hospital and whether penicillin given for intercurrent illnesses may have changed the clinical features of the condition. The records of patients with a neurosyphilitic diagnosis admitted to six mental hospitals between 1950 and 1965 totalled 91, 62 of whom were male. Although these patients do not reflect the true incidence of the disorder in the community, the numbers are substantial, indicating that it is still a material problem. When classified according to type of neurosyphilis and presenting neurological signs, the following facts emerged:

Type	Number of cases
Simple depressed	25
Simple dementing	19
Taboparesis	16
Grandiose	10
Manic	5
Senile	6
Protracted	4
Others	6

Signs	Percentage of cases
Reflex abnormalities	51·6
Slurred speech	24·1
Tremors	21·9
Ataxic	19·7
Diminished or deficient pain sensation	12·0
Alteration in muscle tone	4·3
Hemiplegia	1·0
Epileptic attacks	18·7
Pupillary abnormalities	58·2

DIAGNOSIS

Decline in incidence carries its dangers in that one tends not to think of G.P.I., and while previously routine Wassermann tests were commonly practised, they are now frequently overlooked and Hughes (1959) described 10 cases which were referred undiagnosed to a neurosurgeon. Steel (1960) found that in the 18 months from April 1957 to September 1958, 18 cases of G.P.I. were admitted to an observation ward of a general hospital, and of these, 12 had not had previous treatment. He emphasizes that clinical examination without serological tests was insufficient to exclude syphilis and makes a plea for routine W.R. and Khan tests. Hahn *et al.* (1959) reported on 1086 cases collected from eight hospitals and found the condition to be three times as common in men as in women, with incubation periods of 10–24 years after infection, the outside limits being two to more than 30 years. The simple dementing type of psychosis was much more prevalent than the euphoric, grandiose and expansive or depressive types and the blood W.R. was positive in 92 per cent of the 327 previously untreated cases, but was positive in 100 per cent in the C.S.F. There was no correlation between the initial C.S.F. cell count or protein content and the degree of deterioration as assessed clinically.

The T.P.I. Test

Nelson and Mayer (1949) introduced the Treponemal immobilization test (T.P.I.), in which a living strain of virulent *T. pallidum* is used as antigen, thus providing for the first time a sensitive and specific index of treponemal disease, but it does not distinguish between the individual treponematoses. It is primarily used to verify the presence of treponema infection in patients whose sera have given positive reactions such as the W.R. but where there is not clinical evidence of treponemal infection. Not only will it exclude syphilitic infection but it can direct the diagnostic trail towards other diseases which are associated with 'biological false positive' (B.F.P.) reactions. Catterall (1961) found that in 36 women with B.F.P. and negative T.P.I., only eight showed no clinical or laboratory evidence of disease other than the B.F.P. reaction. In those in whom there was evidence of disease, it was generally serious, such as disseminated lupus erythematosus, rheumatoid arthritis or Raynaud's phenomenon.

Differential diagnosis is from other organic causes of dementia, most of which have their own specific diagnostic criteria. As has already been stated, the serological tests are the final court of appeal, but there is a good case for making them the first court, and erroneous diagnoses such as Alzheimer's disease, Pick's disease, alcoholic dementia, cerebral tumour and the like would not be entertained.

TREATMENT

The development of successful treatment for G.P.I. is one of the romances of psychiatry and it is justifiable to go back a little in time and describe its early history. Febrile episodes had for long been known to influence the course of mental illness and as early as 1887 Wagner-Jauregg had suggested that this phenomenon may be used deliberately in treatment. The agent was not yet available, but in 1890 Koch had produced tuberculin and shortly afterwards Wagner-Jauregg experimented with it and noticed improvement with the general paralytics whom he later treated with typhoid vaccines.

A soldier during the First World War, who was suffering from malaria, was by mistake admitted to Wagner-Jauregg's clinic in Vienna and he took advantage of this error by inoculating on 14th June 1917 three general paralytics with malarial blood. The results were dramatic and though initial response by the medical profession was sceptical, 10 years later Wagner-Jauregg was awarded the Nobel prize. In 1926 a malarial research centre was established at Horton, Surrey, and malaria-infected mosquitoes, as well as malarial blood, were made available for use in hospitals all over England.

Though the advent of penicillin has revolutionized the treatment of syphilis, the undoubted value of malaria therapy still ensures it a place. Many clinics have passed over to penicillin exclusively, but a combination of both gives the best guarantee of success. Furthermore some patients are sensitive to penicillin, or the risk of a Herxheimer reaction may be too great and then malaria therapy alone would provide the only possible effective treatment. For this reason, the technique should not yet be relegated to old editions.

1. *Mosquito.* Four or five mosquitoes are obtained from the centre where they have already been infected with *Plasmodium vivax.* They usually arrive in a glass jar with the top covered with mosquito netting and this is placed next to the patient's skin so that the mosquitoes can bite him through the netting. The skin has been previously cleaned but there should be no antiseptic or spirit on the skin as this may interfere with the 'take'. After the bite, the skin is covered to prevent scratching. The interscapular area is usually

selected as this makes scratching less likely. Though the incubation period is 9–14 days, the patient should be placed on a four-hourly temperature chart, for there are not uncommonly mild pyrexial episodes following the inoculation and it is useful to see them contrasted with the major swings of fever which are the first indication of a 'take'. Initially the swings are irregular but they later stabilize to give the characteristic intermittent fever of quotidian malaria. Thereafter careful recording and nursing are essential and the temperature is noted not only in its degree but in its duration. The time of the first rise is noted, and the following day the patient is placed on a half-hourly temperature chart from half an hour before the time of the first rise. This procedure is continued daily and while the temperature is raised it is recorded every 20 minutes. Although the daily paroxysm of fever is usually accompanied by a rigor, this cannot be relied upon and the main check is a well-recorded temperature chart.

A single dose of sodium bismuth thioglycolate (0·2 g.) by deep intramuscular injection on the fourth day from the onset of the regular rigors will interrupt the fever for 48 hours but thereafter the fever returns every other day. If the injection is given earlier there is a risk that the tertian attacks may revert to quotidian before the requisite number of rigors have been achieved. Sargant and Slater (1954) on whose book this description of the treatment is largely based, emphasize the advantage of the sodium bismuth thioglycolate method of interrupting pyrexia '. . . it interrupts the pyrexia immediately, whereas after the administration of quinine, the next rigor that is due usually still takes place before the fever is aborted'.

Blood films should be examined for parasites on the fourth day of pyrexia, even if this is not high, and repeated daily. Increasing numbers of parasites may indicate a lowering of the patient's resistance. Sargant and Slater state:

> If there is on an average more than one parasite in a thin film for every field of view with a $\frac{1}{12}$ -inch oil-immersion objective and No. 2 eyepiece, the fever should be temporarily aborted.
>
> The aim of the treatment is to give the patient 10 to 12 peaks of fever at 103° (F.) or over (taken by mouth). The patient is nursed between blankets (and from May to September behind mosquito netting).

The general nursing management is that for the acutely febrile patient with particular emphasis on warm even temperature, fluid and electrolyte replacement and dry bathing to mop up the perspiration. Should the temperature rise above 105° F. (40·5°C.) it should be immediately reduced by tepid sponging.

There are a number of indications for termination of the pyrexia and these are conveniently listed by Strecker and Ebaugh (1940):

1. Continued hyperpyrexia refractory to sponging.
2. Shock, extreme exhaustion between chills, foreshadowed as a rule by restlessness and insomnia, rapidly falling blood pressure.
3. Convulsive seizures especially when generalized.
4. Tabetic crises and lightning pains.
5. Rising urea nitrogen in the blood.
6. Haemorrhage from mucous membranes or in the skin (purpura).
7. Jaundice, not to be confused with icterus of anaemia.
8. Cellulitis developing about abrasions or bedsores.
9. Bronchopneumonia.
10. Acute splenitis, a large firm and tender spleen.
11. Cardiac decompensation, characterized by thready pulse and cyanosis.
12. Severe anaemia–haemoglobin below 40 per cent, R.B.C. below 2 million; marked leucopenia.
13. Sudden overwhelming increase in parasites in blood.
14. Stupor between chills.

All this adds up to one important instruction: 'If things arc not going well, for whatever reason, interrupt the pyrexia'. The treatment is an exhausting one even for fit subjects and fatalities do occur. Interruption should preferably be temporary if the patient has not yet had 10 full pyrexias and sodium bismuth thioglycolate is best for this purpose as it will give two days' respite. One dose of quinine sulphate (0·3 g.) will interrupt after one further pyrexia but it will reassert itself in 10–20 days. During this time some of the reasons for termination can be corrected and it has been found that patients are thereafter less susceptible while the fever becomes tertian instead of quotidian. Full interruption is achieved by 15 daily doses of quinine sulphate (0·3 g.) by mouth.

2. *Malarial Blood.* This can be transferred from one patient who is having malarial therapy to another, and in units where a number of these patients are collected, this is feasible. Generally there is only one patient in need of treatment and in that case the blood is obtained from the Malarial Centre which in England is at Horton Hospital, near Epsom, Surrey. A message is received stating the train on which the blood is arriving and a messenger is sent from the hospital to meet it; the patient is meanwhile being prepared for the injection. The blood is delivered at even temperature in a 'Thermos' flask and 2·5 ml. are injected intramuscularly between the scapulae, the same precautions for skin being taken as for the mosquito bite; the syringe should be dry-sterilized and free of spirit or other antiseptic. The incubation period is from 9 to 16 days and full interruption in this case will require 0·3 g. of quinine for seven days.

Because of the introduction of blood which is a foreign protein, some patients may show early pyrexia, but this can readily be distinguished from the major one produced by the malarial parasite.

3. *Penicillin.* This has very largely superseded malaria in therapy and many recommend it as the sole treatment. Hahn *et al.* (1959) found that with early diagnosis and prompt administration of penicillin, clinical improvement and ability to work occurred in more than 80 per cent of patients and that deaths from neurosyphilis were very rare. Even in the severe cases in mental hospitals, 30 per cent could be improved and returned to work, though complete recovery is not common, there being residual impairment of judgment and speech. A course of 6 million units in repository form was as effective as the aqueous solution and further courses were required only if there was deterioration after initial improvement, or if the C.S.F. cell count was greater than 5 per cu. mm. after the first post-treatment year. Though the Herxheimer reaction has been considered by some to be part of the mythology of antisyphilitic treatment, it is worth noting that these authors found a febrile form of this reaction in 14·9 per cent of 629 patients treated with penicillin alone and in 5·8 per cent there was a 'clinical' Herxheimer with exacerbation of the psychosis or epileptic attacks. One patient died from the Herxheimer, but in the others there was no evidence of permanent damage, and these reactions were more common in patients with a high C.S.F. cell count. Such a cell count is said to carry a more favourable prognosis, while a low count indicates a more static process which is less likely to respond to treatment, though also less likely to deteriorate. 'Clinical' Herxheimer reactions were much less frequent in patients who had their penicillin combined with fever therapy, so there would still appear to be some place for malaria therapy, if only to reduce the incidence and danger of Herxheimer reactions.

In Dewhurst's (1969) series patients who received ECT did less well than those who did not as did those who received only penicillin as against those who had penicillin and malaria.

Grandiose delusions were less common and the author attributes this to the relative disappearance of the higher social groups with the disease. This could be due to this group being more effectively treated in the early stages and not having to enter mental hospitals, though there is no conclusive evidence that these delusions are commoner in these groups. Prognosis even in this pre-selected sample was encouraging in that nearly half were discharged after treatment.

4. *Kettering Hypertherm.* This is an apparatus which consists of a series of radiant lamps in a container and which envelops the patient.

It was used in centres where there used to be a reasonable number of patients with G.P.I. such as a combined military psychiatric and venereal diseases unit and was soon nicknamed the 'Hot Box'. It required the most skilled medical and nursing supervision, for the temperature was kept raised for considerable periods. It is probably now rarely used.

5. *Social Therapy.* This may be necessary at all stages of the disease, but particularly when the condition is first diagnosed and the spouse and other members of the family have to be interviewed and have serological tests. The patient may react in a calamitous way because of the social stigma, and at the likelihood of disruption in his or her marital relations. Some would suggest psychiatric help at this stage, but more preferable would be intelligent handling by the family doctor, who with his knowledge of patient and family possesses the key to the understanding of the situation, which the psychiatrist does not possess. Furthermore, this calling-in of the psychiatrist for what is essentially a general practitioner problem, indicates a lack of appreciation of the role of the family doctor and the role of the psychiatrist, who in these matters should be a second line of defence called in to support the family doctor, should the patient's reaction or that of his family betray psychopathological factors which he feels beyond his scope.

Prognosis

Untreated G.P.I. is said to be fatal within five years of the onset of symptoms and as has been said, while penicillin can arrest the infection or prolong life in most cases, it may not restore function completely.

Penicillin has however the advantage of eliminating the risk of pyrexial therapy but we do not yet know the risk of depriving the patient of malarial therapy and one could argue that a treatment which could reverse the cerebral pathology without the help of penicillin may with advantage be combined with penicillin which is more likely to attack the infection alone.

Contra-indicated Treatment

References are sometimes made to the use of electroplexy in some of the chronic psychotic forms of the disease and while this may be given in some cases with impunity, the author has seen severe reactions, two with hemiplegia and one with dysarthria following such treatment. The dysarthric patient was a paranoid sergeant-major, who clinically would fit into the group regarded by some as suitable for E.C.T.

Meningo-vascular Neurosyphilis

This differs from the parenchymatous form in that it affects the meninges and vessels. The psychotic features associated with this condition are dependent on focal lesions which may result in confusion and delirium with occasionally disorientation and in many ways do not differ from those associated with stroke, and for a detailed description of the clinical features a textbook of medicine should be consulted.

Other Infections

Every infection of the brain or meninges can produce an acute or chronic organic reaction. The commoner ones are encephalitis, meningitis, brain abscess, malaria, sleeping sickness, and psittacosis.

Encephalitis. Apart from mental deficiency, behavioural disturbances and apparent functional psychiatric illness can be associated with encephalitis. Durton and Milner (1970) reported 7 cases, one of whom was a pathological liar and psychopath; another started with mutism and later developed waxy flexibility, while a third was a Nigerian cook whose reaction was predominantly a cultural one. The authors pointed out that in 6 patients the CSF was, on at least one occasion, normal. Himmelhoch *et al.* (1970) found 8 patients from over 100 cases with sub-acute encephalitis, who had behavioural disturbances.

The most characteristic pattern while the patient was in hospital was a rapid fluctuation in mental state, a clouded sensorium with disorientation on one day and complete lucidity on the next. Periods of assaultiveness and aggression with sexual provocation were followed by periods when the patient apologized profusely for his bad behaviour and reached out pathetically for the human contact recently rejected. Frequently hallucinations and clear-cut paranoid delusions were manifest. Agitated episodes occurred and these had a driven quality when the patient would get up, sit down, wander and display aggressive feelings usually when confronted with some difficult or abstract task or complicated social demand. Bizarre behaviour, at first transient, became increasingly persistent, lasting for 9 to 10 weeks in spite of treatment.

Seven of the 8 patients had originally been misdiagnosed as functional disorders because their behaviour had induced physicians to overlook the neurological findings. As 3 of the patients spontaneously regained normal intellectual function, the authors speculated that some patients treated for behaviour disorders may really be suffering from undiagnosed, mild forms of subacute encephalitis. This is possible but it must be rare.

PSYCHOSES ASSOCIATED WITH CEREBRAL VASCULAR DISEASE

There are a variety of diseases belonging to this group which are associated with psychiatric symptoms. While some have distinctive features, a number overlap in their symptomatology, and differentiation is frequently based on evidence other than psychiatric. Many patients with these diseases are however traditionally cared for in mental institutions, or the psychiatrist may be called out to see them either for consultation or to arrange disposal, so the group has a particular claim on the psychiatrist's attention and he should be familiar with its clinical constituents.

CEREBRAL ARTERIOSCLEROSIS

Though by far the commonest member of the group, the diagnosis of cerebral arteriosclerosis may be made more frequently than is warranted and a number of other conditions are doubtless embraced by this label. As the other conditions are relatively less common these errors in diagnosis do not materially affect estimates of incidence of cerebral arteriosclerosis, but they would of course affect such estimates of the other diseases. Cerebral arteriosclerosis has a wide age distribution and though some would classify it under the diseases of old age, a number (approximately 3 per cent) occur between the ages of 30 and 49 years, but by far the greatest number occur after the age of 55, the peak decade being between 70 and 80 years. At this older age, the clinical picture is of course adulterated with that of senility and it is very difficult indeed then to decide which symptoms are directly due to the vascular disease. Hughes *et al.* (1954), in a review of chronic cerebral hypertensive disease with personality changes and emotional lability, state:

> Although most of the established cases occurred among old people, a sufficient number occurred in middle age, or had a history going back to the third or fourth decade, to suggest that the level of the blood pressure rather than the chronological age was the deciding factor in the production of lesions.

Some have tried to draw a distinction between patients whose arteriosclerosis is based on chronic hypotension and where the disease is the result of advancing years, but in symptomatology they are one disease, though it may be argued there are essential differences in the pre-morbid personality.

Incidence

As far as the psychiatrist is concerned, figures on this aspect are largely based on mental hospital first admissions and Malzberg (1956) reckoned that 21·1 per cent of first admissions were suffering from cerebral vascular disease.

Aetiology

This is complex and different authors stress different aspects. Some see the condition as an extension of hypertension, while others regard it as caused by dietetic factors leading to high levels of cholesterol in the blood with consequent deposition of atheromatous plaques in the vessel walls. Hypertension, which as previously stated is a precursor of arteriosclerosis, is itself hotly disputed as regards causation, so in arteriosclerosis we have considerable speculation over the cause of the end-result. Katz and Stamler (1953) regard cholesterol as primarily involved and that lipids filter out of the blood plasma through the intima of the artery wall. Cholesterolaemia in itself is not the causative factor, for atherosclerosis can occur in its absence, and the amount of phospholipids also has a bearing. The higher level of phospholipids in relation to the cholesterol the less

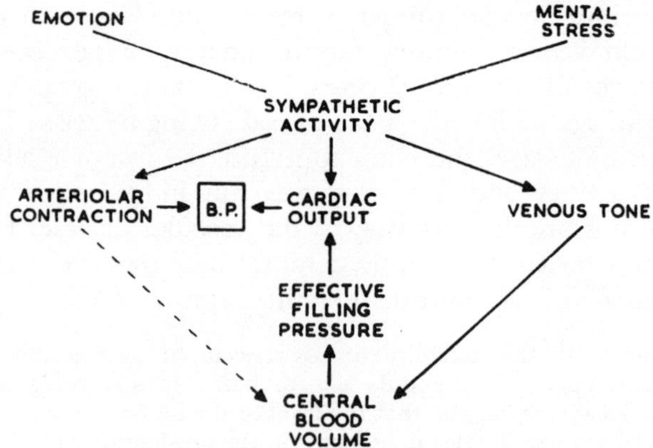

Figure 3 Neural regulation of arterial pressure.
[McMichael, J. (1961). *British Medical Journal,* ii, 1239.]

likelihood there is of atherosclerosis. Certain lipoproteins have a bearing on the presence of the atheromatous plaques and β-lipoprotein which binds with cholesterol is regarded as an important feature in determining the incidence of atherosclerosis. These findings have naturally given rise to considerable interest in preventive diets in order to reduce the levels of cholesterol and β-lipoproteins, but there are exogenous factors which may, irrespective of diet, contribute to high levels. These are diabetes mellitus, hypothyroidism, pyridoxine deficiency and excess of vitamin D as well as situations which precipitate out the cholesterol from the blood stream.

Hypertension, because it is closely associated with arteriosclerosis, is regarded as having aetiological significance. The causes of hypertension already defined are varied yet those of 'essential hypertension' which still account for the largest constituent group have not yet been defined. McMichael (1961) in his Croonian Lectures reviews the aetiological factors in hypertension, emphasizing the effect of the autonomic nervous system and the marked influence of emotion and quotes an instance where in a clinic engaged in research in hypertension the medical staff do not use sphygmomanometers in their out-patient rooms, the pressures being recorded under relaxed conditions 'by pleasant girl technicians who are considered to generate less emotion than a familiar and comforting doctor'. Cardiac output markedly influences blood pressure and McMichael states that '. . . Emotion is one of the most potent of all the influences increasing the cardiac output' and explains the effect of amylobarbitone on a hypertensive subject as being due entirely to its effect of depressing the cardiac output, the peripheral resistance remaining unchanged. He concludes thus: '. . . Hypertension is no more a disease entity than a skin rash, a fever, or an anaemia'. Even 'essential' hypertension which is becoming malignant 'may thus involve some unknown primary humoral disturbance complicated by well-marked neurogenic influences in the early stages, later involving renal factors, aldosterone secretion, electrolyte disturbances, and severe vascular exudative lesions'. Figure 3 illustrates the complexity of the problem. In addition to the causes displayed in Figure 3 there are consitutional and hereditary factors which though not accurately defined have been repeatedly noted.

Pathology

A systematic account must take note of the different arteries in the brain, which can fortunately be grouped under two headings, the large vessels and the small vessels.

Large Vessels. The atherosclerosis in these vessels consists of yellowish patches on the internal surface of the artery, though they are also visible from the external surface due to the relatively thin walls of the cerebral blood vessels. The vessels lose their elasticity and are irregular and nodular with narrowing of the lumen due to projection of deposits under the intima. The constituents of these plaques are a mixture of connective tissue, fatty substances, thickened endothelial lining and thickened internal elastic membrane. As previously stated the lipids in these deposits in the intima are predominantly lipoproteins and also contain cholesterol, and there is frequently fatty degeneration and thickening of the vessel wall with splitting of the elastic membrane and marked reduction of the lumen.

Small Vessels

(a) Diffuse hyperplasia with thickening of the media and later hyaline degeneration of the entire vessel wall with the 'onion-skin' appearance due to concentric layering of the internal cells.

(*b*) Hypertrophy of the muscle of the media with increased collagen deposit. The intima is not thickened.

(*c*) Hyalinization of the intima with deposition of hyaline material in the subintimal layer with progression to complete obliteration of the lumen, and the internal elastic lamina is frequently split and fragmented but may also be reduplicated. This type is seen more frequently in cases with a history of progressive and malignant hypertension.

(*d*) Obliterative cerebral arteriosclerosis is found in the older age group and the intima is mainly affected with proliferation of the sub-endothelial cells and an absence of hyaline and other degeneration.

Wertham and Wertham (1934) favour the classification of Neuburger (1930), who distinguished two forms of cerebral arteriosclerosis, a *hypertonic* and a *senile*, which he linked to two constitutional types. The hypertonic were pyknic in build and developed their arteriosclerosis in the sixth decade. Vascular changes in the kidneys were frequent and invariably there was very extensive hyaline degeneration of the small intracerebral vessels with frequent apoplectic haemorrhages. There was also paling of the cells in the Sommer sector of the *cornu Ammonis* and diffuse changes in the inferior olives. The senile type can be distinguished clinically from the hypertonic type although the pathological changes may not be so marked. Hyaline degeneration of small vessels is less frequent, apoplectic haemorrhages are rare but arteriocapillary fibrosis is common.

The gross pathology will depend on the vessel or vessels affected and whether the lesions are acute or chronic.

The effort by Neuburger and the Werthams to correlate pathological findings with clinical features has been further elaborated by Eros (1951). He found that focal neurological lesions were common in the hyperplastic variety rather than the hypoplastic, while the latter had a higher incidence of mental symptoms and he claimed that some appreciation of the type of arteriosclerosis could be gauged by the early clinical presentation.

Rothschild (1941) has adopted an even more dynamic interpretation, claiming that the severity of symptoms depends on the degree of integration and pre-morbid structure of the personality and that inadequate people of limited capacity had a low tolerance to even small lesions. This is in step with Goldstein's theory of brain function and its reaction to deficit (p. 107).

Symptomatology

As the lesions may be small or large, single or multiple, in areas which are more or less vulnerable and which have their own characteristics either mental or physical, and where arteriosclerosis may exist without causing symptoms, the clinical features of the disease can be most diverse and the diagnosis very difficult. As a general rule, an organic psychosis occurring after the age of 50 years with negative serology and in the absence of other diseases associated with cerebral involvement, should be regarded as cerebral arteriosclerosis, especially if there is other evidence of this condition.

Prodromal symptoms are easy fatiguability, headaches, giddiness, discomfort in the head and neck, inability to concentrate, drowsiness, character changes and intolerance for alcohol. Neurological features such as temporary loss of power in the extremities, paresthesiae, transitory aphasia, pupillary inequalities and spastic gait, may also be prodromal and especially if transitory, may be attributed to spasm of the cerebral arteries, though this phenomenon is still not generally accepted. The presence of supporting evidence such as hypertension, retinal changes of an arteriopathic nature, cardiac (left ventricular) hypertrophy and renal disease will help to establish the diagnosis. A common feature is a confusional episode which may give way to excitement and restlessness indicating cerebral irritation, which is not usually static but can fluctuate with apparently full remission. Frankly psychotic features may present with paranoid ideas, usually of a persecutory nature and auditory hallucinations, the patient changing rapidly from a rational being to one who is mentally disturbed and impervious to reasoning. Those familiar with the patient notice a gradual or sudden falling off in performance which is mainly due to failure to comprehend.

Mental Symptoms

1. *Memory defect* is variable, but initially is usually limited to forgetting of names, places and recent events. A fluctuating course is the rule and there may be surprising episodes of lucidity. Deterioration is usually associated with fresh episodes of what are probably vascular occlusion.

2. *Personality changes* are again varied but certain features are more common. These include a tendency to eccentricity and a deterioration in personal care, with lack of appreciation of one's surroundings and the ordinary proprieties of social conduct. They may result in sexual aberrations such as indecent exposure, which may be in response to provocative suggestions by little girls in the park, and not due to some compulsion but to a failure to comprehend the real situation. Paranoid features are regarded as an uncovering of the individual's pre-morbid personality.

3. *Emotional responses* are labile, but not incongruous. The patient may be easily moved to tears or laughter, but only by situations which would normally evoke a similar response. The term 'emotional incontinence' has been used to describe this change. He is aware of his defects and reacts appropriately, being frequently very distressed by his handicap and occasionally attempting suicide. In fact, a number in the early stages, when dementia is not readily recognized, may be diagnosed as uncomplicated melancholic states and be subjected to a course of E.C.T. which may in certain cases produce a remission of the depressive features, though it is more likely to aggravate the arteriosclerotic changes. The mood may be closely linked with the thought content and in paranoid reactons the patient may be very suspicious, hostile or overtly aggressive and occasionally homicidal.

Course and Prognosis

In a disease whose progress depends on arteriopathy of large and small vessels and supplying parts of the brain which differ in vulnerability, it would be a bold person who would hazard a prognosis. The general physical state must be considered and if the hypertension is severe with retinal and cardiac changes, the prognosis will be poor, but occasionally it can be extremely difficult to say. Rothschild (1956) gave the average duration of stay in these patients in a mental hospital as 3·47 years and when one realizes that a very large number of the older group do not survive the first six months, it sets the extreme limit rather high. Beckenstein and Gold (1945) found that out of 100 consecutive admissions, 42 were dead in three months.

The course of the deterioration may be varied in nature as well as in time and patients may become childish and quarrelsome, elated, hypochondriacal, deluded and hallucinated, but the steady march of a failure in comprehension is common to all and they frequently distress their families by failing to recognize them or by misidentifying, *e.g.* daughter for a wife. This disorientation may be reinforced by hallucinatory experiences, the patient insisting that a close relative is in the ward and he may disturb the other patients in his search for the source of the auditory hallucination. Death may occur from a cerebral catastrophe, but cardiac, pulmonary and renal complications take their toll.

Treatment

There are no specific cures or measures which can materially retard the progress of the disease. A number of treatments have been tried, some of which are based on theoretical views or experimental evidence of the pathogenesis. The one in current vogue is based on dietary regimes for general atherosclerosis, ranging from one which is poor in cholesterol to one which is cholesterol-free. Other measures which lower the blood cholesterol have also been advocated such as thyroid extract and combinations of oestrogens and androgens. It is, however, one thing to show that these agents may depress blood cholesterol and another to assume that the patient with cerebral arteriosclerosis is suffering from these deficiencies and will benefit from their administration. A more old-fashioned controversy is the place of iodides, and intravenous injections of 1·0 g. of sodium iodide three times per week have been recommended. In a condition which is liable to fluctuation with occasionally periods of complete lucidity occurring spontaneously, it is difficult to decide whether these treatments help. Nicotinic acid and lipotropic enzymes as well as vasodilators have also been recommended but there is no conclusive evidence that they are of any value whatsoever. The current obsession of trying to lower the cholesterol level of the blood is in itself open to criticism, for except in grossly high readings, the level is variable and fluctuates in many subjects and has no clinical significance. This is another instance where the laboratory reading may be given greater credence by the psychiatrist than by the Laboratory worker.

There are some positive and rational measures, however, which can help. Many of these patients, through dietary indiscretions, are vitamin depleted and replacement may remove the pellagra-like dementia which occasionally adulterates the clinical picture. Restlessness can be effectively controlled with sedatives like sodium bromide 1·0 g. and chloral hydrate 1·0 g., while tranquillizers such as chlorpromazine can deal with the acute hallucinatory episodes. Dosage will depend on the severity of the disturbance, but 100 mg. t.d.s. may be necessary in very severe cases. Prolonged administration of bromides could lead to bromism which may be difficult to recognize in the presence of cerebral arteriosclerosis. A check on serum bromide levels is therefore necessary.

DYSMNESIC SYNDROME WITH ANTERIOR COMMUNICATING ARTERY ANEURYSM

Talland *et al.* (1967) reported two patients who had been successfully operated on for rupture of an aneurysm of the anterior communicating artery and who later presented with a Korsakoff's (dysmnesic) syndrome. The striking aspect of these two patients was that they were operated on within two days of each other and shared the same room where for weeks they hilariously exchanged the most fantastic and inconsequential nonsense, trading tales neither true nor probable. Immediate recall was reasonable but any task requiring memory after an interruption seemed nearly impossible.

The author has had five patients who were operated on for aneurysm in the same region and while the initial disability was gross it gradually receded and only one has material residual defect. Another after eight years still has a testable dysmnesic syndrome but is functioning adequately in that she does her shopping and runs her home. The last such patient was seen five years ago and as operative treatment is no less popular one must assume that surgical technique has improved.

Anterior Cerebral Aneurysm

The developments of neurosurgery have improved the expectation of life following rupture of cerebral aneurysms and in a follow-up of 79 survivors at intervals of 6 months to 8½ years after the haemorrhage, Logue *et al.* (1968) found that 52 were neurologically unimpaired, and 44 had returned to their previous work level. Of the 79 survivors, 66 were treated by proximal occlusion of the anterior cerebral artery which was mainly responsible for feeding the aneurysm. The authors were concerned with the quality of survival and a principal component analysis extracted from independent components: (a) intellectual impairment; (b) elation/depression; (c) affective release or flattening; and (d) language impairment.

In 9 instances both patient and informant agreed that there had been a personality change for the better, which resembled that seen after a favourable leucotomy, although there was also mild memory impairment. As a number of these haemorrhages may have been precipitated by the prescribing of monoamine oxidase inhibitors for depression, the accidental leucotomy has an added significance, though still not to be recommended.

When the obstruction to the cerebral circulation is due to atheroma in an accessible vessel, surgical intervention can be very successful and such patients should be referred for neurological investigation. Should the stenosis be demonstrated by arteriography, thromboendarterectomy, and occasionally resection and graft replacement may be successful, especially if the common carotid is involved.

As the progressive dementia is a major factor in both the behaviour disturbances and the patient's personal handicap, it would be helpful to create an atmosphere which makes as few demands as possible. There should be a scrupulous preservation of the location of articles of furniture and clothing. Those experiences which are most recently acquired are most readily forgotten, so it is important to see that the patient is not exposed to new learning and frequent changes, for not only will he be incapable of assimilating them, but the catastrophic reaction ((p. 109) may be readily provoked with consequent deterioration in performance and the precipitation of acute behavioural changes. This has practical importance in advising the family, for they frequently suggest that they share the problem of the sick parent by taking him or her for specified periods of the year. Such a commendable sense of responsibility should not be discouraged but the difficulties of this proposed arrangement explained and the alternative of one member of the family being responsible for the domicile, but supported by the others, if suggested, is frequently accepted. Similarly, when the family is unable to cope and disposal is considered it should be of a permanent nature and any temporary, though immediately more attractive alternative, should not be advised.

SENILE PSYCHOSES

It is not strictly correct to include all senile psychoses in a chapter on Organic Psychiatry. This point is emphasized by Macmillan (1960) who considers that the majority of senile psychoses are functional. Nevertheless a number are either organically determined or have an organic component but it is still not possible to appreciate their nature without a knowledge of the psychological process of ageing.

The Psychology of Ageing

Much has been written, many tests have been devised and though no clear picture has emerged, some features commonly appear in a material sample. Welford (1962) summarizes the changes in performance with age thus:

1. *Slowing of Sensorimotor Activities.* This occurs over a wide range of tasks though it can vary to the extent that some who are 60 or 70 years old perform as fast as the average man in his 20s.
2. *Impairment of Short-term Memory.* This does not usually declare itself with the common tests such as digit span. Welford regards this failure of short-term retention as the key factor limiting certain types of abstraction in older people, particularly the 'manipulation of data in the abstract' which is required by many intelligence tests.
3. *Difficulty in Relating what is Perceived to the Required Action.* This is shown experimentally when old people have greater difficulty in carrying out actions observed in a mirror, the mirror destroying the directness of the relationship between perception and action.

All changes with ageing are not disadvantages. An increased ordering of knowledge with a rise in 'information' scores and improvement in vocabulary are commonly found. Neither does ability to learn decline with age to the extent commonly supposed.

Organic Senile Psychoses

These can depend on the underlying pathology. If this be cerebral the symptomatology is similar to that in the younger age groups; vitamin deficiencies such as nicotinamide produce a pellagra-like state; anoxia produces its periods of confusion as does uraemia, hepatic involvement, drugs, etc.

The Ageing Mind

The impairment of memory sets in motion a chain of events which produces the stereotype of the ageing mind: (1) there is increasing difficulty in recognizing persons and objects; (2) defective orientation for time and place; (3) illusionary states regarding surroundings and even his own person; (4) sudden amnesic crises may develop and the individual may be found wandering about the street with no knowledge of his name or address; (5) dreams are not separated from the waking state and the patient literally lives in a dream world mixing dreams with reality; (6) disturbances in sleep rhythm further confuse the patient's orientation for time; and (7) as a result of these developments, frank delusions and hallucinations supervene but these are in a setting of confusion rather than that of clear consciousness found in the functional states.

Affective Disturbances. These are commonly grafted on to the senile process and should they present early the differential diagnosis between a severe depressive illness and early senile dementia can be very difficult. Depressive delusions are similar to those seen in senile depression, with hypochondriasis, poverty and persecution high on the list. Suspicions of being robbed, which are partly based on impaired memory and partly on the unmasked psychotic process, are also common. These suspicions may become frankly paranoid, the patient accusing his life-long partner or his devoted children of trying to rob and to murder him and frequently embarrassing his family by repeating these allegations to complete strangers.

Behaviour Disturbances. These may either accompany the initial psychotic features or develop later. Aggression and violent behaviour may supervene. Deterioration in habits, with loss of the patient's normal regard for cleanliness and attention to his toilet, may make it impossible for the patient to remain at home. The condition, like dementia paralytica, may on occasions be ushered in with delinquent behaviour such as indecent exposure, pilfering, mouthing obscenities or sexual assaults.

Classification

This does not contribute very much to the understanding of the problem and, to date, is mainly an exercise in descriptive psychiatry but some lay great store on these things. There have been heated discussions on what constitutes presbyophrenia and on its incidence among the whole group of disorders. The condition can be mixed or present differently on different occasions so it is not possible to divide it into the usual groups of (1) simple dementia; (2) delirious and confused; (3) paranoid; (4) depressed and agitated; and (5) presbyophrenia.

Rothschild (1956) offers the following functional classification which is more meaningful:

1. Where the psychosis is an understandable, if not inevitable outgrowth of long-standing personality difficulties.
2. Where the pre-morbid personality was good but the pscyhosis has been triggered by special stresses of an organic or situational nature.
3. Where premorbid personality is good and no special events can be elicited but there is steady deterioration with perhaps surrender to the changing social situation.

Pathology

Brain shrinkage is common but may not be the cause of the dementia, for normal senile brains are also shrunken with widened sulci. Subdural haematomata are not uncommon, and it is as well to bear this in mind when seeing the patient, for some may respond to surgical treatment.

Microscopically, there is a reduction of cortical nerve cells and granulo-vacuolar degeneration. Alzheimer neurofibrillary changes are also seen, but not to the same extent as in Alzheimer's disease, though enough to raise the possibility that there is some relationship. Counting the senile plaques and trying to correlate them with pscyhological deficit is still popular but evidence is only suggestive and there must be other aspects of brain pathology in terms of site and nerve changes which may be equally if not more relevant. Just as there are some types of pre-senile dementia with no Alzheimer changes or senile plaques, there are probably similar forms of senile dementia which would, of course, be excluded in these counts.

Treatment. The established condition has no specific treatment, but general measures of hygiene and community care can do much to alleviate the problem. (See Chapter 14.)

Prognosis

The psychiatrist is frequently asked by the patient's relatives to give some estimate of the patient's expectation of life. Generally, it is greater if he can be looked after at home. Goldfarb (1969) undertook the exercise of predicting mortality in 1100 persons over the age of 64 years who were institutionalized and followed them up for 7 years. After one year, 23 per cent were dead; this became 42 per cent after the second year; 54 per cent after the third; 65 per cent after the fourth; 73 per cent after the fifth; 79 per cent after the sixth; and 82 per cent at the end of the seventh.

These percentages were higher for subjects with: (1) incontinence; (2) psychiatric diagnosis of severe brain syndrome; (3) 9 or 10 errors on the Mental Status Questionnaire which equates with the diagnosis of severe brain syndrome; and (4) severe physical dependency. When any of these indicators is present, mortality is clearly greater than average after the first year and somewhat greater in the 3rd, 4th and 5th years. When any 2 are present, mortality is greater than average for all years and when 3 or 4 are present mortality is much greater than average for the entire period. Conversely, when none of these characteristics is present, mortality is lower than average for all years. Naturally the quality of nursing care and the social milieu are important factors.

PRESENILE DEMENTIA

'Presenile psychosis' has been suggested by Ferarro (1959) as the generic term for cases of presenile dementia

> possessing characteristic clinicopathologic features not related to any definite already-known aetiology. Therefore, all psychoses related to arteriosclerotic, syphilitic, neoplastic, toxic and traumatic conditions, although occurring in the chronological span of the presenium, should be eliminated from this category.

He does not favour the term 'presenile dementia' for those cases as it is too general and has been used for any type of organic dementia occurring in the presenium. It is still arguable whether 'presenile psychosis' should be reserved for cases of unknown aetiology, for many do not exhibit psychotic features till the condition is well-advanced and the earliest manifestation of the disease is usually some form of dementia. It therefore gives accent to a feature which may be a late by-product of dementia and divorces the group from the phenomenological study of the pre-senile dementias to which it rightly belongs. It also tends to relegate them to the limbo of the undefined instead of, by associating them with the already defined, stimulating investigators to rescue them from their unknown aetiology. A more rational approach would be to regard them to date as the *idiopathic presenile dementias,* in the hope that in the future they will join the others when the pathological processes have been clarified.

The limits of the presenium have been arbitrarily set between the ages of 45 and 65 years but the general definition of a presenile dementia is a state of intellectual and/or emotional impairment due to organic cerebral change occurring before the age of 65 years. A large variety of disorders are responsible and include space-occupying lesions, cerebrovascular diseases, trauma, infections, poisons of internal origin such as liver and kidney disease, poisons of external origin, such as alcohol, barbiturates and carbon monoxide, vitamin deficiencies, such as nicotinic acid, endocrine deficiencies such as thyroid, and degenerative disorders like Huntington's chorea. These will be described under their various headings and the following descriptions apply to the idiopathic presenile dementias of Alzheimer and Pick, or Alzheimer's disease (A.D.) and Pick's disease (P.D.) as they are called.

ALZHEIMER'S DISEASE

Alzheimer's disease (A.D.) was originally described by Alzheimer (1907), in a woman of 51 years, who, in addition to having delusions of persecution and jealousy, had marked memory loss and apraxia to such a degree that she was unable to find her way about her own home. She was perplexed, disorientated for time and place and had phases of delirium with marked impairment of speech and comprehension. She died four and a half years later and the classical histopathology was described.

Histopathology

There is atrophy of cortical nerve cells and within the cortex are argentiphile plaques which are demonstrable by the silver impregnation techniques of Bielschowsky or von Braunmühl. These plaques, which are also seen in senile dementia, though not nearly to the same extent, have a mixed granular and fibrillary structure. The same silver methods also show some irregular thickening and disorientation of the nerve cell fibrils, which form 'tangles' and 'loops'. In recent years, cortical biopsy has been used for diagnostic purposes and the histopathology of this material has been described by Sim and Smith (1955).

> The cortex showed focal loss of neurones, marginal gliosis and an increase in intraneuronal lipofuscin pigment ('pigment atrophy'). With silver impregnation abundant senile plaques and neurofibrillary alterations were seen. The plaques

had the classical structure described by Critchley (1929), and although present throughout the cortex were more numerous in the outer layers. The white matter showed axonal degeneration, hyperplasia of astrocytes and mucoid degeneration of oligodendroglia. No definite relation of plaques to blood vessels could be seen.

Coarsely granular clumps of material staining positively by the periodic acid-Schiff technique (PAS) were seen at the site of the argentophil plaques. This granular PAS-positive material was amylase fast and was superimposed on a diffuse, PAS positive 'background', which corresponded approximately with the size of the plaques seen with silver impregnation. The 'background' was more strongly positive than the faint PAS reaction given by the cortical ground substance. A positive reaction at the site of the plaques was also given by the periodic acid-silver method for neurones (Dixon, 1953): this method, like PAS, also stained the intraneuronal lipofuscin pigment. Substances staining positively with the Alcian-blue stain for mucin, sudan IV (frozen sections) and sudan-black (frozen and paraffin sections) for lipids and the methyl violet reaction for amyloid were less consistently demonstrable. Metachromasia with toluidine blue was also seen at the site of the plaques. Granules of PAS-positive material were noted in glial cells, both in the cortex and white matter.

Hiroisi and Lee (1936) found 'mucin' and Divry (1927) found 'amyloid', and these findings were confirmed by Sim and Smith (1955). They suggested that the positive PAS and periodic acid-silver reactions indicated the presence of a carbohydrate containing material which appears to be in excess of that shown by mucin and amyloid stains. They added that:

Certain non-carbohydrate containing lipid substances, *e.g.* phospholipids, are also said to give a positive PAS reaction and may be present in the plaques. The presence of lipid substances is suggested by our findings that the PAS and periodic acid-silver reactions were more strongly positive in frozen sections than on paraffin sections which had been treated with fat solvents . . . The staining properties of part of the PAS-positive material resembled that of the granules of lipofuscin pigment found in cortical neurones (Dixon & Herbertson, 1950, 1951). Dixon (1953) found similar granular material in phagocytic cells infiltrating necrotic cerebral cortex and suggested that these granules originated in part from lipofuscin that had persisted and been phagocytosed after disintegration of neurones. An increase in neuronal lipofuscin has often been noted in A.D., and it may be that part of the PAS-positive material in the plaques originates in the way suggested by Dixon after atrophy of neurones. It also seems possible that the argentophilia shown by the plaques is partly due to the affinity of focal, intra-cortical deposits of chemical substances for metallic silver . . . The periodic acid-silver methods (Dixon, 1953) on frozen sections demonstrates the Alzheimer plaques so clearly that it provides a useful supplementary technique for the rapid diagnosis of A.D.

Corsellis and Brierley (1954) have described histochemical findings in two cases of atypical A.D. in whom they found an abnormal substance, probably a mucopolysaccharide in the plaque cores, blood vessels and as free-lying fragments. The search for the nature of the lesion goes on and electron microscopy has now given a more detailed picture of the structure of the plaques. The intensity of the histopathological response is such that McMenemey (1940) has postulated: 'All cases, at any age, showing an abundance of senile plaques, neurofibrillary changes and cell atrophy, which cannot be regarded as senile dementia, belong to the Alzheimer category'. Green *et al.* (1952) have underlined this: 'Considering the severity and omnipresence of Alzheimer cells and senile plaques in A.D., it is difficult to imagine that they would be entirely absent in even a small piece of tissue such as a biopsy'.

Macroscopically, the brain is atrophied with widening of the sulci mainly in the frontal and parietal regions, though the rest of the cortex may also be involved.

Differential Diagnosis. This has given rise to considerable controversy, especially over the distinction between A.D. and P.D. At the histopathological level some workers have found similar changes in mongolism (Jervis, 1948), post-encephalitic states (Greenfield and Bosanquet, 1953), amaurotic family idiocy, lateral sclerosis and heredo-degenerative spinal spastic paralysis (Miskolczy, 1959).

Neumann and Cohn (1953) in a study of 210 necropsies in a mental hospital found the plaques and neurofibrillary tangles in a large number of patients diagnosed as cerebral arteriosclerosis and senile dementia, while Raskin and Ehrenberg (1956) in a similar study confirmed their findings. Kreindler *et al.* (1959) reported a case with a histological combination of P.D. and A.D. and Worster-Drought *et al.* (1940) described a family with hereditary presenile dementia and spastic paralysis with a histopathology of A.D. In spite of these findings the postulate of McMenemey quoted above is still generally held, for the intensity of the reaction is nowhere as gross as in A.D. and this quantitative factor has been stressed by Rothschild in Raskin and Ehrenberg's (1956) paper.

The clinical differentiation between A.D. and P.D. has also raised difficulties.

Stengel (1948) emphasized the depressed, anxious mood, the overactivity and the high frequency of fits in A.D. as against the facile hilarity, lack of spontaneity, increasing apathy and rarity of fits in P.D. Sjögren *et al.* (1952) were unable to confirm these findings and in fact emphasized the inactivity and lack of spontaneity in A.D. and they suggested that A.D. was most readily distinguished from P.D. by muscle rigidity and gait disturbance of extra-pyramidal type. This problem of differentiation has been further complicated by the claims of Stern and Reed (1945) and Miskolczy (1959) who suggested that P.D. and A.D. were pathologically two parallel processes hereditarily determined, with Miskolczy going further by suggesting that the clinical symptomatology depends on the age of onset, P.D. being the dominant disease and A.D. the recessive. As the diagnosis of A.D. in most of those cases had been made after necropsy, it was likely that the clinical features described would be those of the terminal stages of the disease and this would include Alzheimer's (1907) original description. Grünthal (1926) had, in an analysis of 14 cases, divided the course of the disease into three stages:

1. A stage of gradual loss of memory and disturbance in perception, carelessness in work and appearance, disorientation in space, epileptic attacks with dysphasia and dysarthria.
2. Disorientation for time, place and person, impaired comprehension, nocturnal restlessness, alexia, agraphia and acalculia.
3. Increased irritability with deterioration in habits, paraphasia and stereotypy of movements.

These descriptions though valid for certain cases of A.D. could not in themselves be regarded as sufficiently comprehensive.

Sim and Sussman (1962) investigated 46 cases of presenile dementia from the Department of Psychological Medicine of the United Birmingham Hospitals by EEG and air studies, lumbar puncture and psychometry, while serum electrolytes, liver function tests, blood and C.S.F. Wassermann, blood count and blood urea were routinely carried out. In the earliest stage of the investigation (1951), pneumo-encephalography had proved very upsetting to two patients, one of whom suffered a transient hemiplegia, so ventriculography was substituted. This produced less intracranial distension and discomfort and offered an opportunity for cerebral biopsy, of which 32 were performed. Although this method was not as reliable as pneumo-encephalography in defining the areas of cortical atrophy, it did give a clearer picture of the ventricular system and in certain cases of presenile dementia this is important in either locating or excluding a lesion in that region.

By plotting the natural history of the patients whose cerebral biopsy was positive for A.D. and comparing these features with those with biopsies negative for A.D. they were able on the basis of 22 positive biopsies for A.D. to define the natural history of the disease. This work has been extended (Sim *et al.*, 1966) and on a basis of 35 patients with cerebral biopsy positive for A.D. and 21 patients with negative biopsies, a clear distinction could be made clinically between A.D. and non-A.D. Paradoxically, the diagnosis was easier to make in the earlier stages of disease, for with the progress of the dementia and the associated neurological involvement the diagnostic margins became blurred.

The following distinguishing features were noted:

Precipitating factors. These were frequently volunteered by relatives who cited surgical operations, bereavements and children leaving home. All these situations involved an interruption in the patient's routine, *e.g.* operations meant admission to hospital, the brief confusion of the anaesthetic, and separation from family and home; bereavement and children leaving home deprived the patient of support which had hitherto concealed the dementia.

Amnesia. This was present in all 35 patients and was the first symptom noted by patients and relatives and preceded changes in mood and behaviour.

Affective symptoms. These too were early but tended to become obscured by the dementing process. Agitation which had been considered by some workers as part of the affective disorder is more likely to be evidence of the organic process and frequently took the form of perseverative hand and forehead rubbing which conveyed the impression that the patient was in a state of agitated depression. It was really part of the 'catastrophic reaction' (p. 109).

Disorientation. This too appeared early, though after memory loss. It would present as inability to arrange objects in space (as tested by Kohs' Blocks) or dressing apraxia.

Speech disturbances. These were intermediate in onset but were variable in that occasionally dysphasia was relatively early while in others it was relatively late.

Preservation of social competence. This persisted even in the presence of severe degrees of dementia. A patient who was unable to dress himself and was so disorientated that he had some difficulty in getting into an easy chair, would find an ash tray in which to place his cigarette end. Raising of the hat in the presence of a lady and standing aside to permit the nurse or sister to pass first through a door also indicated the relatively high level of social competence in otherwise deteriorated patients. Social intercourse in terms of the small talk of the tea table was often so well preserved that the onlooker would have great difficulty in discerning dementia without personally questioning the patient.

Incontinence. This was a very late feature and the patient was able to control his bowel and bladder when other functions had long since deteriorated.

Psychotic features. These appeared late and when mainly delusions and hallucinations of the type found in senile dementia. They were based largely on false impressions due to impairment of comprehension.

Neurological signs. These became gross only in the later stages and consisted of hemiparesis, striatal rigidity and tremor, spasticity and epileptic attacks. Intermediate neurological signs were facial weakness, extensor plantars, increased tone in the limbs, and tremor of the lips.

Special Investigations

(a) *Air studies.* Cerebral atrophy was bilateral and ventricular dilatation was usually confined to the lateral ventricles. Dilatation of the whole ventricular system was associated with the small number of patients who exhibited euphoria.

(b) *EEG studies* showed little or no alpha rhythm with fast beta or slow theta activity and in the grosser cases, delta waves. These findings were usually symmetrical, but if not, they did not show definite foci or multilead preponderance in more than one lobe.

Gordon and Sim (1967) in a study of an augmented series of 80 patients with primary presenile dementia, of whom 36 had been diagnosed histologically as Alzheimer's disease, confirmed these findings. They conclude:

> in primary presenile dementias abnormal E.E.G.s are invariably exhibited in patients with Alzheimer's disease whereas in the other nosological groups there is frequently a normal E.E G.

(c) *C.S.F. findings* were usually normal, though four had a slightly raised protein.

(d) *Psychological tests* (especially the Wechsler Adult Intelligence Scale and Kohs' Blocks) revealed a gross apraxia in the presence of a well-preserved vocabulary. A patient who could converse well and not appear handicapped would fail completely with the first card of Kohs' Blocks even when shown how to do it. Colour recognition was not impaired. It was often impossible to score these tests because of the ready precipitation of the 'catastrophic reaction', the patient becoming completely handicapped when exposed to questioning or tasks which extended him. From then onwards, his performance deteriorated so that he was unable to complete those tests which he had hitherto done correctly. This was almost a diagnostic feature in the psychological testing of these patients.

Psychopathic and Neuropathic Heredity. These are often difficult to elicit and sometimes several members of the family have to be interviewed before a clear and unequivocal statement can be obtained. In the series reported by Sim *et al.* (1966) it was very rare though remarkable family histories have been reported by Feldman *et al.* (1963) and Heston *et al.* (1966). Though the neurohistology of these patients was that of A.D. the clinical features would not have warranted such a diagnosis. Clearly these families belong to a clinical group entirely different from the much commoner nonfamilial form.

Premorbid Personality. This was generally effective in terms of work record and domestic responsibilities. Patients tended to be conscientious and reliable and this social competence was well preserved even in relatively advanced states.

Sex Distribution. It was slightly more common in females but even in a relatively large series of 35 patients, it is not possible to be sure that this is so and previous statements that the female : male ratio is approximately 2 : 1 are probably not valid for the disease as a whole. Much larger numbers are required to make such pronouncements.

The main differences between A.D. and non-A.D. are shown in the following table.

Clinical Features	A.D.	Non-A.D.
Memory loss	Early	Late
EEG changes	Early	Late
Apraxia	Early	Late
Fits	Late	Early
Incontinence	Late	Early
Neurological signs	Late	Early
Confabulation	Late	Early
Personality changes	Late	Early
Psychotic symptoms	Late	Early

The question still to be answered is whether the non-A.D. group is a homogeneous population like the A.D. group. The probable answer is that it is not. It certainly included some patients who histologically and clinically could be diagnosed as P.D. but there were others who because of spinal changes such as wasting of tongue, thenar eminence or arm, fell into the category of corticospinal degeneration and resembled the condition described by Meyer (1929) as the bridge between amyotropic lateral sclerosis and Jakob-Creutzfeldt's Disease. Though the group as a whole did not show uniformity of symptoms as in A.D. there were some that did, and further differentiation would appear possible.

PICK'S DISEASE

Pick's disease (P.D.) was first described by Arnold Pick (1892) as a form of dementia related to the senile psychoses but with circumscribed lobar atrophy. Subsequent reports have described a variety of clinical pictures, some of which are indistinguishable from those of A.D., although pneumo-encephalography may demonstrate the localized atrophy in the frontal and temporal lobes which is said to be characteristic, but this may not always be evident. A variety of specific histopathological features have also been described, including various degenerative cell changes and reactive gliosis. A cellular swelling which is almost a ballooning of the cell with cytoplasm staining poorly with Nissl stain has been regarded by some as specific but this change is found in a variety of states where there has been malnutrition before death and is similar to that found in the 'central neuritis' or 'primary irritation' described by Meyer (1901).

Sim and Sussman (1962) in their second group of patients with cortical atrophy whose biopsies were negative for A.D. found degenerative changes with gliosis, but without the 'primary irritation', and they suggest that these cases may well be those of P.D. The clinical picture differed markedly from that of A.D. in that early features of the disease were incontinence, euphoria and confabulation of the Korsakoff type.

Further evidence for doubting the diagnosis of P.D. as an entity was provided by Sim and Bale (1973) who reported three families with presenile dementia. In one family one parent had a histological diagnosis of P.D. at biopsy and another had the diagnosis confirmed post-mortem, yet in the other families without such pathological findings the clinical features and laboratory findings, including EEG, neuroradiology and psychometrics were in some instances closer to the one with a histological diagnosis of P.D. than with other affected members of the same family. The authors point out that if such a situation existed in cancer pathology where a clinical condition could be readily identified but where the histology was 'positive' in only a very small percentage of cases it would have been discredited. Evidence for doubting the specificity of the histopathology of P.D. is also available from sources other than those of the familial dementias.

JAKOB-CREUTZFELDT DISEASE

The definition of Jakob-Creutzfeldt disease as a clinical and pathological entity is still in process of evolving and there are at least 16 synonyms for the disease (Roos *et al.*, 1972). Nevin *et al.* (1960) who reported on eight cases of spongiform cerebral atrophy distinguished them on pathological grounds from Jakob's pseudosclerosis as follows:

1. The distribution of the cortical lesions in Jakob's pseudosclerosis is maximal in the temporo-central region whereas in the spongiform condition any region of the cortex may be maximally involved with a special predilection for the occipital lobes.

2. Degeneration of the motor nuclei in the brain stem and spinal cord and primary degeneration of myelinated tracts so characteristic of Jakob's pseudosclerosis does not appear to occur in the spongiform disease.

3. Cell shrinkage is more common in the spongiform than in Jakob-Creutzfeldt's disease and it differs morphologically. In J–C shrinkage of the whole cell occurs and the staining is dark, the nucleus is round and oval, while the nucleolus and cell processes may be visible with a corkscrew epicaldendrite. In the spongiform, there is an irregular or triangular, darkly stained nucleus.

4. The 'Verödungsherde' emphasized by Jakob do not occur in the spongiform.

5. The behaviour of the astrocytes differs in that the glial rosettes and neurophagia of J–C do not occur in the spongiform which has wide stretches of the outer layers of the cortex 'embedded' in a richly proliferated mass of gemistocytic-like glia.

6. Status spongiosus in form and extent as seen in the cortex and basal ganglia in the spongiform is absent in J–C.

These distinctions are not merely academic, for there is a strong move to equate J–C with the spongiform variety because of the exciting discovery that the spongiform can be transmitted by a virus from man to primates (Gajdusek & Gibbs, 1971). These authors appreciate the differential diagnosis of Nevin *et al.* and are hoping to resolve the argument by the successful transmission of a case that satisfies Nevin's clinical and pathological criteria. Till this has been done, it would be preferable to discuss the two conditions as (1) Jakob-Creutzfeldt's disease or Creutzfeldt-Jakob's disease and (2) Spongiform Cerebral Atrophy.

It would appear therefore that in idiopathic presenile dementia there are three eponymous diseases. A.D. presents a classical picture which is readily distinguishable from that of P.D. P.D. and Jakob-Creutzfeldt disease have a similar mental and histopathological picture, with the exception that the latter presents with striatal and spinal changes which may precede the onset of the dementia. The paradoxical feature is that it is easier to distinguish A.D. from P.D. in the *early* stages of the disease, for once the dementia has progressed, the margins of differential diagnosis become blurred and it is probably this aspect which has led to the existing confusion and multiplicity of criteria which, though valid for each case reported, do not help in the diagnosis. One is more likely to arrive at a correct diagnosis if a reliable answer to the questions 'How did it start and progress?' can be obtained. A.D. and P.D. are progressive diseases with changing patterns, with later manifestations which are very different from the early ones and therefore considerable divergence of opinion on symptomatology would result if one observer were reporting only early cases and another later and deteriorated ones. The problem of the genetic aspect is still to be worked out, for as the lesion in A.D. would appear to be a biochemical one which is declared at a certain age group and there is a suggestion that families can be affected, a more thorough study of the relatives of these patients is likely to be of interest, but first the biochemical lesion has to be more accurately defined.

NORMAL PRESSURE HYDROCEPHALUS

Adams *et al.* (1965) described a syndrome of progressive neurological degeneration with mental deterioration, psychomotor retardation, unsteadiness of gait and incontinence of urine. Though this syndrome may be associated with well-defined degenerative states, cerebrovascular disease and after trauma, they showed that in their patients the cerebrospinal fluid (CSF) pressure was normal in the presence of significant hydrocephalus. They explained this phenomenon by Pascal's law for enclosed fluid. The *force* on the walls of a container is equal to the product of the *pressure* of the fluid and the *area* of the wall, *i.e.* F = P x A.

An example is the bicycle tyre which carries a pressure of 30 lb while a huge tractor's tyres contain a much smaller pressure. If the ventricular surface is 60 cm^2, the force exerted on the walls at a CSF pressure of 300 mm should be half that for ventricles with surface area of 120 cm^2.: *or* the force on the surrounding brain tissue exerted by a pressure of 150 mm in ventricles with surface of 120 cm^2 should equal that exerted by a pressure of 300 mm in ventricles of 60 cm^2. The condition was labelled by the authors the 'hydraulic press effect' in hydrocephalus, and while a pressure of 180 mm could be tolerated by normal size ventricles, it could prove too high should they enlarge.

Explanations of the cause vary. Trauma and subarachnoid haemorrhage may cause adhesions which impair the passage of CSF to arachnoid granulations in the superior longitudinal sinus, or dilatation of the basilar artery may produce a functional obstruction of the basal cisterns.

Bannister (1970) stressed the dangers of investigating these patients with pneumoencephalography which can result in sudden deterioration and advocates 100μ Ci of I^{131} labelled serum albumin (RISA) in 0·5 ml of fluid which is injected intrathecally. The radiation dose is approximately 100 millirad to the whole body and 1 rad to the CNS. Nevertheless it should not be used in children and women of child-bearing age. The brain is scanned at intervals and in normal patients the albumin passes slowly to the superior longitudinal sinus in 24 to 48 hours but retention of the albumin in the ventricles for 48 hours or more is diagnostic of the condition and would indicate a good response to the treatment which is a ventirculo-atrial shunt. Bannister (1970) reported on 10 patients who fulfilled the above criteria of whom 9 improved, 5 dramatically. Rice and Gendelman (1973) described 5 patients in whom psychiatric disturbances, including depression, confusion, delusions, and intellectual deterioration were the major features with neurological signs being less evident. They all showed the characteristic changes and of 3 who had a shunt, 2 improved substantially.

The successful treatment of this condition is an encouraging development in a field which has, to date, carried a hopeless prognosis. Yet, caution is indicated, for unless a straight X-ray of skull is available for comparison with the RISA scan a number of 'false positives' may be obtained and the patient subjected to needless surgery. The author was at one time prompted to recommend the operation in proven cases of Alzheimer's disease because of a report of successful treatment of these patients by a shunt. None benefited and neither do other patients with cortical atrophy. One patient who did benefit did not have Alzheimer's disease and fulfilled the diagnostic criteria of Adams *et al.* (1965); it would be advisable to restrict the operation to this group.

HUNTINGTON'S CHOREA

Huntington's chorea was originally described by Huntington (1872) in the descendants of three men who hailed from Bures, Suffolk, and who had emigrated to New England in 1630 (Gates, 1946). It is a degenerative disease of the central nervous system which results in choreiform movements and dementia and is said to be inherited as a pure mendelian dominant, though instances have been described where there was no evidence of a family history. Lyon (1962*b*) pointed out that there are non-hereditary cases of chronic adult chorea which may have a superficial resemblance to Huntington's chorea and reported two cases, one of whom was mentally normal but the other showed psychotic features. This is a not unimportant aspect for in advising a patient on marriage or pregnancy, it is helpful if the hereditary nature of the condition can be eliminated. Incidence in a total population is both difficult to gauge and unhelpful for it tends to group in various districts and even in these districts there may be little spread. For example, Lyon (1962*a*) who described a number of families with the disease in the Moray Firth area of Scotland, suggested they were descended from herring fishers who settled there about 300 years ago, yet such was their inbreeding that the local clans were still completely unaffected.

The neuropathology though defined earlier was first systematically examined with a control series by Dunlap (1927). On macroscopic examination, the brain is small, particularly in the frontal regions with marked atrophy of the gyri, and especially of the corpus striatum, which is seen on coronal section. The ventricles are enlarged and the internal capsule is relatively broad. *Microscopically*, there is atrophy of the corpus striatum with degeneration and destruction of the ganglion cells, particularly in the posterior part of the putamen, the globus pallidus being intact. There is also considerable diffuse destruction of nerve cells in the anterior part of the cortex but with no disorder of the cytoarchitectonics. In the areas of degeneration there is a marked increase in glial nuclei and in the spinal cord there is a thick fibrous gliosis which corresponds to the area of demyelination.

Clinical Features

These may vary considerably. It is insidious in onset and may be ushered in either with personality changes or with the choreiform movements or both and usually starts in the 30's or 40's though earlier cases have been described. Early psychiatric features are moodiness, irritability and neglect of home and person. Change of surroundings or even a visit from someone outside the family circle may precipitate a catastrophic reaction (p. 109), and make the patient behave worse. In the later stages, frank psychotic features are evident and they range through delusions of persecution, religiosity, aggression and grandiose behaviour. Dementia is progressive and an intolerance of alcohol may also occur. Huntington described it as 'That form of insanity which leads to suicide' and Bickford and Ellison (1953) observed a high incidence of suicide in their series from Cornwall; they suggest that the awards for gallantry in World War II to some of their patients may have a similar psychopathology.

The choreiform movements may go unrecognized for some time for in the early stages it may be merely an involuntary twitch of a digit or a facial grimace which might pass as a mannerism. These should be specifically looked for during the initial interview for they have a habit of disappearing when the patient is aware he is being observed. It may develop as a hemichorea or be bilateral with grimacing, explosive speech and spluttering as well as athetoid movements of the hands. The gait may become ataxic, and occasionally in the gross case there is a peculiar gyrating movement. A rarer presentation is a respiratory form when the patient's breathing becomes affected. At one time it was believed that the disease was confined to European stock, but there have been reports of its occurrence among other peoples, including a recent one by Singer (1962) of four generations in a Chinese family with 24 affected members.

Treatment. Until recently this has been ineffective, but with the advent of the phenothiazines, a measure of relief has been given to a number of patients. Chlorpromazine was prescribed in doses just short of producing Parkinsonism, and this drug as well as reserpine was able to control the choreiform movements as well as the more florid psychotic features. Lyon (1962*c*) studied the effectiveness of a variety of drugs previously prescribed for his patients and concluded that phenobarbitone had been the most successful, but that thiopropazate (Dartalan) surpassed it in bringing considerable relief to five out of five patients. Dosage was 30 mg. per day and there were no undesirable side-effects except in one case where pseudo-Parkinsonism developed, which he attributed to the delicate adjustment required to relate dosage to body weight. Reserpine has also been used, the first reports coming from Chandler (1955) and Lazarete *et al.* (1955). On the assumption that reserpine acts by depleting the cerebral amines, Sourkes (1965) treated 3 patients with *a*-methyldopa with favourable results. That reserpine should only be used when phenothiazines have failed has been stressed by the work of Mackiewicz and Reid (1965) who compared the brains of 4 patients treated with reserpine with 9 who were not. They found in the former group foci of destruction in the reticular formation with pathological changes in fibre tracts and vessels in this area. The untreated group showed no such changes. In addition 2 of the 4 treated patients died during a heat wave suggesting that reserpine may have interfered with temperature control. Wycis and Spiegel (1956) have had success with stereoencephalotomy and while this method may prove very helpful in controlling the disturbing movements, if conclusions can be drawn from the stereotaxic treatment of Parkinsonism, it is unlikely to affect the dementia.

PARKINSONISM

The treatment of Parkinsonism by L-dopa (L-dihydroxyphenylalanine) has aroused considerable interest not only in its mode of action but in the psychiatric aspects of the disease itself. Mindham (1970) studied retrospectively 89 patients with Parkinsonism and who also suffered from mental illness. He used the usual clinical classification:

1. Postencephalitic, with a history suggestive of an attack of encephalitis lethargica (19 patients);
2. Arteriosclerotic, where there was good evidence of cerebral vascular disease (24 patients);
3. Paralysis agitans where no aetiology was defined (36 patients).

The other 10 patients were of various diagnostic types.

The post-encephalitic group had an average duration of symptoms of 15 years, paralysis agitans 9·8 years, and arteriosclerotic 4·7 years, so that diagnostic category had prognostic significance. When the group was matched with controls for age and sex it showed a significantly higher incidence of 'non-senile organic' diagnosis and affective illness in that 90 per cent of the 3 major diagnostic groups had depression and one-third showed intellectual impairment and the psychiatric illness frequently appeared in the same year as the Parkinsonism.

The author concluded that depression and intellectual impairment should be seen as important accompaniments of the syndrome.

Jenkins and Groh (1970) tested the effect of L-dopa on 90 Parkinsonian patients as regards memory, behaviour, mood, sleep and dreams. Eighteen patients had mental symptoms with a timing and severity that indicated that L-dopa played a significant aetiological role. Twelve patients developed non-reactive depression of whom 4 became suicidal; of the remaining 8 patients, response to the drug was poor in 3 and depression may have been related to dashed hopes, but motor response was satisfactory in the remaining 5 patients.

Twenty-two of the 90 patients reported improvement in memory, 3 reported deterioration and the remainder noted no change. Seventeen patients reported nightmares or vivid dreams which came on in the early weeks of therapy and usually cleared up spontaneously. Insomnia occurred in 19 patients and hypersomnia in 3 patients. There was a slight increase in the average age of those patients who developed mental symptoms compared with those who did not (67·4 years : 65·8 years). Two male patients experienced increased sexual drive, and this, when associated with severely impaired judgment, could be an embarrassing if not dangerous combination. Depressed patients responded well to imipramine and no inhibition of the effect of the L-dopa was observed, but otherwise mental disturbances were dose-dependent.

Celasia and Barr (1970) reported 16 patients with psychiatric disturbances 14 of whom had associated buccolingual or generalized dyskinesia and they regarded the latter as characteristic of L-dopa toxicity and not attributable to any other drug. They suggested that this aspect may be due to a close interaction among basal ganglia, biogenic amines and motor and mental functions though not due to a single biochemical defect.

The difficulties in drawing conclusions from the comparing of groups of Parkinsonian patients with controls was illustrated by Garron *et al.* (1972) who found that akinesia which is one of the commoner features of the disease was more characteristic of those patients in whom the onset was late in life, and that late onset and akinesia tended to be associated with intellectual deterioration and decreased self-care competence. As the critical group for studying the effects of L-dopa on intellectual function consists of the older, akinetic patients, these may well have a motor and intellectual deficit prior to treatment.

In spite of the apparent association of the prescribing of L-dopa and the onset of depression, Goodwin (1972) reported the results of L-dopa in 23 patients with primary depression but without Parkinsonism. The only patients who responded were the retarded group (5 out of 15) when the dose exceeded 3 grammes.

The theoretical implications of the mental effects of L-dopa its direct effect on catecholamine levels and turnover has given rise to much speculation and is already being included in the 'Pantheon' of those who seek a biochemical cause for all mental illness. Much more work is needed, though it warrants the effort.

PSYCHIATRIC ASPECTS OF HEAD INJURY

The psychiatric sequelae of head injury need not be associated with the organic brain damage, yet the term 'post-traumatic neurosis' is so ingrained that it is difficult to separate those psychiatric symptoms which are directly caused by the injury from those which are mobilized by the compensation element, the individual's inadequacy, or a concurrent psychiatric disturbance. So much of the problem is bound up in our society with compensation neurosis, that it would be advisable at the outset to read the appropriate section in Chapter 11 in order to get the matter into perspective and disabuse one's mind of some of the more extravagant and unauthenticated statements with which the subject abounds.

During the First World War, many cases of hysterical paralysis were attributed to spinal cord lesions and many heated discussions took place between neurologists and psychiatrists concerning the aetiology. Some had claimed to find evidence of undoubted organic involvement of the spinal cord and it was even rumoured that in certain patients who had come to necropsy lesions in the cord had been observed. Yet there was eventually no doubt that these conditions were hysterical or even simulated and of the many thousands who were invalided with the disability very few retained their abnormal gait for long. A similar situation has been described in the Second World War. In a hospital in the Middle East, there were about 20 patients from the same locality who had developed a weakness of the spinal muscles which resulted in a crouching stance. An enthusiastic junior medical officer believed he had discovered an interesting example of epidemic myelitis and the consultant in neurology was invited to express his opinion. The retinue of the consultant, commanding officer and others approached the ward and the patients were mustered by their beds. The hospital sergeant-major knocked sharply on the door with his cane and shouted as only a sergeant-major can shout–'Ward–'Shun!' All the backs immediately straightened.

Such incidents are dramatic and therefore unforgettable but it is important to remember that there are diseases and injuries of the spinal cord which do lead to abnormalities of gait, but to diagnose them there should be unequivocal evidence of organic disease which will account for *all* the patient's symptoms. For the neurologist to claim otherwise would be as fallacious as for the psychiatrist to suggest that undoubted organic neurological signs were functionally determined.

Similarly with head injuries, many symptoms have been attributed to organic causes, on the evidence that the patient had such an injury and that such symptoms frequently occur in patients who have had these injuries. That similar symptoms occur in patients who allege they have had a head injury but have not, and also in patients with phobic anxiety, is frequently ignored by those with an organic bias. Nor do they explain why most severe head injuries do not develop these sequelae–why footballers can head goal posts and be unconscious for several minutes, resume the game and be fit for work on the Monday; and why steeplechasers can be thrown from their horses, lose consciousness and then remount; nor do they explain why a housewife can sustain many bumps on the head while at home and be relatively symptom-free, but should she knock her head ever so gently while cleaning at an office or while on a 'bus which brakes suddenly, the post-traumatic or post-concussion syndrome presents in its most florid form. The doctor should confine himself to the unequivocal facts and refrain from readily attributing functional symptoms to organic causes. It is not a question of depriving a patient of compensation to which he is not entitled, though there is no disgrace in that; it is just bad medicine. There are some doctors who cannot accept that psychiatric symptoms, including hysterical ones are functionally determined and must seek an organic explanation, no matter how fanciful. Such an attitude will find plenty to conjecture with in the sequelae of head injuries but debates on these patients are usually not held at meetings of medical societies, where the court of appeal is the hard rock of clinical medicine and the critical opinions of one's colleagues who are trained to assess the medical evidence. They are usually held in courts of law, which in spite of the best intentions and traditions, can hardly be considered the ideal place for the testing of medical hypotheses.

There are, however, genuine post-traumatic brain conditions which are usually divided into acute or chronic.

Acute

Concussion. As has already been said, in the vast majority of instances, this is uncomplicated. The patient loses consciousness after the injury, and when he regains it he may show nothing more than a post-traumatic amnesia. At one time, the duration of this and the presence of an anterograde amnesia was alleged to be correlated with the severity of the injury and the prognosis, but this view is now being seriously questioned. Some may not even be unconscious, but behave automatically, though purposively and even effectively. Many a footballer has been concussed, but has not lost consciousness and has continued to play and scored goals. After the game he has had no memory whatever for the events following the blow on the head. A similar situation has been described in boxers.

The mechanism is still debated. It has been attributed to cerebral ischaemia, but Denny-Brown and Russell (1941) and Jefferson (1944) showed that it could not be interpreted in such terms, the former indicating that the view had been untenable since Witkowski's classic experiment in which he stunned the heartless frog, and the latter advancing the view that brain-stem damage was responsible. The difficulty of drawing conclusions from experimental and pathological data is that these are usually concerned with gross cerebral disturbance, while concussion as recognized clinically, and as presented in the histories of patients, is a readily recoverable condition. For example, Strich (1956, 1961), using the Marchi method, demonstrated widespread, diffuse degeneration of the cerebral white matter in the brains of patients dying 5–15 months after closed head injuries, and considered that nerve fibres are torn or stretched at the time of the accident by rotational force. Symonds (1962) takes an extreme view. He regards it as 'questionable whether the effects of concussion, however slight, are ever completely reversible'. He quotes the example of the punch-drunk boxer as evidence of the permanent damage that can result from repeated concussion. The psychiatrist is rarely called to see the patient with concussion. It is mainly after the event, sometimes long after, that he is asked to give his opinion on the patient's condition which has already been firmly labelled 'post-concussional syndrome', even by those who legally contest it, such as insurance companies.

The Punch-drunk Boxer

This phenomenon has been lifted out of the field of objective medical appraisal and has become the subject of propaganda by those who would abolish professional boxing and by those who have a vested interest in preserving it. The syndrome was first reported by Martland (1928) who described neurological and psychiatric disabilities in boxers and his conclusions are still relevant. He stated 'Punch drunk most often affects fighters of the slugging type, who are usually poor boxers and who take considerable head punishment, seeking only to land a knockout blow' . . . 'I have found the opinion of shrewd laymen, many of whom are making a living by observing the physical fitness, actions and characteristics of the professional fighter, is perhaps more substantial than the opinon of the medical experts'. Since then Kaplan and Browder (1954) have reported on the correlation between the clinical and brain wave (EEG) patterns of professional boxers and found that the latter were more grossly disturbed in the less able boxers, while McCown (1959) doubted the very existence of the syndrome and stated 'No clinical or laboratory evidence would substantiate the so-called punch-drunk syndrome so often identified with boxers'.

Hemphill (1962), who studied the admissions to Bristol Mental Hospital, found no boxer suffering from organic dementia admitted in 1931, and none had been admitted since. The only boxers admitted since then suffered from catatonic schizophrenia with recovery; mania with alcoholism which was regarded at the time as punch-drunkenness; mental sluggishness and impaired vision which was due to a pituitary tumour with acromegaly; and recurrent depression in an old boxer from the bare-fist era, but with no intellectual impairment. Hemphill concludes: 'These few observations show that psychotic changes in boxers may be wrongfully attributed to boxing injury, and severe organic dementia from this cause must be rare'. Spillane (1962) also had difficulty in relating responsibility of neurological disorder of boxing injury, and in excluding a pre-existing brain defect or coincidental disease. He did however find that 3 out of the 5 who had neurological lesions had demonstrable abnormalities of the septum pellucidum by air encephalography. Mawdsley and Ferguson (1963) augmented the study of Spillane with one on 10 ex-boxers with neurological disease and in addition to dementia in 9, in 6 there was a cavum septum pellucidum and they concluded that professional boxing could produce progressive neurological disease. Blonstein (1963) criticizes their conclusions and states that if they had chosen a similar number of ex-professional rugby players, they would have found similar neurological changes.

It is obvious that much more detailed work is required before valid conclusions can be drawn, but it should be borne in mind that many who take up professional boxing already have a suspect mental equipment. The problem, like drug addiction, capital punishment, abortion and the like, arouses controversy and provokes uncritical statements. It is just as well to await the evidence and subject it to the most careful scrutiny. In the meantime the psychiatrist may find a useful role in the medical assessment of would-be pugilists.

Traumatic Coma. This is a frequent result of severe head injury and the psychiatrist's interest is mainly confined to the dysmnesic (Korsakoff) state which may result from it.

Traumatic Delirium. This has to be distinguished from other causes of delirium and this can be a very difficult task, particularly when alcoholic delirium is being considered. A person who has been in an accident and perhaps concussed may be given some spirituous drink by a benevolent bystander and the doctor will then be confronted by a delirious patient who is smelling of drink. Worse still, an alcoholic in the course of a bout may fall and injure his head and then present with delirium. A thorough physical examination and admission to hospital is essential when faced with such a problem. In hospital, the management may be difficult because of the patient's restlessness, but adequate sedation and phenothiazine should control it. Some have suggested that vitamins should be prescribed in traumatic delirium, on the assumption that a depleted brain is more vulnerable. This may well be true in patients who have been taking a lot of alcohol.

Subdural Haematoma. This, in the acute stage, is more likely to be seen by the neurologist or the neurosurgeon, but may be referred to the psychiatrist at a later stage (see below).

Korsakoff's Psychosis. The dysmnesic syndrome has already been mentioned as being a common sequel of head injury, and is generally a later manifestation of post-traumatic coma or delirium and can present with the classical confabulatory state seen in the alcoholic Korsakoff. It usually recedes and there is an interesting phase when the disorientation for time, place and person gives way to an 'as if' phenomenon. The patient begins to appreciate his surroundings but still cannot believe he is in hospital. He may say that he knows he is in hospital, but that he feels he is in a factory and that the doctor reminds him of the foreman and so on. This usually gives way to full insight, though some do become chronically handicapped.

Chronic States

Subdural Haematoma. This is a complication of a number of less severe head injuries. It is said to be commoner now than when Putnam and Cushing (1925) stimulated interest in the condition. Davies (1960) attributes the increase to three main factors: (1) the increased number of head injuries; (2) the increasing life expectancy (most patients are aged 40–70 years); and (3) increased awareness of the complication. Davies reported 11 out of 44 consecutive cases of head injury and the mental symptoms were mainly confusional but two were hallucinated and deluded and one presented Korsakoff features from which he did not recover.

Post-concussion Syndrome. The psychiatric symptoms are inability to concentrate, fatiguability, and impairment of memory with anxiety features. It has been argued that these constitute evidence of early dementia, but they may well represent a purely functional disturbance. Even evidence of severe head injury does not mean that the symptoms are organically determined, for many patients with brain damage completely recover their faculties and there must be a number who hold distinguished office who have at some time sustained a severe head injury, including the loss of brain tissue. The author has known a medical student with such a history who was unconscious for a week and showed extreme irritability with faulty recognition for some time subsequently, but who made an excellent recovery with no demonstrable or subjective handicap. One might say that, as with leucotomy, the person with the best medical equipment is likely to show least deterioration, while people of limited capacity show most, but it is the nature of the resulting handicap which should decide whether it is organic or not.

THE FOLLOWING INVESTIGATIONS MAY BE HELPFUL

1. Electro-encephalography

In patients where brain damage is alleged to be responsible for symptoms, there are usually EEG changes. In the acute stage there may be bursts of high voltage 2–3 c/s waves, while in the chronic stage the voltage is generally low and the frequency is of the region of 2–7 c/s. Williams (1941 *a & b*) has shown that the disturbance is generally proportional to the severity of the injury and the persistence of symptoms.

It is not uncommon for the problem to be adulterated by drugs, particularly barbiturates, which can influence the EEG, either by producing fast waves, or in severe intoxication, slow waves and occasionally fits. The author has seen such a patient who was regarded as a post-traumatic dementia and was awarded a large sum in compensation. He then gave up his barbiturates for alcohol and the signs of dementia disappeared though he died two years later from the physical effects of alcoholism.

2. Radiography

Pneumo-encephalograms are reputed to be abnormal in 80 per cent of patients who have symptoms related to old head injuries. The commonest finding is a generalized enlargement of the ventricles, though this may not necessarily be pathological.

3. Brain Scan

This is being increasingly used for investigating patients suspected of massive lesions of the brain, particularly tumour and abscess. It is safe and technically simple and is about 90 per cent accurate and is therefore becoming an earlier rather than a later investigation. The most commonly used radioactive tracer is 90 ^{m}/Tc pertechnetate given intravenously immediately or one hour before the imaging procedure. Other agents are mercury (^{203}Hg or ^{197}Hg)-labelled chlormerodrin or chelate of radioactive inderium (^{131m}In) and ytterbium (^{100}Yb). Normal brain tissue is relatively impermeable to most substances ('blood-brain barrier') but radioactive tracers as listed above readily diffuse into lesions such as tumours which show against the relatively low activity of surrounding brain.

Lesions of 2 cm or more in diameter can generally be detected thus giving it a greater than 90 per cent detection success in tumours. Multiple views give evidence of shape, size and site of lesion and the clues are building up so that non-cancerous conditions such as cerebral thrombosis, subdural haematoma, and cerebral contusions can also be detected.

4. Psychological Tests

Theoretically these should be of great assistance, but in practice they do not offer much help in diagnosis. The patient may score badly due to lack of motivation and this lack may or may not be caused by his organic mental state. Of greatest help is a comprehensive test like the Wechsler Adult Intelligence Scale (WAIS), which because of its variety of subtests shows whether there is a general depression of performance, which may be due to functional factors, or whether there are deficiencies in certain operational fields. Should the latter prove to be the case, then organic factors are more likely to be operating.

Projection tests may be of some help, but are unlikely to be conclusive. Creativity is said to be impaired after brain damage, but as there is unlikely to be any pre-traumatic standard by which the deterioration can be measured, it is difficult to draw any conclusions, as most creative artists without any head injury or brain damage would score very differently at different times in a test designed to measure creativity.

Personality Changes

It is in this field where there is the greatest controversy. Loss of interest, irritability, moodiness, apathy, outbursts of temper, are all quoted as post-traumatic personality changes and it is extremely difficult at times to say whether these are organically or functionally determined. These changes are often alleged to be progressive, but Denny-Brown (1943) doubted the possibility of progressive personality deterioration after head injury, especially in the absence of other evidence of organic disease, and Kozol (1946) found that those who had a personality handicap after a head injury, had a pre-traumatic history of poor interpersonal relations. Lewis (1942) was also unable to distinguish between the symptomatology of post-concussion patients and those with common neuroses. Ruesch *et al.* (1943) found that in the personality changes following head injury brain damage was of secondary importance and that the pre-traumatic personality was of primary importance in determining the nature of those changes. They also stated that in the absence of neurological signs, there was no personality change which could be directly attributed to the head injury.

At a recent meeting which was attended by a number of medical superintendents of mental hospitals, the speaker, whose subject was 'Traumatic Neuroses', asked if anybody working in mental hospitals could give him some idea of the incidence of post-traumatic personality deterioration in institutions, but nobody could recall a case. Yet one is frequently asked to report on people whose head injuries are alleged to have caused profound and progressive mental impairment. All the reliable evidence to date would suggest that such cases are extremely rare and that the findings of Ruesch *et al.* (1943) are still valid.

Prognosis of Severe Head Injury

Miller and Stern (1965) in a long-term follow-up of 100 consecutive cases of severe head injury (average post-traumatic amnesia 13 days) which were examined after a mean interval of 11 years found only one death attributable to the sequelae of the head injury while none required chronic hospital care. Psychiatric symptoms initially occurred in 10 of the severely injured but only 2 were disabled by them, while in patients with minor head injuries, 40 per cent were severely disabled with such symptoms. In the severely injured 6–13 years later, only one was occupationally disabled and he was a chronically unemployed labourer of low intelligence. Ten patients had organic mental changes of varying degree, 5 of whom were unemployable, though the other 5 were fully employed. The authors conclude: 'In general the outcome in these cases of severe head injury has proved to be much more favourable than was expected or predicted'.

Treatment

As with any disability, early rehabilitation is essential. This is particularly important in brain damage, for the patient should be encouraged to perform up to his capacity as soon as he is deemed capable of doing so. If deficit has resulted from the injury, various adaptive responses will have to be learned and the sooner these are acquired, the less the permanent handicap will be. Drugs should be used with great discretion and although barbiturates are considered a useful prophylactic against the development of post-traumatic epilepsy, they have their drawbacks in that they potentiate personality changes and generally slow the patient down; if excessively prescribed they can produce a state akin to dementia as well as addiction.

DISSEMINATED OR MULTIPLE SCLEROSIS (D.S. or M.S.)

A disease which produces discrete lesions in the brain, some subcortical and others in the region of the brain stem and which is liable to sudden exacerbations, is likely on occasions to be responsible for mental changes. The commonest is emotional lability, and though it used to be taught that euphoria is a conspicuous feature, depression may be at least as common, if not as conspicuous. As with other organic cerebral states, the predisposition of the underlying personality will strongly colour the psychiatric picture and paranoid reactions are not uncommon. The emotional lability with fleeting and at times indefinite neurological signs, used to be responsible for labelling the condition hysteria, but this was before the dawn of dynamic psychiatry with its emphasis on defining an adequate and fully relevant psychopathology, and before the dawn of the Babinski reflex and the more rigid exclusion of the organic.

Attempts to define a specific personality type in D.S., as one would expect, have been unsuccessful, but evidence of progressive intellectual deterioration has been shown by Canter (1951) in 23 out of 41 patients. Although dementia as a sequel of the disorder is recognized, there are many patients of long-standing who do not deteriorate mentally and it would appear that the psychiatric aspect cannot be divorced from the general progress of the disease. This is especially so when intellectual deterioration occurs, but not necessarily when depression presents.

Surridge (1969) studied 108 patients who were as fully representative of the disease as possible and compared them with a control group of 39 muscular dystrophy patients. Almost two-thirds had intellectual deterioration, ranging from mild memory loss to profound global dementia. In general these deficits conformed to those of the common amnestic syndrome with memory loss and defective conceptual thinking. A quarter were depressed and a similar proportion were euphoric, the latter finding being absent in all the controls. The author concluded that intellectual deterioration, euphoria, personality change and exaggeration of emotional expression were directly due to brain damage and suggested that all patients with multiple sclerosis who are euphoric should be regarded as suffering from intellectual deterioration unless there is strong evidence to the contrary.

The problem of depression in D.S. is a most challenging one to the psychiatrist, for here is an eminently recoverable psychiatric disorder associated with an organic disease which is very liable to be aggravated by electroplexy. The author has seen a few depressed patients with D.S. who had been given E.C.T. with unfortunate results to their organic state. One such patient was of particular interest. She gave a history since she started nursing at 18 years of recurring depression following minor upsets, but with excellent performance in the intervening years. She had a very severe depressive episode in her mid-forties, was started on a course of E.C.T. and immediately developed neurological signs which were typical of D.S. One is led to speculate whether in this and other cases, the recurrent depressive phases constituted emotional manifestation of D.S. and were just as symptomatic of the disease as a diplopia, an extensor plantar or ataxia. Fortunately in depression associated with D.S. imipramine hydrochloride has proved effective.

Schilder's Disease

This is generally regarded as a cause of mental defect since it occurs more commonly in children, but adult cases are not unknown. The pathological lesion is that of a diffuse sclerosis, though there may be some discrete areas of demyelinization, which histologically can resemble D.S.

Symptomatology will depend largely on the site of the lesion. It is a rapidly progressive disease and usually presents with cortical blindness, though optic atrophy and papilloedema have also been reported and the differential diagnosis from a cerebral tumour can prove very difficult, especially as headache, vomiting and vertigo may precede the grosser neurological picture. *Mentally,* the features may vary tremendously and diagnoses ranging from hysteria to dementia, by way of schizophrenia, have been made. There is usually impairment of comprehension which deteriorates to confusion and dementia, and mixed psychotic features occur while the patient is still mentally capable of elaborating them. The prognosis is poor, deterioration is rapid and the challenge to the psychiatrist is likely to come in the early phase of the illness, when he may be asked to see a patient presenting with rather ill-defined psychiatric symptoms. A careful physical examination should reveal the organic nature of the condition.

PSYCHIATRIC ASPECTS OF BRAIN TUMOUR

If there is any problem in diagnosis which causes the psychiatrist most anxiety, it is that he will mistake a brain tumour for a purely functional disorder and treat it as such. This is not surprising for the brain is the commonest site of neoplasms which are most likely to present with psychiatric symptoms and frequently these symptoms may be the earliest indication of intracranial disease. It has been claimed that an intimate knowledge of neurology is no more important to the psychiatrist than one of say, cardiology or gastroenterology, but in the everyday work of psychiatric practice, there is no doubt that neurological conditions take pride of place in differential diagnosis. Another factor has made the problem even more difficult for the psychiatrist, for, as many patients with cerebral tumour present with depressive features, he may give E.C.T. which may aggravate the underlying pathology, sometimes with tragic results.

The problem may present after what was an undoubted psychological stress and therefore be regarded by the patient's family and doctor as an entirely psychiatric illness. The following are two examples:

A middle-aged woman went to the garden gate to receive a telegram from the postman. It was from the War Office saying her son had been killed in Korea, and she promptly collapsed and had what would have ordinarily passed for an epileptic fit but in view of the circumstances was considered to be hysterical. It was later shown that she had a meningioma, which was successfully removed.

A man in his 50's had an only child who had got herself engaged to somebody he disapproved of. There was a scene and he struck her for the first time and she left home. He became very depressed and claimed he was unable to get about and it was generally believed that this was a mechanism designed to get her back on his terms. There was, however, a history of deafness of three years' duration and he complained of numbness on the same side of the face; investigations revealed an acoustic neuroma on that side which was successfully removed (many acoustic neuromas do present initially with severe depression).

These examples illustrate how difficult these problems can be and they can prove equally difficult for one's neurological colleagues, who may, after careful and exhaustive investigation, refer the patient to the psychiatrist as a functional problem. E.C.T. may be given for the severe depression and then the condition declares itself with either a fit which may start with a Jacksonian 'march', or urinary incontinence, or localizing signs. A neurological colleague has called it 'diagnostic E.C.T.', for it has on several occasions declared a meningioma which otherwise would have been missed, but the result is not invariably as fortunate as this. One must therefore be alert to the possibility of a brain tumour being responsible for the patient's symptoms and a diagnosis of hysteria should be the last consideration in patients over the age of 40 years.

The patient may voice rather vague complaints and though physical examination is essentially negative, there is an obtuseness and failure of comprehension which should put one on one's guard and raise the question of a brain tumour. This is particularly so when the general attitude of the patient is one of indifference to the difficulty his failure to cooperate is causing the examiner, for it may be due to fluctuation in the level of consciousness or the beginnings of an organic dementia. The symptomatology of temporal lobe disturbances will be described (p. 176) and it is clear that this too can masquerade very effectively as psychiatric illness.

The diagnosis of brain tumours is outside the scope of this book, and the following account is confined to those aspects of brain tumour which may conceivably present in a manner which would involve the psychiatrist.

Scott (1970) observed transitory psychotic behaviour in 6 of 51 patients on whom he operated for tumours of the cerebello-pontine angle, 44 of whom had acoustic neurinomas. The psychosis developed 3 to 10 days after surgery and persisted for 4 to 21 days without recurrence. The features were delusions of persecution, poisoning and hallucinations in a delirium free setting. None had a previous history of mental illness and the psychosis was not related to position during surgery, air emboli, high intracranial pressure, size or position of the tumour, type of anaesthetic, pre- or postoperative medication, electrolyte or fluid imbalance, infection or haemorrhage. In a questionnaire to neurosurgeons, 37 out of 103 who replied had similar experiences. The author was on less certain ground when he speculated on the aetiology of the psychosis.

Dementia. This may extend from slight impairment of memory to gross cerebral deficit including Korsakoff's psychosis and in all cases where dementia presents, cerebral tumour should be carefully considered.

Epileptic Phenomena. These are described under 'Psychiatric aspects of epilepsy' (p. 171).

Hallucinations. In brain tumour these are rarely auditory, but usually visual, olfactory or tactile. In any hallucinatory state which is not auditory, an organic cause should be seriously considered.

Mood Disturbance. Depression and mania may be associated with temporal lobe lesions, and depression, as has already been mentioned, is a frequent early symptom of an acoustic neuroma. Depression is in any case such a common symptom, that before deciding it is entirely functional, a thorough clinical examination should be undertaken, which should include a careful assessment of the patient's mental state, for frequently the depression is a reaction to organic cerebral deficit, and unless one specifically considers this aspect, its presence may be missed.

Disorders of Speech. Dysphasia, which may not present much difficulty to the initiated, can, especially if associated with some confusion on the patient's part, be regarded as mental illness and referred to the psychiatrist. This is particularly so in the early stages of a vascular accident, but it can also occur with brain tumours.

LOCALIZING SYMPTOMS OF BRAIN TUMOUR

There are certain features which are associated with particular areas of the brain, which though presenting with what might be regarded as mental symptoms, declare the local significance of the lesion and assist the psychiatrist in his exclusion of the functional.

Frontal Lobe

This area and its involvement should be familiar to the psychiatrist, through its association with F.P.I. and pre-frontal leucotomy. Personality changes have been described as tactlessness, apathy and *Witzelsucht*. Brickner (1936) illustrated a disturbance of the ability to synthesize perceptions and as with other areas of brain deficit, there is less capacity for abstract or creative thought. Yet, there are patients who after extensive frontal lobe damage, lose relatively little faculty, while some are more handicapped, so it would appear that the mental sequelae are to a considerable extent dependent on the patient's pre-morbid cerebral equipment.

Temporal Lobe

The part this area plays in mental disturbance will be adequately described under 'Forms of Ictal Experience' (p. 176). It carries much of the responsibility for speech and memory and any such disturbances may indicate a temporal lobe lesion.

Parietal Lobe

In Alzheimer's disease, the parietal lobes are particularly involved with consequent apraxia and some of the grossest deterioration observed either in the patient's everyday life but particularly in performance tests is due to parietal lobe involvement. The psychiatrist, who has perhaps the most continuous and intimate experience of dementia, should be able to recognize the difference between a generalized disturbance of parietal lobe function and more local damage, but much will depend on the stage at which he sees the patient. A detailed account of parietal lobe function and dysfunction is to be found in Critchley's (1953) monograph *The Parietal Lobes.*

THE NATURE OF THE BRAIN TUMOUR

This may give some clue as to its presence and rapidly growing ones like a glioblastoma may present as an acute mental upset with depression, but confusion and dementia soon appear. It is the slowly developing meningioma and astrocytoma which, depending on their size, can simulate mental illness, and if there are initially no localizing signs, the patient may be referred for psychiatric opinion. It may on occasions be extremely difficult to differentiate their clinical presentation from an uncomplicated mental disorder, particularly that of depression. Some patients may even attempt suicide and the psychiatrist is then confronted with an urgent therapeutic problem. It is in these cases that E.C.T. may be given with aggravation of the underlying organic pathology and it is difficult to convince one's colleagues that there was no evidence whatever of organic cerebral disease prior to the treatment, unless they themselves had referred the case initially as being free of such disease. Cerebral metastases from bronchial carcinoma may present with mental symptoms and if there is an associated central neuropathy with dementia, the condition may be mistaken for either a functional psychosis or a presenile dementia of non-specific origin. An X-ray of the chest should help to demonstrate the primary lesion in a large number of cases.

The psychiatric manifestations of brain tumour have to be differentiated from those of cerebro-vascular lesions, such as subdural haematoma and also brain abscess. In the latter, the associated 'toxic' state may cause the patient to appear obtuse and confused and present a picture which can be loosely called 'psychotic'.

SPINAL CORD TUMOURS

Epstein *et al.* (1971) reported 27 patients with spinal canal tumours whose first complaints were regarded as hysterical or malingering. There were 18 females and 9 males and the ages ranged from 9 to 65 years. Their chief complaints which were from 1 to 8 years included a variable pattern of back pains, at times associated with leg pain, weakness and difficulty in gait. Absence of objective findings in the face of increasing disability often led to a diagnosis of functional disorder, and only when gross changes became apparent late in the disease were the patients referred for neurological investigation.

The authors underline the obvious conclusion that it is dangerous to diagnose the functional by merely 'excluding' the organic. It is a constant pitfall for the psychiatrist and for the general practitioner and correctives such as those administered by the authors are not only justified but are welcome.

PSYCHIATRIC ASPECTS OF EPILEPSY

The term 'epilepsy' is derived from the Greek and the definition of Hippocrates that it is a chronic functional disease characterized by fits or attacks in which there is loss of consciousness with a succession of tonic or clonic convulsions has stood the test of time. The scope of the disorder has, however, been widened and it is now more correct to talk of *The Epilepsies,* for the Hippocratic definition applies to only one motor aspect. With the advent of electrical recording of brain activity, definitions have shifted from observable motor phenomena to electrical discharges indicating paroxysmal and transitory disturbances of brain function. The field is a wide one, with neurological, metabolic, biochemical, genetic and social implications and it is frequently very difficult to decide to whom the patient should be referred. The psychiatrist has special interests because some epileptic states may closely resemble functional psychoses or even neuroses, or present as behaviour disturbances, which may involve questions of criminal responsibility. Even when the patient is in the care of a neurologist or neurosurgeon, the psychiatric aspect may predominate, the personality problem requiring an understanding and handling of mental mechanisms which may be regarded by one's colleagues as outside their province. The growth of institutional care for the mentally disturbed has brought a considerable number of these patients under psychiatric care, though the causes of their trouble may be trauma, infection, tumour, congenital abnormality and vascular disease, for it is the end-result which has presented the main problem, the aetiological aspect being either irremediable or the patient's condition being such that neurologists and neurosurgeons have not

yet the resources in their own units to deal with them.
The situation may change and the institutional side may become less of a psychiatric responsibility, especially if some of the proposed units for the investigation and treatment of epilepsy are created. These will being simultaneously to the assistance of the patient all those who are working in the field, but the psychiatrist is still likely to be a member of the team.

INCIDENCE

Cohen (1956) quotes the incidence of epilepsy in Great Britain as between 2 and 4 per 1000 of the population, which would represent a total of 100,000 to 200,000 epileptics. These include the whole range of the problem from those with only minor handicap to those who are completely disabled. It is reckoned that 80 per cent can lead a normal life with a minimum of medical attention and the social and educational scatter is very wide. Cohen (1958) estimates that 10 per cent are intellectually above average, and many would benefit from a university education and some, in fact, do, though there are difficulties which are mainly social and professional and are independent of the patient's academic potential. Of course, a number are below average intelligence as one would expect in the ordinary distribution in the population. Eighty per cent, however, of child epileptics can be educated in ordinary schools and the 20 per cent who need special training are not all mentally backward, but may have frequent fits, behaviour problems, urinary incontinence and post-epileptic automatism.

An accurate picture of the incidence of psychiatric disorders in epilepsy is difficult to obtain. At the one end of the scale there are those epileptics in mental hospitals with frank psychotic states and at the other, the immature, explosive 'epileptoid' psychopath who is a social problem but not gross enough to warrant institutional care and may never come under medical supervision. With the increasing recognition of behaviour patterns associated with epilepsy, more cases are being diagnosed, so the incidence is at present growing, but nothing can be said about those who have not yet been diagnosed but still have the disorder.

AETIOLOGY

Genetic

This aspect has for long been regarded as an important factor.

Lennox and his colleagues in a series of papers (1939, 1947 *a & b*) showed that there was a hereditary factor, yet there are also reports of investigations where no such factor can be demonstrated. Lennox and his co-workers did electro-encephalographic studies on the parents of epileptics, and found that they had abnormal brain waves more frequently than a control group and Lennox was able to reinforce these findings with his report on 66 twin pairs affected by seizures. But the hereditary factor requires certain conditions before it can become manifest, such as trauma, tumour, emotional disturbance, hydration, and hypoglycaemia, to mention only a few. So the genetic aspect is not all-important and even though there may be some grounds for considering it in marriage counselling and in compensation claims, the issue is not clear-cut. If somebody with epilepsy has reached the responsible state of being in a position to marry and the good sense to consult a physician, then even should he produce offspring with a similar defect, it is unlikely to be a gross disability, though naturally if both parents have either epilepsy or a marked cerebral dysrhythmia, the risk of the disease occurring in the children is correspondingly greater. The best the doctor can do is to state the facts as he knows them and not actively discourage their marriage or procreation. He should point out that the vast majority of epileptics lead good and useful lives and that should they produce an epileptic child, it is most unlikely to be a disaster. They should also be informed that some workers in the field have been unable to confirm the findings of Lennox *et al.*

Symptomatic

As has been said, a variety of clinical conditions may give rise to epileptic discharges, and behaviour disorders and abnormal mental states can result from such states just as readily as from the so-called idiopathic group. A detailed account of all these conditions would be more appropriate to a textbook of medicine rather than in a guide to psychiatry, and all that need be stressed here is that a thorough physical examination should be made and all the organic possibilities considered before a diagnosis of idiopathic epilepsy with psychiatric associations is made.

ELECTRO-ENCEPHALOGRAPHY

This investigation (EEG) has come to be regarded as essential, though in patients with obvious motor discharge, its value is more in localization rather than in making the diagnosis. Berger (1929) first demonstrated that brain activity could be recorded electrically but his discovery was not seriously considered till Adrian and Yamagiwa (1935) confirmed it and developed and refined the technique. The original resting rhythm of 10–12 cycles per second recorded from the occipital cortex with the subject's eyes closed and which disappeared when the eyes were opened was originally referred to as 'Berger rhythm' but the term has fallen into disuse and Berger who started it all is, unfortunately, practically forgotten. This rhythm is called 'alpha' *(α)* and is considered to be the normal cerebral frequency.

The EEG is usually recorded on six channels, though some machines have eight and even twelve channels. The machine is really a multiple amplifier which enables several tracings to be recorded simultaneously and the areas from which these tracings are obtained can be varied during the course of the recording. Electrodes are placed on the scalp in pairs so that the antero-posterior and transverse sections are obtained of all areas, or special emphasis may be given to a particular area. The record can be read, just as an electrocardiograph, but because of the variety of simultaneous readings, many machines are fitted with an analyser which automatically analyses the EEG tracing every 10 seconds and gives a histogram of the analysis of the selected channel. The height of reading of the histogram is proportional to the magnitude of the particular wave frequency and this form of analysis is called 'Fourier analysis', but an experienced recordist or EEG interpreter can produce a similar analysis by means of the unaided eye. The frequency spectrum is divided into five bands, each named by the following Greek letters: (1) delta (δ) = 1–3·5 c/s; (2) theta (θ) = 4–7 c/s; (3) alpha (α) = 8–13 c/s; (4) beta (β) = 14–18 c/s; and (5) gamma (γ) = 20–30 + c/s. The alpha rhythm is regarded as the normal rhythm and is seen most commonly in the occipital and parieto-occipital regions. In very young children there are difficulties, in that because of their restlessness and distractibility satisfactory records can be made only during sleep. Early rhythms are 3–4 c/s but these increase in frequency with age and the normal adult frequency is usually established by 8–10 years, but there are numerous examples of delayed maturation.

To stimulate the record to yield its abnormal responses various techniques are employed such as (1) *hyperventilation,* which in the epileptic may induce high voltage delta waves of 3 c/s (they cease shortly after the cessation of the hyperventilation); (2) *photic stimulation,* which is performed by a stroboscope which flashes a powerful light into the patient's eyes (either the flicker frequency is reflected in the EEG, or in the epileptic the slow waves seen on hyperventilation are evoked); (3) *chemical stimulation* is usually performed by analeptic drugs such as penta-methylenetetrazol (Leptazol) given intravenously, and occasionally intravenous barbiturate may potentiate an underlying disturbance; (4) *hypoglycaemia,* which may be induced by insulin, fasting, glucogen and tolbutamide (see pp. 217–218).

Abnormal Rhythms

In addition to epilepsy a number of states can give abnormal rhythms and these need not be specific for the underlying pathology.

Epilepsy. In 85 per cent of cases there is a disturbance of the EEG.

(a) *Grand mal.* There is an increased frequency of waves which appear as sharp spikes at 25–30 c/s.

(b) *Petit mal.* The characteristic spike and wave (dart and dome) picture is seen, alternating at the rate of 3 per second.

(c) *Psycho-motor.* The rate is slow (3–4 c/s) with flat-topped waves predominating.

In about 50 per cent of patients with major seizures, the EEG during the intervals may be normal, hence the need to evoke abnormal rhythm by the techniques mentioned above.

Sphenoidal leads are used to record from the base of the skull and are becoming increasingly important in the diagnosis of temporal lobe epilepsy; they are introduced under barbiturate anaesthesia, which potentiates the abnormality from the temporal lobes.

The EEG is of value in treatment as well as diagnosis, for it indicates the efficacy or otherwise of anticonvulsant measures and it is also a popular research tool both in animal experiments and in humans.

Electro-corticography is frequently undertaken in both animals and humans. In the latter it aids the surgeon in the localization of the affected areas and guides him in his removal of pathological tissue such as scarring which may be responsible for abnormal discharges, not only locally but extending sometimes to the other hemisphere.

The Improper Use of the EEG

Hill (1958), writing on this subject, states:

> The EEG is often used as a means of helping to decide whether a given patient's symptoms are epileptic or psychogenic, or are due to some non-cerebral cause, such as syncope. I believe this is an improper use of the technique and

that in fact the results of doing this can be misleading. A single routine normal EEG is not evidence against epilepsy, nor indeed is the finding of epileptic discharges in the EEG evidence that the patient's symptoms are necessarily epileptic in nature. Such discharges occur in the EEG's of some non-epileptic persons, in many with degenerative brain disorders, in some psychotics, and in cases of behaviour disorder. The prescription of anticonvulsants on the finding of such discharges in the EEG is unjustifiable and often illogical, and may lead the clinician to overlook more important issues for his patient.

The recognition of the epileptic nature of any symptom or group of symptoms is, I believe, a clinical task and must remain one. When the clinician requests an EEG to confirm the diagnosis he is not so much interested in the question of whether the EEG demonstrates focal discharge in the expected area—he is merely disappointed but does not alter his diagnosis if it does not—as in the question of whether the EEG demonstrates the presence of a pathological process, either local lesion or a diffuse one, which is of such importance for the prognosis. However, when the question of surgical removal of a focal epileptogenic area arises both these questions are of equal importance.

Hill continues with some advice on the proper use of the EEG. He favours the use of intravenous thiopentone for demonstrating abnormalities in background activity and quotes Pampiglione (1952) who observed that areas of damaged or dead cortex failed to develop the fast rhythms the drug induces in normal cortex. This finding, together with the capacity for thiopentone narcosis to facilitate the fixing of an epileptic focus, makes for greater accuracy in diagnosis, particularly in determining the location of discharge in temporal lobe epilepsy. Here, he advocates the use of sphenoidal leads, particularly in distinguishing between an orbital-frontal, temporal, or posterior temporal focus which may defy recordings from the scalp.

CLINICAL FEATURES

The clinical features are of paramount importance and while there is an EEG classification (see above), it is when the clinical features are understood and itemized that classification becomes helpful in diagnosis. Williams (1958) prefers the term 'ictal experience' to that of epilepsy and states that these experiences 'may include an example or a distortion of every feeling or movement of which the patient is capable, in an infinite number of variations and combinations'. Quoting from a previous paper (Williams, 1956), he gives the following classification:

FORMS OF ICTAL EXPERIENCE

Sensory Experiences

Perceptual. Illusions and Hallucinations.
Special Sensory: light, sound, smell, taste.
Common Sensory: tingling, pain, or loss of feeling.

Conceptual. Illusions and Hallucinations

Proprioceptive.
Body concept:
Partial. Limb: *e.g.* alteration in size or shape; a supernumerary limb; disturbed positions; disordered relation to whole; *i.e.* 'different', 'unreal', 'sinister', unawareness.
Total: *e.g.* depersonalization; detachment of self; autoscopy.

Exteroceptive.
Partial. Visual: *e.g.* Lilliputian, objects receding; space huge or constricted; objects distorted; objects too vivid.
Auditory: *e.g.* sounds distorted; far away; unreal or impersonal; having personal reference.
Total: Derealization; 'dreamy states'.

Mixed Proprioceptive and Exteroceptive (total conceptual disturbances)
e.g., dissonations; derealization with depersonalization; 'dreamy states' which include the person; bizarre examples: *e.g.* 'I feel the room is vast and I am in the top left-hand corner'.

Temporal Disturbances
Disturbances of 'subjective' time; *e.g.* time seems to stand still; time rushes by.
Disturbances of 'objective time'; *e.g.* people seem to move slowly, to rush along, or 'my thoughts rush by'.
Perceptual distortions, *e.g.* familiarity, déjà vu, jamais vu.

Motor Activity

Somatic (skeletal)
Incoordinate
Focal: muscle twitch.
General: tonic-clonic.
Partial: *e.g.* licking, laughing, sucking, grimacing.

Coordinate
General: quasi-purposive, *e.g.* running, striking.
Purposive: *e.g.* aggressive organized outbursts with inadequate cause.

Visceral
e.g. vasomotor, sudomotor, piloerection, cardio-respiratory, alimentary (belching, borborygmi).

Epileptic Hallucinations

Special Sensation
Unitary:
Visual: unformed or formed; stationary or animate; natural or bizarre; coloured or black-and-white; total or against normal perception.

Auditory: unformed sounds, music, words, or words with personal reference.
Olfactory: unformed.
Gustatory: unformed.

Complex:
Special sensory: *e.g.* visual hallucinations that speak. Multisensorial hallucinations.
Special sensory with perceptual change: *e.g.* 'a feeling of blue balloons in the left leg'.
Special sensory with total conceptual change: *e.g.* living an hallucinatory experience in a dreamy state.
Common sensations: *e.g.* an extra limb.
Total sensation with vision and hearing: *e.g.* autoscopy.
Emotion: mood or feeling tone; fear, depression, pleasure, unpleasure, anger—in various settings, degrees and descriptions.
Memory: always, and only as a pattern for an hallucination falling into one of the previous categories.
Thought: 'spontaneous' cognition did not occur alone in any case, though secondary cognition based on the hallucinations is described. 'Forced thinking' should be reconsidered.

It can be seen from the above that there are a large number of symptoms which would appear to be either 'functional' or closely resemble neurotic or psychotic states.

The major attack (or grand mal seizure) is unlikely to lead to any doubt in diagnosis and either a careful report from an experienced observer or personal observation should suffice, though there is still the problem of the hysterical simulation of grand mal. This condition is now quite uncommon and in differentiating the two, one can still rely on Charcot (1877) whose experience in this field was probably unrivalled. Instead of the classical features of the major fit with its tonic and clonic spasms yielding to sleep or a tranquil post-convulsive phase, the hysterical attack usually occurs in the presence of others, the convulsions are 'pseudo' and may be more complicated than the epileptic, with an accompanying emotional discharge consisting of sobbing and trembling and the attack may go on for some time. Injuries in the hysterical attack are rarely sustained and are usually minor, while urinary incontinence is almost unknown. Neurological signs, such as extensor plantars and pupillary inequalities are absent and a precipitating factor such as an emotional upset can frequently be defined. True epileptic attacks can, however, result from psychological factors, and though unusual, should nevertheless be borne in mind.

HYSTERO-EPILEPSY

This is a borderland diagnosis and was used by Charcot for those cases where it was impossible to distinguish between the hysterical and organic nature of the attack. It was not considered a reputable diagnosis and Babinski (1908) insisted that all cases could be put into one group or the other. Krapf (1957) has reviewed the problem and though not solving it, has demonstrated that it still requires further study. The EEG which was initially regarded as the acid test is now recognized to be less certain, for the very patient who would merit the label of hystero-epilepsy is likely to have a non-specific cerebral dysrhythmia. Aggressive and even inadequate psychopaths who are prone to display hysterical features also have 'abnormal' EEGs, which mainly represent defective maturation. The increasing emphasis on temporal-lobe epilepsy has brought to light a large number of EEG records which are not specific for a temporal-lobe lesion, though the patient's behaviour is very close to that of the temporal-lobe epileptic and in fact to Charcot's description of hystero-epilepsy. Furthermore psychological factors may influence the EEG record either in producing or removing abnormal rhythms.

PETIT MAL

These attacks manifest with clouding of consciousness lasting from 1 to 30 secs., with or without loss of muscle tone. The patient suddenly stops any activity in which he is engaged and resumes it when the attack is over. They occur predominantly in children, are infrequent during exercise and rarely indicate gross brain damage. It has a characteristic EEG with synchronous 3/sec. spikes and waves. Although it used to be regarded as not occurring after the age of 20 years, Schwartz and Scott (1971) reported four middle-aged patients without a personal or family history of epilepsy or psychiatric disorder who were admitted to hospital with acute confusional episodes and were diagnosed as suffering from petit mal. The authors conclude that petit mal status is a rare cause of acute confusion in middle age, benign in course and treatable by diazepam.

Another report of 'petit mal status' in adults has been presented by Novak *et al.* (1971) who studied five patients who showed the characteristic spikes and wave pattern on the EEG. The authors suspect that the condition is much commoner in the adult population than had been previously believed and suggest that many adults with petit mal status have been treated solely as psychiatric patients. Their patients differ from those of Schwartz and Scott in that they all had a previous history of epilepsy. Nevertheless their suggestion that an EEG is justified in a confused or disorientated adult with a previous history of seizure disorder is sound.

GELASTIC EPILEPSY

This is spontaneous, unprovoked and apparently uncontrollable laughter which is a rare but recognized feature of a wide range of brain disorders. It has to be distinguished from a primary psychosis as in schizophrenia or the inane giggling of the severe mental defective, or the emotional incontinence of pseudobulbar palsy and multiple sclerosis, or patients with diencephalic or hypothalamic lesions. The epileptic nature was reported by Trousseau (1873) and eventually Daly and Mulder (1937) coined the term gelastic epilepsy.

Loiseau *et al.* (1971) reviewed the literature and reported five cases. Frequently the patient cannot explain the reason for his laughter since he is amnesic for the attack, but patients who do not lose consciousness may experience the laughter as incongruous and disagreeable. The time in the attack when the laughter occurs is variable; it may be the sole or main ingredient or it can be a component of partial seizures with motor symptoms. Gelastic attacks can occur before, during or after general convulsions, flexor spasms, petit mal absences, adversive seizures, or partial temporal lobe seizures. Symptomatology may change in the course of time and occur at any age, day or night, with or without triggering, lasting from a few seconds to half an hour and with irregular and variable frequency. Interictal and ictal EEG features are also widely variable.

Clinically, disorders of laughter may be the result of stimulation due to frontal, temporal or hypothalamic tumours. The authors contend that gelastic epilepsy does not exist as an entity although ictal laughter does. They distinguish between: (1) epileptic laughter in seizures originating in the cortex and where laughter expresses emotion, and (2) epileptic laughter confined to the motor manifestation with no emotional content.

THE CONSTITUTIONAL FACTOR IN EPILEPSY

Lennox *et al.* (1940) found that 54 per cent of first degree relatives of epileptics had abnormal EEGs, compared with 6 per cent of a normal control group. In 94 per cent of a group of epileptics, one or more of the parents had EEG abnormalities. Yet when epileptic attacks are taken as the criterion only 20–30 per cent have a family history of epilepsy. The evidence would suggest that there is an inherited predisposition to fits, but these occur only under certain conditions. Rosenbaum and Maltby (1943) illustrated this in patients with eclampsia, Williams and Sweet (1944) in patients with anaesthetic convulsions, and Jennett (1962) in post-traumatic epilepsy.

ABNORMAL BEHAVIOUR IN EPILEPSY

Williams (1950) considers there are four factors which give rise to abnormalities in thought or behaviour.

1. The Fit

This may be ictal, post-ictal or replacing.

(a) **Ictal.** This is the positive result of abnormal cerebral activity and is usually aggressive and may appear either purposeful or bizarre and illogical. It can be expressed in disturbance of thought, affect or sensation and the patient may describe experiences in these fields which were due to the attack and disappear when it is over.

(b) **Post-ictal** disturbances are mainly due to the impairment of consciousness, with defects of judgment and comprehension which permit him to carry out only simple, routine acts.

(c) **Replacing** disturbances are seen during treatment. They are rare and are usually affective with depression predominating, though irritability, aggression and truculence may also occur. The affective disturbance may assume the quality of an epileptic attack, being sudden in onset, brief and stereotyped with no emotional precipitant.

2. The Causal Disease

Williams does not consider that epilepsy leads to intellectual deterioration though he admits that the intelligence of patients with symptomatic epilepsy tends to be lower than in the normal population. He states: '. . . . when intellectual defect is present in the presence of epilepsy, it is usually the result of the cerebral disorder which has caused the epilepsy'. There is, however, a difference between intellectual defect and impairment of learning, for in young children, petit mal and grand mal may interfere with learning and though not deteriorated in intelligence, their vocabulary is below that of children who do not have fits.

3. Treatment

(a) *Bromides.* These are no longer in common use, because of their low excretion rate and the large dose sometimes required to control the fits, a high serum level can occur with consequent cerebral impairment.

(b) *Barbiturates.*

(c) *Hydantoinates.*

The effect of these drugs and others are described in greater detail on page 191–200.

4. Related Neurosis

This may aggravate the frequency of attacks which in turn may make for greater difficulty in social adjustment.

The Aura

This may precede a grand mal or other attack and possesses either motor, sensory or psychic qualities and is regarded by the patient as a warning signal of an attack. It is now recognized that the aura is in fact part of the attack, but because consciousness is not lost, the patient may remember it in detail. Furthermore, it may not develop into a fully developed grand mal and the 'aura' is in fact the attack itself. The classification of Williams (1958) described above is comprehensive, though specific examples or elaboration of some of the categories may make their meaning clearer, *e.g.* 'visual; formed' could be a vase of gaily coloured flowers; 'depersonalization' is when the face of his wife and children and the sound of their voices seem strange and have an entirely new quality and although he knows it is his family he cannot accept that they are the same people. Similarly 'depression' can be elaborated in its intensity by the patient describing the feelings of hopelessness and emphasizing their similarity to those in depressive psychosis but with the difference that they last for only a few seconds.

Minor Seizures and Behaviour

Geier (1971) investigated minor epileptic seizures in an environment outside the EEG laboratory. He used a radiotelemetry system which recorded the EEG over a working day and 33 patients in all were studied. The author concluded that on the basis of this study, many clinical manifestations were functional disturbances and not deficits; that loss of consciousness is not a clinical manifestation in minor seizures; that clinical manifestations are generally briefer than the accompanying EEG paroxysms; and that all electroclinical correlations are valid only statistically and never on an individual basis.

Episodic Behavioural Disorders

Monroe (1970) claims that intermittent violent and socially disruptive behaviour results from epileptoid mechanisms and psychodynamic factors in varying combinations. He describes two types of abrupt maladaptive response: (a) episodic dyscontrol characterized by an abrupt single act or short series of acts, and (b) episodic reactions, in which there are more sustained interruptions in life flow.

Four hierarchical levels of dyscontrol are identified: seizure, instinct, impulse, and acting out. Dyscontrol at all levels may be associated with excessive neuronal discharges even when seizures are not prominent. Epileptoid mechanisms are more commonly associated with dyscontrol acts that are primitive and diffuse and which are initiated by neutral or ambiguous situations and unproductive of secondary gain. Epileptoid patients show great disparity between dyscontrol behaviour and behaviour between episodes; sensoria are more likely to be clouded during dyscontrol acts; and they are more apt to have partial recall for their dyscontrol behaviour, to accept responsibility for it but also bewildered by it and unable to explain it. Scalp EEG recording may not show excessive neuronal activity and some acute remitting schizophrenic-like psychoses with florid symptoms and intense affect may be epileptoid in nature but with normal scalp EEG.

Many of these patients have limited capacity for fantasy and meaningful introspection. They may develop defences against dyscontrol such as obsessive-compulsive symptoms or phobic avoidance of difficult situations. Long-term follow-up after adequate therapy suggests that they respond well and contribute significantly to society.

CRIME AND EPILEPSY

Though the vast majority of epileptics lead quite respectable lives, a number do commit crimes and the question arises whether this behaviour is due in some way to the epilepsy. True epilepsy in criminals is not very common, but Gibbs *et al.* (1942) found EEG abnormalities in 34 per cent of 100 unselected criminals, while Silverman (1943) reported such abnormalities in 26·7 per cent of the ordinary prison population. Stafford-Clark and Taylor (1949) did EEG studies on 64 prisoners facing charges of murder and divided their crimes into five groups, expressing the EEG abnormalities as a precentage:

	Cases	Percentage
1. Incidental killings (e.g. self-defence)	11	10
2. Clearly motivated murders (including murder during robbery)	16	25
3. Apparently motiveless or slightly motivated murders	15	73
4. Strong sexual element (e.g. rape)	8	—
5. Insane murders	14	86

The medico-legal implications of these findings are discussed in Chapter 20, but there would appear to be some evidence that cerebral dysrhythmia and crime and particularly violent crime are related. There is however further evidence that fetishism and certain compulsive acts may be associated with temporal lobe lesions and Epstein (1960) has discussed the theoretical basis of this. He considers that the temporal lobe is reponsible for organizing sexual behaviour and that instability of its mechanism releases the control and permits earlier and infantile patterns to emerge. Davies and Morganstern (1960) and Entwistle and Sim (1961) have contributed further evidence which supports this hypothesis. The author had another patient who had a compulsion for stealing minor items from a store counter and after being sentenced on more than one occasion, eventually attempted suicide and was admitted to a mental hospital. She was later discharged and as she still had her compulsion was again referred for psychiatric opinion, but on this occasion her husband volunteered that she did occasionally stiffen up in bed and further investigation revealed a tumour of the left temporal lobe. There are many such cases both in the literature and in the files of psychiatrists and neurologists and some are very strange and their fetishism, such as the patient described by Mitchell *et al.* (1954) who achieved orgasm and/or an epileptic fit by gazing at a safety-pin and was found to have a lesion in his left temporal lobe.

An interesting correction to previous studies that have suggested a close correlation between EEG disturbances and delinquency has come from Wiener *et al.* (1966) from the Mayo Clinic. They studied the EEG's of 80 delinquent boys between 13–18 years and compared them with those of 70 non-delinquent adolescents and found no significant differences between the two groups. The main observed differences were between the 13–14 years olds and the 17–18 year olds (*i.e.* irrespective of whether delinquent or not) and these were maturational in type. Age was therefore more significant than delinquency.

Epilepsy, Automatism and Crime

Gunn and Fenton (1971) quote the definition of an episode of automatic behaviour as 'a condition of impaired awareness in which an individual may perform an act or series of actions of a complex kind, the degree of awareness varying insofar as there may subsequently be complete amnesia for the incident, or, if it can be recalled, recollection is imprecise and partial'. This syndrome is characterized by abnormal activity appearing suddenly, lasting only minutes, and usually not violent in nature. The patient will probably not attempt to conceal acts undertaken during automation and there will be no amnesia for events occurring prior to loss of consciousness. It cannot be excluded by its absence during previous epileptic fits or by a normal EEG.

Automatism is frequently raised as a defence in apparently motiveless crimes, and the authors investigated this reputed association by a national survey of epileptics in Broadmoor Hospital which is a security hospital for mentally disturbed criminals. The prevalence of epilepsy in prisoners and borstals was 7–8 per 1000 men and each of the 158 prisoners identified was questioned about the offence and police and prison records were examined. Although the authors found some association between crime and epilepsy, such as seizures resulting from the stress involved in the crimes, or crimes committed during post-ictal confusion, in no case could they find convincing evidence of automatic criminal behaviour.

In Broadmoor, of 32 men with recurrent seizures, 29 were admitted as the result of criminal offences and 3 were transferred from other hospitals because of dangerously aggressive or persistently antisocial behaviour. Of the 29 who had committed offences, only 3 had a seizure within 12 hours before or after the offence. Two of the 3 committed 'automatic crimes', *i.e.* crime occurring during states of clouded consciousness following seizures. They conclude that automatic behaviour is a rare explanation for the crimes of epileptics and thus cannot account for the excess prevalence of epileptics in the prison population.

FACTORS AGGRAVATING EPILEPSY

Epilepsy can be potentiated by various agencies, such as:

1. Hypoglycaemia which either by itself or in a vulnerable person can produce fits. Frequently the blood sugar is not sufficiently low and a constitutional cerebral dysrhythmia must also be postulated.
2. Alkalosis due to excitement with consequent hyperventilation.

3. Hydration which is frequently seen after excessive beer drinking and gives rise to the erroneous assumption that the disturbed behaviour was due to alcohol.

4. Flicker and rhythmic sounds, which may account for some examples of explosive behaviour in trains or on watching a poorly adjusted television set.

Rhythmic stimulation need not always be an irritation, for it can also be soothing and Oswald (1960) has demonstrated that subjects can be sent rapidly to sleep though exposed to intense synchronous rhythmic music, electric shocks to a limb, and flashing lights to eyes glued open. But he emphasizes that the effects of rhythmic stimuli depend not only on their rate, loudness or complexity, but also on the state of the organism at the time of stimulation and the number of ways open to it to react.

Temkin (1945) states that the ancient Greeks used the phenomenon of flicker when slaves were sold in the market place, by rotating a potter's wheel in their eyes, resulting in intermittent occlusion of sunlight, and producing vertigo and seizures in vulnerable subjects. This phenomenon is used to activate discharges in patients having an EEG. Walter *et al.* (1946) were early in the field, and Bickford (1948) studying normal subjects by photic stimulation, noted that in 92 per cent the occipital frequencies could be 'driven', *i.e.* they follow the rate of flashes from the light source or stroboscope and in some the EEG disturbance spread all over the cortex. Hutchinson *et al.* (1958) describe two girls who discovered this trick for themselves and induced seizures by hand-waving against the sun, achieving a frequency of 15 flashes per second which is about that of effective stroboscopic activation. All efforts to wean the girls (aged 7 and 11 years) from the habit failed and the authors point out the erotic aspect in one of the girls.

Iatrogenic Epilepsy due to Antidepressant Drugs

Dallos and Heathfield (1969) analysed the case histories of nine patients who developed epileptic fits shortly after starting tricyclic antidepressant drugs and showed that all had one or more of the following:

(a) previous or family history of epilepsy; (b) pre-existing brain damage; (c) cerebral arteriosclerosis; (d) alcoholism; (e) withdrawal of barbiturates; and (f) a history of having had ECT.

The authors suggest that before prescribing tricyclic antidepressants these factors should be checked and if any are present prophylactic anticonvulsants are indicated. They do not regard chlordiazepoxide as adequate prophylaxis.

OTHER ASSOCIATED STATES

1. Narcolepsy was the term used by Gélineau (1880) to describe an invincible need for sleep, usually of short duration at varying intervals, but frequently several times a day and causing the patient to fall down or to lie down in order to avoid falling. The episodic nature of the condition has suggested to some an epileptic basis, but EEG studies do not show the characteristic tracing and in fact the record would pass for normal sleep. It occurs usually in young males and various aetiologies have been postulated including encephalitis, pituitary disorders and psychological factors. The standard treatment was dextro-amphetamine sulphate and doses of 50 mg. b.d. were prescribed, though it was usual to start with a smaller dose and work up as required. The danger of amphetamine addiction which is now widely recognized has led to a re-appraisal, not only of the use of amphetamine in the treatment of narcolepsy but of the nature of the condition itself. The author has had 'undoubted' cases of narcolepsy referred whose symptomatology was not as discrete as had been previously considered. There were, in addition, marked depressive features and the hypersomnia was a refuge from the depression. More effective anti-depressant treatment cleared the narcolepsy, though such was the dependence on amphetamine that hospital admission was necessary. It is the sound of the term rather than the nature of the disorder which has the greater resemblance to epilepsy.

Rechtschaffen *et al.* (1963) studied 9 narcoleptics for 1–3 nights with EEG monitoring. They showed Rapid Eye Movement periods (R.E.M.) at onset of sleep instead of 90 minutes after as in normals. They did not differ from normals in other major cyclical variations. It is difficult to know what interpretation to place on these findings, for even though there is evidence of precocious triggering of the pontine reticular formation, as the authors suggest, it does not mean that the condition is not a functional one.

Critchley (1962) described 11 adolescent males with periodic hypersomnia as well as megaphagia and claimed that only a few showed neurotic of psychopathic traits previously. The attacks occurred, on an average, every six months and would last from 5 days to a month (average, 17 days). During the phase the patients were truculent especially when aroused or even in spontaneous waking. There was also confusion which ranged from depersonalization to disorientation with upset in judgment of time and occasionally incongruous speech. There were visual and auditory hallucinations, and waking phantasies often had a crudely sexual-sadistic character and these symptoms could continue for days or weeks after the hypersomnia ended.

The feeding problem was more that of compulsive eating rather than bulimia. The EEG was diffusely abnormal. The author admits the difficulty in defining an aetiology and does not rule out the possibility that it may all be functional.

2. **Cataplexy** is related to narcolepsy and the two may co-exist. The patient suddenly loses power and tone in skeletal muscles and sinks helplessly to the ground and although not unconscious, may be unable to speak. It is frequently precipitated by strong emotional experiences, particularly laughter, though it can follow anger and irritation.

3. **Epileptic Psychoses.** This term has been applied to patients who have established epilepsy and who present psychotic features, and also to episodic psychotic states as described by Kleist (1926). Before the advent of EEG studies many of these patients would not have been classed as epileptic but as periodic psychoses. But some did show disturbances of consciousness followed by amnesia, though the psychiatric picture varied, with hallucinations, grandiosity and catatonic features predominating. Gibbs *et al.* (1938) investigated some of these episodic psychoses with the EEG and found that when affective and schizophrenic forms were present, a temporal lobe lesion could be demonstrated, and Hill (1952) found paroxysmal EEG patterns in periodic catatonia. In these patients it was frequently impossible to distinguish them clinically from the 'functional' psychoses, mainly schizophrenia, yet 'process schizophrenics' do not show such gross cerebral dysrhythmia. There may be other factors operating, for Crammer (1959) has shown that many of these periodic psychoses are associated with water retention. Unsuitable drug therapy may also produce psychotic patterns with abnormal EEG patterns.

Slater and Beard (1963) made a detailed study of 69 patients with epilepsy and schizophrenia and arrived at the following conclusions.

1. The combination of the two conditions was not an accidental one but was indicative of a true relationship.

2. Pre-morbid personality was in general normal and there was no predominance of schizoid traits as one would expect to find in a group of schizophrenic patients.

3. Mean age of onset of psychosis was 29·8 years and the mean duration of the epilepsy was 14·1 years. The duration of the epilepsy

was related to the onset of the psychotic features.

4. There was an inverse relationship between the frequency of fits and the psychotic symptoms. In fact, many did not become psychotic until the epilepsy was controlled.

5. The onset was insidious in 29 and the psychosis was episodic in 20. In 31 the psychosis became chronic.

6. In all but 2 there were typical schizophrenic delusions while hallucinations, mainly auditory, in a setting of clear consciousness occurred in 52. Flatness of emotion was present in 28, thought disorder in 31, disturbed volition and catatonic features in 40. The authors state there was '. . . not one of the cardinal symptoms of schizophrenia which has not been exhibited at some time by these patients'.

7. Forty-five had their origin in the temporal lobe and of the 11 who had temporal lobectomies, all benefited as far as the fits were concerned but in only a few did the psychosis improve, while there was a heavy incidence of organic personality changes.

8. The 7 patients with centrencephalic epilepsy were predominantly hebephrenic.

4. **Epileptic Personality**. This concept has arisen largely from observation on institutionalized epileptics and it is difficult to decide whether the features associated with the condition are all based on the epilepsy or the prolonged stay in the institution. Some are undoubtedly associated with the epilepsy such as explosive and violent behaviour with frequent quarrelling and fighting, although unsuitable drugs, particularly barbiturates in temporal lobe epilepsy have been incriminated. Some are very religiose, avid readers of their Bibles, and ingratiating to the medical staff, but may be extremely troublesome, if not violent towards the nursing staff.

Deterioration in intellect and behaviour may be an accompaniment of epilepsy though it is generally considered to be due to the pathological process causing the epilepsy. The psychotic features are frequently schizophrenic-like and the deterioration in behaviour may be put down to this process rather than to the epilepsy. It is possible, however, by treating the latter aspect to effect occasionally some improvement which may even be dramatic, again emphasizing the need for full investigation, including EEG, in patients who may be labelled as chronic schizophrenics.

Patients with epilepsy have much greater difficulty in social adjustment than other sick people and even though employers may be enlightened and seek to offer them sheltered work in industry, their workmates are frequently hostile and cannot tolerate the spectacle of an epileptic fit and demand their removal, which means dismissal. It is not surprising that some epileptics are therefore resentful of society's attitude and this may well condition their own attitude and contribute to their social misconduct. They frequently attempt suicide, usually by taking an overdose of their anti-convulsant drugs, but occasionally by other methods such as gassing, and they constitute a fair percentage of habitual attempters of suicide, thus indicating their general insecurity, isolation and longing for a milieu where they are treated with loving care and understanding. It is a pity that their 'appeals' must produce a state of dangerous loss of consciousness in order to achieve this objective. A few may become addicted to their anticonvulsants, particularly the barbiturate group, and some cases of 'attempted suicide' in epileptics may result from over-indulgence.

Déjà Vu

This is a symptom which occurs in a variety of conditions but it is becoming increasingly identified with disturbances of the temporal lobe. Efron (1963) studied 12 patients with left hemisphere lesions and considered that it may be attributable to a disturbance of the 'time-labelling' mechanism. If the delay in transmission from right to left hemisphere were, for a period of a minute, delayed by several hundred milliseconds, the left hemisphere would receive information (essentially the same) twice, once directly and the second time relayed after this delay from the right hemisphere. The data are essentially identical and it does not seem unreasonable to assume that the person may believe unconsciously that everything he is presently perceiving has already occurred.

When delayed transmission has persisted for a few seconds, the subject has more information and then realizes that a series of events is apparently occurring twice or that he is merely anticipating what will occur. The author suggests that this could explain some acts of clairvoyance and that his theory could be tested during neurosurgical operations with local anaesthesia applied to the corpus callosum. It is certainly a most plausible explanation of the phenomenon and will no doubt be put to the test

TREATMENT OF EPILEPSY

The pharmacological era in the treatment of epilepsy started about the middle of the nineteenth century and Merritt (1958) reminds us that on the occasion of the presentation of a paper on the treatment of epilepsy by E.H. Sieveking before the London Medico-Chirurgical Society on 11th May, 1857, '. . . Sir Charles Locock, the presiding officer, remarked that, since the seizures in epilepsy were often related to hysteria or the menses, he had been led to try bromide of potassium. . . In 14 or 15 additional cases bromides had failed in only one' (Sieveking, 1857; Locock, 1957). Bromides held the field till Hauptmann (1912) introduced phenobarbitone which in its turn was considered supreme till Merritt and Putnam (1938) introduced diphenylhydantoin. Merritt (1958) divides treatment into three parts: (1) removal of any factors, organic or psychological, that may be contributing to the seizures; (2) regulation of the physical and mental hygiene; and (3) administration of anticonvulsants, but adds that the ideal anticonvulsant, namely, one which would control all types of seizures, have an established dosage and have no undesirable side-effects, is not yet available, so combinations of drugs have to be used.

A wide choice is available, but those most commonly used are derivatives of barbituric acid, hydantoin or oxazolidinedione. The first two are cyclic derivatives of urea, while the third resembles hydantoin, though not a urea derivative.

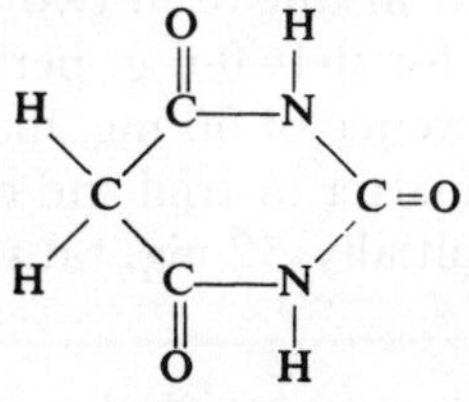

Malonylurea
(Barbituric acid)

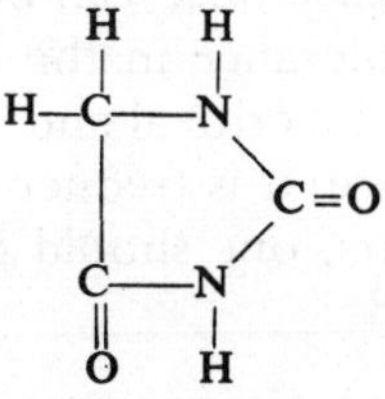

Glycolyl urea
(Hydantoin)

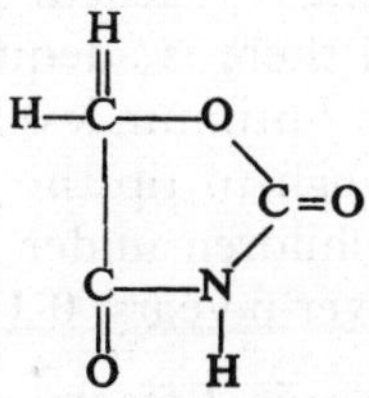

Oxazolidinedione

ADMINISTRATION OF DRUGS

Bromides have gone out of fashion, but there are still some who claim that they should remain the sheet anchor of treatment and they are certainly comparatively safer, less expensive and not as likely to be used in the impulsive attempts at suicide to which some epileptics are prone. Those drugs which are now in general use are phenytoin sodium and phenobarbitone as they are considered to be relatively free of undesirable side-effects.

Phenobarbitone

Dosage. *For adults:* Start with 0·1 g. as a single dose before bed-time and increase to 0·4 g. in divided doses if necessary. More than this is likely to produce toxic effects.

For children: If over 2 years the regime is as for the adult. Below 2 years the dose is computed on body weight.

Toxic Effects are: (a) Drowsiness and lethargy, for which dextroamphetamine can be given (5–20 mg. per day).

(b) Rashes on various parts of the body or at times generalized. Antihistamines are effective in their control.

(c) Ataxia.

(d) Nystagmus.

Armitage and Sim (1960) describe some of these symptoms in patients who are hypersensitive to barbiturates and where the condition had simulated labyrinthine disturbances and mesencephalitis.

Phenytoin Sodium

Dosage. Give 0·1 g. two to three times per day, preferably after meals, and increase by 0·1 g. at weekly intervals till the optimum effect is reached. The daily dose can be given in one or in two parts and there is adequate tolerance in the adult for 0·4–0·6 g. per day. The optimum level may be critical and a difference of 50 mg. may be enough to tip the balance; it is frequently a matter of trial and error. In children under 6 years, one should give initially 32 mg. t.d.s. and if over 6 years, 0·1 g. b.d.

Toxic Effects are: (a) Gastric upset with nausea in the initial stages, but giving the drug at meal time may help to counteract it.

(b) Transient insomnia with unsteadiness of gait occurs in the first few days, but later subsides.

(c) Nystagmus is common, but it is only when associated with diplopia and ataxia that the dose need be reduced to half and then gradually built up again at just below the dose which produced the toxic signs.

(d) Hypertrophy of the gums which varies from slight puffiness and sponginess to severe hyperplasia. Dental hygiene can help and occasionally gingivectomy is necessary.

(e) Hirsutism, which can be very distressing to young girls as it does not disappear with cessation of the drug.

(f) Allergic reactions, including rashes which are either morbilliform and generalized, occurring 10–14 days after the start of treatment, or an exfoliative dermatitis which can occur at any time.

The emergence of these rashes would suggest withdrawal of the drug, as does pyrexia and polyarthritis.

(g) Megaloblastic anaemia.

Methoin

Dosage. When used alone 0·4–1 g., starting with 0·1 g. t.d.s. and increasing by 0·1 g. daily. If used in conjunction with other drugs 0·1 g. per day and increased by 0·1 g. per week till the desired effect is reached. In children under 6 years, half doses are prescribed.

Toxic Effects are: (a) Drowsiness, which may be severe enough to discontinue the drug.

(b) Allergic skin reactions which can also indicate withdrawal.

(c) Blood dyscrasias, including agranulocytosis, pancytopaenia and aplastic anaemia, usually occurring in the first few months of treatment and occasionally fatal. Frequent blood checks are therefore essential.

Primidone

Dosage. Start with 0·25 g. per day and increase by 0·25 g. weekly and an effective dose is usually 0·75–1·5 g. daily. Children require half the adult dose.

Toxic Effects are: Drowsiness, nausea, vomiting, dizziness and ataxia, which usually settle in time, withdrawal being rarely necessary. The drug is generally used in combination with phenytoin sodium.

Acetazolamide (Diamox)

This is a carbonic acid anhydrase inhibitor as well as being an acidifier and dehydrator.

Dosage. Start with 0·25 g. t.d.s. and increase by 0·25 g. weekly to 1 g. t.d.s.

Toxic Effects are: Drowsiness, agranulocytosis, thrombocytopenic and renal lesions.

Phenacemide (Phenurone)

Dosage. Start with 0·5 g. t.d.s. and gradually increase to 2–3 g. per day. Children require half the dose of adults.

Toxic Effects are: Personality disturbance with psychotic features, toxic hepatitis and blood dyscrasias which may be fatal. Frequent blood examinations and liver function tests are essential, and previous liver damage or mental disturbance would contra-indicate its use. Nausea, vomiting, rashes and drowsiness may also occur, but these are not nearly so serious as the previous group.

Troxidone (Tridione)

Dosage. Start with 0·3 g. t.d.s. and increase gradually to 1·5–3 g. per day. In children under 2 years start with 0·15 g. t.d.s. and increase gradually by 0·15 g.; it is primarily used in the treatment of petit mal.

Toxic Effects. (a) Photophobia, drowsiness and nausea which are minor in nature and usually settle.

(b) Rashes are common and may be morbilliform or urticarial and would suggest withdrawing the drug, although it may be resumed, but cautiously.

(c) Aplastic anaemia, agranulocytosis and nephrosis which may be fatal, therefore frequent medical, including blood, examinations are essential.

(d) Transient leucopaenia may settle without withdrawal, but careful supervision is required.

Carbamazepine (Tegretol)

This is a dibenzazepine derivative of the following constitution:

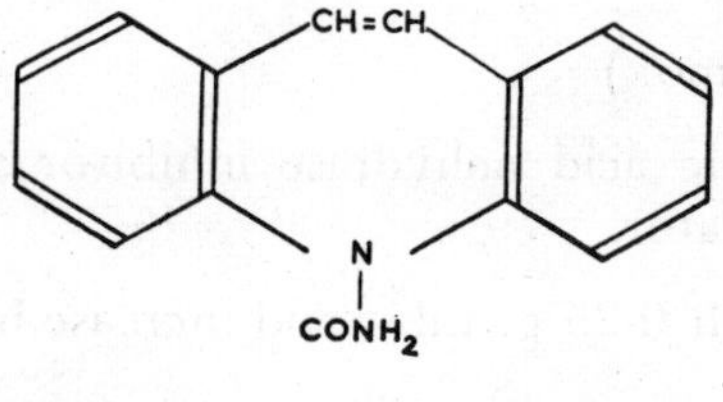

CH=CH

N

$CONH_2$

This drug has proved useful in the treatment of grand mal and temporal lobe epilepsy as well as of trigeminal neuralgia but it is reputed to be less effective in the treatment of petit mal. It has been used as a substitute for other drugs when these were proving ineffective but it has also been used as an adjunct to therapy without any evidence of incompatibility. It has proved helpful in the control of a hitherto intractable problem, the epileptic personality, with aggression, suspicion, hostile and paranoid features. This psychotropic effect has been attributed to its chemical resemblance to imipramine.

Dosage. *For adults:* Initially ½–1 tablet (200 mg.) once or twice a day, followed by a slow increase until the best response is obtained. In some instances this may need 1600 mg. daily but the usual adult dose is 4–6 tablets (800–1200 mg.) daily.

For children: Age up to 1 year–½–1 tablet per day.
1– 5 years–1–2 tablets per day.
5–10 „ 2–3 „ „
10–15 „ 3–5 „ „

Side-effects. Dizziness may occur especially if dosage is not graduated. Other side effects are drowsiness, dry mouth, diarrhoea, nausea, and vomiting but these are rare and seldom severe. Three per cent of patients may be sensitive to carbamazepine and react with a generalized erythematous rash and one case of light sensitivity has been reported but it disappeared on stopping the drug. Three cases of jaundice have been recorded but these too cleared on cessation of therapy. Two fatal cases and one non-fatal case of aplastic anaemia have been reported in elderly women receiving treatment for trigeminal neuralgia, so blood counts should be carried out routinely.

Other drugs which can be used in the treatment of petit mal should tridone fail are paramethadione (Paradione) and phensuximide (Milontin) and new ones are constantly being produced. It is a matter of debate whether the psychiatrist should concern himself with the specialized treatment of the epileptic for most do not present as psychiatric problems. In Britain where psychiatry is separated from neurology, epileptics tend to be referred to neurologists, though some psychiatrists who have become expert in electro-encephalography do practise as 'epileptologists' and while one can appreciate some of the reasons for this, it should be realized that epileptic seizures result from an infinite variety of pathological processes which the neurologist should be more capable of investigating and treating than the psychiatrist. In those countries where the two specialities are combined as neuro-psychiatry, practitioners no doubt have the necessary training to investigate and treat expertly all forms of epilepsy.

RECENT DEVELOPMENTS IN DRUG TREATMENTS

Calne (1973) reviews the mechanism of action, the pharmacokinetics, the drug interactions and estimations of anticonvulsant concentrations in the blood.

Mechanism of Action

The ability to induce experimental models of epilepsy in animals allowed new compounds to be tested for anticonvulsant activity. Methods used are: (a) the application of electric shocks to the head; (b) systematic administration of drugs that produce fits, *e.g.* bicuculline, leptazol and picrotoxin; and (c) the implantation of irritative material into the cerebral cortex, e.g. penicillin and metallic cobalt. While these methods help in developing new drugs, more elaborate techniques are required to elucidate the mechanism of drug action.

Two categories of activity must be considered:

1. Effects on pathological neurons (the epileptic focus), discharge of which initiates the seizure.
2. Effect on normal neurons to prevent their activation by the epileptic focus.

There is no convincing evidence that anticonvulsants significantly inhibit discharge from the pathological neurons that constitute a seizure focus, but anticonvulsants such as phenytoin suppress post-tetanic potentiation, *i.e.* the enhancement of synaptic transmission normally observed after a rapidly repetitive volley of impulses. Such action may help to block the spread of an abnormal discharge from an epileptic focus. Certain anticonvulsants stabilize the normal axonal membrane and suppress the increased irritability induced by hypocalcaemia.

They can also modify the concentration of neurotransmitters in the brain, *e.g.* phenytoin augments gamma aminobutyric acid (GABA) concentration which is a probable transmitter associated with inhibition. This reduces the concentration of glutamic acid which may also be a transmitter with excitatory actions. The convulsant alkaloid bicuculline blocks the inhibitory action of GABA suggesting that further investigation of neurotransmitter function may prove a useful approach in the development of new anticonvulsants.

Pharmacokinetics

Absorption. The majority of anticonvulsants have high lipid solubility and a pKa that allows absorption of non-ionized drug by passive diffusion through the mucosa. The site of absorption for individual anticonvulsants is determined by local pH changes in the gastrointestinal tract, phenytoin being largely absorbed in the distal duodenum.

Distribution. After absorption, anticonvulsants enter the blood stream and a proportion becomes bound to plasma protein. Phenytoin is rapidly taken up by the central nervous system, fat and skeletal muscle, the concentration being higher in the brain, where it is bound to microsomes, than in the plasma. While it is largely metabolized by the liver, 10 per cent is excreted unchanged in the bile, and this fraction together with some excreted in the saliva is reabsorbed from the duodenum.

Metabolism. Phenytoin and phenobarbitone are extensively degraded to inactive products and are metabolized in the liver mainly by hydroxylation in the para position of the phenyl group. The hydroxylated products do not suppress fits though other metabolites are active, *e.g.* primidone is metabolized to phenobarbitone.

Excretion. The major metabolites of phenytoin and phenobarbitone are formed in the liver and discharged via the bile into the gut. Reabsorption from the intestine leads to their ultimate excretion in the urine.

Drug Interactions

Shared Enzymes. As the hepatic hydroxylation pathway is shared by many drugs there are two important sequelae:

1. Chronic administration of certain drugs, such as phenobarbitone, can induce increase of the enzymes concerned with their own metabolism (augmented hepatic hydroxylation) and as the same enzymes are employed in the metabolism of other drugs, such as phenytoin, repeated administration of phenobarbitone to a patient receiving phenytoin can lead to an increase in the rate of metabolism of phenytoin with a consequent fall in its plasma concentration. There are wide individual variations in enzyme production.
2. Drugs may compete for available enzymes with increase in plasma concentration and resulting toxicity. Drugs which reduce the rate of metabolism of phenytoin are sulthiane, isoniazid, aminosalicylic acid and cycloserine.

Protein Binding. Salicylic acid, sulphafurazole and phenylbutazone may produce a transient increase in free phenytoin by displacing it from protein in the plasma.

Estimation of Plasma Concentrations

This allows the monitoring of drug interactions as well as the detection and quantification of toxicity due to overdosage. The epileptic who is not taking his drugs can be easily detected, though a low plasma level does not necessarily mean that the patient is failing to take his drugs. The relationship between dose ingested and plasma concentration displays very considerable variations between patients because of individual differences in the rate of drug metabolism. The usual therapeutic, non-toxic range for phenytoin is 10–20 mg per ml.

Practical Therapeutics

Calne puts forward the following principles:

1. A history of one fit is an indication for investigation (EEG, skull X-ray and possibly brain scan). It is not usual practice to start treatment until a second seizure occurs, because of the difficulty in predicting the risk of repeated attacks on the basis of a single episode.
2. Once drug therapy has been started, it should be continued for 2-3 years.
3. Any change in treatment should be gradual. Anticonvulsants should never be stopped abruptly because of the risk of status epilepticus.
4. A minimum number of drugs should be employed because of the risk of interactions.

SUGGESTED TREATMENT
(for a 70 kg. adult).

Grand Mal and Focal Epilepsy (including Temporal Lobe Epilepsy)

Phenytoin (200 mg. daily) or phenobarbitone (90 mg. daily) is usually given initially. The dose is slowly increased till seizures are controlled or adverse reactions are encountered. If neither drug is satisfactory alone, they may be combined.

If these drugs fail, primidone may be added or substituted for phenobarbitone. Sedation may occur on low doses of primidone, so the effect of a single dose of 125 mg. should be observed before building up to normal levels (750 mg.–1·5 g./day). Other drugs which may be useful in refractory grand mal or focal epilepsy include carbanazepine, methylphenobarbitone, methoin and ethotoin. Pheneturide, phenacemide and sulthiane are occasionally helpful but are more likely to produce adverse reactions. Women who have fits associated with menstruation may benefit from short courses (5 days) of chlorothiazide or acetazolamide starting three days before each period.

Adverse Reactions. Sedation, depression, posterior fossa signs, *e.g.* nystagmus, intention tremor, ataxia and even external ocular palsies, gingival hypertrophy and hirsutism are frequently encountered on prolonged phenytoin therapy. Megaloblastic anaemia and low serum and red cell concentrations of folate may be found, though the exact mechanism of this induced folate deficiency is not known. It was reported that if folic acid were given to patients receiving anticonvulsants, the fits increased in frequency, but this has not been confirmed. Folate deficiency should be corrected by supplements, having excluded B_{12} deficiency.

Hypocalcaemia and osteomalacia may occasionally be found because of the accelerated breakdown of calciferol in the liver consequent upon enzyme induction, and calciferol supplements are helpful. Occasionally allergic adverse reactions occur, such as skin eruptions, blood dyscrasias, lymphadenopathy (occasionally acute, like glandular fever), systemic lupus erythematosus and pulmonary fibrosis. CSF protein may be raised in phenytoin intoxication. Although phenytoin, phenobarbitone and primidone are not without toxic effects they are comparatively low risk drugs and are therefore the most popular.

Petit Mal and its Variants

Dose Regimens. Ethosuximide is the most satisfactory drug. An initial dose of 250 mg. twice daily may be built up to 1·75 g./day if necessary. It may aggravate grand mal which would therefore require treatment as described above. Should ethosuximide be ineffective, troxidone or paramethadione may be tried (300 mg.—2·1 g./day for either drug). Short courses of acetazolamide (250 mg.—1·0 g./day are sometimes useful.

Adverse Reactions. These are rare with ethosuximide but troxidone and paramethadone often cause sedation, skin eruptions and hemeralopia (blurred vision in bright light). More rarely they can induce blood dyscrasias and hepatic or renal damage.

The aim in treatment is to reduce the attacks to an acceptable level. Attempts to abolish petit mal completely often result in complex toxic drug reactions.

Major Status Epilepticus

This is the occurrence of fits in which the patient fails to regain consciousness between attacks, and is different from *serial epilepsy* where consciousness between attacks is regained, which is treated as for grand mal. Paraldehyde 5 ml. by deep intramuscular injection in each buttock using a glass syringe (plastic may react adversely) is effective but reactions at site of injection may produce sterile abscesses or even sloughing of tissues.

Diazepam is the modern alternative or supplement. Intravenous injection of 10 mg. at a rate of one minute should be followed by an intravenous infusion of 100 mg. in 500 ml. of normal saline at a rate which is just sufficient to control the fits. Particular care of the airway is indicated to avoid lingual obstruction due to the muscle relaxant action of diazepam.

If other attempts fail, thiopentone given slowly (25–100 mg.) followed by infusion of 1 g. in 500 ml. at a minimal rate to control the fits is very useful. Facilities for tracheal intubation and assisted ventilation should be at hand when using intravenous diazepam or thiopentone. Should cardiovascular or respiratory depression result from a prolonged status epilepticus, curarization with intermittent positive pressure with continuing anticonvulsant therapy and EEG monitoring will be necessary. Phenobarbitone 50–100 mg. by repeated intramuscular injection may be used to supplement treatment.

From the above description it is obvious that status epilepticus can be a grave medical emergency with a mortality around 10 per cent. The commonest errors in management are: inadequate anticonvulsant dosage, premature change from parenteral to oral therapy and failure to define the underlying cause, which is often a cerebral tumour, infarct or infection.

Infantile Spasm and Hypsarrhythmia

These responded poorly to conventional anticonvulsants but now prednisone 10–40 mg./day or ACTH have been encouraging. Nitrazepam up to 1 mg./kg./day has also been successful, particularly with hypsarrhythmia.

SURGICAL TREATMENTS OF EPILEPSY

These can be divided into three major groups:

Ablation

(a) *Local Decortication and Gyrectomy*. This is used for epilepsy of focal origin, and Penfield (1947) stressed the importance of removing not only the cicatrix, if any, but sufficient surrounding area of brain to ensure that all actual or potential epileptogenic neurones had been ablated.

(b) *Hemidecortication or Hemispherectomy.* The latter implies the removal of all the cortex and white matter lateral to the basal ganglia, and was first introduced in 1926 for the treatment of selected cases of malignant cerebral glioma. The first operation for an epileptic was done in 1936 and Krynauw (1950) laid down the classical indications and contraindications. The ideal candidate would be an infant, child or young adult with a severe infantile hemiplegia, crippling and drug-resistant epilepsy and unmanageable behaviour disorder, but also educable, of stable social and domestic background, and either not institutionalized or with a high potential for socioeconomic reintegration. There should also be neuroradiological evidence that only one hemisphere is diseased.

The pathology can be diverse and is prognostically unimportant unless the diffuse nature of the damage from anoxia or infection may have affected the other hemisphere. Results can be most rewarding, and the author has seen a good result in a 17-year-old youth who fulfilled the above criteria for selection. Unfortunately there is a high incidence of late morbidity and mortality, in that a third of patients operated on develop chronic intracranial haemorrhage with hydrocephalus of the remaining hemisphere and in a few instances haemosiderosis of the CNS. These sequelae affect good and bad results alike, and may not occur for many years; they are lethal if unrecognized or untreated so careful follow-up is essential.

2. Callosotomy

As the corpus callosum is the largest and most obvious pathway for spread of ictal discharges from one hemisphere to another, open division of part or all of it would appear logical, and the operation was introduced by Van Wagenen and Herren (1940). Luessenhop *et al.* (1970) advocated stereotaxic callosotomy for children, since patients without severe hemiplegia need not be excluded. The operation is well tolerated apart form 'split-brain' deficit which is more apparent under the artificial conditions of psychometric testing, because of the blocking of interhemispheric transfer of auditory-verbal and visuo-spatial information. Less extensive attacks have been made on the fornix and commissures.

3. Stereotactic Procedures

The use of these methods in the treatment of epilepsy has been described as the destruction of a dispensable volume of excitable neurones. Popular targets include thalamus, globus pallidus, ansa lenticularis, amygdala, fornix and the field of Forel. Lesions in one area can be combined with lesions in another, unilateral or bilateral, congruous or incongruous and even enlarged subsequently. Wilson (1973) commenting on these procedures states: 'Cases are so far rather few, so that reports tend to be anecdotal. Clinical protocols are heterogeneous. Techniques are idiosyncratic. Criteria for post-operative assessment are sometimes imprecise or elastic. Periods of follow-up are as yet short. The very lesions are for the most part presumed rather than proved to be on target because, despite lesion monitoring by target stimulation, microelectrode recording, and microbiopsy, the only unassailable evidence of the size and accuracy of any stereotactic lesion is that provided by autopsy'.

SURGICAL TREATMENT OF THE TEMPORAL LOBE

This is used in the treatment of focal epilepsy and Penfield (1958), in an autobiographical note, said that he first made experimental wounds to study the healing process in 1922, did his first operation to remove an area of scarred brain in 1927, and in 1928 visited and collaborated with Foerster in Breslau. He states '. . . Most neurosurgeons have learned to live dangerously. They seem to like it. But the surgery of atrophic epileptogenic lesions has a special set of hazards. . . .'

As far as the psychiatrist is concerned, it is the surgical treatment of *psychomotor* epilepsy which is of interest, for he is frequently consulted on these problems and it may occasionally be his responsibility to diagnose and refer them to the neurosurgeon. Before one can begin to understand the implications of surgery, a knowledge of the neuroanatomical and neurophysiological background is essential and the following description is quoted from the account by Turner (1962) who in addition includes a helpful historical note.

The first descriptions of psychomotor epilepsy by Hughlings Jackson laid the foundation for many of the subsequent developments. The clinical manifestations of sensory hallucinations, disturbances of consciousness, dreamy states, automatisms and amnesia were described and were related to focal lesions in the antero-medial portion of the temporal lobe. It had been appreciated that epileptic 'variants' could include affective, psychical and visceral disturbances (Wilson, 1955), but it was not until the recognition of the EEG changes denoting focal epilepsy affecting the temporal lobes (Gibbs, Gibbs & Lennox, 1937; Gibbs, Gibbs & Fuster, 1948; Gibbs & Gibbs, 1950), that the full variety of epilepsies attributable to focal disease of the temporal lobes became apparent. Diagnosis was further clarified by the use of sphenoidal electrodes impinging on the outside of the skull over the temporal poles (Jasper, 1949*a*; Jones, 1951; Kerridge, 1952). Barbiturate anaesthesia was helpful or necessary to demonstrate the presence of focal discharges (Gibbs & Gibbs, 1947) while the absence of pentothal fast activity in an area denoted underlying damage (Pampiglione, 1952).

The methods of surgical investigation and treatment pursued over many years by Penfield (Penfield & Jasper, 1954) involved operations under local anaesthesia, corticography, recording from deep electrodes, and stimulation to produce the actual type of attack complained of. Wider excisions to prevent recurrence led to unilateral removal of the anterior third of the affected temporal lobe (Bailey & Gibbs, 1951; Bailey *et al.*, 1953; Green *et al.*, 1951). Bilateral lobectomy was considered to be unwarranted after reports of severe personality changes by Terzian and Dalle Ore (1955) and Petit-Dutaillis *et al.* (1954), though limited bilateral anterior temporal lobectomy did not always give rise to marked personality changes comparable with the Klüver-Bucy syndrome in monkeys (Klüver & Bucy, 1938). Effects on memory were described by Scoville and Milner (1957), if bilateral damage to the hippocampus were caused posterior to the uncus. Recall of recent memories was grossly impaired, though associative memory was preserved. Because of the impossibility of always limiting operative damage to the particular structures aimed at in the deeply-placed region, bilateral temporal lobectomy on the medial structures is still considered to be unsafe by the majority of surgeons in this field.

Pathological studies clarified some problems, but introduced fresh difficulties. Falconer *et al.* (1955) surveyed 31 cases treated by unilateral lobectomy and concluded that the beneficial results were due to inclusion of the uncus, Ammon's horn and possibly the amgydaloid nucleus in the resection. It was in the anterior and medial structures of the lobe that the main pathological changes were found (Earle *et al.*, 1953; Meyer *et al.*, 1954) and the importance of removal of these deep structures was stressed by Penfield and Jasper (1954) and Rasmussen and Jasper (1957). The pathological changes described consisted of either diffuse sclerosis or small tumours or glial hamartomas, large tumours being excluded from most series (Earle *et al.*, 1953; Falconer *et al.*, 1958). . . Kennedy and Hill (1958) reported on the results of lobectomy in 50 cases, and found that sclerosis of Ammon's horn, the uncus and the white matter of the temporal lobe was correlated with reduction of barbiturate-induced fast rhythm as shown by sphenoidal leads. Pathological changes in the uncus and Ammon's horn were accompanied by a less active contralateral spike focus (less than 1 to 4 in frequency) at the other temporal lobe, but this did not alter the favourable prognosis attached to operative treatment by unilateral lobectomy. Kendrick and Gibbs (1957), however, stated that in general only one out of four cases was rendered free of seizures by unilateral lobectomy. Falconer (1961) described seven cases in which a verified tumour in one temporal lobe gave rise to bilateral independent spike-discharging foci. This underlined the difficulty of determining by EEG means whether a focal discharge arose in the place where it was detected or was arriving there by reason of an abnormality elsewhere. Presumably in these cases the path of spread was by the anterior commissure, as otherwise it should have been picked up also in frontal or midline structures.

Concepts of neuroanatomy were evolving following the critical review of Bailey and von Bonin (1951) which replaced unsupportable subdivisions of tiny cortical areas by wide cortical zones with constant distinctive histological characteristics. One of these was the allocortical areas which MacLean (1952) grouped together as the limbic lobe or 'visceral brain'. They included the frontal base, medial and anterior temporal cortex, hippocampus and the cingulate gyri. From them, autonomic changes could be elicited by stimulation. The discovery of a diffuse projection from caudal structures to wide if not ubiquitous areas of cortex (Forbes & Morison, 1939; Morison *et al.*, 1941; Morison & Dempsey, 1942; Jasper, 1949*b*; Moruzzi & Magoun, 1949) supplied one essential connection for the development of a dynamic theory of total cerebral function. Demonstration of descending influences from cortex to diffuse projections (Wall & Davis, 1951; Segundo *et al.*, 1955; French *et al.*, 1955) completed the circuit. The concept that emerged was of different cortical areas competing for the central neuronal pool of the diffuse projection systems. Many of the descending pathways came from cortical areas that had also an autonomic effect on stimulation and a connection with temperamental traits when ablated. Interest was directed for a time on the amygdaloid nucleus, but it emerged that the most profound effects of stimulation on autonomic functions and aggression were not elicited from this nucleus (Chapman, 1958; Jasper & Rasmussen, 1958), but from adjacent parts including cortex over the uncus, hippocampal gyrus, the tail of the caudate nucleus, stria terminalis and radiations of the temporal lobe (Poirier & Shulman, 1954). A single small lesion placed symmetrically in the fibres passing through the temporal isthmus through the tail of the caudate nucleus dorsal to the temporal horn produced marked loss of aggression, whereas lesions in the amygdaloid nucleus had comparatively little effect (Turner, 1954). In addition to temporothalamic connections (Fox, 1949) this area contained connections between temporal lobe structures and the tectum of the mid-brain (Poirier, 1952; Whitlock & Nauta, 1956; Bucy & Klüver, 1955). Known connections included those from the amygdaloid nucleus via the stria terminalis to the septal region by the inferior thalamic peduncle to the dorsomedial nucleus of thalamus and by Arnold's fasiculus to the pulvinar; also from the temporal pole to the superior colliculus, zona incerta, tegmentum of the mid-brain (Klingler & Gloor, 1960), ventral parts of the putamen and the pulvinar. Medical and lateral temporo-tectal tracts were thought by Poirier (1952) to pass from the inferior temporal and hippocampal gyri.

Implication of posterior basal frontal cortex in the abnormalities discovered in psychomotor epilepsy was found by Kendrick and Gibbs (1957) who found spike discharges in these regions also in schizophrenic patients. Both areas form part of the same allocortical region of Bailey and von Bonin. Kennedy (1959) described attacks resembling psychomotor epilepsy from pathological changes in parasagittal regions on the medial surface and superior border of the hemisphere in the limbic lobe of MacLean. The hippocampus itself was thought for a time to subserve emotional and temperamental functions, but this was not confirmed by certain experimental observations with stimulation (Jasper & Rasmussen, 1958) or ablation (Pribram & Fulton, 1954). Its relationship with recall of especially recent memory, however, was not seriously questioned by reports and experience subsequent to that of Scoville and Milner (1957) and further support for this view was given by Russell and Esper (1961) in their study of penetrating wounds of the brain.

Turner (1963), the author of the above extensive quotation,

reports *bilateral* temporal lobotomies on 38 cases of psychomotor epilepsy who had proved intractable to medical treatment and who nearly all presented severe temperamental disturbances. The social history of many of the patients was poor with impaired work records, long spells of unemployment and disturbed relations with society, sometimes to the point of impending imprisonment or confinement in a mental hospital. He used three types of operation, reporting most fully on the first, which was performed on all cases and which consisted of a quadrantic cut through the roof of the temporal horn one centimetre from the tip. The criteria for operation were focal discharges at one or both temporal bases, together with a clinical history of major psychomotor attacks intractable to thorough medical treatment, often with temperamental or personality disorder in the form of ungovernable rage, or less commonly with attacks of fear and depression in the post-ictal periods.

Results showed a 'substantial though not spectacular improvement in grand mal attacks', but the work records did not usually improve. The unemployed usually remained unemployed and some who had an aggressive and energetic attitude to work seemed to lose their stimulus. Temperamental effects were on the whole beneficial and 'spouses who had previously been viciously assaulted' were now grateful towards the operation, but other psychiatric features such as hypochondriasis, depression and psychopathic trends 'were not improved or were assentuated'. He concludes that lobotomy through the temporal isthmus in the roof of the ventricle virtually abolished temperamental disturbances, especially in the form of attacks of uncontrollable rage and violence.

SOCIAL ASPECTS

Brief reference has already been made to the social problems of epilepsy but Cohen (1958), who discusses the problem according to the age groups affected and the social implications, underlines the practical issues.

The Infant and Pre-school Child

The doctor should be able to discuss treatment and prognosis with the parents. Not every fit in childhood means life-long epilepsy and 75 per cent of children who have fits lose them in adult life, and even if they do persist, it need not be a serious problem. Over-protection by parents should be discouraged and calculated risks accepted, though sensible precautions, such as the use of fireguards, the avoidance of sharp edges and corners to furniture, as well as of tablecloths which can be readily pulled off, should be taken to prevent accidents. The handles of pots and pans on the stove should point inwards and teapots should not be left on the edge of the table.

Parents frequently feel guilty and reproach themselves or each other for the use of contraceptives, abortifacients, masturbation, intercourse after getting drunk and past venereal infection, and it is the doctor's duty to deal with this ignorance. If the child is either ill or mentally defective, the appropriate social agencies should be informed, with the parents' approval.

The School Child

The Education Act (1944), Section 8(2), makes the local authority responsible for providing the necessary special schooling for pupils suffering from any disability of mind or body. Epilepsy was included under Section 33 which gave the Minister of Education responsibility for making provision for special categories but this was modified in 1953 by the School Health Service and Handicapped Pupils Regulation, which defined epileptic pupils as those 'who by reason of epilepsy cannot be educated under the normal regime of ordinary schools without detriment to themselves or other pupils'. Eighty per cent can be educated in ordinary schools and the 20 per cent who require special provision are the mentally subnormal, behaviour problems, those with frequent fits, post-epileptic automatism and the incontinent of urine or faeces. The usual practice is to give the ordinary school a trial first unless the reasons for not doing so are compelling.

These children can do the school work commensurate with their intelligence and play games, but certain obvious restrictions in the gymnasium are necessary, and cycling should be forbidden. Special schools are usually residential and under medical supervision, so there is every chance of the fits being adequately controlled in a constant environment.

University Students

There are certain restrictions necessary here, such as working with chemicals, electricity, radioactive materials and engineering plant, and in the practice of medicine and nursing, but Cohen suggests as suitable outlets, administration, domestic and social science and librarianship.

Employment

The Disabled Persons (Employment) Act (1944) stipulates that employers of 30 or more workpeople should include up to 3 per cent who are in some way disabled. There is a register on which the patient may be placed after the suitable form (D.P.I.) has been completed and the D.R.O. (Disablement Rehabilitation Officer) informed. This not only ensures the sheltered work the patient requires, but in many instances gives him the best chance of a job. The Ministry of Labour in July 1953 issued a pamphlet, *Notes for Guidance on the Employment of Epileptics* which lists the hazardous occupations, including those involving fire, water, vats, ladders and machinery, in fact any occupation which would be dangerous if the worker had a sudden attack with loss or reduction of consciousness. Accommodation can be a difficult problem for the worker who is not living at home, as the incontinence may tax the patience of the landlady; for these patients and others emerging from institutional care, the hostel or 'half-way house' is valuable and some local authorities provide them. Employers' fears *re* litigation resulting from accidents at work should be no greater than those arising from non-epileptic patients, provided that he has taken the necessary precautions, for both groups are covered by the same National Insurance (Industrial Injuries) Act, 1946. Industrial Rehabilitation Units (I.R.U.) offer epileptics vocational training and they are usually taught skilled crafts which do not depend very much on machinery; such labour is at present in great demand. Cohen states that within six months of leaving an I.R.U. 84 per cent of epileptics were gainfully employed. For those who cannot live in the community, colonies have for long been established and while these have always provided some form of work, this is now matched with employment on the outside so that inmates can see a way to full rehabilitation.

Epilepsy and Marriage

Under genetic considerations a brief reference was made to this, but Cohen (1958) deals with the matter in greater detail and the following is a précis. In some countries, epilepsy is a statutory bar to marriage on the grounds of heredity, possible mental deterioration and economic uncertainties. 'But for obvious reasons, in those countries, the illegality of the marriage of an epileptic has proved ineffective as a deterrent.' In England, though epilepsy is not grounds for divorce, the Matrimonial Causes Acts, 1937 and 1950, make it a ground for *nullity*. The 1937 Act states that '. . . a marriage shall be voidable on the ground . . . (b) that either party to the marriage was at the time of the marriage . . . subject to . . . epilepsy'. The 1950 Act restricted the decree to those cases where the Court was satisfied: (1) that proceedings were instituted within a year from the date of marriage; (2) that the petitioner was at the time ignorant of the facts alleged; (3) that marital intercourse with the consent of the petitioner has not taken place since the discovery by the petitioner of the grounds for a decree. The marriage is 'voidable' and not void until the non-epileptic partner has taken successful legal action. The children of such a marriage, despite a nullity decree, are legitimate. Though the law may be fair by including epilepsy in the Matrimonial Causes Act, it perpetuates the prejudice against epilepsy by not including much more damaging factors in marriage such as alcoholism, gambling, sexual perversions or even persistent snoring.

Occasionally pregnancy increases the severity and frequency of fits, but this is not sufficiently serious to be considered a general indication for abortion and sterilization. Non-epileptic parents have a 1 in 200 chance of having an epileptic child; one epileptic parent increases the risk to 1 in 40; but as Cohen points out, general rates are of little value in attempting a prognosis in individual cases.

Driving a Motor Vehicle

Under the Road Traffic Act, 1930, the applicant for a driving licence must state whether he suffers from epilepsy and the Motor Vehicle (Driving Licences) Regulation, 1950, No. 333, precludes anyone suffering from epilepsy from claiming a driving test. The difficult problem facing the doctor is when to permit a patient to drive again. A calculated risk may have to be taken and some stipulate a period of three years without fits or treatment, or two years without treatment, and that a public vehicle be absolutely excluded. With the use of the EEG more reliable advice can be given, for the fit is the expression of a cerebral dysrhythmia and it should be helpful to take this evidence into consideration in assessing the efficiency of treatment and the quiescence or otherwise of the condition.

When all the agencies have been consulted and have done their best, there still remain those with impulsive and aggressive behaviour, the attempted suicides, the paranoid reactions and the like and though their number is not large, like their 'first cousins' the aggressive psychopaths, they have a disproportionate impact on the community. Their answer has not yet been found.

MENTAL SYMPTOMS AND ORGANIC DISEASES NON-CEREBRAL

That the recognition of organically induced psychoses should lead to the acceptance that all psychoses are organically induced, is a bigger step than most psychiatrists are prepared to take. This does not relieve them of the responsibility of keeping abreast of current thinking on these topics. The theories may be incomplete, and the evidence may be inadequate, but there are some relevant and established facts which must be considered, if not in the common psychoses, then in the less common and selectively induced states. Smythies (1960) in a frank confession on the subject states:

> Two years ago I suggested (Smythies, 1958) that progress had been made because various workers had reported positive features in the metabolism and physiology of schizophrenics which differentiated them from normal people. Most of these claims have since had to be abandoned. . .

The adrenochrome hypothesis was given much support from the work of Osmond and Hoffer (1959) who claimed that adrenochrome and adrenolutin were psychotomimetic agents, that adrenochrome was a normal constituent of the blood and that schizophrenics were less able to destroy injected adrenochrome than normals. Subsequent experiments have failed to substantiate these findings. Similarly, disturbed adrenaline metabolism, which was considered an important factor in schizophrenia, has also failed the confirmatory tests. Serotonin levels which are influenced by reserpine and amine oxidase provided the basis for a hypothesis proposed by Woolley and Shaw (1954), that a naturally occurring substance resembling LSD 25 (presumably serotonin) was concerned in the genesis of schizophrenia. Feldstein *et al.* (1959) who measured 5-hydroxytryptamine levels in the blood and 5-hydroxylindole acetic acid (5-HIAA) in the urine, concluded that there was as yet no evidence to link defects in serotonin metabolism with schizophrenia. Other hypotheses which are unproven are those implicating toxic factors in the plasma, abnormal indoles, serum coeruplasmin levels, adenosine triphosphate and glucose metabolism, and tryptophan metabolism. Smythies concludes that 'the results of all this work are a collection of negative findings that do not themselves contribute to knowledge of a positive kind, as well as a large series of contradictory reports'.

The search for a metabolic aetiology for mental illness continues unabated and reports are constantly being published. Such a report by Shaw (1966) with the alliterative title 'Mineral metabolism, mania and melancholia' is in some ways representative. A careful and detailed study of electrolyte changes in mental illness is presented with the premise, but the author poses the question: 'Are the physiological and biochemical events accompanying the affective illnesses primary or secondary phenomena'? With commendable honesty, he replies 'Only further research can provide the answers'.

The lesson for the clinician is that although physical agents can aggravate or relieve mental illness, that does not necessarily mean that they cause it or that the manifestations of what are still regarded as functional states are organically induced.

Yet a large variety of organic states are associated with mental illness and though the mechanisms are imperfectly understood, the phenomena can usually be recognized, the essential features being those of the underlying organic abnormality.

ENDOCRINE DISTURBANCE

Though it is popular to regard one type of endocrine disturbance as responsible for one type of mental illness, it is axiomatic that hormones do not act in this way, but in association with each other and that in any endocrine disease, more than one hormone is involved (Beach, 1948). Yet, when the adverb, *predominantly*, is introduced, it is usually possible to identify mental symptoms which are associated with disease of one endocrine gland. Minor endocrinal abnormalities can produce overt physical changes which influence physique, mental energy and facial appearance and these may in turn draw the attention and comments of schoolmates and others and cause increasing sensitivity on the part of the patient. Such situations are frequently quoted in the case histories of schizophrenics suggesting that the endocrine abnormality produced the mental illness via psychological channels rather than physical ones. Klinefelter's syndrome, Frohlich's syndrome, gynaecomastia, masculinizing tumours in girls, dwarfism and giantism are all obvious examples. But there are endocrine diseases which produce mental symptoms directly and it is these that will now be described.

THE THYROID

The thyroid gland can hypo- or hyperfunction and in each instance mental disturbance can arise.

Hypofunction (Myxoedema)

This is associated with depression of mood and psychomotor

retardation, the mental component frequently deteriorating to a state bordering on dementia. Asher (1949), in a paper entitled 'Myxoedematous Madness', described the classical slowing down of the mental processes which tends to isolate the patient from social intercourse and even family conversation. He quotes a report by the Committee of the Clinical Society of London (1888) that had been appointed five years earlier to consider the subject of myxoedema, which stated:

> Delusions and hallucinations occur in nearly half the cases, mainly where the disease is advanced. Insanity as a complication is noted in about the same proportion as delusions and hallucinations. It takes the form of acute or chronic manias, dementia, or melancholia, with a marked predominance of suspicion and self-accusation.

Asher deals with the question as to whether there is a specific type of psychosis associated with the myxoedema and states:

> Cases in the literature record a very wide variety of mental changes, and certainly in the series I have observed there has been no constant type of psychosis, though general confusion and disorientation with persecutory delusions and hallucinations, and occasional bouts of restless violence, have been common. I have made the diagnosis on the myxoedematous appearance of the patient and not on the kind of mental symptoms. No physician would attempt to diagnose lobar pneumonia or typhoid by the delirium they may produce, and likewise in myxoedema it is the disease which is the characteristic feature, not its mental manifestations.

Other forms of presentation may be hypothermic coma or psychotic features of a paranoid type with perhaps an element of confusion. The first condition can be missed if a special low-temperature recording thermometer is not used. In fact, this instrument is essential for the diagnosis. When the temperature is very low, coma is common, but as it rises, that is, when the patient is beginning to respond to treatment, psychotic features as described above with restlessness may supervene. Easson (1966) in a study from the Mayo Clinic of 19 patients with myxoedema and coincident psychosis was also unable to demonstrate a specific myxoedema psychosis though paranoid features and irritability were common. He found that thyroid replacement, if not done slowly, could aggravate the mental state.

Treatment is as for myxoedema with adequate dosage of thyroid. In the ordinary case, cautious dosage of oral thyroid is indicated and 30 mg. daily for the first two weeks should suffice, but in insensitive patients one may have to give as much as 300 mg. per day as a maintenance dose. In myxoedematous hypothermic coma, oral thyroid is too slow to be effective, and an intravenous preparation such as sod. laevothyroxine is necessary. As the patient emerges from the coma, she may become restless and present psychotic features just as she may have done in her descent into coma, and if the problem is not recognized the psychiatrist may be tempted to use chlorpromazine to control the mental state. There is a danger here, for chlorpromazine is itself a hypothermic agent and may aggravate the condition. The answer to myxoedema in all its manifestations is adequate doses of a thyroid preparation.

The alliterative title coined by Richard Asher and his impressive style of writing may have given undue emphasis to the incidence of this problem. In a busy psychiatric department of a general hospital where patients are routinely screened for thyroid dysfunction, the author has found the condition to be rare, and the mental symptoms are more likely to be those of depression than of a paranoid state.

Hyperthyroidism

This is not infrequently associated with mental symptoms and Dunlap and Moersch (1935) collected 134 cases of thyrotoxic psychoses from the Mayo Clinic. The clinical picture may vary; in some it presents as an acute mania with motor restlessness and excitement, while in others auditory and occasionally visual hallucinations may predominate. Depression and paranoid reactions may also occur and it would appear that like the myxoedematous condition, the individual is reacting to a situation in a manner which is partly dictated by his basic mental equipment, except that the maniacal state is probably a natural extension of the severe hyperthyroidism.

Apart from these florid psychotic states, which may occur in about 20 per cent of severely hyperthyroid patients, nervousness is almost a universal finding in hyperthyroidism. It may show as undue irritability, jumpiness and over-anxiety and in some instances, clinical assessment alone may be unable to distinguish the disease from the symptoms of an anxiety state, for they may have sweating, tremor, rapid pulse and loss of weight in common. The problem may be further complicated in that hyperthyroidism can be precipitated by an emotional shock or follow a period of stress. It is this psychosomatic aspect which has led some to speculate that all cases of hyperthyroidism are psychologically determined and that the disease is virtually a psychosomatic disorder. More responsible contributors, however, recognize other stress agents and seek only to establish parity for emotional factors. Lidz (1949) found a denial of feelings of rejection and isolation in the childhood of these patients and explained the onset of the acute episode as following on the loss of the mother or her substitute or through rejection or desertion. Obsessional features are utilized to ward off the impending disaster and these may colour the symptomatology. These findings have a very familiar ring and are found in patients suffering from a variety of conditions like asthma, ulcerative colitis and peptic ulcer.

Dewhurst *et al.* (1968) studied 20 schizophrenic patients and 44 with affective disorders and showed that emotional stress could cause an increase in the serum levels of TSH (thyroid stimulating hormone) and PBI (protein bound iodine).

PARATHYROID DISEASE

Hyperparathyroidism has for long been associated with depressive illness. Anderson (1968) studied 30 patients with primary hyperparathyroidism of whom 20 had a history free of psychiatric illness prior to the onset of the organic disease. Of these, 7 gave a definite history of depression with loss of energy concurrently with the hyperparathyroidism. Two weeks postoperatively, 23 were certain that they felt better mentally, being less depressed and with more energy than before the operation. On the other hand, Christie-Brown (1968) compared 6 patients admitted for parathyroidectomy with 6 euthyroid patients with non-malignant goitre admitted for thyroidectomy. He found that the observed difference between the two groups could be accounted for by premorbid factors.

Flanagan *et al.* (1970) studied a family with a high incidence of primary hyperparathyroidism. They compared 10 of those affected with 10 other members of the family with a normal serum calcium and with no history of symptoms of the disease. Eight of the 10 with the disease had experienced major psychiatric symptoms for a prolonged period, yet only one of the controls had had such an experience. The clinical features varied, although they were largely characteristic of affective disorders, but no temporal relationship could be determined between psychiatric symptoms and the physical manifestations of the disease. Six of the 7 who had parathyroidectomy of one to three glands had psychiatric syndromes, 3 prior to and 3 after the operation. There was no clear correlation between calcium level and psychiatric symptoms, although calcium levels were available in only 2 cases at the height of their psychiatric symptoms.

The authors postulate three bases for an association between psychiatric symptoms and the disease.

1. Psychiatric symptoms are a direct manifestation of the disease,

related to the same metabolic abnormalities that presumably explain the skeletal and renal lesions.
2. The genetic factor leading to hyperparathyroidism is also linked to the cause of the psychiatric illness.
3. Hyperparathyroidism is a 'psychosomatic' disorder in which the emotional factors contribute causally to the pathogenesis of the disease.

They concede that the third possibility is exceedingly remote. The author has had four patients with mental illness associated with primary hyperparathyroidism. All had depression and one, a male aged 23 who had severe depression preoperatively, became manic postoperatively when his calcium was very low. As most of the author's in-patients have their serum calcium assessed, the incidence in general psychiatric practice is rare. What is needed is a systematic study of a large series of patients with primary hyperparathyroidism.

MYASTHENIA GRAVIS

This organic condition, which is characterized by weakness of voluntary muscles, as with other organic states, has its psychological overtones. The main interest to the psychiatrist is that hysterical conversion states can stimulate the disorder to a remarkable degree. The author has seen two patients thus diagnosed and who had been treated unsuccessfully by thymectomy, who presumably did not have the disorder, for they both recovered following a course of E.C.T.

Two other patients have been seen by the author who were also wrongly diagnosed for years as myasthenia gravis. Both were suffering from severe phobic anxiety and were parading their weakness and fear of collapse as a defence against exposure to situations which they could not tolerate. All four patients were female. The strictest criteria for the diagnosis are essential if the patient is not to be subjected to lengthy treatment for a condition she does not have while her basic disability remains unrecognized and untreated.

Fullerton and Munsat (1966) list the following criteria for the 'pseudo' diagnosis.

1. A history not consistent with myasthenia gravis, either in course, distribution of weakness, relation of weakness to motor activity or response to cholinergic agents.
2. Evidence of significant emotional illness.
3. Absence of weakness on physical examination and inconsistencies

on muscle testing.

4. All laboratory findings within normal limits.
5. Lack of uniform improvement in strength following neostigmine and Tensilon.
6. Bulb ergographs of normal or hysterical pattern.
7. Normal motor response to repetitive nerve stimulation.

PITUITARY DISORDERS

These can influence a variety of 'target' organs and the resulting mental states are virtually due to the dysfunction of these organs. Such a condition is *Cushing's syndrome* which is traditionally associated with a basophile adenoma of the pituitary gland and produces its mental and physical changes mainly by hyperactivity of the adrenal cortex. It is not necessary to postulate a primary pituitary disorder, for the syndrome can be produced by adenoma and carcinoma of the adrenal cortex, or by the administration of corticoids. The physical features are typical, with obesity showing a characteristic distribution. The face and trunk are most affected with pads of fat at the back of the neck and females are more commonly affected with hirsutism of the face and a masculine distribution of pubic hair. The skin is atrophic with purplish abdominal striae and there may be widespread acne. Blood pressure is high and menstruation is suppressed; in the male there may be diminished or absent libido. Osteoporosis, particularly of the vertebrae, results in collapse with kyphosis and pain.

The psychiatric features are varied and can range over the whole field of psychotic reactions, though in the less florid states, depression and irritability are common (Trethowan & Cobb, 1952; Rees, 1953). In addition to the mental symptoms resulting directly from the biochemical changes of the disease, it is claimed by some that there are mental reactions to such physical changes as the hirsutism, 'moon-face' and acne. These are more likely to affect patients who are already hypersensitive, for a number of these patients are apparently unperturbed by these changes. The author has seen one such patient demonstrated at a clinical meeting, who apparently delighted in the reference to her 'buffalo hump' and her hirsutism, and proudly displayed a series of photographs taken at different times, including a recent one which showed the grosser features of Cushing's syndrome. In those states induced by therapy, consideration should be given to underlying disorders for which the steroids were prescribed and the effects of addiction and withdrawal of these steroids.

Regestein *et al.* (1972) commented on the wide range of mental symptoms observed in 7 patients with Cushing's syndrome with elevated levels of 17-hydroxycorticosteroids that were now lowered by dexamethasone. One was normal, 2 had organic brain syndrome only, 2 had brain syndrome with marked paranoia and 2 had endogenous depression. Similar symptoms had been present in 2 patients (one paranoid and one depressed) during periods of stress, postoperative and postmenopausal. The authors suggest that there is a tendency for steroids to arouse previously expressed mental disturbance, and that the nature of the illness is not dependent on the steroids. Drugs in addition to steroids have produced similar reactions in that two patients presented with acute psychoses within a day of taking diuretics. The brain syndromes were acute in onset and all occurred in patients over the age of 65 years. They conclude that steroids may be enough to upset the balance between adequate functioning and breakdown in a marginally compensated system.

Blau and Hinton (1960) describe a case of *hypopituitary* coma and psychosis in a woman who had developed hypopituitarism 10 years previously following pregnancy and who had deteriorated rapidly following an acute infection. Her mental state fluctuated between apathy and noisy and aggressive outbursts. Euphoria, undue suspicion, memory disturbance and disorientation were all in evidence at different times and persisted for three months but she was restored to her pre-pregnancy level with cortisone treatment. Sheehan and Summers (1949) had already observed mental torpor, depression and delusions in hypopituitarism, while Hughes and Summers (1956) reported loss of alpha-rhythm in the EEG in such cases.

An interesting condition with pituitary associations is polydipsia with polyuria. As these features are found in diabetes insipidus, they have been regarded by some as evidence of disturbance of post-pituitary function. The problem is not so simple. Firstly, the polydipsia is frequently for sweetened drinks, so a raised blood sugar may be dietetic rather than pituitary in origin. Secondly, polydipsia of long standing and even when functionally determined can produce a depression of posterior pituitary function which can be very difficult to distinguish from the true organic state. In functional polydipsia there is usually other evidence of psychiatric disturbance. As the polydipsia is essentially compulsive drinking, there should be other obsessional features, though others have preferred to incorporate such obsessional features into an organic syndrome (Barton, 1965). A number of these patients are mentally subnormal.

Mental Symptoms of Adrenocortical Insufficiency

Since Addison (1855) described the clinical conditions associated with adrenal failure, it has been known that mental symptoms frequently accompany the physical changes. Usually these are anergia and loss of interest with mild depression and when these are coupled with hypotension which causes the patient to take to bed, a diagnosis of neurasthenia may be erroneously made. The author has also seen severe depressive reactions in these patients and in one instance there was a serious suicidal risk. This reaction followed a bilateral adrenalectomy for uncontrolled cancer of the breast and it was found that the patient had been having inadequate corticoid therapy. When this matter was corrected, the depression cleared dramatically.

PSYCHIATRIC ASPECTS OF HYPOGLYCAEMIA

The hypoglycaemic symptoms of hunger, restlessness, sweating and weakness, which occur after the administration of insulin or after partial gastrectomy, are uncommon in most varieties of endogenous hypoglycaemia due either to endocrine disturbance or to an islet cell tumour of the pancreas. Patients in the latter group frequently have a long history of progressive mental disturbance with periods of amnesia and confusion, which may lead to a diagnosis of hysteria, schizophrenia or organic dementia. Morley (1952) stated: 'It is possible that many neurological and psychiatric clinics shelter one or more of them undetected, for they are undoubtedly more common than the published records would suggest'. The mental symptoms are so protean that a vareity of psychiatric diagnoses are made. An EEG may be ordered and yield a record which is suggestive or even confirmatory of epilepsy. Occasionally the patient, if a housewife, may relate that her attacks were prone to develop on days when she undertook extra work, such as spring-cleaning or washing. Automatism and aggressive or childish behaviour may occur and occasionally hallucinatory episodes.

Greater awareness of hypoglycaemia as a cause of chronic mental illness and the development of tests with glucose oxidase to determine the level of blood glucose and estimation of circulating insulin have led to improvements in diagnosis. There are, however, a variety of causes of hypoglycaemia which should be capable of definition. These have been listed by Todd *et al.* (1962):

1. Hypoglycaemia due to functional (stimulation) hyperinsulinism.
2. Hypoglycaemia due to organic hyperinsulinism (islet cell tumour or hyperplasia).

3. Hypoglycaemia due to extrapancreatic factors such as hepatic, adrenal, and pituitary insufficiency.

Diagnosis

This usually depends on Whipple's triad of (1) neuropsychiatric symptoms after fasting, (2) a concomitant blood-sugar level below 50 mg./100 ml., and (3) banishment of symptoms by the administration of glucose (Whipple & Franz, 1935). Some patients may suffer symptoms despite a normal blood sugar, and in others, fasting may have to be continued for 48 or even 72 hours and be accompanied by bouts of exercise in order to provoke an attack.

Marrack *et al.* (1961) have reported on the use of glucagon and tolbutamide as provocative hypoglycaemic agents. An intramuscular injection of 1 mg. of glucagon is followed by the normal hyperglycaemic response which does not occur in hepatic hypoglycaemia. The blood sugar then falls to levels below 45 mg. as measured by the glucose oxidase method. Intravenous injection of 1 g. of tolbutamide results in prolonged hypoglycaemia, and the blood sugar does not return to normal levels after the first hour. In both cases hypoglycaemic symptoms may be provoked and 50 per cent dextrose should be at hand to end the test if necessary. False-positive tests may occur if the hypoglycaemia is due to hepatic disease or endocrine disturbance and in idiopathic hypoglycaemosis in infancy, but if these causes can be excluded then laparotomy should be undertaken. A careful search is necessary, because a pancreatic adenoma may be extremely small and if none is found most surgeons carry out a partial pancreatectomy in any case.

It can be very difficult to distinguish 'functional' hypoglycaemia from that due to an islet-cell tumour of the pancreas, though the latter usually occurs after fasting while the former may occur 2–3 hours after a meal. Now that plasma insulin can be reliably measured it is likely that this problem will be solved, but it still leads to many fruitless investigations including laparotomy. An interesting aspect of 'functional' hypoglycaemia is that when it occurs in the presence of phobic anxiety states, it can right itself when the psychiatric condition has been successfully treated.

DIABETES MELLITUS

Bale (1973) investigated the incidence of brain damage in 100 patients (57 males and 43 females) with not less than 15 years' insulin-dependent diabetes mellitus and who were under the age of

65. These were compared with a control group matched for age, sex and social class. The screening test for general cortical damage was the Walton-Black Modified New World Learning Test, and those subjects who were suspect were subsequently tested on the Wechsler (WAIS).

Seventeen diabetics scored in the brain-damaged range in the Walton-Black, while none of the controls did, and the difference was significant. There was a significant relationship between scores indicating brain damage and apparent severity of past hypoglycaemic episodes. Examination of the employment records of the 17 brain-damaged patients showed that only one retired on grounds of dementia. Although severe brain damage is rare in diabetics, dementia of a mild degree secondary to hypoglycaemia is not uncommon.

ANAEMIC STATES

These, whether due to haemorrhage or iron-deficiency, can, *in susceptible subjects,* be responsible for marked mental changes. The author had such a patient, an elderly man with an iron-deficiency anaemia (Hb. 74 per cent). Correction of the anaemia with oral iron resulted in the disappearance of a gross delusional state, in which he was accusing his wife of infidelity with a young labourer nearly 50 years her junior, who he alleged gained entry to the house at night by climbing through the window. A relapse in the mental state was associated with a corresponding deterioration in the anaemia. It might be postulated that the same factor which contributed to the anaemia caused the mental deterioration, but his recovery on two occasions was associated with no treatment other than oral iron.

Bronchial Carcinoma

This has been associated with changes in the central nervous system and Greenfield (1934) and Brain *et al.* (1951) have described instances where mental symptoms occurred. Charatan and Brierley (1956) reported three cases, where severe mental disturbance either preceded or overshadowed the presence of the bronchial carcinoma. They were all male with no evidence of cerebral metastases and clinically they presented the features of a fluctuating toxic-confusional psychosis with lucid intervals. In two cases the EEG showed little abnormality, and there were no associated neurological signs.

The frequency with which mental illness may be the presenting feature of a bronchial carcinomatous neuropathy has been emphasized by Jeri (1963) who found that 21 of his 48 patients with neuromyopathy had mental abnormality manifested in confusion, depression, stupor, dementia or emotional instability.

Carcinoma of the Pancreas

Jacobsson and Ottosson (1971) compared the initial symptoms of 50 patients with carcinoma of the pancreas with 50 patients with carcinoma of the stomach, by interviewing close relatives. Eight patients with carcinoma of the pancreas had initial mental symptoms without somatic complaints lasting 3–18 months, while with carcinoma of the stomach there were 2 such patients of 6 months' and 2 years' duration. Once somatic symptoms supervened the incidence of mental symptoms in the two types of cancer approximated (32 per cent in pancreas and 26 per cent in stomach).

The main symptoms in both diseases were irritability, weakness and *mild* depression and belonged more to an organic psychosyndrome rather than to a depressive one, and there was no difference in these symptoms whether they preceded or were concerned with the somatic ones. It is of significance that once somatic symptoms appeared the condition ceased to be regarded as functional and a correct diagnosis was made.

The authors therefore do not regard carcinoma of the pancreas as a special type, even though initial mental symptoms appear more commonly. There is one reservation on this conclusion: carcinoma of the pancreas is commonly associated with a thromboembolic phenomenon, and the author has had referred to him 3 such patients as suffering from a functional disturbance. Two were behaving in a way which might be regarded as crudely hysterical, but the clinical picture was that of hemiballismus which was later demonstrated to be due to embolic involvement of the *Corpus Luysi.*

VITAMIN DEFICIENCIES

WERNICKE'S ENCEPHALOPATHY

Thiamine, which is essential for the proper metabolism of carbohydrates and fat and for the normal functioning of the nervous system, may, when deficient, cause neurological and psychiatric disturbances. The onset is more acute in children, but in adults it can follow an insidious course which may begin as a neurasthenic syndrome, consisting of anorexia, irritability, emotional lability, lack of concentration and preoccupation with visceral sensations. These may be followed by neurological changes, particularly a polyneuropathy which is bilateral and symmetrical, which initially consists of paraesthesia of toes, burning feet, particularly at night, calf muscle tenderness, and eventually loss of vibration sense and of the ankle jerks, the upper limbs later becoming involved. In the more advanced states, there is ophthalmoplegia which is part of the *Wernicke* (1881) *syndrome,* which includes clouding of consciousness, ataxia and even delirium, though the level of consciousness may appear normal and the patient present a confabulatory state or Korsakoff psychosis. Although Wernicke's original cases included two alcoholics and a patient with persistent vomiting, it has since been described in cases of gastric carcinoma, pernicious anaemia, hyperemesis gravidarum and in malnourished prisoners of war. The ocular signs consist of nystagmus in the horizontal and vertical directions as well as paralysis of conjugate gaze. There may be associated cardiac involvement ('beriberi heart') with an enormous enlargement of the heart, oedema and serous effusions, and sudden circulatory collapse. The cerebral lesions consist of a haemorrhagic polioencephalitis with the mamillary bodies being particularly affected. The laboratory findings include a raised fasting blood pyruvic acid level, but it may be induced by the metabolic stress of 100 g. of dextrose or after exercise.

Treatment lies, as for pellagra, in prevention by giving an adequate diet containing yeast, whole grains, meat, eggs, vegetables and reinforcing the bread ration with a complement of thiamine 1·5–2·5 mg. per day. A therapeutic dose is 10–100 mg. per day, but in an acute Wernicke state 50–100 mg. subcutaneously or intravenously twice daily should be given until a therapeuric result is obtained or the urine indicates tissue saturation by the strong smell of thiamine.

PELLAGRA

Pellagra is traditionally said to present with the classical triad of diarrhoea, dermatitis and dementia. The dementia is not necessarily a mental state exhibiting intellectual deficit for it more frequently comes to the notice of the psychiatrist because of the behaviour disturbance or psychotic and neurotic features. It is still endemic in certain parts of the world where there is a deficiency of the essential food factors, niacin or nicotinic acid, niacinamide or nicotinamide, and the amino acid precursor, tryptophan. Protein containing tryptophan can compensate for a low niacinamide intake and this explanation is given for the greater protection derived from tryptophan-containing proteins like wheat, eggs and milk, as against corn protein which is deficient in tryptophan. Countries where the inhabitants live on a high-maize diet are likely to have endemic pellagra, and in areas where corn is the main cereal, a toxic niacin-neutralizing factor in the corn may be responsible. Gregory (1955) lists a number of factors which singly or in combination may produce pellagra. These are:

1. Dietary deficiencies due to poverty, famine, food fads, ignorance, alcoholism and drug addiction;
2. Low-intake due to anorexia, vomiting, disease of the alimentary tract or psychiatric illness including dementia;
3. Impaired bio-synthesis due to inadequate intake of tryptophan or the bactericidal effects of antibiotics, since the intestinal flora is responsible for processing much of the body's niacin;
4. Malabsorption;
5. Interference with its use because of generalized impaired cellular metabolism;
6. Interference with storage as in cirrhosis of the liver;
7. Increased excretion as in lactation, diabetes and renal disease;
8. Increased requirements as in pregnancy, rapid growth, high metabolic rate, fever and motor excitement;
9. Extensive post-operative use of dextrose infusions without preventative vitamin therapy.

Leigh (1952) pointed out that 'pellagra' includes several nutritional deficiency syndromes, which would explain the frequent adulteration of the clinical picture, particularly with features produced by thiamine deficiency.

The neuropathology in advanced states shows the histopathological picture of 'primary irritation' in the Betz cells of the motor cortex. The nucleus is altered in form and position and the basophile substances in the cell body are present only around the nucleus and at the point of departure of the processes. The cell centre is opaque, stains lightly and is free of Nissl bodies.

The mental symptoms may present in three ways:

1. A non-specific neurasthenic syndrome may masquerade as a neurotic disorder. The patient may complain of fatiguability, headaches, irritability, inability to concentrate and forgetfulness.

2. An organic psychosis with memory impairment, disorientation, confusion and even confabulation may supervene. It may be associated with excitement, depression, mania or delirium, but paranoid reactions are also common and in countries where mental hospital accommodation is scarce and pellagra is endemic, most admissions with paranoid states are pellagrins and many of these have been homicidal.

3. The encephalopathic syndrome is commonest after a period of

delirium and consists of clouding of consciousness, cog-wheel rigidities of the extremities, and uncontrollable sucking and grasping reflexes.

Treatment should be mainly preventive to ensure that everybody has an adequate intake of the vitamin, and niacin-enriched bread has proved to be successful. In institutions there was a tendency for the disease to become endemic and this was due to a lack of care in seeing that those patients who were apathetic or mentally deteriorated were not being deprived of their proper food intake by the more aggressive and voracious patients. It is not enough to issue each patient with his ration of food; it is essential to see that he eats it. The average requirements for an adult are 5 mg. of niacine per 1000 calories or approximately 10–15 mg. per day. When the disease is present 300–1000 mg. of nicotinamide per day should be given in divided doses, depending on the severity of the disease. In the presence of diarrhoea or when the patient will not cooperate with oral therapy, 100–250 mg. should be given by subcutaneous injection two to three times per day, while in the encephalopathic state 1000 mg. by mouth and 100-250 mg. by injection per day may be necessary. Once the condition is under control, the dose can be reduced to a basic level. Nicotinamide is preferable to nicotinic acid as in large doses it does not cause vasomotor disturbances. A liberal diet including a generous supply of milk and adequate meat, liver, peas and greens, and which is low in carbohydrates and fats, is also recommended.

PERNICIOUS ANAEMIA

'Megaloblastic Madness'

This is a term coined by Smith (1960) to describe those psychotic states associated with pernicious anaemia. He reported six illustrative cases from a much larger series in which the mental symptoms preceded evidence of a megaloblastic anaemia. In some, the clinical picture was almost indistinguishable from a functional psychosis. The author summarizes the situation thus:

> Apart from the mental state, an abnormal EEG may be the only positive finding and suggest exclusion of the diagnosis.
>
> Much larger doses of vitamin B_{12} are needed when treating this type of case, and care must be taken to ensure that an associated encephalopathy is not missed in a patient who presents with severe anaemia. Attribution of the mental symptoms to the anaemia may result in under-treatment, with subsequent cerebral demyelination as the physician's reward. . . .

The mental symptoms are generally those of depression though paranoid reactions have also been reported while in patients with organic cerebral involvement, confusional features may also occur. There has been recently considerable interest in the incidence of this disorder and it has been suggested that more patients would be identified with B_{12} deficiency if more refined screening tests were used. Strachan and Henderson (1965) described three patients whose peripheral blood, bone marrow and nervous system showed no evidence of B_{12} deficiency but with tests which included labelled vitamin-B_{12} absorption, serum-B_{12} levels and gastric parietal-cell antibodies, the diagnosis was made. The mental changes can precede the clinical picture by up to 8 years (Holmes, 1956). As the condition generally responds to treatment the case for a more refined screening test for all psychiatric patients is at least as strong as the routine use of the Wassermann reaction. This is particularly important in patients who have a history of gastric surgery. Hunter *et al.* (1967) found that 5 out of 20 patients with partial gastrectomy admitted to a mental hospital were seriously deficient in vitamin B_{12}. They reckon that 1 per cent of mental hospital admissions are B_{12} deficient.

Shulman (1967), in a carefully controlled prospective investigation into the psychiatric aspects of pernicious anaemia, came to different conclusions. He compared the psychiatric status of 27 patients with pernicious anaemia with 21 anaemic patients. Approximately one-third of both groups had psychiatric symptoms rated as moderate or severe. These were depression and memory impairment, but only memory impairment was related to B_{12} deficiency. He found no evidence to support the routine screening of psychiatric patients for pernicious anaemia but B_{12} deficiency may be suspected in patients:

1. at risk clinically, *e.g.* with anaemia or after gastrectomy;
2. with unexplained fatigue;
3. with confusion or dementia of unknown origin.

This work is probably the most helpful guide to practice, to date.

Folic Acid Deficiency

Reynolds *et al.* (1970) reported on 22 patients with low serum folates who were admitted to a clinical investigation with a diagnosis of depression and found that severity of depression was unrelated to low serum folate concentration. The authors consider whether the incidence of low serum levels could be a result of poor diet but could find no supporting evidence, though they admit that reliable data on diet were difficult to acquire. In general psychiatric practice, it is very common to find that depressed patients are indiscreet with their diets and this is a more tenable hypothesis than attributing severe depression to folate deficiency. Raising the level of folate does not relieve the depression.

POST-OPERATIVE PSYCHOSES

These are not very common and before drawing conclusions from pre-operative personality studies, an accurate estimate of the serum biochemistry is essential. Potassium deficiency in particular is a likely factor and when corrected the psychosis may disappear. The mental picture may vary but is usually that of the traditional infective or toxic exhaustive psychosis with delusions, usually of persecution, and hallucinations which are usually auditory but may occasionally be visual or tactile. Illusions are common, the patient misinterpreting auditory and visual experiences sometimes of a trivial nature, such as the rotation of the hands of the ward clock, which they may insist is going backwards and must therefore have some sinister significance. Certain operations have a greater tendency to precipitate psychotic symptoms than others, and most ophthalmologists are familiar with 'black patch delirium' following cataract removal.

Chest Surgery

An operation which has attracted attention is mitral valvotomy for mitral stenosis. Dencker and Sandahl (1961) reported on a consecutive series of 61 patients who underwent mitral surgery and encountered three who became psychotic soon after operation. They also found a high incidence of mental illness before operation (six patients) and they postulated an early cerebral injury of rheumatic type predisposing to mental disease or a joint predisposition to mental and cardiac disease. The author was also struck with the relatively large number of patients referred from a thoracic surgical unit, which was more than all other post-operative psychoses in the hospital, and found it tempting to explain the problem as the crippling effect of the disability on the personality, the magnitude of the operation, the patient's apprehension and the like. An analysis of the data showed that they were not all cardiac cases and a number were lobectomies and pneumonectomies. The sister in charge of the ward was convinced that her thoracotomy patients reacted as a group in a more disturbed way mentally than the others and it may be that the opening of the chest with its resulting upset of the cardio-respiratory system was a contributory factor. It is not only the 'surgical' heart and lungs which produce their crop of psychoses, for a number of these problems arise in medical cardiac units when patients *emerge* from congestive heart failure. A satisfactory explanation for these phenomena is still awaited.

The problem still arouses interest. Matarazzo *et al.* (1963) who found a higher incidence of anxiety/depression reactions following operations in patients with mitral stenosis compared with other surgical patients attributed this to the severity of the operation and pre-surgery illness. Egerton and Kay (1964) reported delirious states in 17 adults out of 60 who survived open heart surgery, but in only 1 child out of 36. The delirium was attributed to the post-operative environment, including abnormal sensory experience. The author's colleague (Davies, 1965) conducted a controlled study into post-thoracotomy patients and compared them with other surgical patients. He was of the opinion that the attitude of the surgical team was an important factor in excluding post-operative delirious states, for in one unit where there was a positive and optimistic approach with scrupulous supervision by the surgeon of the pre- and post-operative states, in a series of 50 patients, there were no such sequelae. The pre-morbid personality of the patient is also relevant and Knox (1963) found that the hysterically prone were likely to react in a similar manner post-operatively and therefore carried a poor prognosis.

Layne and Yudofsky (1971) compared the incidence of psychiatric sequelae in 42 patients over 14 years of age who had intracardiac surgery, who were extensively interviewed the night before surgery, with 19 similar patients who had only a neurological examination. These two groups were compared with a vascular control group who had major surgery on either the aorta or coronary vessels.

Of the 58 patients who survived cardiotomy (40 in the experimental and 18 in the control group) 8 developed post-operative psychoses, but no patient in the vascular control group did so. Those who did were male and older, four had 'obvious organic concomitants or abnormal neurological signs'; one was on steroids but 3 had no obvious organic factor. Four from the experimental group had organic predisposition to post-operative psychosis but did not develop it.

The authors found that psychosis was more frequent in patients with low pre-operative anxiety and attribute this factor, which was based on psychological testing, to the use of denial as a defence. These patients therefore retained serious unanswered questions about the competence and motivation of their surgeons. Denial is, of course, a common mechanism in hospitalized patients, but evidence for its presence and contribution to psychosis should be more strongly based that on a pre-operative psychological test for anxiety. The authors' claim that pre-operative psychiatric interview and personal attention reduces the frequency of post-operative psychosis is ambitious, certainly as far as the psychiatric interview is concerned.

Blacher (1972) gave support to the denial theory. He described 'hidden psychoses' which were not declared at the time but which troubled the patient. He too recommended reassurance in the pre-operative phase.

Portacaval Anastomosis

This is another manoeuvre which has neuropsychiatric complications (Read *et al.,* 1961). As patients with a pre-operative history of hepatic pre-coma or coma were excluded, the complication could not have been due to pre-existing liver failure. Out of 21 patients with portal hypertension, eight had portal-systemic encephalopathy culminating in episodes of hepatic coma. The clinical features varied widely and included disorders of sleep rhythm, apathy, inability to concentrate, emotional lability, bizarre behaviour and constructional apraxia and were commoner in the older patient. The EEG showed slowing of the mean frequency in 15 patients.

As psychiatrists may have charge of such patients, they should be familiar not only with medical treatment consisting of dietary protein restriction, antibiotics and regular purgation, but with recent advances in surgical treatment. Walker *et al.* (1965) reported 8 patients with chronic portal-systemic encephalopathy who were treated by surgical exclusion of the colon of whom 4 improved considerably in mental function and well-being which they maintained for 13–24 months. The authors recommend that the operation be reserved for patients with relatively good liver function accompanied by severe mental dysfunction.

Hourigan *et al.* (1971) reviewed a series of 64 patients with elective end-to-side portacaval shunts performed for liver disease. The success rate, defined as survival of operation with a patent shunt, free of subsequent haemorrhage and severe encephalopathy, was 48 per cent. Among survivors, the most serious late complication was encephalopathy which occurred in 38 per cent and was associated with patients who were over 40 years of age, had a pre-operative history of diabetes mellitus, and with continued drinking in the alcoholic. Most who developed it in the first pre-operative year became chronically and severely disabled.

Hysterectomy

That certain operations have more significance than others is understandable. For example, a woman of child-bearing age is more likely to be affected by a hysterectomy than one who has passed the menopause. It is, however, difficult to draw conclusions from this particular operation for the factors involved are very complex. A number of patients undoubtedly have the operation for psychological reasons and post-operatively are bound to constitute a different group to those who required it for strict and well-substantiated organic causes.

Haemorrhoidectomy

An operation in the male which has produced its interesting quota of post-operative psychoses is haemorrhoidectomy. Again, pre-selection may be operating, for the male who comes to surgery with his haemorrhoids is in some respects a volunteer and is not representative of the much larger male population who are content to live with their haemorrhoids. Yet, at a British Medical Association meeting where operations (including heart surgery) were being relayed in colour to a medical audience, a number of doctors passed out when the haemorrhoidectomy was being shown.

PORPHYRIA

Porphyria which is an inborn error of metabolism presents as three types, the congenital, the acute intermittent and the mixed, the first being mainly found in childhood, while the acute intermittent is the one most commonly associated with mental symptoms. Ever since Gunther (1912) described the condition and pointed out that the attacks are usually preceded by periods of nervous tension and that the acute episodes may masquerade as neurotic or psychotic states, it has fascinated the psychiatrist and has at times occasioned him a diagnostic triumph. As women are more commonly involved than men and the abdomen may be opened without discovery of organic disease, the patient may be referred to the psychiatrist, especially as she may have a hysterical demeanour. In the psychotic phase the patient may be admitted to a mental hospital because of disturbed behaviour. and again the psychiatrist has the responsibility of diagnosing the condition and, if not being able to cure the patient, at least of not making her worse. In the six cases reported by Whittaker and Whitehead (1956) three were discovered in mental hospitals.

Some knowledge of the condition is essential, but its biochemical aspects have become so involved that they can no longer be regarded as the province of the psychiatrist, though Ackner *et al.* (1961) have intensively investigated 12 such patients in the Maudsley Hospital and write most informedly of porphobilinogen and δ-aminolaevulinic acid excretion and the correlation between this and the changes in physical and mental states. The acute intermittent type which is usually associated with mental changes is said to be due to a Mendelian dominant and is familial while the congenital type is said to be transmitted by a Mendelian recessive. The classical triad of abdominal pain, neuropathy and psychotic symptoms is not always present and the diagnosis may have to be made on two or even one of these criteria, with of course a positive urine test, though this may be negative except in the acute attack.

The biochemical lesion is said to be due to an incomplete synthesis of purines with overproduction of porphyrins and their precursors due to interference with the succinate glycine circle. Neuropathologically there are patchy areas of demyelinization with at times destruction of axis cylinders.

Ackner *et al.* (1961) have the following to say on diagnosis:

> From the clinical point of view porphyria is a deceptive and frequently undiagnosed condition. The early symptoms are both varied and variable, and are often unaccompanied by physical signs. Being a rare disorder, it is seldom diagnosed at an early stage. The abdominal pain, vomiting, nausea and constipation may, even in the absence of pyrexia, leucocytosis and abdominal rigidity, lead to a tentative diagnosis of a surgical emergency; and an exploratory laparotomy with negative findings usually results in the diagnosis of a functional disorder. Complaints of weakness of the limbs, with variable aches and abdominal pain unassociated with demonstrable physical signs, commonly cause hysteria to be diagnosed; and this diagnosis has been retained even when advanced paralysis due to porphyria has been present for some time. The impression that the complaints of the porphyric patient are functional rather than organic is often reinforced by the accompanying signs of emotional instability; and if these give way to a frankly psychotic state, admission to a mental hospital is the usual outcome. It is therefore proper that the literature relating to the clinical aspects of porphyria should repeatedly contain warnings of the dangers of dismissing certain phenomena as hysterical, and so failing to make the correct diagnosis.
>
> On the other hand, our results indicate that the finding of porphobilinogen in the urine of a patient with suggestive symptoms does not prove the diagnosis of acute porphyria for quite a high excretion-rate may occur in symptomless cases and mild attacks may be accompanied by no increase in output . . .some workers have claimed that emotional factors can precipitate attacks . . . in many such

patients either the stress is coincidental or the attack itself is largely a hysterical reaction to the stress with the porphyric process playing little or no part.

The diagnosis of the mild attack presenting with no demonstrable physical signs is therefore a matter for clinical judgment, often requiring skilled psychiatric assessment.

Hereditary Coproporphyria

Goldberg *et al.* (1967) report a number of such patients with massive excretion of coproporphyrin 111 in the urine and faeces but predominantly in the faeces. It is hereditary, transmitted by a Mendelian dominant character and is hepatic rather than erythropoietic in type. It may present as an acute intermittent form and it would be advisable to examine the faeces for coproporphyrin as well as the urine for porphobilinogen. As four of their patients had mental symptoms (mainly depression) without other features of porphyria, this variety should also be borne in mind especially as it may be provoked by the administration of barbiturates and possibly tranquillizers and anticonvulsants.

Aggravation of porphyria can be due to a variety of drugs which may be given to a patient during an attack. Most of these act on the liver and include barbiturates, alcohol and sulphonamides. In spite of this well-known vulnerability of the liver, chlorpromazine has been given with benefit and electroplexy too has been recommended as a life-saving measure (Lemere, 1954). It is important that barbiturates be not used to produce anaesthesia prior to the administration of the electroplexy.

The mechanism whereby the nervous system is affected is still obscure but Dagg *et al.* (1965) have compared the clinical, biochemical and pathological features in 50 patients with lead poisoning and in 50 patients with acute intermittent porphyria. There was a remarkable similarity in everything except that anaemia was present in 47 of the patients with lead poisoning but in only 1 patient with porphyria. The way is now clearer for further investigations of the biochemical abnormalities in the nervous system which are present in both conditions.

An historical contribution was made by McAlpine and Hunter (1966) who after a careful analysis of all available evidence 'diagnosed' the recurrent insanity of George III as being due to acute intermittent porphyria. It is not surprising therefore that his physicians at the time were unable to understand this strange illness. Even today, its course and duration makes it the most unique case on record.

DISSEMINATED (SYSTEMIC) LUPUS ERYTHEMATOSUS

With the increasing recognition of the 'group disorder', and the consequently more intensive investigation of 'rheumatoid' states, more cases of disseminated lupus erythematosus (DLE) are being diagnosed. The condition is classified under the 'collagen diseases' and the diagnosis is frequently made, and certainly more frequently excluded by the presence or absence respectively of the 'LE cell' in the blood.

The Clinical Picture

This is one of fever with leucopenia, purpura and progressive wasting. There may also be polyarthritis, polyserositis and endocarditis but symptoms and signs may be referable to every system of the body. In some patients there is a scaly rash which does not itch and may be localized to the cheeks, neck, chest and upper extremities. A characteristic renal lesion, which is responsible for haematuria and proteinuria in two-thirds of patients, consists of a hyaline thickening of some of the glomerular capillaries giving a 'wire-loop' appearance.

Pathological Findings

These are said to be due to a denaturation of nuclear material which is manifested by the presence of 'haematoxylin bodies' in the lymph nodes and in the lesions. This denaturation has been attributed to abnormal gamma globulin and most patients show a high gamma globulin fraction with a relative decrease in the albumin fraction of the serum protein. The ESR is raised and the globulins react with intact nucleoprotein in a manner which suggests an antigen-antibody reaction and this is the basis of the LE phenomenon. There is frequently a false-positive W.R. and the negative Treponema immobilization test (T.P.I.) is regarded as a pointer to the presence of DLE.

Mental Symptoms

These are varied and may be those of anxiety, depression, and even schizophrenia, as well as confusional and delirious phases. These have been described by McClary *et al.* (1955) and O'Connor (1957), and Noyes and Kolb (1958) report that in a series of patients followed up at the Presbyterian Hospital in New York, 50 per cent presented delirious or psychotic features at some time during the course of their illness. A number show neurological features and Malamud and Saver (1954) have been able to demonstrate neuropathological findings.

As the condition is treated with corticoids, these were blamed for the mental symptoms, but Noyes and Kolb (1958) point out that this is not so and that if after recovering from the delirious state further corticoids were given, there was no recurrence of the mental symptoms. Further support exonerating corticoids as an aetiological factor has come from Ganz *et al.* (1972) who subjected 68 patients with S.L.E. to a structured interview and found that psychiatric symptoms predominated in the group who were not on steroids; they were also an older age group and had the disease for 10 years or longer. The role of corticoids is therefore still not entirely solved and more conclusive evidence is awaited.

The prognosis of the psychiatric features is that of the physical illness, which is generally, even with corticoids, guarded.

PSYCHOSES DUE TO TOXIC AGENTS

Toxic psychosis is a term which is frequently invoked to describe those states where there is a definable toxic origin. In this category are two large groups: (1) those cases where the patient is so susceptible that even trivial amounts of the agent will precipitate a psychotic illness, and (2) those cases where the agent itself has earned a reputation for precipitating psychosis. In the first instance there is little to be gained in listing all the agents to which susceptible people may react, though individual examples may be useful in explaining some unexpected events. In the second instance, it is helpful to classify those agents that may be responsible for the psychosis.

EXOGENOUS POISONS

Drugs. These may be responsible either in therapeutic doses or in accidental or deliberate over-dosage.

Bromides

These were widely used as mild sedatives and in the treatment of epilepsy. For the elderly they are useful in procuring sleep and as there is practically no risk of suicide, there is much to commend them. They are believed to be relatively harmless, and the prescription is frequently repeated; as the drug is slowly excreted, a concentration may be built up which can produce a psychotic state. Normally serum bromide is < 3 mg. per 100 ml. and symptoms of intoxication rarely occur below a level of 150 mg. per 100 ml. though in senile and arteriosclerotic patients or those with renal damage a lower figure may suffice. The bromide replaces the chloride in the blood, but it is doubtful if this factor alone is responsible for the ensuing mental state.

In mild cases there may be irritability, sleep disturbance and slight impairment of comprehension which may progress to restlessness and confusion. Unfortunately this picture may persuade the physician or the patient to increase the dose and thus aggravate the condition. Other features are slurring of speech, dehydration with dry skin, ataxia, tremor of tongue and acne. In the severe cases, the clinical picture is one of delirium with disorientation and altered consciousness. Levin (1948) has described four psychotic patterns.

1. Simple intoxication, which is manifest by a dull and sluggish mental state with forgetfulness, but correct orientation. These features with tremor of hands and tongue and sluggish pupils can simulate dementia paralytica.
2. Delirium, which is associated with disorientation, confusion, motor restlessness and insomnia.
3. Transitory schizophrenia, which resembles the 'functional' variety in that the patient is withdrawn, aloof and negativistic. Leven claims that it is very different from ordinary delirium or hallucinosis and considers that it is a true schizophrenic state which has been uncovered in a person with a schizoid personality.
4. Hallucinosis, which presents in a clear and well oriented setting.

The auditory and visual hallucinations of bromide intoxication have been differentiated from those in alcoholic delirium by Curran (1944) in that they seem to be more distant, but there are more reliable criteria in differential diagnosis.

Diagnosis

This is established by estimating the serum bromide, though it may be low if the drug were discontinued a few days before the test. An EEG may give useful information about the organic nature of the illness, for the record is sensitive to bromide and intoxication produces a preponderance of slow waves. Levin (1959) points out that repeated serum bromide levels give no reliable guide to prognosis. 'Recovery does not depend on serum bromide level but, rather, on the extent of cerebral damage and on the capacity of the brain to recover from injury.' The delirium may last for several weeks after the cessation of the drug, while in alcoholic delirium the duration is usually four or five days.

Treatment

This consists of stopping the bromide, fluid replacement for the dehydration, and sodium chloride, 2–4 g. four-hourly. Some patients are unable to take this dose and it may have to be given in enteric-coated tablets, but ammonium chloride which is also a diuretic is now regarded as a more rational treatment and is said to be better tolerated. As with other organic psychoses, electric convulsant therapy has been suggested but there are insufficient reliable reports to support its use.

Because it can be readily diagnosed and a number of patients, particularly in mental hospitals, have been given the drug freely, with resultant intoxication, there has been in recent years a reluctance to prescribe bromides. It is questionable, however, whether those drugs which have replaced it, among which were the barbiturates and thalidomide, are any safer.

Methyl Bromide

This substance is used in refrigeration and in disinfestation. Toxicity is not due to the bromide ion which in bromism produces blood levels of over 100 mg. bromide per 100 ml. It is the methyl element which does the damage and levels as low as 5 mg. bromide per 100 ml. may be toxic. This level can produce a mild euphoria and lack of concern in handling the substance. This in turn can lead to major over-exposure or chronic recurrent intoxication with irreversible brain damage. Neurological signs consist of coarse tremor, generalized hyperreflexia and incoordination of limb movements. Drawneek *et al.* (1964) describe a patient who complained of severe depression, with loss of initiative, concentration and confidence. As there was an impending compensation case and the patient was also complaining of nightmares which centred round his works manager, these psychiatric features should not be regarded as specific.

Barbiturates

(See Chapter 18.)

ACTH and Cortisone

These have since their inception had psychiatric overtones. As they are both apt to be euphoriants, there is a tendency for some patients to become addicted to them, particularly so in dermatological, asthmatic and rheumatology clinics. In view of the very large number of patients who have received the drugs and their specific effects on electrolyte balance, surprisingly few cases of overt psychosis occur. Rome and Braceland (1952) and Ritchie (1956) have described cases which range over the whole spectrum of psychiatric symptomatology. Elation and depression and inappropriate affect have been described and the author has seen a patient develop acute maniacal excitement with hallucinations and delusions which fortunately responded readily to large doses of chlorpromazine. In some instances it may not be possible to discontinue the steroid and it should therefore be given together with chlorpromazine.

OTHER EXTERNAL POISONS

Lead

This is the commonest of the metallic poisons which are responsible for mental disorder. Its place in the mental disturbances of childhood by reason of 'pica' is described in Chapter 17, but it also affects adults, particularly through its use in industrial processes, where inhalation of toxic compounds may produce psychiatric symptoms of either an acute or chronic nature. The commoner jobs which carry the risk of exposure are lead paint spraying, lead burning as in the destruction of old batteries or other salvage work, lead enamelling and lead glass blowing. The symptoms and signs in the milder states of poisoning are anorexia, abdominal discomfort, constipation, headache and pallor. The more severe features are abdominal cramps, paralysis of the extensor muscles and the 'lead line' round the gums. Blood examination reveals a microcytic anaemia with increased basophilic stippling of the red corpuscles. There is an increased coproporphyrinuria, the blood lead is above 0·1 mg./100 ml. and the urinary lead is above 0·1 mg./litre.

The mental symptoms may be acute or progressive. In the acute stage there is delirium of sudden onset with confusion, tremors, visual hallucinations and delusions and occasionally convulsions. In the progressive form there is an apathetic state which may masquerade as depression, memory impairment, speech difficulties and confabulation of a Korsakoff type. A milder form presents a neurasthenic picture with irritability, physical weakness and giddiness, but these symptoms may be due to the anaemia. The author had a patient who developed hypertension which was considered to be of renal origin. He was evacuated to U.K. from India and on the hospital ship was given a milk diet; several days later his mental state was affected. He became dull, apathetic and depressed and was admitted on arrival at Southampton to a psychiatric unit instead of a general medical one. A reliable history was not obtainable from the patient, but his wife when she visited supplied the information that he had worked with lead paint for nearly 20 years. A lead intoxication was confirmed by chemical tests and it was presumed that it was due to the recent mobilization of the lead deposits in the skeleton.

Treatment is firstly prevention and all industries are now alive to the hazard, and rigorous precautions are laid down. For cases of acute poisoning due to ingestion of lead in children, gastric lavage with magnesium, sodium or aluminium sulphate solutions followed by plain water to remove the lead sulphate that has been produced should suffice. Generally the treatment of the established poisoning is by deleading with calcium disodium versenate (ethylenediaminetetra acetic acid), a chelating agent which forms a stable water soluble compound with metals. It is given by slow intravenous drip, the maximum dosage not to exceed 0·5 g./30 lb. body wt./hr.; 1·0 g./30 lb. body wt./24 hr.; 5·0 g./30 lb. body wt./7 days and 7·5 g./30 lb. body wt./10 days in divided doses (Merck, 1961).

A course of treatment should be limited to 10 days with a week's rest between courses and two courses should suffice. In severe lead encephalopathy, it may be necessary to resort to surgical decompression to relieve intracranial pressure. Dimercaprol is of no value.

Mercury

This is not nearly so common as a cause of mental disturbance as lead. It was traditionally regarded as a hazard of the hatter's trade because it was used in the preparation of fur and felt, but whether Lewis Carroll selected the Mad Hatter because of this relationship is a matter for speculation. The psychiatric symptoms are those of a neurasthenic state with irritability and loss of confidence, though it may produce excitement followed by depression. The neurological features, which include a coarse tremor of the orbit, lips, tongue and hands, may be mistaken for a striatal disorder of unknown aetiology, and mercury poisoning should be borne in mind, for it is used in such a variety of trades that it may well provide the answer to an otherwise obscure problem.

Treatment is by dimercaprol (BAL) which is said to be of value in severe cases of nephrosis and in mental disturbance. The regime recommended by Merck (1961) is 3 mg./kg. intramuscularly every four hours for two days, every six hours for one day, and every 12 hours for the next 10 days or until recovery is complete. Haemodialysis by the artificial kidney is of value.

Manganese

This is used in many industrial processes and prolonged exposure may produce neurological and psychiatric symptoms. The former are of an extrapyramidal nature due to involvement of the basal ganglia.

Flynn *et al.* (1940) and Fairhall and Neal (1943) have described mental sequelae which include outbursts of uncontrollable laughing and crying, and general emotional lability of a less dramatic nature. There is, as yet, no specific treatment but removal from exposure may result in an abatement of the mental symptoms, the neurological ones tending to persist.

Carbon Monoxide (CO)

This is both a cause and a result of mental disturbance, for it is one of the commoner methods of attempting suicide. It is produced by car exhausts, mine explosions, incomplete combustion of carbon in its numerous forms, and where there is poor ventilation a toxic or lethal concentration may develop. It is present in acetylene, illuminating (coal), furnace and marsh gas, and it is easy to see how a gas which is so prevalent and so readily accessible has played such an important part in the cause of death from poisoning in Great Britain and North America where it is by far the commonest cause. In 1957 in England and Wales, out of a total of 4902 deaths due to poisonous agents, 3588 were due to CO; 808 were presumed to be accidental and the remainder suicidal. In piped gas for household purposes, the percentage of CO is between 10 and 30, while in motor car exhausts it may reach 25. It combines rapidly and easily with haemoglobin to form carboxyhaemoglobin. Cumming (1961) states:

> A given mass of haemoglobin combines with the same volume of CO as of oxygen, and the resulting compounds both dissociate readily into their constituent parts. If these were the only factors, then the realtive amounts of carboxyhaemoglobin and oxyhaemoglobin formed in blood would be directly

proportional to the partial pressures of CO and oxygen respectively. Under these conditions, breathing quite high concentrations of CO would be compatible with life. In fact this is not so, because CO has an affinity for haemoglobin which is some 200 times greater than that of oxygen. Consequently equal proportions of carboxyhaemoglobin and oxyhaemoglobin will exist in the blood when the partial presence of CO is 1/200 that of oxygen. Since the partial pressure of oxygen is about 150 mm. Hg, the partial pressure of CO to give 50 per cent carboxyhaemoglobin will be only 0·75 mm. Hg. Expressed in percentages this would be brought about by a concentration of CO in air of 0·1 per cent or one volume in one thousand. The adverse physiological effects brought about by the carboxyhaemoglobin are primarily those of anoxia due to deprivation of oxyhaemoglobin, the carboxyhaemoglobin having no oxygen carrying capacity.

Meigs and Hughes (1952) reported that 98 out of 103 patients admitted within 24 hours of acute CO poisoning showed some mental abnormality, though this may have been present prior to the poisoning. Neurological features are common and include abnormal reflexes, increased or diminished, involuntary movements (the author had a case with hemiballismus), spasticity and incontinence. If the neurological signs are gross and persist for several days, then there is likely to be severe mental impairment when the patient regains consciousness. The cerebral pathology consists of ischaemic changes in the nerve cells with areas of softening in the globus pallidus and cortex. Patients who have residual mental deterioration following the stage of recovery are relatively few in number and are invariably associated with severe intoxication with several days of loss of consciousness. The author, who had been seeing large numbers of cases admitted with coal-gas poisoning over a period of 12 years, found only four patients with residual deterioration. One had written a suicide note and when she recovered she was grossly demented and had no recollection of her previous conduct. She had forgotten how to read and her speech was also deficient, but after several months she regained a modest level of performance but was still much below her normal level. She was given a trial at home and by some strange macabre twist, wrote a similar suicide note, her first piece of spontaneous writing since she was resuscitated. Her level of intellectual progress has remained arrested, and this is what usually happens.

Mental changes may not follow immediately on exposure and Gordon (1965) reported a patient whose behaviour disturbances presented after 21 days. These included drinking out of an empty cup and walking out of the house dressed only in a shirt. There were also neurological signs. As in the previous case there was initial improvement but this was followed by further deterioration and death.

Treatment. Hyperbaric oxygen has been reported to be effective and if so, this is a considerable advance, even though, at present, few centres are equipped to administer it.

Carbon Disulphide

This is used extensively in the rubber and rayon industries and prolonged exposure to the chemical can result in mental changes. In the early stages the patient complains of headache, insomnia and bad dreams, and later there is memory loss with intellectual deterioration and occasionally delirium. The neurological symptoms are varied and include tenderness of the nerve trunks, hyperaesthesia and later anaesthesia. Paralysis may ensue and striatal signs with Parkinsonism and choreoathetosis may also occur. There is no effective treatment of the chronic state, though removing the patient from the contaminated area may result in some improvement.

Analgesic Abuse and Dementia

Murray *et al.* (1971) reported on 9 brains of patients who had analgesic nephropathy and 8 other patients with this condition had psychometric tests. Of 6 of the 7 who took phenacetin, neurofibrillary changes were observed in 4 and senile plaques in 6, but no such changes were observed in the 2 patients who had taken aspirin only. Senile plaques were present in the frontal, temporal and occipital regions but were most obvious in the hippocampal gyrus.

Psychometry showed that the two youngest patients (30 and 44 years) who had consumed the least analgesics showed no evidence of mental impairment, but of the 6 patients between 48 and 60 years, 4 showed definite and 2 possible evidence of organic brain disease. Psychological disturbances in analgesic abusers are common and may be a causal factor, and the EEG is frequently of interest and must lead to a search for analgesic abuse in suspected cases of Alzheimer's disease. Of even greater interest is the possibility of studying the mechanisms responsible for these changes.

Water Intoxication

Alexander *et al.* (1973) reviewed 7 cases which they differentiate from psychogenic polydipsia. Three were schizophrenics and 4 were alcoholics and the diagnosis was made on the low serum sodium (120) and chloride (90). The authors' own patient was almost decerebrate with athetoid movements, but plantars were flexor. All limbs had a fine tremor and muscle tone was noticeably increased.

The infusion of 250 ml. of 5 per cent hypertonic saline produced a marked improvement in consciousness.

MENTAL CHANGES DUE TO INTERNAL POISONS

In addition to the failure to eliminate the products of metabolism with consequent toxic effects, disturbance of electrolyte balance may cause mental changes.

Respiratory Acidosis (Carbon Dioxide Retention)

This can be due to a variety of causes, such as depression of the respiratory centre by drugs or disease; weakness or paralysis of the respiratory muscles; reduction of the alveolar area for gaseous exchange, as is seen in pulmonary emphysema, or other pulmonary and cardiac disease; obstruction to the free flow of CO_2 from the lungs, which can be due to either occlusion or severe emphysema; and breathing an excess of CO_2 as one occasionally finds in closed circuit anaesthesia where the absorbent is exhausted.

Mental Symptoms. These are mainly drowsiness with slow cerebration; the patient may appear demented and occasionally deluded and hallucinated. The condition is liable to exacerbation due to respiratory infection or deterioration in cardiac efficiency and, as cerebral oedema is a complication, the optic discs may suggest increased intracranial pressure. It is not unknown for such patients to be regarded as suffering from brain tumours and to be decompressed. The condition is fairly common in Britain where chronic bronchitis is prevalent and should be borne in mind, particularly in senile and presenile psychotic states.

Treatment. This should be directed to the aetiological factor, though in the severer mental disturbances, phenothiazines may be helpful.

Respiratory Alkalosis

This is usually due to neurotic hyperventilation which is described on page 291. The patient may show the signs of tetany with carpal spasm, Chvostek's and Trousseau's signs. There is usually anxiety prior to the attack, but the result of the attack with its threatened loss of consciousness may aggravate the anxiety with resulting panic and occasionally the patient's behaviour can be very disturbing. As many of these patients are in any case very immature, it is difficult to dissociate the behaviour following the hyperventilation from the pre-morbid personality.

Hyponatraemia

This is due to the excessive loss of sodium ion through renal disease, failure of adrenal function, or profuse perspiration. In addition to the fatigue, which is common to all causes, in adrenocortical insufficiency there may be profound depression which can resemble a true psychotic pattern. Occasionally the hypotension and the marked feelings of weakness may earn the patient a diagnosis of neurasthenia. It should therefore be borne in mind in a patient with loss of weight, hypotensive attacks and severe depression, especially as it usually responds to treatment.

Hypokalaemia

Potassium deficit due to either poor intake as in anorexia nervosa and hyperemesis gravidarum, or excessive loss as in steatorrhoea, can result in mental changes of a delusional or depressive nature. There is also an accompanying confusion, but this may be so slight as to lead the observer to consider the condition to be entirely a functional psychosis. The author, who is occasionally called to see patients with severe hyperemesis gravidarum with mental symptons, asks for the patient's serum potassium to be available prior to the consultation and it is usually low. The house surgeon has been aware of the loss of chloride and sodium through the vomiting, but did not budget for the drop in potassium. Replacement results in dramatic improvement.

Hypercalcaemia

This may be due to excessive intake of vitamin D, production of some endogenous vitamin D-like substance from sarcoidosis or carcinoma, or increased production of parathyroid hormone from a tumour of the parathyroid glands. Mentally the patient may be apathetic, confused or depressed and present the features of neurasthenia. When the psychiatrist is shown one of these patients by a medical colleague, he may wonder whether all the cases of fatigued depression he has seen were really exhibiting the features of hypercalcaemia, so closely do they resemble each other. The author has on occasions had bursts of enthusiasm and arranged for serum calciums on a number of such patients but with no success. It must therefore be a rare condition as far as the psychiatrist is concerned and the diagnosis probably rests on features other than the mental ones.

Hypocalcaemia

This may follow removal of the parathyroids and the patient will show the clinical features of tetany. His nervous system may be equally irritable, particularly during the attacks of tetany when he may be excitable, restless and confused or present with manic features.

Denko and Kaelbling (1962) who made a special study of the psychiatric aspects of hypoparathyroidism found that the idiopathic form could manifest as intellectual impairment, organic brain syndrome, 'functional' psychosis, pseudoneurosis or 'unclassified'. Deficiency due to surgery presented mainly as organic brain syndrome and the authors stress that the diagnosis may frequently be missed by psychiatrists and internists.

Uraemia

Renal insufficiency results in the retention in the blood of nitrogenous urinary waste products (azotaemia). The causes are many and need not be detailed here. The psychiatrist's interest is mainly in the exclusion of a uraemic cause for dementia. The patient may be dull, confused and unduly fatigued, and if there is no other obvious cause for the dementia, a blood urea is a useful screening test.

Hepatic Coma

This condition is found in liver failure due to disease, drugs, alcohol or following portacaval anastomosis. The patient may present with an encephalopathy with behaviour disturbances, confusion or lethargy. This toxic state is alleged to be caused by an increased concentration of ammonia in the blood due to the inability of the diseased liver to detoxicate it, yet the clinical picture is not highly correlated with the concentration of ammonia in the blood and other metabolites have been considered. The diagnosis is supported by other features of hepatic failure, such as flapping tremor of the hands, spider naevi, and 'liver palms'. EEG changes consisting mainly of generalized slow waves are seen during the attacks.

Mineral Metabolism

There is an increasing amount of evidence to show that in people who are apparently physically healthy, psychotic features, particularly mania and melancholia can be associated with fluctuations in sodium when assessed by 'whole-body' techniques. Shaw (1966) found that residual sodium (cell sodium and a small amount of bone sodium) was increased by 50 per cent in depression and by 200 per cent in mania. Support for these observations has been contributed by the effective use of lithium in the treatment of mania (Cade, 1949). Lithium can substitute for the sodium ion and when given in therapeutic doses it disturbs sodium transport mechanisms.

CHAPTER 6

Psychosomatic Medicine

The term 'psychosomatic medicine' has been severely criticized by psychiatrists who declare that it perpetuates a dualism which does not exist, and by physicians, who deny the psychological components of a number of the diseases included in the group. Yet it is now well established that certain diseases tend to be more influenced by psychological factors than others and it is difficult to suggest a better term than that of psychosomatic. As long as it is recognized that it is not a restrictive definition, it should not offend the holistic enthusiast, and as long as it is recognized that it is not all-embracing, but is applied to those conditions where psychological factors have been demonstrated to be important, then sceptical physicians should raise no valid objection.

Halliday (1943) defined a psychosomatic affection as 'a bodily disorder whose nature can be appreciated only when emotional disturbances (*i.e.* psychological happenings) are investigated in addition to physical disturbances (*i.e.* somatic happenings)'. He put forward the 'psychosomatic formula' consisting of the following six ingredients:

1. *Emotion as a Precipitating Factor.* Examination of patients in series shows that in a high proportion of cases, the bodily process emerged or recurred on meeting an emotionally upsetting event.

2. *Personality Type.* A particular type of personality appears to be associated with each particular affection.

3. *Sex Ratio.* A marked disporportion of sex incidence is a finding in many, perhaps most of these disorders.

4. *Association with other Psychosomatic Affections.* Different psychosomatic affections may appear in the same individual simultaneously, but the more usual phenomenon as revealed in their natural history is that of the alternation or of the sequence of different affections.

5. *Family History.* A significantly high proportion of cases give a history of the same or an associated disorder in parents, relatives or siblings.

6. *Phasic Manifestations.* The course of the illness tends to be phasic with periods of crudescence, intermission and recurrence.

It is not essential for all the ingredients to be present for the condition to merit the label 'psychosomatic'. For example, Nos. 1, 2 or 4 even in isolation would be suggestive and some might include No. 5.

The relationship between emotions and body changes has been recognized for countless years and most languages abound with examples such as: 'He gives me a headache', 'the mere sight of him makes me sick', 'I just can't stand it'. Grosser examples are 'to die of fright' and 'to have an apoplectic fit' because of some annoyance. A distinction should be drawn between *body reactions* and *body changes* following emotional factors. In the former, the condition is usually regarded as hysterical and denotes a retreat into functional incapacity, such as being struck dumb, blind or paralyzed, while in the psychosomatic disorder, overt body changes occur, such as skin rashes, diarrhoea, rectal bleeding and asthmatic attacks. The role of the emotions in such disorders has been noted by experienced physicians throughout the ages, but it is only in comparatively recent times that there has been a satisfactory explanation of how some of these changes occur.

Cannon's (1939) studies on the autonomic system and the bodily changes in pain, hunger, fear and rage provided laboratory confirmation of phenomena which were already well-recognized, but more important, they shed some light on how these changes came about. His dictum that sympathetic stimulation prepares the body for fight or flight indicated the importance of the autonomic nervous system and the medulla of the suprarenal glands in these reactions. Experimental evidence of the effect of emotions on the human stomach was available much earlier, when Beaumont (1833) studied a patient, Alexis St. Martin, who following a gunshot wound of the abdomen had his stomach wall exteriorized. Wolf and Wolff (1947) over 100 years later with their patient 'Tom' who also had a gastric fistula were able to show that gastric secretion, motility and vascularity were reduced when the patient was sad or frightened, but they were increased when he felt angry, resentful or anxious.

Theories of the inter-relation between body and mind have not been wanting. Some are comprehensive, some are partial, some are based on sound experimental work, some are purely theoretical.

Selye's Theory of the Stress-Adaptation Syndrome

This is based on an adrenocortical response to physical and emotional assaults producing 'stress'. Confirmation of the former is evidenced by the effect of extreme cold, physical trauma, anaesthesia, anoxia, hypoglycaemia and infections, and of the latter by armed combat, boat racing, disturbing interviews, anticipation of surgical operations and final examinations. These are all accompanied by a variable rise in 17-hydroxycorticoid output. Though most of the theory which postulates an imbalance of adrenocortical secretions as a cause of 'stress' diseases in man is still unsubstantiated, it has served to emphasize the role of the adrenal cortex in resistance to stress. An unfortunate aspect of the theory is the word 'stress' itself, for it means one thing to the physiologist, another to the sociologist and yet another to the psychiatrist. For example, many physicians regard as stress those traditional hazards of man, famine, plague, flood and drought, and the impoverished areas of the world are cited as illustrative of abundant stress with a low incidence of psychosomatic disorders, such as peptic ulceration, while in the more prosperous areas of the world where there is a relative absence of these stresses, there is a high incidence of psychosomatic disorder. This argument misses the whole concept of stress in the psychosomatic sense which is regarded as the result of a frustrating experience which the individual is unable to influence or where there is a mental conflict expressed in somatic form. If famine and the others are to operate as psychosomatic stresses, then the cultural attitude of the victims should be one of burning resentment rather than of patient resignation. Those who criticize the concept of psychosomatic illness on these grounds have projected their own (fancied) reactions into cultures with which they are not and perhaps cannot be identified. It illustrates the fallacy of drawing conclusions from introspection, and from projection into situations to which one is not generally exposed and to which cultural reactions vary, and also by people who are least fitted to indulge in such forms of analysis.

A generally acceptable definition of 'stress' is very difficult to come by and at a conference of the Mental Health Research Fund on 'Stress' held in Oxford in 1958, Sir Geoffrey Vickers (1958), the Chairman, expressed the dilemma of the meeting by issuing a note on the second day on the various meanings attached to 'stress'. It read:

> We require a word to cover all those felt needs which evoke purposeful activity. If this be 'stress', then as Professor Selye says, only death can relieve it. To avoid so wide an application, I will use the word 'challenge' to cover both the need and the signal which evokes action to meet it.

The course of response to these challenges may pass through several stages:

(i) The organism can meet the need.

(ii) The organism can meet the need but only for a period which may not be sufficient.

(iii) The organism cannot meet the need without abandoning, at least for the time being, the effort to pursue or evade some other relationship.

(iv) The organism cannot meet the need at all.

If these stages occur successively, the state of the organism will change along four dimensions, which are not exactly correlated: and all these changes may, in current usage, be attributed to 'stress'.

(i) *It will change physiologically.* These changes will depend partly on the energy requirements of the response and partly on its emotional accompaniment. They may begin at stage (i) and often reach their peak in stage (ii) unless they are later complicated by the indirect effect of subsequent stages.

(ii) *It will change emotionally.* Anxiety may arise irrationally at stage (i) or rationally at stage (ii). The whole gamut of emotional changes may appear in the course of stages (iii) and (iv).

(iii) *It will change behaviourally.* At the end of stage (ii) its behaviour towards some or all of its other goals will change. At stage (iv) or earlier it will give up its purposeful activity towards the relation which is being defeated.

(iv) *It will change structurally.* From the end of stage (ii) it becomes differently structured, as it abandons or modifies one after another of its governing relations.

He concluded thus:

To clarify our discussion I make the following suggestions:

1. We are concerned with four separate objects of attention, for which we need separate words. It is unfortunate that three of these are themselves fourfold.

(i) Four types of (more or less) observable change;
(ii) the situations which cause these changes;
(iii) the processes by which these changes take place;
(iv) the behaviours which accompany these processes.

2. The simplest way, consistent with existing usage, in which we can mark these distinctions, when we want to be precise, is, I suggest, to refer to them as 'stress-change', 'stress-situation', 'stress-process', and 'stress-behaviour'.

The terms 'stressor' and 'stress-response' have such strong physiological connotations that they are best reserved for that field; but they would be included by the wider terms 'stress-situation', 'stress-change', and 'stress-behaviour'.

3. Though the four types of change—physiological, emotional, behavioural, and structural—are intimately related, there is clearly not a one-to-one correspondence between them. We should not assume that they are different aspects of the same 'thing', except in so far as we know them to be exactly correlated.

4. The only valid general use of the word 'stress' at present is adjectival. It connotes a degree of challenge sufficient to evoke the kind of change or

behaviour which interests the particular observer. Its meaning therefore depends not only on the 'dimension' in which he is interested but also on the threshold above which appear the kind of phenomena which he finds interesting.

The reporter to the *Lancet* comments: 'The conference did not achieve a better clarification of terminology than this'—and from a layman at that!

Psychoanalytical Considerations

With the tremendous accent on oral gratification, habit training, unconscious symbolic use of organs to express conflict and regressive body language or 'organ jargon' it is not surprising that psychoanalysis has regarded the psychosomatic disorders as a legitimate object of study. Fenichel (1945) deals with the problem under the following headings:

(a) *Affect equivalents,* where

> the specific physical expressions of any given affect may occur without the corresponding specific mental experiences, that is, without the person's being aware of their affective significance. . . . A certain percentage of what are called organ neuroses actually are affect equivalents. . . . The same holds true for those vegetative neuroses that occur when a compulsion neurotic or a reactive neurotic character gets disturbed in its relative regidity. . . .

(b) *The Disturbed Chemistry of the Unsatisfied Person.* Here Fenichel criticizes Alexander's (1943) opinion that the difference in the hormonal state in conscious and in unconscious affects is merely due to the chronicity of the so-called unconscious affective attitudes. He substitutes the interesting theory that these physical concomitants are also qualitatively different from the conscious ones and even speculates that these hormonal out-pourings may be as specific as the physical syndromes of conscious affects.

(c) *Physical Results of Unconscious Attitudes.* A person's behaviour 'is continually influenced by his conscious and unconscious instinctual needs'. If an adequate outlet cannot be found, substitutes may be sought and physical changes in these alternative outlets may result.

> An unusual attitude, which is rooted in unconscious, instinctual conflicts, causes a certain behaviour. This behaviour in turn causes somatic changes in the tissues. The changes are not directly psychogenic; but the person's behaviour, which initiated the changes, was psychogenic. . . . .

(d) *Hormonal and Vegetative Dysfunction.* Fenichel is in no doubt that in menstrual or premenstrual mental disorders, there is a somatic factor in the nature of a physical change at the source of the instinctual drives and that 'every pregenital fixation necessarily changes the hormonal status'. These tenets lack adequate proof and though they may sound reasonable they are far from experimental proof and must be considered as belonging to the more speculative aspect of psychoanalytic theory.

Ego-weakness has been postulated especially in psychotic illness and as psychosomatic disorders can alternate with psychoses, some have even considered this alternation as evidence that the physical state is psychosomatic.

Ego-regression has also been postulated and some hold that during this phase there is physiological reactivity in the regressed organ, but here, too, speculation is way ahead of experimental proof. There has also been much speculation as to why a certain organ assumes primacy in the individual's reaction and a number of views have been put forward, including genetic weakness, previous illness in the organ, and allergy.

Dunbar (1943), in a very comprehensive series of analytically orientated personality studies which she charted as profiles, concluded that those with the same psychosomatic complaint had a similar personality structure. This work has, however, been criticized as not showing sufficient differentiation. It is now more generally accepted that patients with differing psychosomatic complaints have more similarities in their personality profiles than differences. Alexander (1952), whose name is very closely identified with studies on the subject, emphasized the psycho-sexual development of the individual and the importance of the alimentary tract in the child's early emotional experiences with fear of starvation as the first real insecurity. Psychological attributes such as greed, jealousy and envy were associated with eating and oral incorporation, while repressed sexual desires could be displaced from genital functions to more infantile oral ones, so that alimentary activity would assume sexual primacy. Oral cravings could colour the personality of the individual who, if approval hungry, would over-react to withdrawal of affection and what has been labelled the 'vital supplies'. The wish to be loved became the wish to be fed, but the wish was not a physiological need, but the result of emotional needs. The stomach could, however, respond as if food were about to be ingested with resulting persistent gastric dysfunction such as chronic hypermotility and hypersecretion with eventual ulcer formation. This example of Alexander's theory, though specifically related to the alimentary tract, illustrates how emotional problems can affect function but the exact methods or even the specific emotional factors are not yet generally agreed. Parasympathetic overactivity where the patient regresses to a dependent level is alleged to play a part in the genesis of peptic ulcer, colitis and asthma, while sympathetic overactivity as a result of over-compensation is alleged to lead to migraine, hypertension and arthritis, but the dynamics of these conditions will be discussed under their separate headings.

Ruesch (1951) has pointed out that psychosomatic disorders may be evidence of psychological tension resulting from social change and mobility, which is more common in the middle classes with their ambitions, need to conform and constant repression of instinctive drives, than in a proletarian community.

Physiological Considerations

These are now constantly being associated with emotional and affective disturbances and include the experiments of French *et al.* (1954) who were able to produce peptic ulcer in monkeys by hypothalamic stimulation with implanted electrodes, a modern version of Claude Bernard's stimulation of the floor of the fourth ventricle in dogs. French and his colleagues were, however, able to show the interrelation of the anterior pituitary, adrenal cortex, and the vagus, as well as the influence of the reticulospinal pathways on gastric motility and secretion. The hypothalamus is frequently mentioned *en passant* as the mediator of most of the emotional influences on organ change because of its place in the control of the endocrine and autonomic nervous systems, but Cleghorn (1955) has defined the form of control more accurately by postulating a circular feedback system and MacLean (1955) has shown how the hypothalamus interacts with the limbic system (visceral brain) and the reticular formation. Some regionalization has also been postulated, the fronto-temporal area being concerned with self-preservation and control over ACTH secretion, while the more posterior regions influence sexual behaviour and sex hormones.

Arnold (1970) summarizes the neurophysiological mechanisms involved in the emotions and pinpoints the deficiencies in our understanding. His conclusions are worth quoting:

> It is possible to account for the physiological changes in various emotions, and even to work out the neural circuits that trigger them. But only on the basis of a phenomenological analysis of the psychological activities from perception to emotion and action will it be possible to work out a theory of brain function that provides a neural correlate for psychological experience. Without such a theory, the scores of detailed findings resulting from the massive research efforts

of the last few decades are bound to remain isolated and disconnected nuggets instead of clues to the rich veins of future knowledge.

Another word of warning which has been sounded elsewhere in the 'Guide' is that of Arieti (1970):

Modern civilisation has in many countries increased the opportunities for physical comfort, adequate nourishment, and sexual gratification. And yet, clinical evidence—although not yet validated by reliable statistical analysis—seems to indicate that mental illness and psychological malaise have increased and not decreased in these countries. It must be relatively easy to infer that problems belonging to the higher levels of the psyche are to a large extent responsible for man's psychological difficulties. For this reason comparative studies of animals, although elucidating basic psychological mechanisms, do not enlighten us on many aspects of human psychopathology.

He considers that the factors responsible are closely linked with cognition which has not received adequate consideration in psychiatric and psychoanalytic studies. Emotions are divided into three orders:

1. First order emotions

(a) Tension—a feeling of discomfort caused by different situations;

(b) Appetite—a feeling of expectancy;

(c) Fear—an unpleasant subjective state;

(d) Rage—follows the perception of danger to be overcome by fight;

(e) Satisfaction—an emotional state resulting from gratification of physical needs.

2. Second order emotions. These are not elicited by direct or impending attack on a threatened immediate change in homeostasis but by cognitive symbolic processes of anxiety and anger, wishing and security.

3. Third order emotions. These occur with the development of language, the gradual abandonment of preconceptual levels and the development of conceptual ones. He cites depression as a classical example of a third order emotion and illustrates the trend by saying that first order rage is elaborated by second order anger into third order hate.

Relationship between Physical and Psychiatric Disorders

This has been studied in a variety of diseases, thus leading to the definition of psychosomatic disorders. Eastwood and Trevelyan (1972) studied a randomly determined half of all individuals aged 40-64 years who were registered in a group practice in a London borough. They found there was a positive and significant association between physical and psychiatric morbidity, indicating a differential response among individuals within a community, with some members being more vulnerable then their peers. They suggest that because of this intimate relationship between physical and psychiatric disorder, these should no longer be seen as separate entities but as manifestations of ill-health of the whole organism and as psychological and biological responses to stressful situations.

Schachter (1970) is another protagonist of the major impact of cognitive factors on emotional states. He alleges that if a subject were covertly injected with adrenaline or was fed a sympathomimetic agent such as ephedrine he would become aware of palpitations, tremors, etc. and at the same time would be utterly unaware of why he felt that way. The consequences would be a pressure to understand and evaluate his bodily feelings and either relate it to the emotional situation in which he finds himself, or if inappropriate he would decide it was due to something that recently happened.

PAIN

Merskey and Spear (1967) define pain as 'an unpleasant experience which we primarily associate with tissue damage or describe in terms of tissue damage or both'.

Pain can occur in the absence of trauma or organic disease and is referred to as psychogenic pain. To understand the psychological factors which can initiate and exploit pain, it is useful to consider its role in psychological development. Engel (1962) supplies the following summary.

1. *Body Image.* It is part of the system which protects the body from injury, in that it warns of damage to or loss of parts of the body. It thus contributes to development of body image and plays a part in the dedifferentiation of the ego.

2. *Object Relationships.* Pain in the child provokes crying which elicits comfort from mother and the response is pleasurable. Relief of pain may be equated with reunion with a love object.

3. *Pain and Punishment.* These are linked in childhood (as well as semantically). Pain is suffered when child is 'bad' and is therefore deserved and associated with feelings of guilt. It may be cheerfully endured in order to enjoy the forgiveness and reconciliation which follows.

4. *Aggression and Power.* The child soon realizes he can impose his will by inflicting or threatening pain. He can also control his own aggression by the threat of pain to himself.

5. *Sexual Development.* At the height of sexual excitement pain may be mutually inflicted and even enjoyed. Some may prefer the pain to the sexual experience, the latter existing only in phantasy.

The Pain-Prone

Pain can therefore be utilized as a psychological means of adjustment and certain individuals are 'pain-prone'. They are generally chronically depressed, pessimistic and gloomy with guilty, self-depreciatory attitudes. Engel (1962) describes the pain-prone thus:

> Indeed, some seem to have suffered the most extraordinary number and variety of defects, humiliations and other unpleasant experiences, not simply as consequences of the pain they suffer or just as a result of bad luck; rather, many of these difficult situations have either been solicited by the patient or simply were not avoided. Such persons drift into situations or submit to relationships in which they are hurt, beaten, defeated or humiliated, and, to our astonishment, seem not to learn from experience; for no sooner are they out of one difficulty than they are in another in spite of the most obvious warnings. At the same time, they conspicuously fail to exploit situations which should lead to success; indeed, when success is thrust upon them they may do badly. Unconsciously they feel that they do not deserve success or happiness and that they must pay a price for it. Many of these patients are tolerant of pain inflicted upon them by nature or by the physician in the course of examination and treatment. In their medical histories we commonly discover an extraordinary number of injuries and operations and more than the usual number of painful illnesses and pain.

Precipitating Factors

Engel lists the following:

1. Failure of external circumstances to satisfy the unconscious need to suffer.
2. Real, threatened or phantasied loss. This is usually associated with bereavement or its antecedents.
3. Evocation of guilt by intense aggression or forbidden sexual feelings.

A common precipitating factor in an industrial society is injury. The pain persists long after the physical effects of the trauma have gone and there are cultural as well as personal factors which mobilize the patient's aggression against the responsible party. It is of interest that if there is no responsible and insured party, persistent pain is rarely seen.

BODY IMAGE AND PHANTOM PHENOMENA

Kolb (1954) was a major contributor to the psychological study of the phenomena of phantom limbs, laying great stress on the development of the body image and the factors which impair that development. He cites Schilder's (1935) extension of the views of Head (1920) who elaborated concepts in neurological terms of the 'body schema' or body image. He was primarily concerned with its significance in perception of body function to mobility, localization of tactile stimuli and phantom phenomena. Schilder extended the concept to include a sociological meaning for the individual and society. Schilder defined the body image as that scheme or picture of our own body which we form in our minds as a tridimensional unity involving interpersonal, environmental and temporal factors. He also related body image to curiosity, expression of emotion, social relations, duty and even ethics, thus almost equating body image with the psychoanalytic concept of the ego. He extended the purely perceptive aspect of body image to the expressive. Szasz (1957) reinforced the Schilder viewpoint in the light of development of theories regarding ego functions. Dismemberment and mutilation therefore take on a new dimension when one adds the psychoanalytic concept.

The phantom experience may follow loss of a variety of body parts such as nose, eyes, teeth, penis and breast but the most common is the phantom limb or digit which has been reported in as many as 98 per cent of amputees. It is the painful phantom limb which is troublesome and this does not account for more than 8 per cent. Parkes (1973) assessed 46 amputees 13 months after operation and found that 7 still had severe pain, 7 had moderate pain and 24 had mild pain. Age, sex and socioeconomic status were not significantly different in those with persistent pain as against those without pain.

Persistent phantom pain was found more often following illnesses lasting for more than a year before amputation, and illnesses which continued after operation to threaten life or the remaining limb. It was more likely to persist in those who had stump and phantom pain during the first three weeks after operation and in those with a rigid, compulsively self-reliant personality. The author concludes that the compulsively self-reliant amputee who strives to hide his feelings and tries to present a 'heroic' front is most likely to experience prolonged phantom limb pain, and suggests that this may be avoided if he can be helped to express his real feelings. The author does not deal with the influence of compensation for injury in these cases.

PSYCHOSOMATIC DISORDERS

It now remains to report on the psychosomatic factors in the various bodily disorders, and these are, as in general medicine, classified according to their systems, *e.g.* gastro-intestinal, cardio-vascular, musculoskeletal, endocrine, integumentary, respiratory and so on. This has its disadvantages, for it possesses no psycho-pathological validity, but until there is an unequivocal psycho-pathology, it is convenient to use the familiar classification, though it should be realized that it may in itself lead to a restricted form of thinking which could interfere with one's capacity to recognize relationships.

GASTRO-INTESTINAL

A few remarks have already been made concerning Alexander's contribution to the psychopathology of peptic ulcer, but these must be seen in the whole setting of general psychopathology with oral and anal levels of eroticism and the early experiences of love and hostility in which the alimentary tract from teeth to anus plays a leading part. It is not surprising therefore that there are a large variety of psychosomatic disturbances which are closely connected with the intestinal tract when one considers the infant's early experiences of the world—biting, sucking, being hungry, and the subsequent childhood difficulties associated with feeding and elimination, and how readily the stomach or the bowel can represent an emotional attitude. This level of information is already widely disseminated and need not be elaborated here. The specific problems associated with each organ and the established or hypothetical psychological factors involved will now be discussed.

PEPTIC ULCER

Reference has already been made to Beaumont's 'Alexis St. Martin' and Wolf and Wolff's 'Tom'.

Margolin (1951) undertook a psychoanalytic study of a college girl with a gastrostomy of two years' standing, following a suicidal attempt, and his work was not only psychoanalytical, but physiological and experimental. He found a difference in response of gastric secretion (a decrease) to emotional stimuli such as anger and resentment, compared with that of Wolf and Wolff's patient, suggesting that the unconscious meaning of the experimental procedure was different in his case. He considered that this was probably based on the patient's sex as she had an erotization of the gastrostomy with phantasies of the experiment as sexual violation.

A number of workers have tried to define the specific psychological factors leading to peptic ulceration. Some of the earlier studies dealt with the personality and character traits and included those of Alvarez (1929), Hartman (1933) and Draper and Touraine (1932), while Alexander (1952) and Szasz (1949) tried to define a typical conflict situation which initiated the ulcer or caused relapse in patients with differing personalities. They emphasized unconscious motives and pointed out that the wish to remain dependent conflicted with adult pride and that overcompensation in the form of exaggerated ambition and self-sufficiency resulted. Another group of patients were overtly dependent and demanding and were frustrated by an unsympathetic environment. The wish to be loved was replaced by the wish to be fed and the stomach as a result of persistent stimulation showed chronic hypersecretion and chronic hypermotility.

Mahl (1949, 1950, 1952) in his work casts doubt on the specificity of the dependency conflict, as he had found hydrochloric acid secretion increase with anxiety under any circumstances and independently of hostile or passive-dependent situations. His work was based on the experimental induction of chronic fear in dogs and monkeys and on a study of humans undergoing psychotherapy.

Weiner *et al.* (1957) have attempted to predict the onset of peptic ulcer and suggest the following conditions:

1. A sustained rate of gastric secretion as measured by serum pepsinogen concentration.
2. The presence of a conflict related to the persistence of strong infantile wishes to be loved and cared for, and the repudiation of these wishes by the adult ego or the external world, as inferred from projective and psychological techniques.
3. Exposure to an environmental situation which mobilizes conflict and induces psychic tension.

Their postulates were derived from an assessment and investigation of over 2000 army recruits and they claim some measure of success in their predictions.

French *et al.* (1957) have produced gastroduodenal lesions in monkeys by electrically stimulating, for periods up to three months, the low midline axis in the hypothalamus, and thus provide further evidence of the neural pathways involved. This work lends itself to further experiment with variations in technique.

Sex ratio is still an unexplained phenomenon and the male is by far the more vulnerable (a ratio of 12 to 1 has been reported by Mittelman and Wolff, 1942), yet is is said that at the beginning of the century it was commoner in females. It is not easy to verify the earlier findings because of the disparity in radiological examinations.

Stress in the Selye sense has also been invoked and it has been shown (Selye, 1950 *a & b*) that the repeated administration of corticotrophin can simulate the adrenocortical reactions to chronic emotional stress. Grinker and Spiegel (1945*a*) have demonstrated that peptic ulceration could result from prolonged emotional stress and Spicer *et al.* (1944) and Illingworth *et al.* (1944), in London and Glasgow respectively, showed significant increases in perforated peptic ulcers during heavy air-raids in these areas. Gray *et al.* (1951) have suggested that the reaction to stress of increased acid and peptic secretion is mediated by a hormonal mechanism through the hypothalamic-pituitary-adrenal-gastric axis. Drye and Schoen (1958) feel that there may be depression of the normal healing process of tiny erosions which may form from time to time.

Occupation has frequently been suggested as an important factor in the causation of peptic ulcer and the bus driver has been particularly implicated. Raffle (1959), Senior Medical Officer to the London Transport Executive, while admitting that peptic ulceration, gastritis, duodenitis, disorders of function of the stomach and symptoms referable to the upper gastro-intestinal tract, accounted for a sickness absence rate which is three to four times that of functional nervous disorders, found 'virtually no difference in the incidence of these disorders between motormen and guards and workshop staff'. In fact, according to the table he presents, conductors have a higher incidence of stomach complaints than bus drivers, though this does not mean a higher incidence of peptic ulceration.

Gastrectomy for the treatment of peptic ulcer has its own psychiatric aspects and Whitlock (1961) reports on 25 patients who were admitted for psychiatric treatment following partial gastrectomy, 56 per cent of whom required treatment for alcoholism or drug addiction. He considers there is a special relationship between the operation and the subsequent addictions and suggests that psychosomatic disease 'can in some way protect a patient from a more serious underlying psychotic breakdown if the psychosomatic symptoms are relieved.' He regarded the presence of an ulcer in an alcoholic as an efficient brake on excessive drinking.

It is well known that sedatives play an important part in the treatment of peptic ulcer and a large ulcer demonstrated radiologically can in the space of a week disappear entirely when the patient is adequately sedated. Similarly, relaxation through hypnotic suggestion may relax the spasm around an ulcer in the region of the pylorus and thus relieve pyloric obstruction.

COLITIS

'Mucous colitis', 'irritable colon', 'colon neurosis' are terms used to describe a syndrome, which in Victorian times was prevalent among parent-dominated, cloistered young women. Experimentally, von Bergmann and Katch (1913) had already noted intestinal blanching in the frightened rabbit, while Drury *et al.* (1929) had witnessed the effect of fear on a dog's colonic explant. A systematic study of what they termed the 'irritable colon syndrome', was made by Chaudhury and Truelove (1962) on 130 patients of whom 106 had spastic colon and 24 painless diarrhoea. In 77 per cent of the former and 87 per cent of the latter psychological factors seemed to play a part in either onset or exacerbation and the authors reckoned that with more intensive study these figures would have been higher. Biopsy revealed no abnormality in the irritable colon group. Hypnotic treatment as a means of relaxation was beneficial as were barbiturates. These authors found a ratio of female: male of 2:1 which approximates to that for ulcerative colitis though the conditions are very different.

The patient is usually a female with a marked tendency to hypochondriasis and whose stools contain a lot of mucus and occasional bowel casts but are usually free from blood. She frequently gets referred to the surgeon and in former years would achieve appendicectomy and other unneccesary operations, sometimes with temporary improvement. Attempts to introduce more rational therapy are frequently resisted and referral to a psychiatrist is therefore delayed while many never desert their surgeon. It is the psychiatric handicap rather than the physical one which leads to chronicity and the patient though presenting an air of outward calm, may be very disturbed indeed.

Nervous Diarrhoea

Wright and Das (1973) who had previously demonstrated a tendency for patients with nervous diarrhoea to excrete more vanyllylmandelic acid (VMA) than controls, extended their studies to show that these patients also excreted more homovanillic acid (HVA), and their more recent study was designed to confirm and quantitate their previous observations. They showed that the findings for HVA were valid but not those for VMA. As the former is the equivalent end product of dopamine metabolism, and this is confined to the brain, they assumed that the increase in HVA output was likely to be of cerebral origin. They suggest that HVA excretion may serve as a physical parameter for measuring response to stress.

REGIONAL ILEITIS

The diagnosis of regional ileitis can be difficult, especially in differentiating it from ulcerative colitis. Whybrow *et al.* (1968) studied retrospectively 39 persons with proven regional ileitis and were unable to find that the onset of the illness could be clearly linked with psychic precipitants. This is in sharp contrast to the present author's finding with ulcerative colitis, and using this finding as a differentiate, the author had referred to him 'blind' patients with an established diagnosis of ulcerative colitis or regional ileitis and was able on the evidence from the history to label each patient accurately. On the other hand McKegney *et al.* (1970) claimed that when all demographic characteristics, life events, psychosocial and behavioural vairables were considered, they were unable to distinguish regional ileitis from ulcerative colitis. This conflicting evidence would suggest that further work is indicated.

ULCERATIVE COLITIS

This is a very different problem which can also seriously endanger life. The patient is not usually reluctant to seek psychiatric help and there frequently arises the paradoxical situation where the psychiatrist, while appreciating the emotional factors in the patient's illness, realizes that psychotherapy is not enough to contain the disease, yet is unable to persuade the patient to see a surgeon. It is important, however, to be certain of the diagnosis and a number of instances of diarrhoea with very little else to support the diagnosis have been labelled ulcerative colitis. Diagnosis may be difficult, for the condition may be far removed from the classical severe attack of bloody diarrhoea, colicky abdominal pain, malaise, anorexia, fever and weight loss. Even a barium enema with its characteristic pattern of loss of normal haustral markings, shortening of bowel length and irregularity of its contours is not necessarily conclusive. Sigmoidoscopy is helpful in the less acute cases, for it frequently shows granularity of the mucosa with sanguino-purulent exudates. Firm diagnosis is also important in formulating theories as to personality and causation, for many reports on these aspects assume the diagnosis rather than establish it.

Psychosomatic Hypotheses

Wittkower (1938) undertook personality studies in 40 unselected cases of ulcerative colitis and found that they differed so markedly from the average, that he regarded a special control study as unnecessary. A detailed clinical history together with a dated life history taken independently and verified from relatives showed that disturbing events in the patient's life had preceded the onset, return and increase of symptoms to a degree that exceeded chance. He did not find a specific personality type but divided his patients into two main groups: (1) twenty-three were rigid compulsive characters with a strong sense of inferiority; (2) twenty-two (all women) differed chiefly in a more overt display of strong emotion, were more noisy, petulant, argumentative and exhibitionistic, but in other respects resembled the first group. A residue of five patients fitted into no special group, but were shy, depressed, terrified of transgression and exhibited social anxiety.

Most people who work with patients with ulcerative colitis seem convinced of the specific personality structure, particularly their obsessionality. Sim and Brooke (1958), in a questionnaire sent to 164 members of an Ileostomy Association who had had colectomy for ulcerative colitis, received 142 replies, and a cynical colleague remarked that that would probably prove to be the most significant finding! Theories abound. Some stress the personality structure, some the traumatic experience and some the patient-mother relationship, but for each 'specific' psychopathological theory there is usually one which runs counter to it and many have no doubt been formulated on inadequate and sometimes inaccurate data. Some have been elaborated on a couple of cases, but numbers alone need not make for accuracy and may in fact omit some essential ingredient which could be obtained only by prolonged association with the patient, in other words, analysis.

Engel (1954 *a & b,* 1955, 1956, 1958) has most thoroughly reviewed the literature and lists a number of these theories; the following brief accounts are given not because they are all essential to the understanding of the condition; most are not, but they do indicate the wealth of theorizing that goes on in psychosomatic illness of all varieties and how much of this may indeed confuse rather than clarify.

1. **Alexander** (1952) emphasizes the importance of emotional

factors which from early life are associated with excremental and alimentary functions and, assuming that the disease is ushered in with diarrhoea, gives the following formula:
'Frustration of oral-dependent longings→oral aggressive responses→ guilt→anxiety→over-compensation for oral aggression by the urge to give (restitution) and to accomplish→inhibition and failure of the effort to give and accomplish→ diarrhoea.'

2. **Szasz** (1951) suggests that colonic activation and inhibition, leading to diarrhoea and constipation, represent the physiological sequelae of certain alterations in the upper gastroenteric tract, of which the gastrocolic reflex represents the prototype. Mobilization of strong (unconscious) oral incorporative strivings would be accompanied by constipation while a sudden decrease in such strivings, usually because of guilt feelings, would result in diarrhoea. Accordingly, the bowel symptoms do not express any primary psychological meaning, but are manifestations of a vegetative neurosis, *i.e.* as the remote physiologic sequelae of oral tensions.

3. **Sperling** (1946) who worked with children has concentrated on the mother-child relationship and emphasized the contradictory attitude of the mother, who on the one hand unconsciously tries to maintain the child in a life-long dependence to satisfy her own needs and at the same time shows unconscious destructive impulses towards the child. The latter are particularly likely to become intensified when the child fails to satisfy the mother's needs or when the child, to satisfy these unconscious needs, mobilizes guilt or anxiety in the mother. The colitis develops when a change occurs in this specific relationship with the mother (or her substitute). Once this relationship is discontinued much will depend upon the patient's willingness and ability to find a replacement for the lost or surrendered love-object. When the patient is unable to accomplish this, intense frustration ensues, and there is an acute increase in destructive impulses which, however, remain repressed and are discharged through the sympton of bleeding. 'The destruction and elimination of the object through the mucosa of the colon (bleeding) would seem to be the specific mechanism in ulcerative colitis.' The faeces and blood represent the devaluated and dangerous objects. She compares the behaviour, dynamics and personality structure found in ulcerative colitis to that found in melancholia and sees it as sadism turned inward with the choice of organ determined by oral and anal fixations, the colon being the eliminatory organ.

4. **Lindemann** (1945) emphasizes the loss of a key person and the prominence of morbid grief and he, too, points out the similarities to melancholia, but he offers no hypothesis as to how the psychologic

processes bear on the development of the somatic pathology.

5. **Prugh** (1951) who worked with children stressed the reservoir of repressed anger developing in settings of loss of security, and points out the inverse relationship between symptoms and the expression or acting out in play of aggressive or hostile emotions. He implies that the bowel disorder is in some way related to the inability successfully to discharge aggression.

6. **Karush and Daniels** (1953), on the basis of the psychoanalysis of two female patients, concluded:

> The patients never succeeded in building psychological stability, which normally cushions the blow of a serious loss or frustration. They elaborated a precariously effective adaptive system, and, in the face of an emotional blow, the apparatus for effective action required to cope with the emergency was so disturbed that profound anxiety and rage, long suppressed, now threatened to overwhelm them.

Depression, futility and hopelessness ensued, but organ selection they regarded as an enigma which, in adults, was unlikely to be solved by psychoanalysis.

7. **Groën** (1947) sees the condition developing when persons of certain character traits are in conflict situations which involve an acute love loss.

> The repression of this special kind of defect, the outwardly 'normal' behaviour, the finding of a pseudo-solution, while the insufficiency of their own personality has been so rudely revealed to them, the carrying on while they were standing in life helpless, loveless and without confidence in their own personality—all this appeared to belong to the typical reaction of these personalities.

8. **Mushatt** (1954) suggests that a basic problem is that the relationship to the outside world is made at an oral incorporative level.

> This relatedness is expressed through bodily imagery by means of the gastro-intestinal tract, and from this concept the disorganized gastro-intestinal function can be considered both as a preverbal or visceral communication of primitive psychic activity and as a defence against psychic disorganization.

He, too, sees a similarity with melancholia and considers that the mothers are unconsciously rejecting and using the child for their own ends. He does not attempt to explain how these processes eventuate in colitis.

9. **Grace, Wolf and Wolff** (1951) see ulcerative colitis as part of an ejection-riddance pattern involving the large bowel.

> A subject confronted by overwhelming environmental demands may elaborate a pattern of ejection. Thus, a person who has taken on more than he can handle or feels inadequate to the demands of his life situation, or a thwarted and passive

> person filled with hatred, defiance, contempt, or the unconscious aim to eject a threatening or overwhelming situation, may have diarrhoea. However, the riddance pattern being integrated through unconscious processes, the subject exhibiting violent diarrhoea may be calm, sweet-mannered and seem serene.

The choice of organ, they say, is determined by constitutional factors, some people being 'colon-reactors', 'nose-reactors' and 'skin-reactors'.

10. **Sullivan** (1936), in language most graphic, but embodying a theory which is most tenuous, says that:

> Emotion whips the liquid contents of the small intestine down into the colon. . . . Because the emotional difficulty remains a chronic one, either because the situation cannot be solved or the patient is unable to face his problems, the hypermotility of the intestinal content persists and the constant irritation results in a chronic colitis.

11. **Engel** (1955) himself hazards a formulation:

> . . . when separation is not or cannot be dealt with by psychologic mechanisms (as in normal grief as well as in some types of neurotic or psychotic processes), physiologic changes are initiated in the body which interfere with or disrupt other adaptive or integrative processes, permitting various types of tissue breakdown, disturbances in local tissue growth, invasion by viruses or bacteria.

He also accepts that the colon mucosa may be erotized because of failure of psycho-sexual maturation which may make it the site of physiologic changes of a tumescent nature.

Some of these hypotheses make no attempt to explain the somatic aspects. Of those that do offer an explanation, those of Alexander, Szasz, Sullivan, Grace and Wolf and Wolff depend on hypermotility of the gut with diarrhoea as the first sign, while Sperling apart from Engel is the only one who stresses the importance of bleeding as a first sign. It is traditionally held that diarrhoea usually precedes bleeding apart from that small percentage of cases where constipation is the first symptom and is then followed by bleeding. Engel (1954*a*) pointed out that the assumption that diarrhoea is the earliest sympton was wrong and in a study of 32 patients with ulcerative colitis, declared that 68 per cent started with bleeding, 44 per cent were constipated at some time, and only 37 per cent had diarrhoea as a feature of the disease. Apart from the novelty of this information it has an important bearing on psychosomatic hypotheses, for instead of looking for a mechanism which in the majority of instances produces diarrhoea as an early sign, we should now look for one which initiates bleeding. It is also of importance in case-history taking, particularly in the search for precipitating factors, for if one were looking for an event which preceded the onset of diarrhoea, one may either fail to find it or get information which occurred during the course of the illness rather than before it started. Many patients will not yield spontaneously information about rectal bleeding and answers will only emerge if specific questions are put.

A questionnaire completed by 120 members of an Ileostomy Association who had ulcerative colitis (Sim & Brooke, 1958) yielded the information that 47 presented with diarrhoea as opposed to 37 with bleeding, giving modest support to Engel's claim, but it was subject to the criticism that a questionnaire was not as reliable as an individual interview. A subsequent personal study by the author of 100 patients who had the disease and were subjected to colectomy and ileostomy showed that 40 per cent presented with diarrhoea, 33 per cent with bleeding and 27 per cent with bleeding and diarrhoea. While diarrhoea is unmistakable by the patient, bleeding may be present and go unrecognized and it is likely that if the patient considered that they appeared together, the bleeding may well have preceded the diarrhoea. Bleeding as a first sign may therefore have occurred in 60 per cent of these patients which is approximating to Engel's figure of 68 per cent. Of the 100 patients, 65 per cent yielded at least one close relative with a psychosomatic disorder and this did not include those with a family history of coronary thrombosis or hypertension. The commoner disorders were peptic ulcer, eczema, colitis (mainly mucous), asthma and migraine. Twenty-eight per cent had at some time exhibited other psychosomatic diseases and these included eczema, migraine, asthma and peptic ulcer.

Precipitating factors which preceded very closely the onset of the disease were found in 96 out of the 100 cases and they were mainly following school, work and domestic stress, marriage and honeymoon, bereavement and leaving home. A much smaller number occurred after operations or infections or were associated with pregnancy and childbirth. Of the four who did not yield precipitating factors, two had developed the disease before the age of seven years and the other two consisted of a male of 68 years with a four months' history and a 53-year-old male with seven months' history. These last two would suggest that there may be forms of the disease which are not necessarily psychosomatic in nature. Aggravating factors, like precipitating factors, were found in practically all cases, the commonest being 'excitement' which need not be due to unpleasant events and was in fact more frequently associated with what would be regarded as pleasant experiences. Some of these were passing examinations, promotion at work, moving into a new house and expecting or entertaining desirable visitors.

Too much emphasis has been laid on the adverse environmental factors which precipitate the condition. All these patients admitted to a high level of anticipatory excitement, and it was this factor more than any other which was the major precipitant. To assess this response the author generally asks the patient if he is the type of person who is particularly vulnerable to advertisements such as 'Only another 364 shopping days to Christmas', and the answer is invariably an enthusiastic affirmative.

Patients with ulcerative colitis were members of families with an odd number of sibs to a greater degree than one would meet in a normal population and the popular belief that it tended to occur in only children was not substantiated. In fact the percentage of only children was less than in the normal population.

Changes in Body Image Following Ileostomy

Druss *et al.* (1972) reported on four women with permanent ileostomy for ulcerative colitis. All had been in psychotherapy and at some point in their histories all had desired to be men. The following 5 phenomena were identified:

1. 'Phantom reaction', lasting from a few days to two weeks and manifest by a sense of fullness in the non-existent rectum and a strong urge to defaecate.
2. The stoma as phallus; one patient had the conscious idea that it looked like a penis.
3. Exhibitionism.
4. Erotic feelings towards the surgeon.
5. Changes in personality and life style; depression was absent and they appeared mildly hypomanic and aggressive.

The present writer would confirm the stoma as a phallus observation. He had a patient who referred to it as her 'little Willie'.

Treatment

This can be a very delicate matter. Because there are psychological factors in its aetiology and the condition can be ameliorated by psychological influences, many are convinced that psychotherapy is the best method of treatment. It may be that in the mild cases or in those cases that do not react violently to external stress, psychotherapy, in any guise, is useful, but it should not be forgotten that the condition can be precipitated or aggravated by psychological stresses and that psychotherapy which may court a negative transference may be very harmful. A formal analysis such as one would carry out in a neurotic disorder may be strongly contraindicated in these patients and a benevolent, tolerant and ever-ready-to-help attitude is probably the most reliable. This would explain why some physicians, who have developed a special interest in this problem, have considerable success with their patients. They are kindly and tolerant and place their whole department at the patient's disposal, so that if they are not available, the patient has ready access to their medical assistants or ward-sister. They indoctrinate their staff with their own attitude and the patient can always find a haven when in need. Engel (1958), who stresses this aspect, states: 'I have found it valuable to keep a file of nurses who are good with these patients and to try and avoid nurses who have not been successful'. He lays down four basic psychologic processes which the physician must understand and these are:

1. The colitic process begins or relapses in a setting in which the patient feels, consciously or unconsciously, that he has suffered or will suffer the loss of an important object relationship.
2. He responds to this with a feeling of helplessness, hopelessness, despair, a feeling that this is 'too much' that he cannot go on.
3. By virtue of a lifelong mutually dependent relationship on certain key figures, especially the mother, he has not achieved the capacity for independent function that characterizes the more mature person.
4. He looks to the physician to take over in the areas in which he feels incompetent and not to let him down.

A fifth and obvious rule which tends to be forgotten is that the patient has a very vulnerable colon. Because of the real risk of acute and serious deterioration, the physician who undertakes his treatment should have ready access to a hospital bed, for not only will this add to his confidence in the handling of the patient, but it will also ensure the continuity of treatment and obviate the need to establish too many close personal relationships. Formal analysis is not ruled out as long as the delicacy of the problem is appreciated and there is the closest liaison with the physician but should there be phases of acute relapse, it would be wise not to subject the patient to further psychotherapy but to retreat to a more supportive role. There is another danger which is not yet adequately appreciated and that is the longer the history of severe ulceration, the greater the risk of carcinoma developing (Slaney & Brooke, 1959). It will be seen therefore that ulcerative colitis like asthma should be treated with the greatest respect for if it ever becomes an issue between the patient and doctor, the patient has a trump card—he may die.

OBESITY

Boswell reports in his *Life of Johnson* the following conversation:

> Talking of a man who was grown very fat, so as to be incommoded with corpulency, he said, 'He eats too much, Sir'. BOSWELL: 'I don't know, Sir; you will see one man fat who eats moderately, and another lean who eats a great deal!' JOHNSON: 'Nay, Sir, whatever may be the quantity that a man eats, it is plain that if he is too fat, he has eaten more than he should have done. One man may have a digestion that consumes food better than common, but it is certain that solidity is increased by putting something to it.' BOSWELL: 'But may not solids swell and be distended'? JOHNSON: 'Yes, Sir, they may swell and be distended; but that is not fat.'

After all the endocrinological and metabolic studies have been considered, Dr Johnson has been proved right and it is essentially over-eating which causes obesity. If this term could be substituted for the descriptive one of obesity, we should be nearer an aetiological understanding of the problem. Weiss and English (1943) and Fenichel (1945) regard it an an organ neurosis, the latter stressing the importance of exhibitionistic and pre-oedipal mother conflicts. Oral gratification with emotional immaturity and undue dependence on the 'vital supplies' have also been stressed and Bruch (1940) has pointed out that the child may go in for the pleasures of food if he does not get the pleasure of love from his parents. In a later publication (Bruch, 1957) she stresses that fluctuations in weight measured over a period proved a better index of weight disturbance than any derived from height-weight tables. These fluctuations are important in gauging weight loss as well as weight gain, for not infrequently a well-nourished patient may complain of marked loss of weight and much fruitless searching for a precipitating factor may be avoided if attention were focused on the onset of the preceding obesity as this gives a clue to the earlier disturbance. The usual traumatic experiences are withdrawal or threatened withdrawal of affection and the patient then regresses to an earlier oral erotic level where oral gratification is used to create a feeling of security. The rapid increase in weight in those who give up smoking has also been explained on this basis.

Shorvon and Richardson (1949) describe three and analyse 12 cases of sudden obesity following psychological trauma and define a fairly uniform personality pattern with immaturity, impulsiveness and emotional lability. Precipitating factors were death of mother, an unwanted pregnancy or the near-miss of a bomb explosion. The authors used ether abreaction in their patients to facilitate emotional release and claimed satisfactory results, though supplementary psychotherapy was also necessary. It should, however, be recognized that obesity is evidence of underlying instability which can manifest in other ways such as drug addiction, alcoholism, depression and phobic anxiety. The relief of the obesity should be a by-product of treatment, the success of which should not be measured in kilos, but in the satisfactory adjustment of the patient.

Hunger and Instinct

Bruch (1969) claims that the ability to recognize the subjective experience of hunger, as opposed to the physiological state of deprivation, is not innate but must be learned. Obese and anorexic patients have never acquired the normal ability to tell whether they are hungry or sated or the knowledge of how hunger or satiety feels. She quotes experiments that show that normals can tell much more accurately how much food there is in their stomachs at any time and thus regulate their eating.

The infant acquires this ability by interaction with the mother, and biological needs are at first unidentifiable states of tension which are later organized into patterns the infant can recognize. If the mother offers food in response to hunger signals, the child will gradually develop the engram of 'hunger'. If her feeding is consistently inappropriate by ignoring him when he wails with hunger or just shovelling food in mechanically, he does not learn to discriminate between hunger and other forms of distress, and thus obese patients may mistake anxious or depressive feelings for the need to eat. Even those who have learned to control their weight may lose control in times of stress.

Obese patients may experience dramatic improvements or relapses on almost any regimen, including psychotherapy. It is as if they had merely acquiesced once more to perceptions thrust upon them. The impersonal shovelling in of food, as if the child were an eating machine, denies that he is a human being. If the parents insist he is hungry, tired or cold when he feels he is not, he faces the 'double bind' of denying either their love or his own senses as in a schizophrenogenic family.

Obesity, Instability and Social Class

While obesity is rightly regarded as evidence of instability, this is not universally valid. Holland *et al.* (1970) studied 48 white women from the lower socio-economic class and could find no relationship between instability and obesity in that class. It did not incur the social disfavour associated with middle-class women who risked social isolation for their violation of the standards of beauty and desirability. If every third woman in the lower class is significantly overweight then in this group obesity can no longer be called abnormal and the psychopathology of obesity cannot be accepted independently of social class and ethnic factors.

The Relationship of Gastric Motility and Hunger

The popular belief that gastric motility engenders hunger pains and this leads to eating, or in the vulnerable, overeating, was tested by Stunkard and Fox (1971). They studied 3 normal young women for 24 hours and in a second study, 8 subjects of normal weight, 8 obese subjects with no psychopathology and 8 neurotic obese subjects who showed both disturbance of body image and deviant eating patterns. Only a minority showed a strong association between gastric motility and intensity of reported hunger, and these came from all three groups. Contrary to expectation, the neurotic obese patients did not show a lesser tendency to associate gastric motility with hunger, and the authors conclude that though stomach contractions do play a part in the experience of hunger, the relationship is a weak one.

Earlier evidence of a similar nature was provided by Schachter *et al.* (1968), who studied the effects of fear, food deprivation and obesity on eating. They found that obese subjects ate as much, or slightly more when their stomachs were full as when empty, in contrast to normal subjects, indicating that the actual state of the stomach had nothing to do with the eating behaviour of the obese.

Starvation

Starvation as treatment for obesity has gained in popularity. The rapid loss of weight obtained while the patient is in hopsital can be most encouraging, and there are no doubt other deeper reasons for the success. It is what happens after the patient leaves hospital that usually counts. Swanson and Dinello (1970) followed-up 25 (24 male and 1 female) markedly obese subjects who had lost on average 67 pounds without serious physical complications.

At follow-up, despite starvation, dietary counselling and out-patient attendance, none of the subjects reached an ideal weight. Fourteen (56 per cent.) had regained or exceeded their pre-starvation weight within one year. Seven (28 per cent.) dropped out, but even in their short period of follow-up they showed rapid weight gain and it was assumed that those who failed their follow-up were unsuccessful in their dieting. For most patients a return to obesity was more comfortable than trying to fight their problem in the presence of environmental demands.

Night-eating Syndrome

Stunkard *et al.* (1955) investigated the eating habits of 25 obese patients and compared these with 38 controls. Twenty of the obese exhibited a syndrome consisting of nocturnal hyperphagia, insomnia and morning anorexia. The syndrome was prominent but not invariably present during periods of weight gain and increased stress. The authors pointed out that a reducing regime with weight loss in these patients frequently resulted in depression and anxiety and that the alteration in diurnal eating and sleeping rhythm may be similar to that which occurs in depression. These findings have since been amply confirmed and indicate the difficulties in supervising a diet in the obese.

Psychogenic Polydipsia and Polyuria

This condition may occasionally be confused with diabetes insipidus and some of the tests such as the administration of nicotine or hypertonic saline and dehydration, which are alleged to distinguish them, may prove unreliable and even dangerous. Dashe *et al.* (1963) were able to devise a test which did distinguish diabetes insipidus from patients with psychogenic polydipsia and volunteers who had accustomed themselves to drink 8 litres daily.

The test consisted in witholding water for 6½ hours and taking samples of serum and urine at the beginning, middle and end of the period. The test depends on differences between serum and urine osmolality and it was shown that though the psychogenic group may have a subnormal level of serum-osmolality initially they showed (with the volunteers) a great ratio of urine to serum osmolality than any of the patients with known diabetes insipidus, particularly in the last hour of the test.

The author has, on several occasions, seen patients with psychogenic polydipsia presented at a physicians' meeting as cases of diabetes insipidus and the above test would appear to be a useful screen for the physician. The functional problems are usually associated with obesity, for the preferred drinks are frequently sweetened fruit juices. Associated obesity tends to encourage an organic diagnosis as it is regarded as convincing evidence of hypothalamic involvement. Usually such patients have a history of mental instability prior to the onset of the polydipsia and re-education is possible, though the patient may require the strict supervision recommended for anorexia nervosa (see below).

CARDIOVASCULAR SYSTEM

As with the stomach, the heart has established itself in language as an organ which reflects the emotions and terms like 'heavy heart' and 'light-hearted' are used so freely that their implications may go unrecognized. The heart may be 'sad' or 'merry', 'fickle' or 'sincere' and what is probably a more profound psychological truth, 'in affairs of the heart there is no such thing as reason'. Similarly, the arteries have been implicated, but it is a far cry from metaphor to medicine, though an impressive body of evidence has been accumulated which strongly suggests that emotional factors contribute to cardiovascular disease.

ANXIETY AND PULSE RATE

Sinus tachycardia occurs as a comparatively minor feature of many diseases but in thyrotoxicosis, phaeochromocytoma and anxiety states it may be a major manifestation. In thyrotoxicosis it is produced by an increased sensitivity of the adrenergic receptor system which is independent of the elevated basal metabolic rate. Frohlich *et al.* (1966) described two patients with sinus tachycardia, palpitations and anxiety in whom the suggested cause was an abnormal sensitivity of the beta-receptor mechanism to circulating adrenergic substance. They postulate a 'hyperdynamic beta-adrenergic circulatory state' which theoretically may be controlled by propanolol, the beta-receptor blocking agent. While it is possible that there are interesting variants which merit the above definition, some therapeutic trials of propranolol in anxiety states have shown no more benefit than the usual placebo reaction. The author had such a patient whose tachycardia and palpitations were treated with propranolol with no benefit but who responded to the usual regime for phobic anxiety. Further work is necessary but it is of interest to speculate that anxiety may in some instances be a result as well as a cause of tachycardia.

HYPERTENSION

This may result from a variety of factors, and included in these is emotional stress. At the commonest level, it is well known that taking the blood pressure can yield a variety of readings, the higher ones when the patient is unsettled or unfamiliar with the procedure and examiner, but after the patient's confidence has been gained, a lower set of readings may be obtained. Similarly, a persistently high blood pressure may be materially reduced by dealing with the patient's anxiety either by a psychotherapeutic technique or by the use of drugs such as barbiturates, which relieve tension. From tension to hypertension may be a short step for some to take but the one is a mental and perhaps muscular state, while the other is reflected in a raised blood pressure, and while the two are frequently associated, it is usually in the more labile types of hypertension that such evidence is available. In the more persistent and incidentally more pathological varieties, the evidence is not quite so obvious and has given rise to considerable controversy.

Psychological Theory

Repressed rage or anger is regarded by some as the principal factor. It is not discharged through verbal or motor activity and may take an autonomic and endocrine path which leads to arteriolar constriction and increased peripheral resistance. The precise mechanism has not been satisfactorily demonstrated and the factor of 'the susceptible individual' is an essential constant, but why some should be susceptible in this way is still unknown.

Fenichel (1945) states:

> Cases of essential hypertension are characterized by an extreme unconscious instinctual tension, a general readiness for aggressiveness as well as a passive-receptive longing to get rid of the aggressiveness. Both tendencies are unconscious and are effective in persons who superficially seem to be very calm and permit themselves no outlet for their impulses. This unrealized inner tension seems to be at least one of the aetiological components of essential hypertension. . . .

Dunbar (1943) has stressed a personality profile in patients with hypertensive cardiovascular disease as well as for other psychosomatic disorders from data which she listed under the following headings:

1. General adjustment: *(a)* education, *(b)* word record, *(c)* income and vocational level, *(d)* social relationships, *(e)* sexual adjustment, *(f)* attitude toward family.
2. Characteristic behaviour pattern.
3. Neurotic traits.
4. Addictions and interests.
5. Life situation immediately prior to onset.
6. Reaction to illness.
7. Area of focal conflict and characteristic reaction.

Under the last-mentioned she drew attention to situations involving aggression and passivity, rivalry and self-defeat. Her conclusions have been criticized as being too diffuse and not giving sufficient indication as to the basic psychological theory, yet they were based on a careful analysis of the facts as elicited by a thorough history-taking. The field has since been invaded by wilder speculators. The 'personality profile' is no longer fashionable and emphasis has shifted to very early psychological traumata, usually of a pregenital nature such as have been implicated in a variety of psychosomatic disorders and particularly the difficulty and conflict in the handling of aggressive impulses in dependency relationships. Reiser *et al.* (1957) have shown that these patients tend to insulate themselves emotionally in interpersonal relationships and suggest this may be the result of inborn vascular hyper-reactivity rather than an aetiological factor in hypertension. Hypertension is not uncommonly found in middle-aged patients suffering from psychotic depression, though it is not a feature of such depression. The response to treatment is also erratic. After a course of E.C.T. some undergo a lowering of the blood pressure; in others it is unaffected. Adequate follow-up of those whose B.P. fell has not been undertaken.

Heine (1970) investigated the effects of prolonged emotional disturbances on blood pressure in 40 patients (15 male and 25 female) who had a history of depressive illness. It was predicted:

(a) that the blood pressure of depressed patients on recovery would correlate positively with the total duration and number of spells of illness;

(b) that these patients would have higher systolic and diastolic pressures when ill then a normal population matched for age and sex;

(c) that patients' blood pressures during illness would correlate positively with either severity of depression or accompanying anxiety and agitation.

Systolic blood pressure was found to correlate significantly with the number of spells of illness but not with duration for diastolic pressures. When the experimental group and a control group matched for age, sex, height and weight were compared, both the systolic and diastolic pressures of the patients (mean 147/90 mmHg) were significantly higher than the controls (mean 137/84 mmHg). The mean blood pressure of the recovered patients was also significantly higher than the control group. There was no correlation between the severity of the depression and the blood pressure but anxiety-agitation scores correlated significantly.

It was also found that there were no differences in the background between those patients whose blood pressure returned to normal after recovery and those that did not. The author concluded that repeated spells of depressive illness when characterized by marked anxiety and agitation are accompanied by repeated increases of blood pressure, and that repeated exposure to stimuli that increase blood pressure may well lead to a maintained increase.

While a precise account of how emotional factors can produce a permanent form of hypertension does not yet exist, some speculation is permissible on the established facts that emotional disturbance can initiate vascular changes and produce arteriolar constriction, thus having a direct bearing on the disease.

HYPOTENSION

This may result in attacks of syncope following an emotional disturbance, particularly involving fear or nausea. Sharpey Schafer *et al.* (1958) state that though this is common knowledge '. . . There are great difficulties, however, in obtaining records of the circulatory events which precede the attack, and many situations, such as high flying jet aircraft or the altar steps, are impossible to investigate'. In a study on volunteer dental patients, the well-known fear of the dental chair was exploited and compared with a control group of alcoholics undergoing apomorphine therapy. They confirm that fear was the main cause of the hypotension and syncopal attacks, and suggest that emotional stimulation of the heart beat and a fall in cardiac filling pressure cause virtual emptying of a ventricular chamber during systole which fires the afferent mechanism of the faint reflex. There is strong evidence that subjects with heart failure, whose ventricles are not easily emptied, do not faint. It is of some significance that this study, which produced evidence of the mechanism involved in emotional influence on blood pressure, was carried out by a team whose prime concern was the mechanism rather than any psychosomatic hypothesis. Usually the psychosomatic hypotheses are available in profusion but the mechanism is elusive, and now psychological theorists will, when discussing emotional factors and blood pressure, have to take into account the influence of fear which has now moved from the speculative to experimental proof.

CORONARY ARTERY DISEASE

This is frequently cited as a stress disorder and nearly every form of human activity, such as driving a bus, smoking cigarettes, or taking too much sugar in one's tea, has been implicated. As recently as

1960, a leader in the *British Medical Journal* stated: 'The concept that emotional stress might contribute to the development of coronary heart disease is at present regarded with suspicion and misgiving'. The editorial, however, explained that this was probably due to the difficulty in measuring the effects of chronic stress in one community or occupation and comparing them with another. Russek and Zohman (1958) showed that in 91 out of 100 patients under 40 years of age, who developed coronary heart disease, severe emotional stress preceded the attack and that these patients had an intense desire for recognition, were compulsive about time, over-scrupulous and blind to their own limits. They over-worked themselves, could not relax and felt guilty when trying to do so.

Serum cholesterol levels have been regarded as of importance in the aetiology of the disease and these fluctuate with emotional stress. Friedman *et al.* (1958) in a study of variations in pressure of work in accountants dealing in tax returns found that under greatest pressure, serum cholesterol rose, whole-blood clotting time was accelerated and these changes were independent of variations in weight, diet and physical activity. The serum cholesterol fell and clotting time returned to normal when activity was less. The same authors (1959) reported similar contrasts between men with an intense and sustained desire for achievement who are continually in competition with others and working against time and those who were unambitious and in less exacting occupations. Dreyfus and Czaczkes (1959) reported an increase in serum cholesterol in male medical students during the week of their examinations. While many instances of coronary occlusion follow unaccustomed heavy physical exertion, they are also usually associated with an emotional stress, such as the husband having to get his lawn mown in a certain time so as not to be late for a social engagement to which his wife has committed him. There is still much to learn for the indices of serum cholesterol and whole-blood clotting time have not conclusively been shown to have an aetiological significance, while the mechanism of intravascular thrombosis which is the essential pathology is still inadequately understood.

Some patients develop coronary occlusion following strenuous and unaccustomed exercise. The crop of fatalities which result when there has been a fall of snow, with violent efforts to get the car mobilized, have lent support to the argument that exercise itself is responsible. There is another factor which, for obvious reasons, does not get the same publicity. The coronary following the mowing of the lawn is frequently associated with remonstrations from the housewife that they are expected elsewhere for tea and he has to wash and change and they will be late. He hurries on and the coronary follows. Another situation is the man with his family on holiday. He is laden with heavy suitcases and there is a train to catch. It would appear that heavy unaccustomed exercise with associated anxiety may be instrumental, but this view is based on clinical impressions and has not yet been validated.

SUDDEN DEATH

The histories of 26 men who died suddenly from myocardial infarction or cardiac arrhythmia or both were obtained from their spouses (Green *et al.* 1972). They reported in the 3–18 month prodromal period increased tension due to increased pressure at work, longer hours worked and family or other socially precipitated distress. Sexual incompatibility or impotence was not reported as a source of conflict or as an activity occurring at the time of the final acute illness, though a daughter or especially a son leaving home caused considerable distress. The authors conclude that sudden death occurred in patients who had been depressed for a week to several months and that the catastrophe occurred in a setting of acute arousal.

While the study is of interest, the informants were obviously biased and would look outside themselves for a cause and tend to blame the work situation or other members of the family leaving home, with the wife having to shoulder the full burden.

Psychosocial Factors and Myocardial Infarction

In a series of three papers (Theorell and Rahe, 1971; Rahe and Passikivi, 1971; Rahe and Line, 1971) the authors studied survivors of myocardial infarction in a Swedish in-patient and out-patient unit by preparing a schedule of each patient's recent experience by means of a questionnaire into the 3 years prior to the attack. This listed 42 personal changes in the psychosocial categories of work, residence, economics, personal habits, marriage, family, community, social relationships and recreation. Each change was given a weighting as a life change unit (LCU) and there was a matched control group who had no previous history of coronary artery disease. The infarction subjects with no recent episode of coronary heart disease showed a significant increase in their LCU totals over the two years prior to their infarctions. Those with a history of previous episodes of coronary heart disease showed a significant increase in their LCU totals during the second year prior to the investigated infarctions, and these coincided with the majority of previous episodes of coronary heart disease experienced by this group. Life change data from the comparison group showed no significant alterations in their baseline LCU totals during the three years prior to investigation.

The results from both groups in in-patients indicated that subjects' life changes increased significantly from healthy baseline levels during the two years prior to major episode of coronary heart disease. The second study on out-patients confirmed the finding of increased LCU in the period before infarction and that life change increases prior to infarction are relatively constant and do not vary according to the subjects' memory for life events in the past few years. In the third study, life change pattern in the three years before sudden cardiac death showed a significant build-up in life change intensity during the six months prior to sudden death, and the authors relate this finding to that of Parkes *et al.* (1969) on widowers' deaths from coronary heart disease during the six months following bereavement.

The Stresses of the Intensive Care Unit

With a condition like coronary heart disease, which would appear to select patients who are exposed to excessive psychosocial stresses, it is likely that their reaction to an intensive care unit will also reflect their basic handicap, and this has been reported by Hackett *et al.* (1968). In a further study the same authors (Wishnie *et al.* (1971) reported the psychological hazards of convalescence following myocardial infarction. Of the 50 patients in the study of the coronary care unit, 24 were available for follow-up.

Mood: Twenty-one rated themselves as anxious or depressed or both during the first month at home and in 9 this mood persisted for several months.

Activities: Twenty-three felt frustrated at being inactive in the first few months at home and few undertook hobbies or mild physical exercise such as walking.

Sleep: Fifteen patients had disturbed sleep for weeks to months after discharge and nocturnal pre-occupation with heart function accompanied by some degree of insomnia persisted for months in 11 patients.

Habits: Resolutions to stop smoking, drinking or to lose weight were in general not carried out.

Return to Work: Thirteen patients did so either full or part-time and there was no positive relationship between return to work and the severity of the illness. In fact, among those under 65 years, the most seriously ill were working part-time.

Family Conflict: A steady eroding conflict over the illness was noted in 18 families with arguments over interpretation of the physician's instructions.

Follow-up Care: Eighteen required tranquillizers or anti-depressants and few succeeded in altering habits that might adversely influence their illness. The authors, understandably, stress the importance of attitudes in the post-infarction patient and suggest group therapy for patients and their wives with the physician playing a leading role in prophylaxis.

Psychological Stresses of Nursing in Intensive Care Units

Hay and Oken (1972) list the formidable stresses for nursing personnel in such units. There is repetitive exposure to death and dying, to the frightening, repulsive and forbidden. Stimuli are present which may mobilize every conflictual area at every psychological developmental level. The work load is excessive and unusual as well as intricate and fast, with little if any time for communication with physicians, relatives and administration.

Her psychological experience is one of chronic latent anxiety and tension, for any error may be life-endangering and the machinery she must use becomes more complex. Though she occupies a place among the hospital's élite, her self-esteem is often threatened, for frequently her patients die, while even her major successes are still usually seriously ill and are merely transferred. Attachments are formed to patients and frequent deaths provide a situation of repetitive object-loss, the intensity of which parallels the degree of her attachment.

The intense group loyalty of the unit reinforces work pressure by stimulating guilt about absence from work. The group is self-destructive for it cannot refuse additional work even when the total load is unrealistic, for this would violate group norms and threaten the shared fantasy of omnipotence linked to the concept of being special and to the defensive denial of anxiety about mistakes. The only escape is resignation or flight.

The authors recommend regular group meetings to explore the work experience and its stresses, pay differential, distinctive uniform and periodic brief extra vacation. Transfer to another unit should be easy and free of stigma and staff should be screened for psychological aptitude as well as technical expertise with an initial orientation phase.

Comment: No doubt all this has been said before, but this is an excellent example where dynamic psychiatry can analyse a situation and make valid recommendations as experts.

Patients who Survive Circulatory Arrest

Resuscitation for cardiac arrest has its critics particularly because of the risk of irreversible brain damage. Bengtsson *et al.* (1969) reported on 21 such patients and found that only 3 had marked cerebral organic symptoms and they were all over 70 years of age. Resuscitation was started early in all cases and this must be the major factor. There was no correlation between caridac massage of long duration and grave cerebral injury.

CONGESTIVE HEART FAILURE

This sounds organic enough, yet emotional stress has been blamed for its aggravation or precipitation. Chambers and Reiser (1953) related the onset of cardiac failure to emotional disturbance in 19 out of 25 patients, and found that stimuli which caused rage, frustration, anxiety, depression or feelings of insecurity could precipitate it. Schottstaedt *et al.* (1956) found retention of sodium and water during periods of emotional tension or depression, followed by a diuresis after relaxation of the emotions, and Barnes and Schottstaedt (1960), in a study of eight male patients who had recently emerged from congestive heart failure, found them to be highly sensitive to any suggestions about the prognosis of their heart disease. Emotional tension and depression were associated with a decrease in excretion of sodium, total urine and to a lesser extent, potassium. Reasurrance, relaxation of emotional tension, and lifting of depression were followed by increased excretion of sodium and water. Excitement, apprehension, agitation or anger were associated with a greater output of sodium and water compared with tranquil periods, though potassium output was not significantly increased. Body position affected these findings, but though normally walking would cause a decrease of urinary volume and sodium excretion compared with resting in the sitting or recumbent position, this was altered by emotional stress and a patient could be more relaxed sitting than lying with greater output of sodium in the former position. Emotions could prove more important than physical activity in determining sodium output and in one subject it was 32 times greater during strenuous activity than during a period of sitting when in a tense and anxious state of mind. The mechanism whereby these phenomena occurred is still a matter for speculation and increased secretion of aldosterone as a result of emotional stress might possibly account for the reduced urinary volume and sodium excretion.

SUBARACHNOID HAEMORRHAGE

Penrose (1972) in a review of the literature coupled with his own study of 44 patients, found that where an aneurysm was not involved, life events of a stressful nature which immediately preceded the haemorrhage were more common than in those patients where an aneurysm had ruptured. This is explained by the greater rise in blood pressure required to produce haemorrhage where there is no aneurysm. These patients tended to be more in need of psychiatric treatment, but, as has been mentioned in Chapter 5, this could be due to the location of the haemorrhage in the aneurysmal series which tends to be associated with personality changes as with prefrontal leucotomy.

OPERANT CONDITIONING IN HEART DISEASE

A corollary to the identification of the role of psychological factors in the aetiology of organic disease is the role of psychiatry in the treatment of such disease. Weiss and Engel (1971) studied 8 patients with premature ventricular contractions (PVC's) to see if operant conditioning could produce clinically significant control of this arrhythmia. Three differently coloured lights at the foot of the bed informed the patient about his cardiac function, one indicating high heart rate, another low heart rate and the third, which was the reinforcer, the correct rate. In 10–11 sessions the patient was taught to increase or decrease his heart rate during 1–4 minutes in a session and maintain it between preset upper and lower limits. Gradually the feedback from the coloured lights was phased out and the patient made to become aware of PVC's through his own sensations. In three patients the studies were carried out with the use of all or some of the following autonomically active drugs; isoprotenerol, propanolol, atropine, edrophonium, phenylephrine and phentolamine, administered intravenously. Mean heart rates were calculated from automatically counted heart beats and all PVC's were counted.

The results showed clear evidence of PVC control in four patients, one of whom sustained a low PVC for 21 months and the other three with shorter follow-up were able to detect and modify PVC frequency at home. A fifth patient maintained a low PVC frequency for 5 months after the study. One patient was poorly motivated and the other two had a grossly enlarged and an electrically unstable heart respectively. The authors list six elements for successful learning of PVC control:

1. Peripheral receptors which are stimulated by the PVC.
2. Efferents which carry the information to the CNS.
3. CNS processing to enable the patient to recognize the PVC and to provide the motivation and flexibility necessary for learning to occur.
4. Efferents to an effector organ which can bring about the desired change in the pathologically functioning heart.
5. A heart which is not too diseased to beat more regularly.
6. A homeostatic system in the patient which will tolerate the more normal functioning of the heart.

It is through this type of work that the value of the psychosomatic approach will gain acceptability with our cardiological colleagues.

CARDIAC IRRITABILITY DURING SLEEP AND DREAMING

Rosenblatt *et al.* (1973) correlated changes in the EEG with dream states in 10 subjects with chronic cardiac problems, 8 with arteriosclerotic heart disease with an ECG showing past myocardial infarction, or with a history of angina pectoris. Two subjects had multiple premature contractions during waking EEGs but these were probably benign. EEGs, eye movements and ECGs were recorded for 30 nights. The study showed that the premature ventricular beats (PVB) occurred most frequently during the *D*-state (REM state) and with decreasing frequency in stages, 4, 2 and 3. Most cardiac irritability occurred during the first study night with a marked reduction in PVBs during later nights.

The striking feature in all subjects was the apparent marked cardiovascular demands may be suddenly increased. In the normal these extra demands can be met, but in subjects with coronary heart concluded that *D*-state is a physiologically active period in which cardiovascular demands may be suddenly increased. In the normal these extra demands can be met, but in subjects with coronary heart disease, recent or old myocardial infarction, rhythm abnormalities and hypertension, sudden outflow of sympathetic stimuli may result in increased arrhythmia, angina pectoris, or even frank myocardial infarction and cerebral haemorrhage. Decreasing *D*-time and sympathetic outflow during *D*-time with drug therapy may decrease the risk of developing cardiac arrhythmias in subjects with heart disease.

RHEUMATOID ARTHRITIS

Many authors have reported psychological factors in rheumatoid arthritis and while it has been debated whether these are a cause or a result of the condition, there is considerable evidence for the former and very little for the latter. Ross *et al.* (1961) report their study of 59 patients, 14 of whom were treated in the psychosomatic unit of a general hospital and 45 in the private practice of an internist though the treatment was similar. The following points were noted:

1. All patients presented with a diagnosable psychiatric disorder, depression being the commonest.
2. More than half either presented or had a history of some other chronic physical disorder, the commonest being duodenal ulcer and this was evident prior to treatment with corticoids.
3. They do not readily express anger and they are over-sensitive.
4. Frequent contacts with the doctor together with drug therapy were more helpful than if the same drug therapy were used but consultations were less frequent. Supportive psychotherapy was generally enough but a few patients were able to progress to the stage where they overcame repetitive life patterns which led them into difficulties.

Supporting evidence for the above points has been produced by Shochet *et al.* (1969) who stated that their patients' psychological characteristics, vulnerabilities and life conflicts were remarkably similar and consistent with observations found in the literature. The patients showed, in common, a rigid, passive, dependent personality with strong feelings of inadequacy, a poor self-concept and fear of expressing angry impulses. A striking finding in the history of many was the early effective loss of one or both parents. Other repeated themes were emotional deprivation, disturbed childhood behaviour and early school drop-out. Marital relations were poor with frequent and bitter conflict.

In all cases, life stress was related to clinical changes either in its onset or exacerbation. These crises had in common the threat of or actual loss of a loved object and the resultant arousal of feelings of rage which the patient could not tolerate, express or handle effectively.

The author has, for some years, taught medical students during their medical clerking by asking them to present to him their patients with organic disease and the emotional background is then explored. The physician with whom he is associated has a special interest in rheumatoid arthritis and consequently a number of these patients are presented. The above findings have been confirmed and one patient with a severe depressive illness and relatively minor joint pathology had remained bed-ridden for 3 years.

JUVENILE RHEUMATOID ARTHRITIS (STILL'S DISEASE)

This is a significant disease of childhood in which immunopathy, allergy, infection, trauma, heredity and psychosocial factors have all been postulated as aetiologically significant. Heisel (1972) got the parents of 45 patients with Still's disease to complete a questionnaire and demonstrated that those who develop the disease have experienced a cluster of recent changes in their world greater and more intense than in the average child. Still's disease is, on the basis of this investigation, regarded as a complex disorder with three or more diseases, each with its own mode of onset and natural history, and is in effect a 'final common path' for a number of diseases. Those who had polyarticular onset appeared to fit the distribution of scores of the general population, whereas the monarticular variety with acute febrile onset had high stress densities.

SKIN DISORDERS

These have long been known to reflect the mental state and this phenomenon has given rise to the well-known saying: 'The skin is the mirror of the mind'. Obvious examples of skin changes which are no longer in doubt as to their emotional origin are blushing and sweating, but while, as in other aspects of psychosomatic medicine, there is little controversy over the importance of psychological factors in these transient phenomena, there is frequently considerable opposition to claims that more permanent or structurally altered skin conditions may arise from such causes. McKenna and Macalpine (1951), in a balanced appraisal of the problem, state:

> There is a deep-seated tendency to consider the tangible and visible as more apparent, and hence more true, than the intangible, which is often considered for this very reason to be obscure. . . . It cannot be too strongly emphasized that psychology should not be looked upon as a commonsense adjuvant to dermatologists, but rather as a scientific instrument in dermatological research. . . . A deprecatory attitude to psychology is apt to have serious consequences. The psychologist is likely to be consulted as a last resort when no physical treatment has proved to be of avail. He will thus see only specially selected cases which tend to blur his view, and lead to lop-sided conclusions. The disease mechanism he is trying to isolate will be obscured by superimposed habit formations accumulated during the long period which has elapsed since the onset of the disease. This is the more unnecessary since an early psychological diagnosis can be made by a well-trained psychologist or psychiatrist in much the

same way as a dermatological diagnosis. Quite often this can be done in a short interview, the margin of error in a psychological diagnosis being not necessarily any greater than in medicine generally.

They conclude:

We would like to single out at random three problems where such correlation of approach is likely to be fruitful. The first is an attempt to evaluate the factors that determine whether a skin disease will take an acute, subacute, chronic, recurrent, or intermittent course. the second concerns abnormal skin sensibility; the hyperaesthesia and hyperalgesia which may be demonstrated by a physiologist who investigates many itching skin diseases seems to us closely related to the increased skin libidinization of the psychoanalyst. Thirdly, the phenomenon of itching with its attendant rubbing and scratching seems to present a vast field for investigation, from both the physiological and psychological angle. . . .

They quote Erasmus Wilson:

The limits between the physiological and pathological are barely discernible. The blush of emotion is scarcely to be distinguished from the blush of transient erythema or urticaria, and the too frequent repetition and the permanence of the blush become a confirmed erythema, as in gutta rosea.

Bethune and Kidd (1961) are critical of those who would regard all neurodermatoses as psychogenic and postulate that because schizophrenics and mental defectives exhibit these diseases and yet are 'limited in their means of expressing and repressing emotion' factors other than psychodynamic are at work. They draw on a theory publicised by Eysenck (1947) in their attempt to explain skin phenomena regarded as functional and they postulate three components.

1. A state of emotional high drive, which is an inevitable accompaniment of the induction of the hallucinated stimulus. High drive initiates activity of the central nervous system.
2. The subjective feeling of the physiological response directs efferent nerve impulses to the organ or part which is now the seat of subjective sensation. This initiates ideovisceral or ideovascular action.
3. Ideovisceral or ideovascular action is sustained and reinforced by efferent feedback from the organ or parts involved.

With support from the theory of 'organ inferiority' (Adler, 1924) they postulate an underlying weakness of the organ concerned with continued emotional concern (high drive) in relation to it, with the consequent fixing of the lesion by its morbid ideovisceral or ideovascular responses. By using the method of 'perceptual distortion', which is a form of hypnotic suggestion, they claim that they can remove hitherto intractable skin lesions.

The theory is just as speculative as anything psychoanalysis has devised but still lacks the large body of evidence that the latter has accumulated. It also supposes that the mechanisms of hypnosis and perceptual distortion are understood and though the results may have been gratifying, there is much that has been left out in the assessment, particularly in the doctor-patient relationship, and there has been much that has been accepted at a superficial level. Yet it does offer a rationale for a form of treatment which may be effective and can be carried out by workers with a minimum of training. If this method supplants entirely the analytical approach to skin disorders, the failures will, like the successes, never be adequately understood.

SPECIFIC SKIN DISORDERS

Itching

Wittkower and Lester (1962) state that tense, anxious or agitated skin patients complain of itching or burning sensations more frequently than placid, non-anxious, emotionally well-integrated patients. Furthermore in the same person an unchanged skin lesion would itch more intensely during periods of frustration, boredom or increased tension. Cormia (1952) was able to show, experimentally, the temporal association between itch and emotions. Under psychic stress the wheal and flare produced by an intradermal injection of histamine became larger and the ensuing itching more severe and prolonged.

In certain cases the pleasure from scratching can be so intense that it acquires an auto-erotic activity and may be used as a masturbatory substitute. It can, on the other hand, represent a self-destructive, masochistic action which besides the dermal pleasure, inflicts punishment and lightens guilt.

Ano-genital Pruritus

The psychopathology is similar to itching in that it has obvious erotic but also masochistic overtones. The patients are usually obsessive-compulsive. Wittkower and Russell (1953) remark that in cases of pruritus vulvae 'these women consciously or unconsciously regard their genitals as bad, dangerous or contemptible'. In both sexes it is frequently linked with latent homosexuality.

Excessive Sweating

Fear, tension, rage or concentration in marked degree are

associated with increased sweating. Kuno (1934) distinguished between thermal and mental or emotional sweating, the former being mostly on the forehead, neck, front and back of the trunk, dorsum of the hand and forearm, while the latter is found on the palms, soles and axillae.

The condition frequently leads to secondary skin lesions such as vesiculation, infections (bacterial and fungal) and rashes. The role of the emotions in this reaction has not yet been accurately defined.

Alopecia Areata

This, like other skin disorders, has excited controversy over the part played by psychological factors. Anderson (1950), in a study of 114 cases, found that 23 per cent had a history of mental shock or acute anxiety preceding the appearance of the bald patches, while a further 22 per cent exhibited a variety of mental disturbances. Irwin (1953), in a study of 55 cases, found 23 per cent to have followed mental trauma while a further 63 per cent were classed as neurotic. Greenberg (1955), in 44 cases, found only 7 per cent who were free from mental illness, but Macalpine (1958), in a psychiatric study of 125 cases, found no evidence that mental illness, anxiety or mental shock played a significant part in its causation. She was arguing as a psychotherapist and assumed that because she was unable to influence the condition with psychological treatment, it could not be related to psychological stress. There are numerous examples of diseases where psychological factors are generally accepted as established that could be equally refractory to psychotherapy and indeed there are many instances of psychological disorders which do not respond to psychotherapy. To assume on this criterion that these conditions are therefore not influenced in their causation by psychological factors is just as irrational as the view held by some somaticists, that because insomnia can be relieved by pharmacological agents, it must be organically determined. Reinhold (1960) states:

> Psychotherapy is, as yet, a clumsy and often difficult method of treatment, particularly under out-patient conditions. It is a method of treatment of immense benefit to some and hopelessly inadequate for others. It is surely unwise to come to conclusions on whether symptoms are produced by psychological disturbance or not by judging a patient's response to psychotherapy.

She studied 52 patients with alopecia areata and all had psychotherapy for at least three months; all were found to have either very stressful life conditions or moderately severe neurotic symptoms, or both, before the onset of the condition. It is difficult to reconcile Macalpine's study with that of Reinhold and it may be that the following passage from the former's paper which explains her attitude will help to explain her conclusion.

> It is of course well known that psychological factors can influence any organic illness for better or for worse, but in order to justify it being labelled psychosomatic it must be shown that emotional or psychological factors play the initiating role. Otherwise the term psychosomatic will be extended so far that ultimately no organic disease will escape being labelled psychosomatic and no advance be made in diagnosis, prognosis or therapy.

One would applaud most of this statement, but again it is difficult to see how a psychosomatic label can block advances in the aspects mentioned.

Mehlman and Griesemer (1968) made a detailed study of 20 children with alopecia areata and elicited the following: (a) In several of the younger patients it was associated with a traumatic weaning; (b) In another group it followed actual or threatened abandonment; (c) Some of the older children exhibited a high degree of neurotic anxiety at the heart of which lay themes of abandonment and loss; (d) In some it was associated with the birth of siblings; (e) In others it followed loss of a significant relationship.

This evidence is suggestive of the psychosomatic influence though it is highly coloured with the theory of abandonment and loss.

Chronic Urticaria

This does not appear to result from major psychological crises, but from minor ones. Rees (1957) found emotional precipitation of attacks in 68 per cent of his cases, and his groups showed a statistically higher incidence of neurotic symptoms than in controls. Stressful situations were not specific and neither did he find a specific personality type. Reinhold (1960), in her study of 27 patients with chronic urticaria, as in her series of alopecia areata, found that all had very stressful life conditions or moderately severe neurotic symptoms, or both, before the onset of the condition.

Though urticaria usually has a physical cause, such as allergens, toxins, chemical agents and intestinal parasites, a number especially of the subacute or chronic type fail to reveal such cause. Wittkower and Russell (1953) were able to demonstrate a relationship between stressful life situations and relapses and exacerbations of the condition and that 'repressed aggressiveness and regressed revival of infantile skin eroticism' were often encountered. Graham and Wolf (1950) studied patients in experimental stress situations by using arteriole calibre and the reactive erythema threshold as an index of the tone of the minute skin vessels. They demonstrated that such stress situations induced in the subjects extreme dilatation of both arterioles and minute vessels, or the cutaneous changes associated with urticaria.

Atopic Dermatitis

Although an allergic factor is frequently shown by skin tests and there is frequently evidence of mental disturbance, Wittkower and Lester (1962) state:

> . . . The majority of atopic patients are extremely tense, anxious individuals who are very sensitive to interpersonal contacts. They are emotionally labile, dependent and hostile, withdrawing easily from unsatisfactory relationships.

These authors stress three points in regard to emotional factors:

1. There is a marked difficulty in expressing aggression and self-assertion.
2. Studies in children and adults have shown maternal rejection though in some there was maternal over-protection. The latter may be a reaction-formation.
3. Symptoms frequently had symbolic expressive value as in the case of the man in whom the rash was localized around his wedding ring at a time of marital infidelity.

Brown and Bettley (1971) tried to assess the value of psychiatric treatment in eczema. They selected 82 patients and allotted them randomly to two treatment groups, Group A which received dermatological treatment only and Group B which had it combined with psychiatric treatment. After 18 months follow-up it was shown that though the second group seemed to do better as time went on, this was not statistically significant, though a sub-group of Group A that were not even exposed to an initial interview with a psychiatrist, let alone psychiatric treatment, did very badly, suggesting that full psychiatric initial assessment and follow-up had some therapeutic value which would influence dermatological treatment. Their conclusions were:

1. Psychiatric treatment improves the outcome in cases of eczema independently of the degree of overt psychological disturbance.
2. It improves outcome only when there is overt psychological disturbance.

3. It improves outcome only when emotional disturbance is 'highly relevant' to the eczema.
4. It is more beneficial where motivation is high and may be harmful where it is low.

Psoriasis

It is a widespread disease affecting about 1·4 per cent of the population and alleged to be transmitted through a recessive gene. In spite of the genetic factor, non-specific stressful situations may precipitate or aggravate the condition. Wittkower and Lester (1962) regard pruritus in psoriasis as invariably psychogenic and consider an investigation of the psychiatric factors as mandatory, especially in patients showing pronounced fluctuations of symptoms with acute relapses and persistent itching.

Rosacea

Klaber and Wittkower (1937) suggest that common blushing and rosacea differ only in degree and that both are emotionally determined. The author has had 4 patients with severe acne rosacea associated with severe depression and both conditions cleared completely following a course of E.C.T. The response was dramatic and as the rosacea had been present for a long time, the relationship to the psychiatric treatment was difficult to ignore.

Acne Vulgaris and Seborrhoeic Dermatitis

Increased secretion of sebum (seborrhoea) or alteration of its normal consistency (dyssebacea) are found in acne vulgaris and seborrhoeic dermatitis. As sebum secretion is not under autonomic control, Baer and Sulzberger (1952) discounted evidence based on experimental stress, but Seitz (1954) suggested that the influence may be humoral rather than neuronal. Affective disturbances may aggravate the condition and commonly treatment of these conditions with imipramine can effect a remission.

Treatment

From the psychiatric aspect this will depend on the nature of the underlying disorder. The question is frequently raised with skin sensitive patients as to which drugs may be administered. By some providential arrangement, in the author's experience, the drugs which are effective with the psychiatric illness do not, as a rule, disturb the patient. In those few instances where initial sensitivity threatens continuation of treatment it is permissible to prescribe antihistamines.

Treatment is not restricted to drugs and E.C.T. Relaxation either through psychotherapy or hypnosis has its place and the elucidation and intelligent handling of external and domestic stresses is essential. Some patients with eczema become addicted to corticoids and these may be referred to the psychiatrist for treatment of their addiction.

Warts and Hypnosis

Although warts are defined as common, contagious, benign epithelial tumours caused by a papovavirus, their treatment by hypnosis has been practised for centuries or longer. Various controlled trials have been conducted to decide whether the 'cures' by hypnosis were valid, and a particularly careful one was reported by Surman *et al.* (1973).

Twenty-four patients with bilateral warts of common or plantar type were assigned according to the availability of treatment to two groups: A, the experimental–; or B, the control. All were told to abstain from other treatment including home remedies. Group A (17 patients) ranging in age from 9–38 years were treated by hypnosis once a week for 5 weeks. They were told under hypnosis that they would experience a tingling sensation in the warts on one side of the body (chosen by the patient) and that only those warts would subsequently disappear. All were examined 3 months after the first hypnotic session. Resolution was defined as clinical disappearance of warts within the 3-month period. Group B included 7 patients who served as untreated controls but who were promised hypnotherapy or conventional wart therapy, according to their choice, after 3 months.

The groups were similar in age, sex and dermatological presentation and history. Nine patients (53 per cent) showed significant improvement, but in only one patient did resolution occur exclusively on the treated side, and this patient later reported that the remaining wart on the untreated side resolved a week after the 3-months follow-up. A sudden loss of all lesions occurred in 4 of the 9 patients, 4 reported gradual fading of all warts and one had successive sudden loss of individual lesions. All 9 patients were able to experience tingling in these warts through hypnotic suggestion and 3 could experience vivid sensory imagery. None of the 7 controls improved at the end of 3 months but of 4 who subsequently received hypnotherapy, 3 showed significant improvement.

The authors conclude that warts tend to respond to hypnosis, but there was no evidence that it could influence lesions selectively. They explain the action as a general effect on host response to the virus. They propose studying the depth of trance in relation to wart remission.

RESPIRATORY SYSTEM

Breathing and the emotions are closely related and many novelists have described changes in breathing in order to reinforce the picture of emotional disturbance, particularly in anxiety, passion and rage. The mode of expression is usually pulmonary but on occasions it may be manifest as snorting or sniffing and assume the form of a compulsive act which causes as much, if not more, distress to the family than to the patient. As respiration has both voluntary and involuntary control, some of its functional disturbances, unlike the stomach and the colon, may be of a voluntary nature, though it should be recognized that this may shade into an involuntary extension.

Breath-holding is characteristically a childhood disorder and is dealt with under Child Psychiatry.

THE HYPERVENTILATION SYNDROME

This is found both in children and adults and may be initiated as a voluntary act, though in many instances it is a result of anxiety. It may not be recognized as such, for most do not present with respiratory distress, but with the physical sequelae of the hyperventilation. Ames (1955), in a study of 40 patients, found that 15 denied any respiratory difficulties while only one admitted that his problem lay in that field. Half presented with cardiovascular symptoms and about 20 per cent with fainting attacks which may be mistaken for epilepsy; they are frequently admitted to the casualty department of a general hospital and may only be seen by a psychiatrist when the physical investigations are completed and the emotional disturbance which precipitated the attack is buried in the mass of laboratory reports which have accumulated. The collapsed patient complaining of precordial pain and with pallor, tachycardia, sweating and cold extremities may suggest a coronary thrombosis, but the age group is different, for hyperventilation tends to occur in younger people though in certain hysterical characters the attacks are used as a means of getting into hospital and this form of behaviour, particularly in females, may continue into adult life. The washing out of the carbon dioxide leads to vasoconstriction with what has been estimated as a 30 per cent reduction in cerebral blood flow, which may account for the cerebral symptoms and for the occasional evidence of cardiac ischaemia. There may be acute behaviour disturbance with aggression and violence or other impulsive conduct, but it is difficult to decide whether this is due to the cerebral vasoconstriction or to the underlying personality, for some of these patients have a record of such behaviour during times when they do not show the more disabling physical concomitants.

In a milder degree it may accompany anxiety states, particularly of a phobic nature, and contribute to the general panic, for the patient may fear he is going to pass out and gets the sensation of psychological remoteness or unreality. It also explains some of the complaints of these patients, particularly the tingling in the fingers and occasional loss of power in the limbs and jaws, a situation which is strongly suggestive of hyperventilation tetany.

A careful psychiatric appraisal of the situation may define the trigger situation, but in those with behaviour disturbance this may prove fruitless, and it is possible that in these cases the hyperventilation is initially self-induced and not the result of anxiety.

BRONCHIAL ASTHMA

This is one of the commonest and most challenging of the psychosomatic disorders and has attracted considerable attention to its psychological and physical components.

Psychological Factors

These are still debated and their specificity is questioned. As frequently happens in psychosomatic medicine, what was originally regarded as a typical personality for a certain disease seems to be found in other diseases too, and Neuhaus (1958) in a study of asthmatic and cardiac children did not find any significant personality differences on psychological tests. French and Alexander (1941), who made a detailed study of bronchial asthma from the psychoanalytical aspect, state:

> . . . first that the asthmatic attack is a reaction to the danger of separation from the mother; second, that the attack is a sort of equivalent of an inhibited and repressed cry of anxiety or rage; third, that the sources of danger of losing the mother are due to some temptations to which the patient is exposed.

Wittkower and White (1959), in a study of 10 patients, found that they all expressed marked feelings of ambivalence towards their mothers and had felt deprived of maternal love in childhood. They described the mothers as rigid, insecure and domineering, while the fathers were meek, passive and dependent, and the behaviour of the patients in their life-histories as showing varying degrees of pseudo-independence. The authors conclude that this behaviour:

appeared to represent overcompensation of dependent trends and could be related to (1) maternal rejection by a sick or inadequate mother, (2) inability of the normal mother to satisfy excessive dependent demands of the child, (3) maternal demands for premature independence and (4) maternal overprotection.

The oral cavity and respiratory tract seemed particularly vulnerable in their patients and eight had a history of oral surgery, injury or serious respiratory illness shortly before the onset of bronchial asthma.

The authors refer to the theory of Fenichel (1945) that asthma represents an unconscious attempt by the patient to protect himself from loss of maternal love by respiratory introjection of the ambivalently regarded mother. They also quote the theory of Saul (1946) where union with the mother is achieved projectively, the patient trying to retain the good mother and get rid of the bad one and arrive at the following formulation:

... The individual with constitutional autonomic and endocrine lability, possibly genetically determined, and with a respiratory tract prone to dysfunction on a genetic or acquired basis, who also possesses intense oral drives, either inherited or acquired, that bring him into conflict with an 'unsatisfactory' mother to the extent that she is unable to satisfy normal demands or is a relatively 'normal' mother unable to satisfy excessive demands, attempts to protect himself from separation anxiety by respiratory introjection and projection in psychodynamic terms and by ostentatious pseudo-independence on a behavioural level.

They caution that undue emphasis on any single factor in aetiology ignores the essence of the problem, which is that a 'constellation' of factors, with perhaps one, which in certain conditions may appear to be predominant.

Knapp (1969) repeated the descriptions of the mother and father of the asthmatic child by citing two case histories, one of Marcel Proust and the second a housewife who was still in partial bondage to her mother. On the basis of his physiological researches into asthma, he separates the attacks into: (a) transient responses to immediate stimuli which he equates with the urge to express emotion over pulmonary pathways, and (b) sustained results of several interacting influences which can be psychosocial or physiological. He makes the additional point that pulmonary air conductance, like many other 'involuntary' functions, seems to come under voluntary control when the human or animal subject is informed or reinforced on an appropriate 'response'. Such 'learning' may affect sufferers from asthma.

Rees (1963) compared 170 asthmatics with 160 controls and found a significantly higher incidence of unsatisfactory parental attitudes in those patients whose parents were over-protective. These attitudes usually antedated the asthma and could not therefore have been caused by it. The lesson drawn is that the parent should be counselled to encourage the child to increased self-expression and independence.

Treatment

This is no less varied than the aetiological factors that have been postulated, but it is apparent that in a disturbed and vulnerable personality, psychotherapy has a legitimate place, though as in ulcerative colitis, it should be realized that the greatest delicacy in the handling of the patient may be needed for the condition is likely to literally explode in one's face and status asthmaticus is a frightening prospect on the analytical couch. When the mechanism has really got under way, it is virtually impossible to proceed with psychotherapy and too much emphasis on the dynamics of the situation should not blind the therapist to the fact that the patient is exploiting or is in the grip of a mechanism which can prove fatal. It is in a spirit of compromise that all therapy must be conducted with the concessions coming mainly from the therapist in the hope that the patient will yield his symptoms.

It is in the symptomatic treatment that there has been most controversy. Physicians are prepared to concede that a disturbed personality, even with asthma, may require psychotherapy, but some are reluctant to accept that symptomatic treatment of a psychological nature is superior to other forms of treatment. The argument is usually over the place of hypnosis in treatment. Many are convinced of its efficacy, while others decry it; some claim it cures, others that it merely relieves the anxiety and permits the condition to subside. It is not essential to prove that hypnosis has a benefical effect on lung changes to show that it is of value and there is no cause to sneer at a treatment which produces subjective improvement without any physical change. As asthmatic attack is a crippling state and may even prove fatal, so any form of treatment which can either relieve the acute attack or reduce its incidence is of value. White (1961) has shown that by measuring lung compliance, hypnotic relief of symptoms does not produce any change in lung function and that presumably improvement is subjective. Furthermore, this improvement was not dependent on the depth of hypnosis reached. It was not necessary to induce trance and a number of patients improved with what could only be regarded as suggestion under relaxation. It may be that the relief of anxiety in those patients who already have organic changes in their lungs lowers the demands on a failing respiratory system by lowering the basal metabolic rate and thus accounts for the patient's emphatic report of progress with the treatment and his capacity to perform at a more efficient level. Hypnosis can be used even in cases of status asthmaticus, though the patient may appear a most unlikely candidate. Sinclair-Gieben (1960) reported such a case who was *in extremis* and in whom he achieved complete relaxation. The author had a patient referred who had failed to respond to steroids and was in a persistent state of severe asthma. He had previously had E.C.T. and because of his undue predisposition to bronchospasm, the anaesthetist had written on his case sheet in red ink that he must never have an anaesthetic outside of an operating theatre. With very little justification and even less confidence, hypnotic suggestion was tried with dramatic improvement and he has since returned to factory work which he had been unable to do for two years. Hypnosis is not the complete answer to asthma, but even in unlikely subjects, it may be well worth trying. The treatment may fail with one therapist and be successful with another, and it should not be regarded like steroids or other physical measures which, if once tried and found wanting, should be discarded. The issues are too great for such pseudo-objectivity. Some patients can be trained in auto-hypnosis or be given a tape-recording of the suggestion and induce the state themselves.

A carefully controlled trial of hypnotic treatment by Maher-Loughnan *et al.* (1962) provided the following information.

1. Hypnotic treatment was more effective than anti-spasmodics.
2. Centres using hypnotic treatment had better results than the centres using other forms of psychotherapy.
3. Males and females responded equally and patients under 30 and with a history of less than 20 years did best.
4. Mild cases and those with emotional triggers did best, but good responses were also observed in others.
5. Patients who were easily hypnotized achieved deep trances and, most important, those who could practise daily autohypnosis did best.

Even in the physical treatment of the condition, the psychological approach should never be abandoned. The patient may wish to retain a spray or some nostrum which the physician knows has no specific effect, but he should not be deprived of it. Compromise is the very essence of treatment and the physician who cannot control his aggressive impulses should not get involved with the asthmatic.

PSYCHOGENIC DYSPNOEA

Burns and Howell (1969) noted that 31 patients attending a respiratory diseases clinic were more breathless than airways obstruction warranted. When a psychiatric assessment of these patients was made and compared with a control group of 31 patients with appropriate pulmonary disease the following factors were defined in the disproportionate group: (1) poor relationship of breathlessness to exertion; (2) acute hyperventilation attacks present; (3) breathlessness experienced at rest; (4) main difficulty was getting air in; (5) breathlessness fluctuated even in minutes; (6) fear sudden death in attack of hyperventilation; (7) breathlessness varied with social situation; (8) patient had stopped working; (9) not improved by stopping smoking; (10) breathless during conversation; (11) relieved by sedatives and alcohol; (12) woken at night by breathlessness; (13) worse in the morning and evening and not relieved by expectoration.

Symptoms of a depressive illness or an anxiety state with hysterical reactions were more frequent in this group, as were a previous personal and family history of mental illness. Successful treatment of the psychiatric disorder resulted in a complete or partial resolution of breathlessness. Psychogenic stress was also more common and there was a preponderance of obsessional traits and lifelong excessive health consciousness.

EMPHYSEMA

Dudley *et al.* (1969) studied 40 patients with irreversible, diffuse, obstructive pulmonary syndrome over a 4-year period. Ventilatory measurements were collected on all patients as well as data on their psychosocial adjustment. In addition, the 29 who died (73 per cent) were studied more intensively during the process of dying. The subjects consistently used denial, repression and isolation to protect their failing respiratory systems from environmental influences, and these attempts to insulate themselves psychologically from their surroundings led to numerous misunderstandings with staff, relatives and friends, which in turn led to greater use of the defences. A breakdown of the defences was associated with increasing symptoms and physiological deterioration.

Psychosocial assets were found to be as important as physiological assets in the treatment in that they contributed to the patient's co-operation. A high psychosocial score reinforced the capacity to remain alive and seemed to influence the maximum breathing capacity. During death, all patients found it comfortable and relaxing and exceedingly difficult to give up once it was started, and the authors conclude that death trauma is more in the eyes of the beholder than in the actual experience of the dying patient.

BRONCHIAL CARCINOMA

Cancer in various forms has attracted the attention of psychiatrists and psychologists and in view of the strong association between excessive smoking and cancer of the lung and its rising incidence, this particular form of cancer is of particular interest. A cause which would usurp the place of smoking would in certain quarters be most popular. Eysenck (1965) criticises the statistical evidence which has been mustered against smoking and puts forward his own theory that the extraverted personality is constitutionally predisposed to cancer, is commonly addicted to smoking and that the environmental factors of urbanization and air pollution wreak their havoc.

While Eysenck may have overstated his case and based it on a theory of personality which is of doubtful validity, he was right to point out the personality aspect of this disease. Heavy smoking is in itself an addiction and therefore a form of abnormal behaviour. It is not unreasonable to suggest that the addiction and vulnerability of the bronchial epithelium to cigarette smoke may have a common origin. If more attention were paid to this aspect prophylaxis may be more successful, for to date, by emphasizing the smoking alone, it either leaves the victim uninfluenced or directs him into equally dangerous forms of addiction. The sight of a heavy smoker drawing at his first cigarette and the semantics used—'a drag' or 'a gasper' leave one in no doubt of the addictive component in this disease.

Kissen (1963, 1964) has argued that patients with lung cancer exhibit a particular personality feature which he describes as a 'poor outlet for emotional discharge'. By showing that 150 male, lung cancer patients scored lower on childhood behaviour disorders and on 'neuroticism' scales than 150 men with chest diseases other than lung cancer, he maintained they had a tendency to assimilate rather than discharge emotion. This personality factor was independent of smoking in the two groups. He later extended his enquiries (Kissen,

1966) and showed that a significantly higher percentage of cancer patients had an important adverse emotional experience in childhood or in adult life.

There was a negative correlation between 'neuroticism' and lung cancer irrespective of smoking habits, suggesting that a psychological cause need not be mediated through a physical factor such as smoking. Interpretation of this finding will depend on the importance attached to scores on the 'neuroticism' scale which is part of the Maudsley Personality Inventory. It is fashionable to use this test but the author is finding that it tends to confuse more than clarify and if other factors do not support it, its findings should not be taken too seriously and it should not be used alone to support or refute a theory concerning the psychological aspects of cancer.

Allergic Rhinitis (Hay Fever)

Though this is alleged to be due mainly to pollen and animal fur, it frequently has a psychological component. Wilson (1941) who regarded the nose as a sexual organ considered that repressed olfactory sexual curiosity played a part, the patient having substituted the olfactory organ for the visual one. At a more superficial level, the condition is in some people a distress signal and may appear on specific occasions, such as when making an after-dinner speech or presenting a paper to a learned society.

The Common Cold

This is so common as to make any definition of psychological factors appear well-nigh impossible. Yet some people are much more prone than others and excite in the observer the suspicion that psychological factors may be operating. Children are frequently involved and they usually fit into the category of the nervous child and are prone not only to the common cold, but other respiratory tract infections. The evidence is still not conclusive but Despert (1944) found that children from broken homes, who were attending nursery school, had a significantly higher number of absences which were alleged to be due to colds than those from better homes. But it may only indicate that these children stay away more readily from school.

PULMONARY TUBERCULOSIS

This has always interested the psychiatrist. It was one of the diseases that in mental institutions had a higher correlation with schizophrenia than with manic-depressive psychosis. It was the disease which afflicted artists and writers and was responsible for the phenomenon of *spes phthisica* and therefore was associated in the minds of some psychiatrists with instability. That the cause of the disease was already known and had satisfied Koch's postulates has not deterred psychiatrists and physicians from considering other factors which might predispose to or prolong the disease. Wittkower (1949), who approached the study tentatively, expected to encounter a somatopsychic rather than a psychosomatic problem. As the work progressed his interest shifted from the effects of the disease on the patient's psychology to the effects of the latter on the incidence and course of the disease. He divided the pre-morbid personalities of 300 patients into four main groups: overtly insecure types (39 per cent), rebellious types (12 per cent), self-drivers (29 per cent) and conflict-harassed types (13 per cent). An editorial in the *Lancet* (1949*a*) comments:

> . . . The reader, moreover, may well ask, 'Does the whole of humanity fall within these four categories? (And if so, which am I?) And if not, how would Dr. Wittkower describe the remaining types who are apparently immune from tuberculosis?'
>
> He finds that the outstanding common feature of the pre-morbid personality is an inordinate need (overt or concealed) for affection, coupled with conflicts over dependence. Again it may be asked, 'To what extent is this maladjustment the lot of humanity? Is it as rare (4 per 1000 population) as pulmonary tuberculosis? Or is it so common that the co-existence of tuberculosis might be accidental?' . . . we wonder what happens to the psychology of those millions who arrest their disease and return to more or less normal life, and of those who, five or more years later, have almost forgotten they had ever been in a sanatorium. What has the tubercle bacillus done for them?

These are fair comments.

Earlier, Day (1946), who approached the problem as one working with tuberculous patients, concluded that those who develop the disease in the absence of any of the classical physical environmental causes, often do so 'because of dis-ease in their psychological environment'. He equates this with lowered resistance. In a later paper (Day, 1951) he points out the differences between tuberculosis and other psychosomatic diseases and in refreshingly simple language states: '. . . To develop chronic active pulmonary tuberculosis a person needs some bacilli, some moderately inflammable lungs (not celluloid like the guinea-pig's nor asbestos like the elephant's) and some internal or external factor which *lowers the resistance to the disease*'. After listing a number of the physical factors which contribute he raises the issue of the healthy bodied, living in comfortable material circumstances, who break down with the disease. It is in these cases that he considers psychological factors to be operating. He continues: 'Personally—and in spite of the guinea-pig, the elephant, the negro, and the twin, and all the other reasonable arguments put forward by the sceptics—I am convinced that in some cases, disturbance of the psyche does *precipitate* the active disease process'. It has been said that with the advent of effective chemotherapy, much of the psychosomatic argument has been undermined, for specific personalities and childhood influences are no match for modern drugs, but the psychiatrist will still insist that isoniazid is closely related to the antidepressants and that the drug battery deals not only with the organism but with the disturbed affective state which, as Wittkower pointed out, is usually depressive. In spite of present-day successful treatment, psychological studies are still considered necessary and Kissen (1958) undertook an investigation to meet the criticism that psychosomatic studies are lacking both in controls and objectivity. His conclusions were that the disease was commonest in patients with an 'inordinate need for affection' and 60 per cent were deprived of affection in childhood compared with 16 per cent of controls. The commonest emotional factor preceding the onset was a break in a love link such as romance, engagement or marriage. He uses these data to explain the high incidence in mental hospitals, migrants and displaced persons.

Psychogenic Fever

Pyrexia is traditionally regarded as evidence of organic disease and is a frequent challenge to the physician who, in spite of the most exhaustive tests, may be unable to find a satisfactory explanation. The search for a diagnosis may then be abandoned and defeat accepted by applying the label P.U.O. (pyrexia of unknown origin). Yet there is evidence that fever may be psychogenic. Reimann (1932, 1936) described habitual hyperthermia in young women, many of whom were neurotic and exhibited a low-grade fever for up to 19 years without any evidence of organic disease. Hunter (1947) showed that in such cases where anxiety or tension was responsible, discussion of the patient's problems with solution of their difficulties resulted in a defervescence. Bakwin (1944) reported that slight rises of temperature in some nervous children, when in hospital, disappeared on their return home, while Britton and Kline (1939) produced rises in temperature in mammals and reptiles by inducing fear, anger, rage and sexual stimulation.

White and Long (1958), in an attempt to define the incidence of psychogenic fever among first admissions to hospitals, found in 3·6 per cent of patients a rise of 0·5°C. or greater, immediately after the first admission, which subsided spontaneously after a day or two in hospital. All cases with organic pyrexia were so rigidly excluded that it was possible that some psychogenic ones were also excluded. It was commonest in adult males entering the psychiatric wards and the incidence in these wards was 14·4 per cent, which was four times greater than those admitted to the medical, surgical, obstetric or paediatric service. Many of the psychiatric patients had psychosomatic disorders which were linked with vasomotor instability.

Psychogenic fever is, of course, very different from that found in 'Deliberate Disability' (Hawkings *et al.*, 1956). Petersdorf and Bennett (1957) found psychogenic fever in the tense, anxious, often highly intelligent person who had the background of the good conscientious citizen and, although this may distinguish him from the psychopathic simulator, such a background is indeed found in 'Deliberate Disability'.

PSYCHOSOMATIC ASPECTS OF PREGNANCY

It is understandable that during pregnancy old unconscious phantasies are mobilized. These are associated with introjection, and women with oral fixations and ambivalent attitudes to their pregnancy will revive old conflicts associated with oral strivings. Some have tried to put a physiological rather than a psychological interpretation on the phenomenon of the 'cravings' of pregnant women. Drummond and Wilbraham (1957) suggested that her increased requirement of vitamin C and calcium led her to crave foods which were rich in these substances. Yudkin (1956), however, suggested that the psychological aspect was dominant and stated '. . . the pregnant woman may well demand not oranges but peaches out of season'. The author was faced with a similar problem; a pregnant, almost parturient patient demanded a sherbet drink at 3 a.m. on a Sunday in Edinburgh. Her 'physiological' craving for potassium could not have been more inconvenient!

Harries and Hughes (1958) enumerate the 'cravings' of some pregnant women, basing their findings on the results of letters to the British Broadcasting Corporation, in reply to an invitation at the end of a programme dealing with the subject. There were 991 'cravings' in all, 261 for fruit, 105 for vegetables and 187 for non-food substances. Of the last group, 35 were for coal, 17 for soap and 15 for disinfectant, and there were 193 reports of substances normally liked but disliked during pregnancy. Heading this list were 78 instances of an aversion to tea, 24 to tobacco and 22 to coffee.

Though the letters were written in an amused or amusing manner, the compulsion was very strong and frequently associated with a sense of shame and great secrecy. There was no mention of a 'craving' not being satisfied and though there were many descriptions of how the substance was obtained, there were no reports of failure. Of the total letters, 135 mentioned the stage of pregnancy, 59 in the first four months and only six at full term. One writer had her 'theory', saying it was a desire for something to crunch, the texture being more important than the flavour, and this is supported by the high incidence of pickled foods, confectionery, nuts, dry raw cereal and a preference for uncooked vegetables. Posner *et al.* (1957), in a more detailed enquiry in 600 patients in the third month of pregnancy, found that 394 had such cravings while 196 denied them; 10 admitted to 'pica' compared to seven in the B.B.C. enquiry.

That this is a common feature seems established, but the illogical and occasionally perverse nature of the condition has caused many women to keep it secret.

Marriage and Fertility of Psychotic Women

Stevens (1969) reported on a large representative sample of psychotic women of reproductive age from patients admitted to a London mental hospital and later followed up when community care was established. Before first admission the probability of marriage of schizophrenics was 75 per cent of corresponding normal women but after admission it had fallen to 33 per cent. Fertility of schizophrenics was also slightly reduced before and after illness but much of this was due to hospitalization. Marriage and fertility of women with severe affective disorders were similar to normal. The author concluded that despite a lessening of differentials between patients and normal women since the impact of community care, the probability of marriage of schizophrenics was still significantly reduced.

Dyspareunia

Though frequently due to physical factors such as trauma, inflammation, kraurosis vulvae and endometriosis, it can also result from psychological causes. It can be a defence against sexual intercourse which in turn may be based on phantasies of injury. Treatment can be on analytical lines but simpler methods such as reassurance can be just as effective and speedier in many cases. Mears

(1958) describes her treatment which is capable of being carried out by the family doctor.

> If there is no physical cause for the vaginismus, I explain to her how the vaginismus has come about (muscular spasm due to emotional tension). I reassure her that everything is quite normal otherwise (women are very often worried about whether they are too small inside), and I explain carefully that coitus must not be attempted until she has learned to relax sufficiently and that no one can do this for her. Full explanation and reassurance along these lines usually makes them immediately cooperative.
>
> I then ask the patient to insert something in her vagina, sometimes her finger, sometimes a glass dilator, sometimes a cap. I find it better to leave the choice to the patient: so often patients who have had a surgical hymenectomy followed up with glass dilators, without any explanation, have hated inserting dilators and found them consequently very painful, yet will insert a finger readily. On the other hand, there are some women who cannot bear to touch themselves with their fingers, but are quite happy to insert dilators. . .

The same paper gives details of the mechanics of insertion of an occlusive cap or dilator which the patient is encouraged to practise.

The above description is of a treatment which, though having some psychological overtones, is essentially simple and logical and is indicative of a variety of conditions which respond equally well to suggestions of relaxation. While it is ludicrous to expect that such suggestion could cure all forms of psychiatric disturbances, it is equally ludicrous to apply the lengthy techniques of analytical psychotherapy to conditions which respond perfectly well to simpler and more direct measures.

Hyperemesis Gravidarum or Vomiting of Early Pregnancy

This has aroused controversy as to the role of psychological factors. Robertson (1946) in a personality study of such patients reported disturbed sexual function, undue attachment to the mother, and a history of previous dyspepsia. Harvey and Sherfey (1954), in 20 hospital admissions, obtained a history of gastro-intestinal symptoms (including vomiting in response to emotional disturbance), frigidity and psychological immaturity. Coppen (1959) undertook a controlled study of 50 primiparae, 29 who had vomited during pregnancy and 21 who had not. The series differed from those of Harvey and Sherfey in that none was severe enough to be admitted to hospital. He subjected his patients to a personality questionnaire (The Maudsley Personality Inventory) as well as interview and found no significant difference between the two groups. As the personality inventory was designed by Eysenck (1959) to measure two personality dimensions, neuroticism and extraversion-introversion, many who do not accept these dimensions without considerable reservations will hold similar reservations about Coppen's study. But this does illustrate the difficulty one group of workers who have accepted a principle will have in communicating with an unconverted group. Neither group can expect its tenets to be shared and there is, to date, no clearing house for ideas in psychiatry. Each group assumes it possesses the genuine article and, having established some support, accuses the other of being unscientific. Unfortunately these differences are not peculiar to psychiatry.

Treatment of the mild case is mainly one of sympathetic understanding; the vast majority settle and it is rare now for a patient with severe hyperemesis to be admitted to hospital. Should the need arise, it cannot be emphasized too strongly that there is a real risk to life and that even though the patient does not appear in mortal danger, she can slip through one's fingers like a wet fish. Present-day accent on fluid and electrolyte balance makes this less likely, but the patient with her persistent vomiting and rather wayward mental state due to the fluid and electrolyte loss can excite in the nursing staff a resentment which may blind them to the gravity of the patient's condition. They may see the persistent vomiting as a defiance of their authority or a rejection of their help and join battle with the patient. The psychiatrist must then work furiously on the nursing staff, stressing the difficulty in handling these patients but also emphasizing the terms of reference, namely that the patient has her baby in safety and has not come to hospital for character training. That aspect can wait and be left to the child. It is usually the most competent and self-reliant nursing staff who are most vulnerable in this respect and this makes the psychiatrist's task even harder. As in so many psychosomatic disorders, there is an element of defiance represented by the patient's illness, but there is no future in the attitude thus expressed by a nursing sister 'I'll stop her vomiting, if it kills. . .' But it is 'her' not 'me' that will be killed and this revelation can prove most salutory.

Urinary Retention

In women, though this is frequently due to such organic states as a retroverted gravid uterus, haematocolpos, uterine fibroids, tumours of the ovary or broad ligaments, atony of the bladder and multiple sclerosis, it may also be due to psychological causes. It is commonly reported as a hysterical symptom by textbooks of surgery and gynaecology but psychiatric studies are still sparse. Larson *et al.* (1963) reported on 37 female patients. Most were married and had experienced a physical or psychic trauma such as gynaecological surgery prior to the onset. Childbirth, marital discord and broken love affairs were other common precipitants and the patients were of average intelligence. The authors do not indicate the results of psychiatric treatment but imply that as spontaneous remission is likely, surgical treatment in the form of resection of the vesical neck is contra-indicated. Williams and Johnson (1956) reported a case which was treated successfully by psychotherapy and Chapman (1959) described another where the precipitating factors were sexual trauma, seduction and rape by the stepfather. Under psychotherapy her hostility to the stepfather was explored and it was noted that her episodes of retention occurred when her hostility threatened to become conscious. Psychotherapy relieved her. A further case, reported by Knox (1960), was so upset by the 'primal scene' that sexual relations 'became horrible and disgusting'. In her married relations she was very frigid and this was causing marital discord and her condition improved after she had secured a promise from her husband to make no more sexual demands.

PSYCHIATRIC EMERGENCIES AND THE MENSTRUAL CYCLE

Glass *et al.* (1971) tried to assess whether phases of the menstrual cycle related to specific types of psychiatric emergencies, by evaluating 166 representative female patients seen as such during one year at the Yale-New Haven Hospital. Patients were seen at twice the expected frequency during the premenstrual week but at the expected frequency in the menstrual week. Those with character disorders were seen more frequently in the premenstrual phase than schizophrenics (67 per cent: 44 per cent). Suicide attempts occurred at three times the expected rate premenstrually. The premenstrual group had significantly fewer past psychiatric contacts and fewer admissions to psychiatric hospital, but had a stronger medical and gynaecological history with marital and sexual problems and a greater tendency to hostility, suicide ideation and attempts. The authors propose that these women do not verbalize affect into pre-menstrual symptomatology, and they therefore have an increase in the more direct experiencing of hostility.

PRE-ECLAMPTIC TOXAEMIA

This condition which may develop 'out of the blue' has intrigued psychiatrists. Some have declared that it may alternate with puerperal psychosis and others have hinted at a psychosomatic factor. Pilowsky and Sharp (1971) conducted a prospective study by means of a questionnaire and found psychological differences between primiparae who developed the condition and those who did not. This is not strong evidence and more information is needed.

PRE-MENSTRUAL TENSION AND DYSMENORRHOEA

Pre-menstrual tension. This was first described by Frank (1931). In addition to tension, irritability and depression in the pre-menstrual phase, there may be swelling in the breasts and abdomen and even frank oedema. Psychosomatic concomitants that have been demonstrated are: higher accident rate, increased incidence of suicide, increase in misbehaviour and crime, and acute psychiatric illness.

Though connected with some form of hormonal imbalance and water retention, it is also associated with a marked functional element. The pre-menstrual weight gain has been related by Bickers (1958) to the severity of the symptoms, and the improvement following a marked loss of weight after the administration of chlorothiazide was regarded as confirmatory. Yet Sweeney (1934) showed that a third of normal women gain approximately 3 lb. (1·4 kg.) pre-menstrually and Appleby (1960), who supports this finding, goes further by denying any correlation between chlorothiazide and relief of symptoms. Meprobamate (400 mg. t.d.s.) resulted in some degree of improvement in 77 per cent of the 30 patients as against 57 per cent treated with chlorothiazide, thus suggesting that the functional element was dominant.

Bruce and Russell (1962) who investigated two groups of patients, 24 with few restrictions and 10 in a metabolic ward with water, sodium and potassium balances, also concluded that there was no correlation between the physical changes and pre-menstrual tension. The add: 'neither do such metabolic changes, whether at ovulation or during the pre-menstruum, inevitably give rise to symptoms'.

Coppen and Kessel (1963) gave the ubiquitous personality test (Maudsley Personality Inventory) to women selected randomly and who were also asked to complete a questionnaire on their menstrual function. They found a correlation between 'neuroticism' as measured by the test and pre-menstrual tension, but not with dysmenorrhoea. It would be premature to conclude on the basis of the test that the former is, and the latter is not a psychosomatic disorder. The test may reflect only one aspect of 'neuroticism' or 'neuroticism' as measured by the test may not be synonymous with the psychological component of a psychosomatic disorder.

INFERTILITY

Sandler (1968) studied the effects of emotional stress on fertility. He claimed that it is not sufficiently recognized how often infertility is related to stress and particularly to a disturbance in the marital relations. Many patients are threatened at both conscious and unconscious levels by pregnancy and parenthood and in a series of 268 cases of infertility, stress factors operated in 67 (25 per cent).

Of the mechanisms involved, it has been shown that emotional shock can produce an immediate effect on the endometrium. Emotional immaturity may be associated with tubal spasm and the presence of hypogonadal genitalia, and these can be relieved either by oestrogens or the gaining of insight and the achievement of mature sexuality. Some immature infertile women have bacterial infection of the cervical mucus which clears up with their problems. Many have a dry cervix with scanty, sticky mucus associated with hypogonadism, and the mucus may be related to chronic pelvic congestion due to regular sexual stimulation without satisfaction.

Tubal spasm may be associated with general tension as well as with immaturity, and the author recommends that testing for tubal patency should be done with the patient conscious since the spasm may disappear when the patient is anaesthetized. One patient whose tubes were found to be closed was told a joke and laughed. Her tubes opened and she conceived within the month; another, rejecting of pregnancy, was told her tubes were open and they closed immediately.

The author compared 3 groups of infertile patients: (1) 32 who decided to adopt; (2) 20 who suffered from some form of emotional disorder; (3) 188 who had organic disorders.

Charts of conception rates by trimesters for patients who decided to adopt were the same as those for patients treated for emotional disorders, and different from those who were treated for organic disorders, suggesting that adoption facilitates conception by relieving emotional stress.

ORAL CONTRACEPTIVES

These are so commonly used that they are becoming a normal aspect of human behaviour rather than a drug with dangerous side-effects which can cause death and severe and lasting physical disability in young women who would otherwise remain healthy. While it may be interesting to speculate why such risks should be taken to avoid a pregnancy which previous generations had not regarded as catastrophic and why society will ban the use of a drug which has a fraction of the side effects of the 'pill', the main interests to the psychiatrist are the alleged psychiatric sequelae of their use.

Herzberg *et al.* (1971) rated depression, headaches and loss of libido in 272 women before starting a contraceptive method, 54 of whom were later fitted with an intrauterine device and 218 were on three oral contraceptives. Side effects caused 25 per cent of the oral contraceptive group and 13 per cent of the I.U.D. group to abandon the method. Depression, headache and loss of libido were the most common reasons for stopping the oral method and breakthrough bleeding the most common reason for stopping the I.U.D.

The women who stopped or changed their oral contraceptive during the survey were compared with those who remained on the same oral preparation throughout, and the former had higher mean depression and neuroticism scores at the first visit to the clinic and contained more women with a history of premenstrual weepiness, depression during pregnancy, out-patient psychiatric treatment and treatment with antidepressants. These findings would suggest that adverse reactions to the 'pill' were based mainly on the pre-morbid personality of the patient, yet Grounds *et al.* (1970) in a controlled double-blind trial concluded that the common early side effects of contraceptive pills are due to their chemical action and are not dependent on neuroticism. Clearly there is more work to be done to provide the definitive answers that are needed, though even if the chemical hypothesis is not substantiated there is no doubt that for a considerable number of women the 'pill' is a distressing experience.

HYSTERECTOMY

Many women are referred for psychiatric treatment following a hysterectomy, and the question arises as to whether the operation precipitated the mental illness or whether it was itself a symptom of the illness which antedated the operation.

It is easier to answer the first question, and Barker (1968), who compared the psychiatric sequelae of 729 hysterectomy patients with 280 cholecystectomy patients found that the referral rate of the former was 2½ times that of the latter and almost three times higher than the expected incidence among women of similar age in the general population, the most frequent psychiatric symptom being depression. Referral rate was more than twice as high among patients without significant pelvic pathology and 57 per cent of all patients with a previous psychiatric history were re-referred after the operation, while 35 per cent of all women who were separated or divorced at the time of the operation were referred.

These figures provide part of the answer to the second question even though the author does not raise it. It may be assumed, unless shown otherwise, that women with mental illness after hysterectomy have had the operation for psychiatric rather than organic reasons.

VASECTOMY

This operation is performed for a variety of social reasons. In economically advanced countries it has become popular as a form of family limitation, not least among medical men. In poorer countries, it is part of a general campaign to restrict population growth. The psychiatric complications will therefore depend on the social situation and reports are mainly from the more prosperous cultures. Ziegler *et al.* (1969) tried to assess changes in psychological functioning and marital relations following vasectomy by means of a prospective study of 42 couples and compared their findings with 42 couples who used ovulation suppression pills.

The authors are in no doubt that adverse psychological changes can occur, in that most subjects and their wives react as if the operation had 'demasculating potential', and this led to an increase in psychological upset or in compensatory stereotyped masculine behaviour or both. They suggest that these reactions can be reduced in vulnerable patients by full discussion prior to the operation, but they nevertheless advise more care in selection. They state that if the wife finds sexual relationships pleasurable and desirable, is able to assume responsibility in the family, is not subordinate to her husband socially or intellectually, is conscientious and responsible, and is able and willing to take responsibility for contraception, the couple will find ovulation suppression or one of the 'feminine' contraceptive methods highly satisfactory. Should the reverse hold then a masculine form of contraception will be more satisfactory. If completely effective and permanent contraception is desired by the latter type of couple, then, if the husband is not particularly hypochondriacal or concerned about the health of his wife or himself, and if the husband has no apparent doubts about his own masculinity, vasectomy might well be the method of choice.

A similar conclusion was reached by Wolfers (1970) who found that in 10 out of 82 vasectomies there were psychological problems arising from the operation. Screening of applicants was therefore to be recommended with pre-existing instability as a contraindication.

STERILIZATION

Sim *et al.* (1973) followed up 151 women who had been sterilized for social or gynaecological reasons one to three years earlier. One hundred and forty six were completely satisfied with the results of the operation on their health and on their sexual relationships with their husbands. The five who were dissatisfied either wished they could still conceive or found the operation had not produced the effect hoped for.

As permanent contraception through female sterilization is playing an increasingly important part in family limitation, demand is increasing and adverse psychiatric sequelae have been reported. The inquiry indicates that these may be minimized if the following points are borne in mind:

1. The patient should be over the age of 30, and if younger should have had two or more children.
2. The operation should not be performed at childbirth or in the neonatal period, when the risk to the newborn child is greatest. Sterilization could, with the death of the child, compound the loss and precipitate a severe grief reaction. Furthermore, the mother's decision at that time may not be as valid a one as she may make three to six months later.
3. The patient should not be suffering from a postabortive depression, for a sterilization may reinforce this reaction.
4. The patient should be culturally adjusted to the operation.
5. The operation should not be undertaken for frigidity.
6. Apart from conclusion 3, psychiatric considerations need not be entertained.
7. It should not be part of a 'package deal' as a condition for an abortion.

MIGRAINE

This is frequently held to represent 'an inborn type of reaction to a number of stresses, both psychological and physical' (Critchley, 1950). Psychological factors may precipitate an attack but neurologists are reluctant to accept that migraine is a psychogenic affection curable by psychotherapy. While psychiatrists would agree that migraine may be resistant to psychotherapy, they consider that psychological factors are important. When two specialities like neurology and psychiatry differ over the presence or absence of certain factors in a disease, the explanation is only partly that of different orientation and may be mainly due to differing experiences.

The neurologist is preoccupied with the possible physical causes of migraine and he is usually engaged in a diligent search for these causes and may find them. The psychiatrist usually has the patient in whom such physical causes do not arise or have already been excluded and he is more pre-occupied with an estimation of personality structure and psycho-social factors which influence the condition. Headaches, though not synonymous with migraine, are of course frequently of functional origin and everyday language recognizes that people and situations can produce them. Engel (1956) was able to demonstrate an alternation between ulcerative colitis and headaches depending on changes in the patient's situation. Steinhilber *et al.* (1960) tested 50 patients with 'histamine headaches' with the Minnesota Multiphasic Personality Inventory and compared them with 50 patients with undifferentiated headaches. In each group the proportion of abnormal personality responses was high; conversion hysteria scored high in both, and hypochondriasis was especially high in the 'histamine' cases. The authors found a relation between repressed or suppressed anger and headaches in the 'histamine' group and that these patients were all rigid and meticulous perfectionists.

ANOREXIA NERVOSA

This name was originally coined by Gull (1874). He was very cautious in his statements regarding aetiology and wrote that it might be called 'hysterical without committing ourselves to the etymological value of the word, or maintaining that the subjects of it have the common symptons of hysteria'. His patients were 'wilful, often allowed to drift their own way into a state of extreme exhaustion'. It is traditionally seen in young, adolescent girls though anorexia may also be a feature of psychiatric disorders such as severe depression and schizophrenia; in fact, in the days before catatonic schizophrenia yielded to E.C.T. such patients constituted a regular round of tube-feeding for the junior medical staff in mental hospitals. It could also be a manifestation of a paranoid state, the patient refusing food because of some delusion, *e.g.* that he is being poisoned, and it is seen in hysterical states, the anorexia being directed to secondary gain, or it may be an extension of the slimming habit, so common in adolescent girls. The variety of psychiatric conditions associated with anorexia has led to *obiter dicta* declaring that all cases of anorexia nervosa are hysterical or psychopathic, and there has also been a tendency to see the problem in a superficial light which accepts slimming in adolescent girls as a normal manifestation without asking why some adolescent girls should slim in the first place.

The condition varies in severity and it is not surprising that those cases reported are the more severe, while the numerous mild states which are satisfactorily dealt with in the family circle with or without the help of the family doctor go unrecorded. It is the grosser forms that the psychiatrist has to treat, but whether mild or severe, the psychopathology in the adolescent girl is probably a common one and treatment should take account of it.

Psychopathology

This is mainly concerned with the patient's oral drives. Refusal to eat in children may be used to express negative feelings toward the parents. Orality which is the earliest field of instinctual conflict may reflect other and later ones, including genital, so that eating may be equated with becoming pregnant. The offer of food by a parent to a child has a symbolic meaning, for it represents love, and some parents who feel insecure can only appreciate an acceptance and reciprocation of their love in the child's appetite. The conflicts engendered by these processes cannot fail to operate when eating or the refusal to eat becomes a problem in adolescence. The condition is usually seen in girls and in a family situation where the child conflicts with the mother or where the father is dominant. The girl will cleave to the father and may try to usurp the mother's place by various devices such as following the father's occupation. One such patient took up engineering and the evenings were spent working out problems with the father while the mother became a stranger in the house.

Bruch (1966) reviewed 43 patients (37 females and 6 males) and while generally non-eating had a coercive effect on the responsive relative, she divided her patients into 2 main groups.

1. In 30 (26F and 4M) there was an obvious struggle for control and for a sense of identity and effectiveness, with the relentless pursuit of emaciation as a final step. The following features were common to all:

(a) disturbance in body image, the concept reaching delusional proportions;

(b) disturbance in accuracy of perception of stimuli arising in the body;

(c) paralysing sense of ineffectiveness with negativism and defiance.

2. In 13 (11F and 2M) the primary concern was the eating function which was used in various symbolic ways.

She found traditional psychoanalytic treatment ineffective.

Endocrine Factors. These have at times been invoked and there was a phase when Simmond's disease was regarded as the main issue in differential diagnosis, though how this could have arisen remains a mystery, for clinically the two conditions are unmistakable. There are superficial resemblances in the wasting, amenorrhoea and low urinary ketosteroids, but they are otherwise very different, though in the very severe cases of anorexia, secondary physical changes can occur such as liver damage with reversal of the serum proteins, and disturbances of the serum electrolytes. The latter may initiate a confusional state which gives the picture an organic flavour. The usefulness of chlorpromazine in treatment (see below) has stimulated some to regard dysfunction of the hypothalamus as a factor in aetiology, but there is a simpler and more valid explanation.

Clinical Features

The clinical picture of anorexia nervosa as it is generally understood is sufficiently uniform to permit differentiation from other conditions which cause loss of weight. The patient is usually a young, unmarried girl of good or average intelligence, whose behaviour in other respects has hitherto been impeccable. She is usually a conscientious type with a high moral code and a flair for doing good and may be a member of voluntary organizations like the Red Cross or Girl Guides, and may even hold office. The domestic situation frequently reveals a mother who is less dominant than the father, or may even be absent through death or other causes. In the immediate history there may be a factor which appears significant such as anxiety over examinations, loss of friendship or affection, or a variety of situations which are frequently associated with the onset of depression (Chapter 12). There is often a history of fluctuation in weight, the patient putting on and taking off weight with the speed of a prize-fighter and the obesity is no less evidence of the underlying instability than the anorexia.

The home environment is usually very sympathetic but ineffective in dealing with the problem and the mother may very readily be caught up in the patient's ideas on feeding, ministering small sips of a low calorie meat essence to a girl who is dangerously emaciated or even reinforce the patient's refusal to come into hospital. In one such instance, the mother interjected: 'Don't let them talk you into going back to hospital. Remember, it's your life'. The patient died a week later. Refusal of food is invariably accompanied by all forms of subterfuge to get rid of it and these patients can become most expert in disposing of food. Some may even ask for extra helpings and clear their plates so quickly that one wonders where it has gone and well one might, for it has not gone into the patient's stomach. Even if it does, there is no guarantee it will remain there, for during a visit to the toilet it will be vomited. They hide food in the most unusual places, such as biscuit tins, flower pots or wrapped in soiled linen. One patient who continued to lose weight and was in serious physical danger, was as a last resort put on a milk drip, but she still lost weight. Another patient confessed to the sister of the ward that she put her towel on her locker so that the anorexic girl could disconnect the drip when unobserved, and squirt the milk on to the towel, which she then took nonchalantly to the toilet to wring out and replace for the next drenching. Efforts to get the patient to eat are met with protestations of a desire to get better and promises of cooperation but these are never kept and as has been indicated, other patients in the ward are mobilized to support the poor girl who is being made to eat, a situation which the nursery atmosphere of the ward will not tolerate. Weighing may be preceded by a rapid collection of coins which are wrapped in a handkerchief so that a few ounces can appear to have been gained. When they attend as out-patients, there is frequently a display of weight gain, with heavy woollen jumpers, one of which was a caricature of a seaman's jersey and must have been knitted with rope on walking sticks! Parents, especially the mothers, are not only reluctant to accept that subterfuge is being practised but may violently resist such a suggestion for not only are they deceived, but they deceive themselves. The patient has an air of brightness and sparkle and appears energetic, going to work and showing her usual zest and enthusiasm and compensating for any anaemia with lavish applications of make-up. A staff-nurse had reached a weight of 32 kilogrammes and was still on duty with a haemoglobin of 32 per cent.

Some become almost delusional, insisting that they are overweight, and keep displaying their scaphoid abdomen, to prove their argument. Others develop food fads, but these exclude the nutritious varieties and may be mainly for watery fruits such as melons. Any suggestion that they are not cooperating is met with an air of injured innocence or even tears and later protests from the parents.

Physically. There is gross emaciation which may be camouflaged with clothing. A fine lanugo-like hair covers the body and there should of course be no evidence of disease which could produce such marked wasting. *Amenorrhoea* is almost universal. The B.M.R. is reduced considerably, allowing the patient to subsist on a minimum number of calories, and constipation is the rule. The illness can be dangerous and in units where the severe forms are collected, the mortality rate can reach 20 per cent (McCullagh & Tupper, 1940; Nemiah, 1950; Kay, 1953), though with the milder cases the prognosis is more favourable (Venables, 1930; Ross, 1936).

Treatment

In the milder cases this can be psychotherapeutic. Phantasies *re* oral impregnation can be discussed and in certain instances a more analytical approach with efforts to deal with the unresolved oedipal situation may be attempted. These constitute the majority of cases and it is unsound for the psychiatrist practising exclusively in a hospital, or the general physician for that matter, to advise others with more experience of the earlier and less virulent forms of the illness on the treatment of these patients. In hospital, the type of patient admitted has usually demonstrated her capacity to resist the usual forms of psychotherapy and is presenting the doctor with a deteriorating physical state which can prove fatal. It must be regarded with the greatest respect and this attitude must be inculcated in the nursing staff. The patient is an adept at handling mother and mother-substitutes and the ward sister is particularly vulnerable. The doctor is the father-figure and the patient is likely to recreate the home situation. The ward-sister may have an optimistic opinion of her own capacity to deal with the situation and depend on the patient's promises which will of course be broken, but she may take some time to realize this. In the meantime the patient deteriorates and the revelation to the sister that she has been deceived may excite a hostile reaction with all the ingredients of a first-class family row. Even with a knowledge of the psychopathology, at this stage, realism is probably more important and the patient should be carefully supervised in her feeding so that she is given no opportunity to avoid or get rid of her food. The condition is in the same category as that of 'Deliberate Disability' (Hawkings *et al.*, 1956). These authors found anorexia nervosa commonly associated with patients who indulged in 'deliberate disability', such as faking temperatures and self-inflicting injuries, and drew up the table on page 316 to indicate the similarities in the two states and how they differed from hysteria.

The psychopathology of 'deliberate disability' is not entirely understood, but it is probably the result of an over-determined masochism based on the following factors:

1. The actual infliction of the injury is a masochistic act.

2. These patients usually come into teaching hospitals for investigations and these in view of the obscure nature of the disease are usually exhaustive, again catering for the patient's masochism.

3. They run the constant risk of detection and as many are nursing personnel, they are fully aware of this, yet voluntarily expose themselves to this risk.

4. They are essentially conscientious and reliable people, but during this stage, adopt a form of behaviour with its lies and subterfuge, which is the antithesis of their moral code.

5. They nearly all have inadequate sexual outlets and therefore sexual relations cannot be offered as a substitute for their excessive masochistic needs.

Immediate tube-feeding has been advocated by Williams (1958) in a paper which was severely criticized by Sim and Tibbetts (1958) who objected to the author's advocacy of the 'threat of re-intubation' and the following statement of its advantages: 'Because

	Hysteria (a)	Anorexia nervosa (b)	Deliberate disability (c)
Age	Wide distribution	Majority between 16 and 20 (Kay and Leigh (1954)—onset in 70 per cent before age of 26)	Majority between 15 and 25
Sex	Mainly female but not to same extent as (b) and (c)	Mainly female (Kay and Leigh—34 women, 4 men)	Mainly female
Status	Common in both married and single	Much commoner in single women (Kay and Leigh—32 single, 6 married)	Much commoner in single women
Personality	Often inadequate and with a ready tendency to dissociation	More effective than (a). Obsessional traits are common	More effective than (a)
Intelligence	Broad distribution, but frequently found in the dull	Usually average or above	Usually average or above
Psychopathology	Symptoms commonly directed to immediate gain	Not usually directed to immediate gain	Not usually directed to immediate gain
Suggestibility	Common though often ill-sustained	Rare	Rare
Degree of morbidity	Physical suffering or threat to life may be present, but is not common	Gross disfigurement or even threat to life is common	Gross disfigurement or even threat to life is common

little active cooperation is sought the initial resistance is never as great as to normal feeding, and at this stage the more enfeebled the patient the easier it is in any case to overcome'. In their criticism they state: 'The condition may in part be due to an over-determined masochism, and this process frequently tries to excite a corresponding sadism in the doctor. It would be better to preach a resistance to this impulse, than to exhort doctors to indulge it'. Tube-feeding can never be ruled out, but even though it may be easier and more speedy than patiently observing and encouraging the patient to eat, it should be a last resort. Most patients, once they realize that they are being effectively supervised, become more cooperative and it should not be necessary in most instances to start tube-feeding.

Regular weighing at not more than three-day intervals should be carried out, for a week may be too long and provide the shock of a substantial loss of weight. Strict nursing supervision with an attitude of benevolent neutrality is a good policy under which the patient's anxiety gradually settles. Over-optimism is the cardinal error in treatment and the patient should be nursed in bed with cot-sides up, taken to and from the toilet and allowed to sit up only under supervision. The aim should be to get the patient to replace not less than 6 kilos before there is any relaxation and if this is followed by material weight loss, it should be back to bed till the circle has been broken. During this time, the after-care should be organized, the social worker interviewing and helping the mother to adjust to a situation which she had at first refused to believe. Frequent follow-up is essential with re-admission on the slightest sign of relapse. Like alcoholism, one lapse is invariably the precursor of rapid deterioration and it should not be ignored.

Dally and Sargant (1960) described 'a new treatment of anorexia nervosa', which combined the use of large doses of chlorpromazine, starting with 150 mg. per day and going up to as much as 1000 mg. per day, with modified insulin treatment carried to the point of sweating and drowsiness. The patient was confined to bed till the weight was nearly back to normal. They compare this method with others, but not with a method which used effective supervision, and it is likely that their bed regimen was more effective than the drugs. Leucotomy has also been advised, but it would have to be a most malignant form of the disease to merit such a treatment. It is very tempting to try the short-cuts and teach the patient a lesson, but as has already been pointed out, to yield to this temptation is a betrayal of medical practice. Effective supervision with strict bed regime are probably as important as the chlorpromazine but the drug does have a place by weakening the patient's resolve or literally taking the fight out of her and thus rendering her more amenable. These patients can summon almost superhuman reserves to combat those who are trying to save their lives and chlorpromazine is a humane and effective method of controlling this.

HYPERURICAEMIA

As many sufferers from gout have been men of distinction and the disease tends to occur in patients from the higher social classes, there is a tendency to equate high serum levels of uric acid with social and economic success. Brooks and Mueller (1966) tried to relate the personal characteristics of 113 professors at the University of Michigan with their serum uric acid levels. A psychosocial analysis based on drive, achievement, leadership, pushing of self, range of activities, attitude towards pressure, and emphasis on research was translated to a total behaviour score. They found higher than average levels of uric acid were most closely associated with the personal characteristics of drive, achievement, and leadership. Other correlates were obesity, alcohol consumption, and a good appetite so the problem is probably a complex one.

That uric acid levels alone are not responsible is suggested by a rare but interesting condition of hyperuricaemia in children described by Lesch and Nyhan (1964). It consists of choreoathetosis, lip biting and mental retardation. Production of uric acid is enormously increased and serum levels are high.

PSYCHOGENESIS OF ORGANIC DISEASE

The above title goes beyond the principle that psychological factors may play a part in the precipitation, aggravation and amelioration of certain diseases which are notorious for their emotional correlates. It implies that a number of organic diseases, some fatal, may be initiated by psychological factors. There is experimental evidence for such mechanisms in Richter's (1957) work on wild rats. He cut off their whiskers, so depriving them of their customary reassuring sensory import. A frightening experience then caused their hearts to stop in diastole. Engel (1962) has put forward the concept of the *withdrawal-conservation* response to certain stresses where the organism prepares not for fight or flight but for depletion and exhaustion. He points out our lack of understanding of the biochemical, physiological, and particularly the immunological aspects of this affective state and it certainly has not yet had the attention of the now well-recognized stress disorders.

Schmale and Iker (1966) consider that such a mechanism could play a part in the development of cancer and they studied 40 women with apparently normal cervices whose cervical cytology was suspicious and who were submitted to biopsy. An attempt was made to predict the outcome using an interview and psychological testing. According to the presence or absence of the effect of hopelessness or its potential in the 6 months prior to interview, the prediction of 'cancer' or 'no cancer' was made. The results showed that the interviews were 8 out of 14 correct for cancer and 23 out of 26 correct for no cancer according to the pathology report. The psychological tests were unreliable.

Feelings of helplessness and hopelessness are part of the 'giving-up' syndrome and Engel suggests that there may be a number of organic diseases which are traditionally regarded as entirely divorced from psychological influences which could be profitably investigated from this aspect. We may, one day, understand why people are 'scared to death'.

MULTIPLE SCLEROSIS

Mei-Tal *et al.* (1970) working from the premise that organic disease may be an expression of the 'giving-up' syndrome investigated 32 patients with multiple sclerosis to ascertain:

1. The emotional setting in the transitional period between health and the onset of the disease and the nature of the psychological and its intra-psychic meaning.
2. The personality styles and coping devices of these patients and to evaluate the role of the conversion process or reaction.
3. The psychosocial meaning of the illness in terms of primary psychic gratification.

In this first contribution they tackled the first objective and found that in 28 patients the onset of symptoms leading to the diagnosis coincided with a psychologically stressful situation. This was experienced as difficulty in coping and feelings of helplessness and was provoked by the following:

1. Sudden threat to the patient's own life or to the life of an important object.
2. Recent object loss by death.
3. Removal of body parts or iatrogenic changes in body function.
4. Significant events in the family.
5. Family conflicts.
6. Graduation or promotion.

7. Planned or actual marriage or parenthood.

The above list is very similar to that found in well-established psychosomatic disorders such as ulcerative colitis and must therefore bring multiple sclerosis nearer this category of illness. Of even greater importance are the questions being asked, for these, if more widely applied, are likely to lead to a greater understanding of disease in general.

BEHCET'S SYNDROME

Behçet's syndrome (Behçet, 1937) is a complex consisting of recurrent aphthous ulcers of mouth and genitalia, and uveitis. Arthritis, various gastrointestinal disturbances and non-ulcerative dermatologic manifestations, such as erythema nodosum and pyoderma gangrenosum have also been reported in association with the major symptoms. In over 10 per cent of cases lesions of the central nervous system occur.

Epstein *et al.* (1970) reported their psychiatric findings on 10 patients in whom the condition had been firmly diagnosed. All were found to be excessively dependent on spouse or parents, were oversubmissive and communicated hostility indirectly. The self-image was depressive with intermittent compulsiveness and they expressed multiple neurotic symptoms with a poor psychosexual adjustment. In each patient severe relapses were related to life situations where the reality demands could not be tolerated, and this feature applied to all symptons including the neurological. Minor fluctuations did not appear related to emotional states. Most patients came from families where one or more members had a prominent history of psychosomatic illness, and fathers were generally irresponsible, several dying through violence.

The author has seen three cases and his experience would support the above findings. One patient had a neurological disorder very similar to multiple sclerosis and she would relapse when confronted with life situations with which the average person would cope. She also had a severe obsessional neurosis.

CHRONIC PROSTATITIS

Mendlewicz *et al.* (1971) compared a group of patients with chronic prostatitis who did respond to treatment with a group who did not, and made a special study of the influence of emotional or underlying psychopathological factors. The sample included 50 patients, 30 of whom were recalcitrant and 20 responded in the usual time of approximately one month. In the chronic group a greater number were unmarried though the mean age was higher, were maladjusted to the family, and were unsatisfied with their occupation. They were generally anxious, asthenic and depressive, with feelings of guilt and self-reproach concerning their illness which they viewed as punishment and felt they would never recover. They experienced great satisfaction and relief through prostatic massage and some invested it with magic significance. The authors stress that prolongation of prostatic massage placed the patient in a dependent, passive situation and that if there is no improvement it is contraindicated and the patient should be regarded as in need of psychiatric assessment.

BURNS

Anderson *et al.* (1973) investigated the effect of premorbid environmental personality and physical factors on the burn patient's capacity to make a satisfactory emotional adjustment during hospitalization. Subjects were 20 men and 12 women of age range 20–59 years, total burned surface 8–60 per cent. and average stay in hospital was one month. Sixteen (50 per cent) recovered without serious emotional problems and the remainder adjusted poorly, with severe depression, severe regression, violent or nearly unmanageable behaviour, and delirium. Three of the poorly adjusted group died after one month in hospital. The good adjusters had no significant premorbid psychopathology or physical disability, while the 16 maladjusters had a poor premorbid personality with a general tendency toward misfortune. Twelve had previous mental illness: chronic organic brain syndrome (2); schizophrenia (1); depression (1); personality disorders (5); and alcoholism (3). Ten patients, including the 3 who died, became delirious and 7 of these had a burn greater than 30 per cent and some type of psychopathology prior to injury. Though greater severity of burn was a contributing factor in those who adjusted badly, it was less significant than the psychopathology.

HAEMOPHILIA

Haemophilia is a generic term for bleeding disorders due to inherited deficiencies or abnormalities of coagulation factors. The most common forms, Factor VIII or IX deficiency are inherited as X-linked recessive traits and essentially occur only in males, though female carriers transmit the abnormal gene. Deficiencies of all other factors are inherited as autosomal recessive traits.

The adjustment of parents and victims to what is a most dangerous and crippling disease requiring frequent urgent admissions to hospital, has attracted psychiatric evaluation and support (Mattsson *et al.* 1971; Mattsson & Agle, 1972). A more fascinating aspect has been the consideration of psychosomatic factors in the course of the disease itself. The author undertook such a study on patients treated in the Haemophilia Clinic of the Queen Elizabeth Hospital by his colleague, Dr J. Meynell. A large number of these boys took part in strenuous sports and games, involving risk of injury, such as boxing and football. They were quite emphatic that during these activities, although they experienced at times severe trauma, they did not bleed at all or only slightly, yet a gentle knock in a similar area under different circumstances could produce a severe haemorrhage. Mattsson *et al.* (1971) divided their haemophiliacs into good adaptors and poor adaptors, the former showing a consistently high 17-hydroxycorticosteroid level and the latter consistently low levels. Their poorly adapted group seemed to reduce their emotional arousal by intense, at times careless, motor activity with denial of any risks associated with being a haemophiliac. It would be interesting to know whether such activity as in the author's series resulted in relatively little in the way of severe haemorrhage.

RENAL DISORDERS

The development of haemodialysis and renal transplant has focused the attention of psychiatrists on patients, relatives and staff involved. Major contributors in these studies have been De-Nour and Czaczkes (1968) who reported a two-year study of the emotional problems of the medical team in a haemodialysis unit. Main reactions observed were feelings of guilt, possessiveness, over-protectiveness and withdrawal from patients. Demands that patients should do extremely well on the treatment as well as denial that the patients are ill are believed to depend on these emotional reactions which the authors contended were likely to be present in any dialysis unit. In another paper (De-Nour *et al.* 1968) the hypothesis is submitted that the main adaptive difficulty is not solely or mainly the threat of death but the continuation of life, which is dependent on outside factors such as machines, medical teams and society itself.

De-Nour and Czaczkes (1972) reported a study of 43 patients of personality factors which might be the determinants of non-compliance with the medical regimen of chronic haemodialysis.

Adherence to diet was very poor in that 20 abused their diet, and of the 10 patients who died 8 were abusers, the most difficult item being fluid restriction. The most common factor causing diet abuse was low frustration tolerance. The patients claimed they knew and understood the restrictions but they just could not adhere. These patients were also prone to act out their unconscious hostility or striving for independence. Ten patients used denial as a reason for diet abuse, while 21 patients exploited diet abuse for the secondary gain of prolonging their state of invalidism. A few abused the regimen as a result of suicidal tendencies, and some families encouraged abuse out of a conscious or unconscious hostility towards the patient. The authors rightly point out that a study of the mechanisms causing abuse and non-compliance in chronic haemodialysis may have relevance to other medical situations.

De-Nour (1969) studied the psychological significance of urination in his dialysis patients. They displayed extreme distress at the threat to urination prior to dialysis, but once in haemodialysis they ceased to discuss urination and started to deny the loss of function, some claiming they were still passing urine. When nephrectomy was discussed there were objections because life without urination was unimaginable and not quite human. Following nephrectomy some patients still claimed they were passing urine and were in fact demonstrating a phantom phenomenon, one female patient describing her urge to urinate and her bladder distension. The author regarded these phantom phenomena as a massive denial of the loss of urination.

Theories concerning the aggressive aspects of urination, its pleasurable aspects and its connection with pleasurable excitement gain support from the above study.

Quality of Life after Renal Transplant

Beard (1971) found that the quality of life was seriously affected by the transplant operation. Although generally well-adjusted before the event they had to cope with fear of an untimely death, discouragement, apathy and reduced interest and drive. They suffered damage to their self-esteem in that their relationships with significant people were reduced to hostile, dependent attachments. The first three months were full of anxiety and uncertainty concerning survival and possible rejection; six months afterwards ambivalent conflicts between fear and hope, dependence and independence plagued the patient. After nine months there were reliable indications of a return of hope but these depended on support from a concerned and stable member of the family.

PSYCHOSOMATIC RESEARCH AND CASE SELF SELECTION

In conducting research into psychosomatic disorders, workers generally study those patients admitted to hospital with the appropriate complaints and diseases and then draw conclusions regarding pre-morbid personality for the whole population suffering from this disorder. There are fallacies in this approach and these were highlighted by Rawnsley (1968), his main points being:

1. Patients may be selected during the advice-seeking process in terms of personality.
2. Psychological repercussions of the somatic illness and of the process of being recognized and treated may be reflected in the findings from the measures of personality applied to the declared case.
3. Enquiries which go beyond the clinic or surgery and encompass whole populations encounter problems of a different stamp, *e.g.* certain individuals may be more ready than others to disclose to the survey interviewer symptoms of all kinds, whether neurotic in origin or a manifestation of somatic pathology. Associations may therefore be due to the attitudes or the reporting 'set' of the population.
4. In certain psychosomatic disorders, like hypertension, the situation is again different, for the subject is unaware of his somatic pathology.
5. In any enquiry the detection of somatic pathology must be quite independent of decisions by the subjects as to whether or not to seek advice.
6. The measures of somatic pathology must be insulated from the effects of attitudes and of reporting 'set'.

ACCIDENT PRONENESS

It has long been recognized that certain individuals are more prone to accidents than others, though this phenomenon is not a constant one, but a recurring one, coinciding usually with the patient's affective swings, mainly of a depressive nature. The recent popularity of the motor cycle, particularly in the United States has led Nicholi (1970) to describe the *motor cycle syndrome,* which he found in nine college students. The features are:

1. Unusual preoccupation with the motor cycle.
2. A history of accident proneness since childhood.

3. Persistent fear of bodily injury.
4. A distant, conflict-ridden relationship with the father and a strong identification with the mother.
5. Extreme passivity and inability to compete.
6. Poor impulse control.
7. A defective self-image.
8. Fear of and counterphobic involvement with aggressive girls.
9. Impotence and intense homosexual concerns.

According to the author, the motor cycle serves as an emotional prosthesis with the aggressive, active and competitive aspects of the machine serving as an extension of the masculine self, and providing a sense of strength, virility, potency and power. Such features may also be linked with car drivers and small aircraft flyers.

INCREASED MORTALITY AMONG WIDOWERS

Parkes *et al.* (1969) followed up 4486 widowers of 55 years of age and older for a period of 9 years. Of these 213 died during the first 6 months of bereavement, which was 40 per cent above the expected rate for married men of the same age. Thereafter the mortality rate fell gradually to that of married men and remained at about the same level.

The greatest increase in mortality during the first 6 months was due to coronary thrombosis and other arteriosclerotic and degenerative heart disease. There was also a true increase from other diseases, though numbers in individual categories were too small for statistical analysis. In the first 6 months 22·5 per cent were from the same diagnostic group as the wife's death and this may be greater than a chance association.

CHAPTER 7

Alcoholism

The fermenting of fruit or vegetable matter must have been one of the earliest activities of man, and it is not surprising to read in Genesis ix. 20–21, 'And Noah began to be a husbandman, and he planted a vineyard: And he drank of the wine and was drunken . . . .'

The definition of an alcoholic arouses considerable controversy, not least among alcoholics themselves, for denial of the addiction is a conspicuous feature of the condition. The World Health Organization (1951) definition, while not meeting with universal approval, provides a good working statement:

> . . . those excessive drinkers whose dependence upon alcohol has attained such a degree that it shows a noticeable mental disturbance or an interference with their bodily and mental health, their interpersonal relations and their smooth social and economic functioning; or show the prodromal signs of such development.

It is difficult to distinguish the problem from drunkenness, which though at times presenting as a similar social picture, may, in its essence, be entirely different. Drunkenness was a major social evil in Britain till the beginning of the twentieth century and was largely confined to the poorer sections of the community. This was the age of cheap drink and the gin-houses could advertise 'Drunk for a penny; dead drunk for tuppence; clean straw for nothing'. Over-indulgence on certain social occasions has, in many cultures, been regarded as normal practice and though these celebrations may have at times deteriorated to rowdyism and drunken behaviour, those who were 'under the influence' need not have been, and probably in the main were not alcoholics.

INCIDENCE

It has been very difficult to obtain an accurate statement of the incidence of alcoholism, not only because of the formidable demographic problems involved, but because of the moralizing attitude of many people who actively campaign against it, and therefore tend to exaggerate. On the other hand, there are brewers and distillers who emphasize the undoubted social benefits of alcohol and the independent investigator whose purpose is to seek out the truth, finds himself frequently at variance with both groups. That the problem is increasing, both in Britain and America, is now generally accepted, though accurate estimates of the incidence are still awaited. There is no helpful index in terms of mental hospital, general hospital or even prison admissions, especially as not more than 25 per cent have physical complications and furthermore the problem may be so concealed that it need not come to medical notice, while spontaneous remission is not unknown.

Two studies by Green (1965) and Nolan (1965) demonstrated that unrecognized alcoholism was at least as frequent as had been suspected. They examined 1000 and 900 consecutive admissions to an Australian and American general hospital respectively and found that approximately 14 per cent were, in Green's words, physically, mentally or socially incapacitated by prolonged excessive drinking. In Nolan's series the mortality rate of the male alcoholics was 23 per cent compared with 14 per cent for the rest of the men. Alarming though these figures are, Williams and Glatt (1965) pointed out that they may well be an underestimate of the true incidence, for probation officers and health visitors found additional cases who generally did not attend their general practitioners. The question 'How much do you drink?' seldom gave useful information and female patients were particularly reluctant to admit to heavy drinking.

It has been generally estimated that the incidence in the U.S.A. is 4390 per 100,000 of the population, while in England and Wales it is 1100 per 100,000, but these figures at their best can only be vague approximations. They do, however, suggest that alcoholism is a major mental health problem and this view is gradually gaining ground. The time when it was considered a sin and its victims evil-doers has now passed, and responsible medical opinion is in no doubt that it is a sickness requiring medical treatment *before* the physical and grosser mental effects become evident. Its social implications are greater before it becomes an overt clinical problem, and therefore it is not so much a matter for early diagnosis on the part of the doctor, but of an early appeal for help on the part of the alcoholic.

JELLINEK'S FORMULA

Jellinek (1951) produced a formula which attempts to estimate the incidence of alcoholism with physical complications. It is based on these assumptions: (1) if the percentage contribution of alcoholism to a specific cause of death which is not influenced markedly by changes due to treatment, could be estimated and if from reliable autopsy material one could determine: (2) the relative incidence of that disease in the autopsy sample of the alcoholic population; and (3) the relative incidence of death from this cause among the alcoholics in whom this disease was present; then it would be possible to arrive at the number of alcoholics with complications alive in any given year.

The formula is constructed thus:

d=Disease in which the percentage contribution of alcoholism is known and which is a cause of death,

D=Total reported deaths from d,

P=Percentage of deaths from d attributable to alcoholism,

C_1=Percentage of alcoholics with complications suffering from d (autopsy material),

C_2=Percentage of deaths from d among alcoholics with complications who suffered from d,

$K=\frac{C_1 C_2}{100}$ *i.e.* percentage of deaths from d among all alcoholics with complications alive in a given year, irrespective of whether or not they suffered from some degree of d,

A=total number of alcoholics with complications alive in any given year.

Then $A=\frac{PD}{K}$.

K is regarded as 0.694 and constant for all countries, but P is variable for in some countries, cirrhosis of the liver may be due to parasitic infections and chronic malnutrition.

The formula has a very limited value, but it is an attempt to clarify at least one aspect of a notoriously elusive problem. With the help of Gallup surveys, Jellinek estimated the number of social drinkers in the U.S.A. as over 60,000,000 and these are divided into occasional drinkers (less than three times a week) and regular drinkers. Sex incidence varies, but it is usually greater among men, particularly in the regular drinkers. Urban populations of high density have a higher incidence, and regular drinkers concentrate more in the upper income groups. In America, people of Irish descent are reported to have 75 times the incidence of alcoholism than that found in Jews, though the latter constitute a high percentage of occasional drinkers. Various reasons for this difference have been put forward, including the insecure social status of the Jew who has to be careful not to offend the society in which he lives, and a similar reason has been given for the low incidence among the Chinese in the U.S.A. It may be of some relevance that one of the main occupations of Jews in Eastern Europe (and the mass of American Jews stem from there) was in the distilling trade, which also included sale, distribution and tax-collection. Some have attributed the relative abstinence of alcoholism in Jews to socioreligious drinking which tends to keep it in check, but the problem is undoubtedly a complex one and the situation may well change.

The Jellinek formula estimated that there were 350,000 alcoholics in England and Wales, including 86,000 chronic alcoholics with mental and physical complications. A survey conducted by Parr (1957) showed that 35,000 alcoholics were known as such to their general practitioners, though many did not seek treatment from their own doctor–but this figure can now be doubled according to more recent evidence from probation officers and health visitors (Williams, 1965). Offences from drunkenness (which may not be the same as alcoholism) in 1960 totalled 68,109, compared with 47,717, 10 years previously, which would suggest that more people are drinking more, or that more people are being convicted of driving offences.

Edwards *et al.* (1973) highlight the limitations of the Jellinek formula which gave a prevalence in Britain of 11 alcoholics per 1000 aged over 15 years. A survey based on an epidemiological study in a London suburb did more than produce data. It helped (a) to build awareness of the problem; (b) to differentiate syndromes; (c) to uncover cases which were still unknown to agencies; (d) to highlight the special problems of the vagrant; and (e) to make a start on prevention.

The results of the survey indicated that 61.3 men and 7.7 women per 1000 were at risk making the overall total 31.3. This figure, if dealt with by treatment methods, would prove unbearable for the existing resources, thus stressing the importance of prevention.

CLASSIFICATION

Jellinek (1960) has developed his views since he contributed to the report of the WHO Expert Committee on Mental Health in 1951. He now considers that alcoholism is not a specific but a generic term, being a fairly broad genus with a large number of species, the various alcoholisms described in different countries having only two features in common: (*a*) drinking, and (*b*) the damage (to individual and/or society) resulting from it. The genus can therefore be defined only vaguely, but by considering aetiology, elements of the alcoholic process, and the type of damage, Jellinek differentiated five of the most common species of alcoholism, which he called by the first five letters of the Greek alphabet (see below).

From the aetiological aspect, he found psychological vulnerability, which varied from slight psychological deficits to outright neurosis or psychosis, to be present in all species. Physiological vulnerability was a more hypothetical situation, although he conceded that physio-pathological elements may play some part in the addictive process. Socio-cultural elements, such as the attitude towards drinking and drunkenness, and economic elements, among them the price of alcoholic drink, play varying parts in the different species.

He described *the alcoholic process* as being based initially on an acquired increase of tissue tolerance, which was present to some extent in all regular drinkers, but its rapid development to a high degree was probably a major element in the addiction process, and led to physical dependence. Other addictive features supervene such as increasing dosage, withdrawal symptoms and craving. The addictive process can be associated with loss of control with unimpaired ability to abstain after a bout, or with inability to abstain even for 24 hours, but without loss of control over the amounts ingested. *Dependence* in the various species of alcoholism may be psychological or physical, though in certain species there is neither, and the dependence is largely dictated by social custom such as heavy week-end drinking. Nutritional and physical habits may contribute to the deterioration in some species.

Jellinek's classification is strongly linked to the different species reactions. The WHO Expert Committee on Mental Health (1952), in the report of the subcommittee, distinguished two categories of alcoholic: (*a*) 'habitual symptomatic excessive drinkers' or 'non-addictive alcoholics', and (*b*) 'addictive drinkers' or 'alcohol addicts'. In an appendix to the report, Jellinek explained the main differences between these two categories as being *loss of control* over alcoholic intake, which usually comes on after several years of excessive drinking. This loss of control indicated the onset of the third or crucial phase in the development of addiction, resulting in further drinking until the point of intoxication or sickness. At that time

Jellinek stated: '... strictly speaking, the disease conception attaches to the alcohol addicts only, but not to the habitual symptomatic excessive drinkers'.

The WHO Expert Committee on Alcohol and Alcoholism (1955) later added another criterion to that of 'loss of control', namely *'inability to stop drinking'* to help distinguish 'true' alcoholism. Loss of control was found mainly in the predominantly spirit-drinking countries, such as the U.S.A. and Northern Europe, while inability to stop drinking was more characteristic of alcoholism in predominantly wine-drinking countries like France and Italy, the consumer taking his alcohol every day, from morning to night, without necessarily getting drunk. These two patterns could be found in all countries, but the dominant one might overshadow the other and give the impression that it hardly exists.

Although alcoholism is usually regarded as a progressive condition, Jellinek (1952) pointed out that only in the two true addictive species is there progression from social drinking through the various stages, to eventual loss of control and/or inability to abstain. In other species of alcoholism progress was merely in the development of manifestations of chronic alcoholism. Only the first two species, representing addiction in the strict pharmacological sense, did Jellinek regard as diseases and he labelled them:

1. *alpha.* No loss of control, no inability to abstain.
2. *beta.* No evidence of psychological or physical dependence.
3. *gamma.* Physical and psychological dependence *and* loss of control.
4. *delta.* Inability to abstain but controlled.
5. *epsilon.* Dypsomaniac, *i.e.* excessive long binges.

Female Alcoholics

Although the above criteria apply to both sexes, Thompson (1956) has suggested that the female alcoholic, though less numerous, has special features and lists them:

1. From the onset of moderate social drinking it takes less time for them to become alcoholic.
2. They get drunk quicker and more often than men though initially they drink less. Later they become more severe alcoholics.
3. Their psycho-sexual life appears to be more frequently and completely involved.
4. They 'act out' and 'live out' their underlying problems more than men do.
5. They make more suicidal attempts and commit suicide more frequently.
6. When alcoholism is checked they more frequently develop other grave psychopathic states.

7. They develop more frequently chronic paranoid states and Korsakoff psychoses, requiring institutional care.

These differences are explained partly by the vulnerability of the woman to her changing social role though some have unconvincingly implicated the metabolic aspect. The social impact of the female alcoholic is regarded as more traumatic to the family situation and more likely to lead to alcoholism in the offspring (Strecker, 1946).

Schuckit and Winokur (1972) illustrate the dangers of generalizing on female alcoholics. They were able to divide them into two groups: (*a*) good outcome (G.O.), and (*b*) poor outcome (P.O.). The former were generally younger when they came for treatment and were alcoholic for a shorter period. Unlike the P.O. group, few had a history of school dropouts, arrests, divorces and friend and job losses. Most had an affective disorder which had initiated the alcoholism and its treatment. Those with affective disorders did especially well. The present writer would add phobic anxiety to the list for the G.O. group. Many become dependent on alcohol to give them the confidence they normally lack, and once this is successfully treated alcohol is no longer a necessity.

The general social implications of alcoholism in terms of road accidents, crime, venereal disease, broken homes, ruined careers and medical care, are so well known as to hardly need further elaboration. Wortis and Pfeffer (1950) prepared a balance sheet and estimated that one year's loss to the United States in terms of potential wages, crime, accidents, hospital and medical care, and maintenance of drunken persons in local jails, was 765 million dollars.

AETIOLOGY

Aetiology is still speculative, though a number of factors have been implicated.

Cultural and Social

These have already been mentioned in terms of racial and national differences, and the week-end drinkers, but there are others. *Occupation* plays an important part and alcoholism is an occupational hazard among publicans, salesmen and businessmen who conduct their affairs over a bottle of spirits. Even in people of mature age, the social factor as a recent precipitant should not be underestimated, and the author had a patient who became a severe alcoholic after achieving high office which necessitated many formal lunches and dinners. The consequent increase in alcohol consumption, became an uncontrollable addiction. Society's attitude to the person who drinks may also play a part, for it is where there is a strong temperance movement that there is usually heavy drinking with resulting alcoholism. It is popularly believed that the temperance movement is a reaction against heavy drinking, but the alternative should be given careful consideration. As with the psychopath, righteous society has a need for the sinner in its midst and it can manoeuvre a person from moderate drinking into heavy drinking. It is because he is expected to join his would-be reformers or be damned, that he is forced to protest and his natural inclination to drink is reinforced by the mobilization of stronger emotional drives.

Psychological

Diethelm (1955) states that there is not sufficient evidence to support the claim that specific personality types predispose to alcoholism and the view is generally held that it is not a single disease but a symptom associated with a variety of psychiatric illness. Zwerling and Rosenbaum (1959), while not refuting this hypothesis, criticize it. The presence of a variety of clinical psychiatric states in a population of alcoholics, they claim, does not exclude specificity in its psychopathology, as 'a constellation of traits may well be hypothesized to be basic to the aetiology of addictive drinking, and yet be embedded in such a diversity of character structures as to be obscured to eyes focused only upon the most dominant integration of the total personality'. Furthermore, they argue that non-specificity ignores unconscious processes and criticize the other viewpoint in its favour, namely that drinking is a defence mechanism against anxiety and is a feature of a number of clinical states. They claim that 'alcoholism may be found in the setting of any clinical diagnostic state, and that specific drinking episodes may occur in relationship to conflicts at all personality levels, but that the addictive process does develop in a specific character matrix'. With this claim few will quarrel.

(*a*) *Psychoanalytic.* Rado (1933) uses the term 'pharmacothymia' to group all drug addictions whose victims react to frustration with emotional changes of a tense, depressive nature and are very intolerant of pain. Alcohol bolsters up the ego usually at the expense of sexual potency and the addict in the face of crises seeks relief in this auto-erotic activity with consequent discharge of libidinal tension. Knight (1937) considers that the childhood experiences of the alcoholic have encouraged excessive demands for indulgence which are not met in adult life and frustration results in intolerable disappointment and rage. This is followed by intense guilt over his hostile impulses and an intense need for indulgence. Alcohol acts as (1) a pacifier for disappointment and rage, (2) a means of expressing his hostility to spite parents and friends, (3) a form of masochistic degradation, and (4) symbolic gratification of his needs for affection. The alcoholic's mother is over-protective and indulgent and by resort to oral pacifying, establishes the pattern for intense oral needs. Alcoholics have an impulsive character structure with insatiable appetite for affection and approval which if not satisfied results in further frustration and rage, with further impulse to addiction. Lolli (1956) who has an existentialist background regards it as a diseased-food attitude akin to obesity. The alcoholic has longings (conscious and unconscious) for physical warmth, pleasurable skin sensations, maternal coddling, liquid and warm feelings in the stomach, which are equated with those for 'security and reassurance'. He yearns for the experience of undifferentiated pleasure of body and mind and finds it in alcohol, which is a substitute for the mother's milk.

Zwerling and Rosenbaum see in these theories and others 'a consistent thread' showing that the alcoholic is rendered vulnerable to addiction to a fluid which can dispel tension and depression, relieve loneliness, and provide immediate pleasure and mastery of hostile feelings and by its other actions cater for his masochistic needs. They liken the mechanism to that suggested in psychosomatic illness where the disease process originates in a specific conflict pattern but eventually serves as a channel which drains conflicts remote from the original specific patern.

(b) Learning theory and conditioned reflexes. Much of this work stems from animal studies. Masserman *et al.* (1945) showed that cats when exposed to conflicting fear and hunger situations, could be protected from 'experimental neuroses' by alcohol and Masserman and Yum (1946) reported that alcohol disintegrated neurotic patterns in cats who had been rendered incapable of goal-directed behaviour such as food-getting. While 'neurotic' they preferred alcohol to other fluids but when the 'neurosis' disintegrated, the 'addiction' disappeared. Conger (1951) showed that alcohol in albino rats could diminish the avoidance (fear) response and postulated that this operated as a crucial reinforcement in alcoholic addiction. It is, however, a far cry from these animal experiments to the deeper, unconscious motives of man but these experiments have attracted much attention not merely because of their scientific interest, but because of their entertaining analogies.

(*c*) *Psychological tests.* These are mainly of the standard projective and non-projective personality types and are not particularly helpful in defining specific personality traits. This need not be taken as evidence that these do not exist, but rather that the tests are inadequate. Many psychiatrists are sceptical of the reliability of these personality tests and even when they yield a picture which is close to that presented in fact (*i.e.* after a detailed clinical examination) it does not necessarily mean that the tests are reliable, but that the interpretation may be 'inspired'.

Physiological

It must not be supposed that all controversy concerning the aetiology of alcoholism is confined to the psychological. Physiological factors are even more diverse and contradictory. Some of these theories are summarized by Zwerling and Rosenbaum (1959).

(*a*) *Genotrophic.* Genetically determined and partial enzymatic defects render carbohydrates less readily metabolized and alcohol which replaces them as a source of rapidly available energy is preferred. This theory is used to explain the difference in incidence of Irish and Jews.

(*b*) *Adrenal susceptibility.* This is based on the biochemical and clinical similarities between delirium tremens and Addisonian crisis. The plasma potassium and nitrogen are raised, sodium and chloride reduced and hypotension is present, and they both respond to treatment with corticoids. A genetically transmitted susceptibility of the adrenals to alcohol is postulated and this is alleged to be more common in Celts and Scandinavians. Others have stressed that adrenal insufficiency is a complication rather than a cause.

Mendelsohn *et al.* (1971) studied four male alcoholics prior to, during, and after a period of experimentally induced ethanol intoxication. They concluded that ethanol induces an increased secretion of cortisol from the adrenal cortex and that this response is probably mediated via neural-pituitary mechanisms. No evidence of adaptation or exhaustion of cortical response was found during drinking or after alcohol withdrawal. The same authors (Ogata *et al.* 1971) assessed excretion of catecholamines and their metabolites in a similar population, and conclude that their data strongly support the hypothesis that a state of adrenal activation occurs as a consequence of prolonged drinking, and that such activation is associated with enhancement of anxiety and dysphoric state. The highest levels were obtained when the subjects experienced severe withdrawal signs and symptoms.

(c) Dietary defect. A special factor, N_1, when deficient, causes an increase in alcoholic consumption and the condition is aggravated by a thiamine deficiency.

Allergy, thyroid deficiency, 'tensions', and 'resentment' factors in the blood have all been put forward and though animal experiments can show that with certain disturbances of physiology, animals will *prefer* alcohol, an actual *craving* has not been demonstrated.

Action of Alcohol

Intoxication in its various forms is such a common event that to describe them in detail should be unnecessary. A useful way of remembering the different stages is to group them under the letter 'D': (1) *dry and decent*; (2) *delighted and devilish*; (3) *delinquent and disgusting*; (4) *dead drunk.*

It is customary to itemize the effects of alcohol on the various clinical states, but this method is not particularly helpful except to indicate the effect of alcohol in relieving tension whether the patient has neurotic anxiety, is a cyclothyme in a depressed state, or is suffering from a paranoid state and uses alcohol for relief of either internal or external threats to his security. The foregoing psychopathological considerations and a familiarity with the clinical states themselves and particularly the actual patient are more likely to lead to a greater understanding of the patient's problems than any rule of thumb about what happens in certain diseases. The paranoid state with its basis of latent homosexuality has been labelled as particularly vulnerable, but this may be due to the tendency for such patients to frequent bars, the alcoholism being a secondary problem.

Constitution of Alcoholic Beverages

It is important to have some idea of the alcoholic content of the various beverages, for not only should one be able to estimate the quantity the patient is drinking in order to assess the gravity of the problem, but such knowledge may be expected of the doctor when he is asked to appear in court on behalf of his patient.

Beers contain from 3 to 5 per cent of alcohol, together with solids which are mainly starch derivatives. A litre of beer has the nutritive value of 600 calories and these nutritive factors delay the absorption of alcohol, so that it is absorbed more slowly from beer than from whisky diluted to a strength equal to that of beer.

Natural wines contain 8–15 per cent of alcohol, but **fortified wines**, such as port, sherry and vermouth can contain as much as 30 per cent of alcohol. As wines contain organic acids and red wines have large quantities of tannic acid, they may act as laxatives.

Spirits can be divided into pot-still and patent-still spirits. With the former, all the volatile constituents of the liquid which is being distilled passes over into the spirit, while with the latter, the distillate is fractionated and nearly pure ethyl alcohol is obtained. This has then to be coloured and flavoured.

The term '*proof*' has given rise to some difficulty in calculating the alcoholic content of alcoholic drink. It is strictly 'the strength of a mixture of alcohol and water having a specific gravity of 0.91984 and containing 0.495 of its weight or 0.5727 of its volume of absolute alcohol' (*Shorter Oxford English Dictionary*, 1950). The origin of the term is alleged to be of naval significance and was that maximum dilution of alcohol and water which when poured on gunpowder would still cause a flash when ignited. A hydrometer is a more convenient and less hazardous test. For practical purposes proof spirit is equivalent to 50 per cent of absolute alcohol and as most spirituous drinks are under proof (20–30 per cent) this should enable one to estimate the alcohol consumed. It is not generally realized that a pint of good ale is equivalent in alcohol to a double whisky. Other potent sources of alcohol are tonics and tinctures. The former may have quite a strong concentration of alcohol and as they are frequently recommended by physicians for their relatively innocuous contents like phosphates which are alleged to be good for 'nerves', the patient is given the green light for over-indulgence in alcohol and the subsequent risks of addiction. Tonic wines are particularly dangerous, for they are usually reinforced and, particularly in female patients, can readily induce addiction.

Brain Physiology

Himwich (1956) gives the following account: 'As alcohol is rapidly absorbed from the gastro-intestinal tract it is a readily available form of energy, the oxidation of 1 g. producing 7 calories'. Though some is eliminated in the urine and expired air it is mainly destroyed by oxidation, the rate depending on the concentration in the body. The oxidation process consists of five steps: (1) formation of acetaldehyde with the aid of alcohol dehydrogenase, mainly in the liver; (2) production of acetic acid by enzymes, including xanthine oxidase, aldehyde oxidase and aldehyde dehydrogenase, mainly in the liver and to a much lesser extent in the brain; (3) formation of acetyl-C_0A; (4) condensation of acetyl-C_0A with oxalacetic acid to yield citric acid; (5) oxidation of citric acid to CO_2 and H_2O. Blood levels indicative of inebriation should be higher than 150 mg. per cent while those below 50 mg. per cent should rule it out. The intoxicating effects are greater when levels are rising than when falling and this is accentuated in the novice, for in the experienced drinker habituation reduces sensitivity to alcohol.

The cortex is first affected and later the brain stem and medulla; consequently reaction to or anxiety associated with pain is more susceptible than pain threshold. Memory, reasoning and intelligence are more readily involved than reflex time. Its action is mainly depressant and any excitement the patient may show is due to removal of inhibition and it is this aspect which has, wrongfully, earned alcohol the reputation of a stimulant.

In addition there is a physical dependence on alcohol which is shown when it is withdrawn abruptly and delirium tremens and convulsions may result. Pyruvic and lactic acid blood levels are increased and it is the latter substance which combines with sodium bicarbonate to form sodium lactate and CO_2 leading to hyperpnoea. The depressant action is due to (1) interference with cellular respiration through its oxidation, (2) disturbance in energy storage in phosphate bonds which is essential to CNS function, and (3) interference with neuronal transmission through accumulation of acetylcholine in the brain, but this function is not yet proven.

From 5 to 10 per cent of ingested alcohol is excreted and the remainder oxidized to CO_2 and water at a rate of 5–10 ml./hour, each millilitre furnishing about 7 calories. Since its oxidation rate cannot be accelerated in response to energy demands, alcohol cannot serve as an adequate food. The vitamin B complex deficiency which is frequently associated with chronic alcoholism has been explained as a failure to absorb, but it may just as easily be due to a failure of intake because of dietary indiscretion and this view has gained support in the successful treatment of delirium tremens by massive vitamin dosage.

Experimental Work in Man

An important series of experiments has been carried out by Mendelson and Mello (1966) at the Massachusetts General Hospital. They have produced evidence on the drinking habits and the effects of drink on chronic alcoholics and a number of existing hypotheses have been destroyed. They used an operant conditioning paradigm based on the work of Skinner *et al.* (1954) who had used this method to study psychotic behaviour. Reinforcers in such experiments are usually money tokens which can later be exchanged for money. The authors used alcohol in volunteers who were chronic alcoholics and who had not been drinking because of incarceration for some weeks prior to the experiment. All possible control of variables was exercised; the experiments were conducted in a metabolic ward and the operant performance for alcohol was studied in two situations: (1) chained schedules for reinforcement and (2) a driving task in which both tracking accuracy and reaction-time speed determined reinforcement frequency.

The subjects were not restricted and could apply themselves to the tasks to obtain the alcohol reward at any time of the day or night and there was no restriction on the amount of alcohol they could earn. The following consistent features were observed in patterns of drinking and responses to alcohol.

1. An alcoholic subject, allowed to control the rate and quantity of his alcohol intake rapidly ingests enough alcohol to raise his blood level to between 150–300 mg. per 100 ml. All subjects achieved high blood levels in the first 24 hours of the experiment.

2. Despite high blood levels they were only mildly intoxicated, *i.e.* more talkative and boisterous without concomitant slurring of speech, ataxia or gross behaviour disturbances. No subject was incapable of the operant task because of intoxication. Normally levels of 100–200 mg./100 ml. result in mental confusion, gait disturbance and incoordination.

3. Once these high levels were achieved they were maintained, despite mild fluctuations in the daily pattern of work at the operant task and therefore alcohol intake. The authors suggest that this anomaly may be due to an increase in alcohol metabolism in chronic alcoholics and that alcoholics can titrate their intake to produce stable blood values for long periods.

4. As drinking progressed all subjects showed a significant increase in anxiety with feelings of tension, apprehension, mood fluctuations and sleep difficulties. Some worked at the operant task during the night because they could not sleep.

5. As the frequency of application to the task and therefore the drinking increased, there was an increasing degree of ambivalence about prolonging the drinking experience and all reported that their desire to stop drinking markedly increased.

6. None reduced their intake gradually before cessation, even though they all knew that from past experience withdrawal symptoms were likely.

7. The authors suggest that periods of abstinence may be due to lack of companionship and one of the subjects gave that reason for

abrupt cessation. They speculate on the complex social-environmental factors which shelter the alcoholic from loneliness and suggest that Skid Row may fill this need.

These workers have set a pattern of investigation which is not only productive but against which other work will be measured.

PSYCHIATRIC STATES RESULTING FROM ALCOHOLISM

ACUTE PSYCHOSES

Delirium Tremens

This is said never to occur except in the course of severe alcoholism (Thompson, 1956) but this is too sweeping a statement and it can present in post-operative states when there is a verifiable history of abstinence, though barbiturate addiction may play a part in some. There may be a prodromal period of restlessness and general apprehension with poorly defined ideas of reference and the impression is conveyed that the patient is 'simmering' and may 'boil over' any minute. The popular concept that it starts abruptly, occasionally being ushered in by a convulsion, is certainly not universally true and may be less frequent than suggested. As many of these disorders occur in general hsopitals where the patient has been admitted for an operation or after an accident, the focus of the medical and nursing staff may be diverted from the patient's mental state and the prodromal features missed, though on enquiry, the patient may have been reported as sleeping badly or being unduly quiet with little interest in the other patients.

The part played by vitamin depletion has also been debated and though Thompson (1956) states categorically that it is not due to avitaminosis or other nutritional deficiency, many have been indiscreet with their diets, and vitamins certainly play a part in treatment. The condition may occur during a severe bout of drinking or more commonly several days afterwards, or when drinking is abruptly cut off. When the onset is rapid the patient presents the following classical picture.

Physically. The facies is anxious if not terror struck. The limbs are tremulous, myoclonic jerking may be seen and there is extreme restlessness. If the patient is out of bed, he is very unsteady in his gait and may lose his balance and fall with consequent bruising. The pulse is frequently irregular, weak and rapid and the temperature is generally elevated. Peripheral neuritis may be present, but more commonly the tendon reflexes are brisk, the plantars may be extensor and the patient may exhibit epileptiform seizures. Albuminuria is common.

Mentally. He is usually vividly hallucinated and may describe terrifying situations. An army cook seeing a couple of other ranks carrying a tub of water was convinced they were coming to boil him alive and went berserk. Hallucinations are frequently coloured by the patient's occupation or experience but they may be completely bizarre with the classical pink elephants, coloured rodents running all over the place, or of a lilliputian nature. In the latter instances, the patient may be less agitated and present a benign almost bemused attitude at what he considers to be an entertaining experience and this phase can alternate with as well as replace the agitated state. Auditory hallucinations are not so common, but they do occur and are usually of a threatening or persecutory nature. Memory is frequently impaired and there may be disorientation of a type seen in Korsakoff's psychosis, the patient denying he is in a hospital bed and misidentifying the doctor and nursing staff.

The course of the illness is generally self-limiting. In some hard-drinking communities the patient is left to 'work if off' but this is hazardous for it can be a dangerous disease resulting in death, (5–15 per cent) usually because of heart damage. It may therefore be necessary to support the heart action with cardiac glucosides, and in a modern community hospital admission is advisable.

Treatment. This is mainly by tranquillizers and parenteral vitamins. In spite of the reputation chlorpromazine has as a liver poison, the liver of the alcoholic, in contrast to that of the toxaemia of pregnancy, tolerates the drug well, and adequate dosage (100 mg. t.d.s.) either by mouth or parenterally, increasing if necessary to 1000 mg. in 24 hours, usually cuts the attack short, Once tranquillity is achieved it should be reduced to 50 mg. t.d.s. and this dose maintained for several weeks. Concurrently, vitamin therapy should be given: 100 mg. of thiamine supplemented by nicotinic acid (niacin) and riboflavin should suffice. These emergency measures should be supplemented with adequate fluids, dextrose (intravenously), nocturnal sedation such as amylobarbitone 200 mg., and a nourishing diet. Some add a small dose of insulin (20–50 units) to stimulate appetite and cortisone has also been given to mobilize the body reserves of electrolytes. Paraldehyde, 10 ml. intramuscularly, may be helpful in those few cases that are resistant to chlorpromazine.

The author has recently used Haloperidol (Chapter 18) in cases resistant to chlorpromazine. In acute delirium a minimum dose of

3 mg. t.d.s. is necessary and this should be coupled with Benzhexol 2 mg. t.d.s. to combat the striatal effects of the drug. Dosage may have to be increased to 6 mg. t.d.s. and it can be coupled with chlorpromazine. Paraldehyde which was at one time the drug of choice in the treatment of delirium tremens may still be helpful. Dosage is 10 ml. intramuscularly and this can if necessary be repeated in 4 hours.

Withdrawal Symptoms

These can be identical to delirium tremens and call for prophylactic measures which are essentially similar to the treatment of delirium tremens itself. Adequate vitamin supplements, hypnotics and tranquillizers as described above are routine. Various tranquillizers have their protagonists and Moynihan (1965) recommends chlordiazepoxide (Chapter 18) intramuscularly in doses of 100 mg. 2 hourly to a total of 600–800 mg. per day. He claims that such large doses produced no untoward side effects and eliminated the prolonged hypotension occasionally seen with high doses of chlorpromazine. In terms of sleep, blood-pressure, pulse rate, tremors, hallucinations and delirium tremens he found chlordiazepoxide was superior.

Acute Alcoholic Hallucinosis

This develops more slowly and is less common than delirium tremens, the physical signs of which are absent. The only feature may be the auditory hallucinations and illusions occurring in a clear setting, the patient appearing in other respects perfectly reasonable and even capable of doing his job, say as an innkeeper. He may complain to his wife about things going on and she may try and reassure him and point out his illusionary misinterpretations, but these eventually give way to frank auditory and on rarer occasions visual hallucinations, which may result in violent conduct or complaints to the authorities. On examination all the classical features of a paranoid state are evident and there may be an easily identifiable homosexual psychopathology. Hospital admission is essential.

Treatment. This is similar to that for delirium tremens, and because of the underlying paranoid potential, the patient should be kept on more prolonged dosage of chlorpromazine with adequate social support and frequent follow-up. Relapses are common, especially if the patient remains exposed to alcohol.

Pathological Intoxication

Some people are particularly susceptible to alcohol even in small amounts, and may react with sudden violence which is like an epileptic automatism, ending in a deep sleep with complete amnesia for the attack. This correlation with psychomotor epilepsy has been confirmed by EEG studies (Marinacci, 1956), the epileptic showing a seizure pattern without alcoholic stimulus while in pathological intoxication it is induced by a relatively small dose of alcohol, producing a frequency of 6 cycles per second (theta activity) in the temporal regions.

The medical-legal implications are obvious. The taking of alcohol is a wilful act, yet the patient has an innate sensitivity which contributes to irrational behaviour which may be criminal. Is he legally responsible? Frequently the conduct is poorly motivated or motiveless and this helps to answer this question, but on occasions the conduct appears purposive and organized and all one has to go on is the resulting sleepy state with amnesia for the whole event. Obviously no hard and fast line can be drawn and one must consider degrees of responsibility in such cases.

Wernicke's Encephalopathy (Chapter 5)

CHRONIC ALCOHOLIC STATES

Chronic Dementia

Pathology. There are demonstrable organic changes in the brain with frontal lobe atrophy, though the Purkinje cells of the cerebellum, the periventricular grey matter and the basal ganglia may also be involved. The mammillary bodies and hypothalamic nuclei are particularly vulnerable and are alleged to be associated with the confabulatory state and specific memory disturbance of Korsakoff's psychosis (see below).

The nature of this degeneration is not known but vitamin deficiency, particularly of the B complex, is said to be responsible because of its role in the breakdown of glucose to pyruvate, for in vitamin B_1 deficiency very high pyruvate blood levels are found and this is alleged to cause nerve cell dysfunction and eventually destruction. An additional factor is repeated cerebral trauma due to the tendency for alcoholics to fall and damage further a brain already saturated with alcohol.

Symptomatology. Deterioration is usually slow and as many

alcoholics are of superior intelligence and ability, it may take some time for this deterioration to become evident. Psychometry in the early stages has little place, for the tests rarely measure superior intelligence and it is only when there is deterioration below the average that psychological tests are helpful. The patient is unlikely to complain and may cover up his deficiencies by deliberate lying, making excuses for failure, being aggressive or hostile to the critic or resorting to frank projection by blaming others. Those who have worked with him will have noticed a falling off in performance, reduction in his grasp of affairs and a tendency to get someone else to keep things going. *Memory* begins to fail with cruder attempts to conceal it, and habits deteriorate with vulgarity of speech and slovenliness of dress. *Personality* changes ensue, with irritability, loss of social values and neglect of family, complete lack of insight and with no appreciation of the deteriorating process. The patient may be quite euphoric, optimistic and even grandiose which if associated with some neurological signs can be labelled *alcoholic pseudo-paresis.*

Treatment. Proscription of alcohol in any form plus a highly nutritious diet with supplementary vitamins of the B complex is standard treatment, together with the usual safeguards against withdrawal symptoms (see above). This usually means admission to hospital or nursing home. In a few cases a dramatic improvement may result, but usually permanent damage has been done and though the patient continues to abstain, little improvement beyond the initial stage results. It is not, however, possible to say that no further progress will take place till treatment has been effectively given for several months, and the earlier the patient is treated, the better the prognosis.

Chronic Alcoholic Paranoid State

This is really an extension of the acute hallucinosis and is mainly evidence of an underlying paranoid state. With subsequent organic mental deterioration the picture becomes adulterated.

KORSAKOFF'S PSYCHOSIS

This was described in 1887 by the Russian psychiatrist Sergei Korsakoff (1854–1900) and is traditionally regarded as based on chronic alcoholism and presenting with disturbances of orientation, extreme suggestibility, confabulation and polyneuritis. The classical confabulatory state or dysmnesic symptoms have also been described in cases of head injury and brain tumour in the region of the third ventricle and mammillary bodies. As it is not infrequently found following recovery from Wernicke's disease or associated with pellagra, vitamin B deficiency must be regarded as an aetiological factor, though not the only one.

Pathology

The brain may appear normal externally but on section there is occasionally congestion and petechial haemorrhages in the mammillary bodies which is confirmed by histology. In those cases where the mental changes have been associated with brain tumour there was damage also in this region.

Clinical Picture

It may (in the alcoholic cases) follow an attack of delirium tremens but it can also develop slowly. Consciousness is usually unimpaired and the patient appears alert and cooperative. In superficial conversation he (more usually she) can 'get by' and observe the customary niceties of address, but on specific enquiry there may appear *disorientation* for space, time and person. Emotionally, the patient may present with a benign euphoria, rather similar to that of dementia paralytica and obviously lacking in insight as to the gross degree of handicap he presents. It should be emphasized that the *dysmnesic syndrome* which includes disorientation for time and place and confabulation, is a common sequel of head injuries, which frequently present with the 'as if' phenomenon. This is intermediate between the fully developed Korsakoff psychosis and the stage of recovery and is seen more clearly in the post-traumatic state than in the alcoholic variety (Paterson & Zangwill, 1944).

Allen *et al.* (1971) studied eight alcoholics for about three weeks after admission to hospital for prolonged intoxication, and conclude that a recovery of memory as regards free recall does occur during the first two weeks after withdrawal, and that it is primarily short-term memory that is regained. The present writer has had patients with a much longer history of severe alcoholism show improvement in short-term memory for periods up to six months.

Sex incidence. Though alcoholism is commoner in males, Korsakoff's psychosis tends to occur more frequently in females. The usual history is that of a pleasant housewife who may never have indulged heavily in alcohol till she became somewhat depressed and would have a glass of sherry-wine to cheer herself. After two or three years, the alcoholic process is firmly established and up to two bottles per day are consumed. Because sherry is cheap, can usually be provided out of housekeeping, is considered a 'genteel' drink and is not usually associated with alcoholism, the problem is rarely suspected till it reaches an advanced stage, and it is remarkable how imperceptive husbands can be. In addition, there are dietary deficiencies, and the stage is set for a gross Korsakoff psychosis, frequently with a poor prognosis.

Prognosis. In those states associated with alcoholism it is frequently poor. Improvement does occur, but it may not progress to the pre-morbid level and a number remain deteriorated. They present a considerable problem for their families, for they may be completely lacking in insight; they are therefore impervious to psychotherapy and the efforts of Alcoholics Anonymous, and have to be constantly supervised to prevent further deterioration. For many, it means spending the rest of their lives in an institution.

Though in the medical literature Korsakoff (1887) is credited with the first clinical description of the condition, there is an excellent description of the problem of alcoholism including the 'Korsakoff' features in Emil Zola's novel, *L'Assommoir*, which was published in 1878.

MARCHIAFAVA-BIGNAMI DISEASE

This is a rare form of cerebral involvement due to an alleged toxin which is said to be an impurity in some Italian red wine.

Pathology

The pathology is largely confined to the corpus callosum and anterior commissure which show necrosis. Microscopically there is demyelinization which tends to be focal around the blood vessels.

Clinical Picture

Clinically the condition has been described mainly in Italian males. The patient becomes confused, excited and ataxic, with progressive intellectual and emotional deterioration as well as epileptiform seizures. McLardy (1951) reported a case in this country.

METHYLATED SPIRIT DRINKING

This is a problem which is largely, but not exclusively confined to the poor in those countries which have made the price of ethyl alcohol beverages prohibitive. It may be drunk unadulterated, but more frequently it is used to reinforce cheap wines and it can cause toxic confusional states, blindness and even rapid death. Some of the sources of methyl alcohol indicate the desperate or depraved state of its addicts. It has been extracted from metal polish, which has been filtered through corks, and industrial spirit has been added to 'soft' drinks to give it a flavour.

CEREBELLAR CORTICAL DEGENERATION

This was reported in alcoholics nearly 100 years ago by Samuel Wilks (1868) who noted that heavy brandy and absinthe drinkers were liable to become paraplegic though the symptoms could be confined to the legs, 'resembling in character those of locomotor ataxia'. He believed that the volatile oils in these drinks contributed to the poisonous effects of the alcohol. Romano *et al.* (1940) 'resurrected' the condition and since then there have been many cases reported. Victor *et al.* (1959) reported on the pathological findings of 11 cases, and the clinical features of 46 cases. The atrophy, which is sometimes obvious to the naked eye, is almost confined to the vermis and especially the anterior and superior parts (including the lingula, central lobule and culmen) and so may be missed unless the cerebellum is cut in the mid-sagittal plane. All cellular layers are involved, especially the Purkinje cells, and there is cell loss in the olives and occasionally in the dentate nucleus.

Clinically the condition may progress rapidly or slowly and need not be associated with continued drinking; in fact many deteriorate during a period of abstention. Of the cases described by Victor *et al.*, three-quarters were malnourished and the authors considered this an important factor. In addition to the ataxia, there was in half the patients an associated polyneuritis as well as cirrhosis of the liver. Four had Wernicke's encephalopathy, but otherwise psychotic features were not greatly in evidence.

ALCOHOLIC CARDIOMYOPATHY

It has been known for some time that excessive consumption of alcohol may result in myocaridal disease yet this aspect is frequently overlooked. It can also present the psychiatrist with a formidable problem; the author was once asked to admit a patient with delirium tremens, but who also had severe heart involvement, and although one could appreciate the need for psychiatric treatment of the alcoholism, the associated heart condition was an equally important problem. Two types are usually seen: (*a*) cardiac failure with higher than normal output and based on beriberi heart disease which responds to thiamine; and (*b*) the low-output cardiac failure associated with hypertrophy and fibrosis of the myocardium and not or scarcely responding to thiamine. This latter is more commonly seen in America and has been described by Benchimol and Schlesinger (1953) who caution that it may be overlooked as it resembles other forms of cardiomyopathy or coronary artery disease.

Brigden and Robinson (1964) described 50 patients with alcoholic heart disease. They had all drunk heavily and continuously for 10 years or more and with one exception all were male. One-third drank beer only (average 15 pints per day); one-quarter drank spirits (a bottle or more per day); and 17 were in the liquor trade. Nine necropsies showed no evidence of coronary artery disease. They divide their patients into three clinical syndromes:

1. Associated symptoms and signs of beri-beri which respond to aneurin. This is the least common and least serious (5 patients).
2. Patients with a variety of cardiac arrhythmias of which atrial fibrillation and multifocal ventricular beats are the most common.
3. Hypokinetic heart failure, cardiomegaly and E.C.G. evidence of severe myocardial disease.

The E.C.G. had been considered characteristic by Evans (1959) who in 17 patients described variations in the T wave: (*a*) the 'dimple' T; (*b*) the 'cloven' T; and (*c*) the 'spinous' T. Brigden and Robinson are not so definite but do admit that such changes or an arrhythmia with palpitations may draw attention to the alcoholic heart disease before irreparable damage is done.

ALCOHOL AND THE LIVER

Though the relationship between chronic alcoholism and cirrhosis of the liver is generally accepted and is indeed the basis of the Jellinek Formula, there is still no general agreement on the fundamental biochemical disturbance. An excessive accumulation of fat in the liver cells is characteristic of the precirrhotic phase in man and such fatty infiltration can be induced in laboratory animals by giving them alcohol. Isselbacher and Greenberger (1964) discuss five possible biochemical disturbances which could lead to increased fat within the liver cells. These are:

1. Increased mobilization of fatty acids from the trigylcerides of

the adipose tissues could lead to their increased reformation to triglycerides within the liver. Support for this hypothesis is derived from the high correlation in the alcoholic fatty liver between fat content and the level of linoleic acid, an essential unsaturated fatty acid which is not synthesized in the liver but is derived from the diet.

2. Alcohol increases the synthesis of fatty acids by liver cells both in vivo and in vitro. This is not a major factor however for the same biochemical action can be imitated by glucose without a corresponding increase in intrahepatic fat. Moreover fatty acids synthesized in vitro by liver slices in the presence of alcohol are almost entirely saturated whereas in alcoholism it is unsaturated, indicating that mobilization is more important than local production.

3. Inhibition of intracellular oxidation of fat by alcohol has been shown in vitro, but other substances can be even more inhibitory without the end-result of a fatty liver.

4. Alcohol leads to the preferential incorporation of intrahepatic fatty acids into triglycerides rather than into phospolipids and though the mechanism is not known, it is probably an important factor in the production of fatty liver.

5. The normal release of trigylceride by the liver into the plasma in the form of lipoprotein could be impaired either as a result of diminished formation of the necessary protein or by interfering with its passage through the cell membrane.

In addition to theories of hepatotoxicity, diet is still an important factor and in experimental production of hepatic necrosis in animals the restrictions in diet such as choline and other sources of labile methyl groups, which are necessary to prevent abnormal accumulations of fat within the liver cells, are very close to the diet of the chronic alcoholic. Protein malnutrition which is common in chronic alcoholism may also increase the sensitivity of the liver to hepatoxic agents.

Powell and Klatskin (1968) studied 283 histologically proven cases of alcoholic liver cirrhosis between 1951-1963. Of 93 patients who gave up drinking 64 per cent survived 5 years; of 185 who did not give up drinking 40 per cent survived 5 years. Even severe manifestations of cirrhosis, such as ascites, jaundice or haematemesis carried a 60 per cent survival rate if the patient stopped drinking.

TREATMENT

Medical treatment is indicated where excessive drinking:

(1) is symptomatic of a primary mental or physical illness;

(2) is complicated by evident toxic effects on the brain and body;
(3) follows the special pattern of addictive alcoholism;
(4) is otherwise characterized by dependence on alcohol to such a degree that the diagnosis of chronic alcoholism is medically justified.

These criteria for treatment imply a thorough physical and mental assessment, the latter to include the social background. Treatment may in some instances be confined to the underlying neurotic or psychotic process, but generally, the addictive process requires attention in its own right.

It is advisable, in order to overcome the uncontrolled drinking or the inability to stop, to get the patient initially into hospital. This may prove difficult for the alcoholic presents two features which are almost diagnostic, but unfortunately militate against successful treatment. These are his stubborness and his undue optimism. If there is accommodation available in a unit which gives some degree of privacy, it is usually not too difficult to persuade the patient to come in, and though propaganda may help the patient to accept alternatives, it would be better if the more favoured type of accommodation were more readily available for those that desire it.

(a) **Admission to hospital** has its hazards, for alcohol withdrawal can be a most distressing experience for the patient and the precipitation of delirium tremens is a distinct possibility. At one time, small doses of alcohol were prescribed, but this should not be necessary, provided that adequate sedation (amylobarbitone sodium, 200 mg./nocte), tranquillizers (chlorpromazine, 50 mg. t.d.s.) and vitamins are prescribed. It is helpful to order a further 100 mg. of chlorpromazine as an emergency dose should it be required, as speedy administration of adequate tranquillizers can avert a difficult, if not dangerous situation.

(b) **Correction of the deficiency state** has been mentioned above and consists of vitamin B complex capsules. Cade (1972) stresses the importance of thiamine in massive dosage and illustrates his claim by citing the admission and mortality figures in one hospital over three quinquennia. The routine use of prompt, massive intravenous thiamine caused the disappearance of alcoholism as a cause of death which was probably due to a beri-beri or thiamine deficiency heart.

The procedure consists of administering on admission a multi-B solution containing:

Thiamine	250 mg.
Riboflavin	30 mg.
Nicotinamide	160 mg.
Pyridoxine	50 mg.

With very sick patients this dose may be repeated once or twice in the first 24 hours. It should be supplemented with rehydration and sedation (chlorpromazine, intramuscularly 100–200 mg. every 4–6 hours). For night sedation he recommends diazepam and chlordiazepoxide.

(c) **Psychotherapy.** During the acute phase or even in the early stages of withdrawal, attempts at psychotherapy are unlikely to help. When the patient is settled, private interviews should be arranged and these should be conducted with a view to appraising and dealing with the psychological factors in the background. If a severe depression, schizophrenia or a paranoid state should declare itself, this will exclude a more analytical approach and suggest other measures more appropriate for the treatment of these conditions. Although individual psychotherapy will follow the approach normally favoured by the therapist, there are certain aspects of the alcoholic personality which should be taken into consideration. Many have strong attachments to their mothers with consequent immaturity which may determine a latent homosexuality. These and other family and individual problems may be very apparent to the therapist, but it should be realized that the patient is not consciously aware of them and that in fact his alcoholism and life style has been developed to cope with his unconscious conflicts over these same problems. Interpretation should therefore be cautious.

It should be superfluous to say that in the treatment of alcoholism, there should be no moralizing by the psychiatrist. Yet when in his alcoholic state, the patient may behave in such a reprehensible way that his family and even his personal doctor will bring pressure on the psychiatrist to 'discipline' the patient. It can be very difficult to indicate to others that he does not drink because he likes it but to try and resolve his personal problems. The author has even been approached to supply information about a patient by the wife's solicitor, as she was petitioning for divorce, and was considered insensitive to her difficulty for not complying.

It is important not to be dismayed by failure or relapse on the patient's part, as it is not uncommon for a patient to fail to make the grade after two or three attempts at treatment but to succeed eventually. As well as those who go under, there are a not insignificant number who recover in spite of all the predictions.

A prolonged association between patient and doctor, whether it is based on a deep analysis or not, is most helpful and the doctor should try and be the patient's advocate with his family. While many wives are extremely loyal and give their alcoholic husbands tremendous support, others are very reminiscent of the schizophrenic parent—well-intentioned but ineffective, and they can prove most trying on interview. The author, who makes constant use of A.A., has had to warn the secretary on occasions to be very careful in the choice of members whom he may send to a particular patient, as the wife was so formidable a problem that she could induce a relapse in the less secure. As a general rule it can be said that the more helpful the spouse, the better the prognosis.

(d) **Group therapy** is being increasingly advised for the treatment of alcoholism. This may be because of the relative success of Alcoholics Anonymous (see below), or merely an extension of group techniques into a variety of fields. It is proving to be a valuable method because it can be continued for long periods on an out-patient basis and the limited interpretation required, with the undoubted need the alcoholic has for social support, augur well for its future. Where the scatter of psychiatric, social and physical problems is so great, much care should be exercised in the composition of the group. The latent homosexuality of many alcoholics will also require consideration, for the group situation may heighten guilt and precipitate relapse.

(e) **Alcoholics Anonymous (A.A.).** It is not the first time that a lay organization has made a major contribution to what should have been a medical responsibility. It was founded in 1935 by R.H. Smith and W. William, two alcoholics who found they could help each other and decided that this service should be extended to other alcoholics. William (1949) describes the aims and work of the organization which has a programme largely influenced by a religious ethic, though it is so defined that all denominations can freely join, and they do. Its memberships includes Roman Catholics, Jews, Protestants, Mohammedans, Hindus and others. Twelve steps are laid down for the members to follow and these are:

1. We admitted we were powerless over alcohol—that our lives had become unmanageable.
2. Came to believe that a Power greater than ourselves could restore us to sanity.
3. Made a decision to turn our will and our lives over to the care of God *as we understood Him.*
4. Made a searching and fearless moral inventory of ourselves.
5. Admitted to God, to ourselves and to another human being the exact nature of our wrongs.
6. Were entirely ready to have God remove all these defects of character.
7. Humbly asked Him to remove our shortcomings.
8. Made a list of all persons we had harmed, and became willing to make amends to them all.
9. Made direct amends to such people wherever possible, except when to do so would injure them or others.

10. Continued to take personal inventory and when we were wrong promptly admitted it.

11. Sought through prayer and meditation to improve our conscious contact with God *as we understood Him*, praying only for knowledge of His will for us and the power to carry that out.

12. Having had a spiritual awakening as the result of these steps, we tried to carry this message to alcoholics, and to practise these principles in all our affairs.

Meetings are held frequently and there is a sort of freemasonry about them in that members from one branch may pay 'fraternal' calls on another. Membership is open to all alcoholics who have a genuine desire to abstain. Personal case histories are related and the group tries to support those in need. Many attempts have been made to analyse the sources of the organization's strength and these have been put down to the strong spiritual support, the group morality, and the change in role from being a social outcast to becoming a useful and valued member of society. The author has been most struck with two aspects, one a very practical one and the other probably operating at an unconscious level.

The first is *the daily dedication* not to drink for 24 hours. This is realistic and only an alcoholic could have devised such a simple and effective resolution. In the past, many alcoholics had 'taken the pledge' never to drink again, but 'never' is like eternity, while 24 hours is something tangible which can be overcome. The other is the *anonymity* of the members. Though they call each other by their forenames, it is certain that many are known to each other in everyday life, and the anonymity is meant to conceal identity not from each other, but from society. This is superficially explained as being due to the stigma society reserves for the alcoholic and anonymity is therefore designed to protect them from it. In the early days of A.A. this may have been valid, but now society does not stigmatize members of A.A.; it envies them. Anonymity is therefore a means of concealing from society the identity of people who put in a tremendous amount of voluntary work and who will never gain recognition for it. In all societies there are some who do good deeds and hold office, but they are recognized and even rewarded. A member of A.A. can get up at all hours of the night to rescue a fellow member, he can spend all of his spare time working for the cause, his home can become an office, and his place of business a meeting house, but nobody will know and be able to accord him the usual respect which society reserves for its public-spirited citizens. The author has rung up the secretary of the local A.A. on a Sunday morning asking him to see a patient in hospital. He will have visited the hospital before the morning round is completed and wait to give his valuable advice. It is on such dedication that the success of A.A. has grown. This twelfth step is the one which attracts people of good intelligence and good morale and ensures that A.A. will not lack competent leaders.

Compulsion in the Treatment of Alcoholism

There has been considerable agitation to use statutory powers to ensure that the alcoholic is not allowed to roam at large endangering himself and society while refusing to co-operate in his treatment. There has been strong opposition to the introduction of further legislation to deal with the alcoholic and while one can understand the exasperation of those who have to deal with these people and feel unable to do so, there is much to be said for not extending the doctor's powers. There would be more force to the argument if successful treatment were the likely outcome, but the evidence to date is that under such conditions this is not so. Improving treatment facilities where alcoholics can be sent under present legislation would appear to be a more rational solution.

Loss of Control in Alcoholics

It is part of the creed of members of A.A. that as soon as any small amount of alcohol is taken the quantity cannot be limited and this view has been repeated by objective workers including Jellinek. It has been challenged, not only, as one would expect, by alcoholics but by other workers, one of whom (Merry, 1966) experimented with 'loss of control' alcoholics. He pointed out that a number of them who are on disulfiram (see below) frequently stop taking their tablets for several days prior to a severe bout of drinking, indicating that the loss of control preceded the first drink. His experiments did not support the 'loss of control' hypothesis. Though some alcoholics for a short time are able to withstand the temptations of uncontrolled drinking, the vast majority, if not all, do in fact relapse if they continue. The argument is academic for with the alcoholic, as with most people, the issue becomes one of incorrigible optimism, 'if I can drink one, why not two' and as Morgan (1966) points out this 'can lead to an arithmetical or geometrical progression which is not in keeping with the alcoholic's wish to be able to drink as other men do'. It cannot be emphasized too strongly that total abstinence is the only guarantee against relapse.

Rehabilitation of the Alcoholic

After-care can be the rock on which treatment may founder. The patient when looking for a job may have to invent some story to explain his lack of references or unstamped insurance card, for honesty is seldom successful. The social status of the alcoholic may also determine his chances: a labourer can get another job as easily as picking up a shovel, but a professional man may find it extremely difficult to obtain a re-entry. In London, a voluntary body known as the Helping Hand Organization is concerned with setting up a special alcoholics employment bureau.

Alcoholism and Driving

There is a difference between a drunken driver and alcoholism and driving. In the former instances, the problem is very largely one of blood alcohol impairing driving efficiency together with a variety of social and psychiatric factors which have led to the irresponsible behaviour. In the latter instance, the problem is that of the alcoholic and his driving. Glatt (1964) found that, on their own admission, 80 per cent of chronic alcoholic car drivers have driven, more or less regularly, shortly after heavy drinking. The ratio of alcoholics among convicted drunken drivers has been estimated in Canada as 28 per cent (Schmidt *et al.*, 1962) and in Sweden as 35–48 per cent (Andreasson, 1962) while in Great Britain, Glatt estimates it at about 10 per cent.

The argument that alcoholics have a greater tolerance to alcohol than the average drinker is not a valid defence, for they usually exceed their tolerance, while the moderate drinker rarely reaches his critical level. The British Medical Association has accepted a blood alcohol level of 50 mg. per 100 ml. as 'entirely consistent with the safety of other road users'. Alcoholic pedestrians are also at greater risk and blood alcohol levels in excess of 200 mg. per 100 ml. are very common in pedestrians who are fatally injured in traffic accidents. The doctor who attends an alcoholic must therefore, on the considerable evidence available, advise him not to drive while he is drinking.

Disulfiram Therapy (Antabuse)

Hald and Jacobsen (1948) had been working in the biological laboratories of Medicinalco, Copenhagen, with diethylthiuram disulphide [bis (diethyl thiocarbanyl disulphide)]—formula $(C_2H_5)_2$

$NC(S){-}S.S.C(S)N(C_2H_5)_2$. They found that people who had ingested 0·5–1·5 g. (which was otherwise an inert dose) developed characteristic symptoms when they subsequently drank even small amounts of alcohol.

These symptoms include a feeling of heat in the face, followed by an intense flushing, located principally in the face but spreading in some cases to the neck and upper part of the chest and arms or even to the abdomen. A constant effect is dilatation of the scleral vessels, making the person look 'bull-eyed'. These are followed a little later by palpitations, and sometimes slight dyspnoea. After larger doses of alcohol nausea and vomiting often develop. If nausea is intense, blushing gives way to pallor. These symptoms, which are usually accompanied by headache, are very unpleasant. They disappear, however, within a few hours, generally leaving the person rather sleepy. After the alcohol has been oxidized, the person feels completely well again, and all complaints are usually relieved by a short nap.

The authors considered that disulfiram interfered with the excretion of acetaldehyde, an intermediary product in the oxidation of ethyl alcohol, which accumulates and produces the toxic symptoms. A patient who takes alcohol within 12 hours of taking disulfiram experiences the above reaction in 5–15 minutes, with nausea and vomiting in 30–60 minutes.

Method. The treatment should be given in hospital, to ensure that the patient has had no alcohol for three days. He is then given 0·5 g. daily for three days, and on the third day he has his 'test dose' of alcohol, which should be the type of drink the patient usually favours. An ounce of this (usually gin or whisky) is then given and the reaction develops in 5–15 minutes. Pulse rate is increased, and the blood pressure falls, sometimes to a very low reading, but the reaction can be aborted by intravenous ascorbic acid (4 ml., each containing 250 mg.). If the reaction is too feeble a bigger dose is required. Thereafter the patient takes the drug (0·5 g.) daily for months or years, in order to help him overcome his alcoholism. As with most treatments, motivation towards cure on behalf of the patient is essential, for if he is not so inclined, he can stop taking the disulfiram and in several days the 'protection' wears off.

Undesirable side-effects are acute psychotic reactions of a manic or schizophrenic nature. Disulfiram therapy should also be avoided in patients with cardiovascular disease as myocardial infarction may occur. It is also suggested that severe liver disease is a contra-indication as well as diabetes and diseases of kidneys and thyroid. It should, of course, be avoided in pregnancy.

Ferguson (1956) introduced citrated calcium carbimide which is reputed to give a milder reaction with alcohol, but as the uncontrolled drinker may indulge even with disulfiram, it is unlikely that a milder agent would be adequate to reinforce his resolve.

Other Aversion Therapies

Emetine was at one time the most popular of the aversion therapies, its rationale depending on what was considered to be a conditioned reflex. The patient is given graduated injections of emetine hydrochloride which is a strong emetic and to enhance its unpleasant effects, it is followed by an injection of pilocarpine and ephedrine to promote sweating. A detailed description of the procedure is given by Sargant and Slater (1954) who recommend that when profuse perspiration, salivation and tachycardia have been achieved, the first test dose of 1 oz. of neat whisky is given. Another ounce is given when nausea develops a few minutes later, and then a third and fourth ounce before vomiting commences. 'They should, however, be given with due ceremony, and the patient should be made, to his increasing disgust as the treatment proceeds, to sniff at and smell the drink before swallowing it'. Delayed vomiting is overcome by tickling the back of the throat and while the patient is drinking his whisky some practitioners use alcoholic's jargon such as: 'Have the other half!', 'Knock this back!', 'Here's one for the road!'. When vomiting starts strong suggestions are given that drink is poison; that the first drink is the road to relapse; and a frightening picture is conjured up. This is alleged to eradicate the pleasurable feelings the alcoholic had previously associated with drink. These measures go on for about six days, after which the patient is considered to be deconditioned.

The treatment is not without danger and severe degrees of collapse requiring urgent resuscitation can occur. It is a manoeuvre which could only be carried out with conviction by those with very little feeling for the deeper psychological problems involved, and who can act out the part of the therapist which is that of 'a friendly but fervent and dogmatic preacher'. If it were a very successful form of treatment there would be much to commend it, in spite of the rather cruel technique, for it has a lot of 'it hurts me more than it hurts you' about it. But it has not been very successful, and unless one can find a masochistic subject it is unlikely to be, for the mode of action rarely meets strict Pavlovian criteria and the most one can say is that, as with other aversion therapies, the Pavlovian analogy has only a superficial application.

Apomorphine treatment is used more frequently than emetine, but not as often as disulfiram. Like emetine, it depends on its capacity to make the patient feel sick and vomit and alcohol is given at the time. Dent (1954) has used the treatment on an out-patient basis without the test dose of alcohol.

Some patients prefer these types of treatment, if only for the reason that they have a good excuse for not drinking. This is particularly so with disulfiram (Antabuse), for alcoholics are constantly exposed to pressure to have a drink and this is easier to resist if they have been taking their tablets regularly. Some alcoholics have named the tablets 'anti-booze'. It must, however, depend on the patient's willingness to cooperate.

Other forms of treatment that have been and are still being tried are electronarcosis, E.C.T., massive vitamin therapy and hallucinogenic drugs; for delirium tremens, cortisone and ACTH have their advocates. E.C.T. has been recommended by some as a useful method of clearing up a delirium tremens which is resistant to chlorpromazine.

The Spouse

The husband or wife is an important factor in the treatment of the alcoholic. Some may not only adversely affect the outcome but may have also played a part in its origin. The author when briefing A.A. in such cases had advised, that as policemen patrol a dangerous area in pairs, so it would be advisable to do likewise in such instances, for the spouse could be so frustrating and irritating that the first thing the unfortunate visitor would want on getting away would be a drink. The following statement holds: 'Good spouse; good prognosis; bad spouse or no spouse, poor prognosis'.

Results of Treatment

These are difficult to assess and where one can, relatively few meet the criteria for 'successful arrest' laid down by the WHO Report (1951) which is for a minimum of two years' total abstinence. Davies *et al.* (1956) reported on 50 patients treated at the Maudsley Hospital and only 18 per cent remained totally abstinent after two years. Another 18 per cent were abstinent for a greater part of this time and 42 per cent maintained social efficiency despite light or heavy drinking. Glatt (1959) reported on 94 patients treated at Warlingham Park Hospital and one-third did not relapse, one-third relapsed (usually within six months), but could be rated improved, and one-third were therapeutic failures. Wallerstein (1956) carried out a comparative trial on 178 in-patients and 53 per cent were improved with disulfiram, 30 per cent with hypnotherapy, 26 per cent with group therapy, and 24 per cent with conditioned-reflex therapy.

The prognosis of treated cases is more favourable in males than in females; in older than in younger men; in the married than in the single; and in those whose original personalities were not psychopathic. As with other forms of psychiatric treatment, results depend on factors apart from the so-called specific measures employed. These are the enthusiasm of the therapist, convenient access to the clinic, facilities for follow-up, the cooperation of the general practitioner and the presence and activity of a branch of A.A. on the patient's doorstep, and this too may vary in its efficacy. Special centres for the treatment of alcoholism have been advocated, but it is difficult to envisage what more they could contribute than a well-staffed psychiatric service, based on a general hospital and sited reasonably close to the patient's domicile. Special centres tend to be isolated from the majority of the clientele who may require them, and with alcoholics this has many disadvantages. The problem is so bound up with the general psychiatric services that to separate it, deprives both patients and staff of valuable contacts. Although organic problems in alcoholism account for a relatively small percentage (8–15 per cent) of all alcoholics, and a relatively late manifestation at that, they do account for a larger percentage of those who require in-patient treatment and the resources of the general hospital should be readily available.

Suicide in Alcoholics

Kessel and Grossman (1961) reported on a mean five and a half years follow-up of 131 consecutive voluntary patients treated at the Maudsley Hospital for alcohol addiction, and of a second series of 87 patients admitted to St. Pancras Hospital, London. In the first group, nine men (8 per cent) and in the second group four men (7 per cent) committed suicide, which was 75 to 85 times the expected figure for males of their ages in Greater London. Glatt (1962), commenting on these figures, emphasizes that though there were no female suicides quoted, he himself could recall six cases, and he also stressed the difficulty of distinguishing death by accident from death by suicide, and that in some alcoholics their severe alcoholism is a form of chronic suicide. These valid comments would support Kessel and Grossman's concern with 'the very high risk of suicide for the alcoholic'.

CHAPTER 8

Drug Addiction and the Hallucinogens

The WHO Expert Committee on Drug Dependence (1969) defined drug dependence as:

> A state, psychic and sometimes also physical, resulting from the interaction between a living organism and a drug, characterized by behavioural and other responses that always include a compulsion to take the drug on a continuous or periodic basis in order to experience its psychic effect and sometimes to avoid the discomfort of its absence. Tolerance may or may not be present. A person may be dependent on more than one drug.

The report defines a variety of addictions such as the morphine, barbiturate, alcohol, amphetamine, cocaine, cannabis and hallucinogen types.

Although this definition and its rider is the latest of such definitions, it is not entirely satisfactory as a clinical differentiator, for it may be just as important to know of the psychiatric condition which has led to the addiction as the name of the drug used. Many addicts (or should they be called dependents?) use the lot and a complete list would still tell the clinician very little apart from supplying information which may be useful to a Narcotics Bureau, though dosage would be no less important.

The drugs used by addicts vary considerably and depend on geographical, economic and cultural factors. In some countries it is alcohol, in others it is marihuana or hashish, and in certain social groups it may be heroin. The list is a long one and includes all the opiates, pethidine, barbiturates and amphetamine, as well as tranquillizers. In some cultures addiction is not considered antisocial, *e.g.* opium among the Chinese is not regarded as a socially and morally degrading habit, and similarly marihuana or hashish in the Caribbean and in India does not carry the social and legal censure it does in this country. It is therefore important to gauge the cultural background of the patient before making pronouncements about weak or immature personalities. It is, however, true that in our Western culture, drug addicts, like alcoholics, frequently have personality problems and their addiction may be symptomatic of them.

DRUG TAKING AND DRUG ADDICTION

Until recently, in the United Kingdom, drug taking was generally confined to drug addicts. This is no longer so. From time immemorial man has used plants and their products to give himself pleasure or relieve pain and suffering. Brewing infusions, chewing the bark and leaves of trees, and fermenting fruit and cereals are still popular in the habits of tea, coffee and cocoa-drinking, indulgence in alcohol and the use of tobacco. Young people in their zest for new experiences are less cautious in their experiments and over the years have been conspicuous by their enthusiasm for agents which adults have learned to treat with reserve. In the eighteenth century, it was the laudanum bucket of Lamb, de Quincey and Coleridge, and in the nineteenth century, it was the ether parties. In the twentieth century we have seen 'reefers' (cannabis), 'purple hearts' (dexedrine), mescaline, lysergic and many others. While a few become addicted, most overcome the craze and go on to lead reasonably abstinent lives.

Drug-taking in the young has assumed epidemic proportions. The reasons listed by Dumont (1972) are: (1) Pleasure; (2) Impoverishment of their environment; (3) Use of drugs by adults; (4) Commercials and advertisements in the mass media; (5) Propaganda for sleep; (6) Propaganda against obesity; (7) Doctors' prescribing habits. The author concludes:

> Shall we ever know the full costs of our mania for prescribing medicines? A world of antibiotic-resistant infections and amphetamine and barbiturate dependency, a whole generation incapable of coping with anxiety and grief, and an ambience of pill-taking that induces our children to believe that there is a chemical for everything . . .

Apart from the general tendency to take drugs, some young people are organized into protest groups which regard drug-taking as a condition for membership. With so many taking drugs, there must be a number whose personalities make them vulnerable to addiction.

Psychopathology

This has already been referred to in Chapter 7 where the oral dependence was stressed. Wikler (1952), who had conducted experimental work on humans and animals, concluded that drug addiction caters for the primary needs of the addict, giving him satisfaction in his desire for the alleviation of hunger, his sex urges and his aggression and his need for the removal of anxiety and pain. Wikler considers that these effects distinguish drug addiction from alcoholic addiction, in that the latter releases the inhibitions and the alcoholic becomes belligerent, exhibitionistic and grandiose. While this may be true in considering some drugs of addiction, it does not apply to the amphetamine group, where aggressive paranoid behaviour may result, or in some alcoholics who quietly indulge and do not act offensively.

GENERAL PRINCIPLES

In all cases of addiction certain principles have come to be accepted. These are as follows.

Tolerance

This is said to occur when the effect of the drug tends to wear off with use and this has been amply illustrated in the case of barbiturates where doses of 1·6 g./day were required to give the patient the confidence he craved (Chapter 18). It may mean that the drug begins to acquire an entirely different effect to that when it was originally prescribed. For example with barbiturate, what was meant to be a mild sedative or hypnotic, becomes a confidence pill, and although, experimentally, Isbell *et al.* (1950) regarded 600 mg./day as the critical addiction dose for barbiturates, it could also be defined as that dose where the drug no longer acted as a hypnotic but developed a euphoriant effect. It is not only the patient who may develop tolerance, but also the prescribing doctor. It is all too easy. A troublesome patient is given a drug which relieves her. She is basically a nice person who doesn't want to take up a lot of the doctor's time; all she wants is a presciption, and it did her so much good, more than any other doctor had done for her. She comes one day and says she took an extra tablet as she was very distressed and didn't want to trouble him. Did she do wrong? Relieved that at least one patient considers him, he gives her his blessing. The dose increases and more drugs are requested. She may bring her husband along this time to testify to her progress on the drug and she is given a larger supply. During the holiday the locum takes over, and though he may query the large doses he is asked to prescribe, he sees from previous prescriptions that she has had almost as much before and he does not want to upset a patient. The doctor returns and is regaled with tales of how distressed she had been in his absence and the difficulty she had in persuading the locum to prescribe. The next time he is to go on holiday, she asks for a supply to cover his total absence and he reckons that he will have to prescribe over 200 large capsules for four weeks, and it is then (if then), that he reaches for his telephone and makes an appointment for her to see a psychiatrist.

Tolerance can be established very rapidly and it is suprising how a patient with phobic anxiety who has not improved on tranquillizers will immediately report favourably on amylobarbitone soluble. It is a disturbing thought that when a drug works dramatically as in phobic anxiety, and examples are barbiturates and alcohol, there is a real risk of addiciton.

Theories to explain tolerance are still unhelpful, for they are only analogies, like 'cellular tolerance' and 'hyperirritability' of the cells of the central nervous system which require larger and larger doses to keep them down. As in this problem one person's guess is as good as another, the author would join the speculators with the hypothesis that the problem lies in changes induced in the enzyme systems which handle the drug.

Dependency

This is the name given to the physical manifestations following withdrawal and the syndrome produced is referred to as the *abstinence syndrome*. It varies from drug to drug though there are features common to them all, but that which is most popularly portrayed is morphine or opiate withdrawal. The pupils dilate, and rhinorrhoea, lachrimation, yawning and sneezing occur. These are followed by a more severe reaction with profuse sweating, pyrexia, vomiting and dehydration. Wikler (1952) has been able to induce similar reactions in decerebrate dogs, suggesting that they are physiologically determined.

Relapse

This is a feature which occurs in addicts long since deprived of the drug, yet who behave in a way that would lead one to believe they were showing the abstinence syndrome. As with tolerance, very little is known of the underlying mechanism, but it may well be a psychological reaction associated with the physical concomitants of anxiety.

THE CLINICAL COURSE

This will depend, as in the origin, on social, cultural and economic factors. Too much has been reported on those cases which do not respond to 'treatment', that is, efforts to wean them from the addiction. They relapse, lie and steal in order to get their supply and deteriorate socially and this is considered to be the usual downward path of the morphine or heroin addict. Too little has been written about the patient who is given his supply as part of his medical treatment. There are many instances of the respectable doctor who was successful in practice, was a good husband and father, but who maintained himself in those roles with the aid of drugs. The real tragedy occurs when, because of tolerance, further supplies are required and he falls foul of the law in trying to procure them. He then immediately becomes suspect by his profession and others and has acquired a disease which carries a poor prognosis. He resorts to substitutes like barbiturates and alcohol, particularly the latter, and in a couple of years will not only have ruined himself professionally, economically, physically, mentally and morally, but will have broken up his home and almost ruined his family in the process. This must be the fate of the 50 per cent or more who are not successfully 'treated'.

It is possible for addicts to be put on a register and be given the drugs they require to maintain themselves in reasonable comfort and effectiveness. The time has surely come when we must adopt this course with our colleagues and give them the choice of either being registered as drug addicts with no loss of professional status or rights or being treated for the addiction. It is possible that the knowledge of the alternatives will relieve patient and therapist of much of the anxiety which surrounds this problem and give treatment a better chance of success. The biggest objection to such a policy is the fear that the medical profession will fall victim to an epidemic of drug addiction. Like many such fears, there is every chance that it will prove to be unfounded. It need not, however, interfere with our treatment of the individual addict. Kolb (1925) maintained that only psychopaths used opiates for their euphoriant effect, and stated:

> That individuals may take morphine or some other opiate for 20 years or more without showing intellectual or moral deterioration is a common experience of every physician who has studied the subject. . . . We think it must be accepted that a man is mentally and morally normal who graduates in medicine, marries and raises a family of useful children, practises medicine for 30 or 40 years, never becomes involved in questionable transactions, takes a part in the affairs of the community, and is looked upon as one of its leading citizens. The same applies to a lawyer who worked himself up from a poor boy to one of

the leading attorneys in his country, who became addicted to morphine following a severe abdominal disease with recurrence and two operations, and who continued to practice his profession with undiminished vigor in spite of his physical malady and the addiction.... Such addicts, however, are under the necessity of concealing a practice which is disapproved by the public and proscribed by law. To this demoralizing situation is added the shame most of them feel at finding themselves slaves to a habit from which they would like to be free. This combination of furtive concealment and shameful regret cannot help but bring about some change for the worse in any personality, but the change produced in mature individuals is usually so slight that it cannot be demonstrated or cannot be classed as 'moral deterioration'.

Legal Aspects

Society has legislated for the control and sale of drugs which are reputed to cause addiction. In Britain, the Dangerous Drugs Act and in the United States of America, the Harrison Narcotic Act, control opiates and their synthetic substitutes, while the Pharmacy and Poisons Act and the Federal Food and Drug Act control the sale of sedatives and stimulants which are known to be habit forming but are not controlled by the former Acts. It is unfortunate that there should be this legal distinction, for it creates the impression that there are two degrees of addiction, that for the 'dangerous drugs' which entails severe penalties especially for medical men, and the rest. Yet those drugs which come under the Pharmacy and Poisons Act and the Federal Food and Drug Act can have much more severe social and even medical implications. It also, by exclusion, makes addiction to other drugs appear to be less serious or, to those who have a child-like belief in government legislation, even impossible. Yet there are many drugs which are dealt with by the 'lesser' Acts or not mentioned at all which are more prevalent among the addictions. It is likely that any drug which has an action on the nervous system and which produces an immediate feeling of euphoria, contentment or confidence is potentially habit-forming, particularly if given to an addiction-prone person.

The distinction between Drugs of Addiction and Dangerous Drugs is now being recognized and in Britain an Inter-Departmental Committee on Drug Addiction was set up and first reported in 1961 (H.M.S.O. 1961). At that time the Committee saw no need to recommend positive action in terms of registration of addicts, compulsory committal for treatment, special institutions, special tribunals to investigate prescribing, or additional statutory controls of any kind. Four years later (H.M.S.O. 1965) the Committee issued its second report reversing in almost every particular the advice it gave in 1961. Things had changed. Large numbers of young people were becoming addicted to the Dangerous Drugs such as heroin, morphine and cocaine, and even larger numbers to barbiturates, amphetamines and hallucinogens like lysergic acid. This second report though more in keeping with popular opinion would appear to offer a remedy for a problem which has not yet been diagnosed. Many questions are still unanswered. Does drug taking in the very young (who are responsible for the large increase) result in permanent addiction, and psychopathy? What percentage spontaneously 'unhook' themselves? Is drug-taking the worst social and medical manifestation of instability in the young? How does the long-term follow-up of drug-takers compare with alcoholics? Will compulsion in treatment and restriction in prescribing have the desired effects? Are treatment centres for young gregarious populations likely to reduce or increase their drug-taking activities?

Everybody is agreed that further research is needed, but the publicity that has surrounded this problem is more likely to influence enquiry into the psychopathic and deviant drug-taker about whom much is already known and divert enquiry from the rest.

Misuse of Drugs Act, 1971

Responsibility for the control of drug abuse belongs to the Home Office, but doctors are responsible for prescribing. Some doctors have abused this responsibility and this has led to the passing of the Misuse of Drugs Act (1971). This Act has an open-ended commitment in that it can add to those restricted drugs others as they appear. Medical men are generally concerned with lay or government interference with their freedom to prescribe, but their own professional disciplinary machinery was too ineffective and the government had to act. Already, heroin may only be prescribed to addicts by doctors who are specially registered, and new legislation is beginning to extend the range of drugs and their restrictions.

The Misuse of Drugs Act, 1971, and the 1973 regulations made under the Act, are the first of a new series affecting medicines and poisons to reach the Statute Book.

The Act replaces and extends the existing Dangerous Drugs Acts which are repealed. Drugs formerly referred to as 'Dangerous Drugs' together with some new additions are now known as 'Schedule Two Controlled Drugs' or simply 'Controlled Drugs'. These include Morphine, Pethidine and the other opiates plus the following:

1. Amphetamine, Dexamphetamine, (Dexedrine), Methyl-

amphetamine (Methedrine), Methylphenindate (Ritalin), Phenmetrazine (Preludin). Fenfluramine (Ponderax) is *not* included.

2. Methaqualone and preparations containing it, e.g. Mandrax.
3. Codeine and dihydrocodeine tart (DF118) in injection form only.

From 1st July, 1973 all prescriptions for Controlled Drugs whether written in hospital or in general NHS or private practice must:

1. Be in writing and signed by the person issuing it with his usual signature and be dated by him.
2. Be in ink or otherwise so as to be indelible.
3. Specify the dose to be taken and either the total number of doses required to the total quantity to be supplied. This must be stated in *words* as well as in figures and in the prescriber's own handwriting.
4. Prescriptions written outside hospital must also state the address of the prescriber, and, in the prescriber's own handwriting, the name and address of the patient.

Unless these regulations are observed a pharmacist cannot, by law, supply the drugs.

Opiate Addiction

This usually includes addiction to morphine, heroin and synthetic equivalents. The patient in Britain was usually a member of the dental, medical, nursing, pharmaceutical or veterinary profession, or a patient who had the drug prescribed in the usual way and had become addicted. Most are now psychopathic and obtain the drug from non-medical sources.

Dosage varies enormously and can reach, what to the uninitiated may appear phantastic amounts, such as 1–1·5 g./day.

Clinical Features

As has already been stated, in an otherwise stable individual, it may not be possible to tell whether he is an opiate addict unless he is observed in a withdrawal phase, or after a dose of the drug, when the pupils will be contracted. If the dose has been delayed, there may be overt expressions of relief like that emitted by the cigarette addict who after a spell of deprivation gets his first few puffs. The moral deterioration, which is so commonly regarded as pathognomonic, is probably due to the social ostracism directed at the addict or to the initial psychopathic personality which has resorted to the addiction. Some of the latter group may simulate disease of an acute nature such as perforated ulcers and renal or biliary colic, in order to gain admission to hospital and receive the opiates for relief of their 'pain'. These patients constitute a fair percentage of those who simulate illness and described by Asher (1951) as 'Munchausen's Syndrome'.

Withdrawal Symptoms

These usually appear within 12–14 hours of the last dose and have already been described under the general introduction. They are at their worst at 48–72 hours after the initial withdrawal, but thereafter gradually subside and may eventually disappear in about a week. The physical effects of abrupt withdrawal can be extremely severe, requiring energetic supportive measures for a collapsed patient.

TREATMENT

With the rapid rise in drug-taking and larger numbers becoming addicted, treatment has become a major concern, not only for the medical profession but for governments. Withdrawal of the drug and the patient's eventual independence of it, is the aim.

(a) Treatment Centres. These were set up by the Drug Addiction Treatment Act (1968) largely because of the agitation of a voluntary body called 'The Society for the Prevention of Drug Addiction', some of whose members were the mothers of drug addicts. Although they are called 'Treatment Centres', treatment is not a conspicuous feature of their work. They are mainly licensed or rather 'off-license' premises, for the drugs are not usually consumed on the premises.

Their introduction was hailed by some as a great advance which would spare us the worst excesses of the drug 'scene' in the United States. Jones (1969) urged the vigorous implementation of the Act, and to emphasize his case pointed to the American system which encourages large profits from illegal drugs, income-producing crime, multitudes of under-financed treatment programmes, all of which are unsuccessful, a disproportionately high death rate for addicts and an ever-increasing addict population.

Boyd *et al.* (1971) surveyed the first year's referral of heroin-addicted adolescents two years after the opening of a special treatment unit with in-patient facilities where addicts could stay up to 18 months. Out of 130 patients who presented, 78 were selected for treatment, and when followed up only 27 per cent of them were assessed as 'off all drugs'. Many were found to be taking drugs other than those prescribed, suggesting that they were disposing of their drugs illegally and thus contributing to the general problem. So much for the optimistic forecasts. Clearly, Treatment Centres as envisaged under the Act have not solved the problem.

(*b*) *Methadone*. In recent years, methadone has come to be accepted, rather uncritically, as a new 'cure' for opiate and particularly heroin addiction. Its main advantages are good oral efficacy and long action, which means that one dose can be given in orange juice once daily by a clinic, thus avoiding the risk of disposing of the drug illegally, The heroin or other drugs can be stopped immediately and methadone given in one dose of 120–180 mg. which in tolerance is equivalent to 30 mg. of heroin intravenously. Close observation is essential for the patients are unreliable. Acute signs of withdrawal settle in 7–10 days.

Early results, as usual, were most encouraging, and it was generally felt that an answer to opiate addiction had been found, but its claims are now being questioned. Weppner *et al.* (1972) reported on 336 patients admitted to the Clinical Research Centre of the National Institute of Mental Health: 145 (43 per cent) had used methadone illegally, and 111 (33 per cent) had been in a methadone maintenance programme for some time. Sixty-five (19 per cent) had at some time used methadone illegally while participating in a legitimate programme. Seven per cent had experience with methadone only in a legal detoxification programme. Those who had used methadone matched other narcotic addicts in terms of race, arrests, education, length of addiction and age.

Of the illicit methadone users, 44 per cent got it from their regular heroin pusher, 37 per cent from a methadone maintenance patient, and 19 per cent from some other souce; 78 per cent of all illicit addicts took it intravenously. One third took methadone 'to kick the habit', one third to avoid heroin withdrawal effects and one third for its positive qualities, such as the length of euphoria, its low cost and availability. The authors conclude that illegal methadone may become the drug of choice and thereby create a new class of narcotic abuser.

Ramer *et al.* (1971) ask whether methadone by itself is enough, and point out that its speed in removing the addict's craving for heroin may lead to major disruptions in his life which demand 'crisis intervention'. They reckon that one third required extensive ancillary treatment, and despite this help they still experienced difficulty in adjusting to a non-addict existence.

(*c*) *Chlorpromazine.* (*d*) *Diazepam.* These drugs are just as effective as methadone in dealing with the withdrawal effects, though they lack the euphoriant effect of methadone. This is probably an advantage, for one euphoriant experience may easily become a substitute for another. Dosage will range from chlorpromazine 50–100 mg. t.d.s. or diazepam 10–20 mg. t.d.s.

(e) Group Therapy. This has been hailed as the panacea for all psychiatric problems, and naturally drug addiction is no exception. It is difficult enough to wean an addict from his own group and it is surely the height of optimism to take on a group of addicts and expect a mass conversion. A report of such an achievement is still awaited.

(f) Psychotherapy. If a good relationship can be established with the patient he may derive sufficient support to withstand subsequent temptation. As with alcoholism, the therapist should be prepared for a long period of supervision. It has been suggested that drug addicts should be permitted to join Alcoholics Anonymous in those countries where there are not enough of them to justify their own organization. While there are certain similarities in the problems, there are also differences, particularly in terms of social practice and accessibility to the addicting agent.

Prognostic Factors

These are common to most drug addictions and in the clinical interview of an addict those areas which have been found to be of greatest prognostic relevance in treatment should be explored. A limited though well-established set of factors has been defined, such as patterns of drug usage, age, social stability, motivation and diagnostic category.

Tamerin and Neumann (1971) review these criteria and conclude that they are concrete and easily objectifiable but not dynamically rich. Furthermore, previous studies have been mainly concerned with addicts from the lower classes where social stability such as socioeconomic resources, class and occupational stability, a good police record and a good college education were highly correlated with a favourable outcome. The authors point out the limited value of such findings, as all these characteristics are present in most addicts seen in private practice and in private psychiatric hospitals.

A review of several hundred middle and upper-class addicts indicated that the following ten factors were significantly and favourably related to outcome:

(1) *Self-referral*; (2) *Acceptance of the problem*; (3) *Pain from*

problem; (4) *Willingness to change habits or life-style;* (5) *Prior history of financial independence*; (6) *History of accomplishment*; (7) *Sense of responsibility;* (8) *Capacity to relate to the therapist;* (9) *Good attitude to treatment environment*; (10) *Good relationship to spouse or employer and especially fear of loss of either*.

Noble *et al.* (1972) surveyed illicit drug use among 1088 adolescent girls admitted to a London remand home and identified 227 who were using drugs and compared them with 100 girls who had not used drugs. After follow-up (mean period 3 years) 40 of the 194 who were not on *narcotic* drugs were now using them, while only one of the controls did so. The narcotic users had more criminal convictions, particularly for violence, and a high proportion were admitted compulsorily to hospital and a large number absconded or discharged themselves against advice. Most subjects continued to use illicit sources of drugs except when in institutions, and 10 of the girls have died from suicide or drug overdose, 9 of whom were on narcotics or intravenous drugs.

Cocaine

In large amounts cocaine is an unpleasant drug to take and may lead to convulsions; addicts therefore frequently combine it with morphine. It used to be sniffed and would cause ulceration of the nasal mucosa and septum, but it is also taken by injection. It is alleged not to produce tolerance. It has now been largely supplanted as a euphoriant and stimulant by amphetamine. It may produce similar psychotic features (see below), as well as the characteristic feeling of formication or the 'cocaine bug', which is frequently interpreted in a delusional manner. Withdrawal effects are not nearly as catastrophic as those with morphine and there is no tolerance.

Nalaxone for Diagnosis in Methadone Treatment

Nalaxone hydrochloride is a narcotic antagonist which Blachley (1973) claims may be safely, rapidly and effectively used for the diagnosis of physical dependence on opiates. Used in an out-patient setting, with a minimum of personnel, it will distinguish a person who is physically dependent from one who is an occasional user in 10–35 minutes without precipitating severe abstinence symptoms. Nalaxone, 0·16 mg., is first given intramuscularly in the triceps. Pulse, blood pressure, oral temperature, pupil size (measured to 0·2 mm.), presence of gooseflesh on the thorax, sweating, lachrymation, yawning, rhinorrhoea, and subjective complaints are recorded before and 20–30 minutes after this injection. If there is no gooseflesh, a second dose of 0·24 mg. is given, this time intravenously. Observations are repeated after 15 minutes.

A Nalaxone test was given to 33 patients and a Nalorphine test to 15 patients who applied for methadone treatment, but who did not have documented evidence of relapse after hospital or prison treatment, or did not show gooseflesh, the only abstinence sign that cannot be feigned. A negative response to nalaxone was seen in 11 subjects and in 6 to nalorphine. Six patients showed a negative response to the intramuscularly administered nalaxone, but a positive response to the second injection given intravenously. An additional nine patients had a questionable positive response to the intramuscular injection but an unquestionably positive response to the intravenous injection. No patient showed abstinence features to cause medical concern. These began to settle 20–40 minutes after the injection and had disappeared in 90 minutes. The starting dose of methadone could then be given.

The author concludes that despite the discomfort, the opiate abstinence syndrome is not medically dangerous, and as nalaxone, unlike nalorphine, has no dangerous depressant qualities, it appears to be a safe agent to be used in screening potential addicts to methadone. As one third of those applying to the clinic, who had no prior documentation of withdrawal, showed no evidence of physical dependence, such screening is essential.

Marihuana (Hashish, *Cannabis sativa)*

This is one of the oldest and most commonly used intoxicants in the world, and was until recently mainly confined to the Caribbean, the Middle East and India. The active constituents are tetra-hydrocannabinols (THC's) and a synthetic form has become illicitly available.

The drug produces a dreamy state of consciousness in which ideas seem disconnected, uncontróllable and freely flowing. Perception of time, colour and space is distorted and enhanced. There is also an extreme feeling of well-being, exaltation and excitement which is referred to as 'high'. On the other side there may be depression, panic states and fear of impending death with body image distortion and frank hallucinations. It is popularly believed to increase intellectual function and creativity as well as sexual performance but evidence is lacking. Physical dependence does not develop though cravings during abstinence do occur.

The drug may be taken in a variety of forms. The resinous

substance produced by the hemp plant is most abundant in the leaves and flowering tops at the time of flowering and these dried leaves and tops are marihuana, which is popularly called 'pot', 'grass', 'tea' and 'reefers'. If the resin is concentrated and compressed into cakes it is called 'hashish' or 'ganja' or 'charas'. It is considered that its effects are three times greater when smoked than when taken orally.

In recent years the taking of marihuana has reached epidemic proportions, particularly among the young, and in Britain as in other Western countries it is popular on the university campus and in schools. A great debate is in progress with a marihuana 'lobby' insisting that it is a harmless drug and much less of a social evil than alcohol which is legally available. The opposition, like the 'lobby', has equally cogent arguments which are also to some extent based on prejudice.

Prejudice on the pro-marihuana side stems from a political philosophy which argues that because the drug is illegal, this represents the repressive forces of an illiberal society which interfere with the individual's pursuit of pleasure and must be resisted. Others feel that its restriction is an important bastion of the society which they wish to destroy and in this interpretation they are not far removed from those who wish to maintain the ban.

Medical arguments are put forward on both sides but these are minor issues, for the main argument is really one of a society which wishes to preserve what it feels to be a fundamental aspect of its existence and the forces ranged against that society. One side claims that there is no evidence that it does harm; the other provides evidence that it does, and as the present skirmishes are being fought on the presence or absence of such evidence, it is the psychiatrist's responsibility to be familiar with the evidence.

Medical and Psychiatric Complications. There has been a steady stream of papers presenting data, and the following are a selection of the more objective.

1. Hollister and Gillespie (1970) did a controlled trial, using marihuana and ethyl alcohol and a placebo on normal volunteers. The subjects were tested 1½–2 hours and 3½–4 hours after administration, and the results showed that marihuana was very similar in its effects to alcohol as regards reaction time and other psychometrics, except that alcohol showed changes 1½ hours after ingestion, while marihuana took 3½ hours to produce the changes. In addition, marihuana showed an alteration in time perception.

2. Campbell (1971) compared the EEG's of 11 patients with psychotic reactions following the use of cannabis, with 29 patients

admitted with a diagnosis of schizophrenia and 10 with neurological disorders. He concluded that there was a greater number of abnormal EEG's associated with cannabis psychosis than with schizophrenic and neurological controls. He noted further that cannabis usage without apparent psychiatric sequelae also showed a large number of EEG abnormalities compared with controls. Only two cannabis psychotics had EEG abnormalities prior to taking cannabis.

3. Talbott and Teague (1969) had previously reported on marihuana psychosis among American soldiers in Vietnam and described a 'typical' syndrome which included: burning and irritation of the respiratory tract; impaired coordination and difficulty with fine movements; aching of the large muscles of the extremities; and irritation of the conjunctivae soon after the subjects began to smoke. They then experienced impaired cognition particularly of time and place; some impairment of memory; intellectual impairment with confusion; short attention span and difficulty in concentrating; impaired thinking with tangential and disjointed qualities; and impaired judgment. They all exhibited lability of affect, marked anxiety and fearfulness. Ten showed paranoid symptoms. They all recovered within a week.

4. Keup (1970) reported that among patients newly admitted to Brooklyn State Hospital, those with a history of drug abuse increased from 29 in 1966 to 68 in 1967, and to 165 in 1968. Of 126 fully investigated, 14 (11·1 per cent) had cannabis-provoked symptoms.

5. Clark *et al.* (1970) in experimental studies on controls found that processes involved in selective perception, and conversely, habituation to irrelevant stimuli, immediate recall of preceding thoughts in order to keep on track, and capacity for goal directed systematic thinking, are particularly sensitive to relatively low doses of marihuana.

6. Campbell *et al.* (1971) reported on 10 patients between 15 and 25 years who had been referred because of headaches, loss of consciousness and syncope. All showed significant cerebral atrophy, which is rare in young people, and all had been heavy cannabis smokers; 3 of the 10 had been similarly investigated with normal findings prior to smoking cannabis.

7. Bernhardson and Gunne (1972) reported from Sweden on 46 cases of psychosis in cannabis users, and conclude that there is a likelihood of a genuine psychosis due to cannabis, which should be suspected in young patients without previous psychosis when an episodic psychosis of schizophrenic-like, maniac or confusional type is present.

8. Kolansky and Moore (1971) in a study of marihuana smoking

in 38 young adolescents, demonstrated effects ranging from mild to severe ego-decompensations and diagnosed psychosis in eight patients which was mainly a delusional system designed to restore reality. They conclude that marihuana in adolescents accentuates the very aspects of disturbing bodily development and psychological conflict which the adolescent is struggling to master. This leads to an interruption of normal psychological adolescent growth processes so that the adolescent reaches chronological adulthood without achieving adult mental functioning or emotional responsiveness.

As many who take marihuana do not become psychotic or show other mental handicap, there is some justification for the 'lobby' to claim that it is *relatively* harmless. This is as far as its physical and mental effects are concerned. Yet society legislates to protect its citizens even though the hazard be much less than that of taking marihuana. In Britain, cyclamates, which were a useful substitute for sugar, itself a hazard to health, were banned because it was shown experimentally that a laboratory animal fed on the stuff at a level which in the human would mean consuming gallons of sweetened drinks every day for 20 years, could develop cancer.

An even greater cause for anxiety is the tendency for people who take cannabis to move on to the 'hard drugs' such as opiates and cocaine. Again, all cannabis takers do not go on to hard drugs, but there are very few on hard drugs who did not start with cannabis.

Paton (1973) stresses an aspect of cannabis addiction which is frequently overlooked when people argue from one culture to another. He points out that extensive use of cannabis in a population with high expectation of life, health and wealth is a new phenomenon, and furthermore it is associated with multiple drug use. On the pharmacology of the drug he explains that the making of 'majoun' by extracting the physically active principle with butter and then washing in water, shows the lipophilic nature of the drug. As there are 20–30 metabolites the determination of THC by blood and urine analysis is a formidable problem. Contrary to what many claim, there are withdrawal effects such as restlessness, anxiety, sweating, depression, irritability, excitement and sleeplessness.

Amphetamine Addiction

Amphetamine has been regarded as the modern form of cocaine. It produces a feeling of confidence combined with energy and mental alertness and is frequently resorted to by alcoholics and barbiturate addicts as well as psychopaths seeking an ego-booster or an exciting experience. It is also popular among prison inmates and Monroe and

Drell (1947) described four cases of hallucination and ideas of reference amongst prison inmates who had been ingesting strips of amphetamine from inhalers. Just as the barbiturate addict has obtained his amylobarbitone sodium from compound tablets, so the amphetamine addict has obtained his supply from the same source, and these tablets become a popular form of stimulant among teenagers who are trying to whip up the party spirit.

Psychotic Features. These are more common than is generally appreciated and the possibility of amphetamine intoxication should be considered in acute psychotic states of a paranoid and hallucinatory nature. Connell (1958) described a large series and pointed out the difficulties these patients may cause if admitted to a general hospital. Ordinary doses of sedation are inadequate to control their insomnia and acute excitement may follow. Some patients may be very sensitive to the drug and not all cases of amphetamine psychosis occur in addicts.

In addition to the acute psychotic features, behaviour disturbances can also occur and some patients have indulged in shop-lifting, erotic pursuits contrary to their usual conduct, and irresponsible behaviour, such as turning up late for work and failing to appreciate the consequences. As with other drug addictions, chlorpromazine is useful in dealing with withdrawal symptoms and potentiating the action of barbiturates in procuring sleep.

An early physical sign in addicts is continuous chewing or teethgrinding movements, with rubbing of the tongue along the inside of the lower lip, often leading to trauma to the lip and tongue with ulcers visible to inspection at both sites. Ashcroft *et al.* (1965) report that the sign is useful in suspected addicts and in deciding whether or not addicts under treatment have obtained illicit supplies. The sign is apparently well-known among the 'amphetamine fraternity' and is also seen as an exaggeration of chewing movements in rabbits that have been given the drug.

Assault and Homicide

Ellinwood (1971) reported on 13 persons who committed homicide after taking amphetamines. Recurring factors in the histories were: (1) repeated drug abuse over several years; (2) loss of intellectual awareness of the delusional state; (3) amphetamine-induced suspiciousness, delusions, fear and panic, as well as emotional lability and impulsiveness; (4) a solitary life style with little chance for cross-validation of delusional thinking; mutual enhancement of suspiciousness and paranoid ideas with other 'speed freaks'; (6) carrying a concealed weapon; (7) armed robbery as a means of supporting drug abuse; and (8) conflict over drug dealings.

Three distinct phases leading to the violent act could be identified: (1) Chronic amphetamine abuse; (2) Acute change in a person's state of emotional arousal; and (3) A situation which sets off the specific events. After the first two stages, when paranoid thinking and misinterpretation of the environment develop, a minor incident can trigger a violent act. The author suggests that, as the incidence of assault and homicide by amphetamine abusers is not known, a routine urine examination should be performed on all arrested for a violent crime.

Experimental Study

Griffith *et al.* (1972) investigated the psychotomimetic properties of dextroamphetamine sulphate in nine volunteers who had had previous experience with self-administered large doses of the drug. Each subject received 10 mg. intravenously, and subsequent doses were given orally. Six developed florid paranoid features in a 1–5 day period and in two subjects the drug was abitrarily discontinued during a pre-psychotic phase as manifest by paranoid feelings. All subjects appeared depressed when the cumulative dose exceeded 50 mg., becoming irritable, hypochondriacal, fault-finding, anorexic and over-dependent. All who showed florid paranoid features had a pre-psychotic phase; the psychotic sequel was abrupt in onset and it settled rapidly on stopping the drug.

The authors question earlier hypotheses on the aetiology of amphetamine psychosis. They failed to confirm the sleep-deprivation hypothesis, as four subjects became psychotic after less than two nights without sleep. Pre-drug personality was not important, for though the subjects were not 'normal', none was considered psychotic or even borderline. Also, since only dextroamphetamine was administered, the psychosis could not be attributed to barbiturate withdrawal, multi-drug use, or acute brain damage. As eight of the nine subjects became psychotic or pre-psychotic, the reaction could not be regarded as a rare idiosyncratic response, and must now be viewed as a probable complication of high-dose amphetamine abuse.

Phenmetrazine (Preludin) Addiction

Phenmetrazine is a sympathomimetic drug with an action similar to amphetamine, and like it, is used in the treatment of obesity. It is an oxazine derivative and has a structure not unlike ephedrine or amphetamine.

It is also a euphoriant like amphetamine and it is not surprising that since its introduction in 1953, a number of cases of addiction have been reported, Evans (1959) stated that within six months he had seen 16 patients who had become psychiatrically ill after taking phenmetrazine and of these 12 had a psychotic disturbance. He was unable to distinguish the clinical picture from amphetamine, bromide or alcoholic hallucinosis. The psychotic features were restlessness, pressure of talk, disturbance of mood, delusions, hallucinations and clouding of consciousness. It is more likely to be commoner in

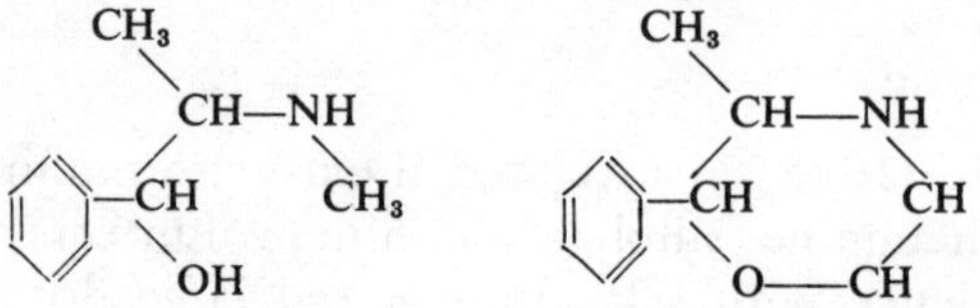

CH_3 — CH—NH — CH_3; CH (phenyl) — OH

Ephedrine

CH_3 — CH—NH — CH; CH (phenyl) — O—CH

Phenmetrazine

females as it is generally prescribed (and at one time, freely bought over the counter) for obesity, and in Evans's 12 cases of psychosis, 10 were females. As with amphetamine it can produce character changes, and the author had a patient who was addicted and whose mother was so disturbed by her daughter's personality change that she actively campaigned to have the drug placed under control, which it now is.

The Punding

Rylander (1972) described a syndrome in 40 addicts who were on large doses of phenmetrazine and amphetamine for 1–9 years. All in reply to a questionnaire had noticed the punding in themselves (75 per cent) or in their fellow addicts. The syndrome is a form of automatic behaviour in which the addict manipulates some object for hours, mostly technical equipment, such as radios, watches and engines, while women comb hair, polish nails and tidy rooms. They generally do something they used to or liked to do.

The addicts described it as a meaningless, protracted occupation in which they got stuck and could not give up, and it would start 1–2 hours after the injection and last for hours or days. All but one found it pleasurable or funny, and efforts to stop would result in anxiety, and it excluded social interactions. It would develop into a jerking syndrome consisting of meaningless, automatic, unwilled movements which were partially choreiform, or sometimes the addict would remain fixed in the same position or staring for hours. It is suggested that this is an organic state induced by the mobilization of excess dopamine into the receptors.

Other Addictions

Seager and Foster (1958) quote examples of addiction to carbromal which is a mild hypnotic and sedative and is frequently included in sedative mixtures sold freely from chemists's shops and to chlorodyne which contains 1·5 mg. of anhydrous morphine in 1 ml. as well as chloroform, alcohol and ether. It is used to control cough, vomiting and diarrhoea and prolonged addiction usually results in peripheral neuropathies.

Petrol sniffing, particularly in children, can become an addiction, especially when it is associated with vivid visual hallucinatory experiences (Bethell, 1965). *Ephedrine* is being used by the young for 'kicks' and has even been taken intravenously.

The large number of immigrants from Asia and the Caribbean are introducing strange addictions (to us) such as poppy heads (unlanced capsules of *Papaver somniferum*, known as 'post'). They can be obtained from a chemist shop and are taken for the purpose of increasing libido and sexual potency. Withdrawal effects are similar to those of opium. *Glue sniffing* is another addiction and has been reported in some who are constantly looking for new experiences. Coloured dreams are a feature and withdrawal can produce delirium tremens.

McCarthy (1971) in a study of 51 members of the 'surfer' sub-culture of South Queensland's beach resorts found a variety of drug abuses which were not generally familiar to Australian doctors:

1. *Psilocybe cubensis.* This is taken for its euphoriant and hallucinogenic effects but regular users soon begin to experience extreme depression, lethargy, loss of the will to live, lasting several days between doses, and occasionally 'freak outs' or terrifying 'trips'.
2. Romilar (containing the opiate alkaloid dextro-methorphan hydrobromide) was used for its euphoriant and hallucinogenic effects, but regular ingestion was followed by a period of somnambulism, lethargy and ataxia.
3. Dimethyltryptamine (DMP) was either smoked or injected subcutaneously. When smoked it produced euphoria and hilarity but when injected it caused visual hallucinations involving coloured patterns.

4. Mescaline-related STP or 'DOM' when used orally was similar to LSD.

5. Methaqualone plus diphenhydramine (Mandrax) caused euphoria, a 'floating' feeling and multi-coloured flashing patterns.

6. 'Mellow Yellow', which is the scrapings of the insides of dried banana skins is smoked and the effects are similar to cannabis.

7. Lighter fluid was inhaled with resulting euphoria, loss of coordination, visual hallucinations, clouding of consciousness and loss of memory for subsequent events.

8. Amyl nitrite when inhaled caused hilarity and euphoria lasting two minutes.

9. Benzhexol (Artane). This is an anti-parkinsonism drug frequently prescribed with phenothiazines and butyrophenones to counteract the striatal effects. In large doses it is a potent hallucinogenic agent.

Gowdy (1972) analysed the use of stramonium powder as an hallucinogenic agent in 212 cases, 54 from the literature and 158 from official sources. Five died as a result of the mental state induced by the drug which is used therapeutically as a sympathomimetic agent in bronchial asthma. Identifiable hallucinatory episodes were present in 99 out of the 212. Amnesia, anxiety and paranoia were present in 34; disorientation related to the degree of intoxication in 45; and hyperactivity and aggression in 22.

The differential diagnosis is mainly to exclude alcohol intoxication, but the absence of alcohol in the breath, the dilated pupils and the pyrexia and a low blood alcohol will clarify the diagnosis.

Analgesic Abuse

As pain is a very common symptom in psychiatric patients, it is likely that analgesic abuse is common in such patients. Murray *et al.* (1970) reported on all patients admitted to a psychiatric hospital over a 3-month period, and out of 181 patients, 16 had ingested more than 1 kg. of phenacetin or salicylate in the six months prior to admission; 26 had ingested these drugs regularly but did not reach 1 kg. and 139 reported no significant ingestion.

Of the 16 analgesic abusers, five had been in hospital for symptoms of peptic ulceration, 3 for renal investigation, and 2 had suffered from symptoms of acute papillary necrosis. The authors conclude that the early identification of analgesic abuse can save needless investigation and treatment of dyspepsia and obscure anaemias and probably arrest renal changes.

It is still debated whether analgesics are addictive, but as their actions vary, the answer is that some are more addictive than others, though it is probable that any drug which can procure immediate relief has effects other than that of analgesia. Drugs which are introduced as pain-killers are initially claimed to be non-addictive, but after a time the reverse is demonstrated. Historically, pethidine is in this category and a more recent one is pentazocine. Inciardi and Chambers (1971) were able to isolate several patterns of pentazocine abuse and addiction in a series of controlled experiments, and with more assiduous searching a number of apparently non-addictive drugs will prove to have addictive qualities.

Ergotamine and Methysergide Abuse

Lucas and Falkowski (1973) described five patients with migraine who abused ergotamine preparations. They conclude that patients who abuse these drugs are subject to rebound headaches when they attempt to cut down their drug intake. They were also unduly anxious, tended to bottle up their feelings, had low stress tolerance and were subjected to prolonged tension which precipitated headaches. Since both ergotamine and methysergide can produce serious complications when taken over a long period and in large amounts, *e.g.* gangrene of the extremities, it is important to reduce their intake. This may require the uncovering of underlying stresses in addition to drug control.

Khat

This drug has similar effects to cannabis and amphetamine. It is mainly used in the South Yemen and its use has spread to the Horn of Africa. Usually the leaves are chewed and produce CNS stimulation with euphoria, rather different from that produced by amphetamine, in that it is associated with a dreamy state. The partaker also becomes garrulous but when the effects wear off there is apathy, depression and loss of appetite.

It is almost impossible for the medical practitioner to keep a check on all drugs which can produce addiction, but he should be aware of the addiction-proneness of his patient and be very circumspect in his prescribing of euphoriants and stimulants.

HALLUCINOGENIC DRUGS

These have been used by man for many centuries and perhaps the most common is mescaline. De Ropp (1958) in language which provides an ideal back-cloth to the topic states:

> On the mesas of Tamaulipas and Jalisco, in the dry infertile regions of Mexico south of the Rio Grande, a cactus grows amid the rocks and sand. It is not erect and magnificent like the Seguaro or the bearer of gorgeous flowers like the night-blooming Cereus. It is, in fact, a thoroughly insignificant little pincushion projecting a bare three inches above the barren soil, a round, dark green protuberance connected to a carrot-like taproot, its surface covered with tufts of silky hair. Though utterly uninspiring in appearance, this humble cactus, *Lopophora Williamsii*, produces in its fleshy top one of the strongest drugs in the pharmacologist's collection. . . .

It was gathered (and may still be) by the Mexican Indians who used it as part of a religious rite in which all the people participated. The dried flesh of the cactus or *peyotl* is chewed and the hallucinotic experience ensues. Its effects have fascinated a number of writers and experimentalists including Ellis (1902) and Aldous Huxley (1954), but more recently it has attracted the attention of psychiatrists, some of whom claimed it produced psychotic states, while others regarded its effects as a model by which the features of a psychosis might be studied.

Synthetic mescaline is given intravenously in doses of 0·4—1·0 g., thus ensuring a pure preparation and avoiding the gastro-intestinal upset that occurs in some subjects who are given the drug orally. Initially, physiological changes are observed such as pallor or flushing, dilated pupils and tremors, which could pass for over-activity of the sympathetic. Later, there is sensory impairment, particularly for pain, spatial perception and body image. After that, the more florid 'psychotic' features emerge against a background of undisturbed consciousness. Some of these hallucinatory experiences are obviously derived from wish-fulfilling phantasies, while others seem to have no obvious relationship to the patient's inner mental life.

Contrary to what one finds in the functional psychoses, visual hallucinations predominate and these tend to vary rapidly in content and in intensity, while somatic sensations, such as feelings of electricity, also occur. Hoch (1951) concludes from his own researches that there are essential differences in the reaction to the drug by schizophrenics and normals and that even those similarities that do exist are only partially similar. Schizophrenics tended to show anxiety and apprehension during the experiment while in normals these features were not evident. Euphoria and sexual content were commoner in schizophrenics and even their reactions which were shared by normals were more intense, with a ready tendency for mental processes to become disorganized. This latter finding is what one would expect in patients whose ego structure even without hallucinogenic drugs was showing signs of disintegration.

Hoch (1955) gave mescaline to three groups of schizophrenic patients: (1) overt schizophrenics in an acute or subacute state of the disorder, (2) chronic schizophrenics with varying degrees of deterioration, and (3) pseudo-neurotic schizophrenics. There was potentiation of the schizophrenic features in the overt group, varying effects in the chronic group, depending on the degree of 'activity' of the disease, but in the pseudo-neurotic group there were the most striking changes. These patients in the ordinary way effectively conceal their psychotic pattern under a mask of neurotic behaviour and complaint, but when given mescaline they disintegrated rapidly and unlike the normals, who took an objective view of their delusional and hallucinatory experiences, they were dominated by them. All this does not add up to mescaline being a psychotomimetic drug as it has been labelled. Just because a drug is a hallucinogenic agent and potentiates schizophrenic symptomatology in schizophrenics, does not mean that its effects in the normal in any way resemble the schizophrenic process. Even at the hallucinatory level with mescaline these are usually visual; in schizophrenia they are almost always auditory.

d-LYSERGIC ACID DIETHYLAMIDE (LSD-25)

This is an alkaloid of ergot and is the essential part of ergonovine. Poisoning from ergot of rye has been known for centuries. The noxious agent is a fungus whose spores are carried to the young ovaries of the rye which are replaced by a curved purple body, the sclerotium or ergot of rye. The toxic states resulting from its ingestion included a convulsive form which was associated with mental changes and was called St. Anthony's Fire, for the victims used to invoke the aid of this saint.

As will be described later (see Chapter 18), Hofmann in 1948 accidentally ingested a minute amount of LSD-25 and noticed a disturbance in his mental state; when he deliberately ingested 0·25 mg. he experienced hallucinations and depersonalization, and others have since confirmed his findings with doses as small as 1 μg./kg. Stoll (1947) was the first to make a serious study of its action in man, and since then there have been numerous reports, including those of Mayer-Gross (1951) in this country and Hoch *et al.* (1952) in the United States. It can produce visual hallucinations of an almost infinite variety and has been used as an adjunct to psychotherapy, especially in those patients who have great difficulty in freely communicating or associating.

Pharmacology

The drug, whose action in some respects resembles that of mescaline, is not derived from it, but is chemically related to sympathin and adrenochrome, the latter containing an indole nucleus which is present in LSD-25.

The mental changes it produces can be antagonized by serotonin (Gaddum, 1953) and this may be due to an interference with serotonin-mediated neuronal function by the LSD-25. The synapse of the cat's brain was studied by Marazzi and Hart (1955) and they found that the action of LSD-25 was similar to that of adrenaline and suggested that thought disorders were due to an imbalance of cholinergic and adrenergic influences on susceptible synapses and that compounds with an indole nucleus like that of LSD-25 can produce these changes.

The effect on a normal subject is to produce initially nausea, headache, palpitation, dilated pupils, sweating, hypotension and occasionally bradycardia. Hallucinations and distortion of visual

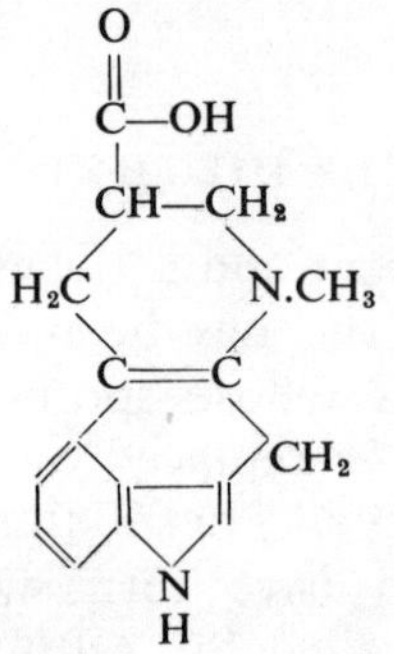

Lysergic acid diethylamide

perception are common and geometrical patterns, brilliant colours and lights with hyperacousis are frequently reported. Emotional lability may result with laughter and giggling or outbursts of weeping. Auditory hallucinations are rare. The whole reaction is usually over in about six hours, starting about half an hour after the ingestion of the drug, reaching its peak after two to three hours, then petering out in four to six hours with a return to normality. In some normal subjects and especially in disturbed patents, the reaction may last much longer and has been known to continue for 24 hours, making out-patient administration hazardous. Some workers (Sandison, 1954; Sandison *et al.*, 1954) have used the drug as an aid to psychotherapy, particularly in those hard-core problems where communication is difficult, such as severe obsessive-compulsive states or psychopathic personalities. These authors stress that the drug is only an aid to therapy and not a treatment in itself though others have used it as a stimulus and permitted the patient to abreact. Sandison and his colleagues have organized the nursing staff to play their role in the patient's regression, nursing them as if they were infants and they, probably rightly, claim that it is this aspect which is therapeutic and not the mere administration of the drug. They stress the dangers of using the drug on out-patients in view of the severe reactions it can precipitate in some patients.

Others have used it in the treatment of habitual offenders and claimed good results. These patients describe a transcendental experience akin to that of a religious conversion which is alleged to lead them to a more peaceful relationship with their fellow men. It may have worked in a few but it has not made any serious impact on the recidivist population. It may be that when the 'prisoner's dream' is given the semblance of reality, it is accompanied by a sense of achievement and satisfaction.

Hatrick and Dewhurst (1970) reported on two female patients who were admitted to a mental hospital because of intoxication with a single dose of LSD. Both had been well-adjusted and unaccustomed to drug-taking. The psychoses developed after an interval of two weeks in one and after two months in the other. Both presented with profound depression and suicidal tendencies while the second patient was homicidal. The first responded to oral chlorpromazine with some residual symptoms, and the second, not at all. Both were given ECT with marked and rapid improvement.

The authors considered the legal implications of a drug-induced delayed psychosis which, with LSD, does not accept a plea of not guilty due to insanity as the person was voluntarily intoxicated. They concluded that the therapeutic use of the drug is not justified especially as it is more likely to precipitate a psychosis in the unstable.

LSD has become in certain circles the basis of a cult. The adherents are to be found mainly on the university campus and extravagant claims are made for its effects. A new dimension to life and a key to the secrets of the universe are some of the virtues of the drug that are extolled and attempts have been made at Harvard to found a national movement for the propagation of its use and the issue has been debated in the national press. One sceptic remarked that alcoholics do not consider that the vivid hallucinations associated with delirium tremens are so valuable to society that everybody should undergo this experience, yet the mechanism of the LSD hallucination is no different. This is sober comment.

Other Hallucinogenic Agents

Other agents, with hallucinogenic properties, have been advocated because they are alleged to be free of some of the undesirable side-effects of LSD-25, either by having a less drastic action or one of shorter duration. One of these is **psilocybin** which is derived from the Mexican mushroom (*Psilocybe mexicana Heim*) and was first isolated in Sandoz laboratories; the findings were reported by Hofmann *et al.* (1958). Chemically it is the phosphoric acid ester of 4-hydroxy-dimethyltryptamine and is related to serotonin and reserpine. An oral dose of 10 mg. caused mydriasis, piloerection, tachycardia, tachypnoea, hyperthermia, hyperglycaemia and hypertension indicating a sympathomimetic effect. Centrally, it had an alerting effect on the EEG and enhanced the spinal reflexes (Weidmann *et al.*, 1958). Delay *et al.* (1958) gave 10 mg. orally or sublingually to four normals and 14 psychiatric patients and reported that it caused hallucinations and dream-like states, recall of affective memories and changes of mood, but that these effects varied from case to case. They concluded that it was not a psychotropic agent, but, like hashish, mescaline and LSD-25 was a 'psychodysleptic', or belonged to the group known as **'phantastica'**.

Isbell (1959) compared its effects in man with LSD-25 and reported that they both elicited abnormal mental states characterized by feelings of strangeness, difficulty in thinking, anxiety, altered sensory perception (particularly visual), hallucinations and alterations of body image. Its effects did not persist as long as those of LSD-25, but the latter was 100–150 times more potent. The author's colleagues (White & Warburton, 1962) recommend an initial dose of 6–8 mg. but it can be considerably increased as tolerance is readily established and they have given doses of 34 mg. without ill-effect. It has a shorter action than LSD-25 and thus lends itself to out-patient treatment especially as its effects can be readily interrupted by 50–100 mg. of chlorpromazine. Their patients showed mood disturbance including depression and euphoria, as well as anxiety and other fears. They also noted excitement, unmotivated laughter and occasionally compulsive movements, but the hallucinatory effect was less marked than with LSD-25. They concluded that it was useful as a therapeutic agent for out-patient treatment in selected cases, but that its action was even less predictable than LSD-25, though as with this drug it was of value in some neurotic patients who had previously defied psychotherapy.

Sernyl has also been used as an hallucinogenic agent and as an aid to psychotherapy. It differs from the *phantastica* in that it is allied to the local anaesthetic novocaine and produces its effect by sensory deprivation.

The search for an efficient intravenous anaesthetic led to the synthesis of a series of cyclohexamine derivatives and l-arylcyclohexylamine (sernyl) was developed.

Although an efficient anaesthetic, some patients in the post-operative period became agitated and showed echolalia and logorrhoea. Luby *et al.* (1959) investigated the drug, using normal subjects and patients, some of whom had chronic schizophrenia. In the latter, there was an intensification of the thought disorder and they became more difficult to manage. Its psychotomimetic effect is said to be

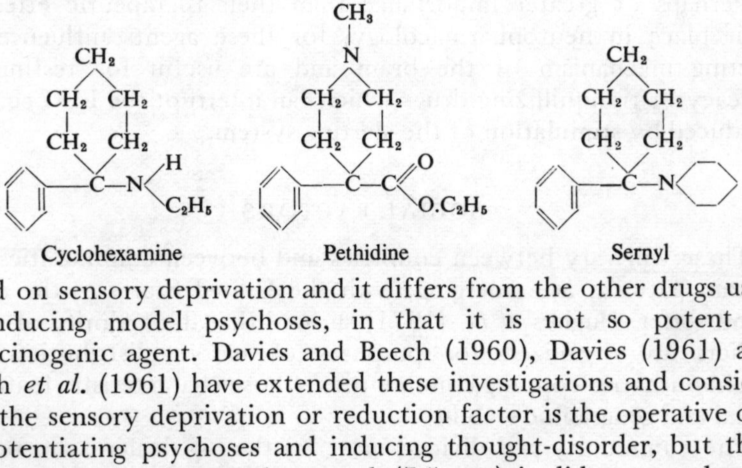

Cyclohexamine   Pethidine   Sernyl

based on sensory deprivation and it differs from the other drugs used in inducing model psychoses, in that it is not so potent an hallucinogenic agent. Davies and Beech (1960), Davies (1961) and Beech *et al.* (1961) have extended these investigations and consider that the sensory deprivation or reduction factor is the operative one in potentiating psychoses and inducing thought-disorder, but they add that in the dosage they used (7·5 mg.) it did not produce a schizophrenic-like disorder.

A Warning

There is now no doubt that these hallucinogenic agents are becoming drugs of addiction and their therapeutic value must now be seen in this light. They have never had more than a limited use, and the added risk of addiction, not to mention the precipitation of a schizophrenic psychosis in the predisposed, places a very heavy responsibility on the psychiatrist who uses them.

PSYCHOTOMIMETIC DRUGS

Psychotomimetic drugs provide a useful means of studying the neuro-physiological association of mental changes and the effects of tranquillizers in cancelling out these changes in animals. To some workers, they suggest the mechanism of functional psychoses, but there are wide discrepancies between the clinical features of schizophrenia and the hallucinatory experiences induced by these drugs.

A number of workers claim that these hallucinogenic agents can produce psychological improvement without the need to enter into a psychotherapeutic relationship, and they have patients attending regularly for their 'abreaction'. There may be some substance to these claims, for the hashish and opium dens must exercise a similar effect on their clients. Most psychiatrists would prefer not to use such drugs therapeutically, for enough information has now accrued to indicate that they may precipitate psychotic reactions and serious antisocial behaviour as well as addiction.

Perhaps of greater importance than their therapeutic effects is their place in neuropharmacology, for these agents influence the alerting mechanism of the brain and are useful for testing the efficacy of tranquillizing drugs which can interrupt the EEG changes produced by stimulation of the alerting system.

SOCIAL FACTORS

These will vary between countries and between communities, but certain patterns are emerging, with the United States as the major trend setter. Hughes *et al.* (1971) showed that the majority of street addicts are organized for purposes of heroin distribution into neighbourhood 'copping communities' whose characteristic feature is social and geographic stability.

The community was divided into: (*a*) the big dealer, who tended to be stable in his interpersonal relationships with relatively little subjective discomfort; (*b*) the part-time dealer scored highly on subjective discomfort but had stable interpersonal relationships; (*c*) the hustlers, who were frequently involved in other illegal activities and were low on all scores apart from subjective discomfort; (*d*) the bag-followers attached themselves to the dealers to support their own addiction and were generally unstable; (*e*) the touts, who, like the bag-followers, were catering for their own addiction; and (*f*) the workers, who had a legitimate job though some were hustlers. They were the best motivated in the treatment situation. The authors conclude that though addicts share the same withdrawal symptoms, they do not share the same psychological disturbances.

Levine and Stephens (1971) analysed the 'Games Addicts Play' in the street-addict sub-culture of typically heroin-using slum-dwelling minority group members who adhere to a deviant set of values. In order to live without heroin the street addict may have to learn a whole new way of life. In order to get money for his drugs his main occupation is 'conning' and this is translated to his behaviour towards the therapist. The rewards of 'gaming' include: (*a*) a sense of accomplishment and self-worth when a 'good con' is made; (*b*) the excitement of a game, with the absence of rewards, adventure and a battle of wits; (*c*) a sense of power from manipulating someone in authority; (*d*) tangible rewards like passes and early discharge; (*e*) respect and approval of his addict peers; (*f*) a sense of security from feeling he is in control of the situation; (*g*) revenge on anyone whom he regards as a tormentor; (*h*) reaffirmation of his identity as a successful 'con man'; and (*i*) avoidance of responsibility for change.

The therapist must substitute new games to replace the old and be consistent in setting limits if the old games are to be rendered profitless.

There are more general issues. Drug-taking has assumed epidemic proportions in countries which, for years, had only a minor drug problem. The evidence is that on the whole it is bad for the individual and bad for the society, yet there is considerable propaganda for drug taking, and entertainers with convictions for being in possession of drugs are lionized and even honoured. The argument that certain drugs, particularly marihuana, are safe and should be legalized, does not stand up to present evidence, and society will have to take stronger prophylactic measures. It is futile to expect the police to apprehend drug possessors, let alone drug takers, and at the same time allow propaganda in the mass media and 'specialist' magazines free rein. The tobacco manufacturers could legitimately claim that they are being victimized.

BARBITURATE ADDICTION

Barbiturate addiction, though having many features in common with other addictions, has some which are specific particularly in the symptomatology, treatment and in that little recognized condition, barbiturate sensitivity. Armitage and Sim (1960) state:

> In the prevailing state of the law and of medical opinion, Goodman and Gilman's statement (1955) that 'addiction to barbiturates is more serious than that to morphine' has all the force of apparent paradox. Morphine addiction may be easier to induce and this, if true, might justify existing restrictions, but

there is now evidence that once developed addiction to barbiturates carries as great risks for the individual addict and the community.

Morphine has long been known to produce psychological and physiological dependence and a striking withdrawal syndrome. Willcox (1934) believed the same was true of barbiturates, but others disagreed. Thus Gillespie (1934), in a paper on 'The alleged dangers of barbiturates', insisted on the safety of their sudden withdrawal from habituated patients. However, Meyer (1939), in the German literature, described the consequences of such sudden withdrawal as including generalized fits and a toxic hallucinatory psychosis. Kalinowsky (1942) confirmed this and commented, like Meyer, on the resemblance of the barbiturate withdrawal syndrome to delirium tremens.

The reported withdrawal syndromes more often than not affected individuals with multiple addiction to narcotics, alcohol, etc., as well as to barbiturates. Definition under experimental conditions of the role of the barbiturates came from Isbell *et al.* (1950) at the Addiction Research Centre, Lexington, Kentucky. They induced in five volunteers (ex-morphine addicts) addiction to either quinalbarbitone, pentobarbitone (max. daily dosage 1·3–1·8 g.) or amylobarbitone (3·0 g.), taking 53 days or more to reach these levels of intake. Mild intoxication symptoms appeared at daily intakes of 0·5 g. (pentobarbitone, quinalbarbitone) and 2·0 g. (amylobarbitone). Further increases gave rise to more serious intoxications, with frequent accidents–fractures, cuts, incendiary incidents, etc.

Electroencephalogram (e.e.g.) changes included an increased voltage of all components and (from the thirty-first day of intoxication) a diminution and final disappearance of delta activity and increasing predominance of fast beta rhythms. On sudden withdrawal after 8 weeks' dosage, all the volunteers improved transiently, losing their confusion and neurological signs of intoxication (nystagmus, dysarthria, incoordination, etc.). After 12–16 hours, however, they experienced mounting anxiety with tremors and increasing weakness and collapse. Between the second and fifth days of abstinence, four of the five volunteers had from one to three epileptiform fits. About the second or third day, prolonged insomnia ushered in a period of delirium and disorientation and terrifying visual hallucinations lasting up to five days and producing a dangerous degree of exhaustion. In another Lexington paper, Fraser and Grider (1935) urge extreme caution in withdrawing barbiturates from known addicts and advocate reductions of not more than 0·1 g. per day, with e.e.g. control, if possible.

Hill and Belleville (1953) following in the work of Soddy (1947), who had established reaction times as a correlate of accident proneness, measured reaction time and muscular coordination in ten quinalbarbitone addicts. Both showed extreme impairment during intoxication, lasting 10–18 days after withdrawal. Hunter and Greenberg (1954) described three cases of barbiturate addiction simulating hyperinsulinism and stated that barbiturate dependence should be considered as a diagnosis in every case of persistent insomnia, irritability and tension, especially when associated with attacks of anxiety, disturbed behaviour and confusion. Total withdrawal in one of their cases produced two epileptiform fits and an episode of organic delirium.

Fenichel (1945) stated that:

Addicts are persons who have a disposition to react to the effects of alcohol, morphine or other drugs in a specific way, namely in such a way that they try to use these effects to satisfy the archaic oral longing which is a sexual longing, a need for security and a need for the maintenance of self-esteem simultaneously. Then the origin and nature of the addiction are not determined by the effect of the drug but by the psychological structure of the patient.

It is this basic factor in the personality of the addict which links the condition with other impulse neuroses and addiction without drugs such as for food or even socially acceptable activities like hobbies which are frequently taken up with 'passion'. The drugs represent to the patient vital oral libidinal supplies, and their withdrawal is followed by intense feelings of insecurity and rejection while their administration is followed by feelings of comfort, satisfaction and erotic pleasure.

Armitage and Sim (1960) described 19 cases of barbiturate addiction and found there were associated addictions, frequently multiple. These included addictions to other drugs (usually only a psychic dependency being involved), to food in general or to particular foods with a special symbolic value for the patient (often with resultant obesity), to various 'health' rituals, or to alcohol. Seven patients were excessively dependent on alcohol without necessarily being alcoholics in the accepted sense—three of them to a brand of stout widely publicized as 'good for you'. (The theme of nourishment and protection, in short, of 'vital supplies', runs through many of these subsidiary addictions.)

The setting in which addiction commenced was in all patients one of neurotic depression and/or phobic anxiety, against which the addiction represented an attempted, often for a time a successful, defence. It is precisely because of this that it is dangerous to prescribe barbiturates for phobic anxiety states. It is true that some will merely carry a token dose around as a sort of talisman, but the danger of addiction is great. Unfortunately some tranquillizers which are now being used as substitutes for barbiturates are just as liable to lead to addiction, even though they are clinically less effective.

Three patients had lost their mothers in infancy or very early childhood and two more were reared from infancy by other relatives after real or seeming rejection by their natural parents. In most of these families the father was a remote or ineffectual figure, and out of the total of 19 cases only one enjoyed a warm relationship with both parents. In 14 cases there was a clearly identifiable stress preceding and related by the patient to the onset of the addiction. Loss of love, loss of self-esteem, and a physical illness severe enough to be regarded as a real threat, were the main stresses involved. The actual events were broken engagements, or liaisons (three cases), stillbirth or death of a child (two cases), death of a husband or parent (four cases), failure in examination or advancement (three cases) and illness or operation (two cases). All had essentially narcissistic personalities with an undue dependence on the approval of others for the maintenance of their self-esteem and were secondarily dependent on any drug capable of substituting for such approval.

Analytical treatment of individual addicts (Crowley, 1939) has adequately demonstrated the psychopathological principles underlying the condition, namely a pre-genital (oral) regression, and Armitage and Sim (1960) confirm that there emerges from their review, persistent and general support for the existing psychoanalytical concept. Although parenteral forms of barbiturate were available to several patients, all preferred the oral route.

Barbiturate Sensitivity

This was exhibited by three patients, but in their repeated recourse to barbiturates and the recurrence of the precipitating stresses, as well as in their immature narcissistic personalities, they differed little from the other cases of barbiturate addiction. Small and occasional doses had produced severe signs of intoxication (confusion, vertigo, diplopia, nystagmus). According to Isbell *et al.* (1950) it normally requires ingestion, in a single dose, of 0·4—0·7 g. thiopentone to produce these features of intoxication. The relationship between their periodic symptoms and their drug taking had been suspected by none of the patients, in whom previous hospital investigations had resulted in such diagnoses as equine encephalomyelitis, bulbar poliomyelitis, third ventricle tumour, acute schizophrenic reaction and acute labyrinthitis. The author was able to remove his own scepticism only after reproducing the symptoms and signs of intoxication in all three patients by the intravenous injection of 0·05—0·1 g. of thiopentone. These persisted for periods varying from 30 minutes to two days after the injection.

Barbiturate Withdrawal

In an addict this must be carried out with great caution. Armitage and Sim (1960) reported that in the five patients where withdrawal was abrupt, usually because the magnitude of the habitual intake had not been appreciated, four developed fits on the third day and the fifth became delirious on the second day. Further experience with another 6 patients has reinforced these findings. In a total of 11 patients now, sudden withdrawal of barbiturates has invariably resulted in epileptic attacks or delirium. These findings again emphasize the importance of Fraser and Grider's (1953) practice of reducing by not more than 0·1 g./day and using an EEG control.

A common, though not generally recognized source of barbiturate addiction are those preparations which combine a barbiturate, usually amylobarbitone sodium, with dextro-amphetamine sulphate. The error is made because some physicians are unaware of the energizing effect barbiturate has on the addict and fondly imagine that the barbiturate will buffer the effect of the dextro-amphetamine, while in effect it reinforces it. One of the author's patients had for nearly four years taken 1·6 g. of amylobarbitone sodium per day and he used the drug to give him the confidence to travel on buses and get to work. On the day that he had to pass a driving test on his motor cycle he felt more insecure than usual and took an extra 400 mg. and passed with flying colours! This patient when admitted and retained for a few days on 1·6 g./day, showed no signs of barbiturate intoxication, indicating the tremendous degree of habituation that can result and illustrating that though much is known about the pharmacology of drugs in the unaddicted, practically nothing is known about the body's capacity to deal with drugs (and alcohol) in the addicted. Obviously, an entirely different mechanism must operate, for most people after the ingestion of 400 mg. of amylobarbitone could not sit astride a motor cycle, and if this were taken on top of 1·6 g., they would be admitted to hospital in coma.

A useful adjunct to gradual withdrawal of the drug is the prescribing of chlorpromazine 50 mg. t.d.s. and fortunately this measure has in the author's experience not resulted in the substitution of another addiction. Withdrawal of the drug is not the whole treatment; it is just the beginning, for such patients require considerable psychological support as well as environmental manipulation. There is, of course, a distinct possibility that they may become addicted to the therapist, but this is a situation which the experienced therapist should be able to handle. Access to the drug is, of course, an important factor, and the problem is much more difficult in doctors, dentists, veterinary surgeons, nurses and chemists, than in others.

DETECTION OF DRUG ADDICTION

More accurate methods are now being devised and it is apparent that ordinary clinical manifestations are now inadequate to identify the presence of addiction and its nature. This is especially so as multiple addictions are now increasingly common. It is possible with chromatography to identify a variety of drugs through urine and blood analysis, and many biochemical departments in hospital are now being equipped for this purpose.

Laboratory Investigations

Most drugs which are abused can be detected in the urine, the notable exception at present being LSD. Thin-layer chromatography is generally used, though some centres are using gas-liquid chromatography. Urine specimens should be sent by the quickest possible route to the laboratory, and, as the investigation may be complicated by the intake of drugs other than those abused, the pathologist should be given a full history of all medicines prescribed, including antibiotics, for these interfere with thin-layer chromatography.

The referral note should state the interval between the last dose of the drug and the taking of the specimen of urine. For example, if heroin has been taken only a few hours before the specimen is obtained, free morphine will appear in the urine. If 36–48 hours have elapsed the morphine will have been conjugated and hydrolysis will be necessary before analysis of the urine will show that heroin has been taken. Specimens should be adequate in quantity, the best container being a 250 ml. plastic screw-top bottle. In thc United Kingdom this is a dcpartmental issue (CS list 3144) and should be despatched in a hard cardboard box. No additive or preservative is necessary unless analysis for alcohol is required, and in that case a fluoridated oxalated blood tube should be used (Standing Medical Advisory Committee, 1972).

GAMBLING

Such problems rarely come to the psychiatrist but are frequently brought to the notice of the family doctor. One should distinguish between gambling as a social convention and gambling as an addiction. Betting on horses, filling in football pools, going to Bingo sessions are only a few of the gambling activities which have an almost universal appeal. It is when the individual develops a passion for gambling that the borderland between what is generally acceptable and what is potentially harmful is crossed.

The excitement of gambling has been likened to sexual excitement, the feeling of winning to that of an orgasm; that of losing to symbolic castration, and the gambler is constantly giving himself as a hostage to fortune to see what fate is to be his. Luck to the gambler means a continuance of the 'vital supplies' which are so essential to the oral erotic group, which has already been described.

Gambling embraces other deep-seated needs. Winning, particularly at cards, involves a certain amount of sadism and one has only to witness the ruthlessness exhibited by friends towards each other over a game of poker to appreciate this. Losing is just as likely to occur as winning, so the masochistic component is also evident. That close friends should constantly expose themselves to these experiences is very reminiscent of sado-masochistic relationships in the physical field.

Some have seen compulsive gambling as an equivalent to compulsive masturbation. Both are used to relieve tension; both are 'playing at' sexual excitement; both are associated with guilt feelings and fears of punishment; for although the youth believes that masturbation is a certain road to disaster be it insanity, disease or even death, he has this compulsion to invite the gods to make a decision about him. So the gambler cannot refrain from 'trying his luck' knowing that the outcome may be disastrous.

The sexual analogy has even greater relevance for it is known that at times when the individual feels most insecure, is tense or lonely, early forms of gratification like masturbation are indulged. Gambling is therefore more likely to become a problem in the insecure and the lonely or may have even deeper significance such as unconscious hostility to a parent. Gambling also provides a 'fraternity' which is guilt sharing and this can offer powerful competition to less hazardous group activities for vulnerable people.

An organization called 'Gamblers Anonymous' has been started but it is too early to comment on its efficiency.

CHAPTER 9

Psychopathia Sexualis

The title of this chapter is borrowed from Krafft-Ebing's (1894) classic monograph which still stands as a landmark in the medical and scientific literature on the subject. Sexual perversions invariably attract controversy and frequently become a battleground between the liberal and conservative elements of a community. Information of a factual nature is not easy to come by, for there are strong social taboos on the subject which operate paradoxically, in that the ordinary citizen has access to a vast literature which caters for his sexual curiosity and entertainment rather than for his education. The professional worker on the other hand has relatively little opportunity for formal instruction in the elements of the problem and is frequently more ignorant than the people he is expected to help. Yet sexual deviations can cause considerable misery and even tragedy to those who practise them and are therefore a proper concern for the doctor and social worker as well as those scientists whose work brings them into contact with the problem. Before the clinical details can be understood, an adequate knowledge of psychopathology is essential and the student should first read Chapter 2.

As the child has been called a polymorphous pervert, it is not surprising that the sexual instinct in the adult should on occasions manifest some of those early infantile practices, or be directed towards earlier love objects. Society has not been constant in its attitude and while some practices may be tolerated by certain sections, they may be condemned by others and even in ancient times Platonic Greece saw no harm in homosexuality and even extolled its virtues, while Judaeo-Christian ethics regarded it as an 'abomination' and deserving of the severest penalties. This conflict within our society has in this country led to the appointment of a Royal Commission which recommended that homosexual behaviour between adult consenting males should no longer be regarded as a crime, but Parliament initially rejected this recommendation on the grounds that the public was not yet ready for the law to be changed. This decision was by a narrow majority and religious leaders, jurists, doctors and others still vigorously campaigned for reform in the law and though their efforts were not entirely successful, the climate of public opinion which permeates the law courts is now one of tolerance and understanding whereas previously it was hostile and repressive (see Chapter 21).

It was not till the end of the nineteenth century that a noticeable change occurred in public opinion and this was to some extent stimulated by the wide circulation of Krafft-Ebing's book which brought the subject to the notice of the medical profession in a systematic and acceptable form. The writings of Havelock Ellis followed and these served to underline the essential psychological nature of the problem, while the publicity associated with the trial of Oscar Wilde ensured that the subject could no longer be ignored. The work of Freud and the analytical school contributed further to our understanding of the aberrations of the sexual instinct and these became a proper subject for medical research and treatment, while the findings of Kinsey *et al.* (1948, 1953) gave the world some startling information of their nature and incidence.

The word 'perversion' has a moral significance which can produce in the patient a profound feeling of guilt which his conduct may not deserve, for there are numerous factors involved. The most important are early influences on the psychological development of the child, while stress and trigger situations in adult life can often determine overt practice in what had previously been a latent tendency. A number engage in perverse practices out of a spirit of curiosity and experiment in a search for ways to revive a failing libido and should not be regarded as psychopathic, yet the female partner may react with alarm at her husband's new approach to sex and seek medical advice. She may even seek legal advice with a view to divorce, yet these practices rarely become habitual and may merely indicate a temporary embarrassment over the loss of normal sexual desire. Though it may be argued that they are disruptive of marriage, the intention is often the reverse in that they constitute an attempt to maintain a sexual interest in the partner rather than seek stimulation elsewhere. These aberrations are not usually permanent patterns of behaviour but a regression to immature forms of sexual expression in the face of insecurity.

In all sexual activity there is the factor of *appetite* which is at least as variable as that for food and the physician should be familiar with the wide normal variations and what controls them. It is only then that he can reassure the impotent or frigid honeymoon partner, or when faced with a wife's allegations of her husband's excessive appetite, distinguish between satisfied and unsatisfied demand for the latter is frequently paraded as an index of appetite, which it is not. In abnormal sexual practices, appetite may be the major problem and incidentally the one most amenable to treatment for it can be reduced with hormones. The actual form of the perversion is psychologically determined, but psychological treatment for the confirmed pervert who has not voluntarily sought help, but has been referred by the Courts, is frequently disappointing. On the other hand a number of patients with similar problems who were genuinely concerned and had sought help before they were too heavily committed, have benefited materially.

CLINICAL VARIETIES OF PERVERSION

SADO-MASOCHISM

Though at one time regarded as two separate perversions, sadism and masochism are now recognized as parts of the same complex, each component varying in degree or dominance.

Sadism

The term is derived from the Marquis de Sade (1740–1814), a French writer of obscene novels whose main themes were lust and cruelty. It should not be confused with aggression during the sexual act where biting or scratching are accepted as being within normal limits, and it need not be expressed in action but can be confined to phantasies and be an accompaniment of masturbation. In certain individuals the impulse to cruelty which accompanies sexual excitement can become violent and extreme and vary in time relationship—either before, during or after coitus or even as a substitute for coitus. Lust murders which, fortunately, are rare, are usually found in people with sadistic phantasies towards the opposite sex and they run to a pattern which is recurrently reported in the literature. For example, Krafft-Ebing's reports of cases in the 1880's bear a striking resemblance to that which occurred in Birmingham in December 1959. A common object for the sadist is the prostitute who caters for this perversion, and she may run the risk of severe mutilation or even death.

In general, however, sadism in the male is a much milder, relatively innocent act which is part of ordinary love play and as Kinsey *et al.*

(1953) have pointed out, is an essential part of the sado-masochism which is a normal feature of this activity. It is not possible to deal with sadism without introducing masochism for the two are complementary and the following line from *Anthony and Cleopatra* (Act V, Scene ii) illustrates this: 'The stroke of death is as a lover's pinch which hurts and is desired'.

Masochism

This term is derived from the name of an Austrian novelist, Leopold von Sacher-Masoch (1836–95), who described men being dominated by women and who in his private life expressed desires that his wife should be unfaithful to him. The sexual feeling of the masochist is controlled by the idea of being completely and unconditionally subject to the will of a person, usually, but not invariably, of the opposite sex, and of being abused by this person in a humiliating way. It may completely usurp the individual's capacity for normal sexual relations and be a cause of impotence. The conduct may vary from the most repulsive to the most trivial, and while the sadist may progress to serious injury or even murder, the masochist is usually content with suffering pain and humiliation though there are instances where the condition has gone further than that.

Flagellation (beating)

This is the commonest masochistic practice, either self-inflicted or at the hands of others, and here again there is frequently found a duality, in that the partners can change roles, though the passive member may experience reflex orgastic experience because of the stimulation of the nates. Phantasies also loom large in the practice and may be the major form of stimulation. A number of prostitutes retain a suitable instrument (usually a whip) for flagellation and among their clientele there are men who prefer to play 'slave' and demand to be trodden on, scolded or beaten. One of Krafft-Ebing's patients wrote: 'A real masochist, without reflection, prefers the kick of a low woman to the embrace of a Venus'.

In the female, however, the role of subjection is regarded as normal and in a number of societies the humiliation and beating of womenfolk is standard procedure.

Fetishism

Most heterosexual males are aroused erotically when they observe the female body or certain parts of it. If the part which stimulates is far removed from the genitalia, such as the hair of the head, or a foot, this reaction is called fetishism. The further removed the stimulating object from the partner's body, the more pronounced the fetishism is said to be, and favourite objects are underclothes, stockings, shoes, brassières, and at the beginning of the century, garters. Some are aroused exclusively by articles such as high heels, corsets or any form of tight clothing or by objects which suggest sado-masochistic relationships. The perversion is almost exclusively a male one and it is of interest that those magazines which cater for the fetishist are directed exclusively to the male customer. The fetishist may also show sadistic trends as in braid cutting which is regarded by some as symbolic castration. Another aspect of fetishism has been emphasized by Epstein (1960) who has drawn attention to the incidence of temporal lobe disturbance in a number of cases and postulates a theory of a weakness of cerebral integration with the emergence of more immature patterns of behaviour.

Transsexualism

Transsexualism is a condition in which the individual experiences long-standing or permanent sex identity opposite to his physical one. This is frequently accompanied by a persistent desire to have his sex reversed by surgical or hormonal means. Some psychiatrists have tried to distinguish transsexualists from homosexuals, in that the sex identity of the homosexual is consistent with his anatomy, in that he accepts his sex organs and derives pleasure from others being interested in them. The transsexual hates his sex organs and desires to have them removed. There is also an intermediate group which includes those homosexuals who have assumed a passive feminine role and apply for sex transformation surgery to rationalize their homosexuality. Those who advocate sex-change surgery would exclude this intermediate group.

Hoenig *et al.* (1970) studied 46 male and 14 female transsexuals. In only 5 per cent was the syndrome well-established before the age of 14 years but by 19 years 83 per cent of the men and 93 per cent of the women were totally committed. Sexual fantasies in all the women and in 76 per cent of the men were entirely homosexual. Prostitution was confined to the men (31 per cent) and as a group they showed a high degree of educational and work maladjustment and a high incidence of promiscuity.

Aetiology. Genetic and endocrine factors have been excluded in the vast majority. Newman and Stoller (1971), in a study of male transsexuals, consider that the disorder starts in infancy as a primitive and pervasive identification with the mother's femaleness, and that by the third year of life the profound femininity of the future male transsexual is already unmistakable. The oedipal period fails to modify, alter or distort the already existing femininity, and evidence of oedipal conflict is not seen because of abnormalities in the family situation, especially the physical absence and lack of emotional involvement of the father and the continuing symbiosis with the mother. She does little to correct it and may even enjoy his femininity. He is not psychodynamically like the oedipal girl who is romantic, seductive or maternal with her father, but is instead preoccupied with outer aspects of the feminine role.

Is Transsexualism Homosexuality? This is denied most vigorously by the patients, but denial is a common mechanism and denial of homosexuality is well-known to psychiatrists. The argument used by the patients and by psychiatrists who have been identified with them is that, as in normal females, their gender identity is female; as such their love objects are males and this is evidence of heterosexuality. It is certainly evidence of Orwellian 'double-think'. Sexual orientation is generally decided on the love object rather than on the gender identity; if a male selects as his love object a male, that is homosexuality; and this also holds for the female.

If this fundamental point is not lost sight of these unfortunate patients would not be encouraged to seek mutilating operations, which, as Green (1970) points out, they have very little knowledge of, and in addition have crude misconceptions as to what can be accomplished by surgery and the use of hormones. For men, electrolysis is necessary for hair removal, and oestrogen will not raise the pitch of the voice nor necessarily create feminine proportions. In women, testosterone will lower the voice and encourage hirsutism but will not reduce breast size. In addition it may create acne. With respect to surgery, the functional results of genitals are highly unpredictable; the capacity for orgasm may be lost, and sterility is unavoidable. Social, family and occupational problems add to the difficulties, but perhaps the greatest of all is advancing years. A swashbuckling Rosalind very soon gives way to a pathetic neuter and the beautiful young man becomes a freak. It is difficult to see how medical men could lend themselves to such artifices. In England the law has come out against it, and even though a sex change be registered, in terms of a marriage contract and divorce proceedings 'it's the chromosomes that count'.

Kubie and Mackie (1968) recommend that the term 'transsexual' be not used because it implies that many of the basic problems related to gender transmutation have already been clearly faced, studied and solved, which they have not. The wish for a sex change is not all that rare, and with the propaganda of organizations devoted to pathological sexuality, many who were hesitant are declaring their interest. It may also have neurotic or psychotic determinants, though most who request gender transmutation are not psychotic.

Even with the limited information available, not all patients who have undergone surgical changes were unalterably convinced of their membership of the opposite sex. The authors use the concept of tranvestism to illustrate the confusion which can be generated by adherence to a term that does not clarify complex ideas. From a purely descriptive point of view only a few characteristics distinguish 'transsexuals' from the similar individuals who are labelled 'transvestites'.

Tranvestism

This is again basically a homosexual equivalent. Men and women do not dress up to resemble the opposite sex in order to attract the opposite sex. It is to attract their own sex, and this is homosexuality. It can shade into overt homosexuality as well as transsexualism and the present writer sees it as a variation on the theme of homosexuality. One has already accepted passive and active partners; one has already accepted the effeminate male and the masculine female; those that dress up share a similar orientation.

One does not hear of transvestites (male) having sexual affairs with females, though many are married and are able to perform sexually with their wives. This has persuaded some that they are not homosexuals. What is not offered in evidence are the sexual fantasies they elaborate when engaging in sexual intercourse with their spouses, and if they have ever sought a heterosexual love object when they put on the DRAG (DRessed As A Girl). Many male prostitutes are transvestites. As with homosexuality there are all grades paralleled in transvestism, from the partially to the fully committed.

Exhibitionism

This is the displaying of genitalia, usually for the purpose of sexual gratification, though it may be done for other purposes. It is not found as a perversion in women but is frequently practised by them in burlesque, strip-tease shows or privately as a means of exciting or entertaining men. The sexes in this respect behave very differently, for women are not in the least stimulated by the sight of the male genitalia, and though they are well aware of the man's interest in watching them cannot really appreciate why, and some professional nudes are frankly contemptuous of those males who pay to see them perform.

The male exhibitionist is frequently a dullard who is otherwise handicapped in his approaches to girls and his behaviour is a form of courtship. It can also occur in elderly men who because of arteriosclerotic or other organic brain changes lack the control they formerly had and may be goaded into it by curious little girls in the park. Others are of good intelligence and have the compulsion to expose themselves not always with erotic purpose but sometimes in order to shame the onlookers. With them it need not be associated with an erection but when it is, it is not usually done for the purpose of inviting intercourse. Some patients have told the author that if the female had responded, they would have been most embarrassed. There is however a tendency when seeing the patient initially to assume that it is done for immediate sexual satisfaction, but this is usually not so and it frequently has a deeper significance.

Voyeurism

This is a predominantly male perversion and is a means of obtaining sexual gratification by looking at sexual organs or others engaged in sexual activity (including animals). Commercialized exhibitions of sexual activity cater almost invariably for the male and take the form of photographs, drawings, coloured pictures built into novelties like a peep-show, and even live performances, and many of these shows cater for sadistic impulses too by showing women in degrading situations including intercourse with animals. But the majority of voyeurs indulge in secret as Peeping Toms, either going out of their way to perch precariously on a ledge of a high building or casually with binoculars from their bedroom window.

Obscenity

This is defined as the use of words or phrases either by mouth or writing as a means of achieving sexual excitement or inducing it in others. The obscene writings on lavatory walls is called *graffiti*. Words used may retain remnants of magical power and refer to the sexual organs, and masturbation is frequently accompanied by the utterance of these words. The modern adulation of four letter words is an interesting phenomenon. It is alleged to emancipate people by removing inhibitions but it has ignored, or failed to see, that these four letter words were never used in the language of intimate and physically uninhibited lovers. They were (and still are) disparaging and debasing words which when spoken by the male to the female could only offend and insult and if used by the female would relegate her in the eyes of the male to a morally inferior role. That these forms of communication may in fact be used in some circles is not necessarily an index of emancipation but may be that of sadism. That these words were made 'respectable' by their free use in D.H. Lawrence's *Lady Chatterley's Lover* does not detract from the above argument, for Sparrow (1966) has clearly shown the perverse nature of the sexual relationship in that novel, and the intense preoccupation of the gamekeeper with shaming and humiliating his mistress.

Obscene Telephone Calls: Psychodynamics. Nadler (1968) reported on the dynamic forces which underlie the selection of this act as a symptom. The perpetrator is similar in his motivation to the exhibitionist, *i.e.* he attempts to deny, at an unconscious level, the morbid fear of his own inadequacy, and to gain, through the response of others, either positive or negative, a transient sense of power and importance. For his purpose the telephone has special advantages: (*a*) he need not physically confront his victim; (*b*) he can call on his imagination and intellect to provide an awesome picture of himself; (*c*) from a safe distance, he can impinge on his victim more actively than the exhibitionist; and (*d*) he may only present himself but he often menaces and threatens.

Of the three cases quoted by the author, low self-esteem and dependence on the response of others for reassurance were the most striking features. No subject could raise his self-esteem by his own efforts. Each needed to impress someone else, and the 'phone call had a meaning symbolically similar to other exhibitionistic acts, although more aggressive and at a greater distance. They all showed profuse self-depreciation and self-derogation and constant conflict with a grandiose self-concept. Each experienced difficulty in getting close to anyone, and had an almost infantile dependency on, fear of and rage at women, whose approbation could keep intolerable feelings of impotence at bay.

The present author had a patient who started his obscene telephone calls after being seduced by a much older married woman at an office party. He felt she was just amusing herself with him, which was no doubt true, and that she had little regard for his sexual competence, which was probably also true. He felt strongly that he had to revenge himself and prove that he could terrify women. It is unfortuante that these patients tend to come to the psychiatrist after being apprehended, for by then they may have become addicted to the practice.

Pornography

The word pornography derives from the Greek, *pornographos* which means writings about prostitutes, describing the life, manners and customs of harlots and their patrons. It is defined in the *O.E.D.* as 'the expression or suggestion of obscene or unchaste subjects in literature and art'.

In recent years, with permissive changes in the law, there has been an explosion of pornographic literature for sale. The size of the market is difficult to gauge, but some idea can be obtained from the seizure of a copy of a magazine which issued a special lesbian number. The printing was 425,000 copies. As these magazines are passed from hand to hand and are left lying around in men's clubs and barber's shops, thc actual reading public must be immense.

The ready availability of this type of literature has aroused controversy. Some actively campaign against it, claiming that it corrupts minors and fixates adults at a more immature level of psychosexual development. Others claim that it does no harm and that any restriction on its publication is an infringement of the basic rights of members of a civilized society. It is difficult to settle these conflicting claims by surveys or by experiments, for it is likely that the vast majority who are exposed to this type of literature will not be *permanently* affected.

The author has had to advise on three court cases and therefore was obliged not only to read but to study the evidence. The literature was freely illustrated, with frontal nudity a prominent feature. The artistic quality of the pictures and the attractiveness of the subjects varied, and these were not particularly noteworthy from the psychiatric point of view. What was much more revealing was the text, for in practically all instances it was concerned with perverse sexual practices such as homosexuality (male and female), sadism, masochism, group sex or orgies and seduction of minors (male and female). Another revealing feature was the advertisements. These are a useful index of the purpose of the publication, for advertisers are interested only in the promotion of sales, and will select a medium which attracts those who are already interested or who can be won over either by the advertisement or the literature or both. Nearly all the advertisements, apart from those for tobacco and spirits, were for the promotion of perverse practices, and in those magazines which provide a gallery of portraits of those who cater for clients, the activities, apart from prostitution, were mainly perverse, sadism and masochism predominating, with the 'tools of the trade' frequently displayed beside the hireling.

It has been argued that such erotica can stimulate the impotent husband to perform adequately, but they do so by providing perverse fantasies to which he is likely to become habituated, and this cannot be regarded as a sound basis for marital sex, especially as any heterosexual portrayal is almost never between husband and wife. The main question for the psychiatrist is, what effect will such literature have on the young and the immature? Psychosexual development in our culture is a very tender plant, and many fail to achieve maturity. Many are mentally disturbed, and in adolescence particularly, the retreat into fantasy is often a precursor of the schizophrenic process. Pre-occupation with sexual fantasies to the detriment of realistic objectives is already common, and such literature, by providing masturbatory material and fantasy fodder, reinforces the undesirable and could precipitate a complete breakdown of ego-defences. It could, and if court evidence can be relied on, has already propelled some into violent and dangerous practices directed either against themselves as in bondage (see below) or against others. It may not be easy to prove that it does harm; it is even more difficult to show that it does good.

Coprophilia

This is usually extended to urethral erotic perversions as well as anal-erotic ones and in fact the former is the more commonly practised and accounts for those men who secrete themselves in female lavatories. The layman as in the case of the exhibitionist can only see this conduct in terms of normal sexuality and does not appreciate the perverse unconscious motive which is alleged to be an attempt to deny the danger of castration (see Chapter 2). The urethral and anal erotic aspects account for those unfortunates who come to the casualty departments of general hospitals with foreign bodies in urethra and rectum.

Coprolalia

This is a combination of coprophilia, exhibitionism and sadism and consists of a compulsion to utter obscenities. Occasionally the impulse is partially controlled and a form of stuttering results, with explosive noises which resemble the obscene words but are prevented from full expression. This is also a feature of Gilles de la Tourette's syndrome (p. 775). The patient may show coprolalia in Spoonerism form and a classic case was reported by Michael (1957) where the patient was obsessed with the name Huckleberry Finn. It may also take the form of obscene telephone calls where the listener chosen is invariably female and the caller is male. The author had a young man as a patient who had been having an affair with a married woman at his office and she had in fact seduced him. Prior to this he had been continent and his conduct overwhelmed him with shame and resentment and he then developed this compulsion to insult women over the telephone.

Oral Perversions

These are not common and are a form of sex play or serve as an occasional substitute for intercourse, though habitual practice is not unknown. Many prostitutes satisfy their clients with *fellatio* (oral contact with the male genitalia) while a number of men indulge in *cunnilingus* (oral contact with female genitalia) and in Kinsey's series 46 per cent of the women with extensive coital experience had permitted such conduct.

Bondage

'Bondage' is a form of masochism in which erotic pleasure is associated with being humiliated, endangered and enslaved, and with being bound, restrained and rendered helpless to a degree that life is threatened. It results in 50 deaths annually in the United States. Litman and Swearingen (1972) describe two such cases where the practitioners actually intended suicide and they also report on nine men and three women who replied to a newspaper advertisement inserted by the authors. The women were only transiently involved in order to please the sadistic needs of a man. The men had in common the erotization of a situation of helplessness, weakness and threat to life which was then overcome in survival. The perversion was a creative and artistic effort to overcome loneliness, boredom, depression and isolation, and the general sexual orientation was towards homosexuality.

Masturbation

This is self-stimulation of the genitalia to effect sexual arousal and is not in itself a perversion but has in some quarters earned this title partly because, in the male, it is equated with *onanism*. Biblical experts are not yet agreed on what the sin of Onan was, but the probability is that spilling his seed on the ground meant coitus interruptus, though until recently certain churches regarded it as masturbation and its practitioners as sinners.

It is usually an adolescent activity though there are age variations in the sexes, in that females tend to be older and it is common in married or previously married women, but this could be explained by the alternative outlets available to the male. In spite of sex education and a growing literature indicating that it does no harm and in the sexually continent is a natural habit, one frequently meets patients who have profound feelings of guilt associated with the practice and believe they have practised a horrible perversion. It makes one wonder whether sex education at a formal rational level has much to commend it for there is no doubt that to the very person who is in need of help, it does not penetrate.

It is in the phantasies accompanying masturbation that the perverse tendencies are declared and these may be sado-masochistic or homosexual. It is just as well to enquire about masturbatory phantasies when exploring the sex life of the patient for these may provide the only initial clue to the patient's real problem. Compulsive masturbation may occur in the over-conscientious and obsessional and seems to serve as a vehicle for the feelings of guilt the patient bears and leads to further obsessional behaviour in other fields. It is also practised at all ages as a means to relieve tension and promote sleep rather than for any specific desire for sexual stimulation and in these cases the accompanying phantasy life is scanty.

In our present society where much accent is placed on genital stimulation in the young, it is likely to be more frequently practised by the female at an earlier age. It is too soon to say whether this will produce its crop of guilt-laden casualties, if only because the prevalence of drug-taking in those groups that are most likely to indulge may mask such reactions.

Sexual Abuse of Children

Swanson (1968) reported on 25 consecutive cases referred by the courts for psychiatric evaluation because of a sexual offence against a child. This type of offence occurs in a wide range of personality structure and psychiatric diagnosis. The following facts emerged: (1) 75 per cent had primarily adult heterosexual orientation; (2) 50 per cent had experienced disruption of their marital situation; (3) 24 per cent had been treated for psychiatric illness; (4) 20 per cent had previous history of sexual deviation, such as exhibitionism and molesting, for as long as 6 years, and some were classical paedophils; (5) 50 per cent had previous criminal charges; (6) 50 per cent drank excessively; (7) 40 per cent expressed remorse or guilt; (8) the commonest psychiatric diagnosis was personality disorder (68 per cent), and chronic brain syndrome and mental subnormality accounted for 16 per cent; (9) 76 per cent of the victims were known and readily accessible to the offender; (10) in 36 per cent no active resistance was reported, and in 60 per cent the sexual offence took place on multiple occasions with the same victim.

The author stressed that the wide range of psychiatric handicap contradicts the implication in certain sexual psychopath laws that sexual abuse of children is based on a specific psychological problem.

Frotteurism

The term is derived from the French, *frotter = to rub*, and means contact with another person in order to obtain sexual excitement. It must be a very common practice among young people and there is usually no objection by the girl who regards this form of behaviour as a safe and pleasurable form of adventure if the boy is a stranger, or a permissible form of courtship if the boy is known to her. It was commonly practised during the dances of the 1920's and some, like the tango, were particularly notorious for this form of sexual expression.

In the above examples, the practice is not necessarily a perversion. It becomes one when the person has a compulsion to rub up against women in bus queues, crowded stores and the like, even at the risk of detection and being reported to the police. The latter event is uncommon for it is very difficult to prove and it is only when the offender appears in the same place on more than one occasion that a store detective or policeman may arrest him. Such patients may have a history of exhibitionism and are frequently compulsive masturbators whose phantasies are sadistic. The difficulty in detection and the long history make treatment unpromising, though if the basic anxiety can be reduced it is possible to effect some general improvement.

SEXUAL APPETITE

It is impossible to define normal sexual appetite, for, like appetite for food, there are wide variations.

Increase in appetite may be due to: (1) latent homosexuality in male and female. This accounts for the Don Juan type, or the nymphomaniac, who are trying to prove their heterosexuality and can only do so by conquest after conquest. The debasing of the female or the male by conquest and discard also accords with their latent homosexuality. (2) Febrile states, as in early tuberculosis. (3) Manic states in both sexes. (4) Schizophrenic states may also predispose to nymphomanic behaviour. (5) Drugs.

Diminished appetite may be due to: (1) age; (2) other interests; (3) latent homosexuality; (4) loss of interest in partner; (5) depression; (6) debilitating diseases.

Unfortunately, many who are themselves sexually inferior over-compensate by boasting, and a perfectly adequate individual may be disturbed by the braggadocio of the 'bar Casanova'. They may feel they are not satisfying their wives and that she may look elsewhere, and, in a susceptible individual—and many frequent bars—a minor problem, or even no problem, is enlarged or created. Until recently such boasting was confined to men, but now women have entered the scene with their records of orgasms, and the same latent homosexuality can be detected in them as in the men. The surprising thing is that one meets more of this in an age when sex education in all its forms has never been so widespread. One may legitimately ask whether sex can be taught in a rational way and whether society's saturation with all things sexual on films, T.V., and in the other mass media, are contributory factors to this ignorance.

There is a strong lobby to make life even more permissive on the assumption that free participation in sexual intercourse even in the very young is not only a therapeutic measure but is a prophylactic against mental illness. This type of thinking derives from a misreading of Freudian psychopathology, when sexual frustration was believed to lead to intolerable tension with a breakdown in the ego-defences. There is no factual evidence to support this, and there are many instances where exposure to sexual behaviour has been harmful. The present tide is not a new one and will no doubt right itself in time, but not before very large numbers of young people and the not so young will have been damaged mentally and in many instances physically.

Ejaculatio Praecox

Cooper (1969) defined three main types:

1. Habitual premature ejaculation with strong erections, present constantly since adolescence.
2. Acute onset premature ejaculation, generally with erectional insufficiency,

occurring in young men, usually in response to a specific psychological or psychophysical stress.

3. Insidious onset premature ejaculation generally with erectional insufficiency and other evidence of declining sexual responsiveness occurring generally in older men.

Five treatment methods were applied:

1. Muscular relaxation for cases with high levels of coital anxiety and/or strong erections and high levels of sexual tension were the rule (Types 1 and 2).

2. Repeated stimulation and interruption of stimulation according to the technique of Seman (1956). This consists of the female partner providing extravaginal stimulation to the instructions of the male when he is fully roused sexually but non-anxious. It is interrupted when the male indicates that orgasm is imminent, and when feeling has faded stimulation is again started and the process repeated for several occasions thus delaying ejaculation and enabling the lesson to be transferred to intercourse. Masters and Johnson (1970) recommend a different technique: The female lies on top of the male, and, when he is about to ejaculate, she firmly pinches the shaft of the penis between her fingers, causing a reflex interruption of orgasm; when it has been averted intercourse can recommence with further similar interruptions when necessary.

3. Sexual education was especially relevant in Type 2 cases in which ignorance or misinformation was common.

4. Provision of novel and excitatory sexual stimulation was effective, especially for Type 3 who experienced premature ejaculation in a setting of sexual apathy, low responsiveness and poor or absent erection.

5. Superficial psychotherapy placed emphasis on explanation, education, reassurance, support and developing and maintaining motivation.

In his reported 30 male subjects, 13 (43 per cent) were improved, while 15 (50 per cent) were unchanged and 2 (7 per cent) were worse. Acute onset (Type 2) had the best outcome (6 improved after 4 treatment sessions). Habitual premature ejaculation (Type 1) did worst: only one after 10 sessions. Insidious onset (Type 3) occupied an intermediate position: 6 improved after 15 sessions.

The New Impotence

Advocates of social change have argued that when harmful repressions are lifted a more successful adaptation will ensue with improvement in the quality of our lives. Ginsberg *et al.* (1972) point out that rapid changes in social mores may also be reflected in changes in psychiatric symptomatology. They select as their theme the effect of increased sexual freedom of women on their male partners. Because of this cultural shift, young men complain more frequently of impotence and young women complain more frequently of initial impotence in their young lovers. There is a reversal of former roles: that of the put-upon Victorian woman is now the put-upon man of the 1970's. It is not necessarily because of the woman's increased need for sexual pleasure, but could be an unconscious transmission of feminine revenge which, by an aggressive manner, enhances a man's castration anxiety.

Frigidity

This is defined as inability of the female to experience sexual satisfaction. For treatment see *Dyspareunia* (Chapter 6).

DISORDERS OF SEXUAL APPETITE

It is difficult to define a disorder of appetite when there is such a wide range in the normal. The definition of the normal range must be open to question too, for men as a rule tend to boast of their prowess while women are more reliable in their statements. Shortly after the publication of the Kinsey Report (1948) a former colleague of the author decided to check Kinsey's findings on his own university campus by questioning his fellow academics. His wife helped him by questioning their wives. The men gave answers which would indicate that they were leading an extravagant marital sex life while many of their wives could hardly remember the last time they had intercourse with their husbands. Even allowing for the male boaster (and there are many) there remain men who perform regularly most nights of the week while others perform only infrequently, yet they are all within normal range.

There is no point in looking up Ford and Beach (1951) and using their figures as a standard to measure one's patients by. So many factors must be taken into account, such as: domestic stress, type of work, wife's physical and mental fitness, husband's physical and mental fitness, ethical and religious standards concerning contraception, hours of work and a host of others. Also the psychosexual maturity of the person may permit only occasional excursions but this does not mean he or she is necessarily abnormal. It is true that in a society which is strongly motivated towards coitus, those who indulge only infrequently may feel they are abnormal, but before reaching this conclusion, it would be necessary to analyse those who do indulge frequently and with whom. Many who have a strong appetite are of the Don Juan type and their sexual prowess instead of indicating a sexual maturity, is in fact evidence of a latent homosexuality which they try to deny. This is particularly so when the sexual outlet (it is not a true love object) is a changing one.

Increased Appetite

This may be due to:

1. Latent homosexuality in male and female.
2. Febrile states as in early tuberculosis.
3. Manic states in both sexes. The increased motor activity and uninhibited sexual expression with general indefatigability account for the excessive performance.
4. Schizophrenic states. These can predispose in both sexes, but not commonly. Nymphomanic behaviour may be an expression of schizophrenia.
5. Paranoid states. Here the latent homosexuality may act as the driving force, either to prove his masculinity (or in the female, her sexual capacity) or it may provide an outlet for hostility to the opposite sex. In the male this may take the form of debasing the partner.
6. Drugs. Many drugs have gained, but not honestly earned, a reputation as aphrodisiacs and potentiators of sexual desire but it is doubtful if any are effective. On the other hand, some drugs like the amphetamines, when taken in large doses, may precipitate a manic state with its attendant sexual overactivity. Hallucinogens like hashish owe their reputation to their capacity to distort time perception and make intercourse appear to last longer, rather than to their ability to increase sexual desire.

Diminished Appetite

This may range from total impotence to serious diminution in performance. The problem should be seen against the patient's normal practice, for if the appetite has never been great and has not changed, it cannot be said to have diminished.

1. Age. Although some elderly men retain their interest undiminished, their performance rarely matches their ambitions.
2. Other interests. Excessive outside interests and work can withdraw sexual appetite and '*barrister's impotence*' is the name given to a condition which though originally applied to barristers is applicable to a whole range of occupations. The industrial worker or bus driver who is putting in long hours of overtime may react similarly.
3. Latent homosexuality.
4. Loss of interest in partner. This can be a complex problem and may cause or be caused by interest in another. A depressive illness which may remove appetite for the wife may provoke a desire for sexual adventure, though this need not be for sexual intercourse and indeed many perverse interests are roused by this situation.
5. Depression. This is one of the commonest causes of loss of sexual appetite which in some patients is so delicately maintained that even a slight degree of depression may remove it. It can therefore be the first feature of a depressive state and may be the last to go.
6. Debilitating diseases.

HOMOSEXUALITY

With perhaps the exception of the sociopath, there is no individual in our society who creates more confusion and prejudice in the minds of the ordinary citizen than the homosexual. This is partly due to the legal and moral issues involved as well as to general ignorance of the subject. It is only about 60 years ago since Havelock Ellis's publication on homosexuality was pronounced at the Old Bailey to be a 'lewd, wicked, bawdy, scandalous and obscene libel'. There is still confusion, even among doctors, between homosexuality as an orientation or attraction and homosexual practice. In Henry VIII's Act, the offending practice was 'Buggery committed with Mankind or Beast', thus penalizing sodomy (homo- or heterosexual) and bestiality, and it was not till late Victorian times that 'gross indecency', which included all the male homosexual practices such as mutual masturbation, was added.

Historical Background

There are two main streams of influence, Hellenic and Hebraic, though the latter was in accord with those laws of the Roman Empire which were adopted by Christendom. Dickinson (1896), reporting the Greek attitude, states:

Personal affection was not the basis of married life; romance took a different form, that of passionate friendship between men. Such friendships among the Greeks were an institution. Their idea was the development and education of the younger by the older man, and they were recognized and approved by custom and law as an important factor in the state.

In Sparta, for example, it was the rule that every boy had attached to him some elder youth by whom he was constantly attended, admonished and trained. The celebrated 'Theban band', consisting exclusively of pairs of lovers, marched and fought in battle side by side, and by their presence and example inspired one another to a courage so constant and high that it is stated that they were never beaten until the battle of Chaeronea, and when Philip, after the fight, came to the place where the three hundred lay dead together, he wondered, and understanding that it was the band of lovers he shed tears (Plutarch, *Pelopidas*, Chap. 18).

Greek legend and history resound with the praises of friends, names that recall at once all that is most romantic in the passion of Greece. Not only, nor primarily, the physical sense was touched, but mainly and in chief the imagination and intellect. The affection of Achilles for Patroclus is as intense as that of a lover for his mistress (*Iliad* XXIV). It was his insistence on friendship as an incentive to a noble life that was the secret of the power of Socrates.

So much indeed were the Greeks impressed with the manliness of this passion, with its power to prompt to high thought and heroic action, that some of the best of them set the love of man for man above that of man for woman. It is in the works of Plato that this view is most completely and exquisitely set forth; among all the forms of love, that one is chief which is conceived by one man for another. Such a love is the initiation into the higher life, the spring at once of virtue, philosophy and religion.

That there was another side to the matter goes without saying. This passion, like any other, has its depths as well as its heights. Still the fact remains that it was friendship that supplied to the Greeks that element of romance which plays so large a part in modern life; and it is to this, and not to the relations between man and woman, that we must look for the highest reaches of their emotional experience.

Even the Hebraic code which is quoted as the antithesis of the Hellenic, does not frown on strong emotional attachments between men, *e.g.* 'I am distressed for thee, my brother Jonathan . . . thy love to me was wonderful, passing the love of women' (II Samuel ii. 26); and it is only the sodomistic practices that are condemned: 'If a man also lie with mankind, as he lieth with a woman, both of them have committed an abomination . . . ' (Lev. xx. 13). Sodomy later became equated with heresy, and the destruction of Sodom, the city of the plain, has in fact given its name to the practice, though this was not the only or major heresy of which it was guilty. The word 'Buggery' is also linked with heresy for the original Bulgarian heretics regarded marriage and procreation as more sinful than promiscuity and the term *Bougrerie* was applied to their supposed sexual practices and jurists claimed that unrepentant sodomists should be burned like heretics and apostates. It is the unnatural practice of anal intercourse which is mainly condemned but the other modifications of homosexual behaviour were included during phases of rigid legislation and were dropped in more liberal moods.

Psychopathology

In Chapter 2 it has been shown that the child goes through a homosexual phase and in adult homosexuality there is a persistence of this element due to a failure in the normal transformations occurring at puberty; these infantile elements instead of being converted into neurotic symptoms persist in unmodified form. The overt perversion is only the conscious part of a much larger unconscious system and owes its presence to the preservation in consciousness of a specially suitable infantile experience on to which the rest of the infantile sexual pleasure was displaced. This process is called 'division'—by sanctioning the smaller part, the rest has been effectively repressed, so that the perversion actually performs a function very similar to that of an eccentricity. The overt part may have been selected because of its own dynamic strength which made it difficult to repress, or because that particular form of experience was not acceptable to the patient's super-ego, which is really the internalized parental imagos.

From the psychoanalytical standpoint, castration anxiety is the basis of most cases of male homosexuality. There is an awareness that the female has no penis and this in itself implies a threat of castration which may be transferred to the female genitalia. Most homosexuals have an overt or latent fear of the vagina and the term *vagina dentata* has been used to express the castration fear the homosexual may have if he attempts intercourse. This aspect is frequently declared in the dream analysis of latent homosexuals and the author had such a patient who had a recurring dream of having to go down a long corridor on either side of which were caged beasts who were baring their teeth and trying to grab at him with their claws.

There are a variety of interpretations for the choice of the male object or over the type of male. Identification with the mother may encourage the patient to seek out adolescents so that he can adopt the maternal role towards someone he can regard as himself, or it may take the form of trying to obtain sexual satisfaction in the manner of the mother. This attitude could also be interpreted as a passive-receptive one to the father and through anal intercourse it can also represent an attempt at symbolic castration of the father with reduction in the patient's own castration anxiety.

Allen (1962) lists four major factors:

1. Hostility to the mother.
2. Excessive affection for the mother.
3. Hostility to the father.
4. Affection for the father when the father himself does not show sufficient heterosexual traits; introjection of an abnormal father.

Female homosexuality is likewise attributed to the arousal of castration anxiety at the sight of the male genitals. But as the earliest love object of the female is the mother, homosexual orientation can be regarded as a regression to a very early state of sexual development and as Fenichel (1945) has pointed out, it carries more archaic traces than in the male. This is said to account for the female's preoccupation with oral rather than genital stimulation, though there is, of course, a simpler explanation.

Biological Factors

Freud (1905) considered that man was bisexual and leaned towards a biological explanation and though there was some support for this from Steinach (1913) in animals, there has to date been no convincing evidence that biological factors operate. Some of the subsequent observations on animals are not without interest. Tinbergen (1951) has shown that the black-headed gull's 'escape' and 'attack' behaviour during early territorial squabbles is frequently carried over into mating with sexual responses instead of combative ones becoming manifest, and he postulated that these two components may provide a basis for ambivalence. He had noted males mounting males at times of sexual frustration (end of season), particularly when the crouching position of the one bird had triggered this behaviour, although the assaulted male repelled the advance. In monkey colonies, males may 'present' to the dominant monkey who may accept this offer of anal intercourse.

The search for an organic factor in the aetiology of homosexuality continues, but to date all one can report are negative findings. Wortis (1937) could find no abnormality in the body build of homosexuals and Sheldon (1949) could find no distinctive features from somatotype photographs. Coppen (1959) tried to find whether they had an abnormal discriminant androgyny score—an index of body build which is said to be related to the sexual development of the individual. The score is thus computed:

3 x biacromial – 1 x bi-iliac diameters (in cm.);

and the term 'androgyny' is defined as the presence of android features in the female and gynaecoid features in the male. When all the measurements had been taken (the bi-acromial diameter being considered the most significant) the homosexuals approximated closer to the control group than the neurotics or psychotics whose sexual development was not in question (Rey & Coppen, 1959). Parr and Swyer (1960) in a seminal analysis in 22 homosexuals found that eight were highly fertile, four fertile, five borderline, three subfertile and two sterile, and the authors conclude that the clinical diagnosis of 'constitutional type' homosexuality was compatible with a high degree of fertility as judged seminologically.

Most studies on homosexuals are handicapped by 'sampling'. It is recognized that not more than 5 per cent are apprehended by the police and of these probably not more than half go to prison, but it is from prison populations and referrals from Court that the majority of those reported stem. Hemphill *et al.* (1958) made a comprehensive study of 64 homosexuals, the vast majority of whom were persistent offenders (56 were at Leyhill, an open prison without bars receiving prisoners serving from three years upwards and of good behaviour). Urine ketosteroid estimations and a comparison between the androgen/oestrogen ratio of the homosexuals and a control group were not significant. This accords with Stürùp (1948) who found that four sexual recidivists after castration were homosexual while castrated heterosexuals did not relapse. Hemphill *et al.* conclude: '. . . The available evidence is that the direction of libido is influenced by psychological and environmental conditions and possibly a genetic factor, and not by sex hormones, which appear only to modify the intensity of sex activity'.

Genetic Aspects

The evidence varies. Kallmann (1952), in a study of 85 twins of whom 45 were binovular, found that 42·3 per cent were homosexual. Of the 40 pairs that were uniovular all were overtly homosexual, including those who were reared separately. In spite of this evidence he concludes that male homosexuality is an 'alternative minus variant in the integrative process of psychosexual maturation comparable with left-handedness in a predominantly right-handed world'. Penrose (1955) is reported as saying that variations in sexual polarity might be regarded as a perfectly normal trait, comparable with variation in stature, hair pigmentation, left-handedness, or visual refractive error. These traits are all probably dependent upon interaction between heredity and environment, and the variation within all of them is one of degree rather than kind and is an example of a natural and probably inevitable type of biological variation. The examples he quotes, however, do not run up and down a scale in the *same* individual as homosexuality does.

Social Factors

These also vary according to the sample investigated but certain general features are emerging. Kinsey *et al.* (1948) found that about 4 per cent of American men are exclusively homosexual while Curran and Parr (1957) in a consecutive series of 5000 patients in private consultation, found 5 per cent were homosexual. Westwood (1960) points out that most of the information (apart from Kinsey's) comes from those either having psychiatric treatment or who have come into conflict with the law. He reports on 127 self-confessed homosexuals of whom only a small percentage belonged to the above two categories and they are therefore more likely to be representative of the vast majority of homosexuals in Britain. The following points emerge from his study which was by personal interview: (1) 30 per cent came from apparently undisturbed backgrounds; (2) the effects of seduction and early sexual experience have been exaggerated; (3) there were a large number who had a sustained love affair in contrast to the Hemphill *et al.* (1958) series where in 60 cases with valid data 83 per cent were promiscuous and the remaining 17 per cent had a succession of partners; (4) most led useful and productive lives and the least satisfactory were most promiscuous; (5) most homosexuals go unrecognized by the public, being neither effeminate in appearance nor attracted to those who are; (6) less than one-third had anal intercourse regularly as against the Hemphill *et al.* (1958) series where 70 per cent indulged habitually in sodomy; (7) there was no evidence that those who indulged in sodomy were worse types than those who did not (Hemphill's figures would suggest that they tended to be more erratic and unstable); (8) very few adult-seeking homosexuals were interested in pre-pubertal boys; (9) the making of contacts in public is only a small part of homosexual behaviour and is mainly restricted to the inexperienced who have yet to form regular habits of association, and the male prostitutes and blackmailers who associate with them. It is the inexperienced who usually get caught; (10) blackmail was regarded as a serious risk; (11) one-fifth of the series had some heterosexual experience but usually light or intermittent; (12) two-thirds had regular girl friends whom they saw fairly often but only half of this group were sexually attracted; (13) those who had come to terms with their deviation were no longer interested in treatment; (14) there was almost unanimous condemnation of male prostitution; (15) the majority disliked feminine characteristics in homosexuals and they criticized the flaunting of clothes and attitudes—the 'pansy' was regarded as an outsider; (16) they showed some of the characteristics of minority groups with strong intra-group loyalty, and 19 per cent engaged in active proselytism as a measure of retaliation against a society which they claimed failed to understand them.

The rating of homosexuals is now generally on the seven point scale of Kinsey *et al.* (1948), which they emphasize is a graduation and not separate types. The place on the scale depends on the amount of overt homosexual experience and the psychic reaction to sex factors. It is impossible to divide people into two categories, homosexual and heterosexual, as people can move to one or the other, and many are in fact bisexual. The ratings are: 0 = exclusively heterosexual, no homosexual experience; 1 = predominantly heterosexual, only incidentally homosexual; 2 = predominantly heterosexual, but more than incidentally homosexual and so on to 6 = exclusively homosexual. A number become homosexual *faute de mieux* and this is (or has been) recognized by some navies where buggery was no longer an offence once the ships had left port.

At times it can assume epidemic form, particularly where men are living together with no access to women and are generally isolated. This occurred on lonely air stations and in prisoner of war camps during the last war. It was not unknown for a partner in one of these 'Stalag marriages' as they were called to refuse repatriation on medical grounds by the International Red Cross, as he did not wish to forsake his homosexual lover for his wife and children who awaited him in England. People can move up and down the Kinsey scale and opportunity is an important factor in determining in which direction the traffic will flow. Stanley-Jones (1947) put this graphically:

> **. . . To commit a cultured invert to the soul-crushing durance of a long term of penal servitude, when his only contact with the opposite sex is an occasional sight of the prison charwomen, is as futile from the point of view of treatment as to hope to rehabilitate a chronic alcoholic by giving him occupational therapy in a brewery. . .**

Passions run high over the problem of homosexuality. Liberals and reformers plead eloquently for its consideration as a normal and harmless practice, and at the other end of the scale Sunday newspapers campaign against 'she-men'. The persistent recidivist is of course a bad advocate, yet it is he who is paraded before the public with great regularity as typical and as has already been said, most knowledge, including that of the medical profession, is about this small group. On the other hand there are some (probably many) highly cultured persons who are homosexuals and it offends many of their friends and admirers that they should be considered criminals. Society's attitude is in itself bound up with the problem, for in addition to Kinsey's rating, psychopathologically all society is homosexual, repressed (and presumably normal), latent (and presumably vulnerable) and overt. Much of the blind prejudice exists among the latent. The overt stir the basic insecurities of the latent who, if they happen to be in a position of authority, may react with extreme hostility.

There are groups of homosexuals who flaunt their perversion in public by their dress, behaviour and talk and unfortunately the public frequently regards them as representative of all homosexuals in the country. It is difficult to see what effect a liberal change in the law would have on these groups, but should it lead to an increase in their number and encourage them in their behaviour, even at present levels, public tolerance may be over-extended. It is likely that the fluctuations in this country's attitude to homosexuality are due to the difficulty in striking a balance in legislation and the over-enthusiastic reformer must take his share of the blame.

The Female Homosexual

In all this controversy the female homosexual or lesbian has not yet been mentioned, not that she doesn't exist, but because her conduct does not bring her into conflict with the law, though she does occasionally present for psychiatric treatment. There is a comprehensive review of its incidence in society as well as its manifestations by Kinsey *et al.* (1953) and there is a very courageous paper by an anonymous female written as part of a series sponsored by the *Lancet*—Disabilities No. 34. Homosexuality (1949). She describes her experiences and how the relationship she had both enriched and impoverished her morally, *e.g.*

> . . . a passive friendship with a colleague flowered into a devotion that gradually absorbed my whole being, until even my identity seemed to merge with hers. We were never lovers, nor was homosexuality discussed between us, for I knew this would have repelled her, but we became inseparable friends . . . In our brief companionship much that was shoddy and second-rate in me fell away under the stimulating influence of this friend . . .

The friend later died of tuberculous pneumonia.

> . . . In this twilight mood I chanced to meet a middle-aged sophisticated woman, who must have been drawn towards me by that attraction which Proust describes as existing between homosexuals. It was with this woman I first experienced sensualism as such, for there was no love between us, only an overpowering physical attraction. With so little mutual regard, the affair soon fizzled out, leaving me still lonely and bereft, but with a new and fearful understanding of what I could become . . . . I decided to concentrate entirely on work, and this I did with renewed energy and with some ambition. I was nearly thirty before I stopped to consider my position again. I knew I was physically attractive and feminine in appearance and I decided to find out something about the world of men. I set out to overcome my physical revulsion from them, and this I succeeded in doing. Experience taught me, though, that this is not everything, for though I learnt to enjoy men physically, emotionally and sentimentally, my satisfaction was still with women. I came to the conclusion that the pattern was too firmly imprinted ever to alter. Once I realized this, I knew also that it was wrong to use my relationships with men as a form of psychotherapy, and I ceased to do so.
>
> Now I believe I have learnt to live with myself, and am reasonably well adapted to my limitations. I have work which I love, and many outside interests in books, music and travel. I have friends of whom I am fond and in whose companionship I am reasonably happy . . . .

Kenyon (1968 *a* & *b*) reported a series of studies on female homosexuals, and some of the details he lists are of interest:

(1) More lesbians had a university education, but more had a poorer work record than controls and proportionately more were in Social class II; (2) there was a greater rejection of religion; (3) fewer were members of a Women's Institute and more had been in the armed forces or police; (4) More (21 per cent) had a poor relationship with their mother and 35 per cent had lost their mothers at the time of the study; (5) More (30 per cent) had a poor relationship with their fathers and fewer (46 per cent) rated their parents' marriage as happy, with a higher incidence of separation and divorce (23 per cent); (6) a positive psychiatric history occurred more frequently in the mothers (15 per cent) but not in the fathers and there was a family history of homosexuality in 24 per cent; (7) apart from a higher incidence of being adopted (6·5 per cent), ordinal position in the family was not significant, but fewer lesbians (56 per cent) reported a happy childhood; (8) more had a positive psychiatric history (19 per cent, controls 6 per cent), the commonest syndrome being depression but only 5 per cent required in-patient treatment; (9) 28 per cent thought parents would have preferred a boy (controls 10 per cent); (10) first awareness of homosexual feelings at mean of 16·1 years (± 5·3 years); (11) first physical experience 21·4 (± 7·6 years); (12) a liking for male clothing in 42 per cent (controls 2 per cent); (13) 29 per cent felt fully feminine (controls 97 per cent).

As with the male, opportunity is an important factor and the condition can become epidemic in the women's services and in institutions where women live and work together. Some adopt a 'masculine' role and may dress and cut their hair accordingly and get jobs where slacks are habitually worn, *e.g.* as railway porters and bus conductresses, but such behaviour has already reached the state of transvestism.

Treatment

It is not possible in the light of modern experience of the problem to specify that any particular form of treatment is indicated in every case. The British Medical Association (*British Medical Journal*, 1955) lists four categories of patients with the appropriate treatment for each category:

1. Well-compensated homosexuals of good character, often greatly helped by psychotherapy.
2. Relatively intact personalities, otherwise well socialized, including young men who have little scruple in living partly at the expense of older homosexuals, and their older counterparts who are promiscuous, but usually know how to avoid blackmail or contact with the law. They are most effectively deterred by the threat of punishment.
3. Young adults and adolescents who require protection from effects which might delay their transition through a temporary phase. Here psychiatric and social treatment could help: hormone sedatives are valuable for short periods only. Approved schools and borstals may help them to mature, but repeated imprisonment may induce a sense of futility and recklessness.
4. Seriously damaged personalities, sometimes intensely lonely, shy and

inadequate persons whose only affectionate and social contact may be in fleeting lavatory offences or minor play with children. Others may be of a very effeminate and essentially narcissistic 'make-up' who like to be admired and feather their nest, and others again may be anti-social and often aggressive characters, with a mixture of other perversions, especially fetishism and sadomasochism, with homosexuality.

The memorandum states that analytical psychotherapy should be used only if the patient is intelligent, young, able to talk about his problem and have the persistence and desire to carry on with treatment. The aims of non-analytical therapy are '. . . to correct those factors in the environment which are producing stress, to relieve anxiety, reduce misunderstanding, and improve insight by some shorter form of psychotherapy . . . ' Group therapy is also recommended, particularly for those in prison. Although these four categories are meant to be comprehensive, it is not difficult to see that they cater in the main for those patients whose problems have brought them into conflict with the law. But these are only a small proportion of all homosexuals, most of whom are genuinely concerned about their orientation.

Psychotherapy

There is far too much pessimism over the results of psychiatric treatment of homosexuality and this has been given wide publicity in the Wolfenden Report (1957) which states: 'We were struck by the fact that none of our medical witnesses were able, when we saw them, to provide any reference in medical literature to a complete change of this kind', referring to a change in the sex object from male to female. Hadfield (1958) does not accept this view and writes: 'The implication of this statement should not remain unchallenged; for it encourages the view that homosexuality is incurable. There must be many medical psychologists who could point to cures of this radical kind'. He argues that because the love object is a person of the same sex, many have jumped to the conclusion that it must have a constitutional basis, but in fact homosexuality differs little from other perversions such as fetishism for objects like corsets or patent leather shoes which could not be regarded as a constitutional propensity. Hadfield says that cure is not (1) the normal transition from the homosexual to the heterosexual phase in adolescence; (2) the ability of the homosexual merely to *control* his propensity, whether on moral grounds or fear of punishment; (3) loss of homosexual desire because of religious conversion, but without full heterosexuality; (4) the ability to have heterosexual relations for these may be achieved through homosexual phantasies. He defines 'cure' as the loss of propensity to one's own sex and its direction to the opposite sex and places on record a number of patients who were cured by psychotherapy of an analytical nature.

The problem may first present when the young man is starting to court and finds he is not 'normal'. Anxiety mounts and this drives the patient back to earlier sexual patterns. Relief of anxiety with analytical interpretation of dreams or situations need not be particularly lengthy and what initially would appear to be a most formidable therapeutic problem tends to settle rapidly. It is important to take into account the masturbatory phantasies for not only do they give an index of the grade of homosexuality, but are useful pointers to progress during treatment. The first sign of improvement may be the substitution of heterosexual for homosexual ones. Phantasies may loom large in psychotherapy and reveal other perverse components, particularly sado-masochism, but these too can settle with relief of anxiety and gain in insight, for such patients are usually young and frequently have guilt feelings over their orientation or conduct.

Psychotherapy for Sexual Deviation. Rosen (1968) defines sexual deviation as 'a habitual departure from normal biological development with adult heterosexual intercourse and procreation as the aim'. Prior to starting psychotherapy it is important to delineate: (1) factors producing the deviation; (2) symptoms or character of the deviant acts; (3) factors preventing a return to normal sexual expression.

Psychotherapy has three tasks: (1) revealing and removing the functional antecedents and defences; (2) inducing the patient to give up a pleasurable and necessary sexual practice; (3) actively fostering development towards heterosexual intercourse by removing the phobic barriers and encouraging heterosexual experiences in reality. It is important, as in psychotherapy in other situations, that the patient be well-motivated. Out of 100 homosexuals, 27 per cent became heterosexual, and this highlights a point which is frequently overlooked, namely, that well-motivated homosexuals do respond to psychotherapy.

The author has found that in well-selected patients a very useful graduation to heterosexual interest and successful marriage can be achieved with psychotherapy, which need not be very prolonged or intensive, though based on psychoanalytical theory. A better guide to prognosis than overt behaviour, are the masturbatory phantasies. If these are even occasionally heterosexual, it is well worth while undertaking psychotherapy. Motivation is equally important and patients should renounce their homosexual interests and practices while undergoing treatment. This may temporarily heighten their anxiety but this can act as a stimulus to the therapeutic situation.

Drugs

Those most commonly used are the oestrogens (stilboestrol and ethinyl oestradiol) which do not affect the basic orientation but do generally reduce or abolish the appetite. There is one disadvantage in that they frequently cause enlargment of the breasts and this has in some instances converted homosexuality to transvestism and even prompted a few to seek surgical intervention to create what they fondly hope is a true sex change. Apart from the financial gain from newspaper articles or from books, there are no psychological or medical advantages and any request for medical help in effecting these changes should be resisted.

Cyptroterone Acetate in Deviant Hypersexuality. This is a powerful new synthetic anti-androgen and progestogen with anti-gonadotrophic effects. Dosage is 100 mg. daily in a single morning dose. Cooper *et al.* (1972) report its use in a 40-year old psychopathic male with a history of uncontrollable deviant sexual behaviour (attempted incest, homosexuality, transvestism, fetishism and compulsive masturbation). He was required to masturbate to his favourite fantasies at 3.30 p.m. each day without fear of interruption and in the security of a single room. After 7 days' medication the patient was unable to masturbate to orgasm and ejaculation. On the 8th day his erection was poor and the volume much reduced. Three weeks after stopping the drug sexual responsiveness had returned to pre-trial levels. There were no side effects or toxic manifestations, no evidence of feminization, and both clinical and endocrine effects were completely reversible after three weeks.

Castration, though practised in some countries for persistent offenders, has nothing to commend it; it does not even reduce sexual appetite and certainly does not affect the homosexuality.

Electric Aversion Therapy. Bancroft and Marks (1968) reported on the treatment of 40 male patients: 16 homosexuals, 3 paedophiliacs, 14 transvestites and transsexuals, 3 fetishists and 4 sadomasochists. Shocks were given to the forearm from a battery-operated shock box, the level of the shock being decided by the patient. Erections were measured by a penis plethysmograph and each had two sessions daily for 20–30 sessions. All patients were highly motivated, and after 1 year's follow-up 6 (15 per cent) were free of their perversion and 23 (57 per cent) claimed they had improved. Transvestites, fetishists and sadomasochists improved most, but transsexuals and homosexuals did badly.

Prophylaxis

This is always referred to as the most important aspect of treatment. To be effective, it should imply a thorough understanding of the problem and the factors influencing it. Platitudinous statments about the good clean life, moral values in the home, and sex education, have been freely voiced for generations with no apparent benefit and one should not confuse what is good with what is good for sexual perversion. There is no evidence that all these highly desirable features make any impact on the problem and they ignore its essential nature. It is an aspect of the development of the sexual instinct and is the heritage of all. It does not die, but is always present, albeit unconsciously, and can seek expression in sublimation. One should realize that society has always accepted that a number of people may not be very interested in the opposite sex and that some will prefer the company of their own sex. Some professions tend to attract homosexuals either latent or overt and it is quite understandable that if a latent homosexual is working as a schoolmaster in a boys' school, and is exposed to temptation or seduction, he may succumb. The same applies to women but it should be made clear that the vast majority of teachers are effectively repressed, and if latent, are sufficiently secure not to lapse. If this were not so, the occasional lapses would not have the news value they do. If a person feels insecure, it would be folly to put himself in a situation which may prove too much for him and it is in this respect that advice from the family doctor would help. A move from a boys' to a mixed school (with mixed staff) may give him the support he needs.

It is claimed that most homosexuals develop their susceptibility in infancy and that parental attitudes are frequently responsbile. Maternal courtship of her 'little man' may interfere with the handling of the Oedipus situation and perversion becomes a means of establishing a compromise with the sex drive. Whether it is possible by special efforts in parent guidance to avoid some of these pitfalls remains to be seen. It would be difficult to effect and even more difficult to assess, yet there would appear to be no alternative now that it is recognized that most if not all homosexuals become fixated in childhood. It is not a simple matter to initiate a prophylactic programme which will cater for the susceptible, for it is frequently the less vulnerable who seek help while the more vulnerable go unrecognized. The most one can do is to help those who can be reached and even then, the necessary skills for recognizing the problem and dealing with it are sadly deficient; and so, the numbers remain high with early prophylaxis an unfulfilled wish. It is still the family doctor who will have to gain the confidence of his adolescent patient and help him over life's hurdles but with more adequate training in these matters, his role can be a very effective one.

CHAPTER 10

Psychopathic Personality

A generally acceptable definition of psychopathic personality is still elusive and the heading of Curran and Mallinson's (1944) comprehensive chapter on the subject, *viz.* 'I can't define an elephant, but I know one when I see one', points out both the variety of recognizable features and the semantic difficulties. The chapter was written when they were serving psychiatrists in the Royal Navy in World War II, and were dealing with a highly disciplined society. Conduct which offended this discipline, particularly if persistent and outside the usual and acceptable forms of mental illness was frequently labelled psychopathic. Such problems are, however, not confined to the Services, and there are many in civilian life who do not appear or even claim to be ill, yet who are unable to conform with or accept the code of behaviour of the society in which they live.

People have behaved like this from time immemorial and their actions have been recorded and their failings recognized. In Genesis there are several examples, beginning with the corrupting effect of the serpent in the Garden of Eden and rapidly followed by the murder of Abel by his brother Cain who, however, expressed some feelings of distress: 'My punishment is greater than I can bear' (Gen. iv. 13) and he was given a commuted sentence which spared his life. This could be regarded as the earliest example of the principle of diminished responsibility and it is again emphasized in the story of the Flood: '. . . I will not curse again the ground any more for man's sake; for the imagination of man's heart is evil from his youth . . .' (Gen. viii. 21). It is this recognition of the 'evil spirit' in man from his childhood which is the basis of the medical study of and responsibility towards the psychopath.

In the modern era of psychiatry which started with Pinel, it is not surprising that he too was soon confronted with the problem of what he called *manie sans délire,* which included those patients who behaved in an irresponsible way without suffering from any established form of mental illness. It was, however, J.C. Prichard (1835), the Gloucestershire physician, who is credited with the first concept of 'moral insanity' and is quoted by Maughs (1941) as saying:

> ... the moral and active principles of the mind are strongly perverted or depraved; the power of self-government is lost or greatly impaired and the individual is found to be incapable not of talking or reasoning upon any subject proposed to him, but of conducting himself with decency and propriety in the business of life.

This excellent definition has not deterred a spate of others which are listed by Curran and Mallinson.

DEFINITIONS

1. Kahn (1931):

> It is impossible to give an exact definition of psychopathic personality (P.P.). By P.P's. we understand those discordant personalities which, on the causal side, are characterized by quantitative peculiarities in the impulse, temperament and character strata and in their unified goal striving activity are impaired by quantitative derivatives in the ego and foreign variations.

2. Schneider (1934):

> P.P's. are those abnormal personalities who suffer from their abnormality or from whose abnormality society suffers.

3. White (1935):

> Psychopathic as a prefix has come to be a wastebasket into which all sorts of things have been thrown. Society has developed machinery—more or less ponderous and creaking and ineffective to be sure, but nevertheless based upon fairly concrete formulations—for handling the so-called insane at one end and the so-called criminal at the other. The psychopaths fall between. They belong in neither group, and they get into either more or less by accident.

4. Henderson (1939):

> The exact term we use is perhaps not very material so long as we define what exactly we mean, but personally I prefer to use the term psychopathic state because it does not stress unduly either innate or acquired characteristics, and does not imply total mental unsoundness, defect or delinquency, but yet allows for modifications of all of them ... it is the name we apply to those individuals who conform to a certain intellectual standard, sometimes high, sometimes approaching the realm of defect but yet not amounting to it, who throughout their lives, or from a comparatively early age, have exhibited disorders of conduct of an anti-social or asocial nature, usually of a recurrent or episodic type, which, in many instances, have proved difficult to influence by methods of

social, penal and medical care and treatment, and for whom we have no adequate provision of a preventative or curative nature. The inadequacy or deviation or failure to adjust to ordinary social life is not a mere wilfulness or badness which can be threatened or thrashed out of the individual, but constitutes a true illness for which we have no specific explanation.

5. Cheney (1934):

P.P's. are characterized largely by emotional immaturity or childishness with marked defects of judgment and without evidence of learning by experience. They are prone to impulsive reactions without consideration of others, and to emotional instability with rapid swings from elation to depression, often apparently for trivial causes. Special features in individual psychopaths are prominent criminal traits, moral deficiency, vagabondage and sexual perversion. Intelligence shown by standard intelligence tests may be normal or superior, but on the other hand, not infrequently a border-line intelligence may be present.

6. Levine (1942):

They tend to act out their conflicts in social life, instead of developing symptoms of conflict in themselves.

A most important feature which many of these definitions avoid is the relative or complete **absence of a sense of shame or guilt** associated with the antisocial conduct.

CLASSIFICATION

Having reviewed the definitions, Curran and Mallinson review the classification which is even more complex.

1. Kraepelin (1909–13): The excitable, the unstable, the impulsive, the eccentric, the liars and swindlers, the anti-social, the quarrelsome.

2. Partridge (1930): *Inadequate*–(*a*) insecure, (*b*) depressive, (*c*) weak-willed, (*d*) asthenic. *Egocentric*–(*a*) contentious, (*b*) paranoid, (*c*) explosive, (*d*) excitable, (*e*) aggressive. *Criminal*–(*a*) liars, (*b*) swindlers, (*c*) vagabonds, (*d*) sexual perverts.

3. Schneider (1934): (*a*) Hyperthymic, (*b*) depressive, (*c*) self-insecure, (*d*) fanatics, (*e*) attention-seeking, (*f*) temperamentally unstable, (*g*) explosive, (*h*) insensitive or anti-social, (*i*) weak-willed, (*j*) asthenic.

Many other classifications are available and there is considerable overlap which is sometimes concealed by using different words, *e.g.* Menninger (1941) lists (*a*) the predatory, (*b*) the sycophantic, (*c*) the histrionic, (*d*) the façade, (*e*) the transilient.

The classification used by the British Army during the Second World War was based on that of the American Psychiatric Association and was sufficiently comprehensive to accommodate the majority of the very large number referred to the psychiatrist, *e.g.*

(*a*) **With pathologic sexuality**–indicate symptomatic manifestations, *e.g.* homosexuality, erotomania, sexual perversion, sexual immaturity.

(*b*) **With pathologic emotionality**—indicate symptomatic manifestations, *e.g.* schizoid, cyclothymic or paranoid personality and emotional instability.

(*c*) **With asocial or amoral trends**—indicate symptomatic manifestations, *e.g.* anti-sociality, pathologic mendacity, moral deficiency, vagabondage, misanthropy.

Henderson's (1939) classification is rather different from the others in that he has only three groups: (1) predominantly aggressive, (2) predominantly inadequate and (3) predominantly creative, and in the last group he included Joan of Arc and Lawrence of Arabia. While this classification has given rise to considerable debate, it does at least emphasize the personality and not the social offence.

CRITERIA OF PSYCHOPATHY

These, unfortunately, vary from observer to observer and again there is considerable overlap but those of Cleckley (1950) are sufficiently comprehensive to convey the range.

Superficial attractiveness, cleverness, facility in talking and often apparently good intelligence; freedom from psychotic and more marked psycho-neurotic symptoms; unreliability and irresponsibility; disregard for truth and honesty; unwillingness sincerely to accept any blame; absence of shame; cheating; lying, thieving often for trivial gains; poor judgment concerning his own welfare; inability to learn by experience; egocentricity; poverty of affect; inability to see himself as others see him; inadequate responsiveness to special consideration or kindness; shocking or fantastic episodes of behaviour often associated with a drinking bout; infrequent sincere suicidal attempts; tendency to create scenes and situations so bizarre and untimely as to seem purposeless; sexual abnormalities, *e.g.* promiscuity; the manifestations of psychopathic behaviour may begin at any time, not necessarily in childhood; lack of perseverance; repeated failure to make good.

AETIOLOGY

As with other forms of mental illness, where there is no well-defined and substantiated cause, theories abound, some based on evidence and some mere hypotheses and these are listed below, together with some critical notes.

Constitutional

It is still popular to attribute aberrant behaviour to constitutional factors even though reliable evidence in the majority of instances is still lacking.

Epilepsy and Brain Damage. Studies have been made on two groups: (1) Epileptics in general, (2) Criminals who are epileptics. In the former there is no evidence that they are particularly prone to antisocial conduct and as Scott (1966) points out neither do they show any particular predilection for murder, rapine or arson and most such offences are not committed by epileptics. Non-institutionalized epileptics have the same incidence of crime as the general population and their crimes are not heinous. Juul-Jensen (1964) reporting on epileptics in a department of neurology found the frequency of crime among males (9·5 per cent) and females (1·9 per cent) identical with that in the general population and there was no correlation between seizures and criminal acts. Scott himself found that out of all admissions to a boys' remand home where magistrates sent 'difficult' cases, the incidence of epilepsy was very close to the general population of boys in a similar age group. Lennox (1943) who surveyed the histories of 5000 epileptics found that not one had been involved in a serious crime of violence.

More positive evidence of constitutional aetiology is provided in the explosive psychopath, and Williams (1941*b*) states:

> An abnormal EEG in an otherwise normal subject is strong evidence of an inborn constitutional abnormality involving the central nervous system. This abnormality appears to be non-specific, and may manifest itself in the subject or his offspring as a behaviour disturbance which may be psychoneurotic, psychopathic, psychotic or epileptic in type.

Gallagher *et al.* (1942) concluded that if the EEG fell within normal limits the chances were that the personality would be normal. Hill and Watterson (1942) stated:

> It is with aggressiveness that the EEG shows the consistent abnormality. The more aggressive the patient, the more likely is the EEG to be abnormal . . . one can have little doubt that an abnormal EEG constitutes for its possessor a handicap in the business of biological adaptation, failure of which may show itself as in our present series, in undesirable social behaviour.

They summarize their own and Williams' (1941*b*) findings in the following table:

Category	*Abnormal EEG*
Highly selected flying personnel	5 per cent (Williams)
R.A.M.C. personnel	10 per cent (Williams)
Mixed controls	15 per cent (Hill & Watterson)
Mixed psychoneurotics	26 per cent (Williams)
Inadequate psychopaths	32 per cent (Hill & Watterson)
Aggressive psychopaths	65 per cent (Hill & Watterson)

These authors favoured the concept of 'cortical immaturity' in that the EEGs of aggressive psychopaths resembled those of young children. There is however quite a difference between the presence of fits and an EEG record which is frankly epileptic, and the 'abnormal EEG' which is frequently an indication of emotional immaturity. One might even argue that the presence of fits acts as a safety valve for disturbed and aggressive behaviour, but it is more likely that there is no real connection between the aggressive psychopath and epilepsy.

Biochemical and Endocrine

As has been pointed out with epilepsy (p. 185) certain biochemical changes can induce a cerebral dysrhythmia with associated behaviour disturbance. Hill and Sargant (1943) reported a case where the EEG became abnormal whenever the blood sugar fell below 100 mg. per 100 ml. and who had been referred because of a psychopathic outburst during which he had murdered his mother. Islet cell tumours of the pancreas are notorious for presenting with disturbed behaviour and a very respectable headmistress of a girls' grammar school was referred to the author as a hysterical psychopath, because of her repeated histrionic outbursts but who on investigation satisfied all the criteria for an islet cell tumour, which was later removed with consequent recovery.

Wittkower and Wilson (1940) found psychological maladjustment four times more common in dysmenorrhoeic women than in a control group. It need not be associated with dysmenorrhoea and is in fact more common in pre-menstrual tension which may be associated with violent outbursts and impulsive delinquent acts.

Prenatal and Perinatal Factors

Most of these studies have been on delinquent children the majority of whom would not necessarily become adult psychopaths, though many adult psychopaths have a history of childhood delinquency. Stott (1957) using retrospective data implicated shock, anxiety and stress in the mother during pregnancy as significant factors in the aetiology of maladjustment in the child. McCord and McCord (1959) could find no such relationship and neither could a number of other workers and Scott (1966) concludes that if such pre- or perinatal factors play any part in the causation of delinquency it is a very small and indirect one.

Genetic Aspects

Abnormal sex chromosome complements have been found to be 5 times greater in mental deficiency institutions than in the new-born population (Court Brown, 1962). As many of these inmates are institutionalized following antisocial acts such as larceny, fire-raising and indecent exposure, it is suggested that the abnormal sex chromosome complement may predispose an individual in a particular environment towards delinquency. Comparable findings have been reported from criminal institutions for the subnormal in Sweden (Forssmann & Hambert, 1963) but Wegmann and Smith (1963) in a study of delinquents in American reformatories, found no such correlation. It would appear therefore that only in the presence of mental deficiency *in males* is there a high correlation between the abnormal sex chromosome and crime.

Psychological

This has a very specific meaning to the psychoanalytical school. Fenichel (1945) in discussing thc 'impulse neuroses' denies that impulsive characters are happy narcissistic psychopaths with no super-ego and are thus able to achieve gratification without considering the feelings of others. Lack of stable object relations in early childhood with oral fixation may prevent the establishment of an effective super-ego and this is borne out by the history of many psychopaths (see below). They can develop frustrations and react to them, but the super-ego is not absent but rudimentary or even pathological. Chronic dissatisfaction may be the main feature in the less severe cases and they constantly seek change and new and 'exciting' experiences to satisfy their chronic need, and Fenichel calls them 'hypersexual and hyperinstinctual' because they are usually dammed up. The more severe cases 'are governed by oral and cutaneous fixations, by extreme ambivalence toward all objects, by the identity of erotic and narcissistic needs, and by conflicts between rebellion and ingratiation'. In this the Oedipus complex and its solutions are disorganized and some have never learned to develop stable object relationships.

Donnelly (1964), while subscribing to the strong oral dependencies of psychopaths, emphasizes their lack of a strong super-ego and a sense of guilt. He postulates that removal of the original object which catered for these dependency needs permits and even compels the energies of hostile emotions hitherto bound to that object to be directed to other activities. These are usually socially constructive but in psychopaths they are generally antisocial and though the precipitating factor, such as death of a parent, may be the same, the resultant behaviour may be very different.

Reich (1925), in his classic *Der triebhafte Charakter* and quoted by Fenichel, describes the 'isolation' of the whole super-ego. Ordinarily the ego either submits to the super-ego or effects some compromise; in the impulsive psychopath, the ego keeps the super-ego at a distance and is free of its inhibiting influence when tempted so that the impulse is acted upon before the super-ego can become operative. He does state that remorse is felt later and in this respect these patients differ from those who have no sense of shame or guilt before, during or after the event. His theory does help in the understanding of these unfortunate offenders who are guilty of impulsive acts such as kleptomania, or indecent exposure. Some patients have a tendency to 'act out' their neurotic conflicts and this may be reflected in their life style. This behaviour frequently ignores reality and is mainly designed to relieve underlying tension and the condition was called by Alexander (1930) 'The Neurotic Character'.

Anti-social behaviour of a criminal nature is, in itself, not a psychological concept, for criminality is action contrary to the penal code and such behaviour need not reflect underlying psychological disturbance and it is likely that the vast majority of crimes come into this category. Fenichel makes the point that 'it is likewise no special psychopathological problem if the content of some normal super-ego is other than the average in a given society or than the rulers of this society demand'. A criminal may have identified with a 'criminal super-ego' which though at variance with society, gives him no grounds for a guilty conscience; in fact he may feel guilty if he breaks his criminal code. This is seen in certain areas of large cities, where the mass of the inhabitants are hostile to the police and admire the exploits of the criminal. Their identifications reveal no abnormalities for they may identify very strongly and consistently.

There are some psychopaths who are in varying degrees 'affectless' and these seem incapable of forming warm relations with any object, criminal or otherwise. They tend to develop 'lone-wolf' personalities and their behaviour may be brutal and sadistic; in addition there is a conspicuous absence of loyalty. They are very disturbed persons who are at a near-psychotic level and many of them do in fact develop paranoid schizophrenic features, especially in a milieu where their anti-social conduct does not excite the usual reaction from society. It is as if they whet themselves against society, and by their behaviour maintain their 'sanity'. During the Second World War the author was impressed by the way a number of these patients, when removed from the prison and put into a hospital ward, treated as the other patients and a permissive attitude shown towards their initial hostility, later developed florid psychotic patterns of illness. There is a corollary to this, in that righteous society has a deep psychological need for the criminal and they are to a certain extent mutually dependent.

Cleckley (1950) has elaborated a psychological theory which claims that the psychopath fails in social adjustment because of his inability 'to grasp emotionally any of the ordinary components of meaning or feeling implicit in the thoughts which he expresses or the experiences he appears to go through'. The P.P. is unaware of the meaning aspect of human life and has a specific dissociation involving mainly emotion and to a lesser extent purpose, and Cleckley has suggested the name 'semantic dementia' and has elaborated a psychopathology which makes use of Freudian concepts, Adlerian theory, *e.g.* the need to escape from inferiority feelings, and Pavlovian and Behaviourist language by referring to faulty conditioning. Most authors who are psychologically minded stress maternal deprivation (Bowlby, 1944), discordant family life, and general insecurity in childhood as aetiological factors.

The Presentation of the Psychopathy

The tendency to equate crime with psychopathic behaviour may make us overlook other forms of social deviance which are just as reliable indices of the psychopathic personality. Gibbens and Silberman (1960) examined nearly 300 men attending a V.D. (Venereal Disease) clinic and found that they fell into similar clinical groups as offenders, yet the rate of crime was no higher (14 per cent) than one would expect in a normal population. When compared with a group of prisoners their backgrounds were almost as disturbed, *e.g.* parental alcoholism was 15:25 while parental discord was greater. The major difference between the two groups was that the promiscuous who contracted V.D. had normal attitudes to work and to the necessity of work, while 200 Borstal boys averaged only 4 out of 10 years in registered employment.

The Natural History of Psychopathic Disorder

Craft (1969) reviewed a number of follow-up studies on psychopaths, having excluded those with psychosis and sex deviation alone and who had I.Q's under 55. He first reported on studies of psychopaths admitted to the Special Hospitals of Britain (Rampton,

Moss Side and Broadmoor) and other units at Herstedvester (Denmark), Patuxent (Maryland) and the Henderson Hospital (England). The general finding was that these patients show more improvement with time than had been expected.

Relationship between Juvenile and Adult Crime

The prison population is a changing one, for as courts tend to use measures other than prison for first and second offenders those who are sent down are more seriously criminal. Gibbens (1966) quotes a study by Silberman which showed that of such a population only 34 per cent had convictions as juveniles, 48 per cent were first convicted between 17 and 30 and as many as 18 per cent were not convicted before the age of 30. This last group were by no means first offenders for nearly one-third had had six previous convictions. These findings suggest either that recidivism and psychopathic personality are not as closely related as one had supposed or that in earlier life other experiences of social deviation had taken the place of crime.

The Firesetter Syndrome

Macht and Mack (1968) regard firesetting as a highly determined behavioural complex or syndrome with important defensive and adaptive aspects. In their analysis of 4 patients (3 boys and 1 girl) the following points emerged:

1. The act of firesetting for these adolescents was not the product of an impulse, but highly determined, as it involved ego operations like planning, timing, fantasy elaboration, undoing and identification.
2. The act had multiple determinants in its meaning to the individual and in its specific association with important human relationships, past and present.
3. The firesetters regarded the act with some guilt and anxiety, but did not consider the behaviour entirely alien to them.

The firesetting phenomenon consists not only of setting the fire but of starting the alarm, waiting for the firemen to arrive, watching and assisting in the extinguishing operation, establishing a relationship with the firemen, using the fire setting as a signal to obtain help and expressing intense sexual excitement and destructive wishes and impulses. In each case the father was absent when the behaviour occurred and this intensified feelings of closeness and excitement in the maternal relationship.

The authors consider that the firemen are father-surrogates and that this particular behaviour is used to help the individual defend against, master, control and discharge the unbearable tension brought about by excessive closeness to the mother.

Comment: The observations are interesting but it reads very much like a case for the defence and rather far-fetched at that. There must be many less hazardous ways of finding a father-surrogate, especially as millions of youngsters are placed in similar positions with great regularity. It is difficult to see such a defence succeeding in a court of law.

The authors have resurrected the following quotation from Walt Whitman's *Poems of Joy* (1860) which confirms the erotic excitement of the fire enthusiast:

> I hear the alarm at dead of night
> I hear the bells–shout!
> I pass the crowd–I run!
> The sight of flames maddens me with pleasure.

The Manipulative Personality

Bursten (1972) attempts to describe in psychological terms the dynamics of a character structure which can account for the antisocial manifestations of what is commonly called the sociopath. He contends that many of the qualities of the sociopath are reflections of the manipulative personality. He defines the key elements of manipulation as: (*a*) the perception of a conflict of goals between the manipulator and another; (*b*) the intention to influence the other by employing a deception of some sort; (*c*) the feeling of exhilaration at having put something over on the other person; and (*d*) he is aware of these activities and enjoys them.

Such a person is driven to manipulate primarily by his inner dynamic position and not because of the situation he meets. He will therefore seek out situations where he can manipulate and will provoke conflict in goals in order to set the stage for his manipulation. This would explain why the sociopath does not learn from experience.

The manipulative personality has an intense but fragile narcissism and a key to the dynamics is the exhilaration of deceit. He feels he is lovable only if he is great and any depreciation or threat of it leads to compensatory reactions designed to support his inflated image of himself. He therefore proves himself on other people. He rids himself of his badness by projection: 'I am not worthless; you are'. This leads to the contempt for others, seen as callousness, superficial relationships, lack of responsibility and outright contempt for society's values. Telling the truth has a low priority in his hierarchy of values, and he will try to cover himself with deceptions and rationalizations in order to maintain a good image. It is therefore not a defect in reality testing which enables the manipulator to lie so easily. There is no guilt about deception because truth and conformity are not significant issues for the manipulative personality.

Comment: This is a very solid contribution to the understanding of the psychopathology of some sociopathic persons but does not qualify as an all-embracing thesis. This is probably because the sociopathic group is composed of diverse constituents.

The Bright Delinquent

Gath *et al.* (1970) studied 50 bright delinquent boys and compared them with 50 ordinary delinquent boys to test the following hypotheses: (*a*) bright delinquents show a greater degree of psychiatric disturbance than controls; and (*b*) these delinquents commit more offences of which the primary determinants are psychological rather than sub-cultural. The findings supported both hypotheses in that the bright delinquents committed more psychologically determined offences, showed greater evidence of psychiatric disturbances, and their peer relationships and general conduct were also disturbed.

The Borderline Patient

He is frequently admitted to hospital because of some self-inflicted injury such as cutting himself, administering painful stimuli to the genitals, or otherwise engaging in daredevil activity. Collum (1972) regards these outbursts as forms of reality testing and a means of maintaining the sense of self when threatened with a stressful situation. These situations stimulate emergency rather than welfare emotions in the following sequence: (1) stressful situations; (2) confusion in thinking; (3) identity diffusion; (4) creation of emergency state; (5) organizing effect in emergency emotions; (6) clarification of thinking; and (7) restoration of sense of self.

Treatment is designed to explain to the patient the reasons for his destructive manoeuvre and helping him to find less destructive ones. The condition is not uncommon and any psychiatrist who works in a general hospital which admits emergencies will be thoroughly familiar with this type of patient.

TREATMENT

With such a wide range of human problems, it is not surprising that nearly every conceivable method has been tried. Some are experimental, some are doctrinaire, and some are expedient and depend more on the character of the therapist than on any preconceived ideas or theories.

There have been some useful experiments carried out in Britain and while their results may not be outstanding, it is a tribute to the maturity of a nation that it can see fit to set aside funds for this purpose. The better-known are:

(a) The Institute for the Scientific Treatment of Delinquency (the Portman Clinic). By its title, it would appear to treat that aspect of the P.P. which involves crime, but in fact a number of patients referred there are not necessarily on charges. It is essentially analytically orientated and it has produced a number of important research publications. It also organizes courses for psychiatrists and others who are interested in or have contact with the delinquent and while the results of analytic therapy for the individual patients referred may not be outstandingly successful, it plays an important part in the campaign for psychological enlightenment and in the training of personnel.

(b) Henderson Hospital. This was originally called the Rehabilitation Centre at Belmont (Surrey) under its first director, Dr Maxwell Jones. It specialized in the adult psychopath who was unable to adjust to his employment, family or society. It has had a strong analytical bias and the administrative side is most permissive, with the patients being very largely responsible for their own behaviour. The group setting is the main therapeutic tool, though some patients are given individual therapy. Much has been learned in the handling of the aggressive psychopath and of group dynamics.

(c) Grendon Underwood. This is a special type of prison hospital for persistent offenders requiring psychiatric treatment. It meets the requirements of a security prison but is well equipped and staffed as a psychiatric hospital and admits selected prisoners of both sexes and has recently added an adolescent unit. Group and individual psychotherapy is undertaken as well as physical forms of treatment but it is too early to assess its efficacy.

(d) Broadmoor. This ancient and famous institution for criminal lunatics has been undergoing some changes in its treatment of the aggressive psychopath. Previously the nursing staff readily distinguished between the 'mad' and the 'bad' and the impulsive schizophrenic was allowed more latitude than the acting-out psychopath. The latter invariably exhibited violence and anti-authority behaviour and fell into two groups: (a) with psychotic episodes and

(b) without psychotic episodes.

A 'system' of treatment was devised for the psychopaths and was based on the principle that if a psychopath was offered rewards he would work for them. Anything good or constructive in the personality was fostered but immediate toughness was shown if a patient stepped out of line, while anti-authority groups were not allowed to develop. With these innovations violence diminished and attacks on staff were rare and the patient responsible was immediately secluded. A tendency towards a more permissive regime with more use of occupational therapy and discussion groups was not always welcomed, for some patients preferred to do nine month's solitary than spend their time arguing about why they had hit someone. Group sessions tended to produce jealousy and disruption, perhaps because of the large proportion of homosexuals.

To some who believe that all aggression is grist to the psychotherapist's mill the above regime would appear harsh, but they should appreciate that some of these patients had 'security' tags which in order to protect the public would have to be enforced for many years if not for life and this fact must condition their behaviour and their response to treatment. Relaxation of supervision or permature discharge could have dire consequences and even if one can develop an indifference to victims of assault, a charge of negligence could be most unpleasant as well as costly. This does illustrate the difficulties our colleagues both medical and nursing have to face in their work.

At Herstedvester in Denmark, Stürùp (1964) has elaborated over the years a programme of treatment for chronic criminals. He agrees with others that the bulk of lawbreakers pass back into the community without too great difficulty. Recidivists however belong to the group of sensitized regressed 'true' criminals of whom some are immature and resent correctional authority. These he labels 'insufficiency of character'. His treatment is styled *Integrating, Individualized, Group Therapy* and has three components:

1. Individualized treatment.
2. Analytic and reconstructive elements in the plan are integrated into the daily learning process of institutional life.
3. Results have to be experienced by the inmate as part of his own personal growth.

Group activity consists of (*a*) the normal daily work, (*b*) special group counselling and (*c*) group therapy. After-care services are run by the institution. He claims that with the above treatment 50 per cent survive in society but comparisons with other or even similar measures in different countries should be made with great caution for the factors involved are legion.

At present there is much debate on what to do with the criminal psychopath. The bold experiment of defining a psychopathic personality in the Mental Health Act (1959) has invested that Act with the power to dispose of such persons to mental hospitals thus creating impossible security problems for these institutions. In addition some hospitals with catchment areas in large cities are liable to accept a disproportionate number of such patients who are unable to receive the concentrated individual attention they require and also tend to disrupt therapeutic efforts in favour of the non-psychopathic hospital population. Rollin (1963) has pointed out this problem in a hospital serving the London area and others have supported his contention that it is futile to send such patients for compulsory treatment to a mental hospital which prides itself on its 'open-door' system and absence of security.

The problem does not lie entirely with the inability of the hospital to cope but in the recommendation itself and psychiatrists before making such suggestions to the Court should seriously consider how they can be implemented and whether the face-saving formula of admission to hospital is preferable to prison where the medical services are no less able to provide the necessary psychiatric treatment.

'Untreatable' Criminals

Stürup (1972) describes his special treatment system called *individualized integrating growth therapy* which he developed at the Herstedvester Detention Centre to provide special treatment for troublemakers rejected by other prisons and mental hospitals. Only psychotics and mental defectives are excluded.

The medical model for a disease with an aetiology is abandoned, and a cure is not expected, as the purpose is to assist criminals to live without further crime. The inmates consider themselves as outcasts and therefore find it easier to relate to other outcasts. They distort reality and live for the moment and these aspects upset normal relationships. He emphasizes that the treatment process is dependent on *adequate* institutional security. If insufficient he will leave, if excessive he will be rightly critical.

The officer of the ward has the closest contact with the inmate, and when the latter is allowed out on leave it is the officer who accompanies him, visits the family, and attends the cinema. Daily conferences between all staff are held. A special psychotherapeutic technique is 'anamnestic analysis' which aims to get the inmate to relive earlier interpersonal conflicts on the basis of his attitude to present interpersonal situations. It is a form of analysis of development, and narcoanalysis and narcosynthesis have been used as *aides*. Drugs are rarely used, though very aggressive individuals have been given tranquillizers.

'Reclaim' is the keynote and it is stressed that life outside will be more difficult, and support extends beyond the institution. In the past 30 years confinement for property offenders has been reduced from 4 to 2 years. For the aggressive offender confinement is often not more than 7–8 years. Fifty per cent of the chronic property criminals return but frequently with lesser crimes, and 10 years after first arrival only 10 per cent are still in or again in custody in Herstedvester. The author regards as his most important contribution the demonstration that it is possible to develop a humane, acceptable way of life inside a penal institution for the most difficult group of offenders.

Comment: Dr Stürùp's experience is unique, as are his facilities. The population in Denmark is another special factor and it is difficult to advocate a transplant from such a unique situation to another culture, but the lesson is there, and no doubt his influence is spreading, though even his modest successes may not be attainable.

Scott (1960), writing from the standpoint of one interested in the psychopath as an offender, lists the available sources of material for research as the 25,000 individuals in prison and Borstal institutions, the 8000 young people in approved schools and children in special schools for the maladjusted and the educationally subnormal, patients in mental deficiency and mental hospitals and State hospitals like Broadmoor and Rampton and also reception centres for the asocial drifters. He stresses that those attending approved schools form a valuable potential for research because:

> (1) there is legal provision for detaining them and for following them up over a statutory period of six years; (2) they are required to pass through (with rare exceptions) a classifying centre where the research team might operate both for initial assessment and for subsequent reassessment during the follow-up periods; (3) their parents will usually be available; (4) these schools are small enough to facilitate the study of every inmate, and sufficiently numerous and differently managed as to vary greatly in the sort of training and treatment provided; and (5) at this age, the approved school is likely to be the first long-stay correctional institution which the inmates have experienced, so that there will be less likelihood of secondary 'processing' by the penal machinery (a complication which may be very important in corrective training or preventive detention).

Scott has elaborated a classification which is different from the others as it is mainly designed to give some clues as to possible lines of treatment. He lists four groups.

1. Trained, but to Anti-social Standards

Treatment here should be restraining and may simply be punishment associated with some advice and assistance. As the offender's personality is intact, his learning processes are unimpaired and a new pattern of behaviour can be superimposed on one which was presumably a subcultural and criminal one.

2. Reparative Behaviour

The crime is a compensation for a sense of inadequacy or inferiority and the offender may be arrogant and sensitive to insult and prone to steal power objects like cars and motor cycles. These offences are goal motivated and gain something in the emotional field with secondary material advantage. Treatment here, too, should be restraining although there will always be a positive defence which will oppose such treatment, so that psychotherapy may also be needed. The pattern is capable of modification, even by punishment alone.

3. The Untrained Offender

He is without standards and weak in character and his behaviour difficulties exist from early life and have frequently been handled by a variety of agencies in an inconsistent manner. Treatment consists of long-term, patient supervision with a background of sanctions. Heavy punishment may tip the patient into a more rigid stage (see below).

4. Rigid Fixations

In these offenders frustration at a critical point in their learning process has resulted in a maladaptive pattern of response. They show a stereotyped, non-adaptive and non-goal directed pattern of behaviour which even after long spells of control reasserts itself and is not improved by severe punishment. Treatment is still unproven, but punishment is useless.

Scott appreciates that this classification is over-simplified and that one offender may fall into more than one category but adds— '. . . Yet such a scheme fits many clinical facts, and may prevent wasteful and fruitless attempts at assessing treatment methods on material of quite different types'. Treatment, he emphasizes, while still largely ineffective, should at least do no harm, and he lists the therapeutic methods available with critical comments.

Wherever possible, therefore, psychopaths should be kept out of custody, for detention carries risks of its own. As soon as offenders or the anti-socially inclined are segregated there is the tendency for staff and inmates to consolidate at opposite poles; a hierarchy tends to develop among the offenders; a threat is thus offered to the staff which calls out a repressive authoritarian regime and the possibility of a vicious circle of resentment and counter-resentment.

As methods of combating the above situation, he recommends:

1. A full programme of constructive and recreational activities with staff participation and with short-term objectives.
2. Some physical hardship which can be overcome by the efforts of the community as lavish material comforts may be harmful.
3. Division into as many different groups as practicable with the staff active in some and in the background in others.
4. Every member of the community must be involved.
5. Free discussion groups for the airing of complaints and grievances.
6. Staff should be of both sexes and be kept up to scratch by staff meetings and have access to those with greater or differing experience, exchanges with other establishments, research projects and refresher courses.
7. Greater use of hostels to help reduce the population and length of stay in closed institutions.

Individual Therapy

Scott recommends the paper by Mackwood (1949) which describes the careful piecing together of the patient's history and holding a mirror before him so that he can see his misbehaviour as part of his life pattern. Getting such patients to cooperate can be very difficult and the indeterminate sentence has been regarded as indispensable by Stürup (1952) and Aungle (1959) in Scandinavia and in the U.S.A. by Boslow *et al.* (1959). Scott doubts its value in his fourth ('rigid fixation') category but considers it may have some value in the others.

Stürup's dynamic growth therapy and the utilization of 'affective moments' (spontaneous catharsis) in changing the patient's attitude and the use of group pressure to bring a new awareness to the patient (Jones *et al.*, 1952) are regarded by Scott as applicable to the second and possibly the third and fourth of his categories.

He also lists a variety of other therapies which are still largely unassessed as regards their efficacy, such as (*a*) non-directive therapy (Rogers, 1942; Snyder *et al.*, 1947), (*b*) group-guided interaction (Weeks, 1958), (*c*) psychodrama (Moreno, 1958), (*d*) closed-group analytical psychotherapy in prisons (Landers *et al.*, 1954), (*e*) Wolpe's (1958) therapy by reciprocal inhibition, and (*f*) Raymond's (1956) aversion therapy for sexual perversion, though he does not expect the last two to be effective with his fourth category. He is critical of pharmacological measures such as oestrogens, disulfiram, tranquillizers and surgical measures such as castration and leucotomy for physically normal people, and considers that they may be regarded as another form of physical as opposed to psychological restriction or control and possessing the shortcomings of such measures. He makes the chastening observation that:

> . . . with psychopaths, highly refined psychotherapeutic procedures, applied by medical men, are often no more successful, sometimes less successful, than the simpler and less esoteric approaches of certain social workers, probation officers, institutional staff, who may have had little or no training apart from on-the-job experience . . . a sympathetic member of the staff capable of winning the individual's respect and able to be with him when day-to-day crises appear is able to effect more than a psychotherapist who sees the individual at stated times. It is an established fact that patients who leave hospital with a bad prognosis after failing to improve as regards their psychopathy may then do well under probationary supervision . . . it may be that those in category four (the fixed pattern) are more responsible to this direct guidance from someone at their elbow and sharing the experience than they would be to many psychotherapeutic procedures. Some workers intuitively obtain good results with certain psychopaths. . . . .

It can be seen that though classification in terms of aetiology is confused, a practical one has been devised by Scott which gives valuable help in deciding which cases should be dealt with by the ordinary corrective measures and which should be given special facilities which will always be scarce and should be used with great discretion. The anti-social behaviour of the psychopath will ensure that research funds and facilities will be made increasingly available and the medical and allied professions have a heavy responsibility in seeing that these resources are intelligently used.

Punishment or Treatment?

Scott (1970) discusses the dilemma facing those who have the responsibility for custodial care of the aggressive antisocial psychopath and has some advice on the subject of *restraint*. He lays down the following criteria:

1. The policy decision to use it should be taken at the highest level.

2. It should be part of the therapeutic intention and not retribution. Segregation should not be for a predetermined time but

for as long as is necessary.

3. Chemical restraint should only be used when there is obvious mental illness and not to subdue disturbing behaviour in the normal. Neither should it be prescribed at the patient's request.

4. A top security institution should be 'saturated' with staff and visiting specialists, students and research workers. It should also be kept in the forefront of public attention.

5. The use of restraint must be constantly scrutinized and discussed at all levels, otherwise it will regress to retributive punishment. He suggests that some mentally abnormal offenders are better kept in prison, which, in addition to being more suitable in terms of physical surroundings, would bring doctors and nurses into prisons to the benefit of the whole prison population.

The reports of Rollin (1965) and Bearcroft and Donovan (1965) have already underlined the difficulties that arise when psychopathic personalities are defined by law and provisions made for compulsory admission to hospital under the Mental Health Act (1959). As there is usually a legal urgency over their admission they take precedence for consultation and accommodation over seriously ill people and when in hospital they frequently disrupt the existing arrangements and prejudice the treatment of recoverable patients. Follow-up studies by the above authors of the efficacy of mental hospital treatment for criminal psychopaths indicate that this milieu is not effective in their rehabilitation if only because so many abscond.

Society and the Psychopath

The provision of units like the Henderson Hospital and Grendon Underwood in Britain and the Chino prison in California are brave and costly experiments to find effective ways of dealing with psychopathic offenders, yet these and future efforts will depend on the public, for these are financed by taxpayers and the climate towards the deviant is hardening. This attitude was graphically put in an unsigned review in the *Times Literary Supplement* (16th February, 1973) of Whiteley, Briggs and Turner's (1972) book *Dealing with Deviants* which deals with the above-named institutions.

> Society is heartily sick of its deviants. The signs of them are everywhere, in the vandalized telephone boxes, the broken glass of road signs, the aerosol paint *graffiti*, the junky washrooms at Piccadilly. In the poorer parts of cities, the alcoholic wrecks crouch in doorways in winter and lie prostrate in summer in the tiny, pocket-handkerchief parks. Meanwhile, back in the tree-lined suburbs, the 'drummers' are about their increasing work of afternoon burglary. In the commercial centres the raiders strike again and pull off yet another successful

robbery. Small wonder that among some social pessimists the accuracy of a police marksman was among the best news items of 1972.

Experiment in reform and treatment can only operate in a social climate which endorses such action and those who wish to continue their experiments may have to cease arguing from the particular to the general if they wish to avoid a complete shutdown. They will also have to produce results which encourage further experiment, and to date these have not been forthcoming. It is good that a society can set aside much-needed funds for experiments in reclaiming the sociopath. It is equally important that those who undertake the experiments should appreciate their total dependence on social climate.

Modern society has many disagreeable tasks and one is the humane rehabilitation of the psychopath. It frequently turns to the psychiatrist for help but all it receives is an acceptable formula. Whether it works or not, does not appear to cause society much concern but psychiatrists should carefully assess their competence in the field and if they are satisfied that they have no competence they should say so and direct their energies into those fields where their work is of proven value. This does not mean that there should be no experiment. It does mean that it was premature to legislate before the factual information was available.

CHAPTER 11

The Psychoneuroses

The psychoneuroses comprise a group of non-organic mental disorders which though particularly distressing to the patient, do not possess the qualities of severe affective change or thought disturbance which are associated with the psychoses. This statement does not constitute an adequate definition, for it merely states what the psychoneuroses are not and still leaves the question unanswered as to what they are. One of the commonest questions concerning this problem put by medical students is: 'What is the difference between a neurosis and a psychosis?' Though teachers of psychiatry for generations now have tried to provide an answer, an entirely satisfactory one is still elusive. It is not only the medical student who is searching for clarification but also the psychiatrist, who has debated the problem at length with his colleagues and rejected one definition after another. Freud (1924*a*) had an early attempt at a definition. He based it on the hypothesis that the ego occupies a mediate position between the outer world and the id and that it has to serve both masters at one and the same time. *Neurosis,* he therefore defined as 'the result of conflict between the ego and the *id*', and '*psychosis* is the analogous outcome of a similar disturbance in the relation between the ego and its environment (outer) world'. He was evidently not entirely satisfied with his definition for he added: 'To be suspicious of such simple solutions of problems is undoubtedly a piece of justifiable caution. Moreover, the most that we should expect from it would not be more than that this formula should prove itself correct in rough outline'. In a subsequent paper (Freud, 1924*b*) he expanded the definitions thus:

> I have recently defined as follows one of the features, distinguishing the neuroses from the psychoses: in the former the ego, in virtue of its allegiance to reality, suppresses a part of the *id* (the life instinct), whereas in the psychoses the same ego, in the service of the *id* withdraws itself from a part of reality.

According to this, the excessive power of the influence of reality is decisive for neurosis, and for psychosis that of the *id*. A loss of reality must be an inherent element in psychosis: while in neurosis, one would suppose, it would be avoided.

In the same paper, he put the alternative definitions: '. . . neurosis does not deny the existence of reality, it merely tries to ignore it; psychosis denies it and tries to substitute something else for it'.

It is possible to argue and undermine each definition, no matter what theoretical basis it may have and many psychiatrists consider the two groups a continuum with similar features and varying only in degree. Bowman and Rose (1951) considered that there was no scientific basis for the distinction and that it depended on symptomatology. It was no doubt easier for psychiatrists to distinguish neurosis and psychosis at the beginning of the century, for most worked in mental hospitals or asylums where nearly the whole population was psychotic and differed markedly from the neurotic patients who attended for consultation. One group had patently demonstrated its inability to exist in normal society by virtue of disturbed behaviour, while the other conducted itself with the propriety of normal citizens.

The end-point of diagnosis has sharpened considerably in recent years, and some conditions which were at one time labelled neurotic have now been recognized as early stages of a psychosis. A classical example is pseudo-neurotic schizophrenia (Hoch & Polatin, 1949) and some psychopathic problems too can deteriorate to schizophrenic levels. Yet even though the theoretical basis is suspect, and the clinical distinctions are questioned, there are still administrative reasons for perpetuating the distinction, though these too are now being disputed. Neurosis centres which exclude patients with psychotic illness were, and may still be popular. Accommodation on hospital ships for the evacuation of psychiatric casualties was labelled 'psychoneurotic' or 'psychotic', though there were many psychotics who could and should have been looked after in the more attractive and less restricted part of the ship, while some neurotics should have been kept in the 'security' section. Psychiatrists who had to label these patients would sometimes perjure themselves so that the patient would not have a 'psychotic' label. Depressives and schizophrenics were therefore labelled anxiety states and thus deterioration on the homeward journey, by reason of unsuitable accommodation, was avoided. It may still be useful to talk of 'neurotic' and 'psychotic' as indicating the severity of a problem or to indicate its contact or otherwise with reality, but the time has now gone when these terms should bear any prognostic or administrative significance. They can help to simplify matters for medical students who, in the early stages of their psychiatric training, may have difficulty in appreciating the finer nuances of symptomatology and prefer a clear-cut classification on which to hang their clinical experience. They should, however, be warned that with increasing knowledge and expertise, they may have to abandon it.

Transition from Neurosis to Psychosis

There is no better way to settle an argument than to provide evidence. Bratfos (1970) followed up for 12 to 22 years patients admitted to a mental hospital with a non-psychotic diagnosis, and of the total of 3,485 patients 333 were later admitted to mental hospitals with a psychotic diagnosis, which is 67 times the expected number in the normal population. Schizophrenia was the commonest diagnosis in young people, while manic-depressive psychoses were commoner in the older age group. The risks varied according to the type of non-psychotic illness; 7·9 per cent in neuroses and 13·4 per cent in the psychopathies. Forty-two of those originally classified as pseudo-neurotic schizophrenics later became psychotic.

A constitutional neurotic type has been postulated (Slater, 1943) indicating genetic determinants for neurotic illness with the corollary that there are genetic determinants for psychotic illness, but while the conclusions drawn from the clinical data may be significant, it is doubtful if the clinical sample of neurotic servicemen who served as the basis for the above study can be regarded as representative either of neurotic illness or of the general population, especially as the period during which the study was undertaken was war-time and many of the neurotic features were heavily adulterated with secondary gain. It is generally accepted that the basis for neurotic reaction, whatever form it may take, is laid down in early childhood and that recent events which trigger off the reaction have attacked a peculiarly vulnerable personality. There have been many attempts to group the aetiological factors together but it would be better to discuss the group as a variety of reactions and deal with each in turn.

Classification

The classification which is in general use is that of the American Psychiatric Association which lists six *reactions:* (1) Anxiety, (2) Dissociative, (3) Conversion, (4) Phobic, (5) Obsessive compulsive and (6) Depressive. It should be noted that these are reactions and not diseases and that one reaction does not exclude another; in fact, several can co-exist, though many disorders are predominantly of one type.

ANXIETY REACTIONS

Anxiety is a very common motive for mobilizing the ego-defences, but it can exist as an entity in itself. From the analytical standpoint, primary anxiety is evidence of unmastered tension and occurs automatically whenever the individual is overwhelmed with excitement. Whenever the ego feels itself threatened, it reacts initially with anxiety. The threat may be external in terms of frustration, danger, or other unpleasant experience, but may also be internal due to the unconscious threatening to overrun the ego with repressed material. Anxiety need not be abnormal, and there are many who regard it as part of the individual's ordinary reaction to his environment. This concept derives from a coterie of philosophical, psychological and physiological works. Kierkegaard (1844), who inspired the Existentialist movement, regarded anxiety as a normal state of life and drew a distinction between it and neurotic anxiety, which was the dread of non-existence. Goldstein (1939) put his views on anxiety and holism thus:

> As manifold as states of anxiety may be, with regard to intensity and kind, they all have one common denominator: the experience of danger, of peril for one's self. To be sure, this characterization is not sufficient, first of all, because it only describes the subjective experience, which is merely a part of the entire phenomenon. Usually, one believes that this exhausts the facts, that the essential aspect of anxiety is given in the subjective experience. However, if we observe someone in a state of anxiety we can disclose characteristic bodily changes as well, certain expressive movements of the face and the body, and certain states of physiological processes, motor phenomena, changes of pulse rate, and vasomotor phenomena, etc. And we certainly have no reason to exclude these changes from an investigation of the phenomenon of anxiety . . .

He considered that the danger which threatens and induces anxiety must have special qualities and that anxiety must be distinguished from fear of an object. Fear derives from an object which confronts and which can be met or run away from, but anxiety 'attacks us from the rear so to speak. The only thing we can do is to attempt to flee from it without knowing where to go. . . .' Fear can be resolved by reassurance and explanation, while true anxiety is not susceptible to these approaches.

Anxiety, Goldstein asserts, serves a useful purpose. On difficult occasions, the normal person exhibits anxiety, such as during examinations, when failure may threaten the existence or self-esteem of the individual. Anxiety therefore has a special significance for the conquest of the environment or for self-realization and a culture which excites this pattern of behaviour is more likely to achieve success in these fields than one which does not. Anxiety in children, he considers, is dissolved by the child's strong tendency to action, which to a lesser extent is also present in the adult. Some not only use this method to deal with anxiety when it knocks, but go out of their way to meet it, by exploration, mountaineering, sailing and gambling. Achievement in these fields cancels out anxiety and may even be of prophylactic value. 'Courage, in the final analysis, is nothing but an affirmative answer to the shocks of existence, which must be borne for the actualization of one's own nature.' Goldstein carries the concept of anxiety a stage further through his observations in the brain-damaged, who because they are not protected against the anxiety situation are therefore particularly vulnerable to it.

Cannon (1915), whose physiological studies on fear and rage defined the biological aspects of anxiety, contributed further (Cannon, 1939) by showing that anxiety should be seen as an expression of interference with homeostatic equilibrium which could be threatened, broken down or try to re-establish itself at a different level. Kelman (1957), who regards the organism and its environment as a unitary system, has postulated that tension in either physical or psychological guise is an essential aspect of the unitary system and that when tension is exceeded, anxiety is declared. In addition to theories and clinical observations, there have been experiments, including those of Grinker *et al.* (1957) who have induced stress experimentally in volunteers and measured the physiological response including serum and urinary cortisol, as well as studying the specificity of the various stress situations. Funkenstein *et al.* (1957) studied the cardiovascular aspects of emotional responses of students to acute emergency. They defined two categories, those who reacted with 'anger out' and showed cardiovascular responses similar to those produced by noradrenaline (norepinephrine), while those who reacted with 'anger-in' or severe anxiety had a response similar to that produced by adrenaline (epinephrine). All responses depended on a variety of factors which, in addition to the nature of the threatening experience, included the personality, cultural status and not surprisingly, the relationship with the examiner. One of these entertained doubts about the experiments he was conducting, and created a response of severe anxiety in every subject tested by him, whereas other experimenters found anger to be the commonest response.

Forearm Blood Flow and Anxiety

Kelly (1967) describes the technique using a water-filled or a mercury-in-rubber strain gauge plethysmograph but considers the former more reliable. With the subject reclining comfortably, recordings are made of forearm blood flow, heart rate and blood pressure during 'basal' (resting) conditions for 15 minutes. Anxiety is then induced by asking the subject to perform a difficult arithmetical task as quickly as possible while trying to keep up with a metronome beating at a two-second rate. He is asked to keep as still as possible while being continually harrassed and criticized. Recordings are made at 30-second intervals for the first two minutes of mental stress, and the B.P. is recorded during the last 30 seconds. The metronome is then stopped and the patient is told he has done very well. Two further recordings are made at minute intervals while the patient is encouraged to relax again.

The differences between 'basal' and 'stress' measurements are calculated as percentage increases and this is considered to be a reliable estimate of physiological reactivity or lability. 'Basal' forearm blood flow is considered to be an approximate measurement of *free-floating* anxiety, whereas 'stress' values are provoked by a specific stimulus and are therefore a measure of *situational* anxiety. The author regards the distinction as important clinically in that chronic anxiety states have persistently high levels of free-floating anxiety with high 'basal' forearm blood flows. Patients with a specific situational (phobic) anxiety, he claims, are generally non-anxious in other situations and have normal 'basal' forearm blood flows. The present writer would contest the latter claim. Many patients with phobic anxiety states have a continuously high level of free-floating anxiety. Gelder and Mathews (1968) found the method a sensitive index to transient increases in arousal but did not prefer it to palmar skin conductance or electromyographic activity.

Sodium Lactate Infusion and Anxiety

Kelly *et al.* (1971) used a half-molar solution of sodium lactate unbeknown to the subject, who had previously been infused with normal saline. In the post-lactate period, which lasted for 12 minutes, stressful mental arithmetic was performed for 2 minutes. Of the 20 patients studied, 16 experienced an anxiety attack during the lactate infusion, one during the post-lactate period, and one during the saline infusion. Only one of the control group, who did not show anxiety symptoms experienced an attack, and this was during the lactate infusion. The authors suggest that the change of clinical state of anxious patients may be reflected by an altered response to sodium lactate, and that this technique can be used to evaluate treatment for anxiety attacks.

Bonn (1973) used one molar strength of DL sodium lactate to the amount of 5 ml./kg. body weight by intravenous infusion over 20 minutes and in patients with anxiety states was able to reproduce panic and anxiety. He used this as a form of treatment, twice weekly for three weeks, and at follow-up relapse occurred in 5 out of the original 33 patients. The symptoms of lactate infusion which occurred 14 minutes afterwards were, anxiety, palpitations, chest constriction, paraesthesia and tremor. Like Kelly *et al.* (1971) he found that only anxious subjects experienced anxiety with lactate infusions, and when saline was substituted the symptoms were less common and tended to disappear.

These and other experiments are but the opening shots in a major attack on the physiological aspects of anxiety. Neurosurgeons have been impressed with its loss after cortical ablations; some experimentalists are studying the reticular formation and its excitatory effects on the cortex, which in turn is regarded by some as having an inhibitory effect on the lower centres and therefore in the control of anxiety. No introduction to anxiety would be complete without mentioning Selye's (1956) work on stress and his accent on the pituitary adrenal axis and its reactions to prolonged stress, but although anxiety may well operate through this axis, there is still no reliable information as to how it affects the target organs.

Aetiology

This is still a mystery and therefore a popular field for idle speculation, ill-conceived experiments, false deductions and extravagant claims. What appears to emerge from the mass of data which has accumulated is that many factors are involved and that it is unlikely that one single aspect will provide the complete answer.

Genetic Studies

These have been more concerned with the neurotic constitution than with anxiety. The fine dividing line between pathological anxiety and the essential normality of anxiety in certain circumstances makes such studies difficult.

Cultural Factors

These are probably of significance as one would expect from the earlier remarks about the social importance of anxiety. In a society where it is fostered, a number will over-react or fail to master the environment and be subject to the disability. In the First World War there was a marked difference in the incidence of anxiety between officers and other ranks. In the former it was common and was almost the only neurotic reaction, while in the latter it was much less common. These differences were again confirmed in the Second World War. Sim (1946*a*) found that the incidence of anxiety states in officers was very much higher than in other ranks. When the psychiatric disease incidence was investigated among the large groups of patients from other cultures, there was a marked cultural variation, the African showing an almost complete absence of anxiety as a clinical entity. There have been many views expressed about this well-recognized phenomenon; some are related to maternal or paternal attitudes towards the child, the cultural pattern and conflicts over values, worship of success and its incompatibility with basic ethics and so on. While, theoretically, infantile experience should be paramount, anxiety can be grafted on in adult life to cultural groups who had previously not shown such reactions.

The Specific Event

This is frequently volunteered by the patient as the cause of his initial anxiety attack and Levy (1950) noted accidents and operations as the most common events, with frights, separations, sudden privations, births of siblings and sudden environmental changes also occurring, though less frequently. He did not consider them the only factor, though the patient who was seeking for a *post hoc propter hoc* explanation, would seize on the event which immediately antedated the attack. With all the distortion and false memories to which such recollections are prone, the patient's information could be very unreliable, and more emphasis is generally placed on predisposition due to psychological, physical and cultural factors, the parent-child relationship being regarded as of special importance. Many patients describe an episode, during which they nearly lost consciousness, as the cause of their trouble, but on closer enquiry, it was really a fear of loss of consciousness. One must therefore go back a step to find the causal factor, for the anxiety must have already existed to produce the fear though it may well have been associated with some physiological change which disturbed the patient.

Psychopathology of anxiety states cannot be divorced from general psychopathology and the reader is advised to refer to Chapter

2, as understanding of the neuroses largely depends on an adequate knowledge of this subject.

Epidemiology of Common Fears and Phobias

It is obvious that those patients with phobias who are referred to psychiatrists are only a fraction of those afflicted, and while probably the most severely afflicted, there are frequently some who are seriously handicapped who do not bring their problem to the attention of their doctors. Agras *et al.* (1969) studied a sample of the population of the Greater Burlington area of Vermont and calculated incidence and prevalence rates of phobic anxiety. The prevalence was estimated at 76·9 per 1000 of population, mildly disabling in 74·7 per 1000 and seriously disabling in 2·2 per 1000. A detailed analysis of the fears showed a high childhood incidence but rapidly declining prevalence as regards fears of doctors, injections, darkness and strangers, showing that they were relatively short-lived, and a slowly declining prevalence of fear of animals, heights, storms, enclosed spaces and social situations, suggesting that once acquired they are long-lived. A third pattern showed a slowly declining incidence extending to the sixth decade, and a prevalence peak in late adult life.

It is just as well for enthusiasts to remember these figures and not dissipate their energies on the milder states which would swamp them and at the same time neglect those who are severely disabled. The decision to treat should therefore be a medical one as it is the doctor rather than the psychologist who is better able to assess degrees of sickness.

SYMPTOMATOLOGY

The symptomatology of the acute anxiety attack differs from the chronic state. The picture is that of over-stimulation of the autonomic nervous system. The heart rate is accelerated and the apex beat is more forcible with in some instances precordial discomfort or pain. Respiration rate is increased and the consequent hyperventilation produces its own syndrome (p. 291). Dyspnoea, dysphagia and a feeling of choking are common and on occasions there is respiratory distress. Urgency of micturition, diarrhoea, weakness of the knees or a total feeling of exhaustion can occur, and the author had a nursing orderly in a military psychiatric hospital, who was a marathon runner, yet who exhibited the above state when a patient became very disturbed and had to be taken to a side-room. It had been very harassing for all concerned but the marathon runner had kept clear of the trouble, yet at the end, he was supporting himself against the wall in a state of complete collapse. Those who have done some boxing need only recall the rapidly exhausting effect of being in the ring with a vastly superior opponent who may not even have landed a blow! Pupils dilate, sweating may be extreme, the mouth is dry, the hands tremble, the knees are weak and the facial appearance is over-anxious.

The Chronic State. This is really a persistence of the acute attack in attenuated form, though liable to periodic exacerbations. These may be associated with 'startle' reactions, which are triggered off by some sudden shock. In servicemen this could be a car back-firing or some other loud noise like an aircraft swooping overhead. The facies is constantly anxious, there is a marked tremor and sweating of the hands, tachycardia and disturbed sleep, the patient being frequently wakened by terrifying dreams. He may complain of the physical concomitants of his anxiety but this is when the anxiety has become 'fixated' and is no longer 'free and floating'. There is a general lowering of efficiency with impaired concentration and a tendency to hypochondriasis.

'Fixated' Anxiety

This is said to occur when the patient focuses his symptoms on an organ or region of the body, and is atrributed to the concomitant physiological disturbance such as tachycardia, dysphagia or pre-cordial pain with palpitations. He is usually seen first by physicians for suspected peptic ulcer, bowel disorders, heart disease, thyro-toxicosis and hyper-insulinism. The last-mentioned is of some importance, for many patients with acute anxiety attacks have an unstable blood-sugar regulating system and low readings in the region of 40–50 mg. per cent are not uncommon and an islet-cell tumour of the pancreas may be suspected. When the anxiety state settles, the glucose tolerance curve may return to normal. A similar picture has been reported by Hunter and Greenberg (1954) in barbiturate addicts, but it could be that the instability of sugar regulation was due to the primary cause of the addiction, namely the anxiety state.

Although these symptoms are described, as if in isolation, in clinical practice this is not usually the case, and there may be anxiety features associated with a large range of psychiatric disturbances. It may be associated with bizarre symptoms reiterated by the patient in an almost perseverative manner and the basic condition is a schizophrenic one. It may also be associated with frank hysterical features, or be part of a depressive or obsessional illness. Not only should the anxiety be seen as a *qualitative* factor in a composite picture, but there should be some attempt made to gauge the *quantitative* aspect, for there is a considerable difference in a mixed case of anxiety and hysteria, where the one is minimal and where the other is maximal. The term 'predominantly' is useful, for symptoms in themselves, if given equal value, can conjure up an entirely erroneous clinical picture. One saw this during the Second World War when an officer and an other rank might both present mixed states with anxiety and hysterical features, yet clinically they differed markedly from each other.

Differential Diagnosis

In the chronic state, this is mainly confined to the exclusion of thyrotoxicosis, which can prove at times very difficult, though radioactive iodine now affords a fairly reliable form of investigation. Even the acute attack can be mistaken for thyrotoxicosis and the presence of an immediate psychological precipitant does not help to exclude it from the diagnosis. Masserman (1955) lists a formidable array of organic states which can be mistaken for an anxiety neurosis, which in addition to hyperthyroidism, include lesions in the region of the diencephalon, carotid sinus hypersensitivity, heart disease and addiction to dextroamphetamine sulphate. It may be associated with organic cerebral states where the patient's deficit may lead to or even heighten anxiety features, for, as has already been stated, they lack the mental equipment to overcome the anxiety and are more easily overwhelmed by it (p. 109).

Course and Prognosis

This is variable for there may be merely one sharp single attack or it may become chronic. Frequently it is periodic, the patient being particularly vulnerable to certain insults such as separation from home and family ('separation-anxiety') or the testing experience of an examination, or public appearance. They usually recover from the acute phase and chronicity should be avoidable.

TREATMENT

As cultural factors are alleged to play an important part, it should be possible by prophylactic measures to prevent the occurrence of anxiety attacks. One can talk of evolving more stable social structures but it is very difficult to do anything constructive. The society is geared to anxiety and the surprising thing is that there are not many more casualties. Psychiatrists get a false impression of incidence and may be persuaded that the problem is a gross one, but severe anxiety attacks which are crippling and long lasting are not common and as in any enterprise, the effects of casualties must be seen against the whole process. Anxiety is fundamental to the social and material progress to which our society is committed, in which it has helped to achieve outstanding success. The condition is rarely permanent and carries a good prognosis and it is doubtful if any tampering with the social structure will in fact make it more stable; it could just as easily make it less so. The doctor's task is still to treat the sick and be highly critical of social experiments, which are alleged to reduce incidence of neurotic illness. 'Man's inhumanity to man makes countless thousands mourn.' Yet it need not produce anxiety. One could argue that these injustices provide the very stuff against which the individual can fight and thus equate his anxiety, but this statement must not be seen as a recommendation!

The acute attack if severe may require very heavy sedation, if not continuous narcosis (p. 464). Generally a useful compromise is amylobarbitone sodium 200 mg. three times a day, though this should not be maintained for more than two to three days and preferably under reliable supervision, for there is always the danger of addiction. With increasing awareness of barbiturate addiction and the relative infrequency of the severe acute attack, continuous narcosis is now rarely prescribed, and the less addictive tranquillizers, such as chlorpromazine, and hypnotics, such as nitrazepam, are preferred.

Some patients may treat themselves with alcohol and become addicted, for it provides effective relief and therefore it must not be recommended. Much of the advertising of tonic wines is directed at the anxiety-prone and their popularity is due more to their alcoholic content than to any special ingredient.

Anxiolytic Drugs

In a society where anxiety is universal and where intolerance of discomfort is the first step on the ladder of affluence, it is not surprising that there is a great demand for drugs to relieve anxiety. There has been considerable activity by pharmaceutical firms to cater for this demand and a whole range of drugs, referred to as *anxiolytic* have been produced and all are supported by clinical trials to indicate their efficacy. The doctor is bewildered by their number and their claims and may be excused if he is a little sceptical and regards them as no better than placebos in spite of the controlled trials to prove the contrary. This subject is dealt with in greater detail under 'Therapeutic Trials' (Chapter 18).

All investigations to date have shown that anxiolytic agents or minor tranquillizers do not perform as well as quick-acting barbiturates such as amylobarbitone sodium but as the latter is a ready source of addiction it is understandable that the search for an effective substitute has a high priority. Unfortunately most of the 'successful' anxiolytic drugs do not in the strictest trials perform better than placebos and reports are accumulating that many of these drugs are also addictive. Minor tranquillizers have therefore very little place in the treatment of anxiety other than as placebos and will not be listed under treatment. Information regarding these drugs can be found under 'Psychopharmacology' (Chapter 18). There are, of course, less expensive placebos which do not carry the risks of hepatic and renal damage, agranulocytosis, persistent hypotension, subarachnoid haemorrhage, Parkinsonism and other complications yet to be described.

Hospital Admission

This need be reserved only for severe cases but as many have their clinical picture adulterated with drug addiction, admission to hospital will then be necessary. This introduces the patient to the stabilizing atmosphere of the hospital where drugs are withdrawn under controlled conditions, sleep is ensured and what was initially an acute if not desperate situation assumes its proper perspective. The forces making for spontaneous remission are allowed free play although in severe phobic states a more positive course of rehabilitation and treatment is needed (see below).

ABREACTION TECHNIQUES

Narco-analysis

If there is any suggestion of a 'specific event', some form of abreactive technique can be useful. This can be narco-analysis, using sodium thiopentone, 0·5 g., dissolved in 20 ml. of distilled water. The drug is given intravenously and injected slowly, the patient being kept at a pre-narcotic level. A thorough knowledge of the patient's history and background should first be obtained, though some workers give these injections and just let the patient abreact, considering that the discharge of the emotional material is the main therapeutic objective and that insight and understanding of the process are not essential. It does work in some instances, but it has its dangers and cannot be recommended. Those who advocate it counter criticism by saying that the major abreactions with narco-analysis may take place after the session is over, when the psychiatrist has gone. This is often true, but the psychiatrist can and does instruct his nursing staff or assistant in the handling of the situation and the recording of data and discusses the problem with them and the patient later. Part of the therapeutic process is for the patient to have someone who can share his problems and help him towards mastering them. A strictly mechanical approach does not provide this help.

Narcosynthesis. This was the name given by Grinker and Spiegel (1945*b*) to a technique similar to narco-analysis in that sodium thiopentone is used, but the patient is encouraged to re-experience the intense emotion accompanying the event which precipitated the attack of anxiety and thus deal with it more adequately. In practice narcosynthesis and narco-analysis are not discrete treatments, but are usually combined.

Agents other than intravenous barbiturates have been used and include ether inhalations, carbon dioxide and the addition to the pentothal of cerebral stimulants such as ritalin and methedrine.

Ether has been known to release inhibitions since its discovery as an anaesthetic almost a century ago. Ether parties, where the guests sniffed the volatile substance and became gay and irresponsible, were popular, but it was not used as an abreactive agent till a century later when it was largely popularized by Palmer (1945) who used it extensively on psychiatric casualties in his unit in Tripoli during the North African campaign in the Second World War. While many of his patients were predominantly hysterical, a large number were suffering from anxiety states with a nuclear situation, such as startle reaction or battle dreams, and the results he reported from the treatment were very encouraging, in that symptomatic relief was obtained and the patient was able to return to duty in a relatively short time, though a more sheltered category was frequently necessary.

An open mask is used and the ether is dropped on to it gently and the patient asked to inhale. Naturally, a thorough physical check, particularly to exclude chest disease, is necessary, and any suggestion of epilepsy would also be a contra-indication. The treatment as with narco-analysis and narcosynthesis should not be undertaken without an extensive knowledge of the patient and his background. The ether stimulates the patient to talk and may even have a slight hallucinogenic effect so that the patient may vividly experience forgotten memories, and excitement can rise to a crescendo followed by a sudden silence; some regard the latter phase of therapeutic benefit. The patient may become violent and aggressive, shouting, kicking and screaming and generally 'blowing off', but it is followed by a period of calm and feeling of well-being and the pattern may be repeated with subsequent treatments. The total number given and their frequency is variable and will depend on the successful removal of symptoms, though some patients become addicted if not to the ether, to the abreaction it produces, and while the therapeutic benefit may flatter the psychiatrist, this aspect should be borne in mind. The author, who has had experience with the treatment with both service casualties and in civilian life, found that the fresh cases arising during combat were much more responsive to this treatment. Civilian states were usually more chronic and had developed a crust which ether abreaction found more difficult to penetrate, an experience which is also found in narco-analysis. It is perhaps unfair to introduce these techniques to young psychiatrists and expect them to get good results with civilian problems, for success is likely to be limited and they may feel the treatment is of little value, but in the acute problem it undoubtedly has a place.

Carbon dioxide therapy was described by Meduna (1950) for the treatment of neurotic disorders. A mixture of 30 per cent carbon dioxide and 70 per cent oxygen is used and the patient is asked to breathe it through a mask. A word of caution about the mixture is necessary. Carbon dioxide is heavier than oxygen and if the mixture is in one cylinder there is a danger that when it is nearly empty, the percentage of carbon dioxide may be higher than 30 per cent with consequent risk to the patient. It is therefore desirable to have the gases in two cylinders and mix them immediately before inhalation. The patient can attend two to three times a week and after each treatment of 30–40 inhalations a state of altered consciousness is reached and there may also be motor restlessness, with waving of the arms and bicycling movements of the legs. When the mask is withdrawn, consciousness rapidly returns and the patient who is in a regressed state may be much more communicative and abreact satisfactorily. It is not an unpleasant experience and with out-patient treatment, few fail to attend. Its specificity has been questioned and Hawkings and Tibbetts (1956*a*) who conducted a controlled trial found it of no greater value than the placebo. It may be that it would have benefited a clinically more homogeneous group than those they studied and apart from favourable reports from other workers, one would be reluctant to abandon entirely, without further information, a treatment which emanates from a source which gave mankind convulsion therapy.

Methedrine can be used by itself or in conjunction with barbiturates for abreactive purposes. Simon and Taube (1946) used it alone for psychiatric exploration. Sargant and Slater (1954) recommend its use with barbiturates as a substitute for ether and carbon dioxide in obsessional patients who may be made worse by these techniques. Initially 10–20 mg. are combined with 0·5 g. of sodium thiopentone, but the dose may be increased to 40 or 50 mg. if necessary. As with thiopentone by itself, it is given slowly and the patient usually becomes very talkative, a state which may persist for several hours after the injection. It is therefore unwise to return him immediately to the war as he may disclose many of his intimate affairs to the other patients with subsequent embarrassment. If the session takes place in the afternoon the waking effects of the drug will not have worn off by night time and heavy sedation may be necessary to ensure sleep.

Although these pharmacological aids may be of value in the treatment of anxiety states, expertise in their administration is not the sole criterion for their use. The patient should be well-selected and the psychiatrist should be sufficiently experienced in psychotherapy and with a sound knowledge of psychopathology to handle the material which may emerge and the situations which may result.

Continuous Narcosis

This has been used for a variety of psychiatric disorders, including acute schizophrenic and maniacal states, but it is now mainly used in the acute anxiety state. Prior to the introduction of convulsion therapy and the phenothiazines, there was some justification for its use in psychotic states, including the agitated melancholic, but it no longer can compete with these more specific measures, though the patient's demand for sleep, which is symptomatic of his illness, may tempt the physician to resort to heavy sedation instead of recognizing the true nature of the clinical problem. One should now draw a distinction between continuous narcosis as used for psychotic states and that required for the anxiety state. In the former, the aim was to achieve 20 hours sleep in the 24 hours, in order to rest the patient and make his nursing care possible, while in the latter one tries to ensure *adequate* sleep with *adequate* rest in between. The rationale of the treatment, particularly in the psychotic, has been explained in Pavlovian terms. It was (and may still be) popular in the U.S.S.R. and Wortis (1950) states:

> A large part of Soviet therapeutic experimentation is based directly on animal research in Pavlovian laboratories, but with proper appreciation of the fact that

the human organism differs from the dog's. There is an enormously varied literature on the effect of all sorts of conditions, diseases and pharmacological agents on sensory perceptions, conditioned reflex patterns and higher integration functions, with corresponding experiments on correction of these experimental disturbances by various means. . . . Of particular importance in this field of interest is Pavlov's concept of protective inhibition, *i.e.* a state of depressed or suspended nervous activity which has important restorative and regulative effects on nervous functions. It is probably for this reason that in the U.S.S.R. various types of sleep treatment are widely used in the treatment of a number of different conditions.

It would be of interest if this were still the case.

Amylobarbitone sodium, in doses of 200 mg. six-hourly, is the drug now generally favoured and it is usually potentiated with chlorpromazine, 50 mg. three times a day. The patient is kept in a darkened and quiet room (an almost impossible task in a modern general hospital), and all his needs, including feeding and toilet, are catered for in his room. Fluids (intake and output) are carefully controlled, the urine is examined repeatedly for ketones and the patient should be strictly supervised, for the treatment is not without risk. In the deeper and more prolonged forms of narcosis, somnifaine was supplemented by paraldehyde and liver damage was a complication. In a military psychiatric hospital there was a young soldier patient who in spite of a quarter-hourly pulse check, turned his head into his pillow and smothered himself, indicating that special pillows which can be breathed through should be used. Fortunately such extreme degrees of narcosis are no longer necessary and the acute anxiety state can be adequately controlled with amylobarbitone sodium, 200 mg. three times a day, supplemented by chlorpromazine, 50 mg. three times a day, for about three to four days, after which the doses can be gradually reduced and other treatment initiated.

Psychotherapy

Psychotherapeutic procedures in the treatment of anxiety vary enormously from superficial suggestion and a supportive relationship, through hypnotherapy, to the deeper forms of analysis with attempts to effect a basic change in character. The last will obviously not be necessary for those patients who respond satisfactorily to shorter and therefore less costly treatments and may even be contra-indicated in the pseudoneurotic anxieties which are really manifestations of schizophrenia.

'Fixated' Anxiety requires an entirely different approach. The patient is usually not nearly so acutely distressed though he may

have acute exacerbations. He is primarily concerned with the physical concomitants of his anxiety and it may be difficult to distinguish the overt symptomatology from a predominantly hysterical reaction. The diagnostic issue may be decided on the presence or absence of physical features of anxiety, such as sweating and tachycardia, and an interesting example of this difficulty was reported by Jones and Lewis (1941) who, in a study of the psychiatric background to Effort Syndrome, classified 11 per cent of their patients as hysterical and 18 per cent as psychopathic.

Group Therapy

Patients with 'fixated' anxiety respond well to group psychotherapy which need not be particularly prolonged or heavily analytical or adhere to the now traditional leaderless group technique. A talk by the doctor on the physiological effects of anxiety and the reinforcement of seeing a number of other fellow sufferers, apparently healthy, helps to reassure the patient. They are more able to discuss their anxieties among each other and what had become organ-fixated is recognized as emotionally determined with consequent lessening of anxiety and reduction in symptomatology. A number do however prove stubborn and more prolonged treatment either in the group or with individual psychotherapy is needed.

PHOBIC ANXIETY

This is a form of anxiety where the phobia acts as a defence, often an inadequate one, to protect the patient from situations or circumstances which may predispose to or initiate the anxiety attacks. The patient recognizes his fear is an irrational one, but is unable to overcome it and is usually unaware of its unconscious origin, though it is doubtful whether even if he were aware of it, the fear would necessarily be removed. Although the condition has been known since antiquity and had been well described by Westphal (1871), it was Freud (1895, 1909*a*) who clearly distinguished the phobic states from obsessional states and demonstrated their intimate association with anxiety.

In the earlier paper, Freud distinguished phobias from obsessions, indicating that the former were invariably associated with anxiety, and that one does not find, in the course of analysis, substitution as a dominant feature, such as is present in the obsessional group. He subdivided them rather artificially into (1) the common phobias which were exaggerated fears of things that make most people feel uncomfortable, such as darkness, solitude, death, illness and snakes, and (2) the specific phobias which are fears of situations and circumstances which do not affect the ordinary person, such as agoraphobia or fear of public places. Some have classified phobias according to the feared object, but apart from providing an exercise in Greek, it has very little real value for the clinician and tells us practically nothing about the condition itself. Freud considered that phobias originated in childhood and in his later paper (Freud, 1909*a*) he described the classical case of the 5-year-old boy, 'Little Hans', who refused to go out into the street for fear of being bitten by a horse, which Freud interpreted as a castration fear, the horse being substituted for the father. The detailed analysis, which was conducted through the boy's father, was a prototype for child analysis and in this respect is of great interest, but it also gives some indication of the psychopathology of the phobic state.

Fenichel (1945) analyses the various phobias and offers some explanations. In certain instances where there is very little displacement, he states that anxiety is simply felt in situations where an uninhibited person would experience either sexual excitement or rage. Sex phobia occurs especially in women who develop fear in the face of sexual temptation and try to avoid it. Eating fears are alleged to have some historical association as do anal phobias and fighting phobias, and the formula, that what is unconsciously feared is unconsciously desired, is offered in explanation.

Unconscious temptations are represented by open streets which Fenichel states are unconsciously regarded as opportunities for sexual adventure. Fears of being alone are associated with temptations to masturbate—punishment is frequently included in the phobic state; an open street is a place where one may be caught; being alone means being unprotected from assault; and hypochondriacal fears may represent symbolic castration. Included in the punishment group are fears of falling down from high places or being run over. No doubt these interpretations were based on careful analytical studies, but they have very little bearing on the day to day management of these patients, for though they may accept interpretations with enthusiasm, they rarely respond with symptomatic improvement and continue to attend for their psychotherapy suitably escorted, or even by ambulance!

The problem is more common than is generally realized, for many patients are able to organize their lives in such a way that the phobia is least handicapping. The commercial traveller who is afraid of heights may arrange to be given an area with no mountain roads. The patient who has a locomotion or travel phobia may compromise by what is sometimes called 'out-work', which means work which is farmed out by the factories to the patient in his home. This usually requires very little in the way of machinery or equipment and demands certain skills and dexterity from the patient. Assembling of small parts, leather stitching, jewellery mounting, carding of goods, sewing and typing are only a few of the jobs that are farmed out in an industrial city like Birmingham and very often the condition is not declared till such work is no longer available. Another precipitating factor is slum clearance or just moving house. In older property, such as terraced houses, there is a communal atmosphere which has developed over the years which allows a person to enjoy a little world within a few yards of her front door. She has plenty of neighbours who will drop in for a chat, leave their children to be minded, and bring back the groceries; or the little shop at the corner may not be so very far away and within the patient's range, especially if she can have the feeling of security that pushing her baby's perambulator can give her. This last point may appear far-fetched, but the author has had patients who could only attend for out-patient treatment if they were holding the hand of their 3-year-old child.

Symptomatology

They may be protean and extend beyond the declaration of the patient's specific or general phobia. It may be heavily adulterated with the symptoms of actue anxiety attacks which in turn may excite the hyperventilation syndrome and even produce transient loss or disturbance of consciousness. In such cases, depersonalization may be a constant feature, though the diagnosis of temporal lobe attacks should be borne in mind. Roth (1959) described the 'phobic-anxiety-depersonalization syndrome', which was given the name 'calamity syndrome' because in under 50 per cent of the 135 cases, 'calamitous precipitants' had impinged on a sensitized person to produce the clinical picture. It is doubtful whether this syndrome really differs from the phobic anxiety attacks which have been well known for centuries. The word phobia is derived from the Greek (φοβος) meaning flight, panic-fear or terror and the ancient Greeks had honoured Phobos as a deity who could induce fear or panic in their enemies, so it is not necessary to supplement the term phobia with calamity. As one would expect, the condition was also described by Shakespeare in the 'Merchant of Venice':

> Some men there are love not a gaping pig;
> Some, that are mad if they behold a cat. . . .

The patient may not declare his phobic features but complain of secondary depression which, should it resolve with anti-depressant treatment, still leaves the phobic state unaffected, and a number of depressions that do not remit with E.C.T. may well be basically phobic anxiety states. Occasionally one may meet the classical phobic state with evidence of castration fear, such as the young man who dreads going into the barber's chair. It can be postulated that the snipping of the scissors is a sound he cannot tolerate, but usually it is the feeling of being localized, perched on a chair and unable to make a quick dash for freedom which terrifies. This is certainly the feeling that is expressed by patients when they are in cinemas, church, bus queues, large stores and so on. Symptomatology may be masked by drugs, particularly barbiturates and as has already been said, many patients become addicted to barbiturates because of phobic anxiety, the drug acting as a confidence pill. Others resort to alcohol, some having to take a pint or two of beer in the morning to get to work, and there is always the risk that alcoholism may develop. It may be necessary to ask the patient specifically whether he has lost confidence and even then he may be ashamed to declare the degree of phobic anxiety he endures, for many feel that it is so ridiculous that a more sinister interpretation may be placed on their psychiatric state and they therefore camouflage the phobic anxiety with complaints about their physical sensations. It may be very difficult to persuade such patients to enter hospital and even if they are put on the waiting list, a number cancel their admission, as they feel, at the time, more secure in their organized phobic state then they think they would be in the strange atmosphere of a hospital. Obsessional features are not an infrequent accompaniment and may be part of the patient's defences designed to ward off the evil which is feared.

The patient usually fears that she will lose consciousness or control when in a public place and that a crowd will gather with consequent embarrassment. Though it may be the main symptom, it is not common for the patient to volunteer it and it has to be extracted by questions about lack of confidence and what the patient fears will happen, with tentative suggestions. Many patients respond to this approach as if, for the first time, their problem is being appreciated and are relieved to think that the doctor knows about it and that it is not unique, for until then they may have believed that nobody else could have such a strange affliction. The handicap may restrict other members of the household, for it can take the form of being afraid to be left on one's own and the husband or wife will lose time from work to stay with the patient; it is not uncommonly this aspect which produces the crisis and brings the patient for the first time for specialist advice. An unusual but not uncommon defence may be not to venture out till after dark, for then they believe they will not be seen or noticed, and if they feel the panic developing they can rest or support themselves without attracting attention. Some carry magic tokens, such as a bottle of water or spirits or some tablets which they feel will abort the attack should it arise. The author had a patient who carried as a prophylactic a large flagon of cider in her shopping bag. Friedman (1959) quotes two delightful verses which as he says express the ambivalent struggle of an agoraphobic patient as she anticipated her first unaccompanied visit to the therapist:

Which Epitaph Shall be Mine?

She couldn't try
For fear she'd die;
She never tried
And so she died

or

She couldn't try
For fear she died;
But once she tried
Her fears—they died.

TREATMENT

Mention has been made of psychotherapy, but in the classical sense, with free-association and interpretation, it can be a very unrewarding task. Patients can attend for months and months and though they may achieve some insight into the psychopathology, this is not usually reflected in improved performance. Relatives and friends are usually unable to do very much, for they cajole, threaten and bully, and the patient is left more insecure than before. The psychotherapist is frequently deprived of essential information as he may believe the patient attended unaccompanied, whereas she was escorted to the door. King and Little (1959) who treated the patients described by Roth (1959) ('phobic-anxiety depersonalization syndrome') were prompted by reports of the efficacy of intravenous thiopentone in war neuroses to give it a trial but were unable to obtain a satisfactory abreaction when giving the injection (2·5 per cent) at a rate sufficient to produce progressive sedation and light sleep in about 15 minutes. No attempt was therefore made to obtain an abreaction, and psychotherapy was restricted to a discussion of concrete problems, simple reassurance and an explanation that the illness is a response to personal calamity, the patient being permitted to wake spontaneously which occurred in about 5–10 minutes. Two to three treatments per week were given and in successful cases, benefit was cumulative, starting after the third or fourth treatment. They found that if there was no progress after six treatments, it seldom occurred thereafter and no further advantage could be gained after 10 treatments, the greatest benefit occurring three months after the treatment was completed, with 85 per cent improved. The authors considered that the thiopentone acted by altering the activity of the adrenergic arousal system, the functional abnormality of which, they suggest, might lie at the core of the phobic state.

Acetylcholine

The author has been using intravenous acetylcholine in the treatment of phobic anxiety states since 1954 but it would be wrong to suggest that the mere injection of acetylcholine constituted the whole treatment for many other factors require consideration (see below).

Acetylcholine in the treatment of psychiatric disorders was first used by Fiamberti (1950) who, in his treatment of schizophrenia, used large doses (up to 0·6 g. of acetylcholine bromide) which were injected rapidly to cause convulsions and loss of consciousness as a form of shock therapy in the tradition of insulin coma. Ibor (1952) reported his use of the same drug but with smaller doses (up to 0·2 g.) of acetylcholine chloride for selected states of anxiety. Initially the patient is given 0·05 g. which is injected very slowly in case the patient is hypersensitive. A satisfactory reaction consists of coughing, flushing of the face, increased salivation and slowing of the pulse. When the drug is injected too quickly, as in the Fiamberti method, cardiac asystole for a short period may result and this is probably the cause of the loss of consciousness, the mechanism being similar to a Stokes-Adams seizure.

Phillips and Hutchinson (1954) reported favourably on its use in anxiety states but Hawkings and Tibbetts (1965) suggested that it produced no more than a placebo response, as they found a similar recovery rate (60 per cent) in 18 'neurotic' patients who had acetylcholine and another 18 who had distilled water. As however only 5 of the former and 6 of the latter suffered from phobic anxiety attacks it would be unjustifiable to draw conclusions from such a small sample. A report of 191 patients with phobic anxiety treated with acetylcholine (Sim & Houghton, 1967) provided the following data.

All patients were materially handicapped in that they were either totally incapacitated as far as work was concerned or were unable to indulge in normal social activities or get into town to do shopping. Although phobic anxiety tends to be equated with the alliterative title Housebound Housewives, of the 191 patients, 94 were men. Results were graded as follows:

Grade 1. Symptom-free and free from handicap.
Grade 2. Practically symptom-free and free from handicap.
Grade 3. Not symptom-free, but handicap materially reduced.
Grade 4. No change.

Six months after cessation of treatment 85·3 per cent were materially improved and 69·6 per cent were in Grades 1 and 2. In a longer follow-up (2–10 years) of 141 patients by their general practitioners, those materially improved totalled 88·6 per cent which compared with 85·7 per cent in a 6 month follow up of the same patients by the author. Of the 28 who did not benefit, 16 failed to complete the course and were erratic in their attendance and in general did not show the strong motivation towards recovery that one should look for in selecting patients for treatment. On the other hand 3 who failed to complete the course did so because they felt better and saw no need for further attendance. They maintained their progress on follow-up.

Addiction and Phobic Anxiety

Forty patients (20·9 per cent) had developed a dependence on drugs and/or alcohol which was either unable to contain their anxiety or had become sufficiently severe to warrant treatment in its own right. Only 10 failed to improve, but as 6 did not complete their treatment, 75 per cent derived some benefit and of these 18 (45 per cent) were in Grades 1 and 2. These results illustrate that phobic anxiety can be complicated with severe addictions and that the prognosis in such patients may be reasonably good.

Phobic Anxiety and Sex Drive

Roberts (1964) reported that 53 per cent of his patients showed evidence of 'frigidity, painful intercourse, inability to achieve orgasm and other evidence of sexual maladjustment'. In the author's series, there were 97 females of whom 28 gave a history of sexual or marital difficulties of any severity. After treatment only 5 still complained of their initial frigidity. Twelve patients who had lacked the confidence to become engaged or to marry were able to do so while undergoing treatment. Follow-up confirmed their satisfactory sexual adjustment and in 3 who eventually had babies there was no relapse.

Economics of Treatment

Phobic anxiety is common and severely handicapping. Treatment should therefore be available to all and not make too heavy demands on a psychiatric service which has many other commitments. Seventy-four patients (mainly male) were treated as out-patients and of the 117 in-patients almost 77 per cent spent less than 30 days in hospital. Treatment was given 3 times per week to in-patients and twice weekly to out-patients. A full course consisted of 30–40 treatments.

Rationale of Treatment

As has been stated, the acetylcholine injections were only part of the treatment. If the patient were manipulating the home environment to perpetuate the disability, admission to hospital was recommended. The hospital itself (Midland Nerve Hospital, Birmingham, England) is a small intimate unit with a permissive approach. Atmosphere is cosy and patients are encouraged to get out and test themselves with graduated tasks. No accent was placed on specific phobias for these are not as common as patients and some therapists would indicate. The approach to treatment was based on the assumption that there is a general anxiety factor and that its localization while of psychopathological interest, was not of great importance in treatment which had to be directed at the general anxiety state. Furthermore some of the patients' difficulties such as taking the chair at an important meeting or giving a lecture to a scientific society could not be recreated in hospital.

This policy was successful for although in many instances the 'specific' phobia was not treated, it would cease to be a problem once the general tendency to over-react with anxiety was countered. Dependency or transference situations with the staff physician were not a feature of the treatment. The total emphasis from the day of admission or the start of treatment was to render the patient independent and while some tried to recreate their former dependencies this was discouraged. It was not considered that the drug had any central action but its peripheral effect was to cancel the tendency towards overactivity of the sympathetic and thus help the patient towards a new mastery over his problem.

Before treatment started the rationale was explained to the patient thus:

> The panic attacks and the physical accompaniments of anxiety which you dread and keep you housebound or prevent you from going to work or to church or on holiday are due to a sudden outpouring of a substance like adrenaline (epinephrine) into the blood stream. This produces the rapid pulse, dryness of the mouth, blurring of vision and weakness of the knees. Overbreathing which frequently accompanies the attack may in turn produce another crop of symptoms such as tightness in the chest, tingling of the hands and a feeling of losing consciousness or control. The substance you are going to have injected is also manufactured by the body and has opposite effects and with subsequent injections you will gradually realise that these sudden panics need not occur when you are afraid.

In the 20 years the author has used this treatment there have been no serious complications apart from recurrence of bronchitis in 3 patients with a previous history of recurring chest infections. In view of the increased bronchial secretion produced by the acetylcholine, it could have precipitated these lapses. Pseudocholinesterase levels before and after treatment showed no significant difference and in no instance has the effect of the acetylcholine been prolonged though it should not be given to a patient who is currently on prostigmine. Patients with recent history of myocardial infarction or with heart block were excluded. Age is not a bar to treatment and neither is duration or severity of the illness. One female patient, aged 68, with a 30-year history of severely crippling phobic anxiety made an excellent recovery. Some preparations, particularly if made up with a triethyleneglycol base, produced venous thrombosis, but acetylcholine chloride (Roche) is perfectly satisfactory.

In-patients were given a rehabilitation programme. Occupational therapists and nursing staff take the patient in hand and graduate her activities, such as going out of the hospital, initially escorted, and later unescorted. Sorties to post a letter are followed by bus rides to the city centre and later unescorted shopping expeditions, the patient bringing back the goods ordered by staff and other patients, together with the receipts from the specified store. In two weeks, five or six treatments will have been given and the patient is usually ready to be tried out for a week-end at home and if this proves favourable, she can be discharged to continue to attend outside working hours for out-patient treatment twice a week. As many of these patients are also depressed, antidepressants such as imipramine (50 mg. t.d.s.) were given and barbiturates were withdrawn by substituting chlorpromazine in doses of 50 mg. nocte (in addicts 50 mg. t.d.s.). t.d.s).

BEHAVIOUR THERAPY

Phobic anxiety states have received considerable attention from behaviour therapists and though there are certain similarities in the method of treatment with that described under 'Acetylcholine', there are essential differences. Behaviour therapy claims to be based on theoretical constructs which are derived from learning theories, particularly those of Hull. A hierarchical list of problems is worked out with the patient and each is tackled in ascending order till complete emancipation is reached. In the regimen used by the author a common approach to all patients was used on the principle that there was a general factor of increased susceptibility in the patient and that the so-called trigger situation was in itself not the most important aspect.

The most objective studies have been those of Gelder and Marks (1966) who in this and other papers evaluate the desensitization process and compare its efficacy with traditional psychotherapy. They conclude that behaviour therapy of the desensitizing type yields results which are superior to those of psychotherapy (Gelder *et al.*, 1967). As there are probably non-specific factors even in the application of controlled behaviour therapy, it is possible that some of the beneficial effects of this treatment are also present in the rehabilitation programme associated with the in-patient regimen for patients receiving acetylcholine. It would not apply to out-patients receiving acetylcholine and furthermore the duration of in-patient treatment for those receiving acetylcholine is much less, though other factors such as proximity of the hospital to patient's home may be material.

The beneficial effect of the treatment can be explained in terms of behaviour therapy for it incorporates some of the criteria associated with that treatment, but there are many aspects which are incapable of assessment, the main one being the quality of the nursing staff, and the author feels sure that in-patient treatment is so much superior to out-patient treatment because of this factor. It is also much more economical to admit the patient initially for two weeks or so, than to court the risk of failure after months of out-patient effort. This does raise a problem, for a number of these patients are reluctant to come into hospital, particularly a mental hospital, and furthermore, many mental hospitals lack the rehabilitation facilities which do not depend on equipment or buildings, but on close proximity to the hurly burly of the city, or in other words, the patient's normal milieu, where she can be tested out easily and frequently, before being returned to her home surroundings. It should be possible to render the patient independent of her handicap by an energetic and sustained approach to treatment, but the family may prove a problem. As many of these patients are women (though men are by no means immune) the husband may feel it is his manly duty to protect her from her imagined fears by his continued presence and his proximity may fulfil his own needs as well as those of the patient, thus obstructing recovery. If progress on an out-patient basis is slow, admission to hospital should be strongly recommended, for otherwise success cannot be assured, though there may be good reasons for the patient refusing to enter hospital, such as the demands of young children. But, if it is a question of handicap or recovery, as it frequently is, the patient must strike a balance sheet and decide whether the handicap is sufficiently severe to overcome the objections and this is a decision which had better be left to the patient and her family. The best terms for successful treatment is a well-motivated patient who has decided on her own account that it is time something effective was done for her neurotic illness.

Implosion ('The bursting inward of a vessel from external pressure' *O.E.D.*) **or Flooding**

Boulougouris and Marks (1969) reported on four phobic patients treated by the implosion or flooding method. In desensitization treatment the patient is taught to relax while slowly entering the phobic situation and anxiety is kept to a minimum at all times. By contrast, with implosion the patient is asked to enter the worst possible phobic situation and to experience the fear at maximum intensity for up to an hour until he is no longer capable of experiencing further fear. The procedure is first done in imagination and then in real life, so that in successive sessions the patient finds it increasingly difficult to feel frightened in the phobic situation, until finally he can enter it with equanimity. Of the 4 patients reported, 3 became almost symptom-free after a mean of 14 sessions and follow-up of 6½ months.

In a subsequent cross-over study, Marks *et al.* (1971) compared implosion with desensitization in phobic states and concluded that the former did better with severe phobias with many symptoms, while the latter was more suitable for focal phobias. Further reports from the same department confirm the early impressions, and physiological and statistical support have been detailed. In comparing this treatment with the present writer's use of acetylcholine, there are some similarities, in that the patient is introduced to a new situation which he probably fears but the acetylcholine has an entirely different physiological effect. It is also quicker to administer and is more certain in its action. In a series of over 500 patients in the past 19 years the results have continued to be most satisfactory and relapse is infrequent. One factor which is not sufficiently stressed in these treatments and which is of prime importance, is that the patient must be well-motivated, and this goes beyond the mere statement of willingness to co-operate. It must be associated with a determination to get well. Poor motivation will prejudice any treatment.

Treatment with Monoamine Oxidase Inhibitors

This treatment has been reported by Kelly *et al.* (1970). The drug, usually phenelzine, either alone or in combination with chlordiazepoxide or a tricyclic antidepressant, was given not infrequently as a maintenance dose for months or even years, and the authors observe that results were superior to those obtained by classical behaviour therapy. Apart from the general undesirability of combining phenelzine with tricyclics, it is obvious that dependence is a real risk together with the severe restrictions in food and drink. The degree of handicap is another feature which tends to receive scant attention in most of these reported treatments, yet it is one of the more important items in evaluation.

Methohexitone-assisted Desensitization

This is a variation of Wolpe's original method of reciprocal inhibition and is little different from barbiturate-induced relaxation. It has been reported by Mawson (1970) who conducted a controlled crossover trial, comparing it with progressive muscular relaxation over which it had considerable advantages.

There seems to be no end to the ideas for getting patients over their phobias. Kumar and Wilkinson (1971) reported the use of a 'thought stopping technique' to build up the conditioned inhibition of unpleasant thoughts. They do this by inducing a state of peace and calm by using a tape of bird songs or the sound of a waterfall. The latter could, in certain instances induce a feeling of considerable discomfort, if not urgency. Orwin (1971) used a technique of breath-holding to overcome the fear, and also a 'running technique' when the patient is asked to run so many steps while holding his or her breath. The surprising thing is that patients are prepared to do these things at the bidding of the therapist. Other than an index of slavish obedience, and therefore strong motivation, it is difficult to see what else it does.

DISSOCIATIVE REACTIONS OR HYSTERIA

Dissociative reactions have much in common in terms of psychopathology with *conversion reactions* and these two can be dealt with collectively under the older generic label 'Hysteria'.

HYSTERIA

This can assume protean forms including amnesias, tremors, anaesthesias, paralyses of limbs, hyperventilation attacks, mutism, deafness, blindness, somnambulism or attacks resembling those of epilepsy. The name 'hysteria' has an intriguing origin. It is derived from the Greek *υστερα* = a womb, and the condition was alleged to be due to its wandering consequent on frustration at being kept infertile. This sexual aetiology of hysteria was abandoned for over 2000 years and it was not till Charcot, at the end of the nineteenth century, with his clinical demonstrations on hysterical subjects, that the way for a more rational approach to the condition was developed. Charcot was able to demonstrate the effect of emotional disturbance in producing the hysterical symptoms and how these symptoms could be removed, altered or transposed by hypnotic suggestion. At that time the diagnosis rested largely on the exclusion of the organic and it was not therefore surprising that a distinguished neurologist like Charcot should have set the trend, but it was Janet (1893), who had been his pupil, who studied the problem at a psychological level and concluded that it was due to a disturbance of personal synthesis, together with some dissociation of consciousness. Both he and Charcot laid great stress on the hereditary defect which they considered contributed to the inability of the mind to hold together under physical and other stresses with resulting dissociation of parcels of thought from the main mental stream. As has been stated in Chapter 2, Breuer and Freud (1895) advanced our knowledge by showing that the cases they studied contained an element of sexual disturbance in their aetiology which was responsible for the repression which plays such an important part in the mechanics of hysteria.

There are two major clinical groupings in hysteria: (1) *the hysterial character* and (2) *hysterical symptoms.*

THE HYSTERICAL CHARACTER

The hysterical character or personality as a clinical entity must have a very old history, but the label 'character' derives from a more recent approach to personality disturbances and has been popularized by Reich (1933) who describes the hysterical character in his book, *Character Analysis*. A definition of 'character' is difficult to formulate and most definitions approximate to those for the ego. Fenichel (1945) states:

> The ego not only protects the organism from external and internal stimuli by blocking its reactions. It also reacts. It sifts and organizes stimuli and impulses; it permits some of them to find expression directly, others in a somewhat altered form. The dynamic and economic organization of its positive actions and the ways in which the ego combines its various tasks in order to find a satisfactory solution, all of this goes to make up 'character'.

Freud (1908) laid the foundations for 'characterology' in his study of the anal character, showing that orderliness, parsimony and obstinacy were prominent in persons who were formerly anal erotics and that these features were the first and most constant results of sublimation. His last paragraph is a plea 'to consider whether other types of character do not also show a connection with the excitability of particular erotogenic zones'. Reich considered that the behaviour of the hysterical character was flamboyantly sexual with coquetry in women and effeminacy in men. This behaviour could project the individual into situations where the apparent sexual goal is within reach and then the gross hysterical behaviour becomes mobilized. He described their unpredictability, suggestibility, over-imagination, insincerity, compulsive love-hunger, dependency needs for approval, dramatic sense, and sharp reactions to disappointment. They tend to confuse phantasy with reality and are prone to a variety of somatic complaints as well as hysterical ones, particularly skin reactions. The tendency to hysterical conversion has persuaded some psychiatrists that they are relatively benign states but it is important to realize that in these patients it is not simply a defence mechanism, but part of their life-style and is indicative of a very severe personality disturbance, closely allied in its malignancy to schizophrenia. The apparent exuberance that these patients display really conceals a shallow affectivity and the scenes and disturbances which frequently surround them are evidence of reality testing. They may be responsible for unwarranted claims against doctors and though they may realise that these will not stand up to the close scrutiny they will receive in a court of law, their need for publicity drives them to litigation and such is their acting ability that they have little difficulty in getting somebody to take up their case. It may be that in their marginal blurring between fact and phantasy, they have deceived even themselves, which would certainly be a kinder way to see it.

Jaspers (1946) has described the hysterical character thus:

> Instead of contenting himself with his endowments and potentialities as they are, the hysterical personality needs to appear in his own eyes and those of others, more than he actually is, to experience more than he is capable of experiencing. In place of genuine, spontaneous experience rationally expressed, there appears a spurious, theatrical and forced experience, not consciously so, but arising from his ability, and true hysterical attribute, of living entirely on his own stage and for the moment identifying himself entirely with his role, so that the whole act acquires an apparently genuine stamp. From this, all other hysterical traits can be understandably derived. The hysterical personality seems to have lost its core and to consist entirely of a series of shifting masks.

Many of these patients seek refuge in illness, but not all. Some prefer to go on acting out their problems in other situations and they may contribute to the ranks of pathological liars and swindlers, confidence tricksters and impostors. Perhaps the least anti-social of their activities is their resort to conversion symptoms, for with these they localize the problem between patient and doctor and spare society even greater embarrassments. Women are said to be more commonly affected than men, but it is difficult to be sure, for they predominate in the histrionic group with their explosive outbursts and frequent attempts at suicide, while the male counterpart may be found more frequently in the police court, because his conduct assumes an overt anti-social form.

Treatment

This can prove a formidable problem, as the patient has very definite views on the nature of her disability and while willing to try anything once, lacks the motivation and persistence to see things through. Psychotherapy would appear to be the most useful approach for there are no drugs which can specifically influence the condition, though if schizophrenic features are latent, phenothiazines may lower the level of sensitivity and render a patient amenable who might otherwise not be. Group therapy has been tried and found wanting, for they are disruptive of the group, demanding attention and showing off to a degree which the other members find intolerable. Individual psychotherapy would appear to be the best we have to offer at present, and even then the outlook must be guarded. There is one encouraging feature, however, for most are, like the psychopath, immature, and maturation does take place though slowly, and as the years go by the problem should become less acute and may eventually settle.

HYSTERICAL SYMPTOMS

The clinical picture has been itemized by Abse (1950) thus:

1. A group of physical symptoms without demonstrable organic basis.
2. Complacency in the presence of a grossly overt disability (*la belle indifférence* of Janet).
3. Episodic disturbances in the stream of consciousness due to an 'ego-alien homogenous constellation of ideas and emotions' occupying the field of consciousness.

No matter how grossly dissociated the person may be, there is generally no disharmony between mood and thought and schizophrenia can usually, though not invariably, be excluded from the diagnosis. In some cultures, however, the picture may be more confusing for severe regression with incontinence may occur, and occasionally one meets bizarre behaviour such as the patient drinking his urine. The main difference is that schizophrenia is generally a process while hysteria is more likely to be an episodic reaction, or if it persists, does not usually develop into a schizophrenic picture, though many schizophrenics may show hysterical features.

Psychopathology

A hysterical symptom is basically a dissociative phenomenon which is a reaction to an anxiety-producing situation. Glover (1949) lists the following sequence: (1) frustration; (2) introversion; (3) regression; (4) reactivation of oedipal strivings; and (5) failure of repression. A form of somatic compliance follows with localization of symptoms in accordance with body-libido, such as on erotogenic zones as well as libido-disturbance resulting from organic disease. The capacity to dissociate depends on a variety of factors such as age, sex, intelligence, cultural background, material and emotional situations and personality structure. That such forms of dissociation are acceptable in certain situations is illustrated by the words of the Psalmist:

> If I forget thee, O Jerusalem, let my right hand forget her cunning,
> If I do not remember thee, let my tongue cleave to the roof of my mouth . . .
>
> Psalm cxxxvii, 5, 6

These verses lay down the matrix for a hysterical paralysis of the right hand and a hysterical loss of speech. They also indicate the personal nature of the symbolism.

The degree of dissociation is also material for though it is traditionally accepted that conversion symptoms are unconsciously determined, a whole range of dissociation is likely and in some instances the distinction between what is unconscious and what is conscious must be very fine indeed. There is doubt among some authorities as to the unconscious nature of these hysterical symptoms and Szasz (1961) stresses that hysterical symptomatology is a form of language used by the individual to convey his distress and secure from society that which he requires to relieve it. He likens the mechanism to a game in which the individual tries to achieve mastery with coercion and self-help but with little or no accent on cooperation. The language of hysteria permits oblique references to problems where direct statements would not be countenanced and it is therefore a form of 'hinting' *i.e.* dropping clues to those who claim they are experienced in recognizing them. In our society the accepted profession for unravelling the puzzle is the medical profession, for the language used in hysteria is that of illness.

It is equivalent to a distress signal flown from a ship's mast but it does not necessarily convey to the observer the nature of the distress. It can mean that there is fire, plague or mutiny aboard or that the ship is sinking. It may not indicate anything more grave than that the ship's captain has forgotten to post his football coupon, but the triviality of the problem may not modify the urgency of signal. In many instances there is an inverse relationship.

These views have not yet been universally accepted, for just as the patient with hysterical symptoms is playing an accepted role in society, so the doctor follows his role and many have not yet reached the stage of looking past the hysterical display and trying to elucidate the nature and the extent of the problem which has nourished it. Others, who have for years indulged in the complementary role of treating the symptoms, have undergone a violent change and deny that there is an illness present at all and that it is all malingering. This would be unfair to a number of people, for many who are genuinely sick and in need of psychiatric treatment resort to the language of hysteria. There are also some who are not sick but speak the language fluently and it is they who contaminate the reaction with malingering.

Anxiety in Hysterical Conversion Symptoms

Lader and Sartorius (1968) set out to test the psychoanalytical theory that conversion symptoms relieve anxiety. They postulated that if this were so, anxiety levels in hysterics who developed conversion symptoms would be lower than in those with unadulterated anxiety or with phobic states with 'free-floating' anxiety. They used a battery of psychological and physiological tests including the Eysenck personality inventory and the semantic differentiating scales, *i.e.* the patient's self-rating as against the 'man-in-the-street' and palmar skin conductance. The hysterics showed more physiological arousal than the phobics and their self-rating scale of anxiety was higher than the phobics. On the basis of these results the authors conclude that the psychoanalytical hypothesis was not upheld.

As this paper has been accepted as a standard by others (Meares & Horvath, 1972; Rice & Greenfield, 1969) comment is appropriate. The self-rating of any patient is unreliable; in a psychiatric patient even more so, and in an hysteric more than ever. The purpose of hysteria is to exaggerate and draw attention to a predicament and a self-rating scale is likely to be used for this purpose. The increased palmar sweating is an index of the patient's immediate reaction to stimuli and the need for conversion rather than a true reflection of his general level of anxiety. The hysteric would have a high level of anticipatory excitement for unpleasant events, but this is not necessarily anxiety.

Amnesia

This is popularly believed to be a common hysterical symptom, but in actual practice it is relatively rare, and it has been said that every war may throw up not more than a handful of cases of genuine amnesia. But there was a plethora of servicemen in the Second World War claiming amnesia in varying degrees, and in practically every case there was strong motivation to evade duty. In a large number seen by the author, two main categories emerged: (*a*) sailors who had 'jumped' their ship and (*b*) soldiers who had married bigamously. The latter presented an almost stereotyped picture; the soldier would possess a wallet with two photographs inside, one of a young glamorous girl and the other of a more homely person surrounded by three or more children, and he could not remember which was his wife. An army psychiatrist used a very rough screening test for amnesia, which he claimed was most effective. If the soldier maintained that he just couldn't remember, this psychiatrist would remark that there had been a dreadful crime in a certain place and that the police were looking for someone who may have lost his memory; perhaps he should offer himself for interrogation. This approach usually resulted in a rapid return of memory and of self-identification. One could, of course, argue that he had really lost his memory and that the shock of the statement had restored it.

The author had, during the Second World War, a patient whom he believed to be a genuine case of amnesia. This soldier had wandered into a field ambulance in North Africa in a complete daze and wearing New Zealand 'tabs'. He was seen by the medical officer who wrote on his Field Medical Card, 'Appears psychotic; evacuate'. He was put aboard a hospital ship and brought to the base psychiatric hospital, with a further note stating that he was very solitary on the ship and had tried to tear up his diary. It was retrieved but without his personal data, though there were some entries in verse about 'Yanks' stealing the girls. He was of good intelligence and claimed complete loss of identity and no clues could be obtained from the patient or for that matter from anybody else. The New Zealanders could not trace him and Intelligence had some wild guesses, including one that he was a Pole masquerading as a New Zealander and was a German spy. Pentothal narcosis, ether abreaction, even E.C.T. which was alleged to be useful as an aid to recovering identity in the hope that in the post-treatment confusion the patient may give himself away, all failed, as did hypnotic suggestion. He remained in the hospital for over two years and was eventually evacuated to the United Kingdom with a fabricated name and rank. Nothing was heard for about three years, till a report appeared in a national newspaper about a man who became very disturbed following a dental anaesthetic. The dentist said: 'Wake up, Mr. ———'. The patient opened his eyes and looked at the dentist and said, 'My name is not ———, it is ———'. Shortly afterwards the same newspaper published a photograph of a woman with her children who claimed she was his wife. This amnesic state would appear to have lasted for over five years. Amnesia can also be symptomatic of severe depression and Stengel (1941) has shown that fugue-like states in adults can be suicidal equivalents, so one's opinion should not be too strongly coloured by army experience.

Multiple Personality

This is usually linked with amnesia and in some cases the patient has lived a completely different life to his usual one, with no knowledge whatever of his previous existence. The classical example of this link between the two states is that supplied by James (1890) in his *Principles of Psychology*. The Rev. Ansell Bourne had disappeared from a town in Rhode Island and two months later a man calling himself A.J. Brown woke up in a fright asking where he was, and he was told he was in Pennsylvania where he had six weeks earlier rented a confectionery shop. He then claimed his name was Bourne and that he was a clergyman and knew nothing of the shop or Mr. Brown. He was subsequently identified by his relatives. Prince (1906), whose study of multiple personality is the most celebrated reported, described the case of Miss Beauchamp. She at various times displayed three aspects of personality—a self-righteous and a moralizing one which was dominant, but it could be usurped by an ambitious and aggressive one which was very disturbing to the patient. While under hypnosis, a third aspect entered consciousness, calling herself 'Sally', who was very critical of the sanctimonious Miss Beauchamp, yet Miss Beauchamp was unaware of Sally. Prince claimed that after six years of therapy, he was able to integrate the three aspects and restore the conventional character of Miss Beauchamp.

Thigpen and Cleckley (1957) described a modern version of Miss Beauchamp in *The Three Faces of Eve.* A commercial film for public viewing was made of the case history and the lady who played the part of Eve was awarded an 'Oscar' for her performance. The author was privileged to see a documentary film of the patient and her illness which was in colour, and when asked for his comments, could only say that it was the patient who merited the 'Oscar'! A feature of patients who exhibit multiple personality is their sense of theatre and drama, and anybody seeing the performance has difficulty in not thinking he is witnessing an act rather than a clinical demonstration. In the forms described by Prince and Thigpen and Cleckley, multiple personality must be very rare though these states can undoubtedly be induced by hypnotic suggestion.

Hysterical Psychosis

This is a condition seen in hysterical personalities which is of sudden onset, of short duration, and usually follows a period of increasing stress. It includes delusions, hallucinations, depersonalization and disturbed behaviour, frequently of a gross nature, and seldom lasts longer than 1–3 weeks. It is often mistaken for schizophrenia because of the presence of delusions and hallucinations. Siomopoulos (1971) does not consider that the delusions meet the criteria of incorrigibility, for they generally do not believe in their delusional ideas. They describe their hallucinations vaguely as they do their hysterical pains, and the author considers that they are thought contents which are communicated as perceptual experiences without having been previously perceptualized. It is a form of regressive behaviour as in children's play, intended to master difficult life situations, and as in the past fantasy is diffused into reality.

Somnambulism or Sleep-walking

This is associated with the fugue-state, though it need not be pathological in children. In the adult it can be a transient phenomenon of a relatively simple nature, or it can involve quite a complex set of activities, including dressing, leaving home, and walking or travelling to a place many miles away and can thus resemble the amnesic state described above. It may be an indication of an underlying depression, the patient trying to sink his identity or escape from himself, and recovery of memory is not in itself sufficient evidence of recovery. The patient's affective state should be carefully assessed and, if necessary, anti-depressant measures instituted.

The Ganser Syndrome

This was described by Ganser (1898) and it has also been called '*prison psychosis*', because of its frequent occurrence among prisoners, particularly those who are still awaiting trial. Carothers (1947) described a similar state in Africans and the author has observed it in a few Arabs who were transferred from detention barracks or prisons because of their peculiar behaviour. Ganser regarded as the most distinguishing feature of his syndrome, *Vorbeireden* or talking past the point, thus giving the condition an alternative name, viz. the *syndrome of approximate answers.* Most clinical reports have come from America and Europe and, though generally seen in prisoners, a number of instances have been reported in the apparently law-abiding.

The patient seems unable to reason normally and the clinical picture may be confused by his claims that he cannot remember. Answers are often bizarre or even ridiculous and it is this latter aspect which contributes to the diagnosis. When asked to add 2 + 2, he may answer 5. He will misidentify objects that are presented for recognition, saying that a knife is a soup ladle or misconstrue the function of an object, saying that a spoon is to cut bread. Legs of quadrupeds are numbered as 5, 6 or 'about 10' and so on. The amnesic element and the crude caricature of ignorance and dementia has given the syndrome yet another name–*Hysterical Pseudo-dementia* and whatever the psychopathology may be, it does not need a psychiatrist to recognize that the patient is behaving in a way which he thinks will be regarded as insane and some of his acts, like drinking his urine, are examples of what he believes lunatics do. Some claim they can differentiate the Ganser syndrome from malingering by attributing an air of perplexity to the former, but it can be a very difficult diagnosis to make and the most the author would be prepared to say is that the motivation is that of the malingerer, and that there is a personality type which readily resorts to this mechanism, betraying a lesser degree of sophistication than many malingerers possess.

It should, however, be distinguished from schizophrenia, which can present with a picture which has been described as a *'buffoonery syndrome'*. In this condition there is an air of defiance about the patient, his behaviour is incongruous rather than ridiculous and the approximate answers which may be offered are never so crude. Organic brain disease can also present a picture with certain features of the Ganser syndrome and the author had one such patient referred to him because of his peculiar behaviour at home. He was upsetting his wife by breaking all the rules of domestic propriety and when charged with this, shrugged it off by saying she was making a lot of fuss about nothing. Attempts to test his intellectual state produced a series of whimsical remarks associated with an air of ennui, alternating with one of puckishness. He had a large sagittal meningioma which, when removed, resulted in the disappearance of his mental symptoms. Treatment is not usually reported, and the author has adopted a 'wait and see' policy with such patients, who tend to settle down to normal behaviour in several weeks or less. It may be that the tendency for the other patients to isolate themselves from the Ganser patient is the most powerful stimulus to recovery in a person whose affectivity is essentially normal.

Whitlock (1967) has critically assessed the published literature on the Ganser syndrome and commends Scott's (1965) suggestion that there should be a differentiation between Ganser *symptoms* and Ganser *syndrome*. The former are relatively common while the latter is extremely rare and because of its organic and psychotic (schizophrenic) associations it carries a much more sinister clinical significance. He suggests that a diagnosis of Ganser *syndrome* 'should be restricted to patients who, following cerebral trauma or in the course of an acute psychosis, develop clouding of consciousness, with characteristic verbal responses to questions, and whose illness terminates abruptly with subsequent amnesia'.

He appreciates that this all-embracing description is likely to be extremely rare and suggests that if a proportion of the features described by Ganser are present, the term *Ganser-like symptoms* should be used. His reminder of the original text is salutary for generally there has been a tendency to equate Ganser symptoms with Ganser syndrome. As long as it is appreciated that the symptoms may also occur in organic and psychotic states the clinician will not err seriously in the differential diagnosis and clinical care of his patients, though he may interpret the Ganser syndrome rather freely.

Hysterical Convulsions

Though frequently referred to as hystero-epilepsy, these are not really epileptic attacks. They show a marked cultural incidence, being relatively unknown in some countries, particularly in the United Kingdom, yet very frequent in Oriental and Mediterranean peoples. The author was struck by the relatively high incidence among Italian prisoners of war who usually selected an occasion when the greatest disturbance would be caused, such as a hospital inspection by a visiting general. The attacks can be most convincing and simulate a true attack of epilepsy, with the sudden cry, the collapse on the ground, and clonic spasms with frothing at the mouth, but there was frequently an added theatricality for the benefit of the onlookers, which indicated the functional basis. These patients would after the last convulsion assume the figure of the Cross with arms outstretched, much to the wonder of their fellow prisoners. Tests, such as water retention, and cardiazol sensitivity, failed to suggest any epileptic basis; unfortunately the hospital did not possess an EEG machine, which might have been diagnostic. The convulsions were, in these cases, undoubtedly motivated by the prospect of repatriation on medical grounds, and in civilian life, it can, in children, signify a rage reaction with hostility to parents or more crudely a means to achieve secondary gain. Kretschmer (1926) saw in the convulsive attack an atavistic violent motor reaction to situations which threaten life and thought that during evolution it tends to recede, but can be resurrected during catastrophic situations such as an earthquake or other frenzies of nature. This explanation could account for the acute panic reaction occasionally seen during a heavy artillery barrage, where the soldier would leave the relative security of his slit trench, forget all his battle drill, and rush purposelessly all over the place.

MOTOR DISTURBANCES

These are numerous and varied and may range from aphonia to

complete paralysis of all limbs; from blepharospasm to generalized jactitation; from inability to write to inability to walk. Apart from the definition of an adequate and fully relevant psychopathology which is the acid test for all hysterical reactions, there are a number of physical diagnostic aids which may help to eliminate organic disease of the nervous system.

Paralysis

This usually affects one limb or part of a limb and one joint of that limb, though a hemiplegia, paraplegia or diplegia may occur and Brain (1962) points out that as the paralysis represents the patient's idea of what an organic lesion should be, there are almost invariably anomalies of distribution. For example, in hysterical hemiplegia there is no weakness of the face, and paralysis limited to the movements of one joint is unknown in organic disease. When the patient tries to move the affected limb both antagonist and prime movers are contracted, so that an attempt to extend the elbow would be associated with contraction of the biceps and flexion of the knee with contraction of the quadriceps. Muscular wasting and contractures, as well as electrical reaction of degeneration, are absent except in very long standing cases, where these changes can result from disuse. The tendon reflexes are usually equal and the superficial (abdominal) and plantar reflexes are normal. Walshe (1958*b*) states that in a hysterical hemiplegia or crural monoplegia, the patient when asked would appear unable to adduct the affected lower limb, but if asked to keep both strongly pressed together, they both adduct strongly, for it is impossible forcefully to adduct the normal leg without adducting its apparently paralysed fellow. Walshe gives further examples: The patient lies on his back and if asked to press the heel of the paralysed leg down on the observer's hand which has been placed under it, no effort or only a feeble one is made. If the observer's hand is not moved and the patient is asked to raise the sound leg, the heel of the allegedly paralysed leg will be felt to press strongly on the hand. In a true paralysis the affected limb would rise from the bed. The hand grasp in the hysterical paralysis has characteristic features in that there is a sense of power withheld, though the grasp be weak. These patients frequently carry out the opposite to what was instructed, extension instead of flexion, and Walshe quotes this as the 'law of antagonistic effort'.

Tremors and Spasms

These may appear to be sustained but much will depend on the patience of the observer, and the author's practice when demonstrating these problems to medical students is to watch the patient for a longer time than is usual, say 15 minutes, and invariably the spasm or tremor, which is usually a coarse one, begins to tire and may even peter out or be transferred to the other limb. Occasionally the tremor may give a remarkable appearance of Parkinsonism and spasmodic movements can simulate chorea or athetosis. *Gaits* are variable and may assume bizarre forms, such as prancing, shuffling or creeping. A well known, but rare type is *astasia abasia*; the patient shows normal power and coordination in bed, yet walks with the greatest difficulty and may require all the resources of two people to support him, whereas in organic paralysis the patient makes some effort to support himself.

Sensory Disturbances

These, like the motor ones, represent the patient's idea of what an organic lesion should be and are usually confined to a limb which may also show a motor paralysis. Loss of sensation, particularly to touch and pin-prick, is the most common disturbance, and when one tries to demarcate it there is an abrupt margin which encircles the limb. All sensation may be lost over half of the body but there is also loss of smell and taste on that side. The hysterical 'stigmata' of corneal, palatal and pharyngeal anaesthesia may be present, with absence of the associated reflexes. One general practitioner did a survey of patients who came to his surgery with complaints which he suspected of being non-organic and in a very large number there was absence of the 'gag' reflex. A vibrating tuning fork placed over the right half of the sternum in a right-sided hysterical anaesthesia may not be felt at all, although the bone should conduct the stimulus to the opposite side. Deafness may disappear during sleep, so that the patient can be roused with a relatively mild noise, and the blinking reflex may be retained on auditory stimulation.

Pain is the most difficult symptom to evaluate, for it can be very severe in functional states other than hysteria. In hysteria, the patient's complaints seem disproportionate to the general state, for persistent and excruciating pain is a very debilitating experience which with the resulting insomnia can make a patient look very ill indeed, and the appearance is very different from that of the hysterical patient, who is usually well nourished and relatively unaffected by his pain.

Ocular Symptoms

Blindness may be total, but is usually confined to one eye and by putting an appropriate prism on the affected eye, diplopia may be produced. Other 'dodges' are to cover each eye with a red and green lens respectively and ask the patient to read letters which are alternately red and green. As one colour is invisible to each eye, if the patient can read all the letters, he can see with both eyes. It is, however, possible for vision to be suppressed in one eye so effectively that the above tests are not valid. The author had a patient with a dislocation of the eye referred from a plastic surgeon. As the eye could not be put back in place, he had a distressing diplopia and could only manage by wearing a patch over the affected eye. It was possible by hypnotic suggestion to suppress the image from the dislocated eye and thus relieve the diplopia.

Blepharospasm which is usually bilateral is relatively rare, but can prove a very stubborn problem. It can be evidence of a vocational problem, and the author has seen three such patients who were engravers and the disability was symptomatic of their inability to cope, just as aphonia tends to occur in school teachers and elocution tutors. Sometimes it is seen in old ladies who are very depressed and it is then a vehicle to reinforce their need for support and an indication of their helplessness. Treatment of the underlying depression is usually the surest way to effect recovery.

Hysterical Amblyopia (Diagnosis)

It is possible to record the dark adapted visual evoked responses (VER's) over the occipital region, thus comparing objective with subjective dark adaptation. Behrman and Levy (1970) studied 14 patients with hysterical amblyopia, with the VER's obtained by stimulating the retini with light flashes. The small potential changes which appeared on the EEG were summated by electronic averaging devices to produce a record. A segment of a ping-pong ball was placed over one eye to diffuse the light evenly over the entire retina, while the other eye was occluded with the patient seated in the dark. The VER was recorded from low-intensity flashes of blue/green light which was then reduced by neutral density filters, so that VER's just above threshhold were recorded. The experiment was continued as dark adaptation progressed till the criterion for normal subjects was reached, *i.e.* a discernible response was evoked by the standard blue/green light reduced by 4 log units of intensity by 8 neutral density filters. Only in two patients was this criterion not reached, and the authors speculate that this could be due to an ability of these patients to suppress cortical activity. Even with this sophisticated technique, the answer is not 100 per cent satisfactory, though 12 out of 14 is a good score.

Dysphagia

This and air-swallowing are not uncommon, particularly the latter, which is not confined to the swallowing of air, but also to its eructation. It is likely that it is this aspect which is the most significant, for like hysterical sniffing it is a most effective way of punishing those who live with the patient and it is not uncommon for the family to protest that they can stand this habit no longer. *Vomiting* can lead to severe emaciation, yet may be associated with a voracious appetite. The author had such a patient, a man of low intelligence, who ate voraciously and when in hospital could not be given enough to eat, yet when unsupervised would vomit. It had tragic consequences for him, for he would hypersecrete with the heavy meal and lose large quantities of gastric juice in his vomit, with consequent severe electrolyte depletion; twice he was *in extremis* and had to be resuscitated and restored to balance with intravenous infusions. He was strictly supervised and gained weight, but when discharged refused to be followed up, and died.

Respiratory Tics

These are common in children and can be treated successfully with hypnosis. A more disturbing feature is respiratory hyperpnoea, the results of which have been described under the 'hyperventilation syndrome' (p. 291).

Acting Out

This should be clearly differentiated both theoretically and clinically from generally impulsive behaviour which is not therapeutically induced. Wood (1968) claims that each group differs in their psychological make-up as well as in their background. The impulsive has generally a history of severe character disorder while, in the acting-out patient these defects, which the author calls 'genetic' are much less striking and only emerge under the regressive influence of the transference neurosis. In the impulsive patient libidinal and aggressive drives are discharged explosively, unevenly and with poor direction, while in the acting-out patient the behaviour is much more circumscribed and explicit, more ego-alien and neurotic. It also reflects a greater capacity for object relationships and a more successfully integrated system of delays, detours and controls. In his case external controls are not usually necessary, for ego controls are adequate; but the impulsive patient needs an educational programme which sets clear and realistic limits on behaviour.

Sperling (1968) has reported that some patients who receive analytical treatment for acting-out behaviour may develop psychosomatic symptoms during the analysis and she regards them as a transference phenomenon. Unlike the paper by Wood quoted above, Sperling does not draw a careful distinction between somatic complaints of a functional nature and psychosomatic illness, which is basically an organic disease with marked psychological associations.

Nocturnal Enuresis

This is very common in children, but also is seen as a hysterical feature in adults, particularly females. It is alleged to be associated with frigidity, and in one of the author's patients it was based on guilt following a sexual indiscretion.

DIFFERENTIAL DIAGNOSIS

Most of the features distinguishing organic disease from hysteria described above are reminiscent of the methods used by a detective trying to trap a criminal and not a doctor examining his patient. Yet, these forms of examination are presumably a legitimate way of trying to define the true nature of a problem. Some are, however, particularly crude, such as the test for hysterical anaesthesia, where the clinician with a pin in his hand and the patient blindfolded, addresses the patient thus: 'Say "yes" when I touch you and "no" when I don't'. Such tests, which enjoy popularity with medical students, have little place in the modern diagnosis of hysteria and should be relegated to history. One must repeat that it is in the definition of an adequate and fully relevant psychopathology that a diagnosis rests. Exclusion of the organic can only be a presumption even with the most refined tests and cannot mean that organic disease does not exist. It is very rare indeed for hysteria to present after the age of 40 years in a patient with a good pre-morbid personality, unless it is a partially converted depression. Many patients in this age-group who have been given a hysterical diagnosis, turn out later to have had organic disease all the time and the psychiatrist is now being assigned a new role, which is to assist his neurological colleagues in the elimination of the possibility of a problem being functional. This can only be done after taking a full case history designed to establish the patient's life-style, his interpersonal relations, his family background, his general effectiveness, the presence of adequate psychological or situational precipitating factors, and previous tendencies to dissociation.

Suggestibility

Since Charcot's time this was regarded as an essential feature of the hysteric and though Eysenck (1947) has in recent years given the concept of suggestibility more prominence, he does not confirm that hysterics are more suggestible than other types of neurotics. He used Hull's Body-Sway Test which consists of the experimenter suggesting to the subject who stands still with eyes closed, that he is falling forward and the amount of sway is measured and scored. Unfortunately Eysenck compares the hysteric with the 'neurotic' group, and it is difficult to ascertain exactly what that group consisted of. It is possible that if it contained a disproportionate number (as well it might) of patients with a tendency to dissociation or with hysterical predisposition, regardless of what symptomatology they presented, they would have scored highly in the Body-Sway Test. A high score in the 'neurotic' group could be interpreted as being due as much to their hysterical diathesis as to their 'neuroticism', if in fact the two qualities differ.

COMPENSATION NEUROSIS

The term 'compensation neurosis', like its victims or exploiters, is partial to masquerade and is frequently called *accident neurosis* or *traumatic neurosis*, but without doubt in the vast majority of cases the dominant factor is compensation, even to the exclusion of neurosis. The problem is a growing one and is not entirely dependent on the great increase of people injured on the roads and at work (over a million a year in the United Kingdom) but on the increased facilities for compensation introduced by the Welfare State. If one tries to understand the problem purely in terms of the claimant's personal psychodynamics, the essence of the problem may be missed, for social factors are frequently more important. Organized labour was initially (and probably still is) strongest in industrial and mining areas, where it felt exploited and opportunities for economic advancement were few. A boy who left school at 14 years was committed to a life in the mines and exposed to its hazards, with no hope of getting out unless he was prepared to leave home—or had an accident which was richly compensated. In fact there were only two ways whereby he could achieve wealth; either by winning a football pool, or by getting a large compensation award or settlement. The former had predictable odds against him and they were heavy, though that did not deter him from persistently trying. The latter was statistically a better proposition and depended on factors definitely loaded in his favour.

First, the incentive was there in his own community, in the form of the miner who had lost his leg, had been awarded several thousand pounds in compensation, had bought a general store and was able to give his children a better education. He was also better cushioned against adversity such as strikes, lock-outs, short-time and sickness, and enjoyed a higher social status. Second, there was the machinery, in the form of a strong and articulate trade union which would back his case to the hilt, even if they had personal reservations about the validity of his claim. Third, the patient's doctor, who was usually the family doctor, had to be a man of immense courage to refuse to give him some support, refuse to issue certificates of disability, or to volunteer previous medical information which might damage his patient's case. Fortunately for the patient, his doctor is rarely asked for this information, so he starts with the advantage that what should be in his case the best-informed medical opinion, is committed to his support. Fourth, the Court of Law would tend to by sympathetic to the man who could produce medical evidence of his disability resulting from the accident and would have no hesitation in awarding heavy damages against the mine owner or nationalized industry or insurance company who had been negligent. Without saying that the man is a fraud, and judges, like nearly everybody else concerned, are most reluctant to do that, the jury must be directed to find for the claimant. Fifth, and perhaps the least difficult, is the accident itself. In an industry where accidents are commonplace, a trivial injury is always to hand, though some claimants have not been above citing a non-existent one. Sixth, the insurance company is frequently prepared to settle in any case for litigation is costly and they can often be 'persuaded' to pay money out of court, even if they feel they will win their case.

The above is, of course, a one-sided and limited picture and does not indicate the range of problem one meets in compensation neurosis.

CLASSIFICATION OF COMPENSATION NEUROSIS

1. The Genuine Case

This occurs where the patient suffered a terrible or mutilating experience with consequent upset to his nervous state. If the pre-morbid personality was adequate, this psychiatric disability which is usually of an anxiety nature should respond readily to effective treatment, and the general practitioner, if he feels he cannot adequately cope with the problem, should at the outset get specialist help. It is more likely to be useful then than later. The prognosis should be excellent, provided adulterating factors, which will be discussed later, can be excluded.

2. The Sick Claimant

He has a genuine disability, but there are serious doubts as to the part played by the accident. The commonest type is the person with a previously effective employment record, who after a relatively minor injury, becomes totally incapacitated with headaches, depression, loss of interest, irritability and emotional lability. If a reliable history can be obtained, there is usually some evidence of a deterioration prior to the accident and also more appropriate precipitating factors, such as an attack of influenza or bronchitis with post-infective depression, or bereavement. The author had one such patient who had a quite severe depression following a road accident. It was only after the full history was obtained that one learned he was on the way to his mother's funeral and became acutely distressed as he was the only member of the family who was unable to be present. It is true that, under these circumstances, the accident by preventing him from attending contributed to the depression which was essentially post-bereavement in origin. One cannot rule out the possibility, and indeed it may be likely that the depressed mood of the patient may have been a factor in the accident, for proneness to injury may cater for the needs of the patient, not only in the pain and disability which might result, but in providing a way out of a situation which because of his depression he is unable to tolerate.

It is in these patients that the corrupting influence of the social factors mentioned above may operate. A worthy person who has worked conscientiously all his life has sustained a trivial injury and concurrently does not feel well. He is immediately encouraged by his relatives and trade union to attribute it all to the injury and claim compensation. This attitude is due partly to the mobilization of the latent hostility against the employing authority that is present in these communities, and partly to their ready tendency to argue on a *post hoc, propter hoc* basis; the event which preceded the illness must have caused it. Prestige is gained in obtaining compensation and there is a tremendous pressure with much advice brought to bear on the patient who frequently can do no more than play the part allotted to him, namely, the victim of an industrial or road accident. Retribution takes precedence over recovery and this mechanism will cater for any paranoid element in the personality of the individual. The patient, who hitherto had led an impeccably honest life, is thus encouraged to exaggerate and attribute his illness to factors which he may know to be false.

A more pernicious aspect, however, is the failure to seek treatment. There are unwritten rules for the game, such as not yielding information to the doctor which might damage the case, and not seeking or accepting treatment which may remove or reduce the disability. The author has frequently been confronted by a patient who sustained an accident, three years ago or even longer, and whose main disability is alleged to be neurotic, yet who had not been referred for psychiatric treatment. It may be that the general practitioner realizes that while the case is pending, and they do drag on, little benefit will result from treatment, and psychiatric clinics are also reluctant to go through the charade of treating a patient whose dominant interest is compensation and who would therefore resist attempts to remove the disability. Patients have told the author that their legal advisers had suggested that they do not enter hospital for treatment prior to the court hearing, but too much reliance cannot be placed on these statements, though the same legal advisers would insist that everything else their clients say about their disability is gospel truth.

Fortunately, a number of these patients who have not been too heavily contaminated find their depression intolerable and would rather be well than rich, and accept treatment. As with most psychiatric conditions arising in a good pre-morbid personality, they respond very well to anti-depressant measures.

3. The Constitutionally Unstable

He is of course a ripe, if not over-ripe candidate for a compensation neurosis. A life-long history of inadequacy, with indifferent or poor achievement and a ready facility to dissociate and present hysterical features, can hardly fail to seize on an accident in order to project personal insecurities. He is frequently unreliable in his statements and his history is designed to conceal his previous record of erratic behaviour, frequent changes of job, domestic disharmony and poor service record. He tends to exaggerate his pre-accident earnings and describes futile attempts at recovery, such as walking in the park and breathing fresh air for a year or more, and, of course, large doses of rest. There is usually evidence of instability such as hyperhidrosis of hands, chronic nail-biting and, if one can obtain it, a previous history of functional disturbances. This claimant, while handicapped, is not materially affected by the accident, and he comes very close to malingering.

4. The Malingerer

This category includes a number of the constitutionally unstable, but may also include a rather different type of person, *i.e.* the older workman who is in his sixties, and who may be hypertensive with early signs of cardiac decompensation. An accident offers him an honourable escape from an intolerable situation. His transfer to light work, which is really of great therapeutic benefit, is cited as evidence of the degree of disability caused by the accident. He is likely to yield a most unreliable history, deliberately excluding any evidence which might detract from his case.

The psychiatrist is involved in these problems either as an expert opinion or therapist, or unfortunately both. Miller (1961 *a & b*) in his Milroy Lectures gives a comprehensive account of the issues involved and psychiatrists who may have to report on, or treat these patients should study these papers, which are clear, fair and factual. He gives examples of malingering, such as a 'hysterical' gait which disappeared as soon as the patient left the consulting room, nicotine stains on the fingers of a limb allegedly afflicted by a flaccid paralysis, and an 'aphasia' which was frankly simulated. He describes a series of 200 consecutive cases of head injury which were referred for medico-legal examination of whom 47 per cent presented neurotic symptoms. The neurotic features were twice as common in industrial as in road accidents and twice as common in men as in women and there was an inverse relationship between the compensation neurosis and the severity of the injury. He states: 'Gross psychoneurosis occurred, for example, in 31 per cent of patients without radiological evidence of skull fracture, in 9 per cent of patients with simple fracture, and in only 2 out of 25 patients who suffered from compound fractures of the skull.' This inverse relationship was also found between the period of unconsciousness and gross display of symptoms. Analysis of social status and nature of employment showed that only 18 per cent held responsible posts above the level of charge-hand, more came from the large industries than from family businesses, and a higher than average number were from dangerous jobs like steel erecting or coalface working. The aches and pains of which they complain may cause them to be referred to orthopaedic surgeons, and leg irons and other appliances have been prescribed for non-organic states, while physiotherapy, especially of a prolonged nature, is common. It is about the only type of treatment to which the patient voluntarily and regularly submits, and if one had to draw a conclusion it would be that physiotherapy for these patients is singularly ineffective. Miller rightly stresses that the big handicap in assessment is getting reliable information, as the doctor in preparing his report frequently has only the patient's statement of his history and symptoms. Interviewing a relative which is such an essential and helpful aspect of ordinary psychiatric practice, in these cases may only reinforce the deception and, in fact, many claimants bring along a relative, not to supply helpful information, but as advocates of their cause.

In spite of all these handicaps, a very careful history may still frequently yield dependable information about the patient's pre-morbid state, even if in a negative way, for they not uncommonly deny even the slightest evidence of the normal insecurities to which all men are heir. They would have us believe that they have an impeccable family history, a most secure home background, a complete absence of neurotic traits in childhood, a stable and most successful employment record, a happy married life and no history of illness even of a trivial nature, till the accident, when catastrophe overtook them. If all this were true, then the patient should be capable of recovering from the most extreme stresses imaginable, and the relatively minor insult of the accident should hardly be noticed. One useful piece of information which should be readily available is rarely produced, and that is the claimant's pre-morbid sickness record. Specialists are given detailed statements of the amount of time the patient has lost from work since the accident, with 'nervous debility' figuring prominently among the causes, but the equally vital information of the pre-morbid state of health is left for the claimant to disclose or disguise. Just as when the Army refers a soldier for psychiatric opinion, and is expected to furnish the man's complete medical records, selection tests performance, conduct sheet and medical officer's and commanding officer's reports, so it should be routine for the fullest possible information of the claimant to be made available, with his consent. It has always struck the author as odd, that a court which strives after truth and the fullest possible information, is prepared to dispose of large sums of other people's money on an issue which is largely a medical one, on most inadequate and frequently false information. The *Lancet* (1961) in a leader remarks:

... Most lawyers perhaps fails to recognize how far social practice has already sapped away the theoretical basis of the law of compensation for civil injuries. For in most cases it is no longer the party responsible for the injury who pays the compensation, but a particular social group, acting collectively through insurance companies; and this collective responsibility is in some cases enforced by law. ... In fact the motor car insurance companies have so far departed from the idea of justice that when no third party is involved they divide the cost of an accident between them ('knock for knock') even though one party, who may be entirely innocent, is unjustly penalized by the loss of his no-claim bonus. The State itself has an indirect interest in all this since unless an injured person is compensated from some other source he becomes a charge on social insurance; and even then there is a subtle distinction between industrial disease and ordinary illness which is reflected in a difference in the scale of benefit.

These are certainly difficult problems, but it is surely clear that the law of compensation for injury has become in some respects anti-social, and that the development of collective and social responsibility has outmoded legal concepts of justice in this field. Has the time not come for a Government inquiry?

Apart from Miller's Milroy Lectures and Walshe's (1958*a*) paper, very few clear statements of the issues involved have been made in the British medical literature and this may in itself be significant. Physicians were at one time able to practise philanthropy from their personal fortunes. This is now rarely possible, but a new type of philanthropy is being practised, namely, the distribution of favours, which the Welfare State has placed in their charge. These may be admission to hospital and convalescent home, certificates of sickness and a protagonist attitude towards the patient who claims compensation. The doctor therefore unconsciously tends to identify with the patient in his quest and not only will be favourable in his reports, but generally refrain from putting or even considering the other side of the case.

An interesting finding of Miller's which casts even more light on the problem is that in a series of 50 cases that were followed up, only two were disabled by their psychiatric symptoms two years after settlement, which would suggest that for these cases, elaborate treatment is not only useless but unnecessary.

The report to the solicitors or the insurance company can be made only with the patient's consent and it is important to obtain this before starting to examine the patient. A number of these patients are already hostile and suspicious, so questions should be delicately put, yet the doctor is entitled to seek an answer which is relevant and factual. Discussion with the patient about his treatment and prognosis is usually outside the terms of reference and should politely be discouraged, and above all, full and careful notes of the examination should be made at the time.

OBSESSIONAL NEUROSIS

The obsessive compulsive reaction is a state in which the patient unconsciously tries to control his anxiety by means of persistent and repetitive thoughts and acts. Lewis (1935) defined obsessions thus: 'Whenever a patient complains of some mental experience which is accompanied by a feeling of subjective compulsion, so that he does not willingly entertain it, but, on the contrary, does his utmost to get rid of it, that is an obsession'.

The term 'obsessive-compulsive' is an example of tautology. Freud called these states *Zwangneurose* and this was translated 'obsessional neurosis' in London and 'compulsive neurosis' in New York. Freud (1896) included obsessional neurosis under the group of defence neuropsychoses, alongside hysteria and certain cases of acute hallucinatory confusion and his earliest definition was: 'Obsessions are always reproaches re-emerging in a transmuted form under repression—reproaches which invariably relate to a sexual deed performed with pleasure in childhood'. Thirteen years later he considered this definition open to criticism as it was too general and did not take into account the many variations in the obsessional patient's symptoms (Freud, 1909*b*). A few years later (Freud, 1913*c*) he wrote about predisposition in obsessional neurosis and elaborated theories based on his own observations and those of his colleagues, including Jones (1913), who pointed out that once the stage of sexual organization which contains the predisposition to obsessional neurosis is established, it is never really overcome.

PSYCHOPATHOLOGY

The psychopathology of obsessional neurosis is very dependent on an understanding of the *anal character*. Freud (1908), in his paper on 'Character and Anal Eroticism', described the orderly, parsimonious and obstinate attributes of these patients and considered them to be reaction-formations against anal-erotic activities or partial sublimations of them. In the process of habit training the child learns to postpone or even renounce direct instinctual gratification and thus acquires mastery over the instinct. Conflicts arise during the course of the training with resistance by the instinct to environmental demands as well as obedience to, and compromise with, these demands.

Parsimony is an extension of the anal habit of retention and this can be motivated by anal erotic pleasure. Orderliness is considered to be an extension of obedience to the environment, while obstinacy is a form of rebellion against it. The basic aspects of the anal character are represented by a variety of personal qualities which in most instances are socialized translations, although the exact opposite (reaction-formation) may result. For example, orderliness or obedience may be recognized as tidiness, meticulosity and punctuality. Obstinacy may manifest as a persistent challenging attitude, defying authority or radicalism. Faeces which are considered to play such an important part in the formation of the anal character are represented in later life by money and a typical picture is that of the miser counting his gold. An interesting pre-Freudian aspect of this theme is the advice given in *Shulchan Orach* to the man who is enjoined in his waking hours to think of God. The question is put that this could surely not apply when he is at stool, and another ritual is suggested as a substitute, namely, counting money.

The matter of *ritual* is very important in obsessional neurosis, for as Freud (1919) pointed out in *Totem and Taboo*, the superstitions of the compulsive neurosis closely resembled those found in savages and he illustrated this with two examples. The first is a quotation from Frazer's (1911) *The Golden Bough:*

> For a similar reason a Maori chief would not blow on a fire with his mouth; for his sacred breath would communicate its sanctity to the fire, which would pass it on to the meat in the pot, which would pass it on to the man who ate the meat which was in the pot, which stood on the fire, which was breathed by the chief; so that the eater, infected by the chief's breath conveyed through these intermediaries, would surely die.

The second is an account of one of Freud's patients:

> My patient demanded that a utensil which her husband had purchased and brought home should be removed lest it make the place where she lives impossible. For she has heard that this object was bought in a store which is situated, let us say, in Stag Street. But as the word 'stag' is the name of a friend now in a distant city, whom she has known in her youth under her maiden name and whom she now finds 'impossible', that is taboo, the object bought in Vienna is just as taboo as this friend with whom she does not want to come into contact.

Although the above two examples are mainly designed to indicate displacement, the first one does illustrate the chain reaction with which obsessional patients fetter themselves. Freud (1907) drew attention to the resemblance between obsessive acts and religious practices:

> I am certainly not the first to be struck by the resemblance between what are called obsessive acts in neurotic and religious observances by means of which the faithful give expression to their piety. The name 'ceremonial', which has been given to certain of these obsessive acts, is evidence of this. . . . It is easy to see wherein lies the resemblance between the neurotic ceremonial and religious rites: it is the fear of pangs of conscience after their omission, in the complete isolation of them from all other activities (the feeling that one must not be disturbed), and in the conscientiousness with which the details are carried out. But equally obvious are the differences, some of which are so startling that they make the comparison into a sacrilege: the greater individual variability of neurotic ceremonial in contrast with the stereotyped character of rites (prayer, orientation, etc.): its private nature as opposed to the public and communal character of religious observance, especially, however, the distinction that the little details of religious ceremonies are full of meaning and are understood symbolically, while those of neurotics seem silly and meaningless. In this respect an obsessional neurosis furnishes a tragi-comic travesty of a private religion.

He does point out, however, that once one can penetrate by psychoanalytical methods the neurotic obsessions, they become full of meaning and that they are derived mostly from the sexual experiences of the patient. Ceremonial and obsessive acts are partly a defence against temptation and partly a protection against the misfortune expected. Protective measures rapidly become ineffective and are replaced by prohibitions and at an even later stage the performances which were initially defensive approximate more and more to the proscribed actions they were originally designed to prevent.

It would not be inappropriate here to recount Freud's comparison between the obsessional process and religion:

> The structure of a religion seems also to be founded on the suppression or renunciation of certain instinctual trends; these trends are not, however, as in the neurosis, exclusively components of the sexual instinct, but are egoistic, anti-social instincts, though even these for the most part are not without a sexual element. The sense of guilt in consequence of continual temptation, and the anxious expectation in the guise of fear of divine punishment, have indeed been familiar to us in religion longer than in neurosis. . . . Unredeemed backslidings into sin are even more common among the pious than among neurotics, and these give rise to a new form of religious activity, namely, the act of penance of which one finds counterparts in the obsessional neurosis . . . The element of compromise in those obsessive acts which we find as neurotic symptoms is the feature least easy to find reproduced in corresponding religious observances. Yet here, too, one is reminded of this trait in the neurosis when one recalls how commonly all those acts which religion forbids—expressions of the instincts it represses—are yet committed precisely in the name of, and ostensibly in the cause of, religion.

> In view of these resemblances and analogies one might venture to regard the obsessional neurosis as a pathological counterpart to the formation of a religion, to describe this neurosis as a private religious system, and religion as a universal obsessional neurosis. The essential resemblance could lie in the fundamental renunciation of the satisfaction of inherent instincts, and the chief difference in the nature of these instincts, which in the neurosis are exclusively sexual, but in religion are of egoistic origin.

It is however, a long way from obsessional thought or behaviour to obsessional neurosis. Obsessionality is a personality trait which is not only within the normal range, but may be highly desirable. The young doctor in hospital practice, who is punctual, scrupulous in his case-history taking, writes notes conscientiously, and is a perfectionist in his work is likely to go far, and need not be a ripe candidate for an obsessional neurosis. In fact the obsessional features may extend well beyond what one might consider the normal range and be compatible not only with efficiency, but with professional eminence. Ritual hand-washing, 'obsessional' note-taking, 'obsessional' politeness, can all be 'carried' by the individual, without any sign of breakdown. Although it is generally accepted than an obsessional neurosis is based on an obsessional personality and that prior to breakdown there is adequate compensation, while breakdown is a process associated with decompensation, there is no evidence that those with manifest obsessional symptoms are more likely to break down than the others. One might argue that their declarations of some of their obsessional traits fulfil the function of an eccentricity and are a more potent ego-defence mechanism. This aspect requires emphasis, for too often the symptom instead of the patient is regarded as requiring treatment. A need for obsessional behaviour in a person with a limited capacity for physical and mental output renders him much more vulnerable than a similar situation in a person with a great capacity. The latter may rise above it, while the former may go under. The milieu may also be important, for if the person has the capacity and the desire, he can satisfy his obsessional needs with honorary or stipendiary duties as a secretary, chairman or organizer and be in considerable demand, while the less well endowed will have no such outlets. Some of the most pathetic obsessional problems are found in people of limited intelligence, where symptoms frequently consist in a pre-occupation with counting, though their weakest subject is arithmetic.

Another feature of the neurosis is *undoing*, which Fenichel (1945) states is related to reaction formation, which is the adoption of an attitude that contradicts the original one. In undoing, one more step is taken in that something is done, which in fact or magically, is the opposite of something which either in fact or in imagination had been done before. Certain obsessional symptoms consist of two components, the second being a complete rebuttal of the first, *e.g.* the person who first has to turn the gas tap on, in order to turn it off. Expiation too is designed to annul previous acts and represents a magical undoing. It can appear paradoxical when the obsession is not to do the opposite, but to repeat the same act. Fenichel explains the paradox as being due to the first act arising from an unconscious instinctual attitude; this is undone when this same act can be repeated. The aim of the compulsion is to carry out the same act freed of its secret unconscious meaning, or with the opposite unconscious meaning. If some part of the original impulse insinuates itself again into the repetition, which was intended as an expiation, further repetition of the act becomes necessary.

Failure of the mechanism of undoing may result in (1) an increase in the number of repetitions as complete reassurance is not obtained with any one performance; (2) some forms of counting compulsions, the unconscious meaning of which is to count the number of repetitions; (3) the ever-widening scope of the rituals; (4) obsessive doubts which may reflect doubt as to whether the undoing has succeeded; and (5) the futility of all these measures.

Isolation is another common defence mechanism of obsessional neurosis. Although the patient may not have forgotten the pathogenic traumata, he has lost trace of their associations and emotional significance. Any attempt to demonstrate these associations is resisted like the hysteric resists the reactivation of repressed memories, and a counter cathexis is operating, the function of which is to keep apart what should be connected. An idea is isolated from the emotional cathexis that was originally attached to it and therefore when exciting events are discussed, the patient may initially remain calm, but at a later stage show emotions without realizing the displacement that is taking place. Repulsive ideas like murder and incest may reach consciousness as obsessions, but they are securely isolated from action. Fenichel considers that the reduced affect which is common in obsessional neurosis and interferes with therapy is based on this isolation. Obsessive blasphemies may be explained as a failure at isolation in that what was intended to be a religious ritual became debased. Logical thought may also be regarded as a form of isolation and obsessional neurotics produce caricatures of it, thus interfering with free-association, which is really a suspension of the normal isolating or logical processes. This feature can and does make psychotherapy on analytical lines impossible, for these patients with their obsession about order and routine cannot allow their thought processes to emerge spontaneously and are continually censoring and systematizing them.

The *ego* in obsessional neurosis is very dependent on super-ego influences and this is reflected in symptomatology. It explains obsessional pre-occupation with the health of parents and an over-solicitude for the safety of those against whom unconscious hostile impulses are entertained. Occasionally the attitude to the super-ego is ambivalent, in that the patient may indulge the prohibition, and feel guilty for doing so, or it may use an act of atonement as an excuse for indulging in the prohibited act. It is this ambivalent attitude which distinguishes the condition from depression, where there is rarely any attempt at indulgence. Obsessional neurotics are therefore frequently able to meet the demands of a rigid super-ego and at the same time gratify their libidinous urges and this is seen classically in the compulsive masturbator, who may ring himself with a variety of rituals, yet indulge his habit to a greater degree than those who have no such obsessional defence. In addition he may carry out expiation acts to ward off the evil he fears may befall him, such as doing his good deed every day, and rather symbolically the most important of these is to take a blind man across the road.

Thinking in obsessional neurosis as Freud has said is very close to the magical thinking of primitive people and frequently contains archaic references. The magic of words is invoked to ward off evil and symbolism is richly represented.

CLINICAL FEATURES

With the above background, the clinical features of obsessional neurosis should be more meaningful. These are usually divided into three groups: (1) obsessional thoughts, (2) obsessional acts, and (3) obsessional fears. These are arbitrary divisions and have no major psychopathological significance but are convenient for descriptive purposes.

1. *Obsessional thoughts* or *ruminations* may be associated with a whole range of subjects. The commoner ones are persistent doubting (*folie du doute*) as to whether the doors are locked, or gas taps are turned off, or an appointment has or has not been forgotten. Sometimes it may be a pre-occupation with a bad word, oath or blasphemy, or with a hostile intention. In every case, the patient is tortured with his obsession and may indulge in obsessional conduct to relieve the tension. Pre-occupation with depersonalization or derealization is not uncommon, particularly in adolescent girls,

though in recent years some of these problems have been found to be due to lesions in the temporal lobes.

2. *Obsessional acts,* as has been said, may be excited by obsessional thoughts, but they frequently exist by themselves. They may be elaborate rituals, associated with bathing or washing or in preparation for going to bed. They may, like the thoughts, have a primitive or magical component and are designed to placate an omnipotent power. Over-protection, over-solicitude, avoidance of contamination, touching, counting, persistent note-taking and recording of each and every event, no matter how trivial, are only a few of the manifestations.

3. *Obsessional phobias* are usually associated with anxiety, and they are frequent accompaniments of the thoughts and acts described above. Fears of dirt or contamination may lead to frequent washing and avoidance of touching certain objects or people. Some patients with fears of contaminating their loved ones will not bring outdoor shoes into the house, but will leave them outside in a dish of disinfectant. Some with fears of spreading germs will scrub their hands till they are raw and damage them further with frequent bathing in concentrated antiseptic. Fears of harming their children may lead them to undertake elaborate rituals to avoid such misfortune. Knives are locked up and the key secreted in a place which is again rendered inaccessible, perhaps by some magical incantation which makes its hiding place taboo. Certain mannerisms in dress may be due to fears of chills or colds and some patients disturb the office staff with whom they work by insisting that windows are kept tightly shut and they themselves wear sheets of cardboard under their jackets and look quite ridiculous in this protective garb. As has already been mentioned some phobic anxiety states may use obsessional defences to ward off the feared catastrophe, such as carrying around some talisman to give them a sense of security.

4. *Obsessions and Psychosis.* These three subdivisions do not adequately convey the infinite variety of patterns of obsessional symptoms. Those features which border on, or incorporate eccentricity are very near the psychotic or delusional level and indicate the form of breakdown that may occur should the defences be inadequate. Deterioration to a schizophrenic psychosis is not uncommon and a number of schizophrenic patients are decompensated obsessionals, retaining some of their former obsessional features either in their archaic behaviour pattern, perseverative speech, compulsive touching or other mannerisms. Obsessional rumination may be projected, so that the patient thinks that the recurring

thoughts are being placed there by some malign external influence. Ritualistic acts are also seen, but the schizophrenic patient lacks the insight and awareness of their incongruity and may disturb others with his conduct. Decompensation may also take the form of severe depression, and here the super-ego factor is more dominant and the rigid personality breaks wide open with obsessional melancholic features, including feelings of guilt and unworthiness, for the expiatory mechanisms are no longer effective.

The severity of obsessional features cannot be gauged from a mere description of their variety. Apart from the effects they may have on the patient, such as distress and exhaustion, they can be most troublesome to the other members of the family. A patient with a dirt phobia may constantly be insisting that the others copy the purification rituals; a wife who has elaborated a complicated process of orderliness and cleanliness prior to retiring may incorporate her husband in the acts, which can go on till 3 A.M.; and a patient who has obsessional doubts about the health of a parent may constantly ring that person at work up to 20 times per day. Whole families can be worn out by the process. It can therefore, in its malignant form, far exceed the private religion described by Freud and, to carry the analogy further, the patient would appear intent on founding a church.

Diagnosis

The diagnosis of the obsessional features is so obvious that in themselves they present no difficulty. What can be more difficult is to decide what stage the process has reached. Is it well compensated or is it decompensating? In the former, the picture will conform, in the main, to the definition of the obsessional personality given above. In the latter, one should seek for the nuances of schizophrenia in the patient's affectivity, which may be reflected in the mechanism of isolation (see above). Bizarre features with some loss of insight and more generalized disturbances of thought processes would also suggest a diagnosis of schizophrenia, while in the more deteriorated cases, florid schizophrenic features may be evident. The distinction between a severe obsessional neurosis with depressive features and a depression with obsessional features can be a very fine one, yet it is not entirely academic. In the former, even though the depression may yield to anti-depressant measures, the obsessional symptoms may not be affected, while in the latter anti-depressant treatment may be enough to clear the whole symptomatology, the obsessional features being a secondary problem, linked to the major one and perhaps aggravated by it.

Prognosis

In a condition which may be linked with schizophrenia, depression and phobic anxiety, blanket statements on prognosis can be misleading. Goodwin *et al.* (1969) analysed 13 follow-up studies of obsessional neurosis; 2 in the United States, 5 in Britain, 3 in Scandinavia, and one each in Germany and Hong Kong, and they summarize their data. About 65 per cent of obsessionals develop their illness before the age of 25 years, though many have clearcut symptoms by the age of 15, and it may start at 6 years. Fewer than 15 per cent developed their illness after the age of 35 years. Pronounced mood factors (depression and anxiety) accompanied the initial development in 25 per cent, with onset being either acute or insidious; the mean duration of illness prior to psychiatric referral was 7 years.

The course may be unremitting, with or without social incapacity, or episodic, and some enjoy complete remissions with return to normal function. Milder obsessionals requiring only out-patient treatment have a good prognosis with 60–80 per cent asymptomatic or improved 1–5 years after diagnosis. In-patients do less well with no more than a third improved symptomatically several years after discharge.

A favourable prognosis is associated with mild or atypical symptoms, short duration and good premorbid personality. It does not involve an increased risk of suicide, homicide, alcoholism, drug addiction, antisocial behaviour, chronic hospitalization or the development of another mental disorder such as schizophrenia. It is evident that spontaneous improvement occurs frequently, and the patient should be told this and also that his impulses to commit injury will almost certainly not be translated into action. Neither is he likely to lose his mind. Leucotomy produced symptomatic improvement superior to and with greater certainty than spontaneous improvement.

Treatment

This will vary in method and result, according to the purity and severity of the reaction. In the relatively unadulterated obsessional neurosis which is not too severe, analytic psychotherapy is worth trying and it should soon become evident whether it is likely to succeed or not. If severe tension is present, and this is usual in the majority of patients, psychotherapy is unlikely to help, and in the affectively bleached group, the development of a transference reaction, the acting out of rage, and the capacity for psychological work are blunted, again rendering the patient unsuitable for restorative psychotherapy. Many will get temporary relief from attending their doctor, but their improvement will not be related to or dependent on the uncovering of early developmental patterns. If depressive or schizophrenic features predominate, the treatment should be directed at these aspects. While depression is generally easy to recognize and is therefore treated, or even over-treated, the schizophrenic aspect may be missed, so it should always be borne in mind and phenothiazines prescribed in suitable cases. Abreactive techniques have very little place in treatment, for the consequent release of anxiety may be very traumatic and do more harm than good. Prefrontal leucotomy (Chapter 20) still has a place in the treatment of severe obsessional neurosis, particularly where there is considerable tension, but patients with features which are suggestive of schizophrenia should not be selected. Of the various operations which the author has had performed on his patients, bilateral undercutting of areas 9 and 10 has produced the best and most consistent results. Inferior quadrant cuts, which may be effective in recurrent depression, have proved disappointing in obsessionals. A practical point in the management of the post-leucotomy phase is that the operation may release aggressive behaviour which can make the nursing very difficult and a useful prophylactic is to give the patient chlorpromazine, 50 mg. three times a day, immediately after or even before the operation. This may have to be boosted to a dose of 100 mg. thrice daily. The drug should be continued for at least two months and if the patient is well controlled, gradually reduced to zero. In spite of the intractability of obsessional states, they are rarely met after the age of 55 years, which may be interpreted in two ways. First, the condition may change its character in time and declare itself either as a frank schizophrenic illness or a depressive one, and second, it may remit spontaneously and there is no doubt that, in time, some very severe and apparently hopeless cases do remit, though this does not mean that they all do, for there is also evidence that some commit suicide. It would, however, be inhuman to leave patients in their distressed state with the risks of decompensation and suicide, especially when the results of leucotomy in well-selected cases are so encouraging.

Ritual Prevention. Levy and Meyer (1971) report a follow-up study of 8 patients treated behaviourally by interference with compulsive rituals. They call it 'apotrepic therapy' which is another way (Greek) of saying 'aversion therapy'. The method involved continual supervision during waking hours by nurses who were instructed to prevent the patient from carrying out any rituals either by engaging him in other activities, discussion, cajoling and very occasionally the use of mild physical restraint, subject to the patient's agreement. When total prevention was achieved, continuous supervision was maintained for 1–4 weeks during which time the patient was gradually exposed to situations which previously evoked rituals and was again prevented from indulging. Supervision was then gradually diminished and follow-up was at 6-monthly intervals for up to 6 years. Of the 8 patients, 6 were either asymptomatic or much improved, and 2 were improved. It is difficult to assess this treatment on such a small sample, and in a condition which frequently remits spontaneously, and where prognosis depends on factors such as pre-morbid personality.

Neurasthenia

This is now an outmoded term with a variety of interpretations, which can be included under other reactions or syndromes. For example, persistent tiredness and anergia is commonly seen in depressive states, easy fatiguability with complete exhaustion in anxiety states, and the perseverative reiteration of these complaints may be part of a schizophrenic picture. In the First World War, it was a popular diagnosis which was used for the invaliding of many soldiers, and the author, who had to review a number of these patients in recent years, was struck by the depressive symptoms which were included under the original diagnosis, and the depressive features which the patients 40 years later presented. The condition must have been very frequently diagnosed betwen 1914–18, for, in order to cope with its diagnosis, treatment and disposal, the Army instituted a short course of training for medical officers, who graduated with the title, 'Neurasthenic Expert', the precursor of the modern psychiatrist. There are a few cases, the symptomatology of which is predominantly neurasthenic, thus giving the appearance of a disease entity, but it is usually possible to identify the underlying condition, and it is that which has to be treated. There is no place in treatment for the large doses of rest with which these patients used to be assailed, neither should there be indiscriminate stimulation, for only a proper appraisal and the appropriate treatment will produce the desired results.

DEPERSONALIZATION SYNDROME

Some would regard the phenomenon of depersonalization as a

clinical entity while others deny it this status and regard it as merely one aspect of a variety of psychiatric problems. The four salient features which are commonly regarded as the criteria of the syndrome are:

1. Feelings of unreality.
2. An unpleasant quality associated with these feelings.
3. The non-delusional nature of the experience.
4. The associated affective disturbance (predominantly depression).

Aetiology

Many theories have been put forward and Ackner (1954) divides them into 4 categories, each being inadequate:

1. Those which invoke disturbances of a particular psychological function.
2. Those which invoke cortical dysfunction either specific or secondary.
3. Psychoanalytical theories which suggest disturbances in psychological development.
4. Those which regard it as a form of schizophrenia.

The obsessional preoccupation with the symptoms does give some support to the psychoanalytical theory which postulates withdrawal of object cathexis with the resulting hypercathected self which can also lead to hypochondriacal features. It is likely that this explains one aspect of the problem rather than the whole condition.

Shorvon *et al.* (1946) in a study of 66 patients, defined the following features which they found to be associated with the condition:

1. Onset is practically always sudden.
2. Most typically, onset is in adolescence or early maturity.
3. It occurs as a symptom in a very wide range of psychiatric disorders.
4. It can occur in normal people as a fleeting experience, *e.g.* in fatigue, after anaesthesia, and experimentally during mescaline intoxication.
5. It is reversible and can recover completely and spontaneously.
6. It is significantly related to relaxation following intense or prolonged stimulation, psychological or physical.
7. It can be relieved by stimulation.
8. It can be experienced in any psychological field whether cognitive, affective or conative.

9. There is a tendency for it to occur in the more intelligent.
10. There is a tendency for it to occur in the emotionally immature.
11. There is a high incidence of unsatisfactory parent-child relationships.
12. There is a high incidence of non-specific mild abnormalities in the EEG.

Negative findings are:

1. It is not a disorder of visual perception.
2. It cannot be accounted for in neurological terms by any known focal lesion.
3. There is no specific relationship with anatomical disease of the brain.
4. There is a relative absence of olfactory, gustatory, or auditory derealization.
5. It is extremely rare in children.
6. It is practically never found in paranoia.

Ackner (1954) who did not regard the condition as an entity stated:

> . . . It has emerged that not only is depersonalization a loosely organized syndrome, but that the criteria of the salient features themselves are often in doubt or lacking in the clarity necessary sometimes for the establishment of their presence.

The author would agree with Ackner for the symptoms are common to a variety of psychiatric disturbances, particularly phobic anxiety states where the associated hyperventilation during the panic attacks induces the experience. These patients, who usually have strong obsessional features, may hold on to the symptoms tenaciously for months or even years. Some of these young patients have gone through their senior school and even part of their university course with the complaint, yet it is not inconsistent with an adequate performance. The author has followed up one such patient who since his schooldays has complained bitterly about his depersonalization experience. He has since qualified in law and has embarked on a successful professional life and has consistently reduced his golf handicap. At times the distress is severe and one may be tempted to try heroic measures such as E.C.T. or as Shorvon (1947) has advocated, a prefrontal leucotomy. These should be resisted, for the condition does tend to right itself with simple supportive measures.

A difficult problem in differential diagnosis is the distinction between the symptoms and an early schizophrenic state and in a few instances there may be an overlap, but generally the schizophrenic process can be identified.

Davison (1964), on the basis of a study of seven patients with episodic depersonalization, supported the view that there is a primary idiopathic state, and postulates a functional disturbance of cerebral arousal mechanisms. It would be important to exclude the hyperventilation attacks of anxiety before drawing such conclusions.

Temporal lobe epilepsy is usually considered in differential diagnosis but it is rarely established in the absence of fits and other features of the disease. The EEG can be abnormal but is usually an immature record and does not show the focal disturbance of an epileptic nature found in temporal lobe lesions.

THE ATHLETE'S NEUROSIS

Athletes are very conscious of their body image. They train hard and try to achieve a high standard of physical excellence, and one would suspect that they would be very vulnerable to a threat of deprivation. Little (1969) compared 44 athletic neurotics with 28 non-athletic neurotics. The former were somewhat older when they became ill and 32 did so after a threat to their physical well-being through injury or illness. Those injured developed their neurotic symptoms almost immediately, often on the same day. Only three of the non-athletic neurotics were subject to physical stresses and of these one was subject to psychological stress as well. They reacted more commonly to difficulties at work, marital disruption, sexual problems and bereavement or illness in family or friends.

Many of the athletic patients despite previously sound work records remained unemployable for years and the author regards it as a form of deprivation neurosis in which conflict plays little part. It is more akin to a bereavement reaction to loss of part of self, *i.e.* the over-valued physical prowess. Athleticism may not be neurotic in itself, but like exclusive and excessive emotional dependence on work, intellectual pursuits, physical beauty or any other over-valued attribute or activity, it can place the subject in a vulnerable pre-neurotic state.

CHAPTER 12

Affective Disorders

Normal mental functions like feeling and thinking cannot be divided into water-tight compartments, for they are interdependent. In abnormal mental states, these aspects are even more closely compounded, yet a disturbance of the one can predominate and be identified. For example, disorders of feeling or emotion can strongly influence and contribute to thought disorder, but the basic emotional disturbance may be the more obvious clinical feature. The term '*affect*' is used for the emotional or feeling aspect of mental life, or mood, and the clinical states where a particular affect is involved are called *affective disorders.*

Variations in mood are normal and there are great individual differences which do not come within the limits of the pathological. Even severe examples of depression or elation can, in certain circumstances, be accepted as normal. After a bereavement an individual or even a nation may be prostrate with grief and present a picture of profound depression which may persist for some time, yet it can still be within normal limits. Similarly, elation during celebrations may be extreme, but in the cultural setting can be regarded as normal behaviour. It is when the reaction persists for an undue period and becomes either inappropriate or culturally disproportionate that illness is said to be present.

Society does provide outlets for swings of mood and in closely-knit communities these may be shared communally. Bereavement, tragedy and misfortune produce reactions which can be freely expressed and, in fact, the deviant is the one who does not exhibit the appropriate mood change. Similarly, on certain holidays and during festive celebrations, behaviour, which under other circumstances would be regarded as manic, is permitted. The individual who is generally of a euphoric or slightly manic disposition can express himself in a number of activities, such as comic parts on the variety stage, high-pressure salesmanship, or be the local 'cheer leader'. Others can throw themselves with gusto into a range of public works on behalf of political, religious and charitable organizations, though there are naturally limits to community tolerance for these activities and any behaviour beyond the normal range would be rejected. One is, however, occasionally surprised at the degree of manic behaviour some people will stand and a number of individuals who are frankly psychotic do find a socially acceptable outlet in these activities.

Society has also some help to offer the depressed, which may tide them over their milder and less prolonged episodes. The social matrix itself may underpin the grief-stricken by providing them with comfort and affection. Entertainments, tobacco, alcohol and other beverages enjoy their popularity because of their ability to cater for the needs of their consumers, and the role of the inn and the café should not be underestimated. There is also, of course, the comfort and support from religious organizations and membership of a Church frequently provides 'a very present help in trouble'.

It is when these measures fail that the condition is recognized as requiring medical attention but, unfortunately, not before the sufferer has frequently been exposed to much gratuitous advice from well-meaning but misguided relatives and friends. Apart from general exhortations such as 'you've got to fight it'; 'don't give way'; 'stiff upper lip'; and 'I fought and won', which are generally accompanied by positive efforts to cheer the sufferer, there may be even more harmful advice offered. The proffering of alcohol to help 'drown the sorrows' and the suggestion that the individual should change his job, are common lay methods of 'treatment' which have their obvious dangers. But it is not only the well-intentioned relative or friend who has entered the field of therapy. There are a surprising number of agencies interested in the comforting of the depressed, each seeing the problem within its own, frequently narrow frame of reference and mostly incapable of gauging the point where the patient is in need of skilled medical help. As depression is probably the commonest illness in our society and carries a high mortality and morbidity rate in terms of suicide and attempted suicide, it cannot be emphasized too strongly at the outset that this is a medical matter with which the doctor should be thoroughly familiar, and in which the layman should not dabble.

MANIC-DEPRESSIVE PSYCHOSES

HISTORICAL

The term 'manic-depressive psychosis' stems from Kraepelin

(1909–13) who first used it in the 6th edition of his *Lehrbuch der Psychiatrie*, but he did not fully expound his views till his 8th edition in 1913 and the English translation appeared in 1921. The alternation, however, of manic and depressive states is probably the oldest recorded mental disease and was documented in the Homeric epics and in the writings of Hippocrates. A classical description is found in the Bible. Saul the son of Kish, who eventually became the first king of Israel was notorious for his melancholic spells, but it is not generally appreciated that he had also exhibited a manic phase. Prophesying is considered to be akin to the manic state and Saul spontaneously joined a band of prophets and began to prophesy, much to the amazement of the onlookers. 'Therefore it became a proverb—Is Saul also among the prophets?' (I Samuel x. 12). He eventually committed suicide. Another Biblical character who exhibited both a depressive and manic phase was Hannah, the mother of Samuel, who after a spell of depressive stupor during which 'only her lips moved, but her voice was not heard' (I Samuel i. 13), gave birth to her child and swung into a manic phase during which she sang her song whose whole metaphor is one of extreme exultation with oral aggression and gratification. She swings from one to the other—death and destruction to the oppressor and supreme power and glory to the subject. Hyperbole is introduced to the seventh degree—'so that the barren has born seven' (v. 5), though she had given birth to only one child (Sim, 1956).

Although Kraepelin is credited with the term 'manic-depressive psychosis', Falret (1854) and Baillarger (1854) had already elaborated the concept of 'folie circulaire' and Kraepelin was undoubtedly influenced by them. Meyer (1952), who introduced the concept of the *reaction-type*, gave a new impulse to the appreciation of psychiatric illness in general and to the manic-depressive psychoses in particular, in that he stressed the individual variations in response and the multiplicity of the forms of presentation. The psychoanalytic school, particularly the papers of Abraham (1912, 1916), contributed further to the insights into the condition. In his first paper, he reported that ambivalence was the basic characteristic in the mental life in the depressed patient, that the quantities of love and hate that co-exist are approximately equal and that the sadism which the depressive directs on to himself was originally directed outwards. His second paper showed that in depressed patients oral eroticism is enormously increased and that conflicts associated with it played a part in depressive inhibitions, eating disturbances and 'oral' character traits.

Freud (1917) pays tribute to Abraham's work in his essay on

Mourning and Melancholia and demonstrates the role of the super-ego and the economic aspects in the psychopathology of mania. He was obviously influenced by the Kraepelinian concept of the manic-depressive state, though he does remark:

> Not every melancholic has this fate, as we know. Many cases run their course in intermittent periods, in the intervals of which signs of mania may be entirely absent or only very slight. . . . It is not merely permissible, therefore, but incumbent upon us to extend the analytic interpretation of melancholia to mania.

Rado (1928) explained the melancholic's self-reproaches as an ambivalent ingratiation of the super-ego and clarified the connections between depression and self-esteem. Klein (1948), from her studies of the infant, claimed that the depressive position is a normal one in every child and is associated with the weaning process, which occurs at about the age of 6 months. The mother who had primarily been externally both a good and a bad object, now becomes internalized and the child's fear of destroying the good object contributes to his feelings of guilt.

In addition to these psychological contributions, neurophysiologists and pharmacologists have added to our knowledge of these states and perhaps even more remarkable has been the tremendous therapeutic advances, particularly in the form of convulsant therapy, first chemical and then electrical, followed by more effective anti-depressant drugs. Manic states, too, have benefited from pharmacological aids and when the exact mechanism of these treatments becomes known a great advance will have been made towards the understanding of the undoubted physical mechanisms involved in the expressions of melancholia and mania (see Chapter 18).

AETIOLOGICAL FACTORS

Genetic

If genetic studies were limited to manic-depressive insanity where there was clear evidence of alternating mental states, one could compare and even integrate the results of several workers and draw some valid conclusions. Unfortunately the concept of the disease has not been so rigidly defined and one frequently sees included in these studies a number of cases where there was evidence of only one component, and that the depressive one, yet it is this type which may never develop a manic phase. It is probably because of this lack of homogeneity of the group and the differing methods of computing genetic influence that there have been discrepancies in genetic studies. Slater (1944) states that inheritance follows a dominant type which depends on a single autosomal gene and explains the lower incidence than would be expected by such genetic determinism, as being due to the gene having a weak and variable expression. Kallmann (1953) supports Slater's view but substitutes 'the mutative effect of a single dominant gene with incomplete penetrance' for 'weak and variable expression'. He does allow for other factors and states that the dynamics of manic-depressive psychosis 'cannot be considered part of a person's normal biological equipment'; he adds that these psychodynamics are similar to those found in other psychiatric states. Pollock *et al.* (1939) were unable to confirm that the psychosis was transmitted in accordance with simple Mendelian inheritance. It is generally accepted that while genetic factors would appear to play a part in *folie circulaire*, non-genetic factors are more important in the depressive states.

At one time genetic factors were considered to be of supreme importance but they are not now held in such high esteem. It is probable that prior to the availability of effective treatment a genetic theory of causation provided some comfort to the impotent therapist. Today both mania and depression can be successfully treated and frequently the illness is a once and for all phenomenon. It is therefore not only unnecessary but embarrassing to invoke a genetic theory for an illness which responds so readily to treatment and which is so often determined by psychological stresses. Familial incidence need not mean genetic transmission but may only indicate the strong influence of cultural factors and there is increasing evidence that these are more significant in the aetiology of depression than genetic factors. The time has probably come when the small group of true manic-depressive disorders which run an alternating and strongly recurrent course be separated from the very much larger group of depressive psychosis, as the search for a common aetiology in these disparate diseases contributes to some of the inadequate genetic theories that have been put forward.

Constitutional

These will to some extent embrace genetic factors. Kretschmer (1925) described a body habitus which was associated with a 'cycloid' type of temperament and stated that approximately two-thirds of manic-depressive states shared this temperament. The body build he called 'pyknic', a term which was used to describe rather short people with wide costal angle as opposed to the asthenic (leptosomatic) or athletic body build with narrow angle associated with the schizoid temperament. The previous criticism of genetic studies applies here too, for it is difficult to be sure whether Kretschmer's figures were based on the true *folie circulaire*, or on a much wider group.

Sheldon *et al.* (1940) developed Kretschmer's work and elaborated their own theory of physical types; they described ecto-, endo- and meso-morphy and gave to each a rating scale. Patients could therefore be described in terms of all three varieties, the difference being one of degree, the manic-depressives being mainly meso-morphs, or endo-mesomorphs, the mesomorphy predominating. The author has used the following childish example to explain these types to medical students—endomorphy is 'gutsy', ectomorphy is 'skinny' and mesomorphy is 'muscular'. Sheldon's theories have been criticized in that the constitutional type is not an essential factor in mental illness but perhaps a contributory one. A number of schizophrenic patients may present a body habitus which according to Sheldon should be associated with manic-depressive psychosis and *vice versa*. There is also the possibility that the pyknic build may be acquired and be dependent on the personality of the individual rather than the reverse.

Pollitt (1965) has tried to explain the two major groups of depression on a physiological basis. He attributes the symptoms of

diurnal mood swing, early morning waking, weight loss, constipation, loss of appetite, inability to weep, dry mouth, decreased sex desire, impotence, menstrual changes, decreased pulse rate, lowered blood pressure, lowered body temperature, loss of facial flush and cold extremities

to changes in biologic rhythms in metabolism and in autonomic balance which are not found collectively in any other illness. This syndrome, he called the 'Depressive Functional Shift' and implicated the hypothalamus. On this basis he divided depression into two main groups:

1. With depressive shift or type 'S' (Somatic).
2. Without depressive shift or type 'J' (Justified).

The mere collection of a group of somatic symptoms does not in itself prove that the condition has a physical cause, for somatic symptoms can result from psychological causes. What is needed to support Pollitt's theory is evidence of a physical cause. A large number of workers are busily engaged in defining the nature of the physical changes and Coppen and Shaw (1963) showed that depressive illness is associated with a considerable increase in residual sodium (intracellular and a small amount of bone sodium), which returns to normal after recovery. A subsequent study by Coppen *et al.* (1966) showed that mania is accompanied by similar electrolyte abnormalities but the changes in mania are more extreme.

These findings, in themselves, need not be of real significance but recently similar studies on patients treated for mania with lithium salts (see under Organic Psychiatry p. 243) have contributed further to the hypothesis, but the matter is still not solved. The major problems are (1) the distinct possibility that the manic-depressive group contains a small sub-group to which these findings may be applicable and (2) the possibility that mental changes may in themselves be influencing the electrolyte disturbances.

Pre-morbid Personality

Numerous classifications and definitions have been put forward and they are practically all distinguished for their adjectival erudition, rather than for any basic contribution they make to our understanding of the problem. What does emerge is that a person with a hypomanic personality is more likely to exhibit mania in his psychotic illness than a person with a depressive personality. Kretschmer has been a strong advocate of these basic states but they now sound strangely out of harmony with modern psychiatric theory and practice. They do, however, draw attention to the importance of a careful evaluation of the basic pre-morbid personality, though critics of Kretschmer would point out that descriptive words such as sociable, humorous, lively, serious, gentle and calm, would hardly qualify these days for pre-morbid personality assessment. It is sad but true, that what were at one time regarded as world-shattering truths are now commonplace, insufficient and even erroneous, and Kretschmer, who has earned his place in the history of psychiatry, can no longer be regarded as contributing seriously to this aspect. Of greater importance are the psychopathological insights of the psychoanalytic school with their emphasis on super-ego hypertrophy and dependency on approval and love. These are reflected in the patient's background, in that he is usually an effective member of society, over-conscientious and frequently a do-gooder with a high moral code. He is generally well-liked and in fact much of his life-style is directed towards gaining the approval of his fellows. This aspect is dealt with more fully under Symptomatology (Chapter 23).

Biochemistry

With the effective treatment of depression by monoamine oxidase inhibitors and tricyclics and the treatment of mania with butyrophenones and lithium there has been tremendous activity on the biochemical front in order to define the biochemical nature of the condition and the exact mode of action of the effective drugs.

Much of the evidence is of a negative nature; *e.g.* Coppen *et al.* (1971) were unable to find any differences in cortisol levels in the CSF between patients with affective disorders and controls not suffering from psychiatric illness. Shopsin *et al.* (1971) estimated the plasma cortisol response to dexamethasone suppression in depressed and control patients and found no support for the adrenocorticol hypothesis of depression but found higher levels in schizophrenia.

Manic-Depressive Illness and Social Achievement

Woodruff *et al.* (1971) studied 70 patients with primary affective disorder (29 bipolar and 41 unipolar) and their 128 brothers. Patients with bipolar illness had more brothers seriously affected (27 per cent) compared with 17 per cent in the unipolar. In addition they were younger and therefore not so far into the age of risk for such illness. Unipolar subjects had achieved at an average level whereas bipolars were achieving at a higher than the expected level, as were their brothers. It could all be explained on energy plus ability as against ability with less energy.

Neurological

No conclusive evidence has yet been furnished, but Kraines (1957) suggests a dysfunction of the diencephalon which elicits a 'psychic response'. The nature of this dysfunction still gives rise to much speculation but a number of workers consider that the illness is mediated through the diencephalic-rhinencephalic-reticular system but can be influenced by a variety of factors, such as changes in circulation and metabolic disturbances. The depressive and occasionally manic reactions associated with epidemic encephalitis lend support to this speculation and there are other examples of diencephalic pathology associated with affective disorders.

Neuropharmacological studies are likely to contribute further and perhaps elucidate these speculations. The depression which follows the administration of rauwolfia preparations in certain subjects and the euphoria which follows amphetamine and other energizers have triggered off a large amount of experimental work which strongly suggests that brain systems such as the reticular formation and the diencephalon play their part. These factors are dealt with more fully under Psychopharmacology (Chapter 18).

Endocrine

In diseases of obscure origin it is not unusual to implicate a variety of systems and in psychiatry the endocrine system has been particularly invoked. That the thyroid, adrenals and pituitary do affect mental function is undisputed but it is far from proven that endocrine dysfunction is responsible for manic-depressive psychoses or affective disorders. The onset of the psychosis may be associated with surgical or medical treatment of hyperthyroidism or with the development of hypothyroidism, but such precipitating factors play only a minor role in the general incidence of a very common illness. This has not deterred many workers from seeking an endocrine basis for the illness, though their efforts have been mainly directed to the more chronic and therefore more challenging condition of schizophrenia.

Plasma 11-hydroxycorticosteroids in Depression. Conroy *et al.* (1968) studied Circadian rhythm in plasma of 11-OHCS levels in affective psychotics and demonstrated higher values than are found in schizophrenics and other psychotic subgroups and also a less regular rhythm. One patient showed a reduction coincident with clinical recovery, while an accentuated fall and rise in the night and early morning samples respectively was observed in the schizophrenic subgroup. They concluded that their results provided further evidence that plasma corticosteroid values tend to be raised in depressive illness, especially in late evening or night samples and may be obscured in the mornings.

Psychopathology

While its role as an aetiological factor has not been finally agreed there is no other member of the aetiological group which has contributed more to the understanding of the symptomatology of manic-depressive psychosis. Fenichel (1945) links depressive states with the impulse neuroses and addictions in that in all *self-esteem* is constantly under threat and much of these patients' behaviour is directed to heighten it or protect it from damage. They react violently to frustration, for their oral dependence makes them approval-hungry and love-addicted. Both reactions can be condensed in the same act and he points out that 'sacrifice and prayer, the classical methods of ingratiation, are often thought of as a kind of magical violence used to force God to give what is needed'.

Although mania is so much rarer than depression, psychoanalytic theory too has been influenced by the manic-depressive insanity concept of Kraepelin, and Freud (1917) in his classic essay *Mourning and Melancholia* couples the disorders. In it he indicates that if a child loses an object, the libidinal strivings hitherto bound to the object create a feeling of panic. In bereavement or grief the adult has learned gradually to free himself from his tie—a process which takes time and has been called the 'work of mourning'. There is at first an identification with the dead person such as is seen in death and burial customs and this has been likened to *introjection* which is said to precede and then facilitate the final loosening from the introjected object. If the mourner has an extremely ambivalent attitude to the lost object, the act of introjection will in itself create guilt feelings because of its sadistic implications, and in another way, death may represent the fulfilment of an unconscious wish and this too can mobilize guilt feelings. Indentification with the dead can punish the bereaved, as he may fear the dead person will seek revenge or that his own death wish is omnipotent and will include him too. This fear makes much of burial ritual meaningful, *e.g.* not speaking ill of the dead, erecting memorials, and pacifying and placating their spirits with prayers and gifts. Grief therefore is a process which protects us from violent discharges of emotion which are said to be at their strongest in the more ambivalent situations.

Anniversary Reactions. Hilgard and Newman (1959) pointed out the importance of anniversaries in the precipitation of severe mental reactions, including psychotic depression and suicide. The anniversary is usually for a bereavement and it is as if the patient is projected into a recurrence of mourning but without the social support that the real bereavement attracted. It has been shown that physical illnesses like coronary thrombosis are also affected by anniversaries (Fischer & Dlin, 1972).

The affective disturbances associated with the introjection will be greater if:

(*a*) the lost object has been used to satisfy the narcissistic needs;
(*b*) the previous relationship has been strongly ambivalent; and
(*c*) the patient is orally fixated.

Fenichel states that '. . . Depression is a desperate attempt to compel an orally incorporated object to grant forgiveness, protection, love and security. The destructive elements liberated by this coercion create further guilt feelings and fears of retaliation . . .' The equation of the ego with the introjected object may make the patient complain that he is worthless and reproach himself for fancied crimes.

This stage when the ego is ripe for punishment is now reinforced by the super-ego which exhibits a marked degree of sadism and may enlist the introjected object. The personality of the individual undergoes a change, with the super-ego usurping the ego which at times is completely submissive but may also rebel, and in its attempt to rid itself of the hostile introjected object, may take the final step of self-destruction.

Suicide. This is not always the result of a depressive psychosis (Chapter 12) but when it is, it can be seen as a turning in on oneself of sadistic impulses. The patient has lost self-esteem and feels he can no longer regain it and seeks a means of escaping the torture of his super-ego.

Narcissistic Regression. This means that there is a withdrawal from object relationships to relationships within the personality and in psychotic depression this process is marked. It is a regression to the earliest stage of mental development, before the ego had been properly established, and much of the hypochondriasis associated with melancholia can be explained on this basis.

Hypochondriasis. The concept of hypochondriasis is far from clear though recent studies are beginning to define its nature and associations. Kenyon (1965) in a study of 512 mental hospital patients with hypochondriasis found that it was always part of another syndrome either anxiety state or depressive state. A smaller survey by Kreitman *et al.* (1965) suggested as a causative factor advertising which is aimed at hypochondriacal concern, linking bad breath, body odour, constipation, social and sexual failure. Some patients, they claim, reproduce symptoms formerly experienced by their mothers and were prone to psychosomatic illness in childhood and adolescence. These may be important in directing the vulnerable patient towards hypochondriasis, but without narcissistic regression there is no hypochondriasis.

Psychological causes can be very varied both in nature and degree. The result will depend on the meaning the precipitating factor has for each patient and his psychological vulnerability. Early injuries to infantile narcissism predispose and these are usually due to severe disappointment in the parents at a time when the child's self-esteem was intimately bound with their omnipotence. Oral fixation which may have preceded these narcissistic injuries is reinforced by the latter and the vulnerable person is usually oral dependent and reacts to frustration with severe depression.

Engel and Reichsman (1956) demonstrated depression in the infant, Monica, with her congenital atresia of the oesophagus and a surgically produced gastric fistula. The mother was unable to hold and cuddle her baby for fear of disturbing the tube through which the baby was fed and the infant after the age of 6 months was left for long periods to cry fruitlessly. The child, who failed to gain weight, at 15 months weighed only 10 pounds, exhibited a profound state of fretful withdrawal and according to the authors was depressed. The depression was alleviated after a few months in hospital where a nurse and doctor spent a good deal of time with the baby. The authors conclude that depression resulted when the mother was unable to satisfy many basic needs but this was alleviated when a sustained relationship was established with the two adults, though the baby remained liable to depressive reactions. This case has made a considerable impact on theories relating to the depression-prone individual and is in accordance with the views of Spitz (1946) and Bowlby (1960) whose conclusions were also based on their observations on infants and children. While their contributions are valuable, they should be seen in conjunction with super-ego development, for children exposed to these insults may be conspicuously lacking in super-ego functioning and are, according to Bowlby, *affectless* and therefore not prone to depression.

Conscience and Depressive Disorders. Although it is generally assumed that guilt is a striking feature of depressive disorders, Amdur and Harrow (1972) reported on 134 consecutive admissions whom they had previously studied for guilt content. They found that on testing a strict conscience was a more persistent and pervasive feature than guilt in patients whose primary illness was a depressive one. Guilt was also present but not to the same extent.

It is difficult to see the significance of this finding for expression of guilt is merely a gross manifestation of a strict conscience; indeed it is impossible to consider the former in the absence of the latter. It is the present writer's clinical experience that guilt is present only in the severer forms of depression. The authors, on the other hand, found it more frequently in neurotic depressives which casts doubt on their test scales, but it is not unusual for psychological tests to produce paradoxical, if not useless results in clinical psychiatry.

Precipitating Factors

Most depressions are preceded by physical or psychological traumata.

Physical. *Infection* is the commonest and influenza the most notorious, an epidemic being followed by a spate of new cases. Infective hepatitis, bronchitis, pneumonia and pleurisy are other common precipitators, but any febrile illness can induce the depression in a vulnerable patient, though there is no satisfactory explanation for the variability in response even in the same patient, except that when he did break down, he was probably more vulnerable.

Operations are not uncommonly followed by depression, and they need not be a major insult and in fact may be as minor as dental extractions. The symbolic significance of having one's teeth removed will not be lost on the analytically inclined.

Accidents are also frequently quoted in the histories of depressed patients, though as with operations, psychological factors may have played a part in determining the physical trauma.

Other experiences include pregnancy and childbirth.

Psychological. As mentioned under psychopathology, withdrawal of affection or damage to self-esteem can precipitate the psychosis. Bereavement is one of the commonest factors, but loss of office, failure in business, a broken romance or inability to fulfil one's ambitions are often cited. A less obvious factor in women is moving into a new house. Here, superficially there would appear to be every reason for the patient not becoming depressed, but they frequently do and it is probably due to social isolation and missing the friendly reassurance of familiar tradesmen. The new and improved surroundings do not compensate for these psychological deprivations.

Parent Death and Depression. Birtchnell (1970 *a, b, c, & d*) in a series of papers studied the influence of early and recent parent death on mental illness including depression and attempted suicide. The psychiatric patients numbered 500 who were admitted to a mental hosptial over a 5-year period and the controls who were matched for age and sex were from a local general practice. It was found that the age period when the difference between patients and controls was most striking was from 0–4 years (9·8 per cent of patients and 4·7 per cent of controls suffered parent death). He concluded:

1. That it was not so much the trauma of separation from the parent as the continued absence of the parent throughout childhood which was the important aspect of early parent death.
2. A more definite relationship was found to exist between recent parent death and first admission than readmission. The mean parental ages at birth among patients and controls who suffered recent parent death were found to be similar, suggesting that parent death and not parental age at birth is the primary phenomenon.
3. Death of a parent, either in childhood or during the years before admission, is as common in depressed patients as in other

types of mental illness. The finding that early death of one parent combined with the recent death of the other is significantly commoner in severely depressed patients, suggests that patients who lose a parent when young cling excessively to the remaining parent and react badly to his or her eventual death.

4. Of the 104 patients who attempted suicide, significantly more had suffered early parental absence due mainly to an excess of parental deaths from age 10–19 years. This was more marked in those attempted suicides who were severely depressed (66·7 per cent). Significantly more had experienced parent death over a period of 1·5 years before admission.

Overwork is sometimes suggested as a cause, either by patient or family, but when one enquires carefully, the overwork is generally self-administered. For example, a bank manager may take on a number of honorary treasurerships, assume the chairmanship of some charities, begin to indulge a latent interest in amateur dramatics and is shortly producing and directing plays. His ability, good spirits and boundless energy are probably admired and it has not occurred to anybody that he is in a state of hypomania and that the subsequent depression is the downward swing of this cycle.

Occasionally a precipitating factor is not uncovered, but like the needle in the haystack, it does not mean that because it has not been found it is not there. The cycloid nature of these patients may lead one to postulate a spontaneous onset just as one frequently meets a spontaneous remission, but in general hospital and out-patient psychiatry, where depression is by far the commonest psychiatric condition seen, precipitating factors are very commonly found.

Oral Contraception and Depression

Kutner and Brown (1972) attempted a controlled study to establish whether there was an association between oral contraception and depression. 5151 female patients of mean age 35·6 years were studied of whom 33·5 per cent had never used the pill, 27·9 per cent were past users and 38·6 per cent were present users. Of the last mentioned, 85·5 per cent used a combination pill (progestin-oestrogen throughout) and 4·5 per cent used a sequential pill (oestrogen for the first 14 days and both steroids for the next 6 days). All patients were tested with the Minnesota Multiphasic Personality Inventory (MMPI) Depression Scale as well as self-rating mood scales and the findings did not support the hypothesis. Rather there seemed to be considerable pre-menstrual improvement especially with combination drugs. The authors claim that their study provides no justification for withholding oral contraceptives because of depression.

The Mourning Response of Mothers to the Death of a Newborn. Kennell *et al.* (1970) interviewed 20 mothers who had recently lost their newborn in order to determine whether tactile contact between mother and infant was more upsetting than if the mother did not handle the child. All mothers showed mourning reactions and the authors conclude that affectional bonding precedes tactile contact and viewing and touching the newborn is not a specific cause of mourning.

SYMPTOMATOLOGY

This is not confined to presenting features of the disease, but must also include an assessment of the pre-morbid personality. In fact, this may prove more valuable than any single symptom the patient may provide. The deeper psychoanalytic concepts of Abraham (1912) will not be apparent, but their influence on personality structure will. Bellak *et al.* (1952), adapting Abraham's theories, consider that manic-depressives have established an equilibrium on a libidinal level which depends on a sufficient degree of *ego-strength.* This strength is based on super-ego qualities, the patient usually having an effective pre-morbid personality with conscientiousness, energy, ambition and other such qualities. He may even show super-ego hypertrophy and be a 'do-gooder' with a commendable record of public service and voluntary work. It is not difficult to see that such a person whose stability depends on this equilibrium is vulnerable to ego weakening or increased libidinal demands. His way of life is geared to gaining the approval of others but he may fail or, even worse, believe he has failed and then the depressive psychosis asserts itself. Its form will depend very largely on the ego-strength of the patient and his cultural level, for the latter may determine the language in which his symptomatology is expressed, while the former will influence the purity of the response. Adulteration can therefore be derived from both sources and, as it is not uncommon, it is of the greatest importance to assess the pre-morbid effectiveness of the patient in terms of school and work record, a high sense of responsibility and absence of delinquency of a pleasure principle type. One is constantly being reminded in case-history taking that the depressive patient is the 'salt of the earth' type—good husband, good wife, good citizen, at times too good, too rigid, too conscientious, perhaps to an obsessional degree, but leaving one in no doubt that these are the people who run our society and put more into this world then they personally take out. Some 'objective' tests have been devised to measure this ego-strength but a clinical appraisal based on a full personal history supplemented by an interview with a relative is still the best method and excels psychological tests such as the Rorschach, and physiological tests such as the Funkenstein (Chapter 20).

The *classical case* is traditionally regarded as presenting the following triad of symptoms:

1. Depressed mood.
2. Psychomotor retardation.
3. Morbid thought content with feelings of unworthiness and guilt.

Depressed Mood

This can vary in degree and in form of expression, and can develop slowly or suddenly.

(a) **Mild to Moderate.** This can present as a general falling-off in interest with difficulty in concentration. The accompanying relative may have noticed that the patient is not as cheerful as he was and remark that he has lost his smile. When asked if this is so, the patient may deny it, but admit that he has to force himself to smile. The mood is variable, showing a classical diurnal variation, being worse first thing in the morning and getting better as the day wears on. Occasionally the rhythm may be reversed. The laughter and noise of children are no longer welcomed with a tolerant smile but arouse irritation and snappiness and *irritability* is frequently the main presenting feature; the patient may even deny he has any depression. Newspapers are regarded as saturated with bad news and the more light-hearted contributions (which are to be found) are overlooked. It is as if the morbid has an attraction for the patient and he may protect himself by not looking at the papers at all. He may be *easily moved to tears*, initially by situations in which he is not personally involved but with which he readily identifies himself, such as television and radio programmes or a cinema show. This lachrymosity is very much out of keeping with his pre-morbid nature when he was 'always ready for a laugh' and he may reinforce this information by saying, 'They used to call me "smiler"–always singing and laughing'.

(b) **Severe.** The patient looks miserable and occasionally agitated. complains that there is *no joy* left in life and that he has reached the bottom of the pit. When asked how low he got, he will reply as low as possible. He may frankly admit that life is not worthwhile and that he does not wish to carry on; he may in fact have seriously contemplated suicide. Irritability may be pronounced and he may even have struck his wife or children. This behaviour is very much at variance with his normal state for he will probably have been a devoted husband and father. Such conduct is usually followed by remorse and it may even be paraded as his main symptom to impress people as to how terrible a person he really is. He may say he doesn't break down and cry but this is not because he doesn't feel like it, but because he 'just can't cry any more'. His relatives will say that there has been a tremendous change in him and that he is nothing like the man he was.

Psychomotor Retardation

This is not seen to any marked degree in the *mild or moderate cases.* There may be a certain contraction of activities and he may complain of tiredness and inability to do anything on coming home from work. 'I just flop into a chair and don't want to do a thing'—yet previously he was a man who was devoted to his hobbies and had time for everything. His thinking is impaired, ideas come very slowly to him or not at all, and he feels 'all dried up inside'. There may be constipation and loss of libido. In the *severe case*, retardation may reach the stage of depressive stupor and mutism. His responses are extremely slowed and he may be incapable of conducting a normal conversation. His gait is slow, he may be completely inaccessible and the condition may be confused with a catatonic stupor (Chapter 13) but the picture of abject misery is unmistakable. Indecision is also a feature of this stage and trying to obtain a signature to a form of consent for electroplexy can be a wearisome if not fruitless task.

Morbid Thoughts

These are usually found in the more *severe* cases and are really depressive delusions. *Unworthiness and guilt* are frequently expressed, the patient saying that he is letting everybody down, his wife, his employers and the world in general. He feels he is not up to his job and what is more everybody knows it and he is the laughing stock of his office. This feeling of inadequacy regarding work is very common and in the less obviously deranged patient may lead to tragic mistakes such as premature resignation from a post which the patient has held for many years and can practically manage 'with his eyes shut'. A lot of the psychiatrist's time may be spent trying to remedy these psychotically determined resignations because the chances are that the prognosis will be good and that the patient will be returned to full vigour of body and mind only to be out of a job which he has voluntarily relinquished after 30 years or more of excellent service and all the 'good will' which that insures. This resignation problem may also arise in another setting (see below).

Guilt is linked with minor peccadilloes such as not having paid one's bus fare and the passage of time is no protection, for the incident may have occurred many years ago. It may be of a sexual nature but rarely anything which the ordinary individual would regard as worthy of note, such as the man who after his wife died had 'lustful thoughts' about her unmarried sister. These expressions of guilt and unworthiness frequently are designed to place the patient in what he considers to be a most reprehensible light and they therefore vary according to age and cultural pattern. A patient, who was subject to recurring bouts of depression since childhood, at the age of 11 years felt he was a cheat and that he was cribbing at school (in fact, he was very bright, and most of the class were cribbing from him). At 16 years he believed he was guilty of a murder, but it was not going to be an ordinary murder. He was going to be undetected and an innocent man would hang for his crime. Later at 19 years when at Oxford he believed he was abnormal sexually and that everybody could read in his face that he was a homosexual. In a less sophisticated setting, it is not uncommon for a very worthy housewife to attempt suicide because of her 'unspeakable crime' which was drawing her retirement (old age) pension, to which she erroneously believed she was not entitled.

The ingenuity of distortion which patients display is frequently conditioned by this cultural background. An elderly retired history schoolmistress was convinced that a felon's cell was being built for her and that she would be incarcerated without sanitation and in this 'awful mess' her gaolers would violate her defenceless body. All this would be done by law under the Statute of Praemunire which Richard II introduced in 1392 to curb the power of the Church and confiscate its property. She had worked it out that as a retired school teacher she was in principle a cleric in the pension of the state and therefore subject to this law. She insisted that it had not been repealed, and she may have been right! The sadistic and punitive effect of the super-ego in these delusions is very obvious.

While the expression of feelings of guilt is classically associated with the depressive psychoses, Amdur and Harrow (1972) showed that a strict conscience was a much more common finding which they measured. This is merely carrying the argument back a stage for guilt is based on a strict conscience.

Other Features

(*a*) **Sleep.** This is frequently impaired and consists of early morning waking rather than difficulty in getting off. It can lead to total insomnia which is highly resistant to hypnotics and though the answer is in the treatment of the underlying depression, the patient and relatives can't see this and there is much pressure on the doctor to prescribe more powerful drugs—'If only he could be made to sleep. . . . .' Very occasionally the depressed patient seeks refuge in sleep and will drowse all day and not get out of bed but the sleep is never refreshing and not followed by a release of energy.

(*b*) **Appetite.** In *mild* cases this can be increased and it is quite common for the housewife to help herself to tit-bits from the larder. Generally it is diminished and weight loss the rule. In *severe* cases the loss can be dramatic, up to 20 kilos in three months, and it has been said that there is no medical condition which can produce such rapid weight loss as a severe depression. Sometimes this is not always apparent as the loss may have been preceded by a rapid gain and the patient may quote his present weight as his standard one, or it may sound more dramatic than it looks, the patient quoting a marked loss of weight, which under normal circumstances would be drastic, but failing to explain that prior to the weight loss he was 20 kilos or more up on his usual weight.

(*c*) **Libido.** Sexual appetite is frequently though not invariably diminished and many states of depression present as impotence. This can be a very distressing symptom for it means much to the depression-prone and therefore approval-seeking patient, and may warrant anti-depressant measures which the overt depression, which appears mild, would not in itself justify.

(*d*) **Somatic Complaints.** These range from the common tension symptoms such as pain in the head, back and neck to marked hypochondriacal features. The tension can manifest very locally—'It's just this one spot', or it can be very generalized, the patient indicating with both hands and covering the neck and head as with a cowl.

(*e*) **Hypochondriasis** is a manifestation of a number of psychiatric conditions but when associated with depression it possesses certain qualities and has a portent which makes its understanding essential. It is not surprising that in a state of *narcissistic regression* hypochondriasis frequently presents. It is not the bizarre pseudo-

-anxiety complaint of the schizophrenic or the light-hearted triviality of the hysteric, but a strongly held belief that something very serious is wrong. The nature of the illness indicated by the patient's complaint is usually of a socially reprehensible nature such as syphilis, or like cancer, carrying what the public consider the threat of a slow and tortured death. His insistence on the presence of the disease and his refusal to be persuaded otherwise by numerous investigations, should make it obvious that this is not a matter for simple reassurance. In fact this approach can heighten the depression, for what the patient is trying to say is that he must have the disease because he deserves to have it. One might just as well try and argue away his delusions of guilt. In the older age groups these patients are prone to commit suicide and one should see the complaint as a death sentence passed by the patient and that it is only a matter of time before he will carry it out.

Melancholic Violence and Cognitive Dysfunction

Malmquist (1971) presents an analysis of the nature of cognitive dysfunction in depression under five headings:

1. Its implications from tendencies to misinterpret external and internal reality.
2. The heightening of the potential for violence against oneself and others during such depression.
3. Cognitive deficits in depressives at the time of a violent episode.
4. An analysis of violence-proneness in the severely depressed based on dispositional tendencies.
5. Legal implications for such cases when the criteria for criminal responsibility are based on intact cognitive functioning.

In ego-maturation, a threat of loss mobilizes emergency emotions such as fear or rage in the depressive-prone. Parallel to this, depressive thinking emerges which expresses self-evaluations of worthlessness, guilt and self-contempt. Ultimately the way in which the depressive thinks and feels about himself is contaminated. Unlike the schizophrenic he makes a desperate attempt to maintain contact with a world that is construed as unrewarding. Rumination about worthlessness impairs the ego capacity to appraise itself and reality testing and morality may lose the semblance and substance of objectivity.

Given such cognitive liabilities in a regressed ego state, the potential for an act of violence by drive regression is enhanced. Extremes of self-contempt give rise to delusions which are used in the service of pseudo-rationality. Suicide and/or homicide is the ultimate solution in patients whose lack of self-approval has reached such an end-point.

The author contends that such subjects who are convicted of violent acts may not have comprehended the nature of their acts at the time because of cognitive delusional distortions.

There is a distorted use of abstract reasoning which results in thinking more characteristic in the child from 3–5 years; language is restricted to negation, autism or simple referential talk of even earlier developmental periods. He may be led to believe he is performing a noble act in sparing others from a continued existence with him.

MIXED STATES

Ego strength will vary, other patterns of behaviour and complaints will emerge and thus we find the mixed states, which can range from a mild hysterical overlay to the near schizophrenic reaction. Diagnostic criteria should be judged not only on a qualitative but on a quantitative basis. The common varieties are:

Depression with Hysterical Conversion. Depression is basic but the hysterical features are paraded. It may be an aphonia in a schoolmistress who initially denies the depressed state, a blepharospasm in an engraver, or a variety of hysterical complaints in a hitherto efficient and stable housewife. In the last case, her low back pain may well have brought her to the gynaecologist, who for excellent reasons performed a hysterectomy and to the original condition is added the trauma of the operation. It is only by a careful assessment of the personal history and the sequence of events and an enquiry into the patient's affective state that the condition can be defined. Even then, the patient and the family may be so heavily committed to an organic cause of the illness that only observation in hospital for a short period to declare its true nature can satisfy them. In unguarded moments the patient may break down and cry, or show a lack of spontaneity or exhibit the classical diurnal variation. A session under light pentothal narcosis frequently declares the underlying depression and the resulting brisk abreaction leaves the diagnosis in no doubt.

These hysterical conversions of depression usually cluster in certain cultural groups, *e.g.* the busy housewife who is unable to or is afraid to verbalize her emotional state and therefore resorts to a physical expression of her illness, or where there is a rigid communal discipline such as in Nurses' Homes, the Services, and occasionally in convents. The hysterical features may play a sadistic role and some patients upset their relatives with compulsive sniffing, snorting, spitting and other objectionable habits. Sadistic trends may extend to other forms of conduct such as the constant reiteration of hypochondriacal complaints and refusal to admit improvement when it is abundantly clear that this is taking place. It is as if the patient hopes that by making others miserable he will lighten his own burden.

Depression with Paranoid Features. The delusions are themselves of a depressive nature and are evidently the work of the super-ego. He may say the police are after him and that he is suspected of treason, or that his work-mates despise him and know of his former immature sexual practices. All degrees of mixture occur and the stage can be reached where the paranoid features are dominant. The differentiation and measuring of the components is not entirely academic for the treatment will vary accordingly.

Depression with Obsessional Features. This is common, for obsessional personalities frequently break down with depressive illness. The depression may be very severe with suicidal risk and though it frequently responds to the usual anti-depressants, including electroplexy, a disturbing obsessional pre-occupation with memory loss may result. A number remit only temporarily with treatment and some not at all, and they provide a hard core which fortunately may respond to pre-frontal leucotomy (Chapter 20).

Depression with Anxiety Features. This is frequent and is manifest by the usual somatic signs—digital tremors, rapid pulse and hyperhidrosis. It is, however, not enough to treat the anxiety component; like most adulterated states, the less serious condition is often nourished by the more serious and until the underlying depression has cleared, anxiety features will persist. Here, too, a careful quantitative assessment is essential.

Depression with Schizophrenic Features (Schizo-affective State). This is much commoner than is generally reported, because of the tendency for psychiatrists when confronted with schizophrenic features to see the problem primarily as such. This attitude may stem from the well-known sequence in adolescent schizophrenia which is frequently ushered in with a depressive phase. There are, however, a large number of acute reactions, particularly puerperal, post-operative and post-infective psychoses, which do not follow the course of the adolescent schizophrenic. In them, schizophrenic features may be marked with bizarre thought and behaviour patterns, but underlying it is a profound depression which usually responds to electroplexy. The prognosis in these states is good and in the puerperal psychoses is no worse than those with unadulterated depression.

Masked Depression. The protean manifestations of depression are being increasingly recognized. What are more difficult to define are those patients who, though depressed, present as a different clinical entity. Some parade a hysterical picture, some are hypochondriacal, some may be paranoid and many exhibit an anxiety state. Pollitt and Young (1971) found that a large number of patients with the physiological symptoms of anxiety were regarded as anxiety states but they responded well to anti-depressant drugs. They suggested that changes in sleep, appetite, weight, libido and diurnal variation are typical of the depressive state and these are called 'depressive functional shift symptoms'.

Other Mixtures. Although paired states have been described above, the mixture may be more complex and it is not uncommon for a schizo-affective reaction to include marked paranoid features or for both anxiety and obsessional features to be found together with depression. Furthermore the components may vary in their extent at different times in the same patient, and as has been pointed out, may respond differently to treatment, so that what started off as a schizo-affective reaction may after a course of E.C.T. be one of unadulterated schizophrenia.

Involutional Melancholia

There used to be much controversy as to whether this condition merited its own title or whether it should be an integral part of the depressive group. By definition there should have been no previous history of a manic-depressive episode and it should occur in the involutional age group. Some psychiatrists claim that it presents specific features which are not found in other depressive states, such as a malignant form of insomnia, a pre-occupation with death, bizarre complaints with nihilistic delusions. Statements such as 'My blood has turned to water', 'I have no brain', 'My bowels are blocked' have caused some to regard it as being related to the schizophrenic psychoses, but its response to electroplexy is very similar to that of depression and such bizarre depressive delusions are also met in younger people. Much of the argument for the existence of the disease as an entity hinges on the definition of 'involutional'. It has become a most elastic term ranging from the age of 40–80+ and applicable to both sexes. It has even been extended to younger age groups by qualifying it with 'early'. The absence of a previous history does not commend itself as an argument, since positive evidence of such does not necessarily put the condition into the manic-depressive or *folie circulaire* concept. A puerperal psychosis can present many of the features regarded by some as typically involutional, yet such a patient may have had no previous history of breakdown or even if she had a previous puerperal psychosis, it would not necessarily include her in the manic-depressive group. It is not surprising that patients at different ages should present differently and this point has already been stressed.

There would appear to be no real justification for regarding this group as a disease entity, but tradition dies hard and as the womb in its fancied wanderings has given rise to the term *hysteria* it would seem that in its involutional state it will also make a lasting though equally irrational impression on psychiatric nosology.

NEUROTIC DEPRESSION

The above types of depression come under the category of *psychotic depression,* but unfortunately the term depression has been attached to other reactions which have a different psychopathology and symptomatology. As these are styled neurotic, it implies that they do not show the same divorcement from reality as the psychotic variety and neither are they so heavily influenced by super-ego hypertrophy. Deep guilt feelings are not a feature and indeed there is a tendency for a greater display of depression than one usually meets in a severe affective disturbance.

Neurotic depression though not entirely satisfactory as a diagnostic category, has been elaborated as a compromise in order to improve nosology which was even less satisfactory.

It was, and unfortunately in some circles still is customary to divide the depressions into two categories: Endogenous and Exogenous or Reactive. It was believed that the endogenous type was of genetic or unknown aetiology while the latter was caused by external events to which a vulnerable patient reacted. The former category represented those psychotic states for which no rational explanation could be given and though precipitating factors could be found they were considered to be so inappropriate that the illness was primarily a 'constitutional' one. The second category appeared more rational, for precipitating factors were definable but the reaction was of a different quality and though the classification of Endogenous and Reactive is an aetiological one, it is apparent that what was really intended was a classification based on the *nature* of the condition.

Psychotic and Neurotic distinctions avoid spurious aetiological claims and indicate that the conditions are essentially different in their nature. There are unfortunately mixed states which perpetuate the argument.

As with psychotic depression the personality of the individual is of great importance in assessing the type of reaction. Such patients are not nearly so effective, responsible or super-ego laden. If they do present features of super-ego hypertrophy, they do not possess the ego-strength to support them in unadulterated form and although they may even voice feelings of guilt and unworthiness these features do not have the same ring of quality as in the psychotic depression. There is a greater tendency to hysterical communication and they are more demanding and manipulative of the environment. Tears are frequently in evidence and dependency, particularly on the physician and/or his drugs is common. Women are much more commonly affected than men.

This neurotic pattern of behaviour is readily excited by somewhat trivial events, and major crises leave them prostrate. Other neurotic features such as phobic anxiety and obsessional pre-occupations are also linked to the depression but these are not as malignant as those which are attached to psychotic depression. It seems that the ego-weakness which makes them prone to react adversely to minor stress, also protects them from the severe neurotic reaction as well as from psychotic depression. Such patients can frequently be supported by a variety of agents such as social worker, parson, marriage guidance counsellor, physician and psychiatrist.

When well, they have a superficial gaiety and may claim to enjoy the well-being of the recovered psychotic depression, but the ego-strength is not there and they are still very vulnerable. When ill they masquerade as psychotic depression but a careful case history and a critical interview should reveal the essential differences.

MANIA

This represents a narcissistic victory over depression in that the vital supplies which are feared lost are present in abundance, with a heightening of self-esteem. The ego is freed from super-ego dominance with consequent hypersexuality which has a distinctly oral aspect. This state has been likened to the 'feast-days' in many cultures where the super-ego is abolished temporarily either by the prevailing mood which is akin to mania, or dissolved in alcohol, or both. The individual reverts to a state which is governed by the pleasure principle and instincts are indulged in an uninhibited manner.

It is the other arm of the manic-depressive psychosis but as has been pointed out, is very much rarer. It is most frequently associated with *folie circulaire* and much of the positive evidence of genetic and constitutional factors in aetiology is more applicable to this condition than to the much more common depression. It may be ushered in by a period of depression which while under treatment develops into a manic state and gives rise to statements, mostly unsubstantiated, that the treatment (such as E.C.T.) was responsible. It can also occur under conditions of psychological stress and Tredgold (1947) described an epidemic occurring in young Army officers who were undergoing rigorous training for the invasion of Japan. The Japanese surrendered before the invasion took place and these officers rapidly developed acute mania and had to be hospitalized. This setting meets the requirements of Freud (1917) who in his essay *Mourning and Melancholia* discusses the psychopathology and states:

> . . . that the content of mania is no different from that of melancholia, that both the disorders are wrestling with the same 'complex', and that in melancholia the ego has succumbed to it, whereas in mania it has mastered the complex or thrust it aside. The other point of view is founded on the observation that all states such as joy, triumph, exultation, which form the normal counterparts of mania, are economically conditioned in the same way. First, there is always a long-sustained condition of great mental expenditure, or one established by long force of habit, upon which at last some influence supervenes making it superfluous, so that a volume of energy becomes available for manifold possible applications and ways of discharge—for instance, when some poor devil, by winning a large sum of money, is suddenly relieved from perpetual anxiety about his daily bread, when any long and arduous struggle is finally crowned with success, when a man finds himself in a position to throw off at one blow some heavy burden, some false position he has long endured, and so on. All such situations are characterized by high spirits, by the signs of discharge of joyful emotion, and by increased readiness to all kinds of action, just like mania, and in complete contrast to the dejection and inhibition of melancholia. One may venture to assert that mania is nothing other than a triumph of this sort, only that here again what the ego has surmounted and is triumphing over remains hidden from it.

These psychodynamic factors can operate in situations which would superficially appear to be entirely organic, such as in post-operative or postpartum mania which are frequently quoted as evidence of the organic aetiology of manic states, yet such an attitude ignores the tension under which the patient was labouring and the tremendous relief which follows the successful conclusion. The Song of Hannah, which has already been referred to, is an excellent example of the manic outburst following childbirth and the relationship with her previous depression has been pointed out (p. 517). This does not mean that organic factors do not operate in producing these states and the present infrequency of acute mania after pregnancy, and in fact generally, has been attributed to control of infection, better nutrition and prevention of severe degrees of anaemia.

There has been in the author's experience a slight increase in the incidence of mania. What was very rare ten years ago is now merely uncommon. This could be a chance finding but enquiries among one's colleagues have reinforced this impression and it is possible that the increase is real. It is interesting to speculate on the reasons for this and while control of organic factors could with some justification be invoked to explain a decrease, cultural factors may explain the increase. Our society is becoming less inhibited generally and the norms of behaviour have shifted several points to the side of extraversion and boisterousness. To suggest that this shift can account for a modest increase in mania is of course based on no evidence whatever and is pure speculation. It is, however, a matter which will require watching and with more careful records it should be possible in the near future to decide whether in fact there is such a trend and also to define the various factors which may be contributing.

Classification

It is usual to divide the group into *mania* or the *manic attack, hypomania, acute mania, delirious mania* and *mixed states. Delirious mania* though showing some resemblance to the other manic states is more likely to be organically induced, the most typical cases having a toxic or infective basis.

The *manic attack* will be described first as many of its features are applicable to the other types and the differences will be listed under the latter's headings.

Onset. This may be difficult to define and it may just develop out of a natural state of well-being, the patient being normally of a lively disposition and liable to mood swings. On the other hand, it may occur after an attack or during treatment of depression.

SYMPTOMATOLOGY

This is best divided into a process of development and the full-blown state.

Development. The patient becomes more talkative and requires less sleep. His energy increases and he ceases to tire. His mood is euphoric and his attitude optimistic, and his general air is readily transmitted to those around him who can easily enter into his banter which is good-humoured and generous. He may give the impression of having had a drink or two though it is known that he hasn't had any, and his friends may pass jocular remarks such as 'I wonder where he gets it at this time of day'. His company is considered to be good and enjoyable for a short time but it does tend to wear out his companions who just can't keep pace with him. His benevolence may later give way to irritability and when his views are contested he may show a complete lack of respect for other people's feelings, calling them fools and ignoramuses and being entirely uncritical of his own shortcomings.

Clinical Features

By this stage *mania* has developed and the following are the classical features:

Hyperactivity. His energy may appear superhuman and the author has known a patient who let his brother take the bus home to a neighbouring town about nine miles away saying he would catch it up later. While running through the back streets he met a lad on a motor cycle, who was impressed by his running and offered to pace him. After a few sprints the motor cyclist suggested they go along to the sports ground of a large firm who were holding their annual sports and the patient entered for several 'invitation' races—just rolling up his trousers and running in his socks. He won several prizes! At the end, and still full of energy, he passed by the stadium of a well-known athletic club and decided the cinder track needed rolling, so he broke into the shed, got out the heavy roller which is normally pulled by two men, and chased twice round the track. Not content with this he thought the railings needed painting so he got paint and brushes and went round a large section of the ground. His family later found him in bed—he had shinned up the water-spout, poised on the window ledge, opened the window and gained entry. When examined he was still over-active and showed no evidence of fatigue. Other patients are prolific letter writers, writing to all and sundry with hosts of suggestions on how to run literally everything.

Mood. This is usually one of elation but it can give rise to severe irritation and rudeness. In the female this exuberance is translated to dress and make-up, flamboyant clothes being worn; lipstick is heavily and inexpertly applied and the general attitude is one of shameless sexual advance which is in marked contrast to her usual 'sober, steadfast and demure' appearance. There is an over-reactivity to stimuli and the patient may laugh loudly at the slightest jest; he may make himself very conspicuous in a theatre audience and literally steal the show. His mood is volatile and displays of temper are frequent but he readily calms down and is always willing to 'shake on it'. Hand-shaking is common and this expression of mood could just as easily be included under 'hyperactivity'. He loves an audience and can be a natural clown but is frequently lacking in insight and cannot understand why everybody should not share in his euphoria and exultation.

Thought. This differs from the schizophrenic as it is mainly a speeding up of the process and a failure to control its sequence rather than bizarre and archaic mental imagery. He displays a *flight of ideas,* the thoughts coming out in rapid succession with very little connection. It could be argued that apart from the grandiosity expressed, and this can assume a delusional quality, there is very little real thought disorder and it is the speech which is mainly involved. The delusions of grandeur can sometimes be mistaken for the delusions of the schizophrenic and frequently have a religiose colouring. Appointments with important personages in Court, political and religious circles are claimed and the family may have great difficulty in preventing the patient from getting involved in embarrassing situations.

Speech. He is verbose and circumstantial, failing to get to the point and insisting on taking his own time. Lorenz and Cobb (1952) and Lorenz (1953) have studied speech in manic patients and list the following quantitative changes: (1) relative increase in pronouns and verbs, (2) relative decrease in adjectives and prepositions, and (3) high verb-adjective quotient which is based on the first two postulates. It does not, however, require a detailed study to appreciate that there is disturbance in speech form. It is heavily laden with puns and 'wise-cracks', some of which impose a heavy burden on the listener. He may invent rhymes which are really a jingle-jangle and depend entirely on a 'clang association'. He is, however, so uncritical that he may regard these efforts as verses with real poetic virtue.

Memory. This is not impaired and in fact for certain events he may be hypermnesic. He is likely to remember the little confidences that the medical and nursing staff may give him, perhaps out of sympathy when he is in a depressed mood, but out they come in embarrassing detail in his manic phases and he doesn't care who hears.

Attention. This is very distractible. He is for ever noticing and remarking and will constantly interrupt the speaker because something has just occurred to him. He is unable to keep to the point or pursue his work to any conclusion and his disturbance of attention frequently makes his hyperactivity profitless. There is a paradoxical capacity for rapid association and he can frequently take in a situation much more quickly than the normal observer and it may be that this makes his attention flag and seek new experiences.

Physical. Although he does not complain about his health, the hyperactivity may cause marked loss of weight although in some a voracious appetite maintains equilibrium. Sexual desire is increased and may lead to promiscuity in people who are normally continent. Sleep is disturbed in that he wakes early but insists that he is none the worse for it.

The Stages of Mania

Carlson and Goodwin (1973) systematically investigated the course of a complete manic episode in 20 patients suffering from typical manic-depressive illness. The three stages were:

1. *Initial,* characterized by increased psychomotor activity, including increased initiation, rate of speech and physical activity. The accompanying mood was labile with euphoria predominating; the cognitive state was expansive, grandiose and overconfident; thoughts were coherent, though at times tangential.
2. *Intermittent,* with further increase in pressure of speech and psychomotor activity. The mood although euphoric at times was not predominantly increasingly dysphoric and depressed; behaviour was explosive and assaultive; thoughts were increasingly disorganized; and paranoid and grandiose trends became frank delusions.
3. *Final,* seen in 14 out of the 20 patients, was characterized by a desperate, panic-stricken, hopeless state, experienced by the patient as clearly dysphoric. Frenzied and bizarre motor activity was present; thought processes that earlier had been difficult to follow were now incoherent with a definite loosening of associations; and delusions were bizarre and idiosyncratic.

While the sequence of symptom progression was remarkably consistent, some progressed to Stage 3 in hours while others took several days. There was no relationship between the severity of the acute manic episode and the level of function to which the patients returned during the follow-up period.

Six of the manic patients in Stage 2 became grossly psychotic with disorganized thoughts, extremely labile affect, delusions, hallucinations and brief ideas of reference so that a diagnosis of schizophrenia was sometimes entertained.

The authors rightly claim that their use of longitudinal sequential analysis of changing symptom patterns, rather than simple cross-sectional enumeration of symptoms, should result in increased diagnostic clarity.

Sex Incidence. Although the above descriptions have been applied mainly to the male, statistics give the palm to the female—70 per cent according to Arieti (1959*a*). The author, whose personal experience of this disorder has increased in recent years cannot subscribe to this sex ratio. It may have to be revised in the light of further knowledge.

Hypomania

This is a lesser version of the manic attack and in some people approximates to their normal state. Their conduct is more purposeful and sustained yet most of the features listed above are present. It is a fluctuating state and may become fully manic or exhibit depressive features. It is rarely brought to the attention of the psychiatrist unless the patient gets involved either in minor crime, or by repeated venereal infection or when it occurs in the course of a manic illness.

Acute Mania

Extreme restlessness with frankly disturbing behaviour predominate, but shining through are the essential features of the manic attack. Occasionally the patient appears to have hallucinations of a grandiose nature and the differential diagnosis from schizophrenic catatonic excitement can at times be difficult. Some do in fact deteriorate to a schizophrenic illness though the manic features of the first attack were unmistakable. At one time such a statement would provoke the descriptive psychiatrist to challenge the original diagnosis, but we now appreciate that mental phenomena can merge and mutate and there is nothing surprising in a change of presentation in an illness; a change in the label need not be accompanied by argument or apology.

Delirious Mania

This is the most disturbed form and may well be due to organic causes; it can be difficult to distinguish from other delirious states. The patient is wildly excited and requires energetic measures to bring him under control, for death from exhaustion is not unknown.

Mixed States

As with depression it is possible to get a variety of combinations and though they have been given labels, little purpose is served in listing them as it would tend to put a limit on the variety and hinder the accurate observer from recognizing new combinations. The most common variety described is the agitated depression, but the motor restlessness associated with this state is very different indeed from that found in a true mania. A more common mixture in the author's experience is the attack of depression in a previously hypomanic person and along with the classical signs of depression some hypomanic features, such as a perkiness in speech and the remnants of bonhomie shine through.

The 'Switch Process' in Manic-depressive Illness

Bunney *et al.* (1972*a*) conducted a longitudinal analysis on the sequence of change in thought and mood during 10 episodes of spontaneous behavioural switches from depression to mania (in 8 patients) and 7 switches from mania to depression (in 6 patients). They reckon that the activated phase be it mania or depression, is frequently precipitated by environmental stress and that it is generally an almost continuous illness in which mild to moderate retarded depression is the major symptom but superimposed is a switch into and out of mania. In a second paper (Bunney *et al.*, 1972*b*) they suggest that switches into mania may be associated with compounds that increase functional brain catecholamines such as *L*-dopa, and switches out of mania with compounds that decrease functional brain catecholamines, such as lithium carbonate and alpha-methyl *p*-tyrosine.

In a third paper (Bunney *et al.*, 1972*c*) they discern the theoretical implications and put forward the following components of their hypothesis: (1) it is genetically determined; (2) it must be activated; and (3) it is reversible. They postulate a presynaptic membrane dysfunction which could be precipitated by drugs like imipramine, cocaine and amphetamine which block the re-uptake of norepinephrine across the presynaptic membrane. They also introduce into their hypothesis the action of lithium carbonate which first reverses and then prevents the further activation of a membrane dysfunction at the vesicular or presynaptic or postsynaptic areas. If this block in the re-uptake of norepinephrine were reversed at a presynaptic cell membrane it would decrease the norepinephrine at the synaptic cleft and also inhibit its synthesis.

Course and Prognosis

This has been revolutionized by the introduction of lithium salts, phenothiazines and butyrophenones (see under Psychopharmacology, Chapter 18) and all previous treatments are now mainly of historical interest. The prognosis should be good but where schizophrenic features develop it should be more guarded.

Differential Diagnosis

Dementia Paralytica. In the early stages it may simulate the manic state and in all cases of mania a thorough physical investigation, including serological tests, is essential.

Catatonic Excitement. This has already been mentioned and it is only the unequivocal evidence of schizophrenic features which will decide. Fortunately both conditions respond to the phenothiazines and butyrophenones, so the truth may never be known.

Toxic States. The commonest agent which can produce a state resembling mania is *amphetamine sulphate* and as it may be taken for depression prior to addiction, the differential diagnosis can prove very difficult indeed, especially if the patient conceals the fact. Some patients can take 150–200 mg. per day and maintain themselves in a state of benign euphoria, but paranoid features may also occur (p. 376). Preludin (phenmetrazine HC1), which has a similar action to amphetamine, is also a drug of addiction and can produce a similar mental picture.

Acute Hysterical Reactions. These, particularly in primitive peoples, may resemble mania and unless one is able to communicate, it may take some time for the true diagnosis to be established. Some mental defectives are also prone to such outbursts.

Epilepsy. This can lead to excitement states with occasionally exalted behaviour. These are usually temporal lobe in origin and the EEG should help in the diagnosis. One practical point is that some of these patients when investigated with sphenoidal leads react violently to barbiturate anaesthesia and prophylactic phenothiazines may be useful.

Social Considerations

When the genetic, endocrine, constitutional and other aspects have been adequately emphasized, there still remains the social aspects. Unfortunately, most studies combine the manic with the depressive reactions under the group term 'manic-depressive'. This can be very misleading for a rise in the depression incidence can more than balance a fall in the mania incidence and so important changes can be obscured. Studies of incidence in depression which is by far the commoner component are likely to be more reliable and that of Arieti (1959) is important not only for its factual information but for his review of the contribution of Riesman (1950) who described the similarities between the 'inner-directed' person and the manic-depressive patient. These are:

1. The sense of parental duty determines strong introjective tendencies in the child.
2. When the child has to accept responsibility, it will have the traumatic experience of a serious loss.
3. He reacts by hard work and develops strong feelings of guilt.
4. This leads to depression.

This theory would explain the rise in depressive states and possibly a *relative* reduction in manic episodes. There is much confirmatory evidence from anthropological studies (Kardiner, 1939; Mead, 1934) and from psychiatric studies of a variety of less 'westernized' cultures, which point out the gradual shift to a depressive form of breakdown. Even in the same national culture, certain groups are more prone to depression than others. Eaton and Weil (1955) have reported this in the Hutterites, where manic-depressive illness was 4·33 times greater than schizophrenia. Earlier studies by Sim (1945, 1946*a*) showed that in an army population there were wide differences of incidence between privates, non-commissioned officers and commissioned officers, while in personnel from more primitive surroundings such as native Africans, the differences were even more striking. This latter aspect has also been reported by Carothers (1953). Studies on suicide (Stengel, 1952) and on incidence of psychosis (Shepherd, 1957) illustrate the increase of the affective disorders, particularly depression.

Treatment

Pharmacological

(a) *Mania.* Phenothiazines, butyophenones and lithium salts (see under Psychopharmacology, Chapter 18).

(b) *Depression.* Anti-depressants such as imipramine hydrochloride and other tricyclic compounds, and monoamine-oxidase inhibitors (see under Psychopharmacology, Chapter 18).

Electroplexy–Chemical Convulsants

(a) *Mania.* See Chapter 20.
(b) *Depression.* See Chapter 20.

Sedation

(a) *Mania.* See Chapter 18.
(b) *Depression.* See Chapter 18.

SUPERVISION OF THE DEPRESSED PATIENT

In the majority of cases, this is not a major issue and many patients can be permitted to go to work while undergoing treatment. In others the risk of unreliable conduct is so great that the patient should be under strict supervision until the problem has eased and recovery commenced. Most patients, even those who have made serious attempts at suicide, can be treated for severe depression in a general hospital setting, for the response to electroplexy is usually certain and speedy, but occasionally one meets a more malignant form or an unreliable and uncooperative patient and other measures have to be introduced. These will depend on local facilities, and ideally there should be a small security ward in every general hospital where patients can be supervised during the more refractory phase of illness. Under the Mental Health Act, 1959, this does not present a problem, for hospitals are no longer designated for mental illness and any hospital, if it is so inclined, can arrange to detain patients formally. This has many advantages as physical disease does not confer immunity to mental illness and a number of patients with organic disease, who might otherwise have to be sent to mental hospitals because of their behaviour, can be kept in the hospital which can cater best for all their needs. The difficult mental state is usually short-lived and a shuttling of the patient from one hospital to another should be avoided, for it may on occasions prove dangerous to transfer the patients.

Supervision should not be confined to watching the patient to see that he does not have access to dangerous instruments or drugs or slip away and do himself harm. It should consist of a comprehensive programme of occupying the patient during the time he is not undergoing special treatment, such as electroplexy. The occupational therapist will have a major role and the physiotherapist too, but the ward sister will have ample opportunity to get to know her patient and spend time with him. These active components in supervision help to make it more effective and also contribute to the patient's recovery as well as providing the staff with more reliable information about the patient's progress. Relatives should be interviewed and the problem discussed, and any useful information that might arise should be noted.

Psychosurgery. This has a place in the treatment of recurrent depressions which do not respond well to less drastic measures (Chapter 20).

Psychotherapy. There is much debate as to the place of psychotherapy in the treatment of depression. It has no place in the treatment of mania, for the patient is so distractible and excitable and in fact not in the least feeling the need for help, that it is pointless. In severe depressions, too, the intense pre-occupation with feelings of guilt and unworthiness renders the patient impervious, and any attempt at interpretation will either not register or make the patient worse. In the milder cases, there may be a case for psychotherapy. As the patient is in need of personal support and has suffered from a severe loss of self-esteem, regular sessions with a benevolently neutral figure will help to replace some of what the patient feels is lost. He may even become addicted to treatment, insisting on frequent interviews and prolonging those which he obtains. At this 'walking-stick' level, psychotherapy fills a need and can be of help, but it is doubtful whether the full significance of classical analytical procedure gets through. Any assessment of results is adulterated by the tendency for the condition to remit either spontaneously, or with physical treatment which would presumably not be withheld. It could be argued that a person who is vulnerable to depressive reactions might benefit from prolonged psychotherapy as an insurance against relapse, but as so many patients have only one severe attack in their life-time and the follow-up studies of those who have had electroplexy are so encouraging, many will consider this measure superfluous. There are, of course, a number of depressive illnesses which are associated with other psychiatric conditions such as obsessional features, anxiety states and the like and it may be that these features which persist after the depression has cleared may respond to psychotherapy. Each case will depend on a number of factors, some unfortunately economic, *e.g.* where the patient has to pay for treatment, or where the psychiatrist in a State Health Service has to decide how best to allocate his limited time.

Social Measures

The large number of suicides, which in Great Britain are about 6000 per year, and the even larger number of attempted suicides, has stimulated efforts to try and reduce this incidence. A society called the Samaritans concerns itself with patients who have attempted suicide and have been resuscitated in hospital and who usually are friendless and probably homeless.

They are also available for consultation to anybody in distress and though the organization was intended to be an anti-suicide device and its publicity is directed towards that end, most of its clientele are not suicidal risks. Some of the propaganda, including a number in the telephone directory is reminiscent of that of Alcoholics Anonymous, but in a recent survey of attempted suicide (Berry, 1966) very few had contacted the Samaritans about their troubles. An analysis of those who approach them for help shows that many are unstable psychopaths and drifters who would normally seek help from the Salvation Army, which can, at least, offer them a bed for the night. Whether the direction of the patient by the Samaritans to the hospital casualty department is a better solution has still to be proven.

In the true psychotic depression, these measures in themselves are unlikely to make any real impact on the illness and as psychotic depression in any case does not account for the majority of attempted suicides, the work of the Samaritans is more likely to be of help in the 'appeal attempts' (Chapter 15), *i.e.* among the lonely, the destitute and the psychopathic.

There has been a tendency for propaganda through the mass media of radio, television and the press to be directed at the depressed patient, allegedly in an attempt to encourage him to seek medical help and forestall his suicide bid. There has been much controversy about these efforts, some claiming on inadequate evidence that many lives have been saved, while others claim, with perhaps no more evidence, that many mentally sick people are made worse by this propaganda and are driven to the very act which the programme was designed to avert. The information included in these programmes or articles is stated by their sponsors to be educative, though the medium, whether it be radio, television or press, is more likely to be associated in the mind of the public with entertainment. If education can prevent the patient with psychotic depression from committing suicide, one would expect that doctors, or at least psychiatrists, would be immune from this drastic step, but the fact is that they are more likely to commit suicide than those sections of the community with much less education in these matters. These programmes and articles fail to take into account the fact that a person who is psychotically depressed is almost impervious to reasoning, and even if he were capable of concentration, which he often is not, he would be more likely to place a morbid rather than a rational interpretation on what he hears, sees or reads. The advice which is designed to help may be regarded by the patient as advice which carries for him the gravest import.

The whole question of medical education for the laity by these media must be seriously reconsidered, for it is unlikely, as far as the mentally ill are concerned, to stimulate the rational approach that is intended. Even for the physically ill, a programme, say on cancer or heart disease, is going to have a different impact on the person who has, or thinks he has, the disease, than on the person who is secure in the knowledge that he has not got it. To the latter, it is basically a form of entertainment and this was borne out by the vast numbers (up to 8 million) who tuned in to a series entitled 'Your Life in their Hands'. It was a tribute to the entertainment value of a medical programme, provided that it is sufficiently dramatic, but this has been recognized for many years by the cinema trade. There is something basically unsound from the psychiatric aspect in putting over a television or radio programme dealing with individual mental illness. At the best, it provides a macabre form of entertainment for the so-called healthy, while at the worst, it uses a mass medium for dealing with the most personal and intimate of human ills. A psychiatrist when confronted by his patient conducts the interview with great delicacy and finesse, adjusting his tone and his words to the patient's individual needs. In short he 'tunes in' to the patient; he does not and should not expect the mentally sick to 'tune in' to him.

In a society where every patient has a personal doctor and where the diagnosis of depression and its implications is being preached at all levels of medical education, to undergraduates, general practitioners and specialists, and on which the drug houses have concentrated a tremendous and commendable effort, it should not be necessary for medical men to project their image through mass media. The courtesies of medical consultation demand that a second doctor should not enter the patient's home without being invited and accompanied by the patient's own doctor. There can no longer be any justification that this unwarranted intrusion is in the patient's interest.

This still leaves the prophylaxis of severe depression and its attendant suicidal risks unsolved. Many do not consult their doctor and will not be persuaded to do so. The main hope lies in those who do. The early recognition of hypochondriasis with its cancerophobia and syphilophobia and other morbid pre-occupations, particularly in the elderly, should relieve much suffering and save many lives. One must seriously question the effect of group practice or rota systems on these patients, for if they are deprived of a constant personal physician, they may be reluctant to communicate with another at the time when they most need help. Furthermore, the recognition of the depressed state often requires an intimate knowledge of the patient and his pre-morbid personality and this is unlikely to be shared by all members of a group practice. The time has probably arrived when the family doctor should show an equal interest in those who do not regularly consult him, and foster a good personal relationship, so that he gets to know his patient and if necessary can visit him informally in his home. This may be in some instances the only way to recognize early depression and take the appropriate action.

CHAPTER 13

Schizophrenic Reactions

The term 'schizophrenia' is a relatively new one in psychiatry and is applied to a psychotic reaction which usually begins in adolescence or a little later and in which there are found thought disorders regarding concept formation and reality relationships, which are associated with affective, behavioural and intellectual disturbances of varying degrees and mixtures. There is a marked tendency to withdraw from reality with inappropriate moods, interruption of stream of thought, regression to a level of deteriorated behaviour and frequently hallucinations and delusions (*Gould Medical Dictionary*, 1956).

HISTORICAL

The name 'schizophrenia' was arrived at in relatively recent times by way of 'dementia praecox' which was the term used in 1898 by that great systematizer, Emil Kraepelin, for a group of three conditions: (1) catatonia, described by Kahlbaum (1874); (2) hebephrenia, a term attributed to Hecker in 1871 (Bumke, 1932); and (3) vesania typica, a condition also described by Kahlbaum and consisting of auditory hallucinations and delusions of persecution. The term '*demence praecoce*' had already been introduced by Morel (1860) but it did not have the comprehensive meaning that Kraepelin gave it. The latter's intention was to divide those cases who went on to deterioration, from the manic-depressive group who did not. Four types were described: (1) **hebephrenic**, (2) **paranoid**, (3) **catatonic** and (4) **simple**, and their clinical features are listed below. Bleuler (1911), who accepted Kraepelin's thesis but did not think the condition need progress to dementia, considered that the fundamental problem was a difficulty in association and a splitting of the personality. He coined the term 'schizophrenia' after the Greek *schizin* = to divide, and *phren* = mind. He also tried to incorporate the teachings of Freud by recognizing the loosening of associations in the minds of schizophrenics, but in this respect he was anticipated by Jung (1906) whose monograph *The Psychology of Dementia Praecox* contains psychological insights into this condition which are just as applicable today as on the day it was written.

Another concept, to which Bleuler has a greater priority, is that of **autism** (Bleuler, 1913). It is a turning away from reality and a form of illogical thinking which is concerned with a phantasy world and may be saturated with archaic imagery or symbolism. It is found in normal situations too, such as in children's play or artistic activity.

The psychobiological approach of Adolf Meyer, while accepting the above terminology, insisted that the condition be seen as part of a whole life situation with the effects of early experiences taken into account and that 'schizophrenic' be seen as 'schizophrenic reaction-type'. This contribution, which is so fundamental to the modern approach to schizophrenia, with its accent on social factors, was not therefore, as some have considered, an insignificant modification of Bleuler's theory. Moreover, Meyer (1906) had stressed the psychobiological approach before Bleuler's publication, and later elaborated it (Meyer *et al.*, 1911).

The psychoanalytical school, and in the early days this included C. G. Jung, defined the role of anxiety in schizophrenia. Freud's papers on 'projection' and 'narcissism' (see under Psychopathology) gave clearer insights into the psychodynamics of the condition and even though the psychoneuroses have been primarily the field of operation for psychoanalytic therapy, schizophrenia has always claimed a large share of the attentions of the school. Even now, new advances are being made in the psychoanalytic treatment of the condition and in the elucidation of parental influences, and lessons derived therefrom are being applied in the field of social rehabilitation of schizophrenic patients. Existential psychiatrists have devoted considerable efforts to the problem and have already claimed to have illuminated certain aspects of its essential nature (Chapter 19).

The organic side has, however, always fascinated, and continues to fascinate psychiatrists, and physical explanations of its cause are regularly offered though unfortunately none, to date, has justified its early claims. Auto-intoxication, focal sepsis, hypoglycaemia, endocrine imbalance, adrenochrome production and many others have made their appearance, but an organic answer is still elusive, though recent studies of the hallucinogenic drugs may give some insight into the more bizarre perceptual distortions that can occur in the disease.

Though schizophrenia is not the most common psychiatric

disorder, it has been a very stubborn condition especially when admitted to the mental hospital, and till recently provided about 60 per cent of its chronic population. It therefore assumed great importance in terms of bed occupancy and much effort has been expended in the search for a key to its cause. It is now generally accepted that much of the chronicity and the gross deterioration in behaviour were in part due to conditions under which these patients were treated and that smaller and more intimate units, with an accent on personal interest in the patient and an active programme of rehabilitation, are more successful than the large institutions to which those patients are usually admitted. It is also being recognized that some patients who had been labelled schizophrenic could really be suffering from some organic state with brain atrophy, but it required the techniques of pneumo-encephalography and the electro-encephalogram to define them.

The advent of the phenothiazines has also made a tremendous impact on many patients, rendering them calm and amenable and therefore permitting them to make their first steps towards recovery, with resulting discharge from the mental hospital and acceptance by the community. But the complete answer to the problem is much more complicated, for once outside the institution, considerable support is required and apart from community tolerance, which is difficult to create and even more difficult to maintain, there should be a continuing interest by the hospital and clinic with out-patient social club, day hospital, hostel accommodation, family support and re-entry to hospital in times of crisis. An even more important aspect is prophylaxis, which means strenuous efforts in the field of Mental Health. Much is heard about Mental Health and there are national and international bodies dedicated to its objectives; while their interests are diverse and worthy, that of prophylaxis against schizophrenia is probably the most urgent, for if ever a psychiatric condition was amenable to social manipulation, it is schizophrenia.

AETIOLOGY

There is hardly a pathological process which has not been implicated at some time or another. Moreover, theories which had at one time been discarded have been reintroduced in a new guise usually following some physiological or pathological discovery. Just as some speculator will seize on an entirely unrelated event in order to justify his gambling, so many in the field of psychiatry see developments in medical and scientific fields as the beginning of an answer to the schizophrenic problem. Gains have not been significant, but a body of knowledge has accumulated, some of it solid and some of doubtful value, but in a problem which is still with us, it is important to be informed of what has already been done so that future enthusiasm will not be contaminated with the errors of the past.

Social

Schizophrenia is alleged to concentrate in the lowest social class. Faris and Dunham (1939) found a much higher admission rate from the slum areas of large cities than from the wealthier suburbs; Hollingshead and Redlich (1958) found that the prevalence of schizophrenic patients in the lowest social class was nine times that of the two highest classes, their figures being largely influenced by the great number of patients in the lowest class who were in the local mental hospital. Some have explained this phenomenon by the hypothesis of 'downward drift' due to the schizophrenic process which sediments those afflicted, while others have tried to disprove this hypothesis.

Before taking sides in such an argument it is just as well to be sure that the figures quoted do in fact represent the true incidence of schizophrenia in the community. These figures only tell us that among schizophrenics who are *similarly ascertained,* those in the lowest social class predominate. There is an assumption that the process of ascertainment operates similarly in all classes. This is not so for the following reasons.

1. The upper classes, as a rule, do not wish their schizophrenic relatives to be brought to the notice of the authorities and go to considerable lengths to conceal the problem.
2. The individual patient because of his higher social background is less likely to 'act out' or show disturbing behaviour. He carries his schizophrenic deterioration 'like a gent' and therefore does not bring himself to the notice of society.
3. Upper classes have access to a number of employing agencies which on their recommendation can find these patients acceptable employment at a modest salary. The author has had several such patients one of whom was given a sinecure as the 'historian' of the company. This actually proved a sensible disposal for he did some useful work. There must be many like him who are never referred to a psychiatrist.
4. There are no geographical restrictions on disposal and many are sent to relatives on farms and a number may go abroad.

5. Financial stringency brings many schizophrenics, who would otherwise go unrecognized, to the notice of the authorities. The better-off can retain such patients at home doing housework, gardening or even pursuing a harmless hobby. Many are comfortably housed in seaside boarding houses and private hotels, while some live an independent life as recluses.

The ascertainment of schizophrenia in a community even in a total census would be incomplete if some family members had left the area and were not personally interviewed. Any sampling is fraught with error. In a current survey of schizophrenic patients that were treated in the author's clinic, Berry and Sim (1967) out of a total of 265 have so far followed up 94 and the social class distribution is 60·7 per cent for 1, 2 and 3 which is very different from that reported by other observers. In this case it is the nature of the clinic, because of its short-stay policy and lack of emergency accommodation, which has a small number of chronic and behavioural problems. It compensates for this deficiency by attracting a number of the higher class patients whose presence may otherwise not have been declared.

Genetic

There are differences of opinion as to the importance of genetic factors in schizophrenia. For example Mayer-Gross *et al.* (1960) say 'It may now be regarded as established that hereditary factors play a predominant role in the causation of schizophrenia'. In addition to quoting the earlier work of Rüdin (1916) they state that 'the most sensitive single test for the significance of heredity factors in causation is to be obtained from the study of *monozygotic* twins'. Kallmann (1953) reported in schizophrenics a concordance rate of 67-86 per cent (the concordance rate is that proportion of the twin-partners who are observed to fall ill with the same condition, the figure being corrected for age at risk and other factors). Slater (1953) estimated a concordance rate of 76 per cent in his series and explained that those twins that escaped the illness (24 per cent) must have been shielded by a relatively protected environment. A similar reason is given for the differences in the age of onset. Kallmann's work has been criticized by Bellak (1948) for having excluded 'the schizoform psychoses' and by others on his statistical technique. Gregory (1960) has not only criticized Kallmann's work, but also the report of Slater (1953) which had hitherto been regarded as a model of care and scientific objectivity. He questions Slater's criteria for monozygosity and lays down most exacting standards, including complete hand and foot prints, rules out hearsay evidence, and rejects photographs as proof of twinning, a pitfall which Hogben (1931) had pointed out. Gregory concludes that the evidence for genetic transmission has not been proven.

Genetic studies continue. Tienari (1963) using the strictest criteria of monozygosity, analysed monozygotic twins in Finland, and out of 16 pairs where one twin developed schizophrenia, the concordance rate was zero. Kringlen (1964) in Norway, obtained a concordance rate for schizophrenics of 25 per cent in 8 monozygotic pairs. These findings posed the question as to whether environmental factors were more important than genetic factors. Gottesman and Shields (1966) in a prospective study, found that of 24 monozygotic pairs the concordance for schizophrenia was 42 per cent while it was only 9 per cent in the dizygotic pairs and that pairs where the proband had a severe rather than a mild schizophrenic illness were more likely to be concordant.

It is still not possible to draw firm conclusions but it is evident that the previous evidence of a strong genetic aetiology for schizophrenia is no longer valid and environmental factors are probably more important than was previously realized. That some genetic factor is present would appear to be established but this should be seen against the general trend of these studies which is that of a diminishing genetic influence. The evidence to date would therefore favour an energetic therapeutic approach to the problem rather than a eugenic one.

Fisher *et al.* (1969) using the Danish Twin Register and the Danish Psychiatric Register tried to determine whether genetic or environmental factors were more important in the origins of schizophrenia. Diagnosis was based on the criteria for the process type with disintegration of personality and affect, thought disturbance, hallucinations and/or delusions and impaired contact with reality. Out of 70 twin pairs a total of 78 probands with a hospital admission for schizophrenia were selected. The DZ to MZ proband concordance rates were 0.56 : 0.26 but this included partners with 'schizophreniform and atypical psychosis'. The authors concluded that although genetic factors would appear to have some influence the MZ concordance rate of their study was more in agreement with those of Tienari (1963) and Kringlen (1966).

Gottesman and Shields (1973) list these reasons for proposing a genetic basis for schizophrenia:

1. It is logical to expect that great genetic variability will occasionally produce a combination of genes that results in a phenodeviant.

2. It is known that many morphological and physiological traits are under some genetic control, so it would be surprising if schizophrenia were altogether exempted from these influences.

3. No environmental causes have been found which with even moderate probability will produce schizophrenia in subjects unrelated to a schizophrenic.

4. The incidence of schizophrenia is about the same in all countries despite great variations in ecologies.

5. The outcome of stress responses depends on the genotypic and experiential uniqueness of the stressee.

6. There is an increasing risk of schizophrenia to the relatives of schizophrenics as a function of the degree of genetic relatedness.

7. The difference in identical versus fraternal concordance rates is not due to aspects of the within-family environment.

8. Such implicitly causal constructs as schizophrenogenic mothers, double-binding, material skew, and communication deviance, have been found wanting.

Comment: There is hardly one of the above points which has not been completely disproved, but the reader should be familiar with the apologia the considerable number of 'geneticists' put forward. While they reiterate their creed, more and more information of the environmental influences in the aetiology, aggravation and amelioration of the condition is forthcoming and more reliable genetic studies are failing to provide supporting evidence. It is time that the effort expended in proving a genetic theory for schizophrenia were abandoned and the energy directed towards influencing the adverse and formidable environmental factors. It may be harder work but it is much more rewarding.

Constitutional

As with the manic-depressive psychoses, Kretschmer (1925) described physical types who he alleged were prone to develop schizophrenia. These were the **leptosomatic** (asthenic) with narrow chest and costal angle, long extremities and poor musculature, and the **athletic** type with good musculature. These two varieties accounted for two-thirds of his schizophrenics, but these findings have not been generally confirmed, though Sheldon *et al.* (1940) with a more refined technique do lend some support. Kretschmer also included a **dysplastic** type which is alleged to be the result of endocrine imbalance, and under this group he listed acromegaloid, eunuchoid and infantile groups as well as virilism and obesity. The vagueness of his descriptions indicates the tentative nature of the theory.

Personality

The schizoid type is regarded as vulnerable, but he is found not only among those who develop the disorder, but in patients suffering from neuroses, among inadequate psychopaths or even in people with no psychiatric handicaps. He tends to be aloof and emotionally undemonstrative, does not enter into easy social contact or may deliberately avoid it. Arieti (1959*b*) stresses that this emotional detachment is a defence mechanism to combat the inner anxiety, that it is protective of over-sensitivity and that the individual, by reducing his contacts, illustrates his involvement with society and his fear of people. It is when he is projected into a less sheltered environment that he becomes more vulnerable and a significant number of young National Servicemen who were adequately compensating when living at home readily broke down with acute schizophrenia when conscripted.

Arieti (1955) has described another personality type, the **stormy**, who is prone to develop schizophrenia. These people lack the submissive defence mechanism for their anxiety and keep trying to make contact but only succeed in achieving an unsatisfactory and eventually disruptive relationship which precipitates a crisis. It would appear that these crises are the patient's reality testing efforts, but they never quite achieve success. They undertake problematic marriages, jobs, and love affairs, and their lives are consequently stormy with frequent resort to alcohol and drugs.

Bowlby (1940), in a monograph on *Personality and Mental Illness,* demonstrated how fallacious these personality traits could be, for he found many of those features allegedly specific for schizophrenia, in manic-depressive states, and *vice versa.*

Endocrine

Nearly every endocrine gland has at one time or another been regarded as a causative factor. There is some justification for this quest in that the disease tends to develop shortly after puberty, cases occur during pregnancy and the puerperium, and as Kretschmer has pointed out, the dysplastic constitution is common. Yet the clinical varieties of endocrine disease are not prevalent in schizophrenics, and Bleuler (1954), though partial to such terms as 'acromegaloid', was unable to find any conclusive evidence that full-blown endocrine disorders played a major part. Many workers have, however, made such claims, some to have them rejected; for example, Mott (1919) claimed that there was a correlation between the atrophy of the interstitial cells of the testes and the disease, but Morse (1923) showed these changes were due to age, nutrition and terminal disease. Hemphill *et al.* (1944), using biopsy material, confirmed Mott's findings, but in general few consider that these histological changes have anything to do with schizophrenia. Endocrine studies have revealed other changes, particularly in thyroid function (Reiss, 1955), but these are minimal and can be explained as the result of the mental disturbance rather than the cause.

The **adrenals** have also been studied extensively, particularly since Selye's (1956) work on the general adaptation syndrome, and Pincus and Hoagland (1950) have reported changes; but again it is likely that these are secondary rather than primary. Glandular manipulation of every conceivable type, including total adrenalectomy and the administration of pineal extract, has been tried with varying success but it is likely that any beneficial results stem from the enthusiasm of the therapist and the non-specific physical stimulus of the treatment.

Metabolic

The number and complexity of the studies in this field make it difficult to assess their value. Wherever the experimental biologist goes, close behind him will be found the experimental psychiatrist with his group of schizophrenic patients. Minor changes are reported and major conclusions are drawn but we are no nearer to an aetiological answer. The following is a short list of some of the metabolic and autonomic changes reported: (1) liver insufficiency, (2) defective oxidative processes due to disturbances in the enzyme system, (3) hypotension, (4) bradycardia, (5) decrease in blood flow, (6) exaggerated vasoconstriction with predisposition to cyanosis of the extremities, (7) disturbance of water metabolism, and (8) phasic variations in total nitrogen balance. A comprehensive review of somatic aspects of schizophrenia is provided by Shattock (1950).

One of the most frequently quoted metabolic studies is that of Gjessing (1947). He made serial studies over a period of years on a group of periodic catatonics, and found the mental changes coincided with nitrogen retention and in the lucid intervals with increased excretion. He claimed that he could terminate the acute catatonic phase with a low protein diet and the administration of thyroxin. This work has been confirmed by Gornall *et al.* (1953) but it is a very rare type of schizophrenia, subject to spontaneous remission, and though the condition declares itself in its behavioural aspect with comparative suddenness, there is usually a prodromal phase of psychological disturbance which may initiate the metabolic change rather than the reverse. Crammer (1959) has made a study of periodic psychoses, which he claims are not as infrequent as some would believe. He defined three elements in these states: (1) a pacemaker which sets the rhythm; (2) a factor which is required to set off the attack; and (3) a symptomatic pattern of the attack with an ordered sequence of events. He considered that it was the physiological disturbance which provoked the psychological one and gave as an example the failure of antidiuretic hormone with cerebral dehydration. He also claimed that the response of some of these mental states to both thyroid and chlorpromazine was due to the former acting on the general physiological disturbance and the latter on the mental sequelae.

That acute psychotic states can result from physiological disturbances is well recognized. Should the latter follow a periodic course, it is to be expected that the mental sequelae will also be periodic. At the same time, in view of the relative scarcity of these problems, it is equally likely in fluctuating psychotic states, which are common, that *by chance* a few will show a periodicity which has a semblance of regularity. Also as these studies have been almost exclusively conducted on chronic hospitalized patients, whose psychotic states react and probably have already reacted to environmental factors, it would be difficult to dissociate the fluctuations in their mental states from their environment. Furthermore, it would be unwise to argue from a few and at times doubtful instances of periodic psychoses to the vast mass of schizophrenic illness.

The Pink Spot. Friedhoff and van Winkle (1962) isolated and defined a compound from the urine of schizophrenics which excited those (and there are many) who persist in their belief that one day some clever biochemist will discover the cause of schizophrenia. They use 19 schizophrenics and 14 controls and treatment with tranquillizers was suspended for 2 weeks prior to the analysis of a 20 hour specimen of urine by paper chromatography. Their technique was to make the urine alkaline to pH9 and shake with ethylene dichloride which is a standard method for extracting basis organic substances from urine such as tryptamine and other amines. This product was concentrated and a single drop (equivalent to 2 hours' urine production) was put on a paper strip and dried and the paper dipped vertically into a butanol-acetic acid-water mixture and the ingredients were dispersed vertically in line up the paper. Nihydrin stained the spots blue and over-staining with Ehrlich's aldehyde reagent caused the blue spot to fade but a single pink spot stood out about two-thirds of the way up the paper. It was present in the urine of 15 schizophrenic patients but not in the controls.

The authors thought they had defined a new amine in the urine, dimethyloxyphenylethamine (D.M.P.E.), which may be connected with schizophrenia and reported their discovery to *Nature.* A number of others have tried to confirm these findings but the majority have not been able to do so and D.M.P.E. is now regarded as a more significant finding in the urine of patients with Parkinsonism than with schizophrenia. Even this observation has been seized on by the 'faithful' who point out that drugs used in the treatment of schizophrenia like reserpine, phenothiazines and butyrophenones can cause Parkinsonism though it is difficult to see what that has got to do with the argument.

Kety (1959) has described a number of biochemical downfalls in the past and showed that schizophrenics may drink more coffee than nurses who are used as controls. They may get less vitamin C, or smoke more. They may secretly take more patent medicines such as laxatives, pep pills, cough lozenges or use less toothpaste. Visitors may give them sweets and other foods unknown to the staff. Some patients sit or stand a lot, others have a low fluid intake; yet all these factors and more can influence the content of the urine. An attractive facet of the Pink Spot theory was the chemical proximity of D.M.P.E. to trimethoxyphenylethylamine or mescaline which has hallucinogenic properties, but hallucinations are no longer regarded as a *sine qua non* in the diagnosis of schizophrenia.

These 'discoveries' are usually given currency when a psychiatrist dabbles in biochemistry or a biochemist in psychiatry. As long as they talk biochemistry to psychiatrists and psychiatry to biochemists a whole mythology can be dressed in suitable guise and accepted by the medical profession for years. This has happened again and again but fortunately the clinical definition and treatment of schizophrenia is now much more effective and psychiatrists and the general public should be less vulnerable to exaggerated or unproven claims. The Pink Spot has now been declared a Red Herring.

The 'Pink Spot' and Tea. Stabenau *et al.* (1970) conducted experiments to determine the source of the 'pink spot' (3,4-dimethoxyphenylethylamine) in the urine of schizophrenics. They concluded that it derived from an exogenous plant source and was not primarily related to the presence or absence of schizophrenia or a history of schizophrenia. The urine is rendered free of the 'pink spot' by a plant-free diet and reappears when tea alone is given. The use of restrictive dietary measures has been recognized as a powerful tool in determining the exogenous nature of other urinary metabolites, *e.g.* the phenolic acids.

Other abnormal findings in schizophrenia which have been reported in recent years are 'taraxein', an allegedly toxic euglobulin, and low levels of neuraminic acid in the C.S.F. but as with the Pink Spot any relevant association with the disease or even confirmation of these findings has not been generally forthcoming.

Melanosis. Nicolson *et al.* (1966) had previously observed that a steadily increasing number of schizophrenic patients had a peculiar metallic bluish-brown pigmentation of the exposed skin and displayed a striking increase in melanogenesis in these areas. A study of 10 necropsies showed deposits of melanin pigment in macrophages throughout the reticulo-endothelial system and in the parenchymal cells of liver, kidneys and endocrine glands. Similar studies prior to the introduction of phenothiazines showed identical pigment in the same distribution but in lesser amounts. The authors do not minimize the effects of the phenothiazines, though they suggest that increased melanogenesis may reflect a basic defect in schizophrenia which is aggravated by phenothiazines.

They tried to prevent and treat the melanogenesis with a low copper diet and a copper-chelating agent, D-penicillamine, and claimed some success both with pigmentation and mental state. They attribute this success to blocking of the formation of melanine and inhibiting the synthesis of serotonin, and as the pineal is involved in these activities they postulate a pineal dysfunction in schizophrenia.

This work awaits confirmation but it is a fact that many chronic schizophrenics have pigmented skins, though the author has in the past attributed this to faulty hygiene.

Pharmacological

Hallucinogenic drugs are alleged to induce a state which is akin to schizophrenia, but there have been serious criticisms of this view. Experimental catatonia which had been first induced in animals, has been repeated in man by Sherwood (1952) and of course this physical state is also well known to the neurosurgeon, but it is a far cry from this organic neurological picture to the catatonia accompanying schizophrenia.

Neurological

A more intriguing relationship is the schizophrenic-like state associated with lesions of the temporal lobe or temporal lobe epilepsy. Here the behaviour disorder, and even some of the thought disturbances, seem to be very close to schizophrenia, but these are described more fully on page 203.

Slater and Beard (1963) and Slater *et al.* (1963) reported on 64 patients who exhibited epilepsy and schizophrenic features. They concluded that the latter represented a symptomatic psychosis which was aetiologically related to the epilepsy or the pathological causes underlying the epilepsy. Clinically 45 patients suggested a temporal lobe origin for their epilepsy and in a further 10 patients unsuspected foci were located in the temporal lobes by EEG with sphenoidal leads. These patients in their premorbid personality rarely showed schizoid traits and the risk of schizophrenia in the parents and sibs was no greater than in the general population.

The onset of the psychosis was generally insidious and coincided usually with a fall in the frequency of fits. Gross catatonic features were rare and loss of affective response was less marked and longer delayed than in typical schizophrenic illness. The patients also tended to keep their symptoms to themselves and did not present a serious nursing problem. The prognosis was generally better and after a mean interval of 8 years from the onset, 30 were living entirely and 16 mainly at home and only 9 were permanently in hospital. One third had a remission when followed up and a further third were improved. Personality changes in the residual third were similar to the intellectual and affective deterioration found in the advanced stages of chronic epilepsy, which has been given the name *ixophrenia* by Continental authors.

Histopathological studies have not suggested that there are any special features associated with schizophrenia, and Wolf and Cowen (1952), in a study of biopsy material from patients undergoing leucotomy, explained previous reports of histological change as being due to artefact. There are still those who claim that there is a pathological process in the brain, but that our present methods of investigation are too crude to detect it.

Neurophysiological

This aspect is well reviewed by Hill (1957) who found an abnormal EEG record in about 20 per cent of patients but no specific pattern, and he concludes that there is not enough evidence to suggest 'a genetic progressive pathological process'.

The whole question of the biological basis for schizophrenia is still an open one, but if the past is any guide, there will be numerous fruitless experiments which could be avoided if the investigators would only try and learn from previous mistakes and apply criteria to the study of this problem which they would be expected to apply elsewhere.

Horwitt (1956) makes some very pertinent remarks and his article is essential reading for anyone interested in the field. The following are some extracts:

> The manner in which the patient chooses to manifest his difficulties may not be a function of his physiological status . . . . The sum total of the differences reported would make the schizophrenic patient a sorry physical specimen indeed; his liver, brain, kidney and circulatory functions are impaired; he is deficient in practically every vitamin; his hormones are out of balance, and his enzymes are askew . . . .

Yet he has a very high expectation of life, and his rude physical health makes him the greatest security risk in the mental hospital.

PRECIPITATING FACTORS

As physical events can apparently precipitate a schizophrenic psychosis, it has been argued that physical factors have a specific aetiological significance. Similarly psychological precipitants have given support to a psychological aetiology, but these factors can not be understood in isolation and must be considered together with the psychopathology of the disorder (see below).

Physical

A number of physical conditions are alleged to be precipitants, but equally a number of physical changes, such as fever, operation and pregnancy can ameliorate the disease. Unfortunately, however, the latter aspect is rarely included in the balance sheet.

Psychological

There is still much argument as to the relative importance of this factor as a precipitant. There are some who see in it the only possible explanation, while others deny it and attribute the disease to a strong predisposition or in fact to an existing psychosis which is aggravated by psychological factors (Mayer-Gross *et al.*, 1960). This attitude places considerable emphasis on the assumption of a constitutional basis for a schizophrenic psychosis. As usual the truth lies somewhere in between and there is ample evidence that large numbers of young people who in fact were selected by medical boards because of their freedom from mental illness and capacity to withstand stress, broke down with acute schizophrenic psychoses when conscripted. They also tended to recover quickly and on follow-up showed a very small relapse rate. These cases would admirably fit into the concept of the **schizophrenic reaction-type** of Adolf Meyer.

Psychological precipitating factors should be appreciated in a psychopathological or dynamic setting and stress should be seen not as war, famine or hunger, but as separation from a familiar environment, and the personal issues that arise therefrom. Most schizophrenic psychoses in National Servicemen did not occur abroad or in battle areas but at home and frequently in the earliest and physically most protected stage of their service. In the Second World War it was not uncommon for young men serving in the Middle East during an active stage of the campaign to remain reasonably well. Shortly after the emergency has passed they reported sick with vague anxiety symptoms and were placed in more sheltered circumstances and later still were seen with fully developed schizophrenic psychoses. It was therefore regarded that external events such as physical hardship were ego strengtheners and when these stimuli were withdrawn there was ego-disintegration with the advent of psychosis. This point is not one of mere academic interest, for many a young man who developed schizophrenia during his military service was denied a pension for an attributable or even aggravated disability as the constitutional aspect of the disease was considered paramount and the absence of enemy action would be cited as evidence of lack of military stress. Yet the mere fact that he was inducted and removed from the environment in which he was normal mentally, may have proved the greatest stress to which he could have been exposed.

Another example of the condition developing in the absence or withdrawal of the original 'stress' is found in prisoners. A number of soldiers with pre-service criminal records usually of the 'lone-wolf' type but free of any psychotic features, would after a few months in a military psychiatric hospital, where their challenge to society could not be whetted either by a police hunt or the fancied persecution of the warders (for they were treated as other patients with all Red Cross comforts), began to break down with florid schizophrenic psychoses complete with auditory hallucinations. In these instances, the 'stress' was admission to hospital and the substitution of a kindly regime for the harsher one. Such is the difficulty of interpreting psychological stress and its meaning for the individual, a difficulty which is seen not only in schizophrenia but in psychosomatic disorders.

PSYCHOPATHOLOGY

As schizophrenia is manifest by ego-disintegration, it is likely that a number of ego defence mechanisms will have already been employed and that the broken ramparts of these ineffective defences will be discernible. Thus evidence of dissociation or hysteria, projection or paranoia, ritualism or obsession, eccentricity or perversion, may appear in its symptomatology. All that psychopathology can do is to explain the vulnerability of the ego and why certain defence mechanisms are more in evidence than others.

The common factor is **regression** which frequently extends to the early narcissistic level, which is caused by a withdrawal of the libido from external objects and its direction into the ego. Fenichel (1945) subdivides the regressive symptoms in schizophrenia into the following:

World-destruction Phantasies

In the early stages of the disease, the phantasy that the world is coming to an end is frequently expressed. This may take the form of a partial experience, the patient in his delusion saying that someone is dead, indicating that the libidinal connection with the person has been withdrawn. Statements such as the world appears to be 'empty' or 'changed' are indications of more total withdrawal of object-libido. This withdrawal of libido also takes place in neurotic illness, but here it is directed to childhood phantasy objects or their substitutes, while in schizophrenia the patient abandons objects altogether. Fenichel explains that the *apparent* object interest shown by these patients is of a temporary nature and is really part of another schizophrenic feature—'restitutional activity' (see p. 571).

Body Sensations and Depersonalization

Hypochondriacal sensations are common and it is considered that **organ cathexis** takes over from **object cathexis.** Narcissism increases the 'libido tonus' of the body or of its organs and this paves the way for hypochondriasis. The infant recognizes its body by superficial and deep sensations but in the incipient psychosis the feeling need not be one of heightened sensation, but lack of it. This explains why certain organs or the whole body may be regarded as not belonging or having changed. These changes in sensation of a plus or minus nature result in a feeling of strangeness, and reactions like **depersonalization** occur. Fenichel states that these are due to a type of defence which is a counter-cathexis against one's own feelings which had been changed by an increase in narcissism. Depersonalization can also occur in other settings such as a defence against feelings of excitement. **Perplexity** which is a common feature in schizophrenia can also be regarded as a reaction of the ego to the awareness of an increase in narcissistic libido.

Feelings of Grandeur

Withdrawal of object cathexis can result in ego inflation with even manic or ecstatic experiences. Some patients react to narcissistic hurt as they did in infancy, by the realization that they do not enjoy omnipotence. The hurt is denied, over-compensation results and narcissistic regression is equated with omnipotence, the loss of love being replaced by increased self-love and without reality testing, delusions of grandeur are elaborated.

Schizophrenic Thinking

This is not as illogical as it would appear, except that the logic is that of primitive magical thinking and is, according to Jungian theory, **archaic** like that which is found to a lesser degree in obsessional neurosis. It has also been described as **prelogical thinking.** These patients show a remarkable familiarity with **symbolism** and in them it is not a distortion of ordinary thinking but a form of archaic expression. Ideationally, they freely express what others repress, such as material associated with the Oedipus complex.

Hebephrenic Features

This aspect of schizophrenic illness is regarded by Fenichel as an example of a specific form of regression, thus giving it a psychopathological validity. It is a form of 'schizophrenic surrender' (Campbell, 1943) where failure in newer types of adaptation results in seeking refuge in older, infantile or even intra-uterine ones. Restitutional attempts (see below) are absent, but transitional states occur with explosive outbursts of rage.

Catatonic Features

Negativism, echolalia and **echopraxia** are considered archaic forms of expression and are suggestive of a blurring of ego boundaries, while **passivity** is also a primitive reaction, indicative of early ego experiences. Fenichel, quoting Bernfeld (1928), equates **automatic obedience** with the imitative 'fascination' in infants. Catatonic postures and movements are rather speculatively regarded as 'impulses from the period of intra-uterine existence'. In **stereotypes** and **bizarre attitudes** 'the original purposeful intention which failed and became automatized by the disintegration of the personality and the deep motor regression, is still recognizable'. **Disharmony between mood and thought** such as incongruous smiling is explained as an attempt to deny fears, including that of being mentally ill.

RESTITUTIONAL SYMPTOMS

Restitutional symptoms are subdivided as follows:

World Reconstruction Phantasies

These are found in the early stages of schizophrenia, the patient insisting the world is all wrong and that he has been chosen by God to put it right. Hidden meanings are seen and a prophetic role may be assumed.

Hallucinations

These are impressions of sensory vividness without the appropriate stimuli. Fenichel's dynamic definition is '...substitutes for perceptions after the loss or the damage of objective reality testing. Inner factors are projected and experienced as if they were external perceptions...' In sleep, with its isolation from object reality, thought gains a sensory vividness which is close to that of hallucination and Fenichel considers that in schizophrenia a withdrawal of the object cathexis has a similar effect. The content of the hallucination is seen as a wish fulfilment and reality is denied, but it can also be an unpleasant experience; in this case anxiety is also present, and the repudiated super-ego may enter into the picture.

Delusions

These (*a*) are false beliefs, and are therefore not true to fact, (*b*) cannot be corrected by an appeal to the reason of the patient and (*c*) are out keeping with the patient's cultural background. They have a similar psychopathology to hallucinations and may be wish-fulfilling or frightening, or an effort to replace the repudiated reality. The classic example is the analysis of Schreber (Freud, 1911) who tried through his delusion to protect himself from passive homosexual phantasies, a situation frequently found in paranoid schizophrenia. The denial formula is 'I do not love him, I hate him': then, 'he hates me' becomes the denial of 'I hate him'; the stage is then set for delusions of persecution and it is often possible to see the patient's own unconscious problem in his delusional system. The super-ego too can be projected and gives rise to **ideas of reference and influence** which may be punitive and chastising.

Object Relationships and Sexuality

'Object-addicts' are those who require constant reassurance of their contact with the objective world. Ideas, inventions, in fact anything which represents a connection with the objective world is clung to tenaciously. These may prompt the schizophrenic to become a member of organizations whose aims are the salvation of mankind, though it would be wrong to consider that all, or even a majority of such members, are potentially schizophrenic. Impulsive and occasionally violent behaviour can be an attempt at restitution, as if to prove that contact with reality can still be made, that people can be touched, struck or frightened.

Peculiarities of Language

Freud (1915), quoted by Fenichel, pointed out that the schizophrenic may use words as an attempt at restitution.

> The patient often devotes peculiar care to his way of expressing himself, which becomes precious and elaborate. The construction of the sentence undergoes a peculiar disorganization, making them so incomprehensible to us that patients' remarks seem nonsensical. Often some relation to bodily organs or innervations is prominent in the content of the utterances. In schizophrenia words are subject to the same process as that which makes dream images out of dream thoughts, and one we have called the primary process.

The patient, in his attempt to regain his object relationships, regains only their 'shadows' or word representation.

Catatonic Symptoms

Stereotypies and mannerisms as well as being regressive phenomena can also be evidence of restitutional activity. They are vestiges of emotional attitudes but have lost their original emotional feeling; they are an archaic form of expression and constitute primitive attempts to regain contact. Autocastration, which is occasionally seen in schizophrenia, is likened to the similar act in religious mystics, who, by removing the organic source of lust, seek to establish a community of spirit with God.

The foregoing summary of the psychopathology of schizophrenia is based on Fenichel's (1945) *The Psychoanalytic Theory of Neurosis* which, with its more detailed descriptions and liberal references, provides an excellent introduction into the understanding of the condition, as opposed to its mere description.

A DYNAMIC MODEL FOR THE UNDERSTANDING OF SCHIZOPHRENIA

The author has found the following model useful in explaining to students the protean symptomatology of schizophrenia:

EGO-WEAKNESS		EGO-STRENGTH
DECOMPENSATED	EGO-DEFENCES	COMPENSATED
	1. Dissociation (Hysteria)	
REGRESSION	2. Rituals (Obsessional neurosis)	
Thought	3. Projection (Paranoid features)	
Speech	4. Eccentricity (Perversion)	
Behaviour	5. Hypochondriasis	

In explanation of the above scheme, schizophrenia can be regarded as the process of breakdown of the ego-defences which have been erected to preserve the ego from erosion or disintegration. The common ego-defences have their counterparts in clinical symptomatology and should these prove adequate to the task and the ego is basically preserved, the situation can be said to be well-compensated. If they are inadequate, decompensation is said to occur. We can thus describe a schizophrenic process as a decompensated obsessional state, and many illnesses start in this way. In the very early stages of such an illness the neurotic defence would appear dominant but if there is a beginning to the loosening of ego-boundaries and a withdrawal from reality then the term 'pseudo-neurotic schizophrenia' would be applicable.

If the paranoid defences were to break down with the beginnings of ego-disintegration, the term 'paranoid schizophrenia' would be applicable. Similarly, some schizophrenics exhibit hysterical and hypochondriacal features, and, to develop the analogy, the broken down ramparts of the old defences colour the clinical picture which may display some or all of them in greater or lesser degree. Even eccentricities present as mannerisms.

When disintegration is evident this can be slight, moderate or severe. When slight, only the features of simple schizophrenia are present, but in more severe forms with marked disintegration, not only are the broken-down defences strongly in evidence but regression also takes place with thought, speech and behaviour disturbances. With this schema it is possible to see a schizophrenic illness as a process with neurotic defences, and deterioration into a florid psychotic state with a protean symptomatology. The accent on ego-weakness and ego-strength directs the observer to these factors which may have contributed to ego-weakness and those which require attention to rebuild ego-strength. It may mean that a schizophrenic process will be recognized before it becomes florid, which is all to the good, for it is a condition which lends itself to prophylaxis. It may also mean that a condition which may not become schizophrenic in the clinical sense will be treated as such. While some psychiatrists regard such a possibility with horror, and which should be avoided at all costs, the author would commend it. If it should prove to be unnecessary, there is no harm in having treated a condition with sinister implications with respect. At the same time it prevents the graver if not the gravest error in psychiatric practice, which is to fail to treat in the early stages a treatable condition like schizophrenia because of blind prejudice.

CLINICAL FEATURES

These are usually grouped under the classical divisions of (1) **hebephrenic**, (2) **catatonic**, (3) **paranoid**, and (4) **simple**, and while these categories have considerable validity, they tend to convey the impression that they are discrete conditions, while in fact there may be considerable overlap. There is also very little in this classification to suggest the psychopathological processes at work. It is, however, important to recognize these states because on them is based the official nomenclature and they also represent identifiable clinical groups. Before embarking on a description of their details, it would make their symptomatology more meaningful if the schizophrenic process with its ramifications were described.

Ego-disintegration and **regression** are the main features of this process, but they are only one side of the ledger for on the other side are the mechanisms invoked as **ego-defences**. These usually fail but even in failure they contribute to the clinical picture and can frequently be recognized either in the early stages or throughout the process. The common defences employed are:

1. **Anxiety**, which is usually somatic with increased hyperhidrosis, digital tremors and rapid pulse, but it may become fixated to some organ or function and result in complaints which are labelled **pseudo-neurotic schizophrenia** or present as frank hypochondriasis.

2. **Projection** which manifests as delusions and which at one time may have been well-systematized, may persist in this form. The resulting clinical picture would be that of **paranoid schizophrenia.** Hallucinations may also be elaborated.

3. **Ritualistic acts** are designed to ward off the threat to the ego and form the basis of **obsessive compulsive features.** It is when these defences break down or decompensate that schizophrenia develops. Even when they have failed in their purpose, they can still be recognized as obsessional features, but without their usual drive and intensity.

4. **Dissociation** is one of the commonest defence mechanisms resorted to by a loosely knit ego but instead of strengthening the ego, as it would in a simple hysterical conversion feature, it merely adds **hysterical symptomatology** to the already involved clinical picture.

5. **Ego-mutilation** is a compromise mechanism which entails a degree of **ego-sacrifice** to preserve its greater part and may be manifest in **eccentricities** or **perversions** or both. These features or their underlying origins are frequently found in schizophrenic illness and can account for the blatant homosexual caricaturization, the mannerisms and unusual poses these patients occasionally present.

The schizophrenic patient may therefore show a variety of psychiatric features, including paranoid, obsessional, hysterical, anxiety and eccentric or perverted, all the result of ego-defences which have failed in their purpose.

There are certain traditional aspects of the schizophrenic process, some of which have been treated under 'Psychopathology', but which will now be enumerated and where necessary described in greater detail.

REGRESSION

In addition to those features mentioned above which were primarily Freudian in concept, the term can be applied to a return to lower levels of functioning as postulated by Jackson in the neurological field. Symptoms can be divided into their **form** and **content.** In the latter, earlier experiences may be manifest either symbolically or in prototype, while in the former, early phylogenetic mechanisms may be employed. Some regard the regression as purposeful and progressive and no matter which level it reaches, it does not finally adjust at that level but is still in a state of disorganization, and deterioration may continue.

Arieti (1959*b*) describes the following specific aspects of schizophrenic regression:

Concretization of the Concept

This is illustrated by the ideas of reference and delusions of persecution of the paranoid schizophrenic, which are essentially a conversion of abstract feelings of inadequacy and despair into a more concrete and perceptible form and the identification of certain individuals as being hostile. Arieti states: 'The "they" is the concretization of feeling; later, "they" are more definitely recognized as F.B.I. agents, neighbours, or other persecutors'. This aspect was pointed out much earlier by Goldstein (1943) but Arieti has modified it and considers that abstraction though grossly imparied is not lost, but is represented differently at a lower level. He (Arieti) regards hallucinations as 'the most typical example of perceptualization of the concept' and the olfactory one of a bad odour symbolizes the rotten person the patient thinks he is. The auditory hallucination is described as the culmination of a process starting with anxiety and going on to the adoption of a 'listening attitude' for derogatory remarks which he feels he deserves, and then he actually hears.

Paleological Thought

This is a lower level of rational thought and Arieti quotes von Domarus (1944) whose principle is stated with modifications as follows: '. . . Whereas the normal person accepts identity only upon the basis of identical subjects, the paleologician accepts identity based upon identical predicates. . . .' This form of thinking is not invariably present, but Arieti regards von Domarus' principle as a useful one in interpreting bizarre and complex delusions. The schizophrenic tends to see what are loose links as identifying ones, and this extends to his language, where a related word may be used for the real one—not unlike the metaphor, but much more obscure in its relevance. This disorganization of language has led Cameron (1938) to itemize it as follows:

(*a*) Asyndetic—lacking essential connectives.

(*b*) Metonymic—lacking precise definitive terms for which approximate but related terms or phrases are substituted (*e.g.* the patient who said he had three menus instead of three meals).

(*c*) Interpenetratative—where parts of one theme appear as intrusive fragments.

(d) Overinclusion—where remotely related material is included.

(e) Non-correspondence—no relationship between what is done and what is said.

(f) Transformation in the Rules in order to justify failure.

(g) Generalizations are freely shifted in relation to inadequate solutions and hypotheses.

While this classification is useful as an aide-memoire and is also illustrative, it should not be regarded as contributing materially to the theoretical aspect of verbal regression or paleologic thought.

Desymbolization and Desocialization

Symbols are regarded as derived from adults during childhood, and during the schizophrenic illness these tend to be lost. Desocialization is equated with withdrawal which implies a change in symbolizing in that the early introjected ones are replaced by more primitive ones. There are **signs, images,** and **paleosymbols** and much of their meaning is associated with the evolution of words from their early paleo-symbol to abstract meaning. Arieti goes into this evolutionary aspect in some detail and for a fuller account of this important topic, his section on 'Schizophrenia' in Arieti (1959*b*) with its useful bibliography, should be consulted. The following is a much abridged account:

Primitive words have two characteristics: *(a)* **denotation** which is the object meant and *(b)* **verbalization** which is the word applied to the object and is independent of symbolic value. In primitive societies the word is equated with the object and has a magical significance. Later the word acquires **connotation,** thus representing the concept of the object it names and can be used to **categorize.** 'Ma-ma' is no longer the individual's mother but all mothers and further concepts are developed with more complex word forms and various subtleties of meaning and interpretation accrue. In the schizophrenic, this development is seen in reverse but it is a disorganized retreat and various aspects overlap. The first to go are symbols referring to self and therefore those aspects which had been absorbed from others are rejected or even projected, and adverse criticism, which had previously been built into the personality, is seen as outside interference. The foregoing is seen as three phases: (1) **introjection,** (2) **assimilation,** and (3) **projection.**

In the use of language the schizophrenic is more concerned with denotation and verbalization and there is an impairment of ability to connote which Arieti calls **'reduction of the connotative power'.** This is seen when the patient is asked to interpret a proverb, for instead of the symbolic meaning he gives a literal translation. This applies to quite simple sayings such as: 'a bird in the hand is worth two in the bush'; 'people in glass houses shouldn't throw stones'; 'birds of a feather flock together', and so on. The patient is greatly concerned with the sound of words and alliteration, and gradually, paleosymbols replace symbols, and this is regarded as a form of regression which has been likened to childhood autistic expressions.

Thought disturbance may show less regression and the anxiety features which are so common in the early stages of the disease may contribute to a vagueness of expression which may give the patient difficulty in describing his 'complaints'. He may show **'thought-blocking'**, *i.e.* the stream of thought, such as it is, is suddenly interrupted and he may explain this as being due to thoughts 'crowding' him so that he can no longer think clearly and his stream dries up. Another common thought disorder is the 'knight's move' type. This is based on an analogy with a game of chess, the patient's thinking showing a devious or indirect approach which makes comprehension difficult.

Emotion in schizophrenia is traditionally regarded as being **blunted** and this is certainly the picture the patient may convey in that a good rapport is very difficult if not impossible to establish. This has given rise to the saying that 'these patients are of us, but not with us'. The patient himself may say that he has lost all feeling and all capacity to react emotionally, but his statement may be accompanied by such a marked display of distress, perplexity and somatic anxiety that the terms **disharmony between mood and thought** or **incongruity of affect** are frequently applied. These are also used to describe the situation where the patient appears superficially cheerful, but describes the most disturbing mental tortures. The 'far-away look' of the schizophrenic may be mistaken for emotional blunting whereas it may really signify pre-occupation with day-dreams or phantasies or even hallucinatory experiences.

Emotional lability may be a feature though it is not the lability itself, but the apparently inappropriate remark or situation which touches it off. In taking a case history where the deaths of relatives or unfortunate early experiences are discussed, the patient may maintain an external calm but later, when a rather ordinary situation is mentioned, there may be a flood of tears. Similarly, during interview there may be the odd giggle which does not ring true or there may be bursts of incongruous laughter.

Self-mutilation or even attacks on others may be made without provocation and apparently without passion and on the rare occasions these do occur, the observer is invariably impressed by the callousness or lack of feeling the patient displayed. It is not possible to say whether there was a lack of feeling or not, because the patient is not likely to communicate his emotional state; what appears to be absent may, in fact, be present, and apparent indifference may be a mask for acute awareness. This latter fact may be confirmed by recovered patients, and it has been postulated that this display of apathy is a defence mechanism and a means of protecting the patient from emotional contact with others.

Maturation is an aspect of emotional development which does not necessarily depend on intellectual development. In schizophrenia, **emotional immaturity** is a common feature and may be striking. It could be called a form of childish regression, in that the patient may show a lack of the usual adult reactions to situations, and chatter away in a manner which belies his years. It is an important diagnostic factor, for many of these patients look, and may even dress, younger than their years and convey the impression that they are intellectually less well endowed. Their difficulty with abstract thought and the general air of childishness may provoke a diagnosis of mental dullness but the previous intellectual achievement gives the clue to the real condition. A number used to find themselves in mental deficiency institutions because their emotional immaturity was mistaken for intellectual handicap.

Volition is frequently impaired and this may be the main presenting feature. The relative absence of the usual schizophrenic features coupled with social ineffectiveness has given rise to the term **'schizophrenic existence'**. The patient may talk intelligently and establish a good rapport but just won't get out of bed. The author had one such patient who spent four years at home; he only left his bed to go to the bathroom, and would try and justify his lack of will to go to work on grounds of physical weakness. A remarkable corollary is the way in which families adjust to these situations, and mothers particularly, will struggle upstairs many times a day, to cater for the needs of their able-bodied sons. This aspect is discussed more fully under 'Families of Schizophrenics' (p. 603).

Volition may be more dramatically disturbed, as in **negativism** or its reverse, **passivity**, or by **impulsive movements** which may constitute extreme agitation or frenzy. It should be appreciated that these are discrete phenomena and though capable of psychopathological interpretation (p. 570) are not necessarily related other than in their presentation as disturbances of volition.

Negativism is a resistance to suggestion and can be either undue stubbornness or a complete refusal to move when physically guided. The patient may stiffen under the hand of the nurse and the impression is rapidly gained that further effort may result in frank hostility. It can extend to other bodily functions such as eating and excretion and give rise to severe anorexia or retention of urine, faeces, saliva, and bronchial secretions. The last can be so severe, due to the failure of the patient to cough, that bronchial aspiration is needed.

Passivity may be expressed as ideas of influence which are applied to thought, speech, behaviour and feelings, and are believed by the patient to be directed by a variety of agencies. Telepathy, invisible or atomic rays, radio signals and special gases, are some of the older methods, but fashions change and the schizophrenic is usually about 10 years ahead of 'science fiction'. Paradoxically, some of the impulsive movements are the result of the patient reacting to influences or obeying commands which may or may not be hallucinatory. In the former case a voice is actually heard while in the latter it is his thoughts which are being controlled by a non-verbalized agency. An extreme form of passivity is **flexibilitas cerea** or waxy flexibility, in which the limbs can be moulded into a variety of positions according to the whim of the manipulator and the patient will maintain these grotesque postures for long periods without apparent fatigue. It is a rare phenomenon and is usually associated with the catatonic form of schizophrenia, but is also found in post-encephalitic states. Such is the dramatic impact of the demonstration of this phenomenon, that teachers cannot resist showing it to students and the latter will remember it as an essential feature of schizophrenia, which it is not.

Echopraxia or the repetition of actions and **echolalia** or the repetition of words may also be seen in catatonics and post-encephalitics and with **flexibilitas cerea** are aspects of **automatic obedience.** The patient may at times assume bizarre postures such as that of a crucified Christ or the curled up 'intra-uterine' position, or the repetition of movements such as touching or pointing, and although some regard these as spontaneous with no psychological significance, they may, like other forms of automatic obedience, be in response to influential experience. They are labelled **stereotypies of posture or movement**, a term which is non-committal as far as aetiology is concerned and include tics, mannerisms, grimacings and pursing of the lips (*Schnauzkrampf*).

Catatonic Features

Though these by definition should belong exclusively to catatonic schizophrenia, they can occur in the course of the other types and some have already been described. The rest will be described under the appropriate heading, but they are noted here as features which are considered characteristic of schizophrenia.

Primary Delusions

These are regarded as fundamental to the schizophrenic process (Mayer-Gross *et al.,* 1960) and are basically a disturbance of symbolization. They are seen most clearly in the very early cases, for once secondary delusions have been elaborated the primary ones become obscured. Many now doubt the importance or even the existence of the primary delusion. That such experiences occur and are commonly described by patients is undoubted but it is not possible to say that the patients were perfectly well before the primary delusion occurred. They may have been labouring for some time with ideas of reference and were able to contain them but a more vivid experience tipped the balance. It is a useful rule to regard the presence of any delusion, primary or secondary, as the tip of an iceberg with nine-tenths below the surface.

They have also been called **autochthonous ideas** where the patient feels that a bizarre thought has suddenly been implanted in his mind and while he may appreciate it is strange, he cannot doubt its reality and a whole chain of secondary delusions may be elaborated to account for it. This phenomenon could rightly have been included under the 'thought disorders' and is really associated with the phenomenon of **desymbolization** (Chapter 23). It is a description of an isolated event rather than a contribution to the theoretical basis of the disease, and in fact can only be understood in the light of the psychopathology already described.

Hallucinations

These have been traditionally associated with schizophrenia and their psychopathological basis would link them with the delusional aspects of the illness (see p. 571). The commonest are auditory and though visual ones have been reported, they are very rare. In frankly disturbed cases the evidence is easily obtained, the patient being very much pre-occupied with the voices he hears; he may in fact answer them, either out loud or by moving his lips. Nights are disturbed, the patient getting out of bed and roaming the house to make contact with or escape from the hallucinatory voice, which is not always an unpleasant experience, for though frequently accusatory or persecutory, it may also be flattering and instil an air of grandiosity in the patient. An equally important diagnostic aspect may be the exclusion of auditory hallucinations rather than their confirmation, for some hysterical patients frequently say they hear 'voices' but on close questioning these 'voices' become 'noises'. An auditory hallucination is an unmistakable experience and the voice should sound as clearly as the examiner's; it is well to ask the patient if the voice possesses this quality, for an illusion in the highly suggestible subject may be regarded as an hallucination. It must again be emphasized that schizophrenia can occur without hallucinations and hallucinations may occur, though rarely, in the absence of the schizophrenic psychosis.

Consciousness is characteristically unimpaired, even in the 'stuporose' states, where the patient appears to be withdrawn and apparently out of touch. In lucid intervals, he may remind the doctor of what was said or done and make it plain that he was very much aware of what was going on.

Schneider's First Rank Symptoms of Schizophrenia

Schneider (1925) classed the following as of first rank importance in diagnosis:

(1) Hallucinatory voices that conduct a commentary on the patient's actions; (2) Hearing thoughts spoken aloud or *écho de pensée;* (3) Broadcasting of thoughts; (4) Bodily feelings of influence; (5) Thought withdrawal and thought being directed; (6) Passivity feelings in relation to affect, instinct and volition; (7) Primary delusions.

All other types of hallucination, emotional change and catatonic features he classes as second rank symptoms.

These criteria are hallowed in some circles so that diagnostic criteria have not only become frozen but fossilized at the 1925 stage and all advances since then are completely ignored. Schneiderian disciples, and there are many, do not recognize the concept of pseudoneurotic schizophrenia or schizo-affective psychosis. They do not take into account the concepts of ego-disintegration with decompensation of ego-defences. They do not ask the question: 'What is going on here'? They are content to describe what they see, and as a result they can only diagnose schizophrenia when it is an entrenched condition with a hopeless prognosis, and even little children could recognize such a caricature in the streets. This is not the sharp end-point of diagnosis that skilled psychiatrists should strive to develop, if only for their patients' sake. A Schneiderian adherent would diagnose schizophrenia when it was too late and not recognize and therefore treat an earlier state ineffectively till it deteriorated to an irreversible degree. The more dynamically orientated psychiatrist would recognize the problem in its beginnings and control and reverse it with some certainty with the techniques and agencies already available. It cannot be stressed too strongly that Schneiderian criteria have no place in the *practice* of clinical psychiatry. It will be a happy day for our patients when this 'tribute' to Schneider can be omitted from future editions of the 'Guide'.

CLINICAL VARIETIES OF SCHIZOPHRENIA

With the above as a background, it should now be possible to describe the main clinical types without much duplication. The ingredients have nearly all been described and what remains to be done is to bring them together into their recognizable forms, but in such a complex condition as schizophrenia, it would not be possible in the compass of even a larger book to list the host of variations of presentation, yet the student should be able to identify the process and its components, no matter how it presents. One type can shade into the other or features of one may be present in another, but if all phenomena were plotted, the graph would probably show clusterings approximating to the clinical types about to be described.

SIMPLE

Hallucinations are rare and delusions are not a prominent feature. It usually begins in adolescence and the first signs may be a falling off in school performance, a tendency to day-dream, secretiveness and withdrawal from social contact. Parents become exasperated, for the patient will not do what he is told and their remonstrances leave him unmoved. He may act impulsively—sleep out or shut himself in his room—and although he may not admit it, he is having **difficulty in concentrating** on his studies and may become pre-occupied with obscure literature and develop a loose interest in fringe political or religious groups. If at work, his efficiency drops and he may leave voluntarily for inadequate reasons or because he fancies he is being picked on by the others. It is true that these adolescents because of their extreme sensitivity become a butt for their colleagues who may mercilessly rag them. Some leave home, try and join the Services or the Merchant Navy or become drifters and accept the jobs handed out to them by the Labour Exchange, and because of their tendency to neglect their appearance, and inability to parade what may have been a good educational background, they gravitate to unskilled jobs, where they may surprise and amuse their less talented colleagues with their erudition.

The condition may become arrested or deteriorate. In the former instance, he may continue in his 'dead-end' job, marry a worthy and maternal figure who looks after him and may present him with children at regular intervals, but he is a relative stranger in his own home. He provides the weekly wage but she manages the home and children. He may entertain some unusual ideas on religion, the political system or some philosophical question, but these are not held with any intensity and the whole picture is marked by emotional blunting, lack of volition, withdrawal and ineffectiveness, which makes his former class-mates who enquire after him rather surprised that a lad of such promise could so deteriorate.

The above is a common enough picture but is not the only form of presentation of simple schizophrenia. Some become vagrants, prostitutes, callous criminals or paupers, while others exhibit a variety of hypochondriacal complaints with repeated attendance at the doctor's surgery. It may be difficult to distinguish simple schizophrenia from the schizoid personality, but generally the latter does not show any deterioration and can be recognized as a personality type with none of the oddities and incongruities associated with the disease which may, however, 'burn itself out' and the resulting picture could be labelled 'schizoid'.

HYSTERO-SCHIZOPHRENIA

This is a recognizable clinical condition which is seen more commonly in the less sophisticated. It tends to be an acute reaction and it is frequently difficult to decide on the proper label. It can also present in a less acute form in patients whose ego-defence was largely in the hysterical field and this may mask the relentless process of ego-disintegration. Some may even masquerade as hysterical characters and the schizophrenia may go unrecognized for years. There is no real advantage in using this diagnostic label for it is no more helpful than tagging on any other ego-defence mechanism to the schizophrenic process. It is true that paranoid reactions have earned their place, largely because of their high incidence, but hystero-schizophrenia is not so common and it is to be hoped that it will not intitiate a trend for a multiplicity of labels. A schizophrenic process or reaction cannot be adequately labelled; it should be understood.

PARANOID

Though this type can be superimposed on the Simple, there are some distinguishing features:

(*a*) **Age.** It usually begins later in life, after the age of 30 years, though it can occur earlier. In the older age groups, 40-60 years, there is very little of the schizophrenic process in evidence and the delusions are held with greater emotional intensity and may be labelled a *paranoid state,* though paranoid-affective state would be more appropriate.

(*b*) **Intelligence.** They appear to be more intelligent, though this may be a false picture due to the relatively better integration of personality and the application of their total available intelligence to support their delusions.

(*c*) **Social Status.** The older age of onset with relative preservation of intellectual capacity usually ensures a higher social status. The 'anal character' with its thrift and fastidiousness which is frequently associated with the condition and the unmarried state would also confer a higher economic status.

(*d*) **Delusions.** These are, of course, the key feature in the condition. They are persistently held and are fairly well systematized, but because of the schizophrenic component, there is frequently a loss of affectivity and intensity and they may, if the schizophrenic aspect is dominant, tend to become disorganized. They are most frequently of a persecutory nature with ideas of reference and are much more prominent than in the *simple* type. Their content is usually dominated by thinly disguised homosexual references, which may range from the belief that frank accusations are being made, to symbolic allusions such as interference through rays, and instruments which assault the anal orifice. If the opposite sex enters into the delusions, the patient is being actively hounded and loudly protests his or her innocence and resentment.

(*e*) **Hallucinations** These are common in the *paranoid* type, but are by definition usually excluded from the *simple* type. They are very similar to their content to the delusions already described and are, as a rule, auditory.

(*f*) **Progress** is variable. It can deteriorate to a severe degree with the paranoid element barely detectable, the patient presenting as a disintegrating hebephrenic state (see below). On the other hand, it can either remain static for many years, especially if it develops later in life, or it can fluctuate and a relatively fixed state may give rise to exacerbations with acute hallucinatory episodes.

(*g*) **Behaviour Disturbance** This is rare in the *simple,* but is traditionally regarded as a feature of the *paranoid* type. It is also relatively uncommon in this variety, though a number, because of the vividness of the hallucinations or intensity of the delusions, are impelled to take action over them. This usually takes the form of complaints to people in authority such as the police, who with their characteristic good humour put up with their regular visits to the police station and listen patiently to their complaints about what the neighbours are trying to do to them or how some sinister spy is threatening the security of the country. A chief inspector told the author that his station had a bigger clientele than the hospital out-patient department, which is more than likely.

Occasionally, letter writing which can be a nuisance, or the carrying of placards, declaiming their persecutors, can result in a charge being made. Very occasionally, they may physically assault either their fancied arch-persecutor or some innocent bystander from whom the accusatory voice or indecent suggestion would appear to emanate. There is a rooted conviction among laymen, and some doctors too, that every paranoid schizophrenic is potentially homicidal, but this is far from the case, although it is true that they are responsible for a number of such crimes. This, of course, places a heavy burden on the doctor who has to decide what action should be taken. A useful rule is that if the patient is not unduly suspicious, if he is prepared to cooperate with treatment and if he takes adequate prescribed doses of tranquillizers, he can reasonably be treated either on an out-patient basis or in the general hospital, but if there is a deep suspicion or hostility with refusal to cooperate, then the chances of unreliable conduct are considerably increased and the appropriate action should be taken.

HEBEPHRENIC

This is the classical variety which starts in early adolescence. It usually comes on slowly with a tendency to withdrawal reminiscent of the *simple* type, but personality disintegration is more rapid and extensive. It can frequently present as a depression with tearfulness and expressions of inadequacy but this aspect is soon overshadowed by the florid schizophrenic features with disharmony between mood and thought, regression with archaic forms of expression, auditory hallucinations and deteriorated behaviour which in the acute state may progress to incontinence. Delusions are commonly grandiose, the young girl insisting that she is going to give birth to two Messiahs or the young man proclaiming loudly that he has a cure for the world's ills and incoherently either by mouth or pen trying to demonstrate his theories. Language loses much of its capacity for representing abstract thought and at times the patient will stop in his tracks and exhibit **thought blocking.** Thought disturbance of the **knight's move** type is common and this leads to difficulty in understanding the patient's conversation. Such patients frequently look very young for their years, the girls possessing an Ophelia-like quality, or rather the air with which actresses tend to portray her. Rapport is difficult, the patient now being in touch, and then lost to the company of his hallucinatory experiences and phantasies.

Obsessional features or **compulsive rituals** may be freely demonstrated with little inhibition and they appear grotesque and poorly coordinated, with the patient showing no embarrassment or attempt to conceal or control them. In fact, all the broken ramparts of the ego-defence mechanisms (p. 573) may be evident and each can assume a dominance in symptomatology. One therefore sees paranoid or projective mechanisms, hysterical forms of behaviour which, however, do not have the ego-integration of unadulterated hysteria, anxiety states which appear bleached, and depressive reactions which lack the depth and persistence of a true melancholia. Hypochondriasis of a bizarre and shifting nature may be the main feature and is impervious to reassurance.

The **course** may be acute, subacute or chronic, the last being punctuated by exacerbations and remissions. **Precipitating factors** may appear specific such as in those acute reactions developing among National Servicemen, or in the sensitive adolescent who is apprehensive regarding a forthcoming examination or interview. Less obvious stresses are those associated with guilt over masturbation. Speech is frequently pre-occupied with sex and the patient's drawings may constitute a parade of sexual symbols. One young schizophrenic lad would frequently fashion a huge phallus and testicles out of plasticine and proudly show them to the matron on her rounds. This behaviour may appear to the onlooker as an attempt by the patient to appear funny. At times the whole picture can consist of literally 'acting daft' and has been called by some the **'buffoonery syndrome'.** It can be mistaken for insolence in a disciplined community like the case of the young soldier who when faced with an insecure superior would appear 'smart' and 'cheeky'. Charges would be preferred and detention and even beatings result if the conduct persisted. It would eventually dawn on the custodians that the lad was definitely odd for he would not respond to punishment and a hebephrenic soldier would later be admitted to a psychiatric hospital. This was fortunately not common, but is mentioned because the diagnosis could so easily be missed. Clowning may represent the patient's effort to make contact with society, and his acceptance by his comrades in this role may even act as a support and prevent further disintegration. **Inappropriate laughter and giggling,** which are common features, are not usually regarded as clowning or enjoyed by the company but are seen as evidence of an affective disturbance.

It may be difficult to get a straight answer from the patient for he may side-step all the issues raised and one is faced with a differential diagnosis of **'pseudo-dementia'** or **Ganser syndrome** (p. 486). **Depersonalization** and **derealization** are commonly seen in early hebephrenia and they may be mistaken for neurotic features, indicating another pseudo-neurotic aspect of the disease.

Differentiation between Process and Reactive Schizophrenia by B-Mitten EEG

The B-Mitten pattern consists of a sharp transient, usually formed by the last wave of a 10-12/sec. frontal spindle, followed by a slow wave. It occurs bilaterally over the frontal and/or fronto-parietal areas. Struve *et al.* (1972) on the basis of two studies, the first, a pilot one, on 21 schizophrenic men (10 with process and 11 with reactive schizophrenia) and the second on 190 subjects, 83 of whom were schizophrenic, found that only two patients with process schizophrenia (one from each study) had the B-Mitten pattern. This incidence (65 per cent) approaches that in normals (0-3.4 per cent depending on age). Among the reactive schizophrenics there was a 72.7 per cent incidence in the first study and a 41.3 per cent incidence in the second study and the authors suggest that this difference could be dependent in part on different age structures of the samples.

CATATONIC

Catatonic features have already been described and their psychopathology discussed. The commonest is *stupor* which may extend to complete physical immobility, though all grades are seen. Consciousness is, however, not impaired and the patient can obey commands sometimes to a fantastic degree as in automatic obedience. This aspect can be demonstrated as **flexibilitas cerea** (p. 580) or by telling the patient 'Put out your tongue, I want to prick it with a pin' and he may comply. It never fails to impress medical students, but it has little real value as a diagnostic measure and after seeing the performance one is left with a strong suspicion that the unfortunate patient regards the examiner with disdain if not disgust for practising such cheap showmanship. *Catalepsy* or failure to initiate movement and the maintenance of rigid postures is also seen but automatic obedience can give way to **negativism** and stupor to **excitement.** Behaviour in the latter is wild and uncontrolled and impulsive attacks on people or property may result. It is as if the patient has gone berserk and has lost all capacity for civilized behaviour. He will shout and struggle and have to be controlled by drugs which fortunately are now rapidly effective. Previously a catatonic outburst in hospital was difficult to get under control, with consequent disturbance to the whole ward and these acute outbursts have been likened to excitement states in different cultures (Chapter 14). Stuporose states are not nearly so common or protracted as they used to be and this interesting change has been attributed to modern methods of treatment and nursing and the changing social structure of the mental hospital.

Catatonia–Retarded and Excited Types

Morrison (1973) analysed both types in a series of 250 catatonic patients admitted over a period of 50 years to the Iowa State Psychopathic Hospital, 110 of whom were predominantly retarded and 67 predominantly excited and 73 were mixed, that is, alternating. There were no significant differences in age, sex, religion, environment (rural or urban) or education. Symptoms which significantly differentiated the two groups were combativeness, nudism and impulsiveness in the excited group, with rigidity and catalepsy in the retarded patients. With the exception of retention of saliva or drooling seen in the retarded, no symptom was confined exclusively to one group. There were differences between the groups in the course of the illness. The excited were generally of sudden onset, and were treated with ECT or tranquillizers; the retarded were generally of gradual onset and received milieu therapy. Although duration of stay in hospital was approximately the same for both groups, the retarded were more likely to be unimproved. The author questions whether catatonic excitement may be more closely related to the affective disorders than to schizophrenia, for 28 per cent of the excited could have qualified for a diagnosis of an affective disorder.

A closer study of the mixed group could assist in the answer.

SCHIZO-AFFECTIVE STATES

These now merit a place in the classification of schizophrenia. It is not enough to say that the hebephrenic variety may be ushered in with depression or the paranoid may be severely depressed with suicidal risk, for the schizo-affective reaction is now common and as a clinical entity easily identifiable. It frequently follows a precipitating factor such as pregnancy, operation or a social or psychological trauma like moving into a new house, or a broken romance. In fact, nearly all the situations which can lead to a depressive psychosis can precipitate a schizo-affective one. The pattern may be constant for the same patient, even if the precipitant should vary, and the author has seen an exactly similar picture present in the same patient after an appendicectomy, and three years later after pregnancy.

Both schizophrenic and depressive features are in evidence, the former frequently of a paranoid type with persecutory delusions or hallucinations, but catatonic features may also present, the patient at times being stuporose and apparently confused and inaccessible. A study of these patients leads to a greater understanding of the schizophrenic and depressive processes, for they show a mutation of symptoms and **quantitative** differences and help to sharpen one's end-point of diagnosis. It is not enough to say that there are two features present, but one should also try and estimate their relative proportions and which is likely to yield to which treatment. The schizophrenic features, although developing acutely, can give the appearance of being of longstanding and the author has seen puerperal patients with a very short history show catatonic features with verbal disintegration, or systematization of delusions which one would usually associate with the chronic state. Some have shown the cramped, bizarre handwriting and even more bizarre messages, the page being covered with words and phrases, with the corners filled in as in a child's letter. Archaic expressions are common and primitive religious ideas may be freely expressed. Delusions are usually depressive and conduct may be unreliable because of them, the patient finding the persecution intolerable. The condition exhibits a whole range of both depressive and schizophrenic features and predominance of one over the other need not be closely related to the pre-morbid personality though in some instances this is the case. It is very tempting to try and place the patient in one category or the other, but that would be ignoring the essential nature of the condition, which is a mixed state, which in fact is not static, but may fluctuate wildly. The variability of the quota of depression and schizophrenia in the same patient is one which should be carefully estimated for it is by serial readings that the need for and success of specific treatments may be gauged.

As has been stated, a quantitative estimation is more meaningful than the mere statement that both factors exist. The author, who was impressed during the Second World War with the number of mixed psychotic states that occurred among servicemen, could not, with any justification, squeeze these patients into the pigeon-holes of official nomenclature. At first the predominant element was given the label, though it was plainly not a valid description of the patient's illness for the condition changed its nature; what had been more dominant would become less dominant and the diagnosis had to be changed. The author suffered the inconvenience of having to change the diagnosis on a number of occasions and was stimulated to overcome this problem by designing a 'vignette' which could permit fluctuation in diagnostic components by including the use of a rating scale (Sim, 1946*b*). The advantage of such a system, apart from intellectual honesty, was that, if the vignette were clearly dated, a trend in the psychotic process could be detected. Either both components receded or one would become more persistently dominant and, whichever it was, the treatment of the patient would to some extent be based on this information. It had the advantage that when a soldier was being evacuated down the line, he could be assessed at each staging post and comparisons drawn. It also improved the inferential or diagnostic aspect of clinical assessment by making diagnosis a quantitative exercise.

Depression following Acute Schizophrenic Episodes

Roth (1970) defined two phases following an acute schizophrenic episode in 11 patients studied intensively:

(1) The compensated-transition phase which is associated with loss of open psychotic symptoms and an impressive return of ego strength with return to work or school. It may last from 1 - 8 weeks (average 4.5 weeks) but all 5 such patients had to give up the activity.

(2) The depression and neurasthenia phase then developed. They desired more sleep, would not continue with psychotherapy, and then relapsed into a second acute schizophrenic phase.

The author considered these phases 'ubiquitous' and under-emphasized in treatment. These findings illustrate the dangers of seeing psychiatric illness as pure reactions and failing to treat patients for what they have got.

PSEUDO-NEUROTIC SCHIZOPHRENIA

Pseudo-neurotic schizophrenia (Hoch & Polatin, 1949) is a relatively new term, though a number of neurotic patients in the 'classical' literature, including those described by Breuer and Freud

(1895) in *Studies in Hysteria,* were in retrospect not neurotic but schizophrenic. Rado (1959) points out that Freud (1918) suspected that the obsessional neurotic he was describing was really a schizophrenic, which is certainly borne out in Freud's 'Introductory Remarks' to the case:

> The patient with whom I am here concerned remained for a long time unassailably intrenched behind an attitude of obliging apathy. He listened, understood, and remained unapproachable. His unimpeachable intelligence was, as it were, cut off from the instinctual forces which governed his behaviour in the few relations of life that remained to him.

Rado adds that the patient from whose observations Ferenczi (1950) abstracted his concept of *pathoneurosis* was subsequently treated by him (Rado) in a mental hospital where he was for months in a catatonic stupor.

Hoch *et al.* (1962) have stressed the importance of this group and have illustrated the psychotic nature of the illness by both long-term follow-up and the vulnerability of these patients to lysergic acid diethylamide (L.S.D.). Some psychiatrists working in the mental hospitals have questioned the validity of the diagnosis and implied that there is nothing 'pseudo' about schizophrenia. This attitude ignores the psychopathology of the schizophrenic process and different rates of progress of the illness. The author is in no doubt that it is a valid diagnosis and what is more, it responds to treatment for schizophrenia. To ignore such a diagnosis exposes the patient to the risk of avoidable chronicity and the hazards of ineffective treatment.

SCHIZOPHRENIA AND SCHIZOPHRENIC-LIKE STATES IN THE ELDERLY

Kay (1972) criticised the traditional reluctance to diagnose as schizophrenia those psychoses that occur late in life because they usually lack certain 'nuclear symptoms' regarded as typical of the illness found in younger people. The later varieties have been bracketed with the organic psychoses of old age with a similar poor prognosis. It has been increasingly observed that persistent paranoid psychoses unrelated to senile or arteriosclerotic dementia can arise for the first time after the age of 60 years and be indistinguishable from paranoid schizophrenia.

It is generally a more or less organized delusional system, usually with hallucinations in a setting of well-preserved personality and intellect and the sex is predominantly female. Onset may be acute but usually follows a prodromal phase lasting months or even years with increased isolation, irritability, suspiciousness and depression. If there is another living at home, the stage is set for *folie à deux*. Hearing has been found to be impaired in 30–40 per cent.

Premorbid personality may show paranoid or schizoid traits and they are often unmarried or have spouses who can tolerate their idiosyncrasies. Indiscretions in diet may aggravate or in some instances precipitate the condition through vitamin deficiencies, particularly nicotinamide. Response to phenothiazines and vitamin therapy is usually good but a long period of follow-up is essential.

PARANOID STATES

The term **'paranoid'** is usually applied to psychotic disorders, whose symptomatology is primarily that of persistent delusions of a persecutory or grandiose nature, and with an absence of hallucinations. The intellect is well-preserved and the patient's behaviour is consistent with his delusions, there being no marked personality deterioration. Although the term has been incorporated in paranoid schizophrenia, this disorder is not usually associated with, and may even be excluded from, the paranoid states. This generally accepted definition indicates how arbitrary the label is, and how its application to mental disorder must frequently be based on a phase of illness which is not as immutable as the definition suggests. A systematized delusional state need not always be persecutory or grandiose, yet other delusions are excluded from the generic term 'paranoid'. For example, the severely depressed patient with marked hypochondriacal delusions may have them just as well systematized and hold them with as much intensity, but he is never referred to as suffering from a paranoid state. Even when the delusions are associated with guilt and unworthiness, nomenclature excludes these patients by saying that they suffer from *feelings* of guilt and unworthiness and they are included in the affective disorders. Yet should the delusion be of grandeur, they qualify for the definition 'paranoid'. It is difficult to see why there should be this incongruous distinction other than that the social evaluation of delusions has influenced nomenclature. It would appear to be less pathological to walk ever so humbly with one's Maker; but let the patient dare to exhibit undue pride or boast himself of tomorrow and there is no hesitation in ascribing to him delusions of grandeur. The term 'paranoid' does not therefore depend on the presence or absence of an affective component or in the holding of delusions, but on the nature of the delusion and whether it conflicts with the nonconformist conscience.

Paranoid reactions are frequently associated with organic disease and events and probably constitute their greatest mental adulterating factor. They are therefore seen in anoxic states, pernicious anaemia, alcoholic psychoses, post-operative psychoses, puerperal psychoses, electrolyte imbalance, and cerebral arteriosclerosis, to mention a few. They can also provide a secondary diagnosis in affective disorders or may be grafted on to a background of mental subnormality. This wide range of precipitants which can induce a severe paranoid reaction in patients who had previously not exhibited psychotic disorder, suggests that the potential for these reactions is more common than is generally appreciated. In a chest surgery ward, the sister-in-charge had learned that a large number of her patients post-operatively exhibited paranoid features, which yielded to chlorpromazine. It would appear that the nomenclature of the various paranoid reactions is tainted in the same way as in the other psychotic disorders, in that their original definition was elaborated from the mental hospital population and thus the incidence and full range of these disorders were not appreciated, while rigid criteria were laid down which in the present-day wider knowledge of psychiatric reactions are no longer applicable. The phenomena to be described do exist, but they must be seen, not as clear-cut clinical entities, but as part of the general process of mental breakdown and they can be so intimately associated with other forms of psychotic behaviour that the margins may be blurred.

The term **'paranoia'** was first used by Kahlbaum in 1863 and it was interpreted differently by various authors till **Kraepelin** tried to systematize the disorder by dividing it into three types: (1) **paranoid schizophrenia**; (2) **paraphrenia**; and (3) **paranoia**. This naturally led to much controversy, particularly over the inclusion of paranoid schizophrenia, and the arguments which have not yet abated are more reminiscent of those of medieval schoolmen than of medical scientists. In view of the relative artificiality of the clinical sub-divisions, these will be described first, after which the dynamics of the paranoid process will be given in some detail.

PARANOIA

Paranoia is the name given to a well and sometimes elaborately systematized delusional state, which is intractable and where the personality is well preserved. It is considered to be extremely rare, but this only means that it is rarely brought to the notice of the psychiatrist or is rarely admitted to mental hospitals. In fact, it can occur in a relatively encapsulated form and may not declare itself unless a specific topic which impinges on the delusional system is raised. If the patient is sufficiently capable of controlling his behaviour, he may never come to anybody's notice. The author had a patient who was severely depressed. He was a man of considerable ability and until his recent breakdown was a captain of industry. After interviewing his wife one learned that for a number of years he had entertained delusions about people spying on him and when they stayed in an hotel he would remain in the lounge till it was empty and sometimes not retire till the early hours of the morning, to make sure that nobody entered his room after he had retired. He would tap the panels of the room and refuse one with communicating door. All this was done in an affable and inoffensive manner and his wife felt that as the hotel managers did not express any surprise at what she considered his inordinate demands or strange behaviour, her husband's ideas could not have been unique.

Again, in the course of conversation on general topics, a certain subject may be raised and a member of the company begins to express ideas which are frankly delusional. The others may laugh it off or dismiss it in a good-humoured way and invite the protagonist to have another drink. The author on these occasions has been intrigued with the possibility that a well-encapsulated paranoid system had been declared, but because of social considerations was unable to explore the matter further. Many who belong to 'fringe' political and religious groups, whose whole creed consists of the elaboration of certain premises which most would consider untenable, are very close in their symptomatology to the patient with an encapsulated paranoia. They do not let their beliefs interfere unduly with their everyday life and are not regarded as abnormal. Even when delusions are held on an individual basis, they may never reach the psychiatrist, other than fortuitously. The author has on occasions met the husband or wife of the patient who entertains delusions about the spouse's conduct, usually relating to fidelity. They may go into long explanations and offer to supply proof of a certain event and one is left in no doubt as to the paranoid nature of the accusation; it need not, however, be associated with loss of efficiency and it obviously does not pervade the other aspects of their lives. One such husband ran his business successfully, was keenly interested in his children and grandchildren and was generally popular with his friends, yet he entertained a marked delusional state about his wife's infidelity which he alleged had been going on for over 30 years. He would then proceed to relate trivial events which according to him could only be interpreted in one way and it was only when one queried the validity of his statements that his otherwise genial presence took on a more vindictive colouring. Yet he protested that he was genuinely fond of his wife and that his persistent attempts to get her to confess to misconduct were in order to re-establish their relationship on a basis of mutual trust. Many wives (and husbands), to keep the peace, may acquiesce and admit to acts they have not committed with occasionally disastrous results.

THE CASE OF DR. SCHREBER

The classical case of paranoia in the literature is that of **Daniel Paul Schreber,** who had been a presiding Judge of the Appeal Court in Dresden. His place in history was assured, firstly by his eminence, secondly by his autobiography (Schreber, 1903) and thirdly, and most decidedly, by Freud's (1911) psychoanalytic study of Schreber's autobiographical account of his illness. The elaboration of delusions of the paranoiac can be very intriguing and one can be lost in admiration of their ingenuity, but generally they follow a pattern which is common to most of them. Freud quotes the account of Schreber's delusions from the report drawn up in 1899 by Dr. Weber, the physician in charge of the sanatorium where Schreber was a patient:

The culminating point of the patient's delusional system is his belief that he has a mission to redeem the world, and to restore mankind to their lost state of bliss. He was called to this task, so he asserts, by direct inspiration from God, just as we are taught the Prophets were; for nerves in a condition of great excitement, as his were for a long time, have precisely the property of exerting an attraction upon God-though this is touching upon matters which human speech is scarcely, if at all, capable of expressing, since they lie entirely outside the scope of human experience and, indeed, have been revealed to him alone. The most essential feature of his mission of redemption is that it must be preceded by his transformation into a woman. It is not to be supposed that he *wishes* to be transformed into a woman; it is rather a question of a 'must' based upon the order of things, which there is no possibility of his evading, much as he would personally prefer to remain in his own honourable and masculine station in life. But neither he nor the rest of mankind can win back their immortality except by his being transformed into a woman (a process which may occupy many years or even decades) by means of divine miracles. He himself, of this he is convinced, is the only object upon which divine miracles are worked, and he is thus the most remarkable man who has ever lived upon earth. Every hour and every minute for years he has experienced these miracles in his body, and he has had them confirmed by the voices that have conversed with him. During the first years of his illness certain of his bodily organs suffered such destructive injuries as would inevitably have led to the death of any other man: he lived for a long time without a stomach, without intestines, almost without lungs, with a torn oesophagus, without a bladder, and with shattered ribs, he used sometimes to swallow part of his own larynx with his food, etc. But divine miracles ('rays') always restored what had been destroyed, and therefore, as long as he remains a man, he is not in any way mortal. These alarming phenomena have ceased long ago, and his 'femaleness' had become prominent instead. This involves a process of development which will probably require decades, if not centuries, for its completion, and it is unlikely that any one now living will survive to see the end of it. He has a feeling that great numbers of 'female nerves' have already passed over into his body; and out of them a new race of men will proceed, through a process of direct impregnation by God. Not until then, it seems, will he be able to die a natural death, and, like the rest of mankind, have regained a state of bliss. In the meantime not only the sun, but trees and birds, which are in the nature of 'bemiracled relics of former human souls', speak to him in human accents, and miraculous things happen everywhere around him.

The patient's own description of his mental state is also worth recording and is of particular interest when seen alongside that of his doctor. Freud quotes extensively from Schreber's *Denkwürdigkeiten:*

In this way a conspiracy against me was brought to a head (in about March or April 1894). Its object was to contrive that, when once my nervous complaint had been recognized as incurable or assumed to be so, I should be handed over to a certain person in a particular manner. Thus my soul was to be delivered up to him, but my body—owing to a misapprehension of what I have described above as a purpose underlying the order of things—was to be transformed into a female body, and as such surrendered to the person in question with a view to sexual abuse, and was then simply to be left where it was—that is to say, no doubt, abandoned to corruption.

It was, moreover, perfectly natural that from the human standpoint (which was the one by which at that time I was still chiefly governed) I should regard Professor Flechsig or his soul as my only true enemy—at a later date there was also the von W. soul, about which I shall have more to say presently—and that I should look upon God Almighty as my ally. I merely fancied that he was in great straits as regards Professor Flechsig, and consequently felt myself bound to support him by every conceivable means, even to the length of sacrificing myself. It was not until very much later that the idea forced itself upon my mind that God himself had played the part of accomplice, if not of instigator, in the plot whereby my soul was to be murdered and my body used like a strumpet. I may say, in fact, that this idea has in part become clearly conscious to me only in the course of my writing the present work.

Every attempt at murdering my soul, or at emasculating me for purposes *contrary to the order of things* (that is, for the gratification of the sexual appetites of a human individual), or later at destroying my understanding—every such attempt has come to nothing. From this apparently unequal struggle between one weak man and God himself, I have emerged triumphant—though not without undergoing much bitter suffering and privation—because the order of things stands upon my side.

The range of delusional expression is infinite and there is very little to be gained by relating a series of case histories, other than to emphasize the pre-morbid personality of the paranoiac, the critical experience or the battery of events which triggered off the reaction and its subsequent development with invasion of the whole personality. The essence of paranoia is that there is no intellectual or personality deterioration and the patient does not exhibit hallucinations. Whether this is really so, is very difficult to decide. Even the classical case of Dr. Schreber was reported as being subject to auditory hallucinations. Hallucinations are subjective experiences and if the patient does not admit to them, the psychiatrist will be ignorant of their presence. Furthermore, in case histories of patients described under paranoia, only a sector of their lives is reported, usually not longer than the third to fifth decades, and all that can be said is that they had not yet deteriorated to the stage where auditory hallucinations and personality disintegration have supervened. The rigidity of the definition of paranoia is therefore highly artificial and only succeeds in distinguishing a small group of patients who for part of their psychotic history do not deteriorate as rapidly as others. That so much attention has been paid to this subgroup is due more to their social impact, than to their clinical identity.

PARAPHRENIA

Paraphrenia was divided by Kraepelin into four types: (1) **systematic,** (2) **expansive,** (3) **confabulatory,** and (4) **fantastic.** It is a very difficult if not impossible to distinguish paraphrenia systematica from paranoia, except that the latter does not deteriorate to the stage of auditory hallucination. The expansive type is usually grandiose and megalomanic and is well portrayed by Schreber (1903) though he was listed as paranoia. When hallucinations appear is a matter of individual differences, though Kraepelin considered that they generally appeared earlier in the expansive than in the systematic group. The confabulatory type is where pseudo-memories predominate, though Henderson and Gillespie (1950) did not believe that this type existed by itself but could be a feature of other delusional states. The fantastic group displayed a luxuriant growth of highly extraordinary, changing delusions, but Kraepelin admitted that these patients exhibited a number of features which were more commonly associated with what is now called paranoid schizophrenia.

There is an old-fashioned term for all these varieties which is no less scientific and at least is more meaningful and for descriptive purposes more generally applicable, and that is **chronic delusional insanity.** Such is the magic of Latin that a classification based on inadequate observations is eagerly adopted, while a perfectly valid and superior descriptive term is discarded.

Psychopathology

Psychiatry would be in a very primitive state indeed if one could see the paranoid reaction (including paranoia) only in terms of Kraepelinian nosology. There are, however, considerable psychopathological contributions to the subject, which help us to understand these vagaries of the mind.

In paranoid states these are largely concerned with the origins of delusions and their interpretation. The mental mechanism which is responsible is **projection** (p. 40) and delusions are misinterpretations based on this mechanism. They are frequently wish-fulfilling and though they may not always be pleasant and in fact are more often terrifying and hostile, they still represent an attempt to replace reality and thus contain elements of repudiated reality and the projected demands for the super-ego.

Freud's analysis of Schreber's delusions is still valid and apart from some minor modifications and elaborations by subsequent workers, it still is the prototype for an understanding of the psychopathology of the paranoid state. Schreber's delusions showed that he had an ambivalent attitude toward God, and also that he was much pre-occupied with being emasculated. This was explained by Freud as an attempt by Schreber to surmount the passive-homosexual aspect of his relationship with his father, the delusions being designed to protect him from these passive-homosexual temptations. This homosexual or negative aspect of the Oedipus complex, with the consequent elaboration of delusions, is a general finding in most paranoid states, where the unconscious conflicts tend to be over homosexuality. Regression in these patients to a narcissistic level brings them to the intermediate stage between love of oneself and love of the heterosexual object, a situation which can be met by homosexuality and it is this compromise which is frequently reached.

The denial of homosexuality in Schreber's case led to Freud's formulation 'I do not love him, I hate him'. This is converted by projection to, 'He hates me'. The patient's own hatred is further rationalized into 'I hate him because he hates (or persecutes) me' and as in schizophrenia, there is a defect of reality testing and the persecutory delusions are tenaciously held. Schreber's delusions also admirably displayed the deep regression of the ego with the emergence of symbols of magical and archaic ego levels. The extreme sensitivity of the paranoid patient enables him to seize on any trivial incident on which to crystallize his projection and give his delusions, to him at least, a semblance of reality.

Anal-sadistic phantasies are frequently recognized in the delusional content and this aspect has been strongly emphasized by Klein (1948). She attributes the basis of persecutory delusions to a very early developmental phase which occurs in the first two years of life.

The infant feels persecuted by cruel sadistic objects which represent its own projected sadism and its fears of retaliation for the sadistic phantasies it entertained. The infant's super-ego at this stage incorporates these distorted images of the parents and is particularly cruel; anxiety provoked by the super-ego at this stage is according to Klein similar to that found in paranoid states in adults. Between the age of 3 and 5 years, the super-ego goes through some modification and is mollified, and though still harsher than the factual parents is not nearly so aggressive and destructive as in infancy. The super-ego of the infant is the regressed super-ego which becomes apparent in paranoid delusions and a tendency to paranoia is said to be a direct result of the failure of the infant to develop fully beyond the infantile sadistic level or to regress readily to this level in the face of external threats. Should a traumatic situation occur, these early terrifying fears are mobilized and are projected.

Her theory embraces not only the paranoid reaction, but the depressive one and therefore has a certain clinical validity, for the delusions of the depressive have a number of facets in common with those of the paranoid patient; although she rejects Freud's interpretation of homosexual denial as being too narrow, it is precisely on this aspect that the two conditions can, in their psychopathology, be differentiated. Super-ego projection is common to both and in the paranoid state accounts for the patient's ideas of reference and influence. He may feel he is being controlled, criticized and punished. The reality situation may break down completely and projection assume a hallucinatory form with the voices usually being critical of his sexual behaviour, and containing thinly veiled or even overt references to his homosexuality. The difference between directing one's aggression against one's persecutor or against oneself can be a very fine one. The author had one such patient, a naval rating, who was tortured with a voice which called him a 'brown hatter', a term used in the navy for homosexuals. He had at one time in response to the voices made a homicidal attack on a seaman who occupied the berth next to him, but was unsuccessful and received a severe blow on the head from an iron bar which rendered him unconscious. The voice abated for a time, but it later returned. This time he got out his razor but felt that it was fruitless to challenge his persecutor and made a serious attempt at suicide by cutting his throat. The delusional content may be very similar to that found in melancholia and should there be a marked affective element in the clinical picture, it may be very difficult to decide which is the dominant element. A number of these 'paranoid-affective' states respond to E.C.T., thus indicating the strong melancholic aspect of their illness.

This affective component can play a more important part in the understanding and treatment of the condition than the delusions themselves. As has been said, the super-ego can be projected and the delusional content though persecutory can have a marked melancholic colouring. The patient may be tortured by threats of a fate more terrible than death and the delusions may be systematized without the presence of hallucinations, yet the main problem is not that usually regarded as paranoid, but as depressive. On the other hand, the patient may persistently reiterate a systematized delusional story about persecution and plots, but with a certain shallowness of affect and the clinical state is unmistakably a paranoid one, without a vestige of depression. These examples suggest that even though the nature of the delusion is important in diagnosis, its affective colouring is at least equally important, and while projection is an essential mechanism, unless it stems from a denial of homosexual strivings, it is unlikely to be associated with a true paranoid state. Because of this marked regression, ego-strength is also impaired and the picture of the affectively-blunted paranoid state results and in its wake there is a reduction of reality testing with the presentation of more bizarre delusions and eventually hallucinations. This differentiation is of course a gross simplification and in practice clear-cut distinctions do not exist. Mixed states occur more frequently and as in other diagnostic problems a quantitative estimation is required to arrive at a reliable formulation.

Though the range of delusions in the paranoid state shows an infinite variety, certain patterns are more common.

Erotomania is derived from the same formula as that of the persecutory delusion, 'I do not love him', but instead of saying, 'I hate him because he persecutes me', it is changed to, 'I love her because she loves me'. Some patients show a most persistent drive to fall in love with a girl, and the author had a young patient who had to leave school because of his inability to refrain from pestering a girl in his class. He would follow her home and call after her, plighting his troth and writing to her that Heaven had ordained that they should marry. When referred to the clinic, the condition had deteriorated and he was frankly schizophrenic, but for some months he was sufficiently well integrated to achieve a reasonable performance at school and pass several subjects in his G.C.E. (equivalent to University Matriculation). Even in his more schizophrenic state with its marked affective disturbance he still voiced his delusions about the girl's love for him. Erotomania can take an **active** or **passive** form. In the active state, the patient spends much time in seeking and finding women whom he tries to love in order to deny his latent homosexual learnings. He may frequent public ballrooms and this may lead to rather dangerous liaisons with older married women with the extension of the delusion that his strength is being drained away from him and that there is something sinister in his partner's love.

This may lead to the passive form, when he feels that he is being interfered with at night and that nocturnal emissions are being induced by some spell the woman has put on him. These passive features of erotomania are seen more commonly in women. They usually claim that some man is deliberately persecuting them with his amorous intentions. The author had a patient who occupied a flat in a converted house and she was convinced that the man underneath, in response to some pre-arranged signal, was able to identify her presence and would follow her when she sent into the bathroom or sat on the toilet. She later became hallucinated and his movements were then accompanied by seductive and indecent suggestions. She was a young married woman who in other respects could behave quite normally. In the older woman, the erotic persecutions can be most bizarre and unremitting. Various agents such as wires, electricity, and a whole range of machines may be used to interfere with her private parts and keep her awake all night. Complaints are lodged with the police and letters are written but the persecution persists.

Jealousy is another derivation of the formula—'I do not love him'; in this case, it is 'She loves him'. Fenichel (1945) states that in analysis it becomes evident that this type of patient, when suspecting his wife, is actually interested in the other man and strives to overcome his homosexuality by means of projection. This identification with the other man is seen in the patient's obsessional pre-occupation with the fancied love scene in which he unconsciously takes the wife's place. These patients frequently get their wives to confess to a premarital relationship and regularly make them go through the details of their sexual experience. Their insistence on a confession has on occasions led to the wife elaborating a relatively innocent affair, or even admitting to a relationship which did not take place. This has the opposite effect to that expected by the wife, for instead of forgiveness and forgetting, there are more and more demands for repeat performances and for further elaborations. The author had a patient who could only have intercourse with his wife under these conditions and as he put it—'It was really the other man who was with her'.

Litigious Paranoia is not necessarily confined to the courts and must be familiar to personnel officers in industry, senior administrators, members of Parliament and town councillors. Mountains are made out of mole-hills and a relatively minor or trivial incident which in the normal course of events could be resolved in a good-humoured way, becomes a source of lasting conflict and a major point of principle. Anxiety of this nature is not uncommon and there may be just as much fault in the way it is mobilized by external agencies as in its presentation by the patient. Many people, particularly those who are generally conscientious and have a strong narcissistic element in their make-up, project their rigid super-ego and the punitive results which follow cause narcissistic regression and protestations of innocence as to their good name and character. They have to challenge authority and therefore re-enact their early conflict with the father. The fancied insult is elaborated and they are compelled to remove any suspicion of guilt and parade the innocence of a primitive narcissistic state. The latent homosexuality is readily recognized and the author saw a number of such patients during the Second World War. They were mainly regular army officers who had become litigious to such a degree that their efficiency had become impaired, though some had adulterated their problem with alcohol. The usual manner of airing complaints through the Military Secretary had failed, and they had to invoke members of Parliament and other influential people. A word of caution is necessary. Even though a person is in need of homosexual denial and indulges in litigious battles, it does not necessarily mean that his claims are delusional. Each case should be most carefully investigated and access to all the facts is essential. All authority is not benign or even normal and persecution unfortunately still exists. 'Man's inhumanity to man, makes countless thousands mourn!' is as true today as when Robert Burns wrote it.

THE FAMILIES OF SCHIZOPHRENICS

These will to some extent vary as the schizophrenic process varies. The schizo-affective reaction with acute breakdown under stress and with an excellent prognosis will probably derive from a different background than the more insidious and therefore more malignant schizophrenic process. It is in the latter group that the families tend to be more remarkable. Lidz and Lidz (1949) and Lidz *et al.* (1957) made an extensive study of these families, particularly of the parents and concluded that the relationship between father and mother was such as not to create the stable and affectionate background necessary for the healthy development of the child. All combinations are found, the domineering father and the dependent mother; the over-anxious and solicitous mother; and the rejecting mother. One might argue that these types are met as parents of neurotic children, or even where the children do not exhibit psychiatric handicap, but it is the regularity with which they appear which suggests that there is a factor here which should not be overlooked.

In the author's experience, it is usually the mothers who present the problem and they can roughly be divided into two groups: (1) the well-intentioned but ineffective, and (2) the denying. The former are usually over-anxious and try to cooperate but just seem incapable of appreciating the delicate balance and sensitivity of the patient. One can spend a lot of time patiently explaining to them what their role should be and while they obviously try hard, they have difficulty in grasping the situation. The author had a young female schizophrenic patient who had presented with severe behavioural disturbance, in that she was found on a major road in the city in her nightdress and was incoherent, hallucinated and completely disintegrated on admission. She gradually improved and eventually approached her pre-morbid level, which was that of a hyper-sensitive, retiring girl, who readily withdrew into compensatory day-dreaming. The social worker had worked hard on her and had gained her confidence and was about to get her to take a job. The department was pleased with its efforts and the patient and mother were being interviewed prior to the patient's discharge. The mother enquired if there was anything she should do and was politely told that this was the type of problem where positive steps on the part of the family did not help; in fact, it might upset things. The clinic and the social worker would continue to keep the patient under supervision and all one would expect from the mother was an attitude of benevolent neutrality. She turned to her daughter and said: 'You see, Mary, the doctor says you've got to do as you're told'.

The 'denying' type can be even more exasperating and because their behaviour does not appear so naive, it frequently appears like a deliberate act to prevent the patient from getting the treatment he needs. A young boy had to be excluded from school because of his overt schizophrenic features and the general practitioner referred the patient for psychiatric opinion. The mother attended, but protested that it was all unnecessary and that the family doctor was fussing for nothing. The boy was placed on heavy dosage of chlorpromazine and the florid features subsided but he was still very disturbed. The mother insisted he was his 'old sweet self' and reduced his chlorpromazine to zero and decided he required no more help from the hospital. She was a school teacher and was obviously the dominant spouse, her husband sitting there without saying a word but nodding in agreement at her assertions. Another mother whose young daughter had been treated in the department, but shortly after discharge had relapsed into a state of catatonic excitement, was 'calmly' doing her knitting when the author was called by the family doctor. The rest of the place was in chaos; the psychotic girl was screaming her head off at the top of the stairs, the husband was torn between supporting his wife's attitude and concern for his daughter. The mother was decisive: 'She's not going back to hospital; she's just a little upset'.

Although these two parental reactions can be clearly recognized, not infrequently they present at different times by the same parent and it may be that they have a similar psychopathology; in any case, they have the same result, in that they both delay the starting of treatment and contribute to the patient's relapse. Denial could be a self-protective mechanism, for it may be impossible to live with the patient, unless one denies the existence of the psychotic process, and this would explain the overt hostility one frequently meets when one tries to bring home to the parent the gravity of the patient's illness. It is important to take parental attitudes into account when rehabilitation is being considered, for the patient may do better lodging with a 'neutral' family than with his own parents.

Homosexual Tendencies in Mothers of Schizophrenic Women

On the basis of previous studies indicating that the incestuous and homosexual tendencies of schizophrenic patients reflect similar proclivities in their parents, and the parents' failure to maintain their gender-linked roles and the essential boundaries between the generations, Lidz and Lidz (1969) reported four case studies of schizophrenic women whose mothers were both cold and homosexually seductive.

They restate the principle that to achieve stable and coherent ego identity, the child needs to form a proper gender identity with the parent of the same sex and that pathological interactions between a mother and her schizophrenic daughter are worse than for a schizophrenic son, the relationship being colder and more nebulous. In the cases described, one slept with her daughter and kept her as an observer while she gave herself enemas, one had her daughter massage her. In all four cases the father assumed many maternal functions. Analytical therapy of these patients was designed to achieve a comfortable distance for the therapist rather than the therapy become the patient's prime objective. This is an interesting study but it is difficult to decide whether it is representative.

Husbands of Paranoid Women: Willing Victims

Dupont and Grunebaum (1968) studied 16 paranoid women and their husbands and defined a specific psychopathology based on an interpersonal relationship. These women with paranoid states (9) chose husbands who were older men, socially isolated from their own families and friends, reliable breadwinners, deeply committed to maintaining the outward appearance of conventional marriage and unable to express angry or sexual feelings. Their marriages were stable and isolated from outsiders. The husbands of those with paranoid schizophrenia (4) reported many job changes as they were ambitious and thought they were underpaid. They were less stable than the former group and the families functioned inefficiently with more recourse to social agencies, neighbours and other members of the family. Husbands of women with other diagnoses but with a paranoid colouring did not show the syndrome of the first group and the authors concluded that it is therefore specific to the husbands of women suffering from a paranoid state.

TREATMENT

A condition which is protean in its symptomatology, where aetiological factors are only beginning to be defined and whose very concept is a battleground for theorists, must present a formidable therapeutic challenge. What to treat? How to treat? Where to treat? Whom to treat? These are only some of the many questions that can be posed.

If one can see the problem as one of ego-distintegration, a more positive approach is possible and one can begin to ask the following relevant questions.

1. Why is the ego disintegrating?
2. What are the major contributing factors?
3. Which of these factors can be influenced?

The basis of all treatment should be a thorough appraisal of the patient, his family, the environmental demands and his total reaction. It is then possible to begin to answer the above questions. It should also be appreciated that schizophrenic patients are hypersensitive and prone to narcissistic regression and that the therapist who is too anxious to elicit a positive response will only succeed in driving the patient more into himself. The basic psychosexual problem of the patient may make it more difficult for a therapist of the opposite sex, though therapists of the same sex may not fare better if they project their own sexuality into the therapeutic situation. The patient's tendency to withdraw makes contact difficult and it can prove a severe strain for the doctor who persists in his efforts to help somebody who constantly rejects help. No two schizophrenic patients are alike in their responses and the environmental factors which are so important are equally varied.

It is therefore not possible to describe the treatment of all schizophrenic patients but merely to define those areas where treatment is likely to be effective.

1. The Patient's Sensitivity

Schizophrenic patients as a rule are hypersensitive, tend to over-interpret and attribute a personal significance to situations which others would not regard as of even general interest. This hypersensivitity creates its own atmosphere to which others in turn are sensitive and may excite a rejection response. It behoves those who are responsible for young people to be particularly aware of this problem and to adjust accordingly. An attitude of benevolent neutrality is most likely to succeed, for if one is too eager the patient may withdraw further. A quiet persistence with a selection of topics of a concrete nature such as hobby, reading, work, holiday activities is a much more secure base from which to establish a relationship than a probing of interpersonal relationships. As the problem is frequently of long standing, sudden and dramatic improvement is not the rule and modest gains should be considered adequate reward for effort.

The sensitivity may be extreme and deteriorate to the expression of frank ideas of reference, delusions and hallucinations. Under these circumstances something more than personal support is needed and tranquillizing drugs have now securely established themselves in the treatment (see below).

2. The Family Situation

This demands close study for it is generally out of this milieu that the schizophrenic process has arisen. Parents should be interviewed, if neccessary singly, for otherwise vital information may be withheld. The common mechanisms of denial and rejection will be readily discernible and the general 'cluelessness' of such parents can be exasperating. The author has tried varying techniques in dealing with them. A slow and careful approach with the aim of creating insight and acceptance is almost never successful, while a sudden confrontation will not break through and may even increase the denial. Of the two, the latter is to be preferred for it is a useful precursor to action. The family doctor and one of the parents can usually be reached and the denying parent may then yield to the offers of help.

Suggestions as to removal from home have to be made with some delicacy and admission to hospital is a useful compromise. It gets the patient out of a disturbing situation and makes it easier for the parents to accept a more prolonged absence from home especially when an obvious improvement in the patient's mental state ensues. Denial by the parent is nourished by contact with the patient and admission to hospital or attendance at Day Hospital gives the parent a welcome respite.

Laing's Existential Approach. (See under 'The Psychotherapies'. Chapter 19).

3. The Social Situation

This too requires careful scrutiny for the patient may have been projected into a work or educational environment which though acceptable to the parents is positively harmful to the patient. It may be very difficult to effect a change especially if the patient is highly intelligent and the work situation is well within his intellectual capacity. Parents and others become obsessed with educational attainments and would rather settle for a university degree and permanent invalidism than a more modest achievement and good health.

Employers and teachers should be personally approached and the position (with the patient's consent) explained. They are usually most co-operative and only too anxious to help. It is obvious that the psychiatrist assumes considerable personal responsibility for all this manipulation and the rate and degree of reintegration of the patient into the community will depend on his assessment of the social situation as well as the patient's capacity. The help of a good social worker is invaluable and it is a matter for regret that such a service which can demonstrably contribute to the making whole of a broken mind is not a popular one with social workers. It may be that in their training they are not given sufficient experience of this rewarding work.

When the areas have been defined, the effective measures that can be employed are also limited. These are:

1. Social Manipulation

This implies the correction of contributory factors as mentioned above.

2. Hospital Treatment

Acute problems which are very disturbing require intensive treatment which cannot be given at home. There is generally little choice as regards the type of hospital for, to date, the local mental hospital has a monopoly. Standards of treatment will vary with their resources which include quality and availability of staff.

It is a popular misconception, even among doctors, that the treatment of schizophrenia is stereotyped; nothing is more erroneous. Every patient is an individual problem and some require a tremendous concentration of effort, by nurse, doctor, occupational therapist and social worker. Effort pays and there can be no justification for a dilatory approach to the problem of schizophrenia. Early appraisal and institution of treatment is vital for these patients do not complain they are being neglected and do not press the urgency of their problem. To ignore this principle is to court chronicity, an all too common sequel in previous years.

The former tendency of housing schizophrenic patients together tended to foster chronicity for they do not stimulate each other. On the other hand a psychiatric unit where schizophrenics are in the minority provides the stimulating environment which they require. The daily interview with the doctor, the occasional talk with the nurse and the visit to the occupational therapy department are in themselves not enough. It requires a group of patients who are generally outgoing and prepared to make contact to provide the degree of stimulation these people require. The ratio is important for if the unit is too heavily loaded with schizophrenic patients, the others tend to hive off and deprive the schizophrenics of their support, while if schizophrenics are very much in the minority, the others can tolerate them and play an active part in their rehabilitation. Small units of the general hospital variety with the schizophrenic in the minority are, in the author's experience, ideal for this purpose and it is most encouraging to see the schizophrenic patient flourish under these circumstances. From being an outcast, he becomes the aristrocrat of the ward.

Geographical Location. The hospital should be sited near the centre of population from which the patient stems. This permits easy access to the city and its amenities as well as to hostels, places of work, out-patient department, day hospital and social club. To expect a schizophrenic patient to travel long distances to maintain contact with hospital or community is to fail to appreciate the ease with which he can withdraw into himself.

These points may determine the success or failure of treatment.

3. Drugs

The Phenothiazines (see under Psychopharmacology). These have proved the major breakthrough in the treatment of schizophrenia. Their introduction in 1952 at a time when most hospitals were heavily committed to insulin coma treatment caused some delay in their general adoption, but few experienced psychiatrists would now deny their value. It is important to prescribe adequately and this is just as necessary for the general practitioner as for the hospital doctor. It is the general practitioner who sees the patient first and effective dosage at an early stage may abort the otherwise relentless progress of the disease. The patient's co-operation is difficult to secure once the illness has developed, so early and adequate medication is vital. There are now a bewildering variety of phenothiazines, but chlorpromazine, the first to be used, is still the most useful, though others such as trifluoperazine are good substitutes.

Dosage. This will vary according to the stage and degree of the illness. An acute hallucinatory state will require not less than 100 mg. t.d.s. while milder forms can be adequately controlled with 50 mg. t.d.s. Less than this dose is generally inadequate and should not be used unless the patient has remitted and is being weaned from his drugs.

Duration of medication. In a persistent illness, it is difficult to know when to discontinue treatment. Some would urge that the patient should never stop taking his drugs and while in certain chronic or malignant states this policy may be justified, as a rule it is not necessary. On the other hand, abrupt cessation shortly after a remission has been secured will certainly court relapse. Generally the patient should continue on adequate dosage for not less than 6 months and if progress has been rapid and satisfactory and environmental factors have been equated, a gradual reduction of drugs is permissible. Some patients who have been on a maintenance dose for a year or more have abruptly discontinued their medication with no ill effects. On the other side it can be said with at least 90 per cent certainty that if a schizophrenic patient on maintenance therapy relapses, it is because he has stopped taking his tablets.

The side effects of drugs should be borne in mind and the appropriate action taken should they appear. Patients on maintenance dosage are usually fit to drive a car.

Long-acting Phenothiazines. The introduction of long-acting phenothiazines in depot dose by intramuscular injection has made a tremendous impact on the management of the schizophrenic in the community. A major cause of relapse was the failure of the patient to take his drugs; now this has been almost eliminated. Fluphenazine decanoate is usually given in a test dose of 12.5 mg. and if no adverse side effects occur after ten days a second dose of 25 mg. is given and this is usually sufficient to control the problem for three to four weeks. The drug is prone to cause striatal side effects with Parkinsonism and dystonic movements, and these are usually contained by an antispasmodic agent such as benzhexol 2 mg. t.d.s.

Many clinics in Britain are using this treatment with great success for it has almost eliminated the defaulting patient. It also is an absolute indication of the patient who has not had treatment. Attendance for the injection means that he has; failure to attend means that he has not, and positive steps can be taken immediately to ensure that he has his treatment and does not relapse into chronicity.

Hirsch *et al.* (1973) conducted a double-blind placebo trial of fluphenazine decanoate, a long-acting phenothiazine to determine its value in maintenance therapy of chronic schizophrenic patients already established on the drug. In low doses it was significantly more effective than placebo in preventing relapse and admission to hospital. Relapse was accompanied by a resurgence of specifically schizophrenic symptoms and by an increase in abnormalities described by the relatives. The results therefore confirm the usefulness of long-acting fluphenazine.

Other Drugs. Reserpine and Haloperidol have their adherents but their advantages should be weighed against their disadvantages and against the considerable knowledge of the phenothiazines that has accumulated.

4. Drugs and Treatment for Secondary Problems

It is frequently overlooked that schizophrenia is usually adulterated with other psychiatric states, particularly depression, and the drugs used for this condition should be given concurrently with the phenothiazines. The author favours imipramine hydrochloride because of its general reliability of action, its relative freedom from dangerous side effects and its safety in combination with other drugs and anaesthetics. Others prefer the monoamine oxidase inhibitors in spite of considerable restrictions in their usefulness.

Combined Treatment with E.C.T. and Antipsychotic Drugs in Schizophrenia. Weinstein and Fischer (1971) contend that the combination of antipsychotic drugs and E.C.T. can be beneficial and ought to be reconsidered, especially as many schizophrenics are abandoned without even a trial of E.C.T. They give the reasons why in the United States there is hostility to E.C.T.: (1) there has been strong bias in favour of psychodynamically based theory and treatment approaches to all types of mental illness; (2) these were considered superior as they encouraged a 'working through' the psychosis and also the assumption, frequently unwarranted, that it would be conquered for good rather than merely suppressing the symptoms; (3) persons attracted to a career in psychiatry are usually introspective and highly verbal, having great regard for the healing power of insight and understanding, and no intervention could be less 'intellectual' than E.C.T.; and (4) there is a feeling that E.C.T. is harsh and coercive, and some claim that it causes permanent, measurable brain damage, though there is no evidence for this.

The young person with chronic schizophrenia who has been treated with high phenothiazine dosage is most likely to benefit from the combination. If a plateau has been reached in his progress a course of E.C.T. may well produce a dramatic clinico-physiological change. The first few E.C.T.'s will cause a rapid reduction in the patient's tolerance for phenothiazines and this shift is always associated with clinical improvement. In rare cases where no change occurs after 3-5 treatments the prognosis is indeed poor. The authors believe that E.C.T. exhibits a synergism with anti-psychotic drugs.

Multiple Monitored Electroconvulsive Treatment (MMECT) of Schizophrenia. This method enables 2-8 seizures to be induced during a given treatment session which takes place twice weekly with at least two days between. In each session five consecutive generalized seizures are given, except where complications (see below) occur. Each seizure was induced as closely as possible to three minutes after termination of the preceding seizure and the total time for a session was usually 30-45 minutes with an average number of 4.6 (range 2-7); the average number of seizures in a course being 21.9 (range 10-35); the mean total seizure time was 4403 seconds (range 1182-9200); and the average number of days from start to finish was 21.3 (range 4-71).

Bridenbaugh *et al.* (1972) reported a 16-month pilot study of 17 acute schizophrenic patients at the Walter Reed Hospital, of whom 14 showed marked improvement and were discharged to their own care. While clinical response did not correlate significantly with total seizure seconds, each of the three patients who required further hospital care had a total seizure time well below the mean for the entire group, and after transfer two of the three had further E.C.T. with benefit. Seizure length was found to be longer during hypocapnoea than with hypercapnoea. The only major complication was one case of pulmonary aspiration, so endotracheal intubation was thereafter used routinely without further incident of this nature. There were 17 instances of cardiac arrhythmia and 16 prolonged seizures (i.e. lasting longer than 15 minutes) and in 11 of the latter group the treatment was terminated. Long term follow-up showed no recurrence in those who improved and the writers conclude that it is at least as safe and effective as conventional E.C.T. and shortens the time space for giving a course of treatment.

Comment: It takes too mechanical an outlook on the treatment of schizophrenia, and though there are economies in saving time in hospital, there are also disadvantages in restricting rehabilitation. Good remission can be obtained without such heroic measures but there may well be the odd patient who has not yielded to more conventional treatment who would benefit from such a measure.

5. Rehabilitation

Brown *et al.* (1968) discuss the rehabilitation of the schizophrenic patient. At different stages a patient may need to be under full supervision in a hospital ward, in a ward under less supervision, in an unsupervised settlement villa, in a hotel outside the hospital, in supervised lodgings or specially registered hostel, in the care of a family not his own or at home. Similarly he may require an undemanding occupation quite different to his usual one, a re-education routine, a course at an Industrial Rehabilitation Unit (I.R.U.), work in supervised occupations, Remploy, special departments of industrial firms or vocational guidance. There should also be an emergency service to deal with situations which arise when other aspects of the service are not working or out of order.

6. Group Therapy

This is popular in mental hospitals for various reasons. It is in accord with the modern idea of the therapeutic community and some units (including staff) are run on a group therapy basis. It is economic in that the doctor meets all his patients and is able to observe them in the group situation. It is claimed to be intrinsically beneficial in that patients are helped to relate to each other and lose much of their sensitivity. Furthermore if one patient raises a problem in discussion, it is likely to be common to the others and therefore the patient who cannot volunteer his own problem before the group gets this vicarious benefit. Its value has not been adequately demonstrated and one suspects it is an expedient or a treatment fad, rather than an established and successful form of treatment.

7. Individual Psychotherapy

This varies from intensive psychoanalysis to superficial support. Most psychotherapists would not advocate analytical psychotherapy in schizophrenia but there are some enthusiastic exceptions.

Rosen (1953) advocates a form of 'Direct Analysis'. He 'assaults' the patient with free interpretation of what he considers to be his (the patient's) unconscious processes. With this method which is combined with prolonged personal contact outside the consulting room there is alleged to be a gradual 'tuning-up' by the patient and the formation of a relationship which is followed by more coherence and social competence and eventually a remission of symptoms.

This process requires considerable time and effort from the therapist and very few have the competence, enthusiasm and stamina to follow it through. If schizophrenia were amenable only to this method there would be much to commend it, but a variety of techniques, including other forms of psychotherapy are at least as effective. Rosen's method had attracted considerable attention because when he published his book in 1953, the phenothiazines had not yet made any impact and the various forms of social manipulation were still inadequately understood. Such is the power of the cult of individual psychotherapy for schizophrenia that many will still recommend this doubtful method in preference to others which are more reliable.

The personal supervision of the patient's general treatment by the psychiatrist which includes frequent interviews, is a form of individual psychotherapy. The patient readily learns that here is someone who is interested in his welfare and with whom he can begin to form a relationship. The author has a large number of schizophrenic patients who have been supported in this way on an out-patient basis and who have made a successful social adjustment.

8. Out-Patient Social Club

This is a very useful agency in the rehabilitation of the schizophrenic. The patient is introduced to the club even when an in-patient though many are initiated directly from the out-patient department or the Day Hospital. Any organized group for the treatment of the schizophrenic becomes less effective if the numbers of schizophrenic patients become too large to be adequately integrated with the more stimulating atmosphere engendered by recovering depressions, phobic anxiety and obsessional states. The Social Club should therefore not be swamped by schizophrenics and unless a healthy balance is maintained a helpful measure can be rendered useless if not actually harmful.

The Club also permits access to relatives and the patient who is not living at home can also meet them under supervision. This could help to improve family relationships but evidence to date is not conclusive. The full potential of the out-patient social club has not yet been exploited but already it has made great contributions to recovery and has helped a number of patients to adjust to life outside hospital.

9. Family Therapy

The demonstration by Alanen (1958) of the disturbance of the mothers of schizophrenics in that they tended to be domineering, excessively possessive and lacking in understanding of the patient's needs and feelings, has stimulated many to treat the schizophrenic in his family setting, Bowen (1960) actually admitted to hospital the relatives together with the patient but others are content to see them together on an out-patient basis. It is difficult to evaluate such measures for even the known factors that are brought to bear are numerous and there are many that are still unknown or unrecognized.

While it is important to help the parents and relieve them of feelings of guilt, the prime responsibility is to the schizophrenic patient and isolation from the family may be more valuable than contact with it. Brown *et al.* (1962) followed up 128 male schizophrenics between 20–49 years, mostly short-stay cases. A 'key' relative (wife or mother) was identified and estimates made of the amount of emotion, hostility and dominant directive behaviour shown by relative and patient to each other. Two hypotheses were tested.

1. That deterioration in the patient would occur if he were discharged to such a home.
2. That if returned to such a home relapse would be less likely if personal contact with family were small.

'High emotional involvement' homes were associated with 76 per cent of those who deteriorated as against 26 per cent in 'low emotional involvement' homes. The authors suggest that social isolation may therefore be sought by the patient as a form of prophylaxis. In young schizophrenics, where such isolation is difficult to arrange, a better start can be made on the problem if the patient is removed from the home background. Family therapy, though challenging and attractive, is a measure that should be approached with considerable reserve in schizophrenia. It could make the patient worse.

Influence of Family Life on the Course of Schizophrenic Disorders. Brown *et al.* (1972) tested the hypothesis that a high degree of expressed emotion (mainly negative) is an index of characteristics in relatives which are likely to cause a florid relapse of symptoms in schizophrenics, independent of other factors, such as length of history, type of symptomatology or severity of previous behaviour disturbance.

They found a significant association between relapse and high Expressed Emotion (EE) in the families as indicated by the number of critical comments, presence of hostility and the presence of emotional over-involvement. Warmth expressed by the family towards the patient showed a curvilinear association with relapse. The authors suggested that the influence of the EE factor can be reduced by regular phenothiazine medication and avoidance of a too close contact (35 hours per week or more) with a highly emotional relative.

10. Non-specific Healing Techniques

Ludwig (1968) on the assumption that certain non-specific elements are common to many types of therapy designed a treatment programme to exploit these influences. The subjects were 30 chronic schizophrenics (16 men and 14 women) with poor prognosis, and after a 2-week period when psychotropic drugs were withdrawn, there was a 10-week period during which deviant behaviour was dealt with through psychosocial techniques, followed by a 10-week period when 15 patients (Group A) were exposed to the treatment programme and 15 were not (Group B) followed by a 10-week period during which Group B was in the programme and Group A was not.

The experimental programme included: (1) emotional arousal meetings, in which patients were confronted, challenged, ridiculed and belittled by the group leader in an effort to provoke protest, anger and self-assertion; (2) suggestion-inspiration meetings, at which tapes were played dealing with self-confidence, self-mastery, willpower etc; (3) 'moral suasion' and re-education meetings, at which instruction was given on etiquette, personal appearance, social conversation and job seeking, with weekly quizzes on the material presented; (4) dynamic-interpretative meetings, at which patient behaviour was interpreted within the framework of psychoanalytic theory; and (5) a behaviour and privilege clinic at which patients were told their ratings on a 7–point scale and what their privileges for the week would be. Behaviour was usually encouraged or discouraged by these weekly changes in privilege status but certain 'Mortal Sins' such as absconding, or 'Venial Sins' such as breaking privilege restrictions, were punished immediately by imposition of restrictions.

The patients on assessment showed more constructive behaviour change during the experimental treatment programme than during the control phase. The author concluded that concentrated application of non-specific healing techniques can significantly improve patient behaviour, at least temporarily.

PROGNOSIS

This will depend on the nature of the schizophrenia and it is customary to describe two categories (Langfeldt, 1937).

1. *Process schizophrenia* which is regarded as the 'hard core' problem.
2. *Schizophrenic reaction* or *schizophreniform psychosis* which carries a more favourable prognosis.

Leonhard (1957) elaborated eight principal groups but this does not contribute much more than Langfeldt's two categories. Krauss (1961) regards schizophrenia as a vast field of pathogenetically varied reactions consisting of a hard core, a number of surrounding layers produced by biological modifications, and of random groups. In addition to psychobiological factors, there are family dynamics, social class and inter-personal communication which 'chisel on the shapes of these groups'.

Prognosis must be varied but the psychiatrist should not seek refuge for his failure in a diagnostic label or even an aetiological factor. There is enough known about the nature of the condition and its treatment to suggest that the place and circumstance of the treatment and the efforts and expertise of the psychiatrist and his staff are vital factors in prognosis.

CHAPTER 14

Social Psychiatry

Coe (1970) quotes Virchow (1849), who, in his *Scientific Methods: Therapeutic Standpoints* stated:

> . . . if medicine is the science of the healthy as well as of the ill human being (which is what it ought to be), what other science is better suited to propose laws as the basis of the social structure, in order to make effective those which are inherent in man himself? Once medicine is established as anthropology, and once the interests of the privileged no longer determine the course of public events, the physiologist and the practitioner will be counted among the elder statesmen who support the social structure. Medicine is a social science in its very bone and marrow.

While much of this can be attributed to the spirit of radicalism which swept Europe in 1848, it is essential to take stock of the social outlook on disease and the way in which organized medicine has responded. This involves a definition of disease itself; its characteristics; the response to illness of the patient, the doctor and society; systems of medical beliefs and practice; the development of western medicine and the forces responsible; the professionalism of medicine; other practitioners of the healing arts; the development of the modern hospital, and its social structure; the meaning of hospitalization to the patient and the community; the web of medical organization; and the cost of financing medical care. Coe (1970) deals with all these topics in a systematic manner which puts the whole sociology into a meaningful perspective.

Social psychiatry, though to a certain extent dependent on contributions from social psychology, embraces a different field. The latter is primarily a social science which uses the techniques of mass observation, studies the nature, similarities, differences and interaction of groups, and draws much of its theoretical support from the biological researches of Tinbergen (1951) and the anthropological studies of Malinowski (1929) and Mead (1928, 1931, 1936, 1950).

Social psychiatry includes all those facets of psychiatry which have social implications such as community care and public health measures including legislation and hospital development. This wide sweep has so far eluded a unifying theory, though a number of theoretical considerations are already incorporated, while others are emerging. The subject has been given greater prominence in recent times, because of the disintegration of the mental hospital and the emergence of effective psychiatric treatment in general hospitals, out-patient departments and in general practice, and there are now conflicting claims for the privilege of treating the mentally ill, inside and outside the mental hospital.

Both sides are engaged in experiments most of which are likely to benefit the patient, but as the mental hospital is still our largest capital asset in the treatment of mental disorder, it is dominant in the minds of governments who are more likely to think in terms of what institutions they possess and maintain, than in terms of hypothetical development. As most psychiatrists, at least in Britain, still work in mental hospitals, their views are more likely to influence the responsible government department. The small minority, who are breaking new ground and whose plans envisage the liquidation of large institutions and their replacement by much smaller units which are better staffed, have still to convert the strength of their arguments into a proportionate capital investment. To some, the mental hospital is a sacred cow which should be above criticism, while to others it is an anachronism which should never have been allowed.

HISTORICAL BACKGROUND

A few words on the historical background should provide a sense of perspective and a basis for comparison. Asylum for those suffering from diseases of the mind had been made available for many centuries both in the ancient world and in medieval times. If the lofty ideals of Platonic Greece and Christian charity played a part, as indeed they did, the patients must have been well cared for. It was when the State and other agencies took over from the Church that standards began to deteriorate and periodically the disclosure of the conditions under which some of the insane were housed produced a crop of reformers. Zeal for reform may be a mixed blessing, for it frequently sows the seed for the next reaction which may be as violent as the reform preceding it. This phenomenon has bedevilled progress in psychiatry and instead of a continuous line of development and enlightenment, one finds a chequered history.

The middle of the nineteenth century is often regarded as a particularly unenlightened era in psychiatry, yet this was a time when the extent of asylum building exceeded by far anything the National Health Service has done, to date, for all branches of medicine. Our present-day reformers have been severely critical of the buildings, pointing out that in some instances the architects were the same people who designed the county prisons. Yet most were attractively and certainly very well constructed and were surrounded, in many instances, by 500 acres of high quality farm land, stocked with pedigree cattle and with beautifully landscaped grounds which would have done credit to Capability Brown. In addition, they were designed to accommodate 200 patients and not the 1000 or more we pack into them today. The annual reports make interesting reading. Patients' rations were 6 oz. of meat, 2 oz. of cheese and 1 pint of ale per day, plus an extra 4 oz. of cheese and a second pint of ale if they worked on the farm. In an early report from one of these institutions, the medical superintendent replied to local criticism. Some of his patients while out for their Sunday walk had gone into the local inn and emerged the worse for drink and made a nuisance of themselves. He wrote to this effect: 'It has been suggested that they be deprived of this privilege. I would sooner resign my appointment than deprive my patients of privileges which are enjoyed by the ordinary citizen.' There can be very few such patient-orientated hospitals in present times; the more enlightened boast of being community-orientated and medical superintendents no longer talk of resigning. A final word about architecture should be reserved for the beautiful St Patrick's Hospital, Dublin, endowed by the celebrated Dean of St Patrick's, Jonathan Swift. The charter was obtained in 1746 and the first patients were admitted in 1757; it is still doing good work.

When Dr John Snow removed the handle from the parish pump, he set the pattern for the control of epidemics and it appeared natural that, with the subsequent success of isolation hospitals, mental illness should also be regarded as one of the plagues. Consequently the mentally ill, afflicted with the most personal of human ailments, were embraced by the great public health measures of the nineteenth century and came under the control of the epidemiologists and the public health departments, and the mental hospital era had arrived.

When one works in a large institution, one can become over-impressed with the size of the buildings, the stores, the farm, the workshops, the laundry and the staff quarters, and it may be difficult to envisage a comprehensive psychiatric service without such backing. This is especially so when the institution is under the direction of a medical superintendent who is regarded by the staff as the fount of all knowledge and the holder of all power. It is often more comfortable to accept the situation than to challenge it and even though the medical superintendent may try and destroy this image, such is the need for people working in an institution for an authoritative figure, that they recreate and maintain the image and will not allow the holder to forsake it.

Germany invaded Poland on 1st September 1939 and on 3rd September war was declared on Germany. Massive conscription created a large army and since putting a man in uniform did not confer on him immunity to psychiatric illness (rather the reverse), there was soon a great demand for doctors with psychiatric experience. A Director of Medical Services would decide that the army required a psychiatric hospital, would look at a map and put it —there! It had to have a Commanding Officer who was either a regular soldier or a member of the Territorial Army and therefore unlikely to be a psychiatrist. Such a unit was stationed in the Sinai Desert. The Commanding Officer knew no psychiatry and what was more important did not pretend he did, and as long as patients were well and efficiently treated there was no interference and the Army organization though not liberal was considerably less feudal than that existing in the civilian mental hospital. The clinical material was interesting, the staff adequate, certainly according to mental hospital establishments, and the standards of treatment, case conference and discussion were high. The closed wards were a bit of a joke, but with the Suez Canal on one side and the Sinai desert on the other, most patients preferred not to leave. In a short time, the mystique of the mental hospital was broken. If the Army could create a psychiatric unit, admitting and treating every kind of mental illness occurring in divers nationalities, enemy and allied, male and female, and retain patients for periods up to three years and run it efficiently, similar experiments could be successful in civilian life. It was apparent that there was nothing magical in the physical structure or personnel arrangements of the mental hospital; all that was needed were adequately trained staff and suitable accommodation. The work could be done practically anywhere; in the wing or ward of a general hospital, in a hospital community or in fact at the edge of the Sinai desert. The Army sited its hospitals near to population centres, encouraged out-patient consultation and treatment, pioneered group therapy, psychodrama and continuous narcosis in this country and developed abreactive techniques, and in the six years of war created the medium for a continuous stream of original publications.

This new experience, however, was not the sole factor in promoting psychiatric services outside the mental hospital. As frequently happens, lay people were earlier in the field. In 1912, a group of Birmingham business people called a meeting which was attended by the Lord Mayor, who said that in this age of the internal combustion engine and the telephone, their workpeople were being subjected to stresses which caused illness which should be treated elsewhere than in the asylum. Medical opinion as represented by the British Medical Association opposed the creation of a new hospital, saying there was no need as everything was already provided, but the lay people were unconvinced and decided to go ahead for an experimental period of one year and founded the Midland Nerve Hospital. After a year, they declared they were satisfied there was a real need. Just before the Second World War, some London teaching hospitals started their own psychiatric departments and provincial medical schools followed suit; in a few years there were general hospital administered psychiatric departments in most medical centres. The introduction of effective physical treatments and the discovery of readily recoverable psychiatric illness accelerated the process and as beds were in short supply and most of these units had started as Out-Patient Clinics, they readily developed services which would save admissions. The teaching of psychiatry improved as medical students had access to patients who were representative of psychiatric illness in the community, while the patients had the benefit of treatment near their homes, in clinics which were adequately staffed with both nurses and doctors.

There are now two main streams of reform: (*a*) the mental hospital, which is undergoing a change, and (*b*) the development of psychiatric services within the general hospital. Between them lie many intermediate schemes but when the whole picture is surveyed, reform in a National Health Service, which presumably allocates an equal share of finance and resources to each area, depends on a variety of factors not all designed to meet the patient's needs. In fact, in mental hospital legislation, the patient has usually been the 'forgotten man' in the administrative arrangements for his psychiatric treatment. He has been regarded as a member of a catchment area and has been directed to the institution which has assumed responsibility for that area. He has never been asked if he would prefer these arrangements and has had to wait till a medical administrator has had a change of heart before an alternative could be provided. Where there is a choice, he and his family usually prefer the less elaborate, and frequently less physically attractive facilities of the general hospital. No persuasive propaganda is required, for he is going where the vast majority of sick people go for treatment. Planning authorities are just beginning to realize that in an enfranchized community they cannot and should not ignore the preferences of patients and their relatives.

Expediency is the main issue in determining the nature and location of psychiatric services and this can depend on such factors as existing buildings, population density, transport arrangements, regional and local organizations, size of city or town, and personalities both in the lay and medical fields. Patients' needs, though obviously the most important, unfortunately do not enjoy the highest priority and there are still anomalies such as towns with populations of 100,000 and even 300,000 with no in-patient psychiatric services and patients and their relatives having to travel to some outlandish spot miles from their homes. An obsession with available buildings can create a situation where patients from mental hospitals in busy industrial areas are removed for rehabilitation to an inaccessible place remote from relatives and the very industries which formerly employed the patients and which could play an essential part in their rehabilitation.

Comprehensive community mental health services are the delight of public health administrators and some medical superintendents, who believe they can satisfy the needs of all the patients within their area. They pre-suppose that all psychiatric illness will be referred to their centres as directed, and though they may claim to be liberal, at the same time they deny patients the privilege of choice. It is an interesting aspect of what is called a free society where patients are neatly parcelled off in catchment areas and served by a central authority which decides where and by whom the patients will be treated. When the war-time expedients of national food and clothing rationing have long since been abandoned, and no one would dream of inaugurating a national housing, entertainment, holiday, school or church service, people still talk in terms of a national mental health service, assuming that the most personal problems of the people are amenable to the public health approach. But in a free society, alternatives eventually become available, the more enterprising use them, and the neat catchment area is broken. Apart from those who seek treatment elsewhere, there must be large numbers of psychotic citizens in boarding houses, private hotels and in their own homes, who, thanks to the liberties we still possess, can live out their psychotic lives without having to declare themselves. It is not without interest that where there is a semblance of a comprehensive service, it is located in a medium-sized city, with a population of 200,000–300,000, with one mental hospital under the direction of an energetic medical superintendent, whose authority has prevented the development of alternative services.

DEVELOPMENTS IN SOCIAL PSYCHIATRY

INSIDE THE MENTAL HOSPITAL

'Breaking up the Mental Hospital'

Baker (1958, 1961) criticizes the size of present mental hospitals and suggests an optimum size of 200–300 beds which could be divided into small functioning units. The measure would be a temporary one till new and smaller units could be built, but in the meantime, by breaking up the mental hospital, instead of one large unwieldy hospital, there would be the equivalent of three or more complete units each with its own administrative and independent medical staff. He predicted, correctly, a reduction in the need for beds once the out-patient services were developed and a new and enthusiastic mood had swept through the hospital. While the general hospital psychiatrist might consider this dividing up of the mental hospital as a very limited approach to the problem, it was probably as much as could be done under the circumstances and paved the way to further developments. That the time for experiment was ripe had been emphasized by the studies of Garratt *et al.* (1958) who after assessing the medical and social needs of 3555 patients in Birmingham mental hospitals, concluded that only 13 per cent needed the full range of hospital facilities; 75 per cent needed only limited hospital services such as supervision because of their mental state or basic nursing; 12 per cent required none of the facilities traditionally associated with hospitals. They suggested that these classes should be accommodated in separate units and in view of the high proportion of ambulant patients, proposed an entirely new concept of hospital structure. Tooth and Brook (1961) in an analysis of mental hospital population concluded that there had been a running down of long-stay patients and a more rapid turnover of short-stay patients and that total bed needs was likely to continue to fall.

The structure of the population in mental hospitals was also changing and Norton (1961) supported the view that total numbers would fall because of the decrease in the number of schizophrenics becoming chronic. He demonstrated that dementia had now replaced schizophrenia as the commonest cause of a stay in hospital of more than two years. He predicted that 'If, in addition, changes in national policy are effective, mental hospitals may perhaps be reduced to one-quarter of their present size'. While much of the decline in the mental hospital population was due to the energy and devotion of medical and nursing staff, it should be appreciated that there were other developments which were having their effect and these will be dealt with in detail later.

Administrative Therapy

This is the term given by Clark (1958) to the role of the medical superintendent in the modern mental hospital. He defines it as:

> the art (perhaps some day to be a science) of treating psychiatric patients in a mental hospital by administrative action. Group therapy developed from individual therapy; administrative therapy is treatment of a much larger group—the hospital. It draws on the knowledge and skills of psychiatry and group psychotherapy, the experience of the professional administrator, and the accumulating contributions of the social anthropologist.

He lists four main facets: (1) organization of the patient's life, (2) staff organization, (3) medical organization, (4) community leadership. In a later paper (Clark, 1960), he elaborates this theme and states:

> Do something new every three months—it doesn't matter what you do, but do something new and keep them thinking! The administrative therapist's task is not to be a creator but a selector, seeing which projects are to be encouraged and which given scope and which deferred; he acts like a telephone operator, selecting those communications which are of immediate value and passing them through, choosing which are to wait for a time and which should be ignored.

The background for this movement is not confined to recent advances in psychiatric practice, but also stems from the challenge to the authority of the medical superintendent, particularly with the grading of some medical staff as consultants and their insistence that they have complete charge of their patients. Medical superintendents have varied in their reactions; some have welcomed the sharing or delegation of responsibility, while others have resisted any encroachment on their authority and have produced a variety of arguments in order to maintain the *status quo*. There are no doubt certain situations which may arise in a mental hospital, where one designated person should have the authority to make a decision, but it has been suggested that if it has to be a medical man, he should be the chairman of the medical staff, elected by them and accountable to them. The last has not yet been heard of this controversy and 'administrative therapy' is probably the most plausible apologia yet offered, but a system where rank is conspicuous has its dangers. This point was well illustrated by Fox (1951) in his Croonian Lecture: '... In a hierarchy where everyone is clearly labelled and wears a uniform, it is difficult for the bishop to believe that he may be less valuable than the parish priest'.

When large institutions are replaced by smaller general hospital units, the administrative therapist will become redundant. Until then, an energetic and talented medical administrator still has a role to play, but he need not claim that an unfortunate anachronism in our modern society is something desirable and worth preserving.

The Therapeutic Community

As it is recognized in Britain the therapeutic community is usually an adaptation, sometimes very free, of experiments conducted at Belmont Hospital by Jones (1952). He made a brave effort to rehabilitate the hitherto incorrigible psychopath by trying to develop a group morality which would prove acceptable. The following summary of his techniques is taken from Crockett (1960):

1. A relatively ordinary and familiar social environment is provided for the patient so far as relationships are concerned. This means minimizing any social factor in the process of hospital care or treatment which emphasizes differences from social life outside the hospital.
2. The patient is made increasingly aware of the effect of his behaviour on other people, and so obtains some degree of social insight.
3. The whole population of the clinical unit concerned takes part in regular community meetings as a matter of therapeutic technique.
4. Trained staff enter into as many as possible of the diverse and fluctuating group situations, including informal (and unplanned) as well as formal social and therapeutic groups. By this means, together with the unifying influence of the community meetings, psycho-therapeutic treatment is applied over the whole 24 hours, and is not limited to, say, a formal daily, or perhaps weekly, psychotherapeutic session.
5. The authority structure of the unit is 'flattened' in such a way as to allow patients and staff members with lesser responsibilities to share authority. This process involves blurring of staff roles, when seen from the uninformed point of view of the patient, but requires sharper understanding of role-playing by the staff.
6. The freest possible channels of communication are created between the individuals, both staff and patients, who make up the community.

Crockett (1960) remarks that 'A permissive interpretative agnostic regime of this kind is almost the opposite of the administrative therapist's approach', and, in an effort to reconcile the two roles of the clinician and the administrator has drawn up the table on the following page. Crockett concludes that there are three types of administration in medicine:

1. Clinical, which is every doctor's responsibility.

2. Supportive, which should be lay and is designed to facilitate clinical administration.

3. Administrative therapy which he defines as 'the expression of a doctor's personality in the control of therapeutic situations at second hand' and which he considers is out of place in a hospital.

Obligations of the Clinician	*Obligations of the Supportive Hospital Administrator*
To establish good understanding with the patient, and use it as profitably as possible on his behalf.	To ascertain the requirements of the clinician, and provide the resources requested.
To judge the material and psychological needs of the patient.	To advise the clinician on, and take delegated responsibility for, the day-to-day administrative arrangements within the hospital.
To satisfy these needs (*i.e.* treat).	
To inform the administrators what is required for proper treatment, and of any imbalance or deficiencies in the resources available.	To advise the clinician on any established administrative circumstances which may affect clinical work (mainly policy, or financial limitations).
To decide the order of priority for administrative action when necessary.	To collaborate with the clinician in modifying such established administrative limitations when clinically appropriate.

The therapeutic community has now gained a vogue with the result that it is being introduced into all manner of situations such as admission units in mental hospitals and into mental hospitals themselves. Martin (1962) was the trend-setter in the mental hospital world and Lightbody and Jacobson (1965) reported the adaptation of his experiment to the acute admission unit of a mental hospital and conclude that it provides an open forum for emotional conflict, for role-playing and for venting disgust, aggressiveness, negative opinion and for all the varied play of social activity and its effects upon the individuals. They advise the importance of steering a middle course between excessive permissiveness and excessive direction.

Stallard (1966) gives the following excellent definition of the role of the therapeutic community:

> By having a structure which allows a considerable degree of control and which counteracts forces of disruption, and which at the same time allows considerable understanding of the forces at work, whether in an individual, in a particular group, or from faulty staff performance, crises can be used constructively and can be important learning experiences for participants.

As with intensive psychotherapy, it was claimed that all patients would benefit, and the structure of the therapeutic community is now being advocated for all psychiatric disturbances. It may be a useful manoeuvre in getting a variety of people to live together for some time but it will have to justify itself as a *therapeutic* agent in comparison with other techniques. Does it get depressives, phobic anxieties, schizophrenics, obsessionals, etc. better quicker and for longer? It is the answer to this question which will decide its future in psychiatric treatment, but the answer is not yet available.

Industrial Therapy

This is the name given to a variety of measures designed to fit the long-stay patient in the mental hospital for work in the community. As is so common in this field, it is really a new name for an old idea. In a country where the major industry was agriculture, farm work was regarded as the logical means of rehabilitation, but in a machine age, the factory is the greatest employer of labour and the accent has been shifted from the farm to the workshop. The question may be asked why in the 1960's this emphasis on industrial therapy should become very popular, when it would have been equally applicable half a century before. In fact there has been a steady development over the years with changes in types of occupational therapy, but now it is more highly organized and, with the blessing of the trade unions, more highly publicized. During the Second World War, it was offensive to some military surgeons to see soldiers who were recovering from wounds, going through the usual motions of remedial exercises or indulging in the traditional activities of the occupational therapy department. They devised a series of exercises which had a military or para-military flavour, such as throwing dummy hand-grenades for stiff shoulders or stripping a Bren gun to mobilize fingers and wrists. These became popular in convalescent depots and were claimed to speed up recovery and return to duty. It may be that the patients were imbued with the tremendous zest and enthusiasm which accompanied such a regimen or were in a hurry to get back to the comparative peace of real soldiering. It certainly gave to the organizers a feeling that they were playing a positive part in the war effort, which, in a unit remote from the battle area, had its compensations. With the present emphasis on increasing production and international competition in trade, it would appear that some enthusiasts were preparing the mental hospitals of the country for entry into the 'Common Market', and according to reports not without success.

Industrial rehabilitation for the sick and injured was given formal recognition by the passing of the Disabled Persons Act (1944), which permitted registration of people who had physical and mental disabilities, and gave them some priority in employment, in that factories employing more than 20 people had to have 3 per cent who were on the Disabled Persons' Register. The Ministry of Labour and National Service opened its first Industrial Rehabilitation Unit (I.R.U.) at Egham, Surrey in 1943 as an experiment but it was not long before the idea spread to the rest of the country and there were soon 14 other units sited near the major industrial centres. Egham is entirely residential, with 200 places, but most of the others are non-residential and both sexes are accepted with a length of stay varying from 6 to 12 weeks during which time efforts are made to assess the handicaps and potentials of those referred. A form is completed (D.P.I.) by the doctor who is referring the patient, who is then interviewed by a Disablement Rehabilitation Officer (D.R.O.) and when a vacancy has been found, he is given a medical and psychological examination and his progress through the course is carefully supervised. Some may be selected for special training in trades or crafts where there is a national or local shortage of labour, thus giving the handicapped person a real advantage in the labour market. Psychiatric illness is included among those disabilities which are accepted by the I.R.U., though some maintain an unofficial quota system as they feel the unit loses its balance if too heavily loaded with psychiatric patients.

Jones (1956) describes an experiment in which selected mental patients still under treatment in institutions attended an I.R.U. daily. Two hundred and eight were selected and 154 completed the course; of these 130 (84 per cent) were placed either in employment or training, which compares with a national average for all disabilities of 83 per cent. A six-months' follow-up of those national figures yielded a 67 per cent success rate, while the psychiatric figures yielded a success rate of 65 per cent. Of even greater interest were the success rates of the different psychiatric categories. Mental defectives had the highest placement rate (93 per cent) and after six months, 68 per cent of these were satisfactorily settled. Psychotics (including manic-depressive, schizophrenic and paranoid states) had a placement rate of 87 per cent of whom 71 per cent were satisfactory after six months. Psychoneurotics had a placement rate of 75 per cent with 59 per cent as satisfactory after six months. Jones considers that 'there seems to be an excellent case for referring selected mental defectives and psychotics while still in hospital to I.R.Us. to prepare them for the kind of work environment that they will meet when they leave hospital. . . .' It is of interest that psychiatric patients when properly selected benefit as much from the I.R.U. as patients with medical and surgical handicaps.

Mental hospitals have on the whole preferred to do their own 'Industrial Therapy' and this has been dictated by a variety of factors. Some have tried to extend the system to the more unlikely patients who would probably not have been accepted for training by the I.R.U.; others have used it as the modern man's answer to occupational therapy and probably to meet a shortage of occupational therapists, while some, like Early (1960), have shown an enthusiasm for competition in the industrial market that our industrialists might emulate. His unit's administration reads like a board of directors, the chairman being the chairman of the Engineering and Allied Employers' West of England Association, and members of the board include the Lord Mayor of Bristol, directors of leading firms in the city, the president of the Bristol Trades Council and the regional and local secretaries of the Transport and General Workers Union. The whole concern is run in a business-like manner and the Industrial Therapy Organization (I.T.O.) has developed a car wash service in Bristol which has been much admired and envied. Bennet *et al.* (1961) advocate a special resettlement unit which makes use of the local I.R.U. and continues to house the patient after he has found a job. They sensibly state: 'Resettlement is more than discharge; more even than the prevention of readmission. It aims to restore the patient to the most satisfactory way of life of which he is capable, despite his disabilities.' It is all very exciting and symptomatic of the new enthusiasm in the mental hospital and a number of chronic patients have been rehabilitated; but once the slack has been taken up and the recoverable are recovered and only the hard core remains, it will prove a severe test for the method and its enthusiasts. It is of course also dependent on an expanding economy with full employment.

Expansion of Services

This measure has given some mental hospitals a new lease of life. Some of these developments have been in fields which have by tradition become regarded as the legitimate province of the mental hospital, such as the establishment of an EEG department, which serves the general hospital as well, or the provision of a child psychiatric unit with paediatric associations, or those with well-developed laboratories have become the central laboratory service of a hospital group. Geriatrics, epileptic units and neurosurgery have been accommodated by mental hospitals and some have gone further and incorporated whole general hospitals. This last move is again not a new thing, for during the Second World War whole hospitals or special units were evacuated to mental hospitals, but with the cessation of hostilities there was a gradual return to their former location. McKeown's (1958) concept of a balanced hospital community has inspired authorities to group general hospitals in the grounds of mental hospitals and Smith (1961) has advocated and to a certain extent has implemented such a scheme at Lancaster Moor Hospital. This arrangement has much to commend it for it claims to break the isolation of psychiatry from general medicine, to avoid duplication of services such as X-ray, pathology and biochemistry and to ensure a better trained nurse. As long as the patients are not too remote from their homes and relatives, there would appear to be distinct advantages, but there are also disadvantages. It assumes that the present structure of the mental hospital is satisfactory for the needs of a modern community and there is a danger that because of expediency, such as availability of land or out-moded capital assets such as the institutional buildings, a more enlightened policy may be obstructed for very many years.

A balanced hospital community is open to wide differences in interpretation. Should it include all forms and degrees of sickness? Should it be limited to those sicknesses where all the facilities of skilled investigation and treatment are necessary? Should balance and comprehensiveness outweigh geographical and other considerations, which in the long run may have a greater bearing on early effective treatment and recovery? Balance need not mean integration for if one speciality is over-represented, it may be extruded from the hospital community. There is an optimum size of psychiatric unit which can be integrated adequately and one has still to learn what this size should be. Lastly it should not become a device to perpetuate the life of a mental hospital whose size and very existence is now a matter for general regret.

The Open Door

This is an example of an old idea under its old name, but heralded as something which if not new, is at least revolutionary. Tuke (1882) in his *History of the Insane in the British Isles* devoted a whole chapter to the 'Open Door System' and at the beginning of the twentieth century there were hospitals on both sides of the Atlantic where the doors were not locked. A closed door can be a source of irritation or a challenge to a patient and to keep one needlessly behind lock and key is inhuman and therefore unjustifiable. Stern

(1957), in a paper entitled 'Operation Sesame' enthusiastically advocates its advantages and makes a plea for 100 per cent open hospitals.

At this stage, one may ask why, if open doors had a vogue over 50 years ago, they lapsed and had to be revived? One should also take into account that during this half-century there was an increasing number of effective drugs to assist the psychiatrist in controlling the aggressive and impulsive patient. It can only be that the 'Open Door' became a fetish and was divorced from the accurate clinical assessment of the needs of each patient. Tragedies must have resulted as indeed they are occurring today and a reaction set in, which probably swung too much the other way. But reformers are frequently blind to the dangers of their reform; they can only see the benefits and it is not surprising that some tragedies have stemmed from 'Open Door' hospitals. Sometimes the 'Open Door' is an agreeable fiction, for there are enough staff to see that the patient does not take advantage of it; sometimes it can be a danger to the patient who, because of mental infirmity, is incapable of coping with his new found freedom. It should not be regarded as a panacea but as an adjunct to successful therapy, the patient having first been rendered fit for the 'Open Door'. It is true that such a decision is often a very difficult one to make but, in the interests of the patient and the community, it cannot be evaded by adopting a catch-phrase like the 'Open Door'. Because of the high re-admission rate of mental hospitals, the 'Open Door' has been called by some the 'Revolving Door'.

The Team System

This has been advocated by Kidd (1961) in an attempt to bring the mental hospital into line with general hospital practice where the consultant is in charge of beds, sees his own out-patients, does his own domiciliary consultations, and is assisted by various grades of junior staff. Prior to the National Health Act of 1948 there was only one specialist in the mental hospital who was officially recognized, namely the medical superintendent, the other doctors holding only 'acting rank'. This led to anomalies. Some doctors were trained and practised exclusively on the female or male side of the hospital yet would have patients of both sexes referred to them as out-patients. Kidd states:

> . . . The patient is often referred to a psychiatric clinic rather than to a named consultant. If the patient is to have out-patient treatment, he will probably continue to be treated by the doctor who originally saw him. But if the patient

is to be admitted to hospital he will probably find himself under the care of another doctor, and he has to go through the whole business of once again telling his story. If he is transferred to a different type of ward, he will find himself under yet another doctor; and finally, when he leaves hospital, the letters to his general practitioner were, until lately, often signed by yet another person—the medical superintendent.

Kidd used some of the methods suggested by Baker (1958), *i.e.* breaking up his mental hospital into three units of 300 heds, with each medical team responsible for male and female, admission and long-stay wards and doing its own out-patient sessions. The team system extended to nursing staff, social workers and chaplain, and Kidd makes the point that each unit became so independent that the administrative officers felt they were dealing with three medical superintendents. '. . . the chief male nurse and matron felt they were being by-passed and not informed on matters which concerned them.' Authority was restored by again underlining the functions of the medical superintendent. It did not occur to them to try, even for an experimental period, to abolish the posts of the medical superintendent and the other senior administrators. It would be most refreshing to read of such an experiment and study the results.

OUTSIDE THE MENTAL HOSPITAL

At least as much has been happening outside the mental hospital. Some experiments have been initiated by the mental hospitals themselves, while others have stemmed from sources which were entirely independent.

Studies of Discharged Patients from Mental Hospitals

These must take into account the environment to which the patient returns as well as the milieu in which he has spent many years of his life, namely the mental hospital. The subject has become increasingly important for with the development of local authority services and a passion for discharge and reluctance to re-admit on behalf of the mental hospital, one must try and learn whether the recent decline in mental hospital populations is one which is likely to continue and whether community tolerance is adequate to cope with those who have been discharged. Brown *et al.* (1958) in an enquiry into patients who had spent more than two years in mental hospitals found that 68 per cent succeeded in staying out of hospital for at least a year, and of these 66 per cent were rated as showing either full or partial social adjustment. Success was associated with clinical state on discharge, subsequent employment and the social group to which they returned. The vast majority were schizophrenics and those who went to stay with siblings or in lodgings did better than those who went to parents, wives or large hostels. Social liability was also assessed and more than half were rated as minimal or nil, but the authors stress the need for supportive social work with the ex-patients and their families.

Hostel Accommodation

This is now being provided for the discharged patient by many local authorities as part of their responsibility for the prophylaxis and after-care of mental illness as recommended in the Mental Health Act of 1959. The staffing need not be as elaborate as that in the mental hospital and the patient is given an opportunity to test himself out in the community while at the same time being under some supervision. It also ensures that prescribed drugs are being taken, that out-patient appointments are kept, and it provides the patient with a sheltered environment which has been called the half-way house. Such hostels may serve the psychiatric units of general hospitals as well as mental hospitals as they are more economical than hospital beds. Some are run entirely by the mental hospital but generally they are local authority controlled. The need for a half-way house is not only for the rapidly recovering patient who is almost ready to take his place in the community, but is absolutely essential for the treatment of social disability which is usually the greatest handicap in the rehabilitation of the chronic schizophrenic. Hemphill (1960) writes:

> The highly artificial, if comfortable and protective social life of the mental hospital, in which normal motivation disappears, undoubtedly produces an effect, even in the first few days after admission. While this may not be so important in the affective psychoses in which quick or spontaneous recovery is usual, it may be disastrous in schizophrenia.
>
> Thought disorder, verbal disability, and psychotic isolation hinder communication and promote the lack of interest patients have for one another. For example, two intelligent patients suffering from long-standing schizophrenia shared a room for some years but neither troubled to ascertain the name of the other. In contrast, they were both interested in and well informed about members of the staff in whose departments they worked.
>
> In the life of large groups, without responsibility and deprived of the elemental privacies that are characteristic of a normal environment, with continuous exposure to protective mental-hospital routine and the example of others, social sense is stifled and the patient then accepts as his norm the condition in which he finds himself. This seems to be more disabling than prolonged immobilization after a fracture or illness would be in the functional sense. The pattern of the mental hospital, stamped into the patient's mental life

during the acute or plastic stages of the illness, plus disuse, may make it impossible for him ever to re-establish himself fully at a normal level. The life of the patient after the acute stage has passed is determined mainly by domestic conditions, hospital design and administrative custom. If these could be altered realistically early enough, social disorientation might be prevented.

Because of this he makes a plea for the psychiatric half-way hostel. It should not escape the notice of the reader that in this plea there is also a tremendous indictment of the part the mental hospital has played in the past in the aetiology of the socially deteriorated schizophrenic and if not structured differently will carry its malign influence into the future.

Day Hospitals

These are reputed to have been started in Britain by Joshua Bierer (Harper, 1959; Bierer, 1959), when he opened what was called the Social Psychotherapy Centre in Hampstead, in 1947, and attributed the theoretical basis of the unit to Adlerian psychology (Bierer, 1951). Harris (1957) in an account of the history of the day hospital attributes its innovation to Soviet Russia in the 1920's and Dr Ewen Cameron had started a day hospital in Montreal in 1940. The name does not really matter, but it has become popular and though many clinics may have had patients attending daily for treatment and supervision long before Bierer, Cameron or for that matter the Russians thought of the day hospital, it is considered to be something new. It may be that the present enthusiasm is a reaction against the traditional concept of a hospital, *i.e.* a place where patients lie in bed, day and night and doctors stand at the foot of the bed for a minute or so each day. The day hospital concept may do more to revolutionize the general hospital than the mental hospital, for it does emphasize that a hospital is not only a place where patients are treated, but where they live and that it is also a place where staff work and that adequate arrangements for both patients and staff are essential.

Though a number of mental hospitals are now running day hospitals, it has proportionately been used to a greater extent by psychiatric units in general hospitals, and Farndale (1961) in a survey of day hospitals in Britain reported that they were sited mainly in London, Birmingham, Bristol and Manchester, while elsewhere their emergence was scanty or non-existent. Harris (1957) in his report on the Maudsley Day Hospital, found that running costs were approximately one-third of an in-patient unit of similar size and Craft (1959) in a report on the same unit, claimed that the most suitable patients were those with psychoneurosis and depression.

Some day hospitals were an organic growth of the psychiatric units they served. Such was the case in the Department of Psychological Medicine of the United Birmingham Hospitals where it was essential to maintain close supervision on a number of patients who were capable of sleeping at home, and because of a scarcity of psychiatric beds and in the interests of economy, it was decided to have them attend daily. This practice continued long before the formal day hospital was built and was used for the rehabilitation of post-leucotomy patients, the continued treatment of schizophrenics, and the re-education of the severe case of phobic anxiety as well as for depressed patients whose families were at work and could not give them adequate supervision during the day. Here the day hospital proved its worth before it was built and it was the need for extra space and facilities which determined its official creation. Born out of expediency, it has continued to function with a flexibility which has made for economy and efficiency. Patients' attendances are geared to their essential psychiatric needs and social circumstances. There are no rigid times set for attendance; patients may come for one day or five days a week and if progress is rapid, return to work is encouraged even though the patient has hardly been integrated into a psychotherapeutic group. Such flexibility requires other services such as a well-staffed out-patient department with the consultant in charge of the patient attending three or four times per week and preferably on one or two occasions outside normal working hours. These services are described below in greater detail. Nearly the whole range of psychiatric treatment can be undertaken and it would be simpler to state those that are excluded. Apart from leucotomy and continuous narcosis, it is usually the patient rather than his treatment that decides admission to hospital. It may be for observation requiring night as well as day reports; for physical investigations which cannot be done on an out-patient basis; for physical disability such as a recent coronary occlusion or hemiplegia which would make out-patient electroplexy hazardous or for patients with drug sensitivities which may require urgent, intensive, in-patient treatment.

Some psychiatrists prefer to maintain a uniform group in the day hospital and plan the course of treatment over a period of not less than three months. This implies a certain rigidity of attitude, at least as far as time is concerned, but does permit greater use of group techniques which would be disrupted by the more flexible methods already described.

Much will depend on the type of patient selected. Some mental hospitals have used the day hospital almost exclusively as attendance centres for discharged schizophrenics and these will naturally attend for longer than three months. It has been claimed that even if the patient does not achieve full social recovery, it is more economical to deal with him in this way than to retain him in the mental hospital, but it is also better therapy, for he has the stimulus of getting to and from the place, of using public transport and generally beginning to live the life of a normal citizen. There is a danger that these units may become institutions and develop the faults of those they were intended to replace for there is a marked tendency in this country towards 'institutionalization'. Well-intentioned enthusiasts are frequently not satisfied with providing the orthodox treatments, but must extend their activities to cover the whole of the patient's day. The ordinary amenities of society are ignored and in a short time the day hospital is running its own cinema, library, evening classes, dances, whist drives and the rest. Some patients, it is true, are not yet ready to enter into these recreations outside the day hospital, but it is tempting, once an amenity has been created to perpetuate its use. It is better for the staff to take the patients along to the local cinema, museum and library and secure their membership of local societies which generally go out of their way to help. Some training may be required initially, and there is a place for out-patient social clubs, but these must be seen as vehicles for closer integration into the community and not as an end in themselves.

Day hospitals have their problems and Chasin (1967) who based his conclusions on his work at the Massachusetts Mental Health Centre lists some special problems he encountered.

1. Difficulty in evaluating patient who is home for most of the time.
2. The responsibility of supervising patients with potential for destruction and suicide.
3. Some patients found it too easy to remain indefinitely in the comforts of day hospitalization.
4. Difficulty in getting patients to come in the morning and leave in the afternoon.

The 150 patients reviewed consisted of 64 schizophrenics and 35 personality disorders with only 20 affective psychoses. It is likely that this distribution was responsible for most of the problems. Selection of patient is extremely important and the Day Hospital should be seen as an extension of the In-Patient Department and not a special independent unit. In the author's clinic the psychiatrist who sees the patient initially supervises his treatment as out-patient, in-patient and at the day hospital and uses each agency according to the patient's needs. He is aware of the impact the unit will make on the patient and that of the patient on the unit and excludes the incompatible. In consequence the problems listed above rarely apply. There is also a much greater number of affective disturbances treated and this raises the morale of the unit. High morale is one of the most important factors in successful treatment.

Out-patient Departments

These can range from a session held once a week at the mental hospital or in a nearby general hospital, to a fully equipped unit with all facilities for treatment, including occupational therapy department, psychological laboratory, group therapy and out-patient social club. It was realized over 60 years ago that patients with mental illness could not be treated adequately in isolation and the Midland Nerve Hospital, founded in 1912, was originally an out-patient unit.

Adolf Meyer in 1913 (Meyer, 1952) stated:

> The great future of Psychiatry lies in the extension of the work beyond the hospital walls, but with the full experience that only hospitals can furnish. For this it will be necessary to look to the State hospitals not merely as Asylums but as centres of the Mental Health Work of the Community. They must be manned by physicians trained to meet that task. To attract those who are in need of help they must establish out-patient departments to which teachers and physicians can send those who are not at their best but not in need of hospital care.
>
> We want to get out-patient departments and through them create a feeling in the community that our special hospitals are places for help, places from which to get the guidance of experience and directions as to prevention.
>
> In some communities it would be best to organize special mental organizations, using the available dispensaries as far as possible, doing emergency work and work in the form of after-care and placing of patients returned from hospitals, and serving as advisers in the decisions as to where to place patients or where to direct them.
>
> The ideal arrangement would be to have in connection with the dispensary at least one physician able to visit homes, assisted by Social Workers trained for investigation and for giving guidance to the patient and to the family and social unit.
>
> I want to urge upon you especially, that the numbers of physicians must be large enough for the hospitals to spare, once or twice a week, one or more members of the staff who will go out as dispensary physicians to community centres at distances from the hospital. My way of arranging that would be to have every ambitious hospital physician trained so that he can be sent out on certain afternoons to do extramural work in one of the centres of the district, where he will see the after-care and preventive cases together with local members of the profession who might take an interest in these conditions and work as local dispensary physicians.

Adolf Meyer if he were alive today would have mixed feelings. He would be bitterly disappointed with some clinics where the out-patient service hardly merits the name but would be astounded at others where the whole hospital has practically been turned over to out-patient treatment. It would sadden him to see that the earliest and now most comprehensive services did not emerge from the State hospitals as he envisaged, but from general hospitals, which because of their closeness to the community have better understood its needs.

Emergency Treatment Units

The model of short-stay intensive care beds in general hospitals has been transferred to psychiatric hospitals, but the exercise is called 'crisis-intervention'. Weisman *et al.* (1969) established their unit at the Connecticut Mental Health Center and used a 3-day in-patient programme with a 30-day out-patient follow-up. Of those admitted, 82 per cent were able to return to the community, while 18 per cent required transfer to longer-term hospitals. Follow-up showed that a further 19 per cent were readmitted for longer care within a year of discharge. Unless the population were largely a chronic hospital one, these figures are not good and suggest that a rapid 3-day programme cannot possibly cater for all the patients' needs. Management is as important as treatment, and for many, three days as an in-patient are not enough. Another week or two may have been enough to consolidate progress and this is very much the author's experience.

The District Mental Health Service

This approximates most closely to what Adolf Meyer had in mind and it has been described by Carse *et al.* (1958). It is firmly based on the mental hospital and by ignoring local government boundaries, can range over the whole area the hospital serves. The patient is referred to the service by his family doctor. A psychiatrist then visits the patient in his home, or if the patient prefers it, he can be seen at the out-patient department which is held at the local general hospital. Treatment, if necessary, can be conducted either by further domiciliary visits or at the day hospital, and those patients who need hospital admission, such as for prefrontal leucotomy and continuous narcosis, are taken into the base unit which is the mental hospital. It was found that four out of every five could be treated as out-patients and it also helped to keep down the number of elderly people admitted. In a further report on the first two years of the scheme, Dr Carse wrote:

> In the very early days of the Worthing Experiment, I learned somewhat to my consternation, that the man or woman I saw in hospital bore little resemblance to that same man or woman at home. At home, even though he was a sick man, he retained his identity and the sense of belonging; he was with his family and he felt secure because he was still in the community which he knew and which he understood. In hospital, the patient is an enforced member of a group living in an entirely artificial environment bearing no resemblance to anything approaching ordinary home life, but where everything is strange and often frightening . . . I cannot believe that it is helpful in treatment for our patients to be compelled to live as a member of a large group of strangers all of whom are sick people, to be completely deprived of privacy and to have to submit to the segregation of the sexes.

This type of service still has the defects of the 'base' mental hospital. If it is undesirable to admit patients to it for conditions which can be treated elsewhere, then it should be generally undesirable to admit patients to such a unit, and an alternative should be found. In fact with this syphoning off of most of the readily recoverable, it is even more iniquitous to admit those few whose treatment cannot yet be provided outside the institution. It also gives cause for reflection that a whole sector of a population had to wait till 1958 before it could enjoy some of the benefits of out-patient treatment which had been available to other sections of the population for many years.

Measuring Need and Evaluating Services

It is of interest to scrutinize what experts are saying about Psychiatric Hospital Care. With the change in attitude from hospital-based to community-based psychiatry, Matthew (1971) states that a need for medical care exists when an individual has an illness or disability for which there is effective and acceptable treatment or care. It can be defined either in terms of the type of illness or disability causing the need or of the treatment or facilities for treatment required to meet it. A demand for care exists when an individual considers that he has a need and wishes to receive care. Utilization occurs when an individual actually receives care. Need is not necessarily expressed as demand and demand is not necessarily followed by utilization, while, on the other hand, there can be demand and utilization without real underlying need for the particular service used.

Comment: This is a fair statement of the problem but its lessons are, unfortunately, frequently overlooked by clinicians and planners.

Community Care

This is very close to the District Mental Health Service, but is more closely linked to the Local Authority through the Medical Officer of Health. It is likely to become increasingly important especially as the Mental Health Act, 1959, considers the local authority responsible for the prophylaxis and after-care of mental illness and though this duty is not yet mandatory, it may well become so. In certain cities like Nottingham (Macmillan, 1958) and Amsterdam (Querido, 1955) there is very close cooperation between the mental hospital and the local health authority and a comprehensive service is provided. May (1961) lists the services that are offered:

> 1. *General Measures.* These include reassurance and encouragement from general practitioner, from social worker, health visitor or out-patient nurse, and from the psychiatrist; together with tolerance and understanding from relatives.
> 2. *Palliative measures* by means of drugs or psychotherapy which by early alleviation of symptoms will encourage both the patient and his relatives.
> 3. *Specific measures*, with electrotherapy, phenothiazine drugs, and so on, must be undertaken where possible to abolish symptoms and permit stable readjustment within the community. Treatment is usually lengthy, as in chronic physical disease, and patient and relatives must often be prepared to accept a slow recovery.

He stresses that:

> *Positive indications* for community care rest on a firm diagnosis of mild to moderate illness which can be adequately treated outside hospital with the facilities locally available. It should be possible to modify domestic, financial, or other environmental stress without removing the patient. The cooperation of the patient and his relatives must be ensured, and the patient should not be denied intimate and sympathetic social contacts while he is at home.

He sounds a warning that as public interest has been awakened in this approach to mental illness, existing plans may well outstrip what can be achieved. That this is already occurring is stated by Ferguson (1961):

> These people used to stay in hospital and apart from causing a regret to some sensitive and frustrated psychiatrist and some sadness to their families, they did not impinge on the community. Now they are a time-absorbing and often abortive slice of our everyday work. Case conferences discuss them endlessly; social workers support them; they are regular attenders at out-patient departments and as day patients. There is a constant stream of correspondence between disablement resettlement officers and the psychiatric clinic. There are telephone calls from their general practitioners about the difficulties they are causing at home, and so on . . . They are subtly destructive of morale in the clinic and in the unit, and they steal a large part of every working day—much more than they used to do when they were living out their lives in hospital.

These are in themselves not arguments against discharge from the mental hospital, but against premature discharge home without the safeguards of adequate hostel accommodation and this will no doubt in time be rectified. But there is another aspect which does not appear to, but should, give rise to concern. From time immemorial, in civilized communities, man has provided shelter or asylum to his fellow man. He also has permitted a high degree of eccentricity or non-conformity for those who did not seek or need asylum. Now both these concessions are being withdrawn and there is a danger that under the guise of treatment we will inflict further insults on people who are weary of society and crave only for asylum.

The Evaluation of a Community Psychiatric Service

Wing and Hailey (1972) critically examine the psychiatric services for Camberwell, a London borough, which, because of its proximity to the Maudsley Hospital, has received more than average psychiatric attention as well as the preparation of a Register. Conclusions are:

1. Health service authorities should accept responsibility for the whole of a geographical area, coterminous as far as possible with that of a local government authority, though there should be freedom of choice within reason so that services should not be completely area-bound.

Comment: There is a paradox here for the provision of all services implies a monopoly while freedom of choice and the abolition of rigid catchment areas implies a free market. The term 'within reason' can be freely interpreted and gives no guarantee that the consumer will have the promised freedom. Perhaps this is what is intended. Real freedom would permit the consumer to seek those services he particularly wishes and opt out of the State scheme if he wishes and be reimbursed for underwriting his own treatment. In a Welfare State such arguments are no longer tolerated. The proponent would be regarded as anti-social.

2. Health services should be comprehensive and varied with out-patient, in-patient and emergency facilities.

3. They should be integrated.

Comment: Integration is an 'in-word'. It is alleged to be more economical but in practice it means more administration and less efficient service. It would be of interest to see a trial conducted between an 'integrated' service and a 'non-integrated' one with cost analysis and efficiency scrutiny. The modern welfare state has a genius for launching schemes in the name of economy and efficiency which in practice do the opposite. This is generally recognized but there seems to be no machinery in a welfare service for reversing this pernicious process. An enquiry as to the reasons for this phenomenon and its remedy is long overdue.

4. The aims of the service are to decrease or contain morbidity in patient, family and community.

Comment: These are laudable aims but they would be more meaningful if there were definitions of morbidity and the positive (or negative) contributions one can expect from our present knowledge and resources. There is a tendency to apply existing resources to entirely inappropriate tasks on the assumption that to do something is better than doing nothing. The history of clinical medicine is studded with the successes of 'masterly inactivity'.

5. The prevention of accumulation of secondary handicaps.

Comment: These are just as likely to be caused by over-intervention as by non-intervention, and this should be stressed in any programme.

6. Since much psychiatric handicap is chronic, many patients are likely to remain in contact for a long time and there must be provision for them.

Comment: This point reflects the orientation of the writer. In fact, the vast majority of cases of psychiatric illness is of short duration and readily recoverable. There are chronic problems, many of them a legacy from the past, but to start off on the assumption that chronicity is paramount, can only foster an attitude which may itself contribute to chronicity. A healthier attitude is to regard all psychiatric illness as acute and recoverable so that the whole battery of therapeutics is constantly applied, for it is the potential chronic patient who requires this intensive approach if he is to be salvaged from chronicity.

7. The claims made by psychiatrists who define illness in social terms can be very wide. Practically any discontent may be regarded as an aspect of neurosis or psychosis, though these terms are not strictly defined. They may be attributed to such features of modern civilization which the psychiatrist happens particularly to dislike. The reactions by some anti-psychiatrists are correspondingly sweeping.

Comment: Sadly true!

Community Mental Health Centres, a Critique

Holoshin and Pomp (1969) developed the following hypothesis based on their observations on the introduction of a comprehensive mental health programme: 'The greater the degree of separation between planners and implementers, the greater degree of error between needs to be met and the programme required to meet them'.

Their major criticisms were:

1. A professional planning group does not have available a sufficiently wide range or depth of experientially or experimentally validated concepts or data upon which to draw. It is, in effect, several steps removed from the problems and potentialities of operational programmes. Planners, therefore, often rely on hypothetical constructs and generalized demographic data which often do not reflect significant aspects.

Demographic data are important but must be related to the needs of a particular community, its institutions, communication patterns and other factors. The authors define a community as a sample of one that is generally unique and different from other communities possessing similar demographic characteristics. Predetermined models have built-in liabilities, especially poor transfer of concepts from one setting to another. 'Good intent is not the same as good sense'.

The professional planner with his armamentarium of charts, graphs, data banks and expensive data processing equipment is prone to overlook those aspects of soft information which are critical to a reliable and valid understanding of a specific community. He frequently fails to consult those who labour in the field, yet they may be able to provide the very information which the planner needs and has not been able to obtain from his hard data.

2. The professional planner, being several steps removed from the actual or projected scheme, frequently becomes a victim of his own attempts at scientific façade. Even though a projected system of delivery of services appears to be internally consistent, this is not a measure of its validity. It may merely reflect the needs of the planner for order than the needs of the population. A theoretical model which would apparently suit all communities may in fact suit none.

3. In their zeal to plan for the brave new mental health world, the planners often overlook the alignment of the existing services with those that are projected. Competence may not be so easily transferable especially as the community mental health solution is based on unproven theory.

4. 'In the United States there exists a multiplicity of state-owned and -operated mental hospitals. The vast majority of these facilities have become repositories for society's rejects and in general can be described architecturally and programmatically as ranging from medieval Asylum Gothic to Contemporary Schizophrenic'.

Planning proceeds on the assumption that:

(*a*) State hospitals cannot be significantly improved.

(*b*) The imposition of the new models (*i.e.* community mental health centres) will obviate the need for state hospitals.

(*c*) By adding new facilities instead of modifying the old all will be well.

The authors express a general fear that there will be two worlds of mental health care: (*a*) the modern and better staffed for the select few who meet stringent intake criteria, and this will be a showcase; (*b*) the state hospital, which, with even more limited resources, is expected to cope with a heavier load of the more chronic and more disturbed and disturbing members of the psychiatric population. They also point out that these new centres tend to refer a greater proportion of patients to the State Institution, thus refuting the suggestion that they will eventually make the State Institution redundant.

5. There is a considerable gap between the setting up of a community centre and its impact on the mental health of the community. 'Information regarding delivery and performance of a mental health program can be likened to a discordant stereophonic sound system in which each of two tracks is providing a different message. The professional planner's sounds are generally of a utopian nature in which promises are made on a conceptual loudspeaker without clear interpretation of such problems as time schedules, program planning, resource development and implementation'. The authors plead for a factual analysis of results, otherwise programmes will depend on slogans and propaganda.

Comment: These arguments could be summarily dismissed as special pleading for the retention of the old system if it were not that many of the points made are true. Psychiatry is becoming a slave to fashion and any powerful lobby can swing resources its way regardless of need or proven competence. That there should be facilities, especially in densely populated areas other than in the large institution is reasonable, but it is essential that these new services are integrated with the staffs of the older hospitals. It is not a question of either one or the other but of a sharing of responsibility with interchange of staff at all levels. An intelligent planner who really wanted the new unit to be successful would see that by bringing in the staff, medical and nursing, of the old unit, he would be sure that the best would be had from both worlds.

On the other hand, there is such a specialty as general hospital psychiatry, and those who have worked all their professional life in a mental hospital would benefit from a spell in a general hospital unit. The issue is extremely important and yet very little has been done to foster integration.

The Mental Welfare Officer

The Mental Welfare Officer has not merely changed his name from that of Relieving Officer, *via* Duly Authorized Officer, but has also changed his function. At one time he was an un-uniformed constable with certain statutory powers to enable him to remove lunatics to a place of safety, but now he has a much wider role, in that he shares some responsibility for the supervision of patients discharged from hospital and he may now claim that his job is to keep people out of hospital. Changing names and duties does not necessarily give a person the necessary training and until such is available, a number of improvisations have been made to overcome this initial difficulty. Pargiter and Hodgson (1959) describe their efforts to bring the mental welfare officer (M.W.O.) in at the start, by having him attend the local out-patient clinic once in two weeks and sit in with the psychiatrist while he was interviewing patients.

> The M.W.O. calls the patient into the consulting room and seats him near the psychiatrist's desk. The M.W.O. then retires to a chair in a corner behind the patient where as a rule his presence is quickly forgotten. Naturally the M.W.O. has to be discreet and tactful. He quickly learns when the flow of history-taking is inhibited by his presence, and he then makes an excuse and withdraws. Similarly, the psychiatrist can secure his withdrawal by a pre-arranged signal. But need for withdrawal has arisen only two or three times in two years. Again, if the patient objects to the M.W.O's. presence he withdraws, but this has only happened once.

There are distinct advantages in this experiment, for it introduces the M.W.O. to the patient and relatives from the outset and he is accepted as a friend and counsellor and when home visits are necessary, he is invited in, instead of being kept on the doorstep. He can arrange for attendance for our-patient electroplexy, and acts as a link between the psychiatrist and the welfare services of the city. As the authors state:

> With the minimum of formality, he can find out the chances of a patient getting a house, getting a job, or being arrested. . . . . The M.W.O. knows the district in which the patient lives, its culture and its social mores. He usually knows whether there is mental illness or deficiency in the family, who is in debt, or behind with the rent, or which relative is in jail. . . .

It is apparent from the above quotation that though the M.W.O. is a valuable aid, it is with a limited group of patients and he is more likely to be useful in a rural area, than in a large city with a mobile population.

THE SOCIAL WORKER AND PSYCHIATRY

Though lady almoners have been employed by general hospitals for many years, the introduction of the psychiatric social worker to Britain was largely sponsored by the Commonwealth Fund in the late 1920's as part of their programme in developing child guidance clinics. The Fund was committed to the team approach consisting of psychiatrist, educational psychologist and psychiatric social worker. With the proliferation of child guidance clinics there was soon a demand for psychiatric social workers and courses of training were started; eventually an Association (A.P.S.W.) was formed to supervise professional standards of membership.

The psychiatric social worker soon entered the mental hospital field as well as the psychiatric out-patient department, though most were employed in the child guidance clinics. They were found to be very useful in that they were mobile, could visit the patients in their homes, could interview relatives and compile a social history. In some clinics the social history replaced the psychiatric history, and many psychiatrists began to rely on the psychiatric social workers for case-history taking, which was not only a bad psychiatric practice, but was regarded by many social workers as being a too limited exploitation of their skills.

The gradual acceptance of psychoanalytical concepts in psychiatric practice and the accent placed on these in her training, gave the social worker an introduction to 'intensive case work' which in many instances was very similar to psychotherapy. The tradition in the United Kingdom of training lay analysts, and the contribution to analytical theory of distinguished laymen, made it acceptable for certain social workers to undertake formal psychotherapy and even training.

At that time, psychiatric treatment of the mentally ill differed very little from the 'moral treatment' of the insane as practised at the end of the nineteenth century with the notable exception of malaria therapy. In the 1930's the situation began to change. Sakel had introduced insulin therapy for schizophrenia, and while its specificity has since been successfully challenged, there is equally no doubt that a number of early schizophrenics who may otherwise have drifted into chronicity were prevented from doing so by the concentrated stimuli to which they were exposed while undergoing insulin treatment. The daily routine, the controlled diet, the concentration of medical and nursing care, the supervision of games and recreation with attention to such details as the little bag of sweets to counter a delayed hypoglycaemic attack, all helped to renew the patient's contact with society.

The introduction of E.C.T. reclaimed many who would have languished in a state of severe depression, and the modern science of psychopharmacology, nourished by important developments in neurophysiology and neurochemistry, has revolutionized the treatment of mental illness. Depression is now a rapidly recoverable condition, schizophrenia no longer carries the hopeless prognosis, and deterioration to chronicity is a much rarer event. Crippling anxiety states and obsessional states can be cleared with short-term methods of treatment, and even the hard-core manic-depressive psychoses can now be reclaimed with the prescribing of lithium carbonate. With the exception of schizophrenic patients where the manipulation of the environment was still a major factor in successful treatment, all the above methods did not depend to any large extent on the psychiatric social worker. Just as the psychotherapist is being used more infrequently, so the value of intensive case work by the social worker is being questioned, not that in itself it did not produce some benefits, but because it did not compare in speed and certainty with other less expensive treatments.

The social worker was not unaware of these changes. Many were becoming dissatisfied with the impact of intensive case work and felt that social reform was more relevant to their work than intensive efforts to get the patient to adjust to a society which they felt was in urgent need of change. They supported a more militant attitude to social work and regarded the Town and County Halls and their inefficient administration, their parsimony and their system of priorities, as unrealistic and out of harmony with their own political philosophies. They felt their main function was not to waste time in futile efforts with individual cases but to reform or even destroy the present system.

As has been said, the major advances in psychiatric treatment were in fields which were, in general, quite foreign to the social worker who rarely had any training in the biological sciences. Yet psychiatrists were leaning more heavily on these disciplines and the model of patient-care was approximating more and more to that of orthodox medical practice where biochemical estimates and drug reactions and inter-reactions were a major interest and the supervision of the schizophrenic in the community depended as much, if not more, on whether he had the right drugs and the right dosage, than on any dynamic interpretation of his symptomatology.

Supervision of the patient in the community was depending more on the critical appraisal by the psychiatrist who had moved nearer the community into the out-patient department and into the general hospital. The Health Visitor, with her nursing training, and who lived near the patient's home, was frequently more able to supervise domiciliary treatment, especially as she already stood in a professional relationship to the general practitioner who was, in effect, responsible for such treatment. Even where environmental manipulation was required, the social worker, whose training is based on listening and the creation of a permissive situation which would facilitate the flow of 'material' was often disadvantaged when the situation demanded immediate action such as admission to hospital or the correction of faulty attitudes on the part of the family. Such situations demanded the exercise of authority which is counter to the social worker's training. She is frequently anti-authoritarian in philosophy and has elected to undertake social work because it allows her to operate in a milieu where authority is not practised.

The Seebohm Report resulted in the setting up of independent departments of social service under the local authority. These have taken over the responsibility for a number of services, especially mental welfare, which had previously been under medical supervision, either through the Medical Officer of Health or the hospital consultant. The social worker has now become an independent practitioner with responsibilities in an area where her training and skills do not help her much. She no longer has the informal contacts with the psychiatrist who could accept responsibility when things were going wrong and who could advise her on specific issues without any breach of protocol. Her immediate superior is generally an administrator who is not even an experienced social worker, and instead of getting professional answers to what are generally professional questions, she gets an administrative answer, which even if satisfactory at that level, which it need not be, is not likely to be helpful. The practice of clinical medicine is frequently the denial of administrative niceties and regulations. It is based on the principle that rules are meant to be broken rather than kept, for rules do not cater for the infinite variety of human responses.

The demands of the Mental Health Act, 1959, on the departments of social service have also created difficulties for the social worker. Though the local authority, under the Act, is given the responsibility for prophylaxis and after-care, a major and essential function is getting people into hospital who need observation or treatment. Some can be persuaded to go informally, but this frequently demands a degree of clinical skill which the young social worker has not acquired. When patients have to be admitted formally there are other factors involved, such as working within the terms of the Act and frequently with doctors who are not very familiar with the procedure. She is expected to remove the patient to hospital on her own authority, compulsorily and with speed, yet her whole training and her very nature are not geared to the rapid clinical assessment and to rapid decisions. It is a task very far removed from what has now become for her a fictive goal, namely intensive casework based on a strong positive transference and, no doubt, an equally strong counter-transference.

If there were no alternative to this situation, one would have to be invented, for one would appear to be training social workers in generic case work for areas where their expertise is of little value and where they are operating in an administrative structure where even the social worker with 'flair' is unlikely to be able to give of her best. Even those duties which she can perform well, such as job and lodging placement, she finds unattractive, for they do not exploit her skills. She is also handicapped in the supervision of the patient in the community who is probably on long-term pharmacotherapy. In other words, the psychodynamic model is less relevant to the practical tasks of the care and rehabilitation of the mentally ill than her teachers had led her to believe. The emphasis has shifted to the medical and to the nursing model.

Here the health visitor is almost tailor-made for the task in hand. She is professionally trained in patient care with the medical and nursing model strongly imprinted. She is part of the community she serves and, just as the doctor derives his authority and respect from the many services he renders patients, so the health visitor is equally respected and is equally able to exercise authority. Her close association with the general practitioner and the hospital gives her the necessary support should she need it, but she is also trained to, and is capable of exercising independent judgment and taking independent action. Any deficiencies in her experience of psychiatric illness are being supplemented by the accent now given to the subject in nurse training, and her whole professional life is one of adaptation to new developments. There is no rigid body of information from which her philosophy derives. New and better treatments replace the old and the inadequate, and new techniques are part of her life style. Unlike the social worker, she has not been indoctrinated in a philosophy which has universal application and which can never be superseded.

The issue facing the mental health service is one of the social worker employed by the new department of social service as against the health visitor. The changing nature of psychiatric services and treatment emphasizes the considerable advantages of the latter and, sooner or later, a radical reappraisal of social services and their competence will have to be undertaken. The cry for more and more social workers will have to be countered with a better answer than the proliferation of output from schools of social science. For a start, one should ask the simplest question—Why?

The Psychiatric Unit in the General Hospital

Like the out-patient department this varies considerably in its size and scope. In some it is an out-patient clinic for consultation only, while in others it claims to provide a comprehensive service. To rate the scope of a unit by the number of beds it possesses, is most erroneous and it is high time the 'bed standard' was abolished and that does not apply to psychiatry alone. With ambulant patients in a densely-populated area, admission to a hospital bed should be infrequent, and may be not more than one in six referred. With a well-staffed and well-equipped out-patient department and day hospital, admissions can be kept down and duration of stay shortened. A few beds intensively worked can do more than a very large unit where the tempo is slower and ancillary services are less well-developed. This aspect requires stressing for in the development of general hospital units there is a tendency to give the psychiatrist too many beds. He will no doubt fill them, but he will lack the time and resources to get patients out quickly. An optimum tempo of work is reached when there is a head of pressure on accommodation so that patients are soon tested out for week-ends at home and then discharged when they are ready and not weeks later. The capital cost of a hospital bed and its staffing is so great that units should be planned initially for their maximum and most efficient use. A psychiatrist (with medical and other help) should not have to look after more than 20 beds, which with 10–15 day hospital places and several out-patient clinics would keep him very busy and ensure that he was working at optimum efficiency. What is not generally realized is that his 'productivity' goes up with fewer beds, though there is, of course, an irreducible minimum.

In recent years there have been a number of communications describing such units and it is of some significance that most have come from the Manchester Region. Carson and Kitching (1949) were early in the field with a modest beginning of 12 beds which catered mainly for depressive states, which either masqueraded as organic states or had attempted suicide. The beds were in a general ward and treatment was largely electroplexy. Since then, Pool (1959), Leyberg

(1959), Freeman (1960) and Smith (1961) have reported developments and Silverman (1961) entitled his paper 'A Comprehensive Department of Psychological Medicine'. He has both acute and chronic sections and is able to serve a population of nearly a quarter of a million people with 99 beds yielding a crude annual admission rate of 1·92 per 1000. He attributes the success of his scheme to domiciliary consultation, the institution of early treatment, the use of the services of the mental welfare officers, district nurses, home helps and other ancillary personnel, with the M.W.O. as the key worker. He also stipulates that there should be an active and cooperative geriatric department within the hospital. The reasons why the Manchester Region should have developed its general hospital psychiatric services earlier and to a greater extent than the rest of the country are complex. It may be that the mental hospitals in the region had grown to an unwieldy size and some alternative had to be found more urgently. It may be that Manchester is traditionally the home of 'Free Trade'! But the rest of the country is not standing still and it is likely that in the next 10 years there will be an increasing number of general hospital-based psychiatric departments.

The advantages are not all on the side of the psychiatric unit, for the general hospital has also benefited in several ways:

1. It has brought within its walls a branch of medicine which has to cater for the needs of patients who are not bed-ridden and the other branches of medicine are realizing that many of their patients are in the same category and that the psychiatrists can help them in planning their day.

2. It ensures a full-time psychiatric service for the general hospital, with trained personnel immediately available and not based on a mental hospital which may be many miles away. When such a unit is established it is not uncommon for the psychiatrist to have as many, if not more patients in his colleagues' beds, than in his own.

3. This service extends to the out-patient department where large numbers of patients referred for medical and surgical opinion are really suffering from mental disturbance. Culpan *et al.* (1960), using the Cornell Medical Index, found that 'the incidence of emotional disturbance among out-patients attending various clinics can be considerable. This is especially so among gynaecological patients, and also among physical medicine patients and among *women* attending surgical clinics.' Mestitz (1957) found that 27 per cent of patients attending a casualty department of a general hospital had no evidence of organic disease.

4. Physical illness does not confer immunity to mental illness and *vice versa*, and many patients who may have to be admitted as a psychiatric emergency, are really suffering from the effects of physical illness. Asher (1954) based his paper 'The Physical Basis of Mental Illness' on cases of organic disease admitted to a mental observation ward and in a later paper (Asher, 1956) stated: '. . . I have found the work a clinically rich and mentally stimulating addition to my general medical work which I would be loth to relinquish.' Goody *et al.* (1960) who view the problem from the neurological aspect conclude:

> In planning for future neurological and psychiatric services for the country in general, it may be worth considering the possibility of creating regional centres sited in such a way as to serve the combined neurological, neurosurgical, and psychiatric needs of a population group; and to be closely linked with a large general hospital. We consider that such units could be far more economical and productive of improved results than the use of non-integrated specialist appointments, without adequate services.

5. Following on the above, it is self-evident that a number of psychiatric patients require the whole range of investigations associated with a general hospital, and duplication of these services is uneconomic. Many mental hospitals have operating theatres, X-ray, EEG, biochemistry and even bacteriology departments where the basic needs of nine-tenths of their population are no greater than those of the average general practice. Any service, to be efficient and to attract good recruits, should be served by a reasonable proportion of pathological material and be in constant use, but very few mental hospitals could, on these criteria, justify their special departments.

6. On the other hand the psychiatric department by introducing the psychological laboratory, a well-supervised occupational therapy department and the concept of the day hospital, brings services to the general hospital which are needed by other specialties.

7. A doctor whatever his work is under constant training and a psychiatric department in a general hospital permits a two-way exchange of experiences and instruction which is to the advantage of all.

8. Nursing staff are now expected to get experience of the psychiatric patient and while a number of general hospitals second student nurses to mental hospitals, a much better arrangement is to have one comprehensive school which caters for all aspects of a nurse's training. A general hospital unit is then put on the same basis as any other branch of nursing and does not divorce the nurse from her contemporaries and tutors. It is also a more realistic place to train the nurse for the future units in psychiatry which are going to be mainly housed in general hospitals.

9. Lastly, the patients and their relatives should not be expected to go to a different place when treatment can very easily be made available where all other patients are treated. To accentuate this individual difference is artificial and unkind. Some mental hospitals have made superb efforts to attract patients and provide conditions which compare favourably with a good-class hotel or holiday camp. But it is not the purpose of a hospital service to attract people. It should provide the best possible service which is geographically convenient and should not stigmatize one type of illness by keeping it apart from the others or house it, together with a large number of senile and other chronic problems, which constitute up to 90 per cent of the present population of a mental hospital. If people were consulted as to where they would like to be treated for psychiatric illness, there is no doubt that an overwhelming majority would opt for their district general hospital. It is unlikely, however, that they will ever be consulted or even demand to be consulted, for most people do not anticipate such an eventuality as admission to hospital for psychiatric illness. The gradual and now increasing provision of such units will however stimulate the demand and a planning authority should realize that to build a new unit which perpetuates the structure of the mental hospital is socially and medically undesirable and will not meet the needs of a modern community. It would be no consolation to proclaim to the world that we have the best mental hospitals in the world when the rest of the world had abandoned the whole idea of the mental hospital.

A strong defence for the preservation of the mental hospital has been put forward by Lewis (1966). His arguments are presented under the following headings.

1. It serves a useful function in gathering information about psychotics and their behaviour including the terminal stages of illness.
2. It acts as a testing ground for new modes of behaviour.
3. Controlled re-exposure to stress can be effected.
4. It can provide a whole series of therapeutic environments.
5. It is particularly useful in the re-education of the chronic patient.
6. It is able to provide an effective control to patients who 'act out' and who would be too disturbing in a general hospital unit.

These are really arguments in favour of what a good mental hospital can do. They do not say that some of these services may be provided by the general hospital unit which already implements 1, 2, 3, 4, 5 and probably 6. Mental hospitals in the past have tended to provide a one-way street from the medium to the long-stay wards and transfer from the long-stay to the short-stay ward is still a rare event. In a general hospital unit all accommodation is designated as short-stay, and the chronic patient with the acute is exposed to the 'total push' which the resources of the unit can muster and is more likely to be rendered fit for discharge. When the full range and quality of treatment which the general hospital unit provides is eventually appreciated, apologists for the mental hospital may withdraw their opposition.

Effect of General Hospital Unit on Mental Hospital

This is a very controversial matter and should be given serious consideration. An innovation which has apparent advantages but which has created fears among those working in mental hospitals should be subjected to close scrutiny in order to gauge the effects of an alternative psychiatric service. The author's unit does in fact operate within the catchment area of a mental hospital and such a study was undertaken (Orwin & Sim, 1965). A sample year was chosen and the following data not only give some idea of the impact of the author's unit on the mental hospital, but of the numbers and types of patient treated.

Admissions by Diagnostic Category

Diagnostic category	Mental Hospital (745 beds)	United Birmingham Hospitals (31 beds)
Schizophrenia	241	40
Affective states	201	318
Presenile states (including cerebral arteriosclerosis)	18	12
Senile states	58	3
Psychopathic states	50	10
Alcoholism and addiction	17	31
Psychoneurosis } Others }	67	105 28
Total	652	547

United Birmingham Hospitals

Day Hospital

Schizophrenic disorders	18
Manic-depressive states	42
Anxiety states	17
Obsessional states	5
Hysteria	8
Post leucotomy states	5
Alcoholism	2
Drug addiction	1
Others	4
	102

Outpatients

New referrals	349
Subsequent attendances	4479

This mental hospital when compared with other mental hospitals in the region showed the following:

1. A higher rate of compulsory admissions.
2. A much higher increase in patients over 65 years.
3. A greater number of chronic and psychopathic patients were admitted.
4. A substantial number of patients who would otherwise have gone to the mental hospital were treated at the general hospital unit on an in-patient, day or out-patient basis.
5. The general hospital unit with only 31 beds (at the time of the enquiry) had an admission rate approximately five-sixths that of the mental hospital.
6. Twenty-five per cent of the mental hospital's admissions were going to the general hospital.

This particular study may not be universally applicable but it does show that there is a 'creaming-off' of patients by the general hospital and that general hospital units can no longer be seen as one of those extensions of the National Health Service which are designed to meet a hitherto unsatisfied demand (*e.g.* cardiac surgery or neurosurgery) but are competing directly with the mental hospital. Small as their bed numbers may be, they are in many respects providing an alternative service.

Some would argue that this is a good reason for curtailing the experiment, but there is no doubt that it is what the public prefer and the arguments in favour (see above) are sound.

It is obviously not enough to create more general hospital units and leave the mental hospital to carry an increasing load of geriatric and other problems. When the Mental Health Act, 1959, came into force, it was expected that local authorities would shoulder much of the responsibility for aftercare, and that there would be an adequate number of hostels for patients not requiring the full resources of the mental hospital. Unfortunately these have not been forthcoming in anything like the number required. Yet many patients in mental hospitals could be adequately cared for in such hostels. They should preferably be small (about 20 beds), and as such could eventually become a useful accessory in the conduct of general practice, enabling the general practitioner to admit his own patients directly or to receive patients from either the mental or general hospital. As they would probably be near the patient's home, this arrangement would promote a more intimate atmosphere and keep the patient close to his relatives and general cultural background. The patient would also be attended by his own doctor, who is familiar with his previous history. An indirect advantage would be the provision of an outlet for those senior nurses from the mental hospital who may not wish to transfer to the general hospital and who often have a special liking for their long-stay patients.

As these hostels would be substituting for mental-hospital beds, local authorities may, understandably, be reluctant to subsidise the running-down of the mental hospital. This highlights one of the weaknesses of the Mental Health Act, 1959, in that two of the most important functions in mental health, namely, prophylaxis and after-care, are specifically delegated to local authorities which lack the resources to fulfil them. These functions are far removed from the traditional field of public health and cannot be separated from the hospital service. It is difficult to understand why they were ever handed over to the local authority, for it merely frees the Health Service from the responsibility of treating patients once they have left the institution.

There are still patients who will require long-term residential treatment and are therefore unsuitable for the short-stay general-hospital unit. These include psychopathic personalities, unco-operative alcoholics and drug-addicts, and security risks. There are also the younger schizophrenic patients who through many years of institutionalization cannot lead an independent life in the community or in the sheltered conditions of the hostel. All these form only a small proportion of the total mental hospital population which is rapidly becoming geriatric, and therefore do not justify the preservation of the mental hospital in its present form, which, in any case, caters rather ineffectively for their special needs.

The general hospital unit also has formidable problems. Its

development, particularly in the teaching hospital, has been hampered by financial stringency; for, in most instances, boards of governors have had to find the money from their own limited budget. Any expansion could take place only after competing with other more entrenched departments of the hospital. The Minister may say that he would view with favour the extension of general hospital psychiatric services, but until he sets aside special grants for capital expenditure, establishments, and maintenance, these units will be unable to develop to their full potential. Even where a board of governors finds the money from its own budget, it is not always desirable that a new department should siphon off capital to which other departments feel they have a prior claim. This could destroy the goodwill on which the very future of the new department depends. In any case, as has been shown, a general hospital unit does much of the work of a mental hospital and should be given the financial support to continue with and expand this work.

The above suggestions still leave much unsolved. As has already been stated, this study applies to a densely populated urban area only. It remains to be seen what the impact of a general hospital unit will bc in a rural or semirural area. A factual study reveals information which would otherwise not have been suspected, and there is no adequate substitute for the patient assembly of facts. The time has probably come to experiment.

Geriatrics

This has its social as well as its clinical aspects and both have strong psychiatric associations. Roth (1960) tried to put the problem into perspective and was critical of physicians, psychiatrists and social and welfare workers who get a jaundiced view of the picture.

> We tend to think in terms of lonely old people and selfish, irresponsible children, forgetting that 95 per cent of the aged are living outside institutions . . . the bonds within most families are strong and enduring. . . . There is however a large marginal group, whose adjustment if undermined would swamp the welfare services.

He comments on:

> the greater psychological resistance to accepting communal responsibility for old, as opposed to young, dependants . . . reference is rarely made to the valuable but imponderable contributions of the aged in caring for grandchildren, transmitting knowledge about child-rearing and household crafts, and influencing human relationships with their wisdom and experience. . . . The main factor underlying the ageing of population is not greater expectation of life as much as a decline in fertility. . .

He quotes figures from the General Register Office (1952) showing that 1,400,000 people were living alone in 1951, as compared with less than half that number in 1931 and concludes that loneliness is a major factor 'that leans especially heavily on the aged'.

Suburban and new town development has attracted mainly young people while South Coast resorts have catered for the elderly and so instead of a balanced community, we are creating discrete ones for the young, the middle-aged and the elderly. It is frequently stated that a great contribution would be made to the social problem of the aged if ample provision were made for them on new housing estates so that the three generations could live happily together. But this is more likely to prove a fond hope than a practical solution. One of the greatest socially disrupting influences in our time is the ever-increasing mobility of the population. The coalescence of industrial and commercial groups creates huge organizations with a national and international character. Young people move to their jobs and old people away from them and in an expanding economy these movements are becoming more frequent and it is difficult to see what can be done about it. Even if a family unit is initially constituted on a housing estate, movement may soon occur and it is small consolation to aged parents to know that another young family has occupied the home of their children and grandchildren.

It is therefore expedient to provide a service for those aged who require one. Macmillan (1960) described his efforts on their behalf as part of his Community Mental Health Service in Nottingham. He states: 'We can now offer our elderly psychiatric patients community care, joint medical and social domiciliary visits, out-patient services, a geriatric key-centre, day-hospital facilities, short-term in-patient treatment and long-term hospital care'. He stressed the importance of isolation and particularly 'rejection', which he defined as 'the relatives' determination to be free from what has become an intolerable burden', and described its natural history from a grievance, such as the refusal of other relatives to take their share of the responsibility to 'partial rejection' and finally to 'complete rejection'. He made some shrewd comments on the end result:

> Once rejection is fully established, in my experience nothing will alter it. Neither short nor prolonged relief through admission to hospital is of any avail. The relatives are determined not to accept any further responsibility, and will take extreme measures to avoid doing so. In deciding whether to admit a patient to hospital, the relatives' attitude is more important than the duration of the psychosis or the severity of the symptoms. Even in a severe senile psychosis, if the relative is willing to look after the patient at home admission to hospital may

not be necessary; yet it may be essential in a slight psychosis if the patient is rejected by his relatives or the community.

He considered that if effective action is taken early, 'rejection' can be prevented from growing and becoming complete. Temporary admission to permit the relatives a holiday was helpful and he had prepared lists of holiday relief admissions during the summer months and relatives frequently consulted with him months in advance in order to book their holidays.

When discussing prophylaxis, he laid great stress on 'the secondary emotional disabilities' which he considered lead to senile psychosis. 'Deprived of this minimal emotional fulfilment, the old person reacts emotionally be making excessive demands with consequent deterioration in interpersonal relationships.' He made the interesting suggestion that:

> The chief manifestations of what is called senile psychosis or senile dementia are not organic; they are an emotional response to unfulfilled basic emotional needs. It is not the organic memory impairment, but the restlessness, the nocturnal wandering, and the incontinence which bring matters to a head. The greater my experience of non-organic incontinence is, the more I become convinced that it is an emotional reaction—a protest or an expression of unhappiness or dissatisfaction.
>
> Over and over again we have found that geriatric conditions, which used to be regarded as wholly organic and permanent and necessitating hospital admission, are in fact partly organic and partly reactive, and that the reactive symptoms are the more disabling.
>
> Observation over some years of the patients attending the day geriatric centre has shown that conditions diagnosed in hospital as senile dementia gradually improved and the patients became re-socialized.

He instanced the social isolation of a spouse when the partner dies and the development of paranoid reaction as a consequence but considered that most can remain in the community with the help of the social services, social education and community tolerance. The day centre is advocated, for here the physical needs can be met with a well-balanced meal, while the short-stay annexe can put right a number of disabling illnesses.

He explained that:

> The atmosphere of the centre and of the in-patient annexes must be a group one, and the best number for a geriatric group seems to be 6–10. Until the group relationship had developed at our day centre, the old people did not accept it, and persistently stopped coming on one pretext or another. Once the group atmosphere was established, the whole picture changed—they were eager to come, and were disappointed when they could not. If the centre was closed more than three or four days the continuity broke, and the group reaction had to be built up again. For this reason the original arrangement of closing the centre at holiday-time for a week or two was discontinued, and the holidays of

the staff are now staggered. A sympathetic and understanding atmosphere with common activities and a regular routine are the essential for the group relationship....

When one of two isolated old people died, the other tended in a few months to develop a senile psychosis and to prevent this occurring, the health visitor was instructed to arrange for the survivor to attend the day centre as soon as possible. Cases were referred from general hospitals and general practitioners and even old people themselves have called at the centre 'usually quite appropriately'.

Macmillan concluded:

Instead of providing more and more residential accommodation for old people it would surely be logical to provide more and more community services, day-centres, and short-stay in-patient units, so as to give expert help with potential psychiatric illness as early as possible. With this help old persons can often continue to live at home, their relatives are relieved of undue strain and have their emotional needs resolved. A few psychiatric beds will be needed to give short-term relief as well as for some long-stay patients. But by using community methods the pressure on psychiatric beds as well as on long-stay beds for physical illness and on residential accommodation will be relieved.

Macmillan's contribution was an important one to an increasingly important problem. That the community is prepared to shoulder its responsibilities is illustrated by Sheldon (1960) who pointed out that in Britain in 1946, good neighbours provided nearly 20 per cent of the home nursing of old men and 30 per cent of old women. He does, however, emphasize the disrupting influences of social change:

The changes in housing arrangements and in employment tradition have led to the severance of many intangible human ties, and one may, in fact, say that the major problem of the present time is to promote the conditions in which these ties of human affection, whether as kinsmen or as neighbours, can continue to flourish and so support the evening of the lives of our older people.

That the problem is a major one has been recognized by the World Health Organization (1959) in a special publication, and by Colwell and Post (1959) who approached it by trying to assess, not the value of a community service, but the community needs of elderly psychiatric patients. They followed up for two years, 131 patients who were discharged from the geriatric unit of the Bethlem Royal Hospital. They concluded that 'the scope for community action . . . is frighteningly large' and that one-third of all their cases 'without any doubt went through periods during which action by the community might either have been therapeutic or should have brought people back into psychiatric treatment at an earlier date'.

As in other sections of society, in a free economy, with its differentials, it would be futile to try and organize all the elderly into day centres and as has already been pointed out, 95 per cent take care of themselves or do not require help from the social services. Hospital and welfare workers, by the very nature of their work, are unaware of the variety of measures which society itself has designed with a 95 per cent success rate. These may be just as worthy of study as the failures.

Social Class and Mental Illness

This is regarded as sufficiently important for the Registrar-General to draw up five grades for mental hospital admission. Definitions of these grades are:

I. Professional, business and administration.
II. Management and some professional.
III. Skilled occupations (manual and clerical).
IV. Partly-skilled occupations.
V. Unskilled occupations.

In the bulletin from the Ministry of Health and the Public Health Laboratory Service diagnostic categories are listed according to social class and there is a striking difference between that of schizophrenia and the manic-depressive psychoses. The former tend to occur mainly in the last three groups, while the latter occupy the first three groups. These findings are in accordance with reports from other countries. For example, Faris and Dunham (1939) found that schizophrenic patients in Chicago were usually from the more densely populated and socially disorganized areas of the city, a finding which was confirmed from other centres of population by Clark (1949). Hollingshead and Redlich (1958) set themselves the task of discovering whether mental illness was related to social class, and how far social class determined the treatment given. Reviews of their work have been enthusiastic. The *Lancet* (1958) stated:

> . . . the work they have reported and the facts they have marshalled make this one of the most valuable pieces of socio-psychiatric research: clearly set out, thoroughly documented, adequately summarized, it presents one of the best of the 'inter-disciplinary studies' . . . . Anyone working in or around the field of social medicine or psychiatry should keep at his elbow this astringent though objective commentary on some of the ills of our time; and many others (including politicians) will find much to interest them. . . .

The *British Medical Journal* (1959*b*) described it as 'an outstanding contribution to social psychiatry'.

The authors used a five-point social classification which though not identical to that of the Registrar-General, had points in common and was roughly comparable. Classes I and II were induced to seek help by 'gentle and insightful means', whereas in classes IV and V the means were authoritative and compulsory. The first two classes tended to be treated with psychotherapy while the lower classes were given physical forms of treatment. Apart from the information derived from their study, it offered an interesting and fruitful example of cooperation between the sociologist and psychiatrist, but the cynic might remark that not all sociologists are of the calibre of Hollingshead nor all psychiatrists of the calibre of Redlich. As with previous workers, they found that schizophrenia predominated in the lower social groups. Other findings were:

1. The wealthier psychotics had earlier treatment and were discharged from hospital more quickly.
2. Treatment had little correlation with diagnosis and depended more on the psychiatrist to whom the patient was referred.
3. Psychiatrists were divided into two main schools (*a*) the 'psychological and analytic' (P. & A.) and (*b*) the 'directive and organic' (D. & O.). The wealthier were treated by the P. & A. group and the poorer by the D. & O. group.

The authors confined their study to patients who had been treated by a recognized medical agency and presumably missed a fair number who did not present for medical treatment. Even in a Welfare State with no economic bar to treatment, a large number of the mentally disturbed evade the numerous social agencies that are available, so one can expect an even larger number to have eluded the authors' survey of the residents of New Haven (Connecticut). But as in all matters, the variables are legion and it is very difficult to draw conclusions from data. Even the generally accepted correlation between schizophrenia and low social class is open to a variety of interpretations. Hollingshead and Redlich attributed the differences to differences in treatment and the patient's response to treatment. This, at first sounds questionable and to those who regard schizophrenia as an organically determined disorder, it would be dismissed as highly improbable. Yet, we have ample evidence now that social factors are extremely important in supporting the chronic schizophrenic patient discharged from the mental hospital (Brown, Carstairs & Topping, 1958), and it is not difficult to see how a psychotherapist who maintains close contact with the patient and relatives, and perhaps acts as his own social worker in arranging rehabilitation, obtains better results than the hospital psychiatrist who because of his much heavier case load is reduced to infrequent and short interviews, unsupervised medication, and physical treatments. The structure of group V is itself relevant, for it is much easier for the person who is not only himself indigent, but whose relatives are unable to help, to remain in an impecunious state and readily become a burden on the social services with consequent admission to a mental hospital. The well-to-do can 'underpin' their unfortunate relatives either by remittance or by some arrangement whereby they are comfortably lodged and cared for. To get a more realistic appreciation of the true social incidence of schizophrenia every private hotel and boarding house should be scrutinized, but the resources of social classes I and II will have found other solutions which may be even more out of range of the sociologist, for their relatives are adopting methods which are specifically designed to keep their problems away from public view. All data have their interest, but hasty conclusions should not be drawn and the *Lancet's* suggestion that the politicians might find Hollingshead and Redlich's book of interest could be dangerous. Those professionally engaged in the field have still a long way to go before they can offer the politician anything sufficiently concrete.

OTHER SOCIAL IMPLICATIONS

There is now almost a frenzy of experiment and endeavour in the social field and a number of interesting aspects, new and old, have been reported, some of which seem likely to make a lasting contribution to the treatment and care of the mentally ill, while others have little to commend them apart from their novelty.

'Neurotics Nomine'

This is the name given to a voluntary association of psychiatric patients and ex-patients. It has been known for a long time that the sympathy and understanding which a patient or a recovered patient has for a fellow-sufferer is greater than in those who have not had such an experience. The Association was formed towards the end of 1957 by Dr Joshua Bierer and a former patient Mr John Custance, and membership is open to all who share its aims. These have been set out by Housden (1961) as follows:

1. To help patients and ex-patients to meet each other and people outside the Association.
2. To assist the patient in taking the first step towards social readjustment.
3. To support each other by meetings at home or by talking over the telephone in an emergency.
4. To provide a panel available to discuss or answer questions to an audience of G.P's. or members of the social services.

5. To help remove the stigma and fear that still surround mental illness.
6. To help members by providing opportunities for useful work, social contacts and self-expression.

He adds: '. . . some feared that it would become a happy hunting ground for pseudo-psychologists and armchair psychiatrists, but this has not been so, and the group meetings are purely social'. It is not difficult to see the resemblance between this association and Alcoholics Anonymous (A.A.) except that it prefers not to be anonymous yet avoids the more stigmatized term 'psychotic'. At least the alcoholics call a spade a spade.

A friend in need is most precious and if any organization can bring some comfort to the friendless neurotic or psychotic, then its work is commendable. The members seem to feel they have been bolder than the alcoholics in not seeking anonymity, but in doing so, they have missed the very essence of A.A. which offers a man or woman an ample outlet to help his less fortunate neighbours without having to advertise the fact.

Family Care or Foster-family Care

This is alleged to have had its origin in Gheel, Belgium. According to the legend, in the year A.D. 600, Dymphna, an Irish princess, was fleeing from her mad father who had been making incestuous advances towards her. He found her at Gheel and executed her. In consequence of certain miracles she had effected, she was canonized and made the patron saint of the insane. The old Gothic church is dedicated to her, and in the choir is a shrine enclosing her relics, with fine panel paintings representing incidents in her life. Pilgrims, many of them insane, visited her shrine and stayed and were looked after by families living nearby. By the thirteenth century a colony for the insane was established in the farm and houses round about and it eventually was taken over by the state. A small hospital for the essential medical needs is the only formal medical institution and the system has for many years been regarded as the acme of the humane treatment of the insane.

Greenland (1961) quoting Peterson (1912) describes a similar arrangement in the Japanese village, Iwakura.

> The third daughter of the Emperor Gosanjo in the eleventh century, developed melancholia in her eighteenth year. Word was brought to the Imperial household that at Iwakura was a holy fountain, the water of which was healing to mental disease and to disorders of the eyes. The emperor's daughter was taken there nearly 900 years ago and recovered and so brought fame to the temple and well of Iwakura, as a result of which the insane were brought there in great numbers. At first three small inns were constructed to receive them, then later

tea houses and villas and cottages sprang up in which to care for the ever-increasing influx of patients.

In the year 1889 the village had 239 houses, with 1579 inhabitants, and up to that year one or two patients were received into each family to share in the occupations of the household, which were chiefly out-of-door employment in fields, gardens and forests.

In 1887 the Japanese government, evidently under the impression gained from a study of the asylum systems of Europe and America, came to the conclusion that their colony system, that had grown up so naturally was too far removed from our Western ideals as exemplified in our colossal caravanserais for the insane, and so forbade the insane being any longer taken to the village of Iwakura.

The result of this opposition of the government has been to reduce at least temporarily the number of insane in the colony. It is altogether likely that as soon as the authorities learn that out of themselves they have developed through nearly a thousand years the best of all methods of caring for the insane, toward which the West itself is struggling with much difficulty, they will remove the proscription and restore Iwakura to its ancient rights and privileges under State organization and inspection. There is one retreat for about 90 patients at Iwakura built on European models under the care of physicians, to which excitable cases may be brought from the family homes in the neighbourhood.

The principle is now generally accepted but social policy does not appear to be able to initiate the practice where none had previously existed. Criteria may be laid down as to the type of patient and family that are most suitable, but unless the family is forthcoming and sufficient incentives can be provided, it may be that, as the Belgians and Japanese have found, it takes a miracle to get the thing started.

Mothers with Children in a Psychiatric Hospital

These are now a familiar sight. Main (1958) described such a situation as part of an experiment within the hospital community started in 1948 at the Cassel Hospital, 'to see whether it could become less of a social vacuum—more of a place of treatment and less of a retreat from the stresses and strains of domestic and industrial life to which a patient must inevitably return'. Not only did it maintain and promote the positive element in the mother-child relationship, but it high-lighted the negative aspects which might otherwise have been unsuspected. From 1955, the bringing of babies into the Cassel Hospital has been a condition of the mother's admission and according to Main there have been few exceptions and it works well and affords unique opportunities for studying mother-child relationships.

Mothers requiring psychiatric treatment following childbirth are frequently given the opportunity to bring their baby into hospital with them and this has been the practice in the author's clinic since 1950. Some mothers prefer not to do so and the evidence to date is that there is no detectable difference in the progress of the mother or in the development of the child. It is possible to argue that those mothers whose children would suffer from separation have an instinctive knowledge of this and bring them in with them, while those who do not have equally reliable knowledge. One point is clear; babies in hospital are good for the morale of the nursing staff and other patients but in themselves these are not sufficient grounds for admission.

Mental Illness in a New Town

It is alleged that there is a higher incidence of mental illness in new towns and Sainsbury and Collins (1966) undertook a sample survey in Crawley New Town by means of a structured questionnaire. Women had a less favourable attitude to moving than the men but perhaps more significant than their very limited positive findings were the various difficulties in interpretation of data, which the authors acknowledged. A similar study was reported earlier by Hare and Shaw (1965) who compared mental morbidity in a new town with an old district of Croydon. The only notable difference in physical morbidity was a higher prevalence of respiratory diseases in the low-lying old town. In both communities poor mental health tended to be associated with poor physical health, although not so strongly as to justify a revival of the 'miasma' theory of the aetiology of mental illness. As with the New Town Study, this work is another indication that field surveys of mental disorders are clearly burdensome undertakings, particularly when carried out with careful checks on the reliability of findings.

One may ask what these surveys are intended to reveal. They have, in themselves, not revealed much, but they do illustrate the difficulties of acquiring valid information and the danger in interpreting such information. They may also suggest that relevant information is more likely to declare itself without resort to such costly investigations.

Social Mobility

It is now generally accepted that social mobility is contributory to the nature of mental illness though not necessarily to its incidence. These opinions are based on studies of the types of mental illness in various social groups. One such by Michael and Langner (1963) showed that low socio-economic groups contained a relatively high percentage of organic types, psychotic types, psychosomatic problems, character disorders, alcoholism, dissocial behaviour, hypochondriasis, passivity, dependency, and schizophrenia. Higher social groups were twice as often free of symptoms with a high incidence of aggressiveness, while the lower groups scored high in immaturity, rigidity, suspicion and frustration.

These symptoms in the low income groups need not be seen as conclusive evidence of mental disease. In many, mental symptoms are merely a form of communication and an expression of social difficulty.

In the higher income groups symptomatology is more frequently associated with severe disability and this is predominantly in the super-ego laden conditions such as depression, anxiety states, obsessional neurosis and paranoid reactions. Social mobility removes a person from his original culture and in an affluent society this is becoming an increasingly common experience which many find stressful.

Mental Health and Social Policy

The above is the title of a book by Jones (1960). She had already written on the history of the subject in a previous book, *Lunacy, Law and Conscience* (1955) which dealt with developments in the care of the mentally ill between 1744 and 1845. Her second book included an account of the Mental Health Act of 1959 and in addition to describing the changes in legislation she introduced an interpretative note, explaining the stringent legal safeguards of the Act of 1890 as being due to a fear of wrongful detention which in turn led to delays in treatment. This preoccupation with the legalism of the 1890 Act and attributing to it all the disadvantages of mental hospital treatment, was given wide publicity and to a certain extent inspired the new Act, yet from information that is accruing since the passing of the new Act, formal admissions have increased rather than decreased. Some decide from Olympian heights how social policy should be interpreted and while there are considerable merits in intelligent planning, all planning is not intelligent. Mental health may be influenced by social policy, but not necessarily favourably and what can appear to be an enlightened piece of legislation may have adverse effects. For example, compulsory registration of labour was a war-time measure which extended to the post-war years. Ministry of Labour officials would become exasperated by vagrants who moved from town to town and thus defied their efforts to localize and register them. When transport was nationalized, some of these officials felt that by issuing orders to long distance lorry drivers to refuse these vagrants lifts, the problem would be solved. They failed to appreciate that vagrancy was a mechanism adopted by a variety of individuals to solve their emotional problems and that by depriving them of this outlet, they increased the risk of serious mental breakdown.

An egalitarian approach to human problems may be appropriate in a dedicated egalitarian society, but to try and graft it on to a stratified society can lead to much hardship and deprive some whose sensitivities prevent them from sharing the benefits of the Welfare State. It should be appreciated that the treatment and the mental health of individuals are most personal issues, and that grand policy or regimentation has only a very limited place. It is important to ensure adequate provision but having done so, there should be considerable latitude in the development of the services. Some patients will prefer a private consultation or treatment, and to ignore their preferences makes a mockery of other efforts which are alleged to be designed for their individual needs. It is true that some prefer to be organized and derive a measure of support from a communal service, but to others it is anathema. A private service is certainly more economical in administrative costs and is more flexible in practice as well as being a very sensitive instrument, which readily attunes itself to the demands, and which is more likely to encourage profitable invention and experiment. A balanced approach is needed. A mental health service is partly a communal responsibility which demands a certain amount of policy making, but an increasing proportion is a personal service and this is best privately negotiated between patient and doctor.

Social changes may influence the incidence of mental disorder and this has been apparent in dementia paralytica and alcoholism. Our competitive society puts a premium on conscientiousness and obsessionality, which in turn produce their crop of casualties. Should society be modified to prevent their occurrence or should society make provision for their treatment? The answer will be decided by the balance sheet, which at present is heavily in favour of treatment. Once the cost of treating these problems outweighs the benefit such personalities bring to the economy, prophylaxis will assume priority. At present, aside from economics, psychiatry is on more certain ground in treatment than in prophylaxis.

Attitude of the General Public

The public's attitude to mental illness has a considerable bearing on community tolerance to the psychotic patient, and in an enfranchized community may influence the importance a government attaches to the problem of mental illness. Carstairs and Wing (1958) interested themselves in a series of five television programmes by the British Broadcasting Corporation on 'The Hurt Mind'. Belson (1957) had already reported on the subject in what was intended to be a controlled experiment in Audience Research, in that the responses of a group who viewed the programmes were compared with those of a group who did not. Whether it is fair to use as 'controls' a group of people in another part of the country who do not elect to watch a series of programmes which were viewed by 5 millions of the population is open to question, but Belson's conclusions were not very striking. He stated that: 'There was a moderate but broadly based increase in viewer's confidence in the ability of medical men to cure mental illness. . . . There was a small but well-spread increase in the viewers' willingness to associate with the ex-patient. . . . ' Carstairs and Wing analysed 1267 letters, which were written to the B.B.C. in response to these programmes and though appreciative of the uncontrolled bias of the contents of the letters, considered that they offered resounding instances of 'sociological serendipity'. The public seemed ready for an increase in 'community care'. Many letters asked for further information and for titles of good books on psychiatry; very few (17 letters) were concerned with heredity and 'only 7 implied a belief in organic causes'. It could be argued that in some respects the laity were better indoctrinated than the profession! There was considerable criticism of the lack of the general practitioner's capacity to help, and particularly over his tendency to resort to prescribing. Some actually suggested that more attention be given to the teaching of psychological medicine to doctors in training.

CULTURAL FACTORS IN PSYCHIATRY

Introduction

Psychiatric illnesses occur when stresses precipitate biological or psychological changes in susceptible individuals. Experiences which are regarded as stressful depend in part on the individual's culture, as may his methods of coping with these experiences, the form his symptoms will take, the outcome of his illness and nearly every other aspect apart from any basic biochemically induced disorder. Members of a culture may accept or even expect one kind of symptomatic behaviour and label another as deviant. These differences can lead to different forms of secondary elaboration and varying degrees of disability.

Kiev (1972) points out that the patient will not only experience symptoms in a manner consistent with his culture, but if he seeks help from a native healer, he will present his symptoms in a manner he knows will be acceptable. Thus the basic psychiatric syndromes will take different forms in different cultures. He extends his argument by claiming that all mental disorders are forms of the basic syndrome known to Western psychiatry but this is an assumption which may not be valid. It may satisfy the Western psychiatrist to think that any aberration seen in a patient from another culture must be a variant of those he already recognizes, but it may not; it may not even be an illness. Yet the author goes on to say that because symptoms of some disorders are accepted as normal in a given society, this does not mean that the person who displays them is, in fact, normal, but that individuals with similar disorders are permitted to function differently in different settings. One would have thought that with the recent questioning of diagnostic criteria in Western psychiatry there would have been more restraint in applying questionable labels to people from other cultures.

He explains culture-bound syndromes as special forms of familiar disorders; for example, anxiety may take the form of *koro, susto* or bewitchment; obsessional neurosis may appear as frigophobia or *shinkeishitsu*; hysteria may take the form of *latah*; phobic states are represented by fear of the evil eye, voodoo death and the curse; depressive reactions include *Hiwa, Itck, windigo* psychosis and malignant anxiety; and dissociative states include *amok, hsieh-ping, piblokto*, and spirit possession. These equivalents are based mainly on analogy and the present author has run into similar trouble when teaching at the medical school in Salisbury, Rhodesia. There, African patients who presented with hallucinations and delusions were labelled schizophrenia because they showed some recognizable features of a schizophrenic illness, but that is a long way from a diagnosis of schizophrenia, which should be based on a full psychopathological assessment, including ego-defences and ego-strength. It is very tempting for Westerners and also very conceited of them to interpret cultural reactions in terms of their own reference system.

Kiev holds rigidly to his model and relates how pre-scientific healers would agree about which persons in their culture needed help, which they provided on their own theoretical basis, such as soul loss, spirit possession and taboo violations. Preventive measures were advocated such as avoidance of contagion, and their treatments included exorcism, drugs and encouragement of cult membership. He claims that to the extent that these methods worked, the incidence of mental disorder in the culture would be underestimated.

A unique opportunity of observing the reactions of a variety of cultures and subcultures presented during the Second World War, when approximately 48 different nationalities in sizeable numbers were treated in the major psychiatric centre in the Middle East. Sim (1945, 1946*a*) reported on the incidence of mental illness in these groups and divided one group into officers, non-commissioned officers and other ranks. Like other observers, he commented on the relative absence of depressive and anxiety states in soldiers from the less well-developed areas of the world. Yet there were almost as striking differences between British other ranks and officers, indicating that cultural influences on mental illness need not be exclusively racial. Actual incidence did not vary much between the groups, but there were gross differences in the nature of the breakdown. Carothers (1947) in a study of psychiatric illness in Africans confirmed this low incidence of depression and in a later and more comprehensive publication (Carothers, 1953) re-emphasized this point. Carstairs (1958) wrote: 'My own experience in India was on similar lines. When I lived for a year (and practised medicine) in a village of 2400 inhabitants, I was aware of only one case of severe depression—and that did not last long'. Carstairs rightly stresses the importance of psychiatric studies by psychiatrists who belong to those cultures and the dangers of leaning too heavily on reports from outside observers, but better still, the observer, inside or outside the culture should be a good observer and though the one from inside may be familiar with some of the local patterns of behaviour, this does not in itself compensate for inadequate psychiatric training or experience. It can, however, be very difficult to 'tune in' to a specific pattern if one is not familiar with it. For example, the author was completely puzzled by a number of Indians who complained of loss of semen till he read Carstairs' (1956) account of *jiryan.* This syndrome is a chronic anxiety state in males in which patients complain of exhaustion, inertia, and wasting away of the bodily tissues, with no physical evidence of disease. He compares it to effort syndrome except that they are convinced their weakness is due to the leaking away of their semen, and postulates a psychopathology based on relationship with the father which is one of extreme deference with a constant fear of giving offence.

Murphy (1973), who has been a major worker in the field, makes the following *obiter dictum:*

Culture in the sense of transmitted values, beliefs, attitudes and habits, is a major determinant of the experiences which individuals undergo from infancy onwards, and of the interpretation that they put on experiences. If one believes that mental disorder is in any way affected by experience and attitudes, it is logical to believe that it is affected by culture and that the theories linking psychopathology to experience also link psychopathology to culture.

He suggests that the great variety of cultures offers, not only an opportunity to test a theory in different societies, which is becoming increasingly popular, but also the possibility of selecting a cultural setting to give that theory its strongest challenge. Increasing attention is now being given to the question of which theory a given culture is best suited to test. The following four areas are submitted:

1. Diagnostic significance of symptoms and signs.
2. The broader meaning of symptoms apart from diagnosis.
3. The testing of aetiological theories.
4. Studies of the therapeutic process.

While psychotic states such as those of senility and schizophrenia are alleged to be found in all cultures, some conditions are more localized. These are:

1. **Amok**. This is found in Malayans who are said to 'run amok'. The patient, who usually is of schizoid personality and given to brooding, suddenly seizes a weapon and slays anyone within reach and eventually kills himself or is killed. Those who have survived, claim to be amnesic for the whole episode. Similar conditions have been described in Africa and the Philippines and the 'going berserk' of the Vikings has been regarded as a similar condition. It has been suggested that these reactions are becoming less frequent, due to education and general advancement. *Pseudo-amok* is a hysterical simulation of the real thing, but nobody usually gets hurt.

2. **Latah**. This was also described in Malayans, though it is found in other peoples. The patient is usually female, simple and compliant and it may occur following a sudden fright such as seeing or stepping on a snake. Echopraxia, echolalia and coprolalia and occasionally violence may also be present, and these features have been compared by Yap (1951, 1952) to the 'Jumping Frenchmen of Maine' and through them to Gilles de la Tourette's disease.

3. **Koro**. This was called by the Chinese '*shook young*'. It is found among the inhabitants of Celebes and West Borneo. The patient fears his penis will disappear into his abdomen and that he will die, and to prevent this he grips the penis until exhausted. In addition to physical help from relatives including fellatio by the wife, a variety of devices are employed which range from wooden clasps to injection

of a 'male factor'. There is also a female equivalent of the condition with pre-occupation with loss of secondary sexual characters.

4. **Voodoo.** This is derived from the Creole French *vaudoux* = a negro sorcerer; it was the name given to certain magical practices, superstitions and secret rites which were prevalent among the negroes of the West Indies, and especially in Haiti. It has been applied to a form of death which occurs when a primitive person has broken a taboo or feels he has been bewitched. Death may occur in a day or two or even more dramatically, but the exact cause has not been established. In a superstitious community, where accurate diagnosis is not available, it is not difficult to ascribe sudden death to supernatural causes, but there have been instances which were strongly suggestive that death was not caused by any recognizable organic state.

5. **Shamanism.** By definition this is the primitive religion of the Ural-Altaic peoples of Siberia, in which all the good and evil of life are thought to be caused by spirits which can only be brought about by Shamans or priests or priest-doctors. It has been applied to similar religions, especially of north-west American Indians.

Dean and Thong (1972) describe the practice of psychiatry in Bali, an Indonesian island with a population of 2½ millions, mainly Hindu. Many of the psychiatric needs are handled by the village-based Shaman, known locally as the *balian*. He may be a charismatic individual without formal education or an educated, high-ranking government official. An essential feature is the possession of a 'therapeutic personality' and supernatural powers.

The Balinese recognize two main types of mental disorder, *bebainen* and *buduk* which are classified according to symptoms, *e.g. mengil* (mute) or *gadungen* (grandiose). *Bebainen*, ascribed to evil spirits (*kala*) is a culture-bound reactive syndrome ethnogenic to Bali and is said to be caused by the connivance of vengeful persons and angry spirits. Such an illness is the special field of the *balian*. *Buduk* is thought to be caused by the sins of the forefathers (*karma*) or by acute emotional problems; it can manifest as mental deficiency, chronic schizophrenia and organic brain disease, and it is regarded as the province of the physician.

Bebainen is the commonest mental illness. Onset is acute with sudden outbursts of tears, attempts to run away and resistance to restraint. It may just as abruptly cease, but should the attack recur on several occasions, the patient is referred to a *balian* with instant cure once an 'agreement' with the *balian* is reached. Resistant or mute cases are treated by more complicated methods, including drugs. Most recover, but those who do not may be restrained by the use of stocks (*blagbag*), the exact method being carefully defined, as it is believed to have a therapeutic value as well.

The authors state that as Shamanism and its various counterparts are prevalent throughout the world, modern science could gain by devoting more attention to its therapeutic benefit. It removes the stigma of mental illness for it is accepted as an integral part of community experience, and because treatment occurs in the community there is minimal disruption of family and community ties with consequent better readaptation. This prescription may suffice for the minor cases, and indeed many people in Western society do indulge in such 'cures', but in the more severe cases it is doubtful if tying in the stocks would be acceptable no matter how elaborate the ritual.

African Psychiatry. As seen by the African psychiatrist, this subject has been reported in a series of papers by Lambo (1959, 1960). In the 1959 paper he stressed that in planning and organizing mental health services, psychiatry in under-developed countries should avoid the mistakes of more advanced countries and in advising against a slavish application of foreign methods stated: '. . . we are getting more and more convinced that an independent diagnosis of our position may prove more profitable in the end than a borrowed remedy'. In the 1960 paper he illustrated some of the peculiar features of African psychiatry, particularly in the unusual hysterical features, the prevalence of organic syndromes such as trypanosomiasis, encephalitis in children and the complications of ankylostomiasis.

Mental Illness in Maoris. Reports of mental illness in differing cultural groups continue to appear. Some derive from developing countries where resources in diagnosis and treatment have not yet reached an adequate level and few conclusions can be drawn. In New Zealand which has highly developed health services, about 150,000 Maoris live alongside 2 millions of European extraction and all enjoy the same medical and social benefits. This situation provides an opportunity to study contrasting patterns of culture in terms of mental health. Foster (1962) provides some statistical observations of mental hospital admissions. There were differences in age structure in that 58·5 per cent of Maoris were under 20 years of age compared with 39·4 per cent of Europeans, while 12·5 of the latter were aged over 60 years compared with 3·8 per cent of the Maoris. The commonest diagnosis among Maoris was schizophrenia with a crude admission rate nearly 50 per cent higher than that for Europeans. Crude rate for manic-depressive psychosis was twice as high in Europeans.

These figures reflect cultural differences such as different administrative attitudes by society and the mental hospitals themselves, but the differences in disease incidence probably indicate real differences in the pattern of disease, though these too could be culturally determined.

West Indian Immigrants. Gordon (1965) has reported the influence of cultural patterns on psychiatric symptomatology among West Indian immigrants to England and who were admitted to a mental hospital. The striking feature was the 'pathoplastic' effect of their previous culture with reference to witchcraft and other supernatural influences. These findings are not new and Henderson and Gillespie (1950) reported similarly on inhabitants from the Orkney Islands who were treated in a mental hospital in Edinburgh. The author would confirm that such 'pathoplastic' influences extend to other immigrant groups like Hungarians, Poles, Indians, Pakistanis and others.

Psychiatry in the Caribbean. Wittkower (1970) studied the transcultural problems in the Caribbean and found that the major issues were: (1) alcoholism, which was more prevalent among the affluent, and (2) possession states, which included Voodoo and cultural variants of a hypnotic state.

Contributing factors were: (*a*) rhythm of song and dance; (*b*) persuasive and authoritative voice of the *Houngan* (priest); (*c*) his directions; (*d*) the collectively shared experience; (*e*) the anticipation of becoming possessed; (*f*) the desirability of the state of possession.

Symptomatology. The delusional content is influenced by the culture and psychiatrists should learn to decode the culture-specific meaning of the symbols used. Acute delusional states occur in individuals with weak egos and whose super-egos are poorly structured and whose main ego-defence is massive regression. These are culturally acceptable means of escape from intolerable conflicts.

The Upward Mobile Negro Family. McKinley *et al.* (1971) postulated that the middle-class Negro when ascending from one socio-economic class to another finds himself isolated from the white middle class as well as from the black masses in general and although he is financially secure and has a stable family, his mental health may not reflect these conditions.

Despite the apparent stability of family life there was much conflict between the parents, which centred on the sex roles associated with Negro culture in America, where the female parent assumes the leadership role in the family and the male parent is stereotyped as undependable and irresponsible. This led to a power struggle in which each tried to destroy the other's influence on the children. Some patients paraded the importance of racial issues in the development of their personal problems in an attempt to avoid dealing with painful intra-psychic material. Traditional psychotherapy (by a white therapist) was ineffective but 'role reversal' techniques were found to be quite effective in demonstrating to the patient the therapist's willingness to identify and share some of the feelings and frustrations of a patient from a minority group.

SCHIZOPHRENIA

It has been stated that schizophrenia is a universal mental illness with a universal incidence in all areas and cultures (Slater & Roth, 1969). Yet in many cultures, though patients may present withdrawal, hallucinations and delusions, the pre-morbid personality, the precipitating circumstances, the natural history and response to treatment would suggest that it is in general a very different condition to that seen in more advanced cultures. It may be that in a sample of so-called schizophrenic patients there are some who would approximate to the criteria in advanced cultures, but there is an even greater number who do not fulfil these criteria, and that they are labelled such, because one has not tried to attach a more valid label to them. Differentiation of a disease process which entails a careful study of its origins and natural history is not an easy exercise, and it is very convenient to see reactions with even a tenuous link with a recognizable condition as an example of that condition. In clinical medicine this approach would have been discarded long ago.

Murphy and Raman (1971) in a twelve-year follow-up of indigenous tropical peoples with a diagnosis of schizophrenia found: (*a*) that the incidence was close to that in the British Isles; (*b*) that the percentage found functioning normally and symptom-free on follow-up was much higher than a comparable British sample; (*c*) that they showed fewer relapses in the period between discharge and follow-up.

The authors concluded that the impression that functional psychoses in indigenous populations (African and Asian) ran a less chronic course than among European and North Americans was confirmed.

It can now be assumed that even if the disease may still be called schizophrenia, it behaves differently. The next step is to break down the problem and separate those that approximate from those that do not.

General Practice

It is in general practice that psychiatric disorders initially present and much of the earlier manifestations of these illnesses can only be observed in this milieu. The general practitioner will see aspects of schizophrenia and depression which are not seen in the mental hospital and will see processes at work which in the relatively short period of observation in hospital will go unrecognized. The College of General Practitioners prepared a report for the Ministry of Health and its essential features have been published in the *British Medical Journal* (1958). It showed a clear appreciation of the essentials, for example:

> Every good family doctor must be a good psychologist, for psychological medicine is part and parcel of all general practice. To misdiagnose organic disease has long been regarded as a serious error; it is now appreciated that to miss psychological illness is just as bad and may lead to even greater unhappiness.

The report comments on the different estimates of incidence of the problem, comparing Pemberton's (1949) figure of 6·5 per cent with Paulett's (1956) figure of 70 per cent and considers that 30 per cent would be more generally acceptable. The report ends with a plea for more undergraduate and postgraduate training in psychological medicine and for a closer link with the social services. Watts and Watts' (1952) survey of psychiatry in general practice was an early stimulus to their fellow practitioners and Balint (1957) with his book *Psychotherapy in General Practice* showed that it was possible by part-time training and supervision to give a group of interested doctors the necessary insight and technique to deal with some of their commoner psychotherapeutic problems.

Attitude and Prejudice

These may not immediately strike one as having strong medical associations, but as the reporter in the *Lancet* (1962) of a conference on the subject remarked: 'An abnormal mental condition which results in the death of some 6 million people merits a high place among the killing diseases'. The conference was one sponsored by the United Nations Educational, Scientific and Cultural Organization (UNESCO). The following general conclusions emerged:

1. Real differences—perhaps inherent ones—exist between groups and the aim is to modify attitudes towards these differences.
2. Anti-discrimination legislation need not and should not wait upon education programmes, and should run ahead of public opinion. Desegregation of housing estates in the U.S.A., for example, though strenuously resisted at first, was shown to lead to more tolerant attitudes towards Negroes.
3. What public figures said and did was important—the example set by the Queen, for instance, when she visited a leper colony in Nigeria.

Dicks (1963) in an address to a meeting of the Medical Association for the Prevention of War advocated a 'pathology of prejudice' which would enable us to regard discrimination and persecution as material for therapy rather than elevating them to the dignity of political acts. Prejudices had an obvious survival value in that fear of the unknown was a safer guide to man in his individual or social infancy than overconfidence. Emotional security in childhood is advocated as the panacea, for if the child accepts the parent figure as a mainly safe, loving person this would counter any hostile and suspicious aspects of the personality and prevent the distorted image of the hostile, persecuting parent becoming incorporated into the psyche.

Much energy could be used in 'defending' oneself against these hostile images with consequent emotional arrest, lack of independence and lack of creative energy. Fear of the hostile parent-object or the content of one's own feared unconscious became so great that the attitude towards it was one of propitiation and avoidance. Submerged hate and fear is 'projected' and the world is divided into hostile, persecuting, figures and noble, idealized ones—the 'out-group' and the 'in-group'. The more massive the unconscious phantasy the greater the distortion to the point of actual psychosis as is seen in paranoid states. Sexual inadequacy or abstinence not infrequently went with repressed admiration for the supposedly primitive, sensuous, merciless qualities of other races. Greed, too, was expressed deviously: anti-Semitism drew on it, while the wealthy in America projected their guilt on the working classes who were 'greedy and always wanting more'. Even out-group members like Jews and Negroes could take on the mores of the culture in which they lived and become the most anti-Semitic or anti-Negro of all, showing an ambivalence towards their own primary group.

Xenophobic prejudice and behaviour came to the surface at times of threat to a group's economic and social status. Key personalities in institutions would then require watching, for the severely authoritarian tended to propagate themselves and a democratic or tolerant regime could swiftly become totalitarian. This last suggestion brings the argument round full circle for who is to do the watching other than those with a built in suspicion of any encroachment on their freedom.

Some of the theories put forward by Dicks are plausible but are not always borne out in practice. When the severe test comes, it is not the emotionally secure 'liberal' element who stand up to the tyrant and risk their lives. Karl Stern in his *Pillar and the Flame* illustrated this from his experiences in Nazi Germany, where Right Wing and overtly anti-Semitic colleagues lost their lives in their opposition to Hitler while many 'liberals' rapidly became docile Party members. In the conflicts of men, it takes more than infantile emotional security to safeguard justice, and prejudice in itself need not always be evil for there is also prejudice against prejudice.

Prostitution

This is an ancient practice which has flourished in primitive and classical times and in all regions. Social attitudes change in that the temple harlot would be completely out of place in the parish church, but no doubt this transfer from the sacred to the profane can be explained and Henriques (1962) whose first volume of *Prostitution and Society* conveys the sociological implications of the practice, gives promise that in his later volumes, he will explain the phenomenon. Psychological aspects of prostitution have been seriously studied and Havelock Ellis is reputed to have commended the study in this dictum: 'There is more psychology to be learned in the brothels of a large city than in all the universities of Europe'. Deutsch (1946) describes the moral cynicism of prostitutes:

> Even the simplest moral laws have absolutely no influence on these women, because these sanctions express values that are completely alien to them.... Their psychic infantilism makes of the entire world a nursery in which social institutions are personified by their representatives.

She relates the story of a prostitute, Anna, whom she saw regularly for three years. She had been regarded as psychopathic and was very hostile to the male doctors, but behaved better towards the female staff. Her entry into prostitution was for economic reasons but underlying them were her social and psychological difficulties. Masochism plays a great part in their lives and this is shown in their relations with their 'protectors' who defend them from the outside world like a brother or father, but yet exploit them brutally. It is this brutality which sexually excites them, though they are probably frigid with their clients.

These clients are not without psychological interest. Rolph (1955) divided them into two categories: neurotic or disturbed personalities who were only able to obtain sexual satisfaction with prostitutes, and the lonely who wanted temporary companionship. Gibbens and Silberman (1960) in a study based on 230 patients who contracted venereal disease from prostitutes, found 'a bewildering variety of histories and personalities'. In trying to sort out these complexities, the authors considered that generally two factors were at work: a conflict of dependence and independence in their relations with women, starting with the mother, and lack of an adequate father figure with whom they could identify. Superficial explanations, such as lack of more socially acceptable outlets, they reject, and in the case of sailors and long-distance lorry drivers, they suggest that the choice of job is in itself evidence of underlying instability. The person whose sexual outlet is exclusively the prostitute, is usually inhibited, passive, and in a steady job, who probably lives at home and supports his mother. Some, even if they marry, are unable to perform the sexual act with their wives, without invoking the 'prostitution phantasy' and may even seek to reinforce it by insisting that the wife dress and make up for the part.

Patients with no Fixed Abode

In a large urban area with expanding employment there has been, in recent years, an increase in the number of patients who seek the shelter (or asylum) of the mental hospital and who have no fixed address. It is therefore difficult to return them to the community. Berry and Orwin (1966) who reported on the problem in Birmingham, have defined the following characteristics:

> They are usually male; unemployed; no family ties; lived at no fixed abode for over a year; more than 50 per cent have a criminal record; are usually compulsory admissions; 76 per cent had previous hospital admissions; 1 in 4 discharge themselves against advice; a few are schizophrenics but the majority are personality disorders some of whom attempt suicide to gain a lodging in hospital.

It is obvious that the mental hospital is not effective in rehabilitating these patients and society must devise some other arrangement and legislate for their needs, or specifically exclude those who have no intention of collaborating with their treatment from the provisions of the Mental Health Act. At present there is no alternative but to keep re-admitting them to hospital even though everybody knows it is futile.

Priest (1970) compared a group of homeless men in the U.S.A. with others in the U.K. and found a considerable area of similarity in both groups. He quotes the Edinburgh survey of lodging house population where of 77 men, 20 were schizophrenic, 7 were alcoholic, 9 had personality disorders, 6 were mentally defective, 5 had organic brain disease and 4 suffered from depression.

Patch (1970), in his London survey, found that out of 123 men, 18 were schizophrenics, 25 severe alcoholics, 30 moderately heavy drinkers, and 10 suffered from depression. As regards sexual data, 69·1 per cent had never married, compared with 25·2 per cent in the 1961 census; 52 per cent were heterosexual; 5·7 per cent were homosexual and 21·5 per cent said they had no sexual interest.

Dax (1970) quotes Jordan (1963) on the problem of the social misfits:

> They have forced themselves upon the attention of society by scavenging, begging, theft, drunkenness and persistent reliance upon public and private charity. They have been regarded as the epitome of the undeserving poor, the embodiment of crime and vice, and a terrible example of God's judgement upon sinners.
>
> The way of life and even the physical setting is remarkably persistent and widespread—the doss-house and mission, the begging, the drinking of cheap fortified wines and non-beverage alcohol and the endless pitiful procession through the police courts. Nevertheless, two things stand out. Firstly, no-one has invented an effective solution to the problem. Secondly, there is a curious lack of serious literature on the subject.

Problem Families

In addition to containing a fair quota of psychiatric problems, the problem family is in itself a problem in social psychiatry. Scott (1958) in a survey of London's problem families, lists the following factors which are likely to be found:

1. *In a Parent*
   - (*a*) Low intelligence or mental deficiency.
   - (*b*) Mental illness.
   - (*c*) Physical handicap or illness which prevents work or permits of light work only *e.g.* tuberculosis, heart-disease.
   - (*d*) Long-continued or recurrent unemployment of main wage-earner from other causes than physical handicap or illness.
   - (*e*) Excessive drinking.
   - (*f*) Excessive gambling.
   - (*g*) Sexual promiscuity.
   - (*h*) Serving, or has served, a prison sentence.
   - (*i*) Suspected cruelty to or neglect of children.
   - (*j*) Known cruelty to or neglect of children.
2. *Other Parental Shortcomings*
   - (*a*) Persistent quarrelling.
   - (*b*) Failure to call doctor for major illness.
   - (*c*) Leaving young children unattended.
3. *In a Child*
   - (*a*) Repeated hospitalization of one or more children for gastroenteritis or respiratory disease, or two or more children for minor accidents.
   - (*b*) Persistent truancy.
   - (*c*) Juvenile delinquency (court cases only).
   - (*d*) Attendance at child guidance clinic.
   - (*e*) Under Probation Officer or committed to care by a court.
4. *Housing*
   - (*a*) Statutory overcrowding.

(*b*) Living in intolerable conditions (while not overcrowded) because of either lack of amenities such as piped water, damp or insanitary conditions, and/or enmity of other occupants of dwelling.

5. *Poverty and Mismanagement*
   (*a*) Chronic family debt.
   (*b*) Lack of minimal necessities of furniture and bedding.
   (*c*) Inadequate and irregular meals.
   (*d*) Domestic filth and disorder.
   (*e*) Wilful damage to property.
   (*f*) Lack of, or inadequately maintained, clothing of children.

6. *General*
   (*a*) Unnecessary crowding at night.
   (*b*) Gross personal uncleanliness.
   (*c*) Failure to take advantage of necessary help and service proffered.
   (*d*) Child or children taken into care other than as the result of court action, and who are frequently taken into or out of care.

In an analysis of aetiological factors in 1000 families, he found emotional instability in 54·5 per cent of the potential problem families and 71·6 per cent in the hard-core problem families, with mental deficiency or low intelligence in 42·2 and 67·3 per cent respectively. He defined the potential group as 'those in which there are early signs of failure which may lead to disruption of normal home life with consequent risk to the children', and the hard-core group as 'those which are unable, by their own efforts, to raise themselves from the state into which they have fallen or to take advantage of the social services of which they are in need'. He advocates handing over these families from health visitors to social workers because of the short time the former can spare for this work; the average was 20 minutes per week for a 'potential' and 28 minutes per week for 'hard-core'. He suggests that: 'If such selected families could be passed on to social case-workers who might *on average* give up to ninety minutes a week to them, some progress might be made'. In spite of concentrated effort by armies of social workers little progress has been made. It seems that these families almost thrive in their inadequacy when exposed to social workers. A more promising approach is the provision of nursery training for the children so that the young are reclaimed and in turn influence their parents.

MENTAL HEALTH CONSULTATION

Caplan (1970) has become the doyen of mental health consultants and the main protagonist of the concept of preventive psychiatry (Caplan, 1964). He admits that '. . . we have little scientific evidence to prove that mental health specialists and psychiatric clinics and hospitals are more helpful to the mentally disordered than other professionals and nonprofessionals'.

Characteristics of the Mental Health Consultation:

1. Mental health consultation is a method for use between two professionals in respect to a lay client or a programme for such client.

2. The consultee's work problem must be defined by him as being in the mental health area, relating to (*a*) mental or personality disorder of the client; (*b*) promotion of mental health of the client; and (*c*) interpersonal aspects of the work situation. It is assumed that the consultant has expert knowledge in these areas.

3. The consultant has no administrative responsibility for the consultee's work or professional responsibility for the outcome of the client's case. He is under no compulsion to modify the consultee's conduct of the case.

4. The consultee is under no compulsion to accept the consultant's ideas or suggestions.

5. The basic relationship between the two is coordinate, there being no built-in hierarchical authority which is expected to potentiate the influence of ideas and their easy adoption.

6. The coordinate relationship is fostered by the consultant being a member of another profession and a visitor.

7. Dependency is avoided as consultations are few, brief, and intermittent.

8. Consultation is expected to continue indefinitely in that consultees are expected to encounter unusual work problems throughout their careers and increasing competence makes them more likely to recognize problems and demand more consultations.

9. A consultant has no predetermined body of information that he intends to impart to a particular consultee. He responds only to that segment placed before him, though other areas may be submitted at subsequent consultations.

10. The twin goals are to help the consultee improve his handling or understanding of the current difficulty and thus improve his capacity to master similar problems in future.

11. The aim is to improve the consultee's work and not his sense of well-being.

12. Consultation does not focus overtly on the consultee's personal problems and feelings. It respects his privacy. The consultant does not allow the discussion of personal and private material.

13. This does not mean that the consultant does not pay attention to the feelings of the consultee, but he deals with them in a

special way such as the form in which the consultee has displaced them on to the client.

14. The consultant should be free to abandon the above rules if he decides that the consultee's actions are endangering the client by overlooking the risk of suicide or serious mental breakdown. This breaks the coordinate relationship, but in favour of a higher goal.

15. Mental health consultation is not a new profession but merely a special way in which existing professionals operate.

Types of consultation: (1) client-centred; (2) consultee-centred; (3) programme-centred administrative; (4) consultee-centred administrative.

Comment: To one who is not committed to the value of this approach (and without 'scientific' proof, who should be?) there is much about the proposals which suggests a cult rather than an effective and economic method of bringing appropriate skills to appropriate problems. If this were a pilot scheme to see how it works, one would applaud the enthusiasm of the experimenters and anxiously await the opportunity to scrutinize their results. But it has been going on now for nearly twenty years, and the Director of the National Institute of Mental Health, U.S.A. (Dr Stanley Yoller) in a foreword to Dr Caplan's book, is enthusiastic about the preventive aspects of mental health consultation; this is now included as one of the five service components that are established as 'essential to each community mental health centre' and this is now mandatory for the funding of these centres. Dr Caplan states that 'by the end of 1970 five hundred community mental health centres will have been funded by the National Institute of Mental Health and it is projected that two thousand centres will be funded by 1980'.

A question which springs to the mind of an outsider is: Why this tremendous rush to spend huge sums of money and deploy scarce skills and syphon off from the community a large sector of university and college production in a field where the results are not even obvious, yet alone validated? It is being too cynical to suggest that only politicians could be so profligate of human and fiscal resources?

FAMILY PSYCHIATRY

Because of the present accent on environmental factors and family influences in mental illness, there has been considerable attention, in recent years, to what is called family psychiatry. Another stimulus has been the common experience that one member of a family is referred to the psychiatrist, but it soon transpires that other members are more disturbed. The original patient was really a symptom of a family disturbance and treatment directed at the patient alone would not solve the patient's or the family's problems.

Some see the family as a group and include them all in group psychotherapy sessions. MacGregor (1964) describes his variant which he calls *Multiple Impact Therapy with Families.* He claims it is successful with neurotic and schizophrenic adolescents and is based on the therapy team consisting of psychiatrist, psychologist and social worker who are intended to serve as a model of healthy group functioning; presumably they have been well selected! The family interactions within itself and the team provide cumulative and converging data which the team has constantly on view and utilizes as it works with the family to define and resolve issues. Channels of communication are easier to keep open and the family becomes a partner in therapy while more energies are released for the task in hand.

Titchener and Golden (1963) claim they can predict therapeutic themes from their observations of family interaction evoked by using the 'revealed differences' technique. Families (parents, patient, sibs down to age 11) are observed, the subjects presenting mainly with symptomatic neuroses or character disorders. The family is asked to complete a questionnaire with 15 moderately controversial but homely items regarding family life and adolescence in our culture. Papers are marked and returned and the experimenter points out the differences and agreements and the family are asked to reconcile their differences and explore agreements. Oneway screen and tapes are used and each response is carefully evaluated. The family's life style is then defined and a pattern or series of patterns are found to be highly specific for the family. One such pattern was when parents spoke directly to each other; another was when they did not, but through their children. The authors claim that this avoidance of direct parental communication was of unfavourable prognostic significance.

Esterton *et al.* (1965) report their results of family-orientated therapy with 20 male and 22 female hospitalized schizophrenics. All patients were discharged within one year of admission and the average stay was three months. Seventeen per cent were readmitted within a year of discharge, but 70 per cent of the rest were earning their living during the whole of the year after discharge. They adhered to the following principles in their treatment:

1. A systematic clarification and undoing of patterns of communication which they regarded as 'schizogenic' in the family.
2. A similar clarification and undoing of such patterns of

communication between patients and between staff and patients.

3. Continuity of personnel working with the family during and after the patient's stay in hospital.

4. No individual psychotherapy was given.

5. None of the so-called shock treatments were used, nor was leucotomy.

Patients received comparatively small doses of tranquillizers; 25 per cent had none at all; no male patient received more than 300 mg. of chlorpromazine per day.

Social therapists were trained and the wards re-organized to create a human context which avoided so far as was possible any situation which had been shown to precipitate psychotic behaviour. Each patient was ensured a relationship with at least one other person significant to him and this was the role of the social therapist.

These are impressive results and indicate the extent to which manipulation of the environment can help in the treatment of schizophrenia.

Social Functioning as the Prime Aim of Treatment

The above tenet will not be generally accepted for many are now concerned with the patient's 'well-being' and 'happiness', although they may have given little thought to what these terms imply and whether they are permanent states or not. Ruesch (1966) in an analysis of duration of patient's stay in hospital concludes that it usually has little bearing on economics or social functioning and strongly recommends short-stay rehabilitation with intensive treatment as these give better results than prolonged insight therapy. He limits the aims of treatment to adequate social functioning and has this to say about the State's responsibilities:

> As social and psychological functioning are passibly well-restored, the obligation of government and group to their less fortunate members ends. The 'pursuit of happiness' and the refined psychological methods used to bring about self-improvement and self-realization are optional tasks that may be undertaken at the discretion of the individual.

SOCIAL PSYCHIATRY AND SOCIAL SCIENCE

Social science has rapidly grown to the level of a major exporter from our universities and colleges and pervades many fields which were previously dominated by the medical profession. Much of this growth is due to the word 'science' which social studies bear, and while the use of this word has frequently been questioned, serious criticism by sociologists has not been prominent.

Social Sciences as Sorcery

Stanislaw Andrewski (1972), who is a professor of sociology, is a critic from within the ranks, and while his case is vigorously and even indelicately presented, his expertise and status are such that medical men can learn from him. Andrewski's main thesis is that power to manipulate the natural world lies in exact science. Power to manipulate the human world lies in sorcery. He likens the social scientist to a witch doctor who judges his work by the effect it will have rather than by the truth it embodies and that this tends to spawn an obfuscating morass of pseudo-scientific inanities which insidiously succeed in serving various ideological ends.

The difficulties inherent in the studies of society such as the sheer complexity of the human brain and the ability of man to react, either positively or negatively, to statements about himself, do not mean that we cannot know more (as opposed to everything) about social life. But he regards social scientists as a group as ill-informed, unaware of basic rules of grammar, and tempted into charlatanry by being faced with a subject utterly beyond their mental powers in fields where it pays better to mislead or conceal than to reveal. Under the guise of scientific objectivity, they can bedevil their victims by the selective dissemination of information and the smuggling of value judgments disguised as facts or impartial concepts. By giving descriptions of 'normal' behaviour they can influence behaviour in this direction.

The denigration of the concept of responsibility based on the unwarranted dogma of psychological determinism has, he considers, contributed significantly to the undermining of our civilization. The use of cybernetic models is not only an ingenious method of studying politics by overlooking the subject matter but also, by stressing the resemblance between cybernetic machines and human society, may convince people they are nothing but cogs, leading them to behave accordingly. He comments that psychology leaves us in 'the void between quantified trivialities and the fascinating but entirely undisciplined flights of fancy'. Enthusiastic welcomes are extended to 'verbal fads consisting of new labels for old and often worn-out notions'.

Comment: Medical students are rarely exposed to a critique of the social sciences. They are generally regarded as one of the influences for good, like the nursing profession, and it is as well that their shortcomings should be exposed, especially as in the community the doctor is being asked to forsake the nursing model for that of the social worker. In one respect the enthusiasm for the social sciences may confirm another of Andrewski's claims: 'Even a cursory survey of human beliefs reveals that man has no innate inclination to seek the truth and that absurdity and obscurity, far from repelling, have for most people an irresistible attraction.'

Social Stress and Psychiatric Disorder

Eisler and Polak (1971) assessed the social and situational stresses that preceded the admission of over 1500 patients to a Crisis Intervention Service. The 15 social stresses listed were: marital, work, migration, medical, financial, separation, bereavement, sexual, pregnancy, legal, school, family, child and adolescent, ageing and interpersonal relationships. An average of nearly three stresses was experienced by each patient in the 2-year period prior to admission. Nearly half had experienced marital and/or family stress, and nearly one third actual or threat of separation. Specific diagnostic patterns were not related to specific antecedent stressors.

CHAPTER 15

Suicide and Attempted Suicide

Because every successful attempt at suicide results in death, it has been assumed that it was the intention of the individual to die. Similarly, unsuccessful attempts have been regarded as frustrated efforts at self-destruction. Neither of these assumptions is warranted. Some commit suicide without really intending to do so, while many more attempt suicide without the slightest intention of dying. On the other hand most people who commit suicide fully intended taking their lives, and a number who attempted it, intended to destroy themselves but are unsuccessful because of chance happenings outside their control, such as the heroic measures in hospital which resuscitated them. This overlap between the suicide and the attempted suicide has led many to regard them as similar, if not identical problems. Indeed, the Act which deals mainly with those who *attempt* suicide is called the Suicide Act (1961). In this Chapter the two conditions will be dealt with separately for their differences are greater than their similarities.

SUICIDE

Incidence

There are some facts available but these may not give a reliable picture. Even in a highly organized country like Britain with a legal system which has for many years required a Coroner's inquest on every case of suspected suicide, the figures are not reliable and some investigators have claimed that not more than 50 per cent of suicides are recorded as such. Much of this discrepancy is due to the Coroner's reluctance to record such a verdict, in order to spare the sensitivities of the recently bereaved family who are often present in his Court. There are also religious, legal and insurance complications and many coroners lean over backwards not to bring in a verdict of suicide. A more reliable index of the incidence of suicide might well be the number of inquests held where suicide was suspected.

Incidence varies from country to country and even in different parts of quite small countries, so national figures, which initially may well be unreliable, may also confuse, in that essential differences such as those between urban and rural areas can be obscured in the final figures. The World Health Organization derives suicide rates per 100,000 of the population from these unreliable figures and if one were so minded a 'league table' could be drawn up, of which the following is an example for 1961:

Suicide deaths per 100,000 population in 1961.

West Berlin	37·0	Denmark	16·9
Hungary	25·4	Sweden	16·9
Austria	21·9	France	15·9
Czechoslovakia	20·6	Belgium	14·8
Finland	20·6	S. Africa (European)	14·1
Japan	19·6	Australia	11·9
West Germany	18·7	England and Wales	11·3
Switzerland	18·2	United States	10·5

N.B. It would be very rash to draw any conclusion from these figures.

Stengel (1964) in his analysis of suicide rates in Western communities found a positive correlation with:

male sex; increasing age; widowhood; single and divorced state; childlessness; high density of population; residence in big towns; high standard of living; economic crisis; alcohol consumption; broken home in childhood; mental disorder; physical illness.

A negative correlation was found with:

female sex; youth; married state; large number of children; low density of population; rural occupation; religious practice; low socio-economic class; war.

These factors do not tell us all we need to know, for the relationship may be a casual rather than a causal one. The suicide rate itself, even if reliably assessed, does not necessarily mean what it would superficially suggest. A high suicide rate is generally regarded as an index of a disturbing social situation and countries with a low rate are quoted as enviable examples of a desirable social matrix. High rates are generally found in the more prosperous countries which also achieve a greater expectation of life, and which leads to more people being in the age groups at risk. Unless rates are reconciled to age structure of the population, an entirely erroneous impression may be gained. As Stengel says; 'A low suicide rate may conceal more human misery than is revealed in a high rate'.

Social Isolation

In British studies, this would appear to be an important factor in suicide and may well tip the balance in elderly people living alone or in the university student living in Hall or in lonely lodgings.

This aspect of suicide had long been recognized for Durkheim (1897) showed that the loss of a feeling of identity with the social group was an important factor and this view has since been confirmed by Sainsbury (1955). Districts of a large city with many hotels and lodging houses are also likely to have a higher suicide rate.

Religion

It is popularly assumed that Roman Catholics because of their Faith are less likely to commit suicide. This may be so, but in non-Catholic communities, it is found that those who are actively practising their religion are less liable to suicide, while in Catholic countries there are wide discrepancies, *e.g.* Austria (21·9) and Eire (3·2) which could be due to differing attitudes to religion, or to entirely different reasons.

Age

The 70-80 decade has the highest suicide rate *per unit of population at risk,* though most people commit suicide in their 50's. That this age distribution can adulterate surveys on suicide was shown by Stengel and Cook (1958) in their study of suicide in two industrial cities in the North of England. One had a suicide rate several times the other and the authors attributed this to a decline in the local industry resulting in emigration of the young people and a consequent over-representation of the elderly.

Social Class

The Registrar General's classification is based on the individual's employment (see p. 662). Suicide rates are highest among classes I and II with doctors and dentists high on the list. This could be due to ease of access to dangerous drugs, skill in their use and knowledge of medicine. The last factor is regarded as especially important in doctors for they are able to assess the prognosis of any physical condition they may have. Of perhaps more importance is the tendency for doctors (and medical students too) to put the worst interpretation on relatively harmless symptoms. If there is a depressive element as well, and there usually is, hypochondriasis of a delusional intensity supervenes and the death sentence is executed.

Black Suicide

Hendin (1969) studied the incidence of suicide in young urban blacks in New York and found it occurred twice as frequently between the ages of 20-35 years as among white men of the same age. Homicide rate among black men reached its peak during the same period, indicating a relationship between suicide and violence. The author regards the subjects as hovering between depression and rage, between conscious overt violence and self-destruction. He drew conclusions about the psychopathology of black suicides from studies of 25 blacks who attempted suicide. Such deductions are fraught with many pitfalls, and while the author's raw data are impressive, they merely indicate the need for further study and cannot be accepted as a satisfactory analysis of the problem. Questions which spring to mind are the reporting habits of suicides in black and white communities, and the influence of drugs, blackmail and other selective agencies. It is tempting to seize on a set of figures and make a meal of them by incorporating attitudes and prejudices and even though these be favourable, they do not compensate for a more thorough and objective enquiry.

Suicide and Pregnancy

Since Sim (1963) reported the infrequency of suicide in pregnant women, a finding which had already been noted by Durkheim (1897), there have been protests disputing the finding but very little of any evidence to refute it. Whitlock and Edwards (1968) in a search of records in Brisbane, Australia, and in their own study, failed to discover a pregnant woman who had taken her life. They did report on 30 women who had made a 'suicidal attempt' but even in these the pregnancy was not the only or even the most important cause of the suicidal act.

Suicide in Students

This is greatly in excess of the national average for similar age groups with marked differences between 'provincial' universities and those of Oxford, Cambridge and London, the former being not much greater than the national average. Though in number they are very much less than among the lonely aged, they have received much greater publicity. This is largely because promising young lives are cut off and the community is rightly concerned. It is to be hoped that the less publicised groups will not be forgotten.

Parnell (1951) was one of the first to emphasize the extent of serious mental illness among undergraduates at Oxford where the suicide rate was 11 times that of a comparable population. Rook (1959), in a study of morbidity in Cambridge undergraduates over a period of 35 years, found that out of 103 deaths, 41 were due to accident, 35 to suicide and 27 to disease. These older universities had a much higher rate of suicide than the provincial universities and Rook put forward the hypothesis that this difference may be due to the smaller number in residence in the provinces. He states: 'The college staircase may facilitate study but it can also lead to loneliness and can encourage brooding'. A similar picture has been reported from Yale (Parrish, 1957).

There is now strong pressure for additional psychiatric services for students because of their high risk and while there is probably a case for extra attention, a proper perspective should be maintained, otherwise even higher risk groups, such as the lonely elderly will be further deprived of the limited resources available. If Halls of Residence do contribute to the instability and eventual suicide of some students, it would be more rational and much more economical for universities to reverse their present policy of recruiting students from outside their area and give priority to young people who live locally.

Seasonal Incidence

This has intrigued many investigators from Durkheim onwards. Suicide is commoner in European countries in the Spring while in Australia the season is December and January. In Israel, suicide in the elderly tends to occur during the hottest season and may be an expression of an inability to cope with the added physical discomforts. Obviously high temperature alone is not enough, as is convincingly demonstrated in Britain. It does tend to follow the pattern of incidence of depressive psychoses and in the author's experience these are commoner at holiday times when everybody else is enjoying themselves and the patient feels more and more isolated and eventually gives up.

Motives

These are difficult to define with certainty especially as the main witness is unable to testify. Occasionally a 'suicide note' is left but even this is not a reliable indication of motive. It may express hostility or love or plead forgiveness but rarely is the true motive mentioned. If it expresses self-depreciation and guilt this would indicate an underlying depressive psychosis.

The Suicide Pact

This is allegedly an agreed arrangement for mutual self-destruction. Usually one of the parties is murdered by the other who then commits suicide. The amount of agreement is difficult to decide though occasionally suicide notes are left by both which may confirm that there was a pact. Although attempting suicide is no longer a crime, the survivor of a suicide pact can be charged with either murder or manslaughter. Generally, such pacts involve spouses or cohabiting adults.

Suicide Notes

As mentioned above these are not uncommonly left by the parties of a suicide pact, usually to exonerate the murderer. A study of such notes has been reported by Shneidman and Farberow (1957) who tried to distinguish the genuine notes from the simulated ones. The simulated notes were produced by a control group who were asked to write a note as if they were about to take their own lives. The genuine ones referred more to persons, things and spatial relationships than the control group. Capstick (1960) reported similarly in that 15 per cent left notes, more were over 60 years of age and they were concerned with those they were leaving behind.

Method

This varies and may even follow the trend of fashion. Availability of resources such as the Eiffel Tower, bridges over rivers or gorges, skyscrapers and cliffs explain some local preferences, but poisoning by domestic gas is still the most popular with both sexes in Britain. Other forms of poisoning like drug overdosage come next and then hanging, drowning, firearms, etc. In America, probably because of more easy access, firearms or explosives are by far the commonest cause. Coal gas used to be commoner in the United States, but it has now been replaced by a less toxic variety which is unsuitable for suicide.

The Suicidal Risk

Sainsbury (1968) laid down the following criteria for the bad risk for suicide: (1) he will have a psychotic depression and be over 40 years of age; (2) he will have lost one of his parents in childhood from suicide and will himself have threatened or attempted suicide; (3) the illness will be of short duration or he may have recently been discharged from hospital and will be living alone; (4) he is more likely to harp on his feelings of hopelessness and worthlessness and loss of energy than on his adverse circumstances; loneliness rather than physical illness in the elderly depressive will increase the risk; (6) he will be drinking heavily.

He adds the following hints. Suicides frequently give a clear warning to their family doctor or to a psychiatrist. Treatment should be thorough, for half-treated depressives can become certain suicides and there should be precise and set procedures for after-care and follow-up. The worst time is the six months following discharge.

Causes

In human behaviour, normal or otherwise, it is difficult even to talk in terms of causation for so many factors are involved. All one can do is to define what appeared at the time to be the most dominant factor. This was done by Sainsbury (1955) in his North London survey of 390 cases of suicide. Social factors as contributory or principal (60 and 35 per cent respectively) were highest on the list, with mental disorder (47 and 37 per cent respectively) next in order. Physical illness (29 and 18 per cent) was not a negligible factor. The relatively high number with a social factor could have been due to the higher rate of suicide among the unemployed in the area. All investigators have remarked on the relative infrequency of pregnant women among suicides and Sainsbury found only 2 in the 390 cases he studied.

THEORIES OF SUICIDE

Psychoanalytic

Freud postulated a death instinct or 'Thanatos' to balance the life instinct or 'Eros', and the former may seek expression in suicide. The patient has usually identified with somebody he both loves and hates and this ambivalence may be directed on himself and the aggressive or hate impulse may assume sadistic or suicidal dimensions. Zilboorg

(1936 *a & b*) stated that suicide could be a method of thwarting outside forces which the patient finds unbearable and that by dying the patient can find immortality and fame. O'Connor (1948) has pointed out that in depression, suicide is a return to an early power narcissism, giving the victim omnipotence through the act. Escape from the unbearable situation is a dominant theme in children's suicide and suicidal attempts, and this is coupled with an 'overflow' aggression directed at the parents. Bender and Schilder (1937), in a study of 18 children under the age of 13, found that spite operated in nearly every case.

The types of suicide have been differentiated on analytical lines by Bergler (1946), who lists three types:

1. **Introjection.** The patient has guilt feelings against which is mobilized pseudo-aggression.
2. **Hysteric.** An unconscious dramatization of how one does not wish to be treated is accompanied by a childish belief that death is not final.
3. **Miscellaneous.** These include a variety of psychiatric disorders such as paranoid schizophrenia where the super-ego is projected outwards in the form of hallucinatory voices which command the final act.

Menninger (1938) in his book *Man Against Himself* takes a wider view of the suicide act and includes all kinds of behaviour which are harmful to life, such as alcoholism, drug addiction, and martyrdom, self-mutilation and accident proneness. He emphasizes the life and death instincts of man and makes use of the sado-masochistic complex in his interpretation. Three elements in suicide are defined:

1. The desire to kill.
2. The desire to be killed.
3. The desire to die.

All are alleged to be present in the suicidal bid, though only one may predominate. Obviously if the desire to die is not strongly represented the attempt will be only half-hearted and is unlikely to result in death. The first two elements are expressions of the sado-masochistic needs of the individual.

SUICIDE AND MENTAL ILLNESS

Though most people would regard self-destruction as indisputable evidence of mental illness, there are cultures which accept suicide, under certain circumstances, as normal behaviour. Ceremonial suicide is represented by *hara-kiri* in Japan and in the state of *amok* where the individual, as a result of wounded honour, loss of face, and a desire for revenge, includes homicide in his stormy passage to death. In India, *suttee* which demands that the widow seek death with her husband is a gentler version of a similar attitude to death. Even in our own culture, where honour is still highly regarded, suicide could, under certain circumstances, be condoned and not regarded as evidence of mental illness.

Suicide is not specific to any particular type of mental disorder, though *psychotic depression* is the commonest precursor. The feelings of guilt and unworthiness, the intense hypochondriasis, the general attitude of hopelessness, and the agony of living with the torturing thoughts and self-accusations cause many to attempt suicide, and, if unsuccessful after the first attempt and left untreated, to try again. *Schizophrenic patients* occasionally commit suicide in response to a hallucinatory command or to a delusion.

Psychopathic personalities though almost the polar opposites in their mental make-up to patients with psychotic depression, do occasionally commit suicide. The author had one such patient who was sentenced to life imprisonment for stabbing a fellow naval rating to death. He murdered a fellow-prisoner a few years later and then was found hanging in his cell. While a patient, his behaviour, as one frequently finds, was exemplary.

Alcoholics are prone to commit suicide, thus supporting Menninger's contention that they are intent on self-destruction. Many alcoholics start as symptomatic drinkers, the psychiatric disturbance being a depressive one and this may still drive them to suicide. The sadistic component of the alcoholism which results in the ruination of their families' lives as well as their own may reinforce the masochistic needs which then seek expression in death

Suicide and Homicide

This is found in the suicide pact (see above) but it may occur without the consent of the other party or parties. It is usually based on depressive delusions though persecutory ones may also be responsible. The author had a patient who was suffering from a psychotic depression and thought she was too wicked for this world. She did not want to leave her aged mother to face the world alone, so she murdered her and then tried to commit suicide but was discovered in time to be resuscitated. Though these cases are rare, it does add to the responsibility of the doctor in assessing a patient's risk for suicide; he or she may also be liable to homicide.

Plural Attempts

These are generally indicative of a serious bid to commit suicide and imply using more than one method simultaneously. In the author's experience it is becoming commoner with an overdose of tablets as the common denominator. Associated methods are gassing, hanging and lacerations of throat and wrists. These have no special significance apart from showing the patient's determination.

Chronic Suicide

Such problems are usually undramatic but no less lethal. It is found in those patients described by Menninger (see above) and to them can be added severe cases of anorexia nervosa, diabetics who ignore their diet and insulin requirements, obese cardiac patients who refuse to reduce their weight, severe hypertensives and coronary invalids who insist on exposing themselves to a stressful existence which would prove too much for fitter men. There are numerous other examples, such as the patient who conceals her malignant condition because she knows that if untreated it will surely kill her. Not enough is known about these problems, though many physicians and surgeons have individual experience of them.

Erotized Repetitive Hangings

Resnik (1972) described the syndrome of erotized repetitive hangings in which adolescent males and young men engage in masturbation titrated to increasing self-manipulated neck pressure. It is reckoned that at least 50 deaths annually result from this practice in the United States.

The elements of the syndrome are ropes, belts and other binding material which are so arranged that compression of the neck may be produced and controlled; evidence of masturbation; partial or complete nudity; solitude during the act; attempts to insure that there will be no visible mark on the person; absence of any apparent wish to die; the presence of erotic pictures or literature; binding of the body and/or the extremities and/or the genitals with ropes, chains or leather; and in some cases, female attire. Neurocirculatory mechanisms, especially cerebral hypoxia, reinforce the hanging behaviour by enhancing the masturbatory pleasure. Unexpected death may result from unconsciousness due to carotid sinus reflex and gradual asphyxia resulting from complete body suspension.

The author adds an amusing quotation from Dorothy Parker's *Résumé:*

Razors pain you;
Rivers are damp;
Acids stain you;
And drugs cause cramp;
Guns aren't lawful;
Nooses give;
Gas smells awful;
You might as well live.

Newspaper Influence on Suicide.

Motto (1970) studied the suicide rate during a 268-day period of complete cessation of newspaper publishing in the major metropolitan area of Detroit and compared it with the mean rate for the same calendar period of the prior four years and subsequent year. There was a dramatic decrease in female suicides (60 per cent) and the following year it rose again; male suicides were relatively unaffected. The author concluded that newspaper reports of suicide do influence suicide behaviour and recommended less emphasis in reporting the details.

ATTEMPTED SUICIDE

The above title unlike that of SUICIDE begs the question for it assumes that everybody who has deliberately harmed himself by injury or noxious agent intended to take his life. At one time this may have been generally true, though Shakespeare recognized the importance of the threat of suicide in manipulating the environment (*A Midsummer Night's Dream,* Act V, Scene 1). Today the vast and increasing number of instances of deliberate self-damage are not intended as serious suicidal attempts but have other significance. Labels, other than attempted suicide, for such gestures have been proposed. Lennard-Jones and Asher (1959) who were impressed by the lack of desire to die in these patients, suggested the term 'Pseudocide'. This has been criticized by the pedants who point out that the term can mean pseudohomicide as well as pseudosuicide, but it is attractive, not only because it bears the hallmark of the good pun, but because it accurately interprets the patient's intention. Kessel (1965 *a & b*) who was impressed with the high incidence of self-administered poisons in these patients suggested the term 'Self-Poisoning' but this by definition would exclude the considerable number who resort to self-wounding. Attempted suicide includes 'self-poisoning', 'pseudocide' and, of course, attempted suicide, and few investigators have tried to disentangle the individual members of the group.

There have been careful studies of patients admitted to hospital for self-damage and those of Dahlgren (1945), Ettlinger and Flordh (1955) and Sainsbury (1955) are of particular importance. More recently Parkin and Stengel (1965), Kessel (1965 *a & b*) and Greer and Gunn (1966) have added further to our knowledge of this subject, but the problem has by no means been exhaustively investigated for there is still this pre-occupation with total numbers and the act itself. Though the data are subjected to analysis, not enough is yet known about the increasing popularity of 'pseudocide' and the factors contributing to it. When controls are used as in Greer and Gunn's they are 'non-suicidal psychiatric patients as well as medical, surgical and obstetric patients without psychiatric disorder'. The first group would assume that all the patients studied were in fact suicidal; this we know is unlikely. The second group is even more difficult to interpret, for admission to hospital for a general medical or surgical condition frequently has major functional overtones which require considerable probing to elicit. These authors concluded that their patients 'differed significantly from both control groups in having a greater incidence of childhood parental loss . . . a significantly higher proportion . . . had experienced recent disruption of a close relationship due to interpersonal conflict'. It is difficult to know what these factors really mean in terms of attempted suicide and 'pseudocide'.

Parkin and Stengel (1965) tried to establish the incidence of non-fatal suicidal acts in a city with a population of slightly under half a million. Their definition of the suicidal attempt is worth quoting:

> A suicidal attempt is any act of self-damage undertaken with the apparent intention of self-destruction, however half-hearted and ineffective. The patient may have been only vaguely aware of his intention, which sometimes has to be inferred from his behaviour.

They drew their sample from hospital admissions, casualty departments and estimated those seen only by their general practitioners, but they were unable to ascertain the number who did not attend their general practitioner. They concluded that approximately 9·7 patients attempt suicide for every one who is successful. As far as it goes this report is factual and therefore valuable. As the gesture of self-damage is becoming more popular, their work is likely to be of historical interest, but it still fails to differentiate the intentions behind the act.

Kessel (1965 *a & b*) tried to get away from the idea that all acts of self-damage have suicidal intent. He divided his sample as follows:

Predictable Outcome of Act	Males (170)	Females (352)
Death	19%	19%
Death probable	11%	11%
Death unlikely	28%	21%
Certain to survive	40%	49%
Unclassified	2%	0

There are still minor criticisms, for a number included under 'death' or 'death probable' may not have intended to die, and all cases of wounding have been excluded. This enquiry has clearly shown that there is no point in lumping together all patients who resort to self-damage as if they were a homogeneous group.

An interesting finding was the increase of 'other drugs' among agents used. The traditional forms of poisoning are coal gas, barbiturates and aspirins but Kessel found that 23 per cent of his patients were using drugs prescribed for their mental state such as tranquillizers and anti-depressants.

Motives

He lists the following:

Motives for Self-Poisoning	Males (1963)	Females (348)
*Troubled relationship with other people	39% (51%)	59% (65%)
*Distress arising from within	45% (66%)	37% (49%)
*Material problems (money, housing, etc.)	15% (18%)	14% (16%)
'No reason' or 'don't know'	23%	16%

*These factors are not exclusive of each other.
Figures in parentheses are the clinical assessments based on interviews with relatives as well as patients.

Background to Attempts

This can only be dealt with in a general way:

1. *Sex.* Females are more common among the 'pseudocides'.

2. *Age.* This used to be between 30-39 years but is now much less and many adolescents are admitted to hospital with overdose of drugs and self-injury.

3. *Marital Status.* Many are young and unmarried, but of those who are, particularly in the Swedish study, there is a high incidence of divorce.

4. *Loneliness.* This is difficult to assess in our changing culture. It

is a common factor leading to suicide, but in the self-damaging, there is frequently a history of a break-up of a relationship, suggesting that the loneliness was very recent.

5. *Financial Embarrassment.* Ettlinger and Flordh found that 15·3 per cent were on public relief compared with 5·4 per cent of the general population. Other financial stresses such as a sudden reduction in income due to unemployment or the inability to meet hire purchase commitments may precipitate an attempt.

6. *Employment Status.* Ettlinger and Flordh found nothing significant in this aspect apart from an increased number of wives who go out to work. They conclude that working married women are more exposed to mental stress, though they do not suggest what these stresses are. The subject is obviously open to free interpretation.

7. *Alcoholism.* This varies from country to country, and it is to be expected that where the problem is common this will be reflected in the background of attempted suicide. The incidence of alcoholism in Batchelor's (1954) Scottish series was 21·5 per cent compared with 28·6 per cent in Ettlinger and Flordh's Swedish group. Kessel's figures, which were mainly derived from the same source as Batchelor, also indicate the strong influence of alcoholism. There are of course countries with a lower incidence of alcoholism than Scotland and Sweden.

8. *Previous Psychiatric Illness.* Up to 50 per cent of the Swedish group gave a previous history of having attended a psychiatric clinic or having been in a mental hospital for treatment. This figure will depend on the availability of such services, but it can be concluded that at least 50 per cent have shown evidence of previous instability.

9. *Criminality.* The sex distribution will influence the number of patients who have a history of criminal behaviour, for women are less likely to get into such trouble. Batchelor and Napier found that 13 out of 25 males had a criminal record, while Ettlinger and Flordh found that 24·8 per cent of their males had such a history but only 2·8 per cent of their females. These figures are liable to be influenced by the nature of the treatment unit. It would be, if a public institution, the first port of call for the impecunious and particularly the vagrant groups, for it is unlikely that many such people would put themselves out to secure their treatment privately, or for that matter conceal their attempts from the authorities. It is apparent however that instability, while manifest in criminality, can also manifest as attempted suicide.

10. *Previous Suicidal Attempts.* In Batchelor and Napier's patients 17 per cent had made previous attempts, while Ettlinger and Flordh's group showed a 29 per cent incidence. Some patients earn

the label of habitual attempters and they frequently coincide with the criminal or psychopathic group. In them the motive is not an isolated attempt to seek refuge from an external threat, but a chronic and recurring effort to solve an internal and personal problem. It is their way of drawing society's attention to themselves and experiencing a different role—that of the cared-for, rather than the hunted.

11. *Broken Homes.* This factor is dominant in the psychopathic group, and Batchelor and Napier's (1953) series produced a figure of 73 per cent, while in Ettlinger and Flordh's general group the figure was only 29 per cent, and there is no evidence that the national level of broken homes is higher in Scotland than in Sweden.

Attempted Suicide as Language

Kreitman *et al.* (1970) postulate that 'many patients who attempt suicide are drawn from a section of the community in which self-aggression is generally recognized as a means of conveying a certain kind of information. Among this group the act is viewed as comprehensible and consistent with the rest of the cultural pattern, and possibly as appropriate behaviour in some circumstances, even if not formally condoned'. They studied 135 patients and checked data with relatives and friends and found a similar pattern of behaviour especially if they were below 35 years of age, were female and using drugs.

Adolescents who Attempt Suicide

Teicher and Jacobs (1966) postulate three stages whereby the adolescent comes to view suicide as the only solution:

1. A long-standing history of problems.
2. A period of escalation of problems by the introduction of new ones based on adolescence.
3. A final stage; a recent onslaught of problems normally characterized by a chain-reaction which destroys any meaningful social relationships.

The progressive social isolation constitutes 'the problem' and at the same time serves to prevent the adolescent from securing any possible means of resolving it.

Wrist Scratching as a Symptom of Anhedonia

Asch (1971) uses the word 'anhedonia' to describe the inability of an increasing group of adolescent girls to experience pleasure. They complain that they feel empty or dead inside and the striking characteristic is scratching or cutting their wrists. They are usually between 14 and 21 years of age, have histories of eating difficulties, feelings of intense loneliness or boredom and inability to concentrate on school work. Promiscuity and abuse of drugs are common features. They tend to be passive and submissive, though sporadic outbursts of violent and destructive rage can occur. Object relations are poorly developed and are founded on the desperate need to maintain contact and closeness with their objects at any cost. They tend to become involved in overtly sadomasochistic relationships, the source of which seems to derive from their attempts to ward off unacceptable impulses by turning them on themselves. Anxiety rather than depression is the common affect.

The author sees similarities between these anhedonic girls and the 'as if' patient in that they require outside objects to provide value judgements to regulate self-esteem and even to provide reality testing, and they both use denial of aggressive impulses through acting out of passivity. The distinction between the two groups lies in the anhedonic showing sadomasochistic object relations, recurrent anxiety, chronic states of depersonalization and self-mutilation.

The cutting episode was generally premenstrual and pain was never experienced. It followed feelings of rejection and being an outsider; thoughts and impulses of rage appeared, followed by partial or complete feelings of depersonalization and in the majority of instances the cutting was not suicidal. The author suggests that the cutting is a specific technique for dealing with both the rage and the depersonalization.

Comment: Wrist-cutting is common among males, particularly in prisoners and servicemen and there must therefore be a variety of interpretations. In the present writer's experience, girls who cut their wrists are generally from social classes IV or V, of limited intelligence and with a delinquent history, though a few do match those described above.

The Russian Roulette Principle

Some regard this attitude to suicide as specific, where the wish to die is not 100 per cent. The term derives from a mess 'game' played by officers in the Czar's army. One bullet is introduced into the chamber of a revolver and the chamber is spun, the revolver is placed to the head and the trigger is pulled. Theoretically the person has a one in six chance of killing himself, but in practice, if the revolver is well-oiled the weight of the bullet would tend to drag it past the barrel and leave an empty chamber to be struck.

This risk-taking aspect of attempted suicide is very common and may well be a factor in all attempts, even the 'pseudocides'. There is much here of the psychopathology of the gambler rather than that of the depressive psychotic (see p. 394) and this aspect may account for the repeated attempts and eventual success of some of these people. It could also account for a number of 'accidental' deaths in young people who play 'daring' games such as 'Chicken'.

Motives

These are difficult and sometimes impossible to elicit as the patients are frequently untruthful and deliberately misleading and may deny that the attempt was suicidal. They may say that they just could not get to sleep or that they did not know what happened and they are often supported in these statements by relatives. Motives, when volunteered by patients, are generally referable to interpersonal problems such as husband-wife disagreements, broken romances and the like. These have been stressed by Harrington and Cross (1959), but all motives yielded by patients should be seen in the light of dream interpretation—a manifest content and a latent content, and it is the latter which is frequently the more significant.

It is, however, in the motive that the psychiatric diagnosis may lie and one should look particularly for expressions of guilt and unworthiness and in fact enquire directly about them, for in this way the true melancholia can be recognized. Disturbed interpersonal relationships may be an index of the individual's general difficulty in establishing satisfying relations with others, and the schizophrenic patient may have motives which are indicative of his disturbed thought processes, such as those based on delusions or hallucinations. Although women with an unwanted pregnancy frequently threaten suicide, they are very rarely seen as hospital admissions or for that matter in the hospital mortuary.

It is apparent that a variety of mental disturbances can lead to suicidal attempts and the list would read like a psychiatric diagnostic index, and include schizophrenia, involutional melancholia, drug addiction, psychopathic personality, hysterical character, neurotic depression, alcoholism, mental defect, dementia and even cerebral tumour. It is not possible to arrive at any systematized concept of suicide from the mass of clinical data available, and although brief references have been made to Menninger's (1938) psychoanalytic views, these are not comprehensive and other theories and views have been put forward which, though equally incomplete, help towards our understanding of the problem.

Farberow (1950) has reviewed the several theoretical contributions and divides them into two groups, psychoanalytical and non-analytical. A summary of these theories may prove of value to the reader.

Non-psychoanalytical

A number of authors have put forward a variety of suggestions, some of which are based on disturbed cerebral function. The patient suffers a restriction in his field of consciousness because of his despair and is therefore unable to appreciate the totality of the situation and becomes influenced by inadequately monitored information. Crichton-Miller (1931) has suggested that the psychological process is a failure to adapt and a regression from reality. Some attribute the act to an infantile exhibitionist protest or an act of hostility against a harsh restraining figure. The patient may be so insecure that he is unable to complete the aggressive act against himself and an abortive attempt at suicide results. Studies of the influence of the weather, market fluctuations, festive seasons and moon phases have all been claimed to provide 'clues to suicide' (Shneidman & Farberow, 1957).

Ellenberger (1953) provided ethnological support for Menninger's psychoanalytical formulation. The 'wish to die' he equated with the 'biological suicide' found in African and Melanesian cultures in which death appears to follow automatically the violation of religious taboos or as the result of magical practices. The 'wish to be killed' he found in the Tschuktschi Tribes in Northern Siberia where there were two methods: (1) suicide proper, occurring only among boys who were not allowed to meet death at the hands of others and (2) allowing oneself to be killed. These deaths were considered honourable and assured the victim of special privileges in the after-life. The 'wish to kill' is found in states like 'amok' and hara-kiri (see p. 673).

Prevention

This would appear to be the most rational approach to an ever-increasing problem and certain measures have already been instituted in Britain and America. That efforts, to date, have not been crowned with success is not surprising as the problem itself is not entirely understood and there is therefore a tendency to apply remedies in the hope that they will prove effective, yet it is always possible that these 'remedies' may in themselves contribute to the size of the problem.

In Los Angeles, Farberow and Shneidman (1961) formed a Suicide Prevention Center to try and cut down the 6000-7000 attempted suicides per year. Attempted suicide, as has been pointed out, is a very different matter from suicide itself. Many have what Stengel and Cook (1958) called an 'appeal' character, and all a prophylactic clinic can do is to answer the 'Cry for Help' and try and prevent attempts which are in any case unlikely to succeed. There is no evidence that these prophylactic clinics actually reduce the number of suicides. Theoretically they should, at least, reduce the number of attempts, but again there is no conclusive evidence of this.

The Mental Health Research Fund (1962) issued a booklet, *Depression and Suicide,* which puts before the lay public some of the facts in the hope that relatives who read it may recognize the problem in time to do something useful. Unfortunately, relatives tend to deny the gravity of these problems and there is probably no group apart from the patients, who are so impervious to this type of propaganda.

The Samaritans and Suicide

The organization known as the 'Samaritans' provides a telephone number which the patient in distress or his relative may ring and appeal for help. It is unlikely that such measures will make any impact on the incidence of suicide for those intent on committing it are usually psychotically depressed or deluded and are more intent on carrying out the act than avoiding it.

When a lay body enters the field of preventive medicine it may lack the objectivity and scrupulous ethics that one would expect from the medical scientist. The organization gets its clients through advertising and its financial support from government and local authorities; this to a large extent is dependent on persuading these bodies that the Samaritans are making a positive contribution to reducing the number of suicides.

There has been, in Britain, a reduction in the number of suicides in recent years, and the Samaritans have claimed that it is largely, if not entirely, due to their influence. There are certain qualifications which should be stated:

(1) Suicide rates are not a reliable index of suicide, for suicide is a verdict produced by a Coroner's Court and the author knows of many instances where a Coroner has brought in a open verdict or one

of misadventure where on the family's statement it was obvious that suicide was intended, even to the extent of a suicide note left behind.

(2) Psychiatric services have been rapidly developed in recent years, and training has also improved, so that many more skilled personnel are available to recognize and treat the potentially suicidal with effective anti-depressant measures.

(3) General practitioners have also been the target for much education both in their medical schools and at postgraduate training centres, and they are becoming more expert at recognizing and treating the potentially suicidal.

(4) Social services, particularly for the elderly, who form a large population at suicidal risk, with home visiting by health visitors, meals on wheels and day attendance centres have made their contribution.

(5) The change-over from coal gas, which was a killer, to natural gas, which is much less lethal, has robbed the suicidal patient of his most effective weapon.

(6) The drop in the prescribing of barbiturates as a hypnotic and the substitution of Nitrazepam which is very much safer has also deprived many of a suicidal agent which was equal in importance to coal gas.

(7) Improved resuscitation measures in general hospitals have resulted in many fewer succumbing to their suicidal attempts.

(8) If the Samaritans were making a real impact on the suicide scene, there would be an even greater reduction in attempted suicides, but the reverse holds. Samaritans claim that in areas where they operate the suicide rate has fallen; but these areas, usually urban and with better than average general medical, psychiatric and social services meet most of the points stated above. Unfortunately for the Samaritans' claims, they also have a higher than average incidence of suicidal attempts and this figure is rising steeply.

(9) Some Samaritan groups with which the author is familiar do not claim that they are making much, if any, impact on suicide, but provide a counselling service which is needed and appreciated.

(10) Barraclough and Shea (1970) in a study of Samaritan clients found that they were most at risk of committing suicide in the year following self-referral with a rate of 347 per 100,000. Of the 45 suicides studied, 32 (71 per cent) killed themselves within a year of self-referral, and 14 (44 per cent), within their first month as clients. About 4 per cent of all suicides are Samaritan clients.

Radio, television and the Press have been used in the fight against suicide, but it is again very doubtful whether such a personal problem in very disturbed people can be reached by the mass media. The seriously depressed patient who is most at risk is unlikely to be listening, viewing or reading with sufficient concentration to take in the message. It is more likely that his mental aberration would distort it and instead of acting as a prophylactic, it could hasten his end. The author has asked large numbers of depressed patients with suicidal pre-occupation whether they were influenced in seeking help through such programmes or articles. Their answers indicated that they regarded these media as forms of entertainment, which when well they could enjoy but when they became depressed, they either could not summon the interest to read, listen or view, or misinterpreted the message so that their morbid fears were reinforced.

Drugs Left at Home by Psychiatric In-patients

Robin *et al.* (1968) showed that 49 per cent of actively suicidal patients admitted to hospital left drugs at home which could provide the material for another attempt. They recommended that a leaflet be sent with the notification of admission asking that all drugs be brought into hospital and handed to the nurse-in-charge.

The Role of the Family Doctor

He is already making a significant contribution. He is now well-trained to recognize the symptoms of a psychotic depression and institute the necessary treatment. Anti-depressants are now very effective and many severe states have been cut short by their judicious administration. He should have the time to see his patients at regular intervals even when they are not complaining of physical symptoms. There is too much emphasis on the merits and demerits of the routine physical check and it may be that as a screen for serious disease it is not particularly effective. There is one killing disease, viz. suicide, which can be prevented and the routine check, provided it is not over-shadowed by physical investigations, offers an opportunity for the regular assessment of the patient's mental state. Even then, a number will slip through, for severe depression can deteriorate rapidly to suicidal behaviour.

Treatment

It is apparent that in suicidal attempts a variety of psychopathological states are involved which call for considerable experience in diagnosis. In addition, a large number of patients try again, sometimes successfully, so it is important that the appropriate treatment is given and the necessary precautions instituted. While the casualty house surgeon (or his senior officer) may have some psychiatric training, the differentiation of the various conditions is a task which even the expert can find most difficult and he should not assume the responsibility of discharge without getting further advice. This may raise difficulties, for psychiatric services vary in their availability and comprehensiveness.

The following is suggested as the essential psychiatric requirements. There should be a close relationship between the psychiatrist and the hospital and preferably he should be a member of the staff of the special resuscitation unit. He will require the services of a medical or psychiatric social worker, for many patients, as has been shown, will present socio-economic and interpersonal difficulties. It should be his duty to instruct the registrars (medical and surgical) and the casualty house officers in the psychiatric aspects of the problems they are likely to encounter and brief them in case-history taking and interviews with relatives. These should be adequately recorded so that the psychiatrist after examining the patient can formulate his opinion on the fullest possible information, which should include notes from other hospitals.

If the general hospital has its own psychiatric department, specific treatment presents few difficulties, for the resident medical and nursing staff will be familiar with the psychiatrists' needs in the form of trays prepared for electroplexy or abreactive techniques such as pentothal induction. The psychopathic or acute psychotic patient can usually be settled (after resuscitation) with adequate doses of chlorpromazine, up to 100 mg. three times a day, though the presence of liver damage would urge caution and the substitution of another phenothiazine like trifluoperazine (Stelazine) in doses of 5–10 mg. three times a day. Severe depression usually demands an urgent course of electroplexy which can be initiated in the resuscitation unit and later completed in the psychiatric department as an in- or out-patient. In very infirm patients an antidepressant drug may be indicated and imipramine hydrochloride (Tofranil) in doses from 25 to 50 mg. three times a day can be useful, though there is a time lag of 10–14 days before an adequate response is obtained. In the very old, the side-effects of giddiness may be troublesome and cause falling and fractures, and in the male urinary retention can occur.

It is popularly believed that psychotic depression is the commonest cause of suicide and attempted suicide, and while it would be difficult to argue the former, it is certainly not the case in the latter. This is important in treatment, for the very effective measures now in use for psychotic depression would make relatively small impact on the patients admitted. A large number, probably 25 per cent, are neurotic depressions who have over-reacted to conflict situations; a larger number are immature people frequently of limited intelligence who have used the suicidal attempt to draw society's attention to their problems, and there will be the odd case of schizophrenia too. The social support of these patients when they leave hospital is of prime importance and the casualty house surgeon should be familiar with the social agencies who can help.

The Influence of the Law

There was considerable public concern over the criminal aspect of attempted suicide though for years the police were very rarely asked to deal with such patients. Many reformers felt that the mere fact that somebody who attempted suicide could be charged with the offence was enough to have the law changed and the Suicide Act of 1961 was the result. The arguments at the time were that fewer people would commit suicide because of the change in law and that as the social stigma was removed fewer would attempt it. More and more people are attempting it and more are successful; so much for the forecasts.

'Pseudocide' has now become a form of language in our society. It is not always an appeal for help but may indicate a moment of pique or an act of revenge. One must consider whether the change in the law has contributed to the increased incidence. There are, no doubt, other factors such as increased availability of drugs, the climate of our culture which encourages people, particularly the young, to 'act out', and the erosion of the more permanent relationships which had formed a barrier to stormy scenes and frequent breaks.

The law, by withdrawing its disapproval of the act, has made it more respectable and acceptable, so it has indirectly encouraged the young and irresponsible in a form of behaviour which, at an economic level is wasteful of precious medical and nursing resources but also of human lives. The time is approaching when the effects of this legislation should be assessed. It was certainly inaccurately assessed before it was passed.

A minor disadvantage in the change in the law is that a patient who took an overdose and then denied intent to commit suicide and did not appear sufficiently ill to be detained formally in hospital, could be referred to the police and the magistrates court which could order his attendance for treatment as a condition of probation. This was humane, for it stressed the sickness in mind of the person and ensured proper treatment. Now such patients may be allowed to slip away to repeat the act successfully. It is very difficult to initiate formal detention in a patient who denies suicidal intent and can argue his case persuasively.

CHAPTER 16

Mental Deficiency

Mental deficiency is not a disease, but a condition resulting from a variety of causes, inborn or acquired, whereby there is arrested mental development which is apparent from birth or from an early age. Although the terms 'idiot', 'imbecile' and 'feebleminded' (moron) are no longer official in Britain, it will still be necessary to define the different grades or severity of defect, if only on administrative grounds (see Legal Aspects of Psychiatry, Chap. 21).

Idiots are so low-grade that they are unable to protect themselves from common physical dangers such as fire, heights or inedible matter, and have no language.

Imbeciles can learn to avoid these dangers and have a limited vocabulary which permits communication but are usually unable to learn to read or write or be trained to lead an independent existence.

Higher-grade defectives (morons) can benefit from formal education though they are frequently classed as educationally subnormal and have to attend a special school where their handicaps are given due attention, but they *can* learn to read and write and make the necessary social adjustments to maintain themselves independently in the community.

Naturally, these grades tend to merge with each other, with the moron group shading into the duller members of ordinary society. The first two groups at some time will probably require institutional care, though such is the devotion of parents and relatives that a number are retained at home and become a sacred trust, receiving a measure of love and care which no institution can match. The higher grades, in the majority of instances, could live in the community with some support either from the family or the social services. They are, however, vulnerable and can frequently be tempted to petty crime or prostitution and have not the ability to respond to ordinary corrective measures; they may therefore be committed to institutions because their families or society are unable to control their behaviour. Misconduct is not necessarily related to intelligence and in fact it is the higher grades who are more likely to get into trouble, the very low grades having a measure of protection through their social isolation.

The prevalence of the problem will depend among other things on the available facilities for its recognition and the type of community, for in one with highly developed social services, compulsory education and adequate record systems, very few will escape detection, while in less highly organized societies the problem can pass unnoticed. In addition less well-endowed societies tend to be rural and a number of defectives can get by in this less challenging environment but would readily break down in the city. It is not surprising therefore that when the rural area is subjected to more rigid screening, the prevalence would appear to rise. The numbers in institutions or under special supervision from Local Authorities do not give a true estimate, but they do at least tell us what responsibility the community is undertaking on behalf of its mentally defective population and in England and Wales (population 50 million) this amounts to approximately 64,000 in institutions and 85,000 supervised by the Local Authority (1964 figures). These figures are also incomplete, for there is a shortage of accommodation which if available would raise the first figure without necessarily decreasing the second figure, for the social services have more than they can manage and the field has by no means been exploited.

Tizard and Grad (1961) have indicated another factor which increases the demand on accommodation, in their social survey of the mentally handicapped and their families, namely the tendency for middle-class families to seek such hospital care more often than lower-class families. The authors suggest that this would lead to an increased pressure on beds at a time when the service is unable to cope with the current demand.

There is still no general agreement on the place of genetic factors in mental defect apart from some organic and biochemically determined conditions which are described below. Over the role of genetics in the remaining and vast majority of the subnormal there has been considerable controversy which at one time engendered heated arguments over 'the fight for our national intelligence' with the advocacy of eugenic control by sterilization of the unfit, limiting the families of the dull, and encouraging the intelligent to proliferate. While there is some evidence that dullness tends to beget dullness, there are also signs that stocks can mend and it is now not unknown for a person born of defective parents in an institution to have these parents out on licence under his or her care. Social factors too can influence mental development and it is now recognized that the child brought up in a secure and happy home will reach a higher intelligence level than the child who is deprived of such an upbringing. The I.Q. itself has been under fire and is no longer regarded as the accurate and meaningful measure of intelligence it was once thought, and the old saying, 'Give a child a high I.Q. and he spends the rest of his life trying to live up to it; give a child a low I.Q. and he spends the rest of his life trying to live it down' no longer applies. Selection procedure for grammar (high) schools now takes into account the late developer and the emotional and social factors which influence intelligent performance.

The psychiatrist has a limited role in the care of the mental defective though in certain situations, primarily in institutions, he is the administrative director of all agencies—social, educational and medical—that are responsible for the patient's welfare. On the other hand, in large cities such as Birmingham, there are Occupation Centres managed by the Education Committee where ineducable defectives attend daily for training and which between them carry a higher load of low-grades than are housed in the institutions; whether a child attends the occupation centre or is sent to the institution may depend more on factors like the mother's health, housing conditions or social class than on the child's intelligence. Even in the strictly medical aspects there are divisions in responsibility, this time between psychiatrists and paediatricians, and the latter with their more intimate knowledge of biochemistry, and expertize in the organic field have already made their contribution to the understanding of phenylpyruvic amentia and Wilson's disease (see below). In the social rehabilitation aspects, it is again frequently an external situation which determines whether the individual will be sent as a patient to a hospital or to a classified approved school run by the Home Office. All this is healthy, for from being a 'cinderella' subject, mental deficiency is now claiming the attentions of our best paediatricians, psychiatrists, psychologists, biochemists and educationalists, and because of this new emphasis, society too is prepared to play its part by showing a greater community tolerance and by spending more on the service and on research.

DEFINITION OF MENTAL DEFECT

A fully satisfactory one does not exist as it can depend on variable social parameters which are incapable of definition. The following criteria of Doll (1941) are regarded as useful:

1. **Social incompetence** based on lack of prudence, economic dependence, and failure in citizenship.

2. **Mental subnormality** which leads to No. 1 for reasons other than from physical handicap or socio-economic disadvantage.

3. **Developmental retardation** which is not due to deterioration but to arrest.

4. **A condition obtaining at maturity** which is therefore incurable or irremediable other than by habit-training.

5. **Of constitutional origin** either from hereditary lack of potential or through trauma, disease or deprivation, making normal adult status unlikely.

These criteria must not be considered in isolation. For example, No. 4 has been criticized as some do reach normal adult status but Doll has replied that the original diagnosis must have been wrong and the term 'pseudo-feeblemindedness' has been suggested by Clarke and Clarke (1955).

THE I.Q. (INTELLIGENCE QUOTIENT)

The I.Q. (Intelligence Quotient) as a yard-stick of mental deficiency has been seriously criticized (see above) and it would be appropriate to deal with the problem at this stage. I.Q. is measured by tests which have both *validity* and *reliability*.

Validity is the degree to which a test measures what it claims to measure. Although the criteria can be argued, in practice satisfactory validation co-efficients can be obtained either by comparing the test with previous ones 'which, by a sort of apostolic succession, have been correlated with earlier versions of the Binet test' (Clarke & Clarke, 1958), or by designing it arbitrarily to measure abstract thinking. It is necessary to have adequate samples of mental activities which are poorly correlated but whose scores correlate highly with the sum of the total scores. The more poorly the constituent tests are intercorrelated the wider the spectrum of mental activity they measure and therefore the greater the validity of the whole test.

Reliability is the degree to which a test can be gauged by retesting the same person or group or by designing a parallel test (Form M with Form L of the Stanford Binet). The subject may be *unreliable* in the technical sense in that he may vary in himself between one test and the other and this is especially so in clinical problems where emotional factors operate. Clarke and Clarke (1958) pose the following assumptions and add their comments:

1. **'Intelligence can be Measured.'** They claim this to be largely correct.

2. **'Intelligence is Normally Distributed.'** Although the results of intelligence tests in a population follow the classical Gaussian curve of height or body weight, it does not mean that the mental levels are of the same pattern, for these tests were designed to meet a normal distribution, but it is likely that they are. Similarly, curves of mental growth as defined by test results may also be invalid.

3. **'The I.Q. is Constant.'** This is the exception rather than the rule and there is much evidence that it changes. Reasons for the change may be errors of measurement, test familiarity, incorrect testing based on the inexperience of the tester, using the wrong test for the subject, testing in a disturbing situation, or too short a test, and finally, variations in the rate of intellectual growth.

Mental Age (M.A.) is frequently used instead of I.Q. but it is losing favour as it possesses many fallacies such as *(a)* lack of equality between age growth and mental growth, *(b)* lack of meaning of the term in adults, *(c)* the change in the processes measured at different ages, and *(d)* the differences of meaning of the same mental age at different chronological ages. An example of *(d)* is the obvious differences in a M.A. of 8 scored by a child of 6, 8 or 10 years old (Greene, 1941). The Clarkes add that a M.A. at the *same* chronological age may not have the same meaning for different persons since M.A. represents the sum of separate scores which sum could be achieved by a variety of units.

AETIOLOGICAL FACTORS

Environmental

Anthropological studies have shown that when children are brought up in a primitive and/or under-privileged environment they perform worse in mental tests than their genotype who have not been so deprived. Examples are quoted from Negro scores in the U.S. Army which generally were lower than White scores, but Negro recruits from some of the Northern States were superior to White recruits from the Southern States. Children reared in foster homes do worse than those in secure families and Bowlby (1951) rather pessimistically describes the irremediable damage caused by maternal deprivation. Bourne (1955) showed that imbecile children with no evidence of organic impairment tended to have exceptionally adverse homes with in some instances 'pathological mothering'.

Dermatoglyphics

The dermal ridge arrangement of hands and soles of feet can now reliably discriminate between monozygotic and dizygotic twins, between mongols and normals and show characteristic patterns in other karotypic abnormalities. Much importance in the past has been placed on the single transverse palmar (simian) crease but its significance was never clearly understood. Davies and Smallpiece (1963) found the single crease in 80 (5·3 per cent) of 1500 newborn infants, in 30 (3·0 per cent) of 1000 consecutive paediatric outpatients, and in 14 (1·7 per cent) of 811 primary-schoolchildren in the Oxford area. Only 5 of the affected 124 were mongols indicating that though the crease may be useful in the diagnosis of mongolism, most creases have nothing to do with the disease.

Thirteen single creases occurred in 58 newborn children with malformation. Stillbirth and neonatal death incidence was 16 per cent in the group with single creases but only 4 per cent in the normals. Thirty per cent with single crease had a low birth weight as against 11 per cent in normals. The authors suggest that the simian crease should be regarded as an indicator of impaired foetal growth very early in embryonic life and that this impaired growth may later manifest as maldevelopment. In the diagnosis of mental deficiency dermatoglyphics are likely to play an increasingly important part.

Organic Factors and Mental Defect

There are a number of pathological states associated with mental defect which are classified by Penrose (1954) into:

1. Defect presumed to be due to a dominant gene.
2. Defect presumed to be due to a recessive gene.
3. Environmentally determined disabilities, such as those due to embryopathy.
4. Defects whose origin is still obscure.

DOMINANT DEFECTS

These have characteristic pedigrees and in the standard case where each heterozygote carries the gene, three criteria are essential:

(a) Sharp distinction between affected and unaffected members of the family.

(b) Every affected person has an affected parent.

(c) Approximately one half of the children will be affected in every sibship where there is an affected parent.

Tuberous Sclerosis

This was first described by Bourneville (1880), and Sherlock (1911) gave it the name *epiloia* which is an artifice signifying epilepsy, mental deficiency and adenoma sebaceum, the three main features of the disease, but this term is not very popular now and it is mainly referred to as tuberous sclerosis. Several members of the same family can be affected but genetic transmission is not always demonstrable and it is estimated that 25 per cent result from new mutations. It does not invariably present with the classical triad, and in a family one member may show only the adenoma sebaceum and another the epilepsy without the skin rash. The lesions that can appear are:

(a) **Skin**: adenoma sebaceum—a nodular rash of the characteristic butterfly spread on nose and cheeks, though it may also be on the forehead and chin; *peau chagrin* (Shagreen patch) on the lumbar region which does not appear till puberty; subungual (fingers and toes) fibromata and in rare instances it can be associated with neurofibromatosis.

(b) **Visceral tumours** are commonly in kidney and heart, but may also occur in the lung and in fact any organ, and their structure varies accordingly, *e.g.* glioblastoma in the brain and rhabdomyoma in the heart.

(c) **Brain.** Mainly periventricular tumours which calcify and are easily seen on X-ray. A brain lesion may become malignant and show all the features of a rapidly growing glioblastoma. The histology shows very large glial cells.

(d) **Eye.** Grey-yellow-white plaques (phakomata) of varying size are seen on the retina in about half the cases.

Mental Changes. Severe degrees of defect are the rule but cases have been described of either high-grade or normal intelligence (Entwistle & Sim, 1961). Psychotic states mainly of a primitive catatonic schizophrenic nature are not uncommon (Critchley & Earl, 1932).

Epilepsy. This can be very severe and difficult to control and some of the psychotic features noted may be due to temporal lobe lesions. Rate of deterioration varies and frequently depends on the degree of malignancy of the visceral or brain lesions, the latter particularly becoming glioblastomatous.

Neurofibromatosis (von Recklinghausen's Disease)

Clinical Features. Skin lesions (neurofibromata), areas of pigmentation (café au lait) and phakomata. Mental defect is not severe and is present in about 30 per cent of cases.

Rud's Syndrome

Congenital ichthyosis with epilepsy and mental deficiency and occasionally spasticity.

Haemangiomatosis

(a) **Sturge-Weber Syndrome.** Alexander and Norman (1960) record 7 case histories and describe as essential features the following:

> Cutaneous facial angiomatosis (always extending above the palpebral fissure); gyriform calcification (radiographically apparent after the age of two years) underlying an area of leptomeningeal angiomatosis which is unilateral and usually confined to the posterior half of the brain; mental deficiency and epilepsy; buphthalmos and hemiparesis.

The authors found no association between the site of the facial lesion and the distribution of the trigeminal nerve. Since the epilepsy seems to result in mental deterioration and paralysis, they recommend lobectomy (or the removal of the affected area) at the age of two months.

(b) **Von Hippel-Lindau.** Here the angiomata involve the retina and cerebellum with the appropriate symptoms.

Cranio-facial Dysostoses

This is frequently associated with mental defect which may be due either to the mechanical effect of the skull change or to independent brain lesion.

Acrocephaly (Oxycephaly)

An abnormally high or pointed head found in a variety of syndromes associated with mental defect.

(a) **Crouzon.** Exophthalmos with small orbits and narrow optic foramina. Increased intracranial pressure may result.

(b) **Apert.** Ocular hypertelorism (wide separation of the eyes) and syndactyly.

Marfan's Syndrome (Dystrophia Mesodermalis)

A generalized disorder of connective tissue characterized by very long extremities including fingers and toes (arachnodactyly or spidery fingers). Ectopia of lenses, congenital heart defect and aneurysm of the aorta may also be present (Marfan, 1896). Mental retardation is common but may not be severe.

Sinclair *el al.* (1960) point out that long fingers may be a feature of an otherwise normal family, or may even be the subjective impression of the observer. They therefore propose the use of a 'metacarpal index'. The lengths of the right second, third, fourth and fifth metacarpals as seen on a radiograph are measured and the breadth of each metacarpal at its exact midpoint is also measured. A figure for each metacarpal is obtained by dividing the length by the breadth and the average of the four is taken. The authors claim that the normal range is from 5·4 to 7·9 whereas in Marfan's syndrome it is 8·4 to 10·4. An index greater than 8·4 is therefore diagnostic of arachnodactyly.

Sjögren's Syndrome (1950)

Hereditary congenital spino-cerebellar ataxia accompanied by congenital cataract and oligophrenia.

RECESSIVE DEFECTS

These occur when a person inherits the same pathological gene twice (one from each parent). They are said to account for 20 per cent of low-grade mental defect (Medical Research Council, 1956). Penrose cites the following criteria:

1. Affected and unaffected persons in the same family can be sharply distinguished.
2. Parents and all immediate ancestors are unaffected.
3. Father and mother are blood relations more frequently than expected.
4. More than one offspring is likely to be affected.
5. Occasionally cases occur in collateral branches of the same family.

Many of these conditions are associated with disorders of amino-acid transport which since the introduction of paper chromatographic separation have been increasingly recognized. The abnormal amount of amino-acid which is excreted in the urine could be evidence of an 'overflow mechanism' due to an increase in plasma concentration as in diabetes mellitus or a 'renal mechanism' as in renal glycosuria. Until recently the few conditions that were recognized were regarded as discrete but now that the biochemistry is better understood a certain order is being introduced. Milne (1964) approaching the problem as one of the body's transport systems classifies the disorder thus:

1. Pure overflow amino-aciduria. Under this heading he lists four hereditary diseases with the amino-acid involved:

(*a*) phenylketonuria: phenylalanine.

(*b*) maple-syrup-urine disease: the branched-chain amino-acid valine, leucine and isoleucine.

(*c*) histidinaemia: histidine.

(*d*) glycinaemia: glycine.

2. Mixed overflow and renal amino-aciduria. *e.g.* The rare hereditary disease citrullinuria (citrulline).

3. Renal amino-aciduria involving a specific amino-acid transport system *e.g.* Hartnup disease and cystinuria.

4. Renal amino-aciduria associated with generalized proximal tubular damage *e.g.* Wilson's disease and cystinosis. In the former the renal tubules are poisoned by copper deposits.

This classification is not designed to take into account those conditions which are usually associated with mental defect, but is primarily concerned with the behaviour of amino-acids. This would appear to be a more rational approach for it brings certain problems of mental deficiency into close contact with the associated metabolic errors. In this chapter only those conditions with reported mental defect will be listed.

Phenylketonuria (Phenylpyruvic Amentia)

Fölling (1934) described a number of instances of familial mental defect associated with a defect in protein metabolism with an inability to metabolize phenylalanine to tyrosine. Instead it was de-aminated into phenylpyruvic acid which with the phenylalanine and phenylacetic acid were excreted in the urine. As phenylpyruvic acid in an acid medium gives a green reaction to ferric chloride with subsequent colour fade, a simple diagnostic method was available. High phenylalanine levels in the blood have been regarded as in some way responsible but other amino-acids such as tryptophan have been suspected in view of reduced blood levels of serotonin. Urine examination may be negative in new-born babies and become positive after a few weeks.

Clinical Features. Most are low grade but imbecile and feeble-minded cases occur; it is rare in people of high intelligence. Patients are frequently undersized with blonde or reddish-brown hair, reduced head size and widely spaced incisors. Some suffer from a severe and stubborn chronic eczema and occasionally epileptic attacks. Healthy relatives may show a normal phenylalanine level which rises and remains high after its ingestion. The incidence in mental deficiency institutions in Britain is less than 1 per cent.

Pathology. There is demyelinization of the optic, cortico-ponto-cerebellar and corticospinal systems (Alvord *et al.*, 1950), an increase of astrocytes and microglia and a decrease in Purkinje cells. Fellman (1958) found the substantia nigra and locus ceruleus of the brain deficient in pigment and lack of tyrosin and methionin in the adrenals.

The Guthrie Test. This is the test most widely used in screening for phenylketonuria. It is a bacterial inhibition assay method based on the fact that phenylalanine is an essential growth factor for the test organism, commonly *Bacillus subtilis.* An agar plate is prepared in which the culture medium contains a specific phenylalanine antagonist and spores of *Bacillus subtilis;* the antagonist prevents the bacillus from growing. Discs of filter paper impregnated with samples of blood are then placed on the culture plate and the plate incubated and the clinical constituents of the blood diffuse into the surrounding agar.

If the serum phenylalanine level is normal, that is, less than 3·5-4·0 mg. per 100 ml, then the amount of phenylalanine diffusing into the agar is insufficient to negate the effects of the specific antagonist, and when the plate is incubated no growth occurs. If the serum level is high, the spores grow and the test is positive, and in most laboratories positive results can be obtained with serum levels above 4·0 mg. per 100 ml. A drop of blood is obtained from finger, heel or ear lobe and a spot at least $\frac{3}{8}$ inch in diameter is made on the filter paper which is dried in a cool dark place and posted to the laboratory.

Treatment. Bickel (1954) claimed that a phenylalanine-free diet could cure the condition and this has started an enthusiastic attack on the disease; as one would expect first reports were encouraging. It is not difficult to change the metabolism though improvement in the mental state has been reliably reported in only the very young, but it is notoriously difficult to ascertain the value of a single factor in therapy in mental deficiency. Mautner (1959) gives instances where it was not possible to tell whether improvement was due to the diet or to environmental factors.

In some patients when the diet was interrupted there has been no deterioration and some have improved, so the place of the phenylalanine-free diet is not as secure as was originally hoped. That a child develops normally on the diet does not necessarily mean that it is due to the diet for many develop normally without it. In the

Medical Research Council (1963) trial of 25 patients treated before the age of 3/12, 5 failed to develop normal intelligence. Others with the diet did badly, developed a rash and failed to gain weight, yet the addition of milk caused a dramatic recovery. It may take a few more years to get this treatment into proper perspective.

Maternal Phenylketonuria

That untreated mothers with phenylketonuria may damage the foetus was first pointed out by Dent (1957), and Mabry *et al.* (1963) described three untreated phenylketonuric women who had 1, 5 and 8 children respectively. The 7 children who survived were all mentally retarded, though none of the 5 who were investigated had phenylketonuria. Others have reported similarly, and these findings complicate further the effects of treatment of the child with phenylketonuria. Is his retardation due to maternal influence or to his own disturbed biochemistry? If the former, then no diet will suffice even if the biochemistry is corrected.

Maple Syrup Urine Disease

This is characterized by increased excretion of the branched chain amino-acids, leucine, isoleucine and valine in the urine with the smell of maple syrup, as well as high levels in the plasma. The infant fails to thrive, vomits and shows signs of severe cerebral degeneration. It is usually rapidly fatal and treatment is to date ineffective. Dancis *et al.* (1960) supply a detailed description.

Hartnup ('H') Disease

This is a generalized amino-aciduria of renal origin called after the family in which it was first described. All amino-acids except proline, hydroxyproline, methionine and arginine are increased in the urine to 5–15 times normal while the plasma amino-acids are 30 per cent lower than normal. The primary defect is a decreased absorption of tryptophan from the jejunum and diminished reabsorption of tryptophan and other amino-acids by the proximal renal tubule. Urinary excretion of indoxyl sulphate (indican) and indolacetic acid is invariably increased and can be further augmented by injection of tryptophan.

Symptoms are variable and may include a pellagra-like rash, cerebellar ataxia, diplopia, nystagmus and slow mental deterioration. Treatment by oral nicotinamide improves most symptoms except the mental ones. Baron *et al.* (1956) supplied the first full report.

Fructose Intolerance

Froesch *et al.* (1957) reported on a 6-year old girl who was slightly retarded mentally and physically. Since being weaned she was subject to attacks of vomiting, unconsciousness and shock. Her mother had noticed that the attacks were precipitated by certain sweet foods, fruit and vegetables and by trial and error she had arrived at an innocuous diet. A younger brother showed a similar pattern of behaviour from an earlier age and was not retarded. A test dose of fructose by mouth caused the girl to vomit, blood pressure fell and she became sweaty, cyanosed and lapsed into coma. Intravenous glucose revived her. It is now claimed that early diagnosis and the exclusion of fructose from the diet can prevent permanent mental and physical damage.

The condition is quite distinct from fructosuria, which, though associated with a raised blood-fructose is a harmless curiosity. In fructose intolerance assimilation of fructose is halted early by what would appear to be an inborn deficiency in the hepatic-phospho-fructaldolase reaction. This block leads to accumulation of the hexose ester in the cell and as the concentration of this intermediate metabolite increases, it becomes the competitive inhibitor of other enzymatic transformations. These secondary inhibitions rather than the primary defect account for the main clinical and biochemical findings.

The clinical features are essentially those of hypoglycaemia, though the patient's total blood sugar (which includes blood-fructose) may be high and therefore mask severe drops in blood-glucose. Later signs of renal and hepatic damage may appear. Diagnosis is based on the history of fructose-intolerance in patient and family and on a fructose-tolerance test which should be carried out cautiously with intravenous glucose to hand.

The condition should be borne in mind when dealing with the food fads of children; these may not be psychogenic.

Galactosaemia

This is an inborn error of metabolism characterized by a deficiency of the enzyme, galactose-*l*-phosphate uridyl transferase which assists in the formation of glucose-*l*-phosphate from galactose-*l*-phosphate in the conversion of galactose to glucose. This block causes an increase of galactose and galactose-*l*-phosphate in the blood and tissues, as well as in the urine after ingestion of milk or other foods containing lactose or galactose.

The child is normal at birth but soon exhibits vomiting and diarrhoea and fails to thrive. The abdomen is distended and the liver enlarged and occasionally there is jaundice and ascites with hepatic cirrhosis. Proteinuria is invariably present and mental retardation is common. About 50 per cent of the severe cases have cataracts but the less severe may show no more than gastro-intestinal upset. The condition improves with age probably because of the development of an alternative pathway of galactose metabolism. Diagnosis is made by the identification of galactose in the urine, first by a reducing sugar test and then by chromatography. A galactose-tolerance test can induce severe hypoglycaemia with convulsions and should be avoided.

Treatment is mainly by the exclusion of all milk and foods containing lactose and galactose.

Arginnio-Succinuria

Large quantities of arginnio-succinic acid are excreted in the urine (2–5 grammes in 24 hours). This acid is an intermediate in the ornithine-urea cycle and the disease in characterized by severe mental defect and occasionally fits. The hair is unusually friable. There is no treatment to date and the condition was fully reported by Allan *et al.* (1958).

OTHER METABOLIC DISORDERS

Citrullinuria

McMurray *et al.* (1962) during a chromatographic screening programme for amino-aciduria found large quantities of citrulline in all specimens of urine voided by a mental retarded child aged 18 months.

Hyperuricaemia

Lesch and Nyhan (1963) reported a condition in children which is associated with hyperuricaemia. The patients are mentally retarded, and show signs of cerebral palsy, choreo-athetosis and self-biting. The biting which is found in all these patients is continued in spite of the pain and the lips may be chewed away and the end of a finger may be gnawed down to the first joint. If teeth are pulled to prevent biting the drive is directed to picking at the body or abrading the skin. Symptoms start at 4 months and the age group described extends from 2–11 years. The condition is familial and probably due to an inborn defect and it is probably not due to the high level of uric acid in the blood.

Cystathioninuria

The urine chromatogram shows peaks identical with *l*-cystathionine with excretion of 960-1,300 mg./day and a C.S.F. content of 0·21 mg. per 100 ml.

The following picture is described by Frimpter and Horwith (1963):

> Acromegalic features; bilateral grooves in the scalp of the lateral occiput; small ears with pre-auricular fistulae on the left; bilateral conductive deafness; enlarged tongue; thyroid gland enlarged x 2; liver and spleen palpable; poor score on testing (Wechsler); poor concentration and judgment.

The authors suggest urine chromatography screening on all patients with mental deficiency.

THE LIPOIDOSES

These are diseases involving the accumulation of lipids. Those generally associated with mental defect are:

Amaurotic Family Idiocy (Tay-Sachs)

First described by Tay (1881) and Sachs (1887) in the children of Jews of Eastern European descent. It usually starts in infancy with rapid deterioration leading to death at about 2 years and is manifest by failure to develop mentally, blindness, paralysis and characteristic cherry-red spot on the macula, though at times it can be grey. There are other types:

(a) Late infantile (Bielchowsky-Jansky) with cerebellar involvement and occasional absence of the macular spot.

(b) Juvenile (Vogt-Spielmeyer). Visual disturbance appears first at about 5–8 years and in two years progresses to blindness. Convulsions, lack of emotional control, restlessness apathy and speech difficulties follow and then mental retardation progressing to idiocy and paralysis. The disease has been reviewed by Levy and Goodman (1952).

Pre-natal Diagnosis of Tay-Sachs Genotype. Navon and Paden (1971) determined the hexosaminidase activity in cultured and uncultured amniotic fluid cells taken from seven pregnant women who had previously given birth to infants with Tay-Sachs disease. Complete deficiency of hexosaminadase A was confirmed on examination of the foetus after therapeutic abortion. Of the other 6, 3 were considered heterozygous and 3 homozygous normals.

Gargoylism (Hurler's Syndrome)

Though Hurler (1919) gave it his name the condition was also described by Hunter (1917). It may start in infancy or later and develop slowly. The bones of head and face are affected with protruding forehead and broad nose and jaw—hence the term gargoylism. There are other skeletal deformities, particularly of phalanges and metacarpals, and the abdomen may be protuberant with umbilical hernia. There are two forms, one in males, which is sex-linked with clear corneas and deafness, the other with cloudy corneas with autosomal recessive transmission. It is said to be due to a disorder of polysaccharide metabolism with lipid deposit in the brain with ballooning of the cell bodies—a change similar to that found in amaurotic family idiocy.

Treatment. Levin *et al.* (1972) regard the condition as one of the mucopolysaccharidoses and on the evidence of a deficiency of β-galactosidase explored the possibility of restricting dietary galactose. A boy aged 3 years had been on a galactose-free diet for 9 months and while it was difficult to assess whether clinical improvement has occurred, there had been no deterioration and urinary mucopolysaccharide excretion had tended to fall following dietary therapy. No doubt all the pitfalls in the treatment of phenylketonuria will be encountered.

Laurence-Moon-Biedl Syndrome

This starts in early life and is associated with retinitis pigmentosa causing a variety of visual defects; polydactyly of hands and/or feet; mental defect; obesity of the hypopituitary type; hypogenitalism; and diabetes insipidus.

Formes frustes have been found in relatives and recessive gene is regarded as responsible. The mental defect is usually not very severe.

Hepato-lenticular Degeneration (Wilson's Disease)

This is reported to be associated with a defect in copper metabolism in which the bound copper is decreased because of the defective synthesis of ceruloplasmin, a protein used in binding copper (90 per cent in the blood). As a result the unbound copper is increased and interferes with oxidation enzymes which may lead to lesions in brain and liver. Blood copper is low (20-50 mg. per cent) and urinary copper is high (x 100). The liver is cirrhotic and there is degeneration of the lentiform nucleus and cerebral cortex with copper in liver, brain and cornea. It usually occurs in adolescence and presents with choreo-athetosis, mental deterioration and occasionally behaviour disorders. A typical feature is the Kayser-Fleischer ring—a brown copper deposit seen in the cornea. Treatment is to get rid of the copper with the anti-metallic drugs—Versene, BAL and penicillamine.

The Elfin-face Syndrome

Dupont and Claussen (1968) described a condition where the face has a flat nasal bridge, prominence of the maxillary bones and an open mouth which is large and somewhat asymmetric. The lips are pouting, with a prominent upper lip and a highly-arched palate, an alternating squint, malocclusion, recessed mandible and crowded teeth, especially mandibular. The ears are prominent and big, especially in the horizontal level.

It is associated with hypercalcaemia, supravalvular stenosis (aortic) and mental deficiency. The authors, out of 1200 patients in one institution, found a 4-year old, a 5-year old girl and a 40-year old man. In another institution they found a 23-year old man, and he and the others all showed the following features: elfin-face, kyphosis or kyphoscoliosis, mild or moderate mental retardation and a history of failure to thrive in infancy suggestive of hypercalcaemia. The condition was first reported in 1886.

MONGOLISM (DOWN'S SYNDROME)

The name was coined by Langdon-Down (1866) because of a fancied resemblance in the eyes which are almond-shaped with epicanthic folds, but apart from this single feature there is absolutely nothing to identify the condition with the Mongolian race except that it can also occur among members of that race. The alternative name of *acromicria* because of the short fingers and facial bones had been put forward by Schüller (1907) and was revived by Benda (1953) but tradition dies hard and the name mongolism has not been supplanted, although recently there has been a strong move to rename it Down's syndrome.

AETIOLOGY

Genetic Factors. Penrose (1956) postulated a recessive mechanism with the younger woman possessing protective factors which decrease with age. Book and Reed (1950) calculated that a tainted family had an incidence of 4 per cent which is 20 times greater than in the general population. Uniovular twins were invariably affected while one of binovular twins may by normal. Berg and Kirman (1959) considered that the condition was due to an interplay of three factors: (a) maternal; (b) foetal; and (c) environmental, the last to include the effects of ageing.

Jacobs *et al.* (1959) demonstrated that patients with classical mongolism had an extra chromosome (No.21) and since then there has been a veritable explosion of investigations and reports. A disease which till 1959 had an unknown aetiology had now been demonstrated as being caused by a chromosomal abnormality. It became apparent that mongolism was not synonymous with trisomy-21, for Polani *et al.* (1960) described a case due to 15 : 21 translocation, while Clarke *et al.* (1961) described a mongol 'mosaic' having a mixture of two cell lines, normal and trisomic. Dent *et al.* (1963) described 'partial' mongols with very mild stigmata who had only part of chromosome 21 in excess. Other variations described by Valentine (1969), included 'anti-mongolism' where part of a chromosome-21 is absent and a child with 45 chromosomes only (monosomy-21). There are no differences in sex incidence.

CHROMOSOMOMAL ABNORMALITIES

Autosomal trisomy-'G' (Trisomy-21). In this syndrome, the extra chromosome is a small acrocentric numbered 21. Affected individuals are trisomic for this chromosome and the total complement is thus 47 instead of 46 chromosomes. It has been suggested that chromosome-21 carries loci for the ABO blood groups, leucocytic alkaline phosphatase and galactose-*l*-phosphate uridyl transferase. The extra chromosome had been previously regarded as a 21 because it bore a 'satellite' which is a minute speck of chromatic material at the end of the chromosome and separated from the body by a poorly staining zone. These satellites are found only on acrocentric chromosomes and are found regularly on two of the G group though not always on the 21 chromosome, which can now be more clearly distinguished from 22 by the fluorescent banding technique.

Although the parents of mongols do not have detectable chromosomal abnormalities, they are reputed to have an increased incidence of taste abnormalities, such as insensitivity to quinine and some thiourea type compounds. The much greater incidence in older mothers suggests that the abnormality may result from non-disjunction during meiosis of the oocyte when there is incorrect segregation of migration of the chromosomes into the daughter cells of that division.

It accounts for about 85 per cent of cases of Down's syndrome and the overall incidence is 1 : 700 live births with a marked variability according to maternal age; in early child-bearing years the incidence is 1 : 2000 live births, but it rises to 1 : 50 in mothers over 40 years.

There are numerous hypotheses on the cause of this non-disjunction.

1. *Maternal age at birth* has been shown by Penrose (1949) to be higher than the average for all births (37/29 years).

2. *The state of the uterine mucosa* has been questioned. Mautner (1959) states that he has seen some cases where the mother confessed attempts at abortion and quotes Ingalls (1947) who has suggested damage to the uterus at the end of the second month of pregnancy, Husler (1931) who has claimed it may follow ineffective attempted abortion, and Mayerhofer (1939) who has found the condition in mothers with a history of abortion with curettage. Cohen *et al.* (1963) consider that if such environmental factors exist they act on the parental gametes or on the fertilized ovum not later than several days after fertilization.

3. *Endocrine.* Benda (1947) has stressed hypopituitarism due to a deficiency of the gamma cell system with the inability to form chromophilic elements and the chromophine granules in the adrenals have been shown to be poorly developed. The thyroid gland has had much attention and its function is generally depressed but its contribution to the aetiology has not been defined.

4. *Infective Hepatitis.* Stoller and Collmann (1965) in their survey of all infants with Down's syndrome in the State of Victoria elaborated the hypothesis that it was caused by infective hepatitis because:

(a) The annual incidence, in both urban and rural areas, was inconstant; it varied periodically, with an interval of 5–7 years between maximum peaks.

(b) Urban peaks in every case were higher than rural peaks, suggesting higher rates of contact.

(c) Rural peaks followed one year after the urban maxima, suggesting a slow spread of infection out of the high-contact urban areas into the rural areas.

(d) Cases of Down's syndrome clustered significantly in both time and place.

Their study extended over a period of 3 years and they claim they predicted the 1962-63 peak and postulate that the virus affects the ovum before or at about the time of conception. This novel hypothesis will require confirmation but the quality and extent of the survey would suggest that it be seriously considered.

5. *Mycoplasma hominis.* Mycoplasma cause chromosomal damage and mitotic inhibition of normal cells in tissue culture. Deletion of the short arm of chromosomes-21 and 22 as in Down's syndrome has been noted in W1-38 cultures infected with *Mycoplasma hominis* (Allison & Paton, 1966).

6. *Arginine depletion* has also been cited as an aetiological factor (Aula & Nichols, 1967).

Translocations

These are generally found in young mothers and are therefore not related to increasing maternal age. The patient has 46 chromosomes, but one is larger and atypical due to an extra chromosome 21 becoming attached to either a member of the D (13-15) or the G (21-22) groups. It is usually transmitted through the mother but G : G (21 : 21 or 21 : 22) translocation often stems from the father with a mean paternal age of 42·5 years, which is 10·8 years in excess of the overall mean paternal age. Translocation mongols have a high incidence of neck webbing.

Theoretically, the chance is 1 : 3 that a mother with a D/G translocation will have a mongoloid child but the actual risk is lower (about 1 : 5). If the father carries the D/G translocation, the chance of having a mongoloid child is only 1 : 20. In extremely rare instances the translocation involves both 21-chromosomes of the G group, which join to form an isochromosome, and the chance of a mongoloid child is 100 per cent. Some translocations, usually of the D/G type occur spontaneously in the child of genotypically normal parents. In this rare event the chance of a mongoloid sibling is the same as for the more common sporadic trisomy form.

Mosaics

As a result of non-disjunction in the fertilized zygote a few cases have two cell lines, one normal and one with 47 chromosomes. The relative proportion of each cell line is very variable from individual to individual and within different tissues and organs of the same individual. They tend to have a few of the typical characteristics of mongols, and are usually more intelligent with less pronounced physical stigmata and different dermatoglyphics.

Double Trisomics

These patients have 48 chromosomes (usually XXY or XXX together with trisomy 21). The Down-Klinefelter syndrome has other abnormalities of sexual development (Nelson *et al.* 1969). Other associated conditions are Turner's syndrome, trisomy-18, and trisomy 13-15.

Other investigations which have been undertaken to throw further light on the nature and mode of transmission of mongolism, include those of Coppen and Cowie (1960) who reported on maternal health and mongolism, as it is generally agreed that this factor is also a contributory one. They examined 55 mothers of mongols and failed to confirm earlier reports of thyroid abnormality, including a raised serum P.B.I. Body build did not differ from normal generally, but it was found that those who had a mongol child at 27 years or younger had a raised androgyny score and a raised mean biacromial diameter. Obstetric histories showed an extremely high rate of miscarriage which was irrespective of the conception order and unrelated to the birth order of the mongol. A subsequent enquiry by this team (Rundle *et al.,* 1961) into the steroid excretion in mothers of mongols showed that the urinary output of dehydro*epi*androsterone (DHA) was significantly higher in those mothers who had borne mongols at an early age (27 years or under), compared with those mothers who had mongol children in later life. The authors regard this evidence as confirmatory that those younger mothers possessed a specific genetic constitution.

Berg *et al.* (1959) confirmed the statement that children with mongolism are hypersensitive to atropine and considered that it was evidence of genetically determined drug sensitivity. Penrose (1962) investigated paternal age in mongols, comparing the genetic variants. In those mongols whose cells showed chromosomal fusion of 13, 14 or 15 : 21 (or more commonly referred to as 15 : 21) there was no significant difference from that of the general population. In those, with somatic chromosomal fusion of the 21 : 22 type, advancing paternal and not maternal age. proved to be a highly significant aetiological factor. He suggested that selection which acts against unbalanced gametes, ova and sperms, carrying the 21 : 22 fusion, but which was not effective against sperms from older fathers was one possible explanation.

Incidence. It is the commonest condition in M.D. institutions. Penrose (1933) estimates the risk at about 1 per 1000 live births, and mongolism accounts for 10–15 per cent of patients in M.D. institutions. The numbers will vary according to the age structure of the institution's population, being higher in a younger age structure and lower in an older age structure.

Clinical Features. These are numerous, but only several need be present to establish a diagnosis. The patient is short, and exhibits the following features: *skull,* small and brachycephalic with flattened occiput. Fontanelles close late; *eyes,* palpebral fissures are slanting and narrow with epicanthic folds. Strabismus, myopia and cataract are common and the iris shows white or light yellow spots at regular intervals (*Brushfield* spots) which are considered the most reliable guide to the diagnosis in the new-born. As the iris darkens with age, they disappear or become small whitish stripes. Conjunctivitis and blepharitis frequently occur; *teeth* are irregular and small and there is a congenital absence of some permanent teeth, particularly the maxillary and mandibular lateral incisors and the second bicuspids; *ears* are small, rounded and stick out; *palate* is flat at the sides and elevated in the middle and has been called the omega (Ω) palate; *tongue* is large and fissured (scrotal) and often protrudes; *nose* is short; *extremities* are short, particularly the hands; *skin* is rough and dry; *hands* show the little finger bent inwards with a reduction in size of its middle phalanx and the palms show a single transverse crease at the base of the four fingers; *feet* show a cleft between the big and little toes; *hair* is scanty and may be absent in the axillae while alopecia is common; *hypogenitalism; heart* malformations are common and many die at birth because of them. These are usually septal defects (atrial or ventricular) but Esen (1957) has described ostium atrioventriculare commune as the mose common severe malformation which he alleges is almost never encountered in non-mongols; *muscles* are hypotonic; *joints* are lax; susceptibility to *respiratory infection; epilepsy* is *very rare* but has been reported (Kirman, 1951).

The incidence of acute leukaemia is greater than in the general population, with figures from 3-61 times, and is usually lymphoblastic but myelogenous and stem-cell types have been reported. This increased incidence has been linked with the finding of Philadelphic (Ph') chromosome in some cases of chronic myeloid leukaema in non-mongols.

Scully (1973) lists the following immune phenomena that have been observed:

(1) Diminished skin reactivity to multiple antigens; (2) sluggish lymphocytes with a diminished response to phytohaemoglutinin; (3) an apparently innate deficiency of IgM: (4) an excessive rise in IgG when exposed to an institution for the mentally subnormal; (5) IgA is increased in adult mongols; (6) increased basophil counts; (7) increased response to the stress stimulus of adrenaline as shown by a marked leucocytosis and hyperglycaemia; (8) poor response to influenza A/PR8 antigen, with normal response to A2 and B.

Intelligence. The physical signs are usually, but not invariably, associated with mental defect of the imbecile grade but idiocy and feeblemindedness can also occur.

Personality. They are generally cheerful and friendly and good mimics but naturally these features are not universal.

Prognosis. Mortality, especially in females, is very high in the early years, as 40-55 per cent do not survive the first year. Death is due mainly to respiratory infection, the results of the cardiac lesion, or by leukaemia. They are particularly prone to exanthemata.

Treatment. There is no specific measure available and most are ineducable, though the impression is gained that the intelligence level is rising and that a number will qualify for education in special schools. Because of their docile and affectionate natures, many parents are reluctant to commit them to institutions and they tend to form a large part of the population of Occupation Centres. There they can be trained to a high level of social competence but are usually unable to lead an independent existence. Expectation of life was formerly not high, but the picture has changed with the advent of antibiotics in the treatment of respiratory infections and no doubt the cardiac surgeon will eventually make his contribution.

Genetic Counselling

Amniotic cell culture has a high success rate in the pre-natal diagnosis of Down's syndrome (Bain & Sutherland, 1973). The amniocentesis involves withdrawing 10-20 ml. of amniotic fluid between the 14th and 16th weeks of gestation, using the trans-abdominal approach. In familial cases of translocation Down's syndrome each subsequent pregnancy should be monitored. Foetal chromosomes can be readily distinguished in the cultured amniotic fluid cells and diagnosis can usually be made. If the foetus has 46 chromosomes and among them the translocation chromosome, the parents should be told that their child will have Down's syndrome so that they may consider therapeutic abortion. If in subsequent pregnancies there are normal pregnancies then the pregnancy should not be terminated. The whole question of foetal diagnosis with a view to abortion of a handicapped foetus is a very controversial one and recent developments are making it more difficult.

Cowie (1971) stresses the advantages of amniocentesis and the certainty it can bring to a situation which had previously been full of doubts. The odds need no longer be quoted as 1 : 4 but as 100 per cent or zero.

Genetic Disorders Detectable in Cultured Amniotic Fluid Cells

(1) Maple syrup urine disease; (2) Homocystinuria; (3) Cyst-

athioninuria; (4) Galactosaemia; (5) Glycogen storage disease (Types I, II, III and IV); (6) Lesch-Nyhan syndrome (hereditary hyper-uricaemia); (7) Lysosomal acid phosphatase deficiency; (8) Tay-Sachs disease; (9) Refsum's disease; (10) Muco-polysaccharidoses (Hurler's, Hunter's syndromes and other variants); (11) Hyper-valinaemia.

Cri du Chat (Lejeune *et al.* 1963) **Syndrome**

The demonstration of chromosomal abnormalities in mongolism was sure to stimulate a search for other conditions with kindred abnormalities. Lejeune and his colleagues having already reported trisomy-21 in mongolism described such a syndrome which has now been confirmed by several workers.

Clinically the children have a curious weak mewing cry which appears to be due to weakness and underdevelopment of the upper part of the larynx, with a small, soft and very mobile epiglottis. Mental deficiency is usually more severe than that of mongols, but much less so than in the other well-established autosomal defects, trisomy 13–15 and trisomy-18.

Lejeune described the face as characteristically round with wide-set eyes that have an anti-mongoloid slant, low-set ears and small lower jaw with microcephaly. Other workers are not so certain of these facial characteristics. Transverse-palmar creases are common and occasionally there is a congenital heart lesion such as a patent ductus arteriosus.

The chromosome lesion is a simple deletion of the short arm of one of the four 4–5 chromosomes, probably a 5. Usually only one member of the family is affected.

DEVELOPMENTAL DEFECTS OF OBSCURE ORIGIN

These may be genetically determined but no conclusive evidence is available; they are more likely to be due to an interplay of genetic pre-natal influences, and a variety of pathological states ensue.

Agyria (Lissencephaly). There are no convolutions in the brain and mental defect is severe.

Pachygyria. Only a few large convolutions are present and mental defect is severe.

Agenesis of the Corpus Callosum. Usually associated with other malformations, such as spina bifida, meningocele and meningomyelocele.

Congenital Hydrocephalus. This may result from pre-natal influences (see below) but there is a type due to a congenital atresia of the aqueduct.

EMBRYOPATHY

Embryopathy is damage to the child by a variety of agents before birth.

Genetic Microcephaly

This may be due to causes other than the recessive gene, for it is found after X-ray overdosage and rubella in the first months of pregnancy, and is therefore divided into a primary genetic form and a secondary exogenous form. The face is characteristic, being bird-like or Aztec with a low cephalic index (breadth-length). The majority are imbecile.

Rubella

Gregg (1941) reported congenital cataracts in children following German measles in the mother during gestation. Mental defect also occurs, and may be accompanied by congenital heart defects, microcephaly, partial or total nerve deafness with occasionally deaf-mutism. The infection of the mother is in the first three months of pregnancy and the incidence of congenital defect according to Swan *et al.* (1943, 1944) is about two-thirds. The incidence of mental defect and congenital abnormalities following rubella in the pregnant woman is not as clear-cut as was previously believed. It depends on the type of epidemic as some produce a greater crop of defects than others but more so on the time of infection. The earlier the infection during gestation, the greater the risk. It rapidly falls after the second month. Furthermore the degree of defect cannot be predicted; most are not severe.

Syphilis

Infection is usually by the mother through the placental circulation. Early infection produces foetal death and abortion, while later, diffuse or localized meningovascular lesions result. Early pregnancies are more vulnerable than later ones and a history of miscarriages is a frequent precursor to the birth of a syphilitic child. The disease had been regarded as responsible for up to 20 per cent of admissions to mental deficiency institutions, but antibiotics and ante-natal care have reduced maternal syphilis and consequently the incidence in children. The dullness associated with syphilitics may be an expression of familial dullness rather than due to the infection, and Mautner (1959) prefers the label of familial oligophrenia in feebleminded syphilitics but that of congenital syphilis in the idiots and imbeciles.

This would mean that the other stigmata of congenital syphilis could be present without brain involvement. A rare type is juvenile general paralysis which shows rapid mental deterioration with serological and pathological changes similar to those in the adult. Hydrocephalus is usually mild.

Toxoplasmosis

The pathogen is a protozoon, toxoplasma, which has been found in birds, rodents, dogs and cats and is transmitted to the foetus by the infected mother but it can also be acquired in infancy and the young or embryonic brain is particularly vulnerable.

Clinical Features are mental defect, chorio-retinopathy, cerebral calcification, hydro- or microcephaly and epilepsy. The parasites may be found in the C.S.F. and serological tests are positive.

Pathology. Cystic granulomatous encephalitis with ventricular dilatation and cortical atrophy. The brain parenchyma shows areas of necrosis filled with phagocytic *gitter* cells with gliotic and granulomatous scars surrounding. The lesions are near the ventricles and in the cortex, and a 'Swiss cheese pattern' is seen on microscopic examination. Although the condition is considered rare, it is likely to be more frequently reported now that it is generally recognized.

Broad Thumbs and Toes and Facial Abnormalities

Rubinstein and Taybi (1962) described 7 children with broad thumbs and toes and mental retardation, while 5 had beaked noses. They suggested that this was a specific syndrome. Berg *et al.* (1966) reported another 6 cases and because of the facial resemblance and the dermatoglyphic patterns they supported the thesis that a new syndrome had probably been established though not proven. No definite aetiological factor had been implicated and biochemical screening was negative.

Erythroblastosis Foetalis (Kernicterus; Haemolytic Disease of the New-born)

If blood from a rhesus monkey is injected into a rabbit, the rabbit's serum will then agglutinate over 80 per cent of the white population and these people are called Rh-positive, while approximately 15 per cent would not agglutinate and are called Rh-negative; this Rh factor is said to be a complex of antigens inherited as a Mendelian dominant (Roberts, 1953).

In certain cases only an Rh-negative mother whose husband is

Rh-positive may produce an Rh-positive foetus and develop the anti-Rh agglutinins in her blood during pregnancy and these enter the foetal blood stream through the placenta. If the mother has been previously exposed to Rh-positive blood either by pregnancy or blood transfusion, the stage is set for a mass reaction with severe haemolytic disease in the newborn child, who may be born dead or rapidly succumb. Should the child survive, severe jaundice develops, usually before 36 hours. The central nervous system may be permanently damaged, the basal ganglia being particularly vulnerable, hence the name kernicterus (nuclear jaundice).

Pathology. The lentiform nuclei, thalamus, hypothalamus and *cornu Ammonis* are yellow and the *corpora luysii* especially so. The pyramidal tracts are spared.

Clinically the picture is variable and may be one of general athetosis, persistent spasticity, ataxic or atonic diplegia. Nuclear deafness and speech defects have been described, but the commonest feature is mental defect.

Treatment. The early recognition of the possibility of the disease developing has resulted in birth control, the parents hazarding one child, but perhaps not a second. Exchange transfusions as soon as the condition develops have also reduced the incidence and the number of cases of kernicterus entering institutions is dwindling.

Drugs

The world-wide aftermath following the use of thalidomide by pregnant women has spot-lighted the serious risks of producing deformed and defective children by prescribing new drugs to expectant mothers. No doubt, drugs will be blamed for producing all these tragedies, some of which may well have been caused by other embryopathic agents, but it cannot be too strongly emphasized that drugs which are prescribed to such vulnerable patients should be absolutely essential and have no tainting of toxicity. Substitutes for well-tried, efficient and *safe* preparations should have overwhelming advantages to be given a trial.

BIRTH TRAUMA

This may be due to (1) prematurity, (2) Caesarean section, (3) high forceps delivery, and these account for the majority of cases. A variety of causes of anoxia, such as anaesthesia, twisted umbilical cord and protracted labour have been implicated and there are instances of cerebral bleeding and thrombosis (both venous) while oxygen 'poisoning' with resulting retrolental fibroplasia is also included as a birth trauma. Symmetrical spastic paraplegias are found in premature children while in those with a high birth weight, diplegia with extrapyramidal signs, asymmetry of extremities, dysfunction and hypotonicity are prevalent. The range of mental defect is great and is *not* proportionate to the physical handicap. Epilepsy is a frequent concomitant.

Post-natal Trauma

Many parents volunteer a history of head injury in children with mental defect and it is frequently disregarded because head injuries are so common in children with no untoward sequelae. They should not be entirely ignored for just as no permanent brain damage may result from severe injuries, there are a number of instances reported where serious damage and even death has resulted from slight injuries. As with birth trauma, the sequel will depend on the site and severity of the damage, but the grosser physical handicaps are less frequent and there should be a history of normal development till the time of the accident or later. Behaviour disturbances may follow.

Poisons

Children are not only very susceptible to poisons, but are prone to expose themselves to the risk because of accident or pica (p. 785).

Lead. This is especially dangerous because of its affinity for brain tissue. The common sources are lead toy soldiers, lead paint which can be scraped off doors and walls, from brightly painted cribs and nipple shields, and fumes from burning lead-lined batteries. The literature was reviewed by Gibb and MacMahon (1955) who stress that in addition to the hazards of paralysis, anaemia and encephalopathy, there can be serious impairment of mental development and their views are confirmed by Mellins and Jenkins (1955). Moncrieff *et al.* (1964) consider that the traditional diagnostic criteria such as punctate basophilia, lead lines in the gums and X-ray evidence of bands of increased density at the ends of the long bones are no longer helpful as they may not appear till it is too late. Blood levels are essential and of 122 mentally retarded or psychologically disturbed children 55 per cent had blood levels in excess of the normal 36 mg./100 ml. There are two clinical types, acute and chronic, though the latter may give rise to acute episodes. Treatment is with the anti-heavy metal group, such as BAL, versene and calcium di-iodine-ethylene diamine (Ca EDTA). Penicillamine has been favoured as it can be given by mouth. Both penicillamine and EDTA have a chelating action which extends to bone where most of the lead is stored. Prophylaxis should be directed at the exclusion of lead from paints where children are housed, and from their toys.

Infections

Meningitis is caused by a variety of agents, but is primarily meningococcal and tubercular. With the success of antibiotics these cases are less common. Mental defect can be very severe, reaching idiocy and occasionally hydrocephalus can develop.

Encephalitis or inflammation of the brain can be mild or severe yet the subsequent development of mental defect may be unrelated to the severity of the infection. One may therefore be unable to obtain a history of severe cerebral disturbance with the classical features of high fever, coma, convulsions, paralysis of limbs and ophthalmoplegia and all one may get is a history of a severe cold with some features resembling influenza. Although the most commonly contributing encephalitis to mental defect is encephalitis lethargica (von Economo, 1917), other types may contribute and one should enquire about a history of measles, mumps, whooping-cough, chickenpox, scarlet fever, rheumatic fever, vaccination against smallpox, and in patients from appropriate backgrounds, typhus, Rocky Mountain spotted fever, rabies, psittacosis, equine, St. Louis and Japanese encephalitis. The von Economo type was pandemic in Europe between 1917–19 and the resultant aftermath influenced the 1927 amendment to the Mental Deficiency Act of 1913 to include the term 'moral defective' because of the gross behaviour disturbances which followed. It also changed the definition of mental deficiency in terms of age of onset, from 'an early age' to 'before the age of 18 years', because of the lag between the original infection and the onset of mental symptoms.

These are: motor disturbance of an extrapyramidal nature; intellectual defect with learning difficulty; personality disturbance associated with hyperkinesis and deficiencies in social orientation; impulse disorders which may be quite violent leading to suicide and even homicide (Bender, 1950).

Although the causes are many, the clinical picture is fairly constant and does not give much indication of the responsible agent. Neurological signs and severe mental defect are more prevalent when the infection occurred in infancy, while behaviour disturbance with mild mental defect predominates in later infections.

Pathology. Macroscopically, there is depigmentation of the substantia nigra of the mid-brain, with fibrous gliosis which extends to the periventricular grey matter of the mid-brain and diencephalon. The histological reaction will depend on the stage of the disease; in the early stage there is an inflammatory reaction with perivascular cuffing, and in the later stages there is an 'outfall' of nerve cells in the substantia nigra, which is regarded as the most characteristic lesion.

Treatment is mainly education and rehabilitation and some remarkable successes can be achieved. A patient of 9 years who was reduced to an infantile level with loss of language and control of bowel and bladder, and who had remained in this state for several months, regained his previous level in less than two years and was able to resume normal schooling, his residual handicap being occasional epileptic attacks. The impulsive and anti-social conduct may need institutional care and in very severe cases the condition has been labelled the 'Apache type'.

ENDOCRINE FACTORS

Many defectives show features of endocrine dysplasia, but only in a few instances are these causally related and the mechanism is obscure.

Hypothyroidism. Physiological Background

The hormones of the thyroid gland which influence physical and mental development are dependent on an adequate iodine intake which contributes to the production of thyroxine, iodated tyrosine and tri-iodo thyroxine. Thyroxine is stored in combination with thyroglobulin which is the main constituent of colloid and which disappears when the gland is overactive. The above combination is broken down and thyroxine liberated to enter the blood stream where it is taken up by protein and this protein-bound iodine is a measure of the liberation of the hormone, and the pituitary (anterior lobe) controls its production through its thyrotropic hormone. The uptake of iodine from the blood stream can be a measure of the activity of the thyroid gland and is measured by radioactive labelling (I^{131}). The thyroid through its influence on cardiac output, enzymatic processes in the brain, water metabolism and oxygen utilization, can interfere with cerebral function, but its exact method of action is still unknown and is under active investigation.

Cretinism

This is due to lack of function of the thyroid in the newborn and it has a special place in the history of the study of mental deficiency, for it was the first condition leading to severe defect to be remediable. It is not a single entity. The commonest type is **endocrine cretinism** which is found in mountainous and hilly regions remote from the sea and where there is a deficiency of iodine in the diet. The gland may be enlarged and a goitre or struma result and the lack of thyroid function leads to the classical picture of dwarfism; dry skin; myxoedema; low B.M.R.; delayed carpal development; hypothermia; constipation; and severe mental defect which can amount to idiocy. Regions affected are Switzerland, the mountainous parts of New Guinea, Rocky Mountains and Derbyshire, and the condition has been largely controlled by the prophylactic introduction of iodine to the diet by adding it to the salt in the proportion of 5 mg. of Pot. Iod. to 1 kg. salt (Mautner, 1959). When the condition has developed treatment is with thyroid, and Hubble (1953) suggests a daily dose of 1 gr. (60 mg.) as adequate for the first year of life, but increasing to 2–3 gr. (120-200 mg.) in later childhood.

SOCIAL ASPECTS OF MENTAL DEFICIENCY

Social aspects of mental deficiency are now becoming of paramount importance, for not only are the institutions where the patients reside imbued with the new enthusiasm which has permeated the mental hospital, but with the increase in population and the more complete ascertainment of mental defect, there is a consequent acute shortage of residential places. This has focused attention on alternative forms of treatment outside the institution, and more rapid discharge of patients. The Mental Health Act (1959) with its accent on informal admission has helped to ease the burden, for it is now possible for parents with a defective child to get away for a holiday or have several weeks' rest while the child is cared for in the institution (renamed 'hospital' under the Act). Thus, what might have been a strong and persistent application for a permanent place, can be modified to one for periodic short terms of stay, with a tremendous saving in accommodation. One bed, under these circumstances, can serve up to 12 patients while previously it would have been blocked by one patient. The contribution of the Occupation Centres has already been mentioned, and in urban area where access is easy and not time-consuming, they provide a very adequate alternative for a large number of low-grade patients. Local authorities who have a financial obligation for the supervision and after-care of these patients have been quick to see the advantages of procuring employment for higher grade patients, especially in the Parks and Salvage Departments. There they can work under supervision and are cushioned against the fluctuations of the labour market.

In the institutions themselves there has been a change in the types of jobs the patients are trained to do. It used to be mainly a question of using them as semi-skilled labour in crafts which served the needs of the institution, such as bootmaking and repairing, tailoring, brush-making, rug-making, portering, gardening and horticulture. For various reasons, a number of these occupations are no longer in favour, the most important being that they are frequently not available outside the institution and therefore training was geared to keeping the patient in, rather than getting him out. As with the mental hospital, modern industrial training has replaced the traditional crafts but in view of the limited intelligence of the patients, much ingenuity was required in breaking down the jobs to their simplest and 'fool-proof' components. A visit to such a unit can be most refreshing for instead of the dull, apathetic schizophrenic approach one sees in the mental hospital, there is a liveliness, cheerfulness and application which many industrialists would envy. Patients with an I.Q. of less than 50, execute simple industrial processes with consistency and accuracy and the finished products are well up to commercial standards. Contracts are obtained from neighbouring firms and the group enthusiasm is highest when the day's work is despatched. Incentives in terms of money and privileges are used and the whole arrangement is made to resemble as closely as possible modern factory conditions. Patients clock in; tea breaks are organized; overalls are worn; factory hygiene is practised; and through this process, the defective derives an education in living which serves him well outside the institution and increases his chances of holding down a job.

While this industrial training is going on, instruction is also given in the general aspects of living in the community and this is very far removed from conventional ideas on schooling. How to use the telephone, personal hygiene, the counting of money, practice in buying from a shop, are some of the 'subjects' taught. Literacy, while of value to the higher grades, is not essential for some of the lower grades and would in any case occupy a disproportionate part of the curriculum. Instead, the patient is trained to recognize essential items, such as traffic signals, and words like 'canteen', 'toilet', 'men', 'women', 'cloaks', and in several months a considerable body of useful knowledge can be acquired. Trial periods at home or in a hostel are used and the patient, if successful, is then gradually eased out into the community. This entails supervision on the district by welfare officers, who maintain contact with the patient, the family and the employer, while periodic visits to the institution, or preferably its out-patient department, ensure that emotional disturbances, to which these patients are prone, are promptly recognized and treated.

Even for those who do not make the grade, the factory atmosphere which has been incorporated by the institution is a much more stimulating experience than the older system of training, which was frequently to no real purpose. Results should not necessarily be measured in discharges, as these may depend on the degree of defect requiring admission, but on the overall contribution the new scheme makes to the patients' happiness and effectiveness.

Vocational and Social Rehabilitation of the Feebleminded

This has been described by Gunzburg (1958) who lists their deficits as (1) subnormal intelligence; (2) educational backwardness regardless of I.Q.; (3) lack of general knowledge regardless of I.Q.; (4) background of adverse experiences; (5) emotional hunger; and (6) ambivalence to authority. This list is very useful for it indicates the fields in which breakdown has arisen or is likely to occur and to what ends rehabilitation and remedial measures should be directed. His conclusions are very pertinent.

> Generally speaking every feebleminded patient admitted to an institution is socially and often also emotionally maladjusted. The hospital's task is to initiate rehabilitation of the patient, so that an early return to the community has a good chance of success . . . The consideration of the problem of mental deficiency largely in terms of supervision and care, was bound to lead to answers emphasizing the defective's disabilities; the modern approach, which does not consider the hospital to be the only and the best solution to the problem, emphasizes the overcoming of these disabilities—which, on closer investigation, have turned out less formidable than originally thought.

Dealing with the Parents

This can tax the skill of the most experienced psychiatrist. Parents may wish to deny the existence of the handicap, yet have a desire to know the truth. This ambivalence can prove so difficult that a frank statement may excite considerable resistance, and unfortunately a number of doctors, who cannot bear a negative reaction from the parents, mollify them with half-promises which are really half-truths. The truth need not be brutal and it should be possible to gauge whether they really want to know the truth and, if in doubt, it would be wiser to postpone the verdict until they are ready for it.

The issue should not be glossed over with some platitude which raises their hopes, only to have them dashed later. Although the condition may be an obvious one and lend itself to a 'spot-diagnosis', such as mongolism, tuberous sclerosis or some other form of brain damage, it is important to undertake a thorough examination for it is a sound medical principle, and justice must also appear to be done. If the result of the examination, which should include a full history from the parents (see Chapter 23), is unequivocal, then the parents should be told. It is much kinder to settle their doubts than to protect oneself with a vague statement and have them lead the child round to a whole series of doctors, none of whom is prepared to commit himself to a diagnosis, which in fact presents no clinical difficulties.

Answering their relevant questions will demand a thorough knowledge of their domestic and financial circumstances, their plans for more children and the effect of the patient on the sibs. It is frequently this advice that they really need, for they may strongly suspect the diagnosis in any case, and to deny them the information they require, because of timidity in giving them the diagnosis, deprives them of the essential part of the consultation. The most satisfying consultation is one which results in the psychiatrist being given all the relevant facts and being asked about prognosis, effects on other children in the family, the pros and cons of institutional life and advice on the immediate disposal. They may have already seen the Special Schools Medical Officer who has advised them that the child is ineducable, but were reluctant to accept a place in an Occupation Centre. This may well be the real reason for the consultation, and any hedging on the part of the psychiatrist only aggravates what is already a very delicate situation and postpones a decision which is urgent.

Waskowitz (1959), who interviewed 40 parents of retarded children at the Johns Hopkins Hospital, Baltimore, emphasized the difficulty parents have in adjusting to the information about their child's deficiency and has suggested that with some, time was needed for the parents to overcome their anxieties and that more than one consultation was usually necessary. Schulman and Stern (1959), working from the same hospital, asked the parents of 50 retarded children from 3 to 12 years to estimate the developmental age of their child before diagnostic testing. The parents' estimate correlated to some extent with the test results and they conclude that with the older child the parents had a long enough experience to form an opinion, but their awareness of the situation was sensed rather than clearly understood. They however found the parents' estimate a useful springboard for discussion of the whole problem. The Royal

Commission (1957) which initiated the Mental Health Act (1959) recommended diagnostic clinics for severely subnormal children, where the parental problem could be more adequately investigated and treated, but the doctor referring these children would still not be freed from telling the parents why he is sending them to the clinic. In the final analysis it is still the general practitioner's responsibility, though he may seek help with diagnosis and in the handling of the parents.

The Mental Defective and Marriage

There has been considerable resistance on the part of society to permitting mental defectives to marry and this attitude was based on a variety of factors such as theories about inherited defects, inability to care for children, unbridled procreation and the extension of legal prohibitions concerning carnal knowledge of a certified defective. Shaw and Wright (1960) carried out a survey of the married mental defective by following up a random sample in Sheffield. They found that out of an original 242 defectives who had married (120 men and 122 women), 45 (19 per cent) had moved outside the city boundary, but they were able to trace 197 (81 per cent) and the results of their enquiry are grouped under the following headings:

Intelligence. Of the 122 who had been tested, 93 (76 per cent) had I.Qs. between 50 and 69, 13 (11 per cent) were above and 16 (13 per cent) were below this range.

Size of Family. The mean age of marriage was 22·2 years for men and 25·2 years for women, which differed from the national figures which indicated that men tended to marry three years older than women. In spite of this, live births were 50 per cent greater than the national average for women marrying at the same age and the birth rate was also above that of unskilled families in the community.

Infant mortality was high and approximated to 73 per 1000 live births.

Employment. Thirty-four men were in unskilled jobs, but 24 were doing semi-skilled and even skilled work. Of the women, only 14 were employed outside the home. Nine of the men were registered as disabled persons.

Criminal Record. Five men were serving prison sentences and a further seven had been in prison. Another 30 had been before the courts for stealing, sexual offences and minor misdemeanours. Eleven women had been in court for prostitution and theft, but only one had served a prison sentence.

Broken Marriages. Thirty-eight divorces or separations resulted (20 per cent of total families traced). Nine marriages were obviously unsatisfactory. The authors add: 'Nevertheless most of the marriages seemed to be reasonably happy and stable even when the families presented problems to others'.

Child Care. Thirty-four families were known to the National Society for the Prevention of Cruelty to Children, and the Children's Department of the city had been concerned with a further 11 families over reports of neglect. These accounted for one-third of the families with one or more children. The defective parents of the neglected children had themselves had unsatisfactory homes to the extent of 68 per cent, compared with 44 per cent of the parents of the remaining families. Of the total families, 92 were childless. A study of the second generation showed that of the 377 children, 46 were unsuitable for ordinary school and of these 6 were in M.D. institutions, 9 at occupation centres, and 26 at E.S.N. schools.

Of the 10 families where both parents were defective, five were considered problem families, and of the other five, only two could be considered satisfactory, and one of these was a childless marriage. In 40 families where the man was defective (44 per cent) and in 38 families where the woman was defective (44 per cent) they appeared to be living reasonably happy and normal lives and were self-supporting. Of the small families 64 per cent were successful compared with 39 per cent of the larger families. The authors support the view of Sheridan (1956) that temperamentally stable defective mothers can cope with their households fairly well while they have only one or two children, but when their family responsibilities outgrow their capacity they become overwhelmed.

Mattinson (1970) studied 32 marriages in which both parties were mentally handicapped. She found a marked correlation between the happiness and effectiveness of the marriage, based on the partners' own assessment, and their scores for achievement, defined as managing in the outside world. There was no correlation between I.Q. and the ability of a couple to cope with life, particularly when the partners mutually compensated for each other's limitations.

Nineteen were reported as supportive and affectionate, 6 as supportive but showing signs of stress. Only 3 cases were unsatisfactory. Of the 40 children, 34 were in care of the parents, and the majority of the parents were consciously trying to make up for their own deprivation and hardship. The author was on the whole favourably disposed to the old restrictive hospital system in that it contained patients during adolescence and early adulthood which are the peak periods for delinquency and marital breakdown in the community as a whole.

CHAPTER 17

Child Psychiatry

I had six theories about bringing up children. Now I have six children and no theories.

Earl of Rochester (1670), quoted by Rolph (1972)

The subject of child psychiatry which was comparatively neglected till 40 years ago has now become a bone of contention among psychiatrists, paediatricians, social agencies, psychologists and public health services. Much of the controversy is reminiscent of claim-staking by ill-equipped prospectors lacking the necessary appliances to work their claims, and what is now needed are more precise and effective techniques to deal with the problem. Considerable resources in terms of highly-trained personnel have already been invested by the community in the hope that mental illness in adult life can be averted, but there is as yet no conclusive evidence to indicate how effective present measures are.

Though Breuer and Freud (1895) in their early paper on hysteria had affirmed: 'No adult neurosis without an infantile neurosis', the systematic study and treatment of childhood psychiatric disorders did not begin seriously till 1909, when William Healy organized the first child guidance clinic in Chicago, to investigate the causes of juvenile delinquency. His approach was psychodynamic as opposed to the nosological pre-occupation which was prevalent at the time and the publication of his book (Healy, 1915) stimulated wide interest. Another early worker was Arnold Gesell who organized the Yale Clinic of Child Development in 1911, but the impact of his publications did not become significant till several years later. The main impetus came from the Mental Hygiene movement in the U.S.A. which was supported by the Commonwealth Fund of that country and in 1921 the first Child Guidance Clinic was opened in Boston. The *clinic team* consisted of a psychiatrist, a psychologist and a social worker and as the Commonwealth Fund sponsored similar training schemes in Britain, the British pattern has tended to follow closely the American one. The first clinic in this country was established in 1926 and since then, with the availability of trained staff and sometimes even without trained staff, these clinics have multiplied. Education authorities have played the major role in their development and in their administration, though some have been organized by mental or paediatric hospitals.

Some have felt that this emphasis on the educational aspect has narrowed their scope and divorced their work from the main stream of psychiatry and medicine, and Creak (1959) in her Charles West lecture, made a plea for the integration of child guidance with the paediatric hospital.

> Somehow a place, in the geographical sense, must be found for psychiatric work with children—in the children's hospitals. The clinic or the child-guidance centre which has no physical liaison with the other paediatric services will be lost to them, and will itself lose much. Correspondence and even the telephone are no substitute for the means whereby a problem, or the case itself, may be jointly seen or discussed.

A reaction against the concept and even the name 'child guidance' has come from the Association of Undergraduate Teachers of Psychiatry, and in a memorandum submitted to the *Lancet* by Curran and Garmany (1961) it is stated:

> We consider that the term 'guidance' is unfortunate in that, like marriage guidance and vocational guidance, it suggests an activity which can properly be carried out or supervised by those who are not medically qualified . . . it has been our experience that most patients attending them (*i.e.* clinics) have shown pathological anxiety with or without symptomatic behaviour disorder, physical symptoms, psychosomatic disorders, or psychoses; or have been below average intelligence. We have not seen many instances where 'guidance' in any way covered the work that was done.

The Association made the following recommendations:

1. The term 'child guidance' should be abandoned and the alternative 'child psychiatry' should be used in all cases.
2. The director of a child psychiatric clinic should in all cases be a consultant psychiatrist with experience of adult work.
3. A paediatric hospital or department is the ideal site for a child psychiatric clinic, and the out-patient department should be supported by beds under the control of the psychiatrist.
4. We are firmly convinced that, at national level, child psychiatry should be the responsibility of the Ministry of Health.
5. We do not believe that child psychiatry is a legitimate preoccupation of the education authorities.

Paediatricians are showing an increasing interest in the psychiatric problems of childhood and Tizard *et al.* (1959) suggested that:

psychiatry should no longer be looked on solely as a specialty, and should pervade all teaching of clinical medicine. This ideal could be gradually achieved by introducing psychodynamically trained physicians into the undergraduate medical schools. Because psychoanalytical theory is based on the study of emotional development a personal analysis would seem to be a more suitable preparation for this kind of teaching than the conventional training in adult psychiatry which concentrates on diagnosis and physical treatment . . . a personal analysis may in the future become a necessary or desirable part of training for most family or paediatric practitioners. For the present one would at least like to see some paediatricians fitting a personal analysis into their post-graduate training.

It is noteworthy that these authors from the paediatric standpoint have suggested more fundamental changes in psychiatric education than had hitherto been made by psychiatrists in this country. Yet, this full commitment to the psychodynamic model is itself being seriously challenged, for the impact of psychopharmacology and other techniques in child psychiatry is approaching that of the adult.

But not all paediatricians are so committed to a thorough training in dynamic psychiatry and Apley (1960) in an experiment which he admits is 'tentative and preliminary' used psychiatric social workers to deal with 'the common minor emotional disorders'. Most psychiatrists would view this experiment with some concern and while accepting such an approach from analytically-trained paediatricians, would strongly condemn this 'off the cuff' delegation of treatment by one who did not have this training.

While it is not yet decided who should be responsible for the treatment of disturbed children, it is not surprising that there are considerable differences in the treatments practised and in the opinions on diagnosis. As with adult psychiatry, there is much conflict over diagnosis, which is partly based on differing theoretical considerations, but also on the inherent difficulty of the problem. An adult has already established a personality with a recognizable and somewhat fixed pattern of behaviour in certain situations. The child is a rapidly developing organism and in addition to its changing experiences in the family and social setting, there are even greater changes in the child itself. Furthermore, psychiatric diagnostic categories which were barely applicable to adult problems have been transferred *en bloc* to the problems of the child with the result that one looks for these fancied states in the child and either fails to find them or, what is worse, pretends one does. Unless one is familiar with the social and psychological development of the child it is not possible to arrive at a valid formulation as to what is happening.

But the child is a helpless being for the first years of its life and is not only dependent on its parents, but much of its development is influenced by them, so to appreciate the child's problems, a knowledge or even a study of those who gave it birth or nurtured it, is of importance. While these investigations can be divided between the members of a team, it is likely that the psychiatrist may at times have to evaluate, if not undertake all of them.

CHILD DEVELOPMENT

Child development from the psycho-sexual aspects has been dealt with under Psychopathology.

Personality development is intimately bound up with psycho-sexual development, but also incorporates other biological aspects. Though physique, emotion, intelligence and character are inter-dependent, and all contribute to personality, it is possible to study some of thse aspects independently and it helps in the understanding of total personality if one has a knowledge of these constituent items. The concept of *growth* is essential when considering all the child's faculties, yet it has produced its own problems for it has become identified with 'mile-stones', and many parents become unduly anxious over any failure on their child's part to reach these 'mile-stones' at the prescribed time. Gesell *el al.* (1941) 'tersely' summarize these achievements:

> In the *first quarter* of the first year the infant gains control of twelve tiny muscles which move his eyes.
>
> In the *second quarter* (16-28 weeks) he comes into command of the muscles which support his head and move his arms. He reaches out for things.
>
> In the *third quarter* (28-40 weeks) he gains command of his trunk and hands. He sits. He grasps, transfers and manipulates objects.
>
> In the *fourth quarter* (48-52 weeks) he extends command to his legs and feet; to his forefinger and thumb. He pokes and plucks. He stands upright.
>
> In the *second year* he walks and runs; articulates words and phrases; acquires bowel and bladder control; attains a rudimentary sense of personal identity and of personal possession.
>
> In the *third year* he speaks in sentences, using words as tools of thought; he shows a positive propensity to understand his environment and to comply with cultural demands. He is no longer a 'mere' infant.
>
> In the *fourth year* he asks innumerable questions, perceives analogies, displays an active tendency to conceptualize and generalize. He is nearly self-dependent in routines of home life.
>
> At *five* he is well matured in motor control. He hops and skips. He talks without infantile articulation. He can narrate a long tale. He prefers associative play; he feels socialized pride in clothes and accomplishment. He is a self-assured, conforming citizen in his small world.

He describes the child's growth through four major fields of behaviour:

1. *Motor characteristics* include postural reactions, prehension, locomotion, general bodily coordination and specific motor skills.

2. *Adaptive behaviour* is a convenient category for those varied adjustments, perceptual, orientational, manual, and verbal, which reflect the child's capacity to initiate new experience and to profit by past experience. This adaptivity includes alertness, intelligence, and various forms of constructiveness and exploitation.

3. *Language* embraces all behavior which has to do with soliloquy, dramatic expression, communication, and comprehension.

4. *Personal-Social behavior* embraces the child's personal reactions to other persons and to the impacts of culture; his adjustments to domestic life, to property; to social groups, and community conventions.

His analysis of the child's development is detailed and informative; it cannot be adequately summarized and to anyone who is interested in the field his book is indispensable. It also gives a valuable analysis of the test results obtained from groups of children at the Yale Clinic of Child Development and indicates the percentage achievement rates, thus putting the 'mile-stones' into a proper perspective. It should be realized that the findings of Gesell and his colleagues are based on studies which took place over forty years ago. Social factors, which include parental and other family attitudes, can modify the 'landmarks' of child development. It may be that more up-to-date charts will be produced and that additional criteria will be introduced.

Piaget's System of Child Development

Piaget (1953) has made a prolonged and intensive study of how children view the world around them and considers that intelligence develops through a sequence of progressively more complex patterns of action and thinking. Each step is regarded as a stage of development and each new type of behaviour or thinking is generalized to other aspects of reality though with some time lag.

The following is a brief summary of Piaget's System and for a more comprehensive and very readable review the reader should consult Woodward (1965).

Sensori-motor Stage (up to 18 months)

Substage 1 (1st month). Reflex schemata. Looks at light. Attempts to grasp. There is learning within each scheme but no co-ordination of schemata or formation of new ones.

Substage 2 (approximately 1–4½ months). New schemata are acquired and their development is accounted for in terms of

Baldwin's concept of *circular reaction, i.e.* an action by chance leads to a certain result and if the child perceives it, the result is the stimulus for the repetition of the action and so on. These forms of behaviour at this stage do not produce effects on objects. He fixates objects and follows moving ones; develops various hand movements *e.g.* opening and closing fist and moving hand and looking at it; utters sounds and plays with his saliva.

Independent schemata are co-ordinated through a process of reciprocal assimilation and accommodation. Looking in direction of sound co-ordinates visual and auditory sensation. At 2–3 months he gazes in direction at which person disappeared from view but does not search with his eyes.

Substage 3 (approximately 4½ to 8–9 months). Uses vision to direct hands to objects to grasp them. Develops new type of behaviour pattern–*secondary circular reaction* which characterizes this substage. New schemata produce an effect on objects. They produce with each repetition the same sort of effect on the object *e.g.* shaking pram makes toys dangle and he keeps on shaking the pram.

Other examples. Banging a brick on the same surface; shaking a rattle hitting a hanging object so that it swings.

These schemata eventually lead to the development of subsequent ones. At this stage the child does not uncover a completely hidden object. A feeding bottle covered by a hand remained out of sight.

Substage 4 (8–9 months to 11–12 months). Co-ordination of schemata in Substage 3. One is subordinate to another to achieve a goal.

Substage 5 (11–12 months to 18 months). More complex manipulations (*tertiary circular reaction*). Adaptive behaviour in problem solving is now apparent. New ways are developed by trial and error and there is corresponding progress in construction of objective world and in imitation. New schemata are formed if previous ones are inadequate.

Substage 6 (18 months onwards). Solution of problems by invention of new means instead of by trial and error; search for hidden articles; appreciates external forces as cause of movement; distinguishes himself from objects; objects have a separate existence. He has now reached a new *stage*.

The Pre-Operational Stage. *(a) Symbolic and Pre-conceptual Stage* (1½–4 years). When the development of tertiary circular reaction makes possible the imitation of new models, each repetition gives rise to new anticipations which develop the memory image in the absence of the model. This Piaget calls *deferred*

imitation. Symbolic activity is then possible and an image may represent the unperceived object, and combined with other objects and words as in make-believe play and language. *(b) The Intuitive Stage* (approximately 4–7 years).
Concrete Operational Stage (approximately 7–11 years).
Abstract Operational Thinking (approximately 11 years onwards).

HEREDITY OR ENVIRONMENT?

The question of heredity or environment is a constantly recurring one in child development and the mere asking of it indicates an appreciation that the 'mile-stones' of the child are subject to influences outside the organism. Anastasi and Foley (1948) have pointed out the fallacies in the either/or argument. Even the open-minded who are prepared to accept that both factors interact are still unable to provide conclusive evidence of the effects of one or the other, though some of it is very suggestive. Bowlby (1944, 1951) has stressed the importance of maternal deprivation, while Spitz (1946), Bender (1945) and Goldfarb (1943) showed that children reared in institutions are less able to respond adequately to their environment. These issues are relevant and topical, and in modern society are vital where children's homes, adoption, fostering, hospitalization and fashions in child rearing are rapidly extending.

Instinct. This has been regarded by some observers as more important than heredity or environment. They assume that the infant's instinctual needs are uniform and can be measured, and behaviour such as sucking is cited as one example. One worker suggested that every infant requires two hours of sucking per day but others (Davis *et al.,* 1948) could not produce experimental proof in support.

ETHOLOGY

Ethology is the study of behaviour of an animal in its normal environment. Grant (1965) has listed the following contributions which he considers ethology can make to child psychiatry.

1. It brings the help of an observer trained to think of behaviour in quantitative terms and give accurate descriptions. 2. It contains 'a promise . . . that a detailed analysis of human behaviour will provide a biological background against which individual problems can be viewed and permit statements on motivation'.

3. Ethology, which explains behaviour in terms of adaptive value

and evolutionary origin, may indicate possible ways whereby behaviour has arisen.

As examples the ethologist's definition of aspects of behaviour, he gives:

1. *Flight,* which he equates with fear. This results in:

(a) Reduction of incoming stimuli, *e.g.* closing the eyes or covering them.
(b) Reduction of outgoing stimuli, *e.g.* freezing of movement.
(c) Confusion of stimuli, *e.g.* convulsions.

2. *Ambivalence*

(a) Alternating expression;
(b) Simultaneous expression;
(c) Displacement activities;
(d) Redirection of activities.

As an example of the organization of social behaviour, he quotes the work of Harlow (1959) concerning the affectional responses in the infant monkey in which he shows that the actual response during which the mother figure is learned is not feeding, but probably some form of contact behaviour *e.g.* clinging or hugging. Monkeys raised with two forms of surrogate mother, one of wire and one of rough cloth, would go to the cloth mother frightened, even if it were the wire mother that had 'lactated'. Neither did those animals which had only experience of the wire mother go to her when frightened.

Comment

These and other observations are of interest and may even have some bearing on child psychiatry but at present it is difficult to see what this is. *Anthropinism* which by definition is looking at things in relationship to man is more likely to be productive if practised by somebody who is already trained to study man in his normal and abnormal states. One would have thought that a medical education with its great emphasis on observation of the total behaviour of the human being would be the ideal background for a first-class ethologist contribution. Medical men tend to be too depreciatory of their own training as observers of the human species which is unrivalled by any other profession.

If comparative studies are required, then the doctor should join with the ethologist and be responsible for the human side of the study. Apart from ethical considerations, and these are not trivial, it is the author's experience that many non-medical observers tend to see in human subjects an extension of their previous experiences and fail to gauge the complexity of the problem and the capacity of the human being to influence his environment, including the observer. The author, who has conducted such observations on patients with gross dementia, has been struck by the residual operational fields that remain and the discrepancy between his own assessment of intellectual and other functions and those of non-medical observers who generally tend to underestimate performance.

Co-operation between the new science and psychiatry there should be, but the tendency by some psychiatrists to hand it all over is neither in the interests of psychiatry nor ethology.

INDIVIDUAL DIFFERENCES

These are apparent from earliest infancy and have been demonstrated in the autonomic nervous system (Grossman & Greenberg, 1957), which may account for different responses to similar environments. Chess (1959) cites examples which may determine the whole personality structure of the child and warns against the prevalent mood of teleological explanation.

> Actually no-one really knows what an infant is thinking, since he has not yet required to communicate ideas through language. It has been hypothesized that since the infant is incapable of acquiring awareness of the actual chain of events occurring between his hunger cry and the flow of milk into his mouth, he must conclude that his food arrives solely because he cries for it. Consequently, he comes to regard himself as omnipotent, that is, possessed of the power to turn desire into reality.
>
> This jump from a report of behaviour to a statement of the nature of infantile consciousness is based on the arbitrary assumption that the infant is, as a rule, fed fairly promptly after his cry of hunger, that any interval of time which may elapse before a feeding means nothing to the infantile consciousness, and that the infant is capable of thought. Such a concept appears to rest on assumptions which cannot be validated. An infant might have as much reason to regard himself as insignificant and neglected as to believe he is all-powerful . . .
>
> What is being observed is behaviour. The infant cries and sooner or later is fed. One child may be sated and fall asleep. A second child may continue to swallow until he overdistends his stomach and vomits . . . the infant may develop a regular rhythm of satiation, hunger, and satiation again or may regularly become overdistended and vomit. As these patterns of behaviour continue, eating eventually becomes associated with attitudes and emotions: comfort and pleasure in the first case, discomfort and displeasure in the second.

Parent-child Relationships

Parent-child relationships have rightly been stressed as of prime importance in the child's development. Here, too, Chess (1959) makes some very pertinent comments:

> . . . So much has been written about parent-child hostility, the child's resentment of dependency and similar aspects of the subject that the psychologically well-read mother may hope for no more than that she will not show up too badly in her child's analysis when he becomes a maladjusted adult. Such a parent may try to operate on the theory that she must not frustrate a child or do anything that will create conflict for him.
>
> In actuality, neither frustration nor conflict is destructive in and of itself. The child who is never frustrated, whose conflicts are resolved for him by eliminating or easing those factors which militate against the spontaneous expression and satisfaction of his desires, becomes well-adjusted only to an extremely artificial set of circumstances. When such a youngster approaches those later stages of socialization which his parents do not control, as on reaching school age, he will lack the kind of experience that would help him know how to respond to each new situation.

The defining of specific parent-child relationships and their effect on development is one of the most speculative and difficult fields in psychiatry. The child is not a *tabla rasa* who is passively ready to have the ingredients of character traced by its parents. It takes quite an active part in shaping these influences and the subject should be written 'parent ⟷ child' relationships. Difficulties with feeding may excite in the mother feelings of failure and guilt with associated anxiety and this in turn conditions her attitude to the child.

Interparental strife is, of course, a disturbing influence on children but there are other subtle situations, which may be even more influential. Cultural change may isolate the parents from the child's world, and this is usually regarded as a potent factor in immigrants' children. The rapid changes in a modern world are responsible for a battery of social stresses, whose nature is still imperfectly understood.

Unfortunately speculation is more prevalent than fact. It is now popular to talk of parental attitudes to pregnancy and childbirth. The cold, clinical atmosphere of maternity hospitals is being blamed for some of the early problems in childhood and there has been a revolution in the management of these affairs. Bibring (1959, 1961) has stressed the importance of rooming-in as opposed to separating the mother from the child in hospital. Her study is valuable in that it is based on experiment and the assembling of evidence. Fathers are encouraged by some hospitals to attend the confinement in order to support the wife so that she may not feel martyred.

We are very much fashion-ridden, and squeamish fathers nearly or do pass out in the labour wards in order to satisfy the latest psychological fad. Many of these innovations are an attempt to 'humanize' the bacteriological and resuscitative approaches which were primarily concerned with reducing maternal and infant mortality. Yet more and more women are being delivered in hospital because it is alleged to be safer, and efforts are directed to making the hospital resemble as near as possible the home, which is virtually an impossible task. Some have tried to overcome this trend towards hospital admission by having a 'flying squad' with all the essential equipment for safe delivery in the home, but the national, if not international disease of providing more and more maternity beds continues to spread.

The role of the father is being increasingly stressed. At one time he was regarded as the authoritarian figure in the home who took a hand in the child's upbringing after it was weaned, but he is now, literally, in at the birth. He is expected to share in the mothering process and show the child the tender affection it at one time derived exclusively from the mother. There would seem to be no limit to the type of experiment that parents are prepared to make in child rearing and it says much for the adaptability of the child, that most seem to emerge none the worse for their experiences. Mothercraft recipes abound and though now the emphasis is on 'demand-feeding', it was not long ago when 'clock-feeding' was the vogue.

Though many of the theories advanced are not adequately proven, and indeed, some may be incapable of proof, a few are not without interest, particularly for the way in which they incorporate dynamic principles. Levy (1943) stressed the importance of *maternal over-protection* which he explained may be a device for the denial of hate, particularly for the child which was initially unwanted. As an expression of maternal guilt over unconscious hate, it may take the form of an obsessional over-solicitude which extends into the many areas of contact between mother and child, such as feeding, nursing and dressing, and their prolongation beyond normal limits. Some of these mothers have their children sleep with them even in their teens, and make companions of them, thus depriving them of contemporary friendships and blunting their capacity to make easy contact with strangers. The over-protective mother may be either indulgent or dominating and in the former instance the child does not readily relinquish his infantile demands, with consequent feeding problems as well as behaviour disturbances such as impudence, aggressiveness, tantrums and disobedience. In the latter instance, the child may be over-anxious, shy and lacking in independence. The mother's insatiable hunger for love robs the child of positive maternal contributions, such as security, sympathy and love, and the child is then likely to suffer from *'affect-hunger'*.

The infant is considered to have a need, present from birth, for sensory stimuli to its skin and mucous surfaces. When these are deficient or abruptly withdrawn, such as may occur with sudden weaning or too early toilet training, the child's development may become unsettled which may also lead to insecurities, with consequent behaviour disorders or frank psychiatric symptoms. Considerable emphasis is being placed on these early experiences of the infant, particularly in the field of object relationships. The three-to four-month-old child is capable of identifying and relating to an adult and it is considered that at this age, patterns are laid down for the future, though in time these may be modified but are still recognizable and play a part in determining attitudes to others, and in moulding the personality. Importance is attached to suckling and weaning, feeding and toilet training and support for elaborating their influence on personality has come from anthropological studies (Mead, 1928, 1931, 1936, 1950). It is difficult to evaluate the purely anthropological contribution, for many of these studies were made from a psychoanalytical standpoint and though the observers reported what they saw, their interpretation was heavily influenced by psychoanalytical bias.

Other studies have emphasized the role of the family in moulding personality, and Burgess (1926), who was a sociologist, defined the essential features of the family as 'sentiments', 'conceptions of itself', 'social imagery' and 'super-personality'. Here, too, psychoanalytic theory, hitherto regarded as peculiar to the individual norm, was now being adapted to explain the behaviour of the group. These studies and their interpretations did much to modify the strongly held genetic theories which drew much of their support from the incidence and concordance of mental illness in selected families.

MATERNAL DEPRIVATION

This term has been loosely used to define an aetiological factor in a variety of childhood psychiatric disorders. It was time that a more critical appraisal of the term and its application was undertaken and Rutter (1972) in his paper, 'Maternal deprivation reconsidered', admirably fills this role. He proposes that the term includes many different types of experience involving lack, loss and distortion, that little progress is likely till the separate effects of each experience are determined, that different psychological mechanisms account for different types of outcome and that the term itself is misleading in that in most cases the deleterious influences are not specifically tied to the mother and are not due to deprivation.

He considers the specific conditions which are presumed to result from maternal deprivation, namely, acute distress, developmental retardation, intellectual impairment, dwarfism, delinquency and antisocial disorders and affectionless psychopathy.

1. *Acute Distress.* This he regards as due in part to a disruption of the bonding process, but the bonding is not necessarily with the mother. While deprivation is correct in describing this syndrome, the adjective 'maternal' may be misleading.

2. *Developmental Retardation* is probably due to a lack of stimulation rather than its loss and therefore privation would be a more appropriate word than deprivation. Moreover, it is a lack of stimulation which matters and not mother's presence, so that 'experiential' is a better adjective than 'maternal'. While an absolute restriction of a number of forms of stimulation can have deleterious effects on the child's mental development, the single most important factor concerning verbal intellectual development is the child's language environment. It is the conversation that matters and the mere presence of an interested adult is not enough. So again the effect is explicable in terms of 'privation' which is 'experiential' rather than 'maternal'.

3. *Dwarfism.* The balance of evidence suggests that, overall, impaired food intake is the most important factor be it insufficient feeding or poor appetite. This syndrome is therefore attributable to 'nutritional privation' rather than to 'maternal deprivation'. Although Whitten *et al.* (1969) demonstrated that growth failure was due to lack of food intake in 13 infants, Evans *et al.* (1972), who reported on 45 children who failed to thrive and on their families, found support for Rutter's argument in only 14 of the children, the others being exposed to varying degrees of maternal deprivation.

4. *Delinquency and Antisocial Disorder.* These are more likely to stem from disturbed family relationships in general rather than a distorted relationship with the mother.

5. *Affectionless Psychopathy.* This is based on a failure to develop bonds or attachments in the first three years of life leading to attention seeking, uninhibited indiscriminate friendliness, and finally to a personality characterized by a lack of guilt and an inability to form lasting friendships. It is the bond formation which matters and this need not be with any particular person.

Though Rutter, in his criticisms, is not entirely correct, his analysis of what had become a sacred cow of child psychiatry was needed and should lead to more accurate observations in future.

Familial Influence

Familial influence has been described by Spiegel and Bell (1959) under three headings:

1. *Parent-child relationships* which presumably contribute to mental illness. These can be attributed to pathological traits in the parents of which almost a whole alphabet from 'Abusive' to 'Wavering' is listed, or to some interference in the child's emotional development because of pathological attitudes of the parents. Out of these arose the concept of the schizophrenogenic parent (Reichard & Tillman, 1950). These parents present no psychiatric symptoms themselves but were alleged, because of their personality, to foster the development of schizophrenia in the children. Their faulty attitudes have been defined as overtly or covertly rejecting in the case of the mother or domineering and sadistic in the case of the father.
2. *Structural aspects* of the family such as birth order, and the number and sex of siblings have been studied in order to throw light on the aetiology of mental illness. As is commonly found, reports are conflicting and the same holds for broken homes and movements of families.
3. *Genetical aspects* when studied carefully do not yield any conclusions, except that constitution and environment are not as independent of each other as some investigators have maintained. In fact they are interdependent.

As Spiegel and Bell (1959) remark: 'It is clear that it is easier to establish correlations than to interpret them . . .' There are now many reports relating to these and other aspects, and it is important that the information they contain be subjected to the closest scrutiny, for in this field of enquiry a strict and reliable methodology is difficult to maintain.

History-taking

In child psychiatry this differs in some respects from that in adult psychiatry. An obvious difference is the inability of the young child to state his problem or give the essential information about his earlier background. It is the parent or guardian who is therefore the most fruitful source of information, though other agencies with an interest in the child such as school teachers and social and welfare workers should be consulted. The patient collection of facts is fundamental to medical history-taking and the same holds for psychiatry, but there have been some objections. Allen (1942) considered that the collection of facts tended to produce something which was far removed from the living person who should be studied directly and that the assessment of the parent was of more value than enquiry into the past. He stated:

> Some child guidance clinics still operate on the assumption that there is value *per se* in accumulating 'complete' histories; and base this assumption on the false belief that if enough can be learned about situations and happenings and motives, change will take care of itself. Or they believe that a person can be changed by the 'complete understanding' a therapist acquires through having all these facts. It is the actual reality of the troubled parent and his disturbed child and not the historical narrative *per se* which holds the central interest in therapeutic work. The healing values inherent in the present experience in which therapist and patient meet are side-tracked and even lost when we overlook the present and follow only the tortuous and endless task of trying first to evaluate all that has preceded. To understand the present, even though its content may be largely in past terms, is our major therapeutic responsibility, and from that understanding can emerge, actually, a better evaluation of the past.

No doubt such an approach in certain hands and in certain circumstances is perfectly satisfactory, but it does imply that every relationship is primarily a therapeutic one. It may, however, frequently be diagnostic, either because the referring agency wishes an opinion or the examiner himself is satisfied that no treatment by him is required. Medical practice ethics in Britain do not give the specialist the right to undertake therapy with every referred patient; that decision is usually left to the patient, after consultation with his family doctor who has had a report from the specialist. The patient may ignore the advice of the specialist and seek another opinion. This practice is likely to lead to fewer patients receiving psychotherapy, which, if unnecessary treatment is avoided, is not a bad thing. If the patient is obviously in need of treatment, another appointment is usually made.

It is, of course, a simple matter to practise this ethic in Britain but it may be very difficult to try and introduce it into those countries where patients choose their specialists and arrange their appointments without the intermediary of the family doctor. It has, however, much to commend it and where everybody has a family doctor, there are no serious disadvantages. Allen's argument would be more valid with adults than with children, for in the former, the patient is able to state his disability and has some notion of how to present his case, while in the latter, the person from whom the history is obtained is not usually the patient, but a parent. It is, in fact, possible to get the reliable history from a relative and yet establish a good rapport with the patient for therapeutic purposes.

Allen, however, does antedate the present trend in existential psychiatry and his emphasis on the present and antagonism to the historical past has a very modern look which is reminiscent of the importance the existentialists attach to the 'encounter' (p. 555).

Many forms have been designed to provide the necessary information but they are of more value when completed by teachers, social workers and probation officers, than by the psychiatrist who is assuming full responsibility for the examination. They should not be over-elaborate but yet include the essential data in a restricted field, which would not normally be available during the interview with the child or with the parents. Such a form which is specially prepared for completion by the school teacher is reproduced below.

SCHOOL REPORT—CONFIDENTIAL

Name of Child .... Date of Birth ....

School .... Date of Entry .... Class ....

Position in Class: Top Middle Bottom (underline)

Is the child Bright Average Dull? (underline)

Has the child any difficulties with school work? ....

Has the child any special abilities? ....

Conduct

In School ....

Attitude to Teacher ....

Attitude to other children
(*e.g.* friendly, popular, prefers older or younger children)

....

Behaviour in play (*e.g.* likes or dislikes games, takes the lead, is timid)

....

Opinion as to child's character ....

What signs of nervousness or abnormal behaviour have been noticed?

....

Results of any Intelligence Tests with date(s) ....

Other observations

....

Signature ....

Date ....

It can be argued that parents or guardians or those who are emotionally bound up with the child and its problems should not be presented with a standard form for completion. They no doubt possess much information which can be entered on a form, but this information is frequently more meaningful if it is not divorced from its emotional aspects and these can only be gauged at interview. While it is customary to interview only one parent, usually the mother, it is often helpful to see both, if only to extend the enquiry into the parents' attitude to each other. This should not exclude a private interview with one parent either at the request of the psychiatrist who may feel he will gain more knowledge of the problem this way, or at the request of a parent who may wish to communicate something in confidence. Data collected in the history-taking frequently reflect the interest of the examiner and his views on aetiology of childhood disturbances. This may be heavily biased on the genetic side with a fully documented family tree, showing consanguinity, diseases of other members of the family, and presence or absence of twins. On the other hand it may be mainly concerned with environmental influences, ante-natal as well as post-natal, and parental attitudes and ambitions may also be included. Some histories will reflect the latest theories on child psychiatry, such as periods of maternal deprivation which may start with the puerperium. The most recent concern is with the maternity hospital nursery which is alleged to be more traumatic than rooming-in. In the matter of forms, Chess (1959) has sound advice to offer:

> The point is frequently made that no history form is any better than the person using it. Kanner has stressed, for example, that it is more important to be skilled in extracting information than to have an elaborate history form. Merely amassing facts does not automatically lead to their comprehension . . . On the other hand, it is possible to amass facts discriminately and use them purposefully; there need not be any conflict between having a complete form and using it skilfully.

As with adult psychiatry, history-taking and examination of the patient is more likely to be profitable if based on a sound knowledge of child development and factors which may influence it, as well as familiarity with the clinical problems. The subject can be left for the present until the clinical aspects have been described.

DIAGNOSTIC CLASSIFICATION

This is no less a problem in the child than in the adult. There are, however, some essential differences. Child psychiatry is a relatively new branch of psychiatry and the legacy of outworn and irrelevant nomenclature that is so frustrating in the adult section need not be countenanced. Unfortunately, many of these terms have already been adopted. They are now entrenched and are going to prove as difficult to change as their adult counterparts. The plasticity of the child's reactions and the tendency for its behaviour to over-ride psychopathological considerations, has tended to favour a nomenclature where the description of the reaction has perhaps been given undue prominence. A practical diagnostic pattern suggested by Chess (1959) has much to commend it, in that it has some aetiological validity and gives some indications for therapy. Her categories include: (1) normal; (2) organic brain disturbance; (3) reactive behaviour disorders; (4) neurotic behaviour disorders; (5) neurotic character disorders; (6) neurosis; (7) childhood psychosis and schizophrenic adjustments; (8) psychopathic personality; (9) mental retardation.

The Normal Child

He may be brought to the psychiatrist because his behaviour has made parents, teachers or the court suspect that he may be abnormal. Many psychiatrists are reluctant to come to a decision that a child who has shown aberrant behaviour is normal, yet our medical colleagues are regularly issuing negative reports on patients with suspected cancer or heart disease. It is true their diagnostic techniques are more standardized and probably more exact, but it does illustrate that symptomatic complaint or display is consistent with normal physical and sometimes normal psychological functioning.

Chess describes the normal child thus: 'he gets along reasonably well with parents, siblings, and friends, has few overt manifestations of behavioural disturbance, is using his apparent intellectual potential to a degree close to its estimate, and is contented for a reasonable proportion of the time'. It is important that normal qualities such as shyness or boisterousness be not dressed up in words like 'schizoid' or 'hyperkinetic'. If the psychiatrist has reasonable grounds to believe that the child is normal, and he can also apply the time-honoured definition, 'if a child eats well, sleeps well and looks well, he is well', he should not hesitate to say so. It is unfair to continue to exploit the child as a vehicle for parental instability and if it is the parent who requires support, it should be quite in order to send the child back to school and ask the parent to continue to attend the clinic. There are no doubt arguments in favour of having the child attend but they would have to be overwhelming to divorce a normal child from its normal surroundings.

Exceptional or Gifted Children

One would expect the child with superior intelligence to have an advantage over his less well-endowed neighbour in that he will have less difficulty in acquiring skills and will be spared many of the problems associated with schooling. Yet according to Bartlett (1965) there is frequently an imbalance between the varying facets of his development. Emotional maturity in particular is likely to lag behind intellectual growth, since in this sphere there would seem to be no substitute for time. Because of the child's superior vocabulary and reasoning, adults tend to forget the age and expect a greater degree of emotional control. High intelligence with small size may expose him to the hostility of his peers and he may be isolated if not extruded from a group. A number underfunction and do not achieve their full potential and because of this, societies for the gifted child are springing up to ensure that like the subnormal, they are given the educational facilities they require. One can imagine that such societies would not lack applications for membership from parents but it is still to be seen whether modification in the educational system can help these children.

The Brain-damaged Child

Frequently the brain-damaged child is mentally subnormal and most of those conditions which cause brain damage are dealt with under that heading (p. 740). Bender (1956), Strauss and Lehtinen (1947), Strauss and Kephart (1955) and Eisenberg (1957) have all contributed to the definition of what is now regarded as the syndrome of the brain-damaged child. Those symptoms most commonly associated with it are hyperkinesis, distractibility, short attention-span, labile mood, anti-social behaviour, anxiety and limited intelligence. Pond (1961), in the second of his Goulstonian Lectures, sets out the criteria for brain damage:

1. **History,** which may be of a head injury, encephalitis, anoxia at birth, meningitis, or many another trauma or inflammation of the brain and its coverings. This history may be good evidence of brain damage in the past, but there is the obvious danger of *post hoc, ergo propter hoc,* when it is claimed as the cause of subsequent symptoms.

2. **Neurological Signs and Symptoms such as Hemiplegia or Hemianopia.** These symptoms are signs of damage of a particular part of the brain. Their absence does not signify the absence of brain damage elsewhere, nor does their presence necessarily imply that the damaged areas producing these symptoms may also be responsible for the other psychiatric symptoms of which the patient complains.

3. *(a)* **Special Investigations: Physical (AEG and EEG).** The

airencephalogram is a coarse test of brain damage and sometimes shows normality even when surgery or necropsy has subsequently shown clear evidence of brain damage. The interpretation of the EEG contains even more pitfalls, because there is certainly no EEG change pathognomonic of diffuse brain damage. The findings of an excess of slow activity in an EEG of a patient with a past history of brain damage cannot be regarded as unequivocal evidence of a continued physiological disturbance from that brain damage (see Cobb, 1950). Furthermore, in children there is a very wide variation in standards of normality at any one age, making interpretation still more difficult.

3. (*b*) **Special Investigations: Psychological.** An adequate survey of the psychological test investigations in brain damage would occupy a lecture in itself (see reviews of Meyer, 1960, and O'Connor, 1958). There would seem to be three main groups of tests. The first refer to the use of special indices in the standard intelligence tests of Wechsler or Binet. Measures of deterioration in adults by comparing the verbal and performance scores are well recognized and standardized. Their application in children is more difficult, since on the one hand wide discrepancies may be found between verbal and performance scores in patients in whom brain damage is not suspected, and on the other no such discrepancies may be found in children with undoubted brain damage. Educated parents can produce a spuriously high verbal score in their backward children.

The second group of tests are those concerned with special psychological functions, of which those related to perceptual anomalies seem to be the most important—for example, the Bender-Gestalt, various form-board tests, etc. Unfortunately, most of these tests have been poorly standardized with inadequate controls. Moreover, often there are no clear correlations between the test results and, on the one hand, the neurological status, and, on the other, personality difficulties and maladjustment (Cruickshank & Bice, 1955).

The third group of psychological tests are the so-called projection tests, of which the Rorschach is the one most frequently used. Many authors have described specific organic signs in the Rorschach test, but these have been equally often denied, and the whole status of this test, and therefore, by implication, of other projective tests, is at the moment under a cloud.

Pond (1961), in his study of 58 cases of brain-damaged children without epilepsy, found that males were affected twice as frequently as females and that half his patients had an I.Q. of less than 80; birth events were by far the commonest cause. Symptoms in all cases varied considerably and the classical picture of the brain-damaged child covered only a few of those examined. He identified three groups of symptoms which he called neurotic symptoms, abnormal aggressiveness (temper, tantrums, cruelty, etc.) and hyperkinesis or restlessness. He summarizes his findings thus:

In the first place, the brain-damaged child is handicapped as regards those functions, included under the general concept of intelligence, with which are bound up memory and learning. The term dementia is usually applied to older subjects, and implies most typically a loss of recent memory—that is, the capacity to learn new material. Making allowances for the differences produced by age, the difficulty of the brain-damaged child in learning may not be fundamentally different. The poverty of our methods of localizing brain damage makes it impossible to implicate any particular area of the brain, and in general, mental defect has been associated quantitatively with the amount of cortex damaged . . .

Secondly, the psychological reaction of the child to being handicapped manifests itself in symptoms that are related to age, and understandably only when the emotional environment of the child is also taken into account. The brain-damaged child syndrome does not exist in its own right, like an extensor plantar response; but only when the whole situation is considered can the contribution of the intrinsic handicap be assessed. The management of the brain-damaged child requires the fullest and deepest psychiatric approach.

Thirdly, the child who has epilepsy as well as brain damage has an additional handicap in two ways. Firstly, the epileptic activity may intensify the extent to which the brain damage interferes with cerebral activity, particularly when frequent attacks disrupt the activity of the normal parts of the brain. Secondly, the fits are a considerable social and emotional handicap, to which adjustment is difficult.

Though Pond's series included a larger proportion of birth injuries, head injuries in children are on the increase, particularly because of road accidents, and in 1959 more than half the admissions of children to hospital in Britain as a result of injury were because of head injury (H.M.S.O., 1959). Dillon and Leopold (1961) reported on 50 children with head injuries mainly resulting from motor accidents and found that 47 had psychological changes such as aggressiveness, anti-social behaviour, a tendency to withdraw from society, deterioration of school work, anxiety symptoms, hyperkinesis, sleep disturbances and enuresis. The typical adult post-concussional syndrome of headache, dizziness, irritability and fatigue was rarely seen. These findings confirm those of Rowbotham *et al.* (1954) who described the effects of head injury in 82 patients under the age of 12 years, of whom 27 had psychiatric disturbances which were similar to those described. Dencker (1960) carried out a unique study of 128 consecutive patients with closed head injuries in persons of twin birth. The patients were examined from 3 to 25 years after their accidents and the co-twins of the same sex were used as controls. As with many investigations of this problem, prognosis was found to be linked to duration of post-traumatic amnesia, though this can be very difficult to estimate in younger children. The pre-traumatic personality and factors in the child's environment were more important than the nature and severity of the head injury in determining the response to the accident.

Further support for this view comes from Hjern and Nylander (1964) who studied psychiatric sequelae in 305 children who had acute head injuries. They found that such sequelae occurred almost entirely in children with emotional disturbance before the injury and whose parents *and physicians* were anxious and over-protective.

Children with behaviour disorders were also more prone to head injuries.

Chess (1972) has reviewed the relationship between neurological dysfunction and childhood behavioural pathology over a 19 year period. The material consisted of 1400 patients (838 boys and 562 girls) with ages ranging from 13 weeks to 19 years at initial consultation. Eighty-eight neurologically damaged children (60 boys and 28 girls), and matched controls were compared for presenting complaints, psychiatric diagnosis, and the special group of symptoms associated with brain damage, namely, hyperactivity, short attention span, distractibility, mood oscillation, high impulsivity and perseveration. Perseveration was the sole symptom statistically more characteristic of the neurologically damaged child. Clustering of three or more of the special symptoms was significantly related to neurological damage. Other than perseveration, the presence of one or two of the special symptoms failed to distinguish the groups, while absence of all special symptoms characterized the neurologically intact controls.

All workers in the field of the brain damaged child echo the statement of Bender (1953): 'Even an organic brain lesion does not create fundamentally new trends but it merely underscores specific psychological problems'.

Clumsy Children

There are some children whose coordination and control of muscular activity is much less efficient than is usual and whose movements involve excessive expenditure of energy, with inaccurate judgement of the necessary force, tempo and amplitude. Attempts to define organic causes have not been successful, yet the degree of clumsiness can be so severe as to interfere seriously with education and training. Walton *et al.* (1962) studied such children who had been regarded as mentally backward because of failure to progress at school. On verbal tests (WISC) they did well but performance test scores were extremely low; four showed ambidexterity or rather ambilaterality. The authors compared these children with those with congenital dyslexia where the performance scores are high but the verbal scores are low and concluded that the clumsy children have a similar defect of cerebral organization. The ambilaterality would support this hypothesis for congenital dyslexia is attributed to the failure of the establishment of dominance in either cerebral hemisphere. They recommended careful individual teaching and training by teachers experienced in such defects and report impressive results.

Treatment

This at one time was restricted to the physical results of the damage, but has now been extended to the total child in its total environment. Bender (1951) suggests that if hyperactivity cannot be eliminated, it can at least be channelled; early signs of impulsive behaviour are recognized and an outlet provided. The secondary psychiatric features of the brain-damage extend to social attitudes on the part of the child, who feeling rejected and losing self-esteem, may react accordingly. This factor may explain the exhibitionism or extreme withdrawal of these children. Society, too, reacts badly to these children. There is a fear of their impulsiveness and destructiveness and they are frequently excluded from normal society with consequent aggravation of the problem. It is important that the handicap be explained to the child, so that he is aware of it and knows how to deal with those aspects which may lead to his social isolation. Drug therapy is valuable in controlling the hyperkinesis and explosive outbursts (p. 881) but it should be combined with psychotherapeutic approach.

Reactive Behaviour Disorders

These may be a prolongation or reactivation of a normal reaction to a frightening experience and are seen particularly in childhood fears or phobic states, where an almost unrelated experience can trigger off an earlier reaction. A child who may have successfully resorted to tantrums to reach his objective, may use this pattern in less appropriate circumstances. It is for these reactions which can normally be controlled by environmental manipulation, such as reassurance or a more steadying form of discipline, that the above term is used and treatment is a relatively simple matter. Occasionally the problem is more complex, for the child's behaviour may excite in others the very reaction he fears most and his conviction is reinforced. This is seen in a child who feels that people are against him and by behaving accordingly will tend to become even more shunned and isolated with consequent aggravation and perpetuation of his behaviour. When this is no longer amenable to simple explanation and reassurance, the next stage is said to have been reached.

Occasionally disturbed behaviour can be related to an unrecognized organic condition and Harcourt and Hopkins (1972) report four children who presented with progressive disturbance of behaviour due to increasing visual handicap. The relationship went unrecognized for periods of 18-30 months, yet they were all suffering from tapetoretinal degeneration, the diagnosis depending on the electroretinographic response. Transfer to schools for the visually handicapped resulted in improvement in their behaviour disorders.

Neurotic Behaviour Disorders

These usually demand psychiatric treatment of the child, for by definition they are not amenable to reassurance or the modifying effects of time, though in some instances support of the parents alone may prove effective. As these disorders represent deterioration of the reactive state, prevention would appear to be an obvious measure in the earlier stages, but like many psychiatric problems they have a malignancy factor which defies the simple prophylactic efforts which theoretically should be crowned with success. Among those problems which cause considerable anxiety to the parents as well as the child is compulsive masturbation. Sex instruction does not seem to rob the child or adult of guilt over this habit or other forms of sex play. The parent may be too ready to see the habit in quite innocent acts and convey a sense of shame to the child who is virtually unaware of the reason for it. Most compulsive masturbators use the habit as a vehicle to relieve tension and anxiety or just to get to sleep, and the lowering of this tension may in itself be enough to remove the need without making any direct attack on the specific form of behaviour.

Other neurotic behaviour patterns are:

Tics. These are involuntary movements though they may well have been initiated deliberately either by imitation or as an attempt to attract attention. Like hysterical conversion symptoms they are worse under emotional stress or when the child is observed and less when the attention is distracted. Blinking, winking, tossing the head, shrugging of shoulders and arm jerking are commonest, though sniffing, coughing, and other respiratory movements are also seen. Precipitating factors may be obvious and in that case manipulation of the environment may suffice. In others a full appraisal of the child and the family may have to be undertaken as the tic may be symptomatic of a deeper problem. Hypnotherapy often provides dramatic relief.

Thumb-sucking. If this habit persists, it may indicate unfulfilled oral craving or general insecurity. It tends to upset parents who join battle with the child over it, thus heightening rather than relieving the problem. Parental reassurance with attempts to fill the gap in the child's emotional needs may suffice.

Nail-biting. Like thumb-sucking this is an oral craving and the same comments on aetiology and treatment apply.

Neurotic Character Disorders

These are said to be present when neurotic behaviour disorders are so ingrained that they play a major part in the formation of the child's character. Chess states that they are:

> . . . marked by extremely fixed and pervasive attitudes which create distorted impressions of other people's motives, attitudes and conduct. As a result the neurotic behaviour engenders unfavourable environmental response, which in turn further engenders neurotically defensive behaviour in a vicious cycle.

These behaviour patterns tend to be intractable and resistant to psychotherapy. The child may be aware of the results of his conduct but usually does not relate them to his conduct and may even develop a paranoid superstructure. Motivation to overcome the handicap is frequently lacking and this also prejudices treatment.

SYNDROMES ALLEGED TO BE OF NEUROTIC ORIGIN

These include a variety of conditions such as enuresis, encopresis, pica, stuttering, anorexia, and as they constitute a very large percentage of childhood disorders, they shall be treated separately and in some detail.

Stammering

This is synonymous with stuttering, the latter term being more commonly used in N. America. Bloodstein (1958) defined it as 'an interruption in the normal rhythm of speech of such frequency and abnormality as to attract attention, interfere with communication, or cause distress to the stutterer or his audience. He knows precisely what he wishes to say but at the time is unable to say it easily because of an involuntary repetition, prolongation or cessation of sound'.

Metreux (1950) described two types:

1. *Physiological or primary.* This often occurs temporarily during the normal acquisition of speech between 2 and 4 years and consists of hesitations, repetitions and syllabic prolongations. It is not accompanied by awareness or anxiety.
2. *Pathological or secondary.* This applies to the more persistent stammer which appears between 4 and 7 years and may occasionally develop from the primary. Boys are more commonly affected than girls. Andrews and Harris (1965) in a survey of the Newcastle-on-Tyne area found that not only did males exceed females at the outset but that male predominance increased as the

children grew older. Initially 3 per cent of the population stuttered but because of early remission the prevalence seldom rose above 1 per cent. There was a positive correlation with low intelligence.

Emotional factors are important in determining and aggravating stammer and these require attention. Relaxation, speech therapy and hypnosis have all been tried with varying success.

Gilles de la Tourette's Syndrome

Gilles de la Tourette (1885) described eight patients with multiple tics and coprolalia, and since then there has been a continuous debate as to whether the condition is organic or functional. Morphew and Sim (1969) analysed the literature as listed by Fernando (1969). They contributed another six patients and reached the following conclusions:

Of all cases listed, only 37 were capable of adequate analysis, which, with their own six, made a total of 43.

1. Below average intelligence was no more common (10) than average (10), or above (12).
2. Age of onset was 2-18 years, with 7 years most common.
3. Most common first signs were: facial tics (17); limb jerking (7); grimacing (4).
4. There were 14 enuretics, including 6 girls.
5. Other common childhood neurotic traits were: phobic features (8); retarded speech (6); feeding problems (6); nail-biting (5); temper tantrums (5).
6. There was a marked preponderance of obsessional personalities (15 out of 21 recorded).
7. Most precipitating events listed were psychological rather than physical: death or illness of relative (3); beginning school (5); birth of sibling (3).
8. All aggravating factors were psychological.
9. Though phenothiazines and butyrophenones were helpful (17), they also help in functional states and in particular where ego-disintegration in schizophrenia is threatening.
10. Non-organic influences such as psychotherapy (4); leaving home (4); hospital admission (3), helped a total of 14, which was almost as many as responded to drugs.
11. There was a heavy concentration of neurotic features in the parents, in that 10 fathers and 2 mothers were obsessional and 12 had personality problems (insecurity, alcoholism and violence). Mothers tended to be over-anxious and over-protective.

12. None of the cases analysed showed evidence of neurological or EEG abnormalities or a history of encephalitis. Most patients were of average intelligence or higher, and the sex incidence (28 male, 15 female) was more likely to be linked with psychological than organic factors.

13. The syndrome tends to be associated with disguised hostility and aggression, particularly towards a parent or a spouse.

14. Phenothiazines may lower the aggressive impulses and prepare the way for recovery; if there is no longer a need to express hostility, there is no longer the need to contain it with bizarre movements and barking noises.

15. In some ways the condition is close to some forms of stammering and it could be regarded in psychopathological terms as 'a displacement upwards of the anal sphincters'.

Recent reports have stressed EEG changes in the condition (Wayne *et al.* 1972) and suggest that it may be organic in origin. It will require more evidence than this to cancel the formidable body of evidence described above.

SEXUAL ASSAULTS ON CHILDREN

Much has been written about the effect of sexual assault on children and it is appropriate to discuss this aspect here.

The present legal procedure provides three modes of prosecution.

1. Trial on indictment at Assizes which is reserved for the felony of intercourse with a girl under 13 years.
2. Trial on indictment at Assizes or Quarter Sessions which deals with misdemeanours of assault with intent to commit buggery.
3. Trial on indictment at Assizes, Quarter Sessions or, if the accused consents, summarily before magistrates, deals with misdemeanours of indecent assault on a boy or girl.

These trials on indictment take place a long time after the event and the repetition of evidence with the solemnity of the court proceedings are alleged to have a disturbing effect on the child. Because of this, parents and family doctors are often tempted, for the sake of the child, to refrain from reporting sexual offences against a child. The legal correspondent of the *British Medical Journal* (1961*a*) examined medical and parental responsibility of failure to report and stated:

> Such failure to report can only be criminal if it amounts to the crime of misprision of felony. There is no such crime as misprision of misdemeanour, so

that failure to report a sexual crime of the sort under consideration can only be criminal if the crime reported constituted rape, intercourse with a girl under the age of 13, or buggery. The position where a doctor or parent fails to report the commission of one of these latter crimes is uncertain.

Until recently, it was thought that the crime of misprision of felony was practically obsolete, and the Court of Criminal Appeal had indicated that it ought probably to be confined to cases where the person accused of misprision benefited from the concealment. The doctor or parent would, of course, not benefit personally from such a concealment. However, in 1959, Slade, J., held that the element of personal benefit need not be present for the crime to be committed. He defined misprision of felony as the concealment of knowledge of the commission of a felony which a reasonable person would regard as sufficiently serious to report to the police. It is not unlikely, however, that the Court of Criminal Appeal would overrule this decision by holding that some element of personal benefit is necessary to make misprision of felony criminal.

There is therefore still some danger in failing to report.

The views of the late Sir Basil Henriques (1961), a magistrate, of the effect of these assaults on the child are worth recording.

Children in these cases react in different ways. Some seem not to have been disturbed at all, others pretend not to have been disturbed. There are often very strong guilt feelings. There are children who are ashamed of what happened to them and there are those who have a tendency to show off and who are perpetually telling their friends about their experiences. If after a lapse of time a child's general behaviour seems to have changed, parents should be encouraged to seek the advice of a psychiatrist, but if the child remains apparently quite unperturbed, the subject should not be mentioned again unless the child brings it up.

Finally, I must emphasize that it is as important that justice is done to the child as it is to the defendant. Our procedure does not do justice to the child.

Few could find fault with these comments.

It is frequently advocated that those found guilty of sexual assaults should be examined by a psychiatrist, but relatively little attention is paid to the victims of such assaults. They are generally regarded as innocent and the matter is left at that. But close scrutiny may reveal most unexpected situations. Brill (1946) has shown that a 9-year-old girl may be capable of seduction and the author has had a patient who was referred for importuning lorry drivers. She had only recently been the chief witness against her father who was convicted of incest. An older sister had in fact been having an incestuous relationship with the father and the patient was envious and reported the father for having relations with her too. Physical examination revealed the effects of her importuning and medical evidence was conclusive. Gibbens and Prince (1963) in their study of child victims of sexual assault found that two-thirds are sufficiently willing participants to co-operate in assaults more than once or by more than one assailant. The surprising thing is, how little promiscuous children are affected by their experiences, and how most settle down to become demure housewives. It is of interest that Henriques lists two categories—the unaffected and the guilty—and that seems to put the matter in a nutshell.

The witnessing of the 'primal scene', or sexual intercourse between parents is traditionally regarded as a traumatic episode for a child, but it is more likely to loom large as a potent factor in neurotic behaviour in the adult under analysis than in the child undergoing psychotherapy. It is difficult to explain this paradox, for one would have expected those early memories to be more accessible to the child.

Not uncommonly, a sexual assault on a child is interpreted by the parent as a traumatic experience which must lead to neurotic behaviour. This attitude is most prevalent where the parent has a strong emotional interest in the event, such as revulsion against a homosexual assault, or should the father be the culprit, the mother may project all her marital resentments on the child's experience. These can be very difficult problems for the psychiatrist. He is presented with a child who has been assaulted and a number of neurotic symptoms are alleged to have followed. The parent is incensed and consciously seeks support for his or her attitude. Yet to grant this may mean subjecting a relatively unaffected child to a treatment which is counter to what the parents may expect or wish. They do not want the traumatic experience to be resolved or dissolved—it must constantly be resuscitated and the child is expected to behave as an injured party. Several diagnostic interviews should be undertaken before expressing an opinion, for during that time the parents can also be seen and their tensions and anxieties reduced. They may then be in a better position to accept the situation when one is pleased to inform them that the child has been relatively unaffected by his or her experience. This is not merely a dodge in order to get round an awkward situation, but a serious effort to resolve a parental attitude which is more likely to affect the child adversely than the actual sexual assault.

Swanson (1968) studied 25 consecutive cases of sexual offenders and found a wide range of psychiatric disturbance. He concluded that the propensity to have sexual contact with children may be seen as a continuum, ranging from individuals to whom the child represents the sexual object of choice (the paedophiliac), to those for whom it is a matter of convenience or coincidence.

Nocturnal Enuresis

This is probably the commonest childhood problem which

presents to the psychiatrist and particularly if he practises at a child guidance clinic. Yet not all go to the psychiatrist, for many are treated by their family doctors and paediatricians. The condition is said to exist when a child after the age of 3 frequently wets his bed. Organic factors have been traditionally regarded as important and instances of spina bifida have frequently been quoted as causing the disorder; but this aetiology has happily joined those other organic states, the 'floating kidney' and the 'dropped stomach' and one rarely hears it mentioned unless there is obvious cord involvement.

An evolutionary theory has been elaborated by Bostock (1958) who suggests that gestation of the child should be regarded as 'interior' (9 months) and exterior (8–10 months). After that time the sleep pattern of the child changes in that it becomes elective and the child becomes capable of locomotion. The neonate's sleep is quite different to that of the adult and Bostock suggests that the majority of nocturnal enuretics suffer from persistence of this deep primitive sleep into later life. Ninety per cent of his enuretic children were free of organic disease but were less susceptible to stimuli during sleep, and when wakened their actions were automatic. He explains the persistence of the primitive pattern as being due to maternal pre-occupation with toilet training and in his 200 enuretics he found that there was ample evidence of this tendency. An infant, he states, wakes spontaneously only to be fed, and artificial waking for potting is paid for later by deeper sleep and enuresis. He illustrates his argument from the customs of primitive communities where demand feeding and a *laisser-faire* attitude to toilet training are the rule. In addition to the cultural, he postulates a genetic type who suffers from delayed maturation.

Nichols (1956), reporting from his general practice, defines two personality groups:

1. The timid and apprehensive—though often intelligent.
2. The madcaps or tomboys, overexerting themselves physically and mentally. These are often defiant and misinterpret attempts at control as lack of love.

Their reactions to bed-wetting differ and the first group he calls 'the soaker and waker' and the second, 'the saturated sleeper'. He criticizes the 'usual' methods of treatment that have been tried, and his paper is so full of common sense that it bears extensive quotation.

> One cannot emphasize too strongly to the parents that the desire to be dry is much greater in the child than in the parents. Being an enuretic is no bed of roses.

'In future', I say, 'we will do without signs, gestures, bribery, and deprivation punishments of all types.' Throw any calendar you may keep, to show the dry nights, into the waste-paper basket. There will be no whispering at the breakfast table, no lifted eyebrows or gestures of any kind, no frank praise like 'Your brother was a good boy last night' to the other children, and no sighs at having again to wash the sheets.

Next we consider the home treatments to which the child has already been subjected.

'He has nothing to drink after teatime' brings the rejoinder from me, 'What, no fluids at all—no drinks of any kind for thirteen or fourteen hours? Why, that is the worst thing you could possibly do. Having no fluids at all, his urine must become terribly concentrated, and this will make it most irritating. No wonder the lad has to wet the bed so frequently. A small amount of highly concentrated urine causes more desire to evacuate than larger amounts of dilute urine. Think also of the psychological upset. His brothers and sisters are drinking but he is refused. What method could force more attention to his lack of control and make him feel more bitter and resentful?

'What of the second treatment, the dragging of the child from his bed, half or deeply asleep? Has that again produced a dry bed? How many times has the child just pipped the clock? It is much more helpful to encourage the child to hold his water for longer and longer periods through the day.'

I explain that in exercising control, relaxation of the abdominal muscles and diaphragmatic breathing may help.

Talking to the child alone, I explain that the bladder has forgotten at night what it can do in the day. A little urine in the bladder leads to the impulse to empty it. It is misinterpreting its own messages; it is in a state of dither, and can't trust itself to act as it should. We must therefore correct its faults by training it to hold more water for longer and longer periods. I tell the child that whenever he feels the urge to empty his bladder, he must try to hold his water for as long as possible, so that the bladder gets accustomed to being full, and is not so eager to empty itself during the night. Drinking a lot will help the bladder to get used to holding a lot.

Régime

When these explanations have been given to the parents and the child, I tell them that he is to take plenty of fluid, such as orange squash, at bedtime, and I prescribe dexamphetamine sulphate, in doses over 20 mg. if need be, to prevent him from sleeping too deeply. Ephedrine, ½ gr., may also be useful for its sympatheticomimetic action. The dexamphetamine is continued for at least two weeks, and the extra fluid until the patient is dry.

Hypersomnia and nocturnal enuresis would appear to be such an obvious partnership that it is surprising that it has not been given more emphasis. Patients are, however, in no doubt about the relationship, for in the Disabilities Series in the *Lancet* (1949*b*) the writer stressed the heaviness of sleep. Ström-Olsen (1950) described 28 patients who 'showed an absence of anxiety and were free from neurotic symptoms' who were hypersomnic and who responded to a nightly dose of amphetamine. While symptomatic treatment of the hypersomnia is usually crowned with success the problem should not be regarded as a simple issue of lightening sleep, for hypersomnia may itself be a symptom of a deep-seated or more obvious insecurity from which the patient seeks refuge in sleep. This factor should always be taken into consideration and enquired into, for to deal with the hypersomnia without investigating its probable cause is contrary to the best standards of medicine.

For nocturnal enuresis, there are numerous treatments, each claiming its percentage of cures. Ephedrine is alleged to lighten sleep and reduce bladder irritability. Mowrer and Mowrer (1938) introduced the electric alarm which is set off by the contact of urine with a pad placed on the mattress. Gillison and Skinner (1958) reported its successful use from their general practice, but others have criticized it on grounds of expense and its failure to deal with the essence of the problem. Other issues are raised by its use, for the alarm not only wakes the child but the mother too, and may initiate another set of problems. Pituitary snuff which is said to inhibit the secretion of urine has also been advocated, though Jones and Tibbetts (1959) have shown that it is no more effective than a placebo. Hypnotic suggestion may prove successful in that it may help the patient to achieve what has hitherto been an elusive control.

Dextroamphetamine is now out of favour and has been replaced by the tricyclic anti-depressants, particularly imipramine. Dosage is initially 25 mg./nocte, increasing gradually to 75 mg./nocte.

Imipramine, which has proved itself to be a most effective anti-depressant has been given a thorough double-blind, placebo-controlled study with cross-over by Poussaint and Ditman (1965) in 47 patients aged 5-16 years. Dosage ranged from 25-50 mg. each night for children aged 5-7 years, increasing to a maximum of 75 mg. over the age of 10 years. Treatment may have to be continued for 2-3 months.

Though imipramine is valuable it should not be forgotten that there is a large psychological factor in many enuretics and a confidential talk with the patient on the physiological control of micturition and the purpose of the imipramine is likely to reinforce its action. Setbacks following initial progress can frequently be related to unsettling events at home or at school and should be enquired into, for they may be amenable to social support and a long steady pull is much more profitable than a series of jerks. The patient may tend to lose confidence but the doctor should never betray that he too is weakening. He has no need to, for the prognosis in the vast majority of cases is excellent.

The incidence of nocturnal enuresis in children is never fully appreciated till some social change such as evacuation from city to country during the war years or a special survey (Miller *et al.* 1960) brings it to public notice. The survey was made in Newcastle-on-Tyne and yielded a figure of 9·8 per cent in 5-year-olds. It is customary to divide the condition into two types, primary and acquired, the former indicating a failure to develop control by the usual age and the child never being dry for more than two nights in succession, and the latter indicating a relapse into enuresis after having established control. Muellner (1960) has summarized the stages through which every child must pass before full control is gained. Initially there is automatic emptying, but by the age of 12-18 months he is able to tell his mother that he is passing urine or is about to do so. He later learns to inhibit the contraction of the detrusor muscle and hold the urine through the use of the levator ani and the pubococcygeus and then to control intra-abdominal pressure by use of diaphragm and abdominal muscles. The final stage is reached when he can stop or start the flow of urine at any degree of bladder filling. Muellner is of the opinion that primary enuresis is due to improper development of bladder capacity and that these patients have retained an infantile bladder. Encouraging the child to hold the urine for longer and longer periods and forcing fluids are designed to stimulate growth of bladder capacity.

Genetic factors have been postulated by Hallgren (1959) who found another affected person in 70 per cent of families of 203 sufferers and a much higher incidence of enuresis in both siblings of a pair of identical twins than in both siblings of unidentical ones. These familial factors could, however, be due to the effect of similar environmental circumstances. Miller *et al.* (1960) regarded enuresis as a reflection of family relationships and attitudes and showed that there was a strong correlation between the incidence of enuresis and insecurity related to parental deprivation, marital instability and parental crime. It was more highly correlated with insecurity and irritability in the family than with standards of physical care and it predominated in the lower social grades and in children of younger mothers. Cust (1958), in a study on the epidemiology of the problem, found that it tended to arise from a background of poorer homes, more school difficulties, more emotional troubles and lower educational attainments than is found in non-enuretics. As causes, he lists illnesses and admission to hospital between 1 and 3 years as well as mistakes or difficulties in toilet training. This last aspect has not been confirmed by Dimson (1959) and Muellner (1960) who found there was no relationship between the age at which toilet training began and the establishment of control, though Douglas and Blomfield (1958) found that relapse was less likely if training was begun early. Resistance to training is more common if training is delayed (Drillien, 1959) and this aspect of negativism in the child may well be an important factor in the aetiology.

Encopresis

This was the name given by Weissenberg (1926) to involuntary defaecation not directly attributable to physical illness. It is not nearly as common as enuresis and is usually a diurnal rather than a nocturnal event. Control is normally established at 2 years though subnormal children may be more retarded in this function as in others. Burns (1941) described three groups: (1) simple soiling continued beyond infancy in feebleminded or untrained children, (2) neurotic children, and (3) children with associated dysrhythmic or vasovagal conditions. The symptom in the second group is rarely seen by itself and is usually accompanied by enuresis, temper tantrums and feeding difficulties. Precipitating factors can usually be elicited and these may be situations which interfere with the constancy of the environment in a child who is very susceptible to changes. Starting school, the birth of a baby and removal from home such as temporary admission to hospital, are the usual situations and the encopretic may use his symptom as an expression of hostility or retaliation for a fancied insult. Sometimes this hostility may extend to concealing the faeces in paper parcels and introducing it into the parents' bedroom. It is generally regarded as a more severe emotional problem than enuresis, although the two can co-exist. It can prove a very stubborn problem, for these neurotic children can be very reticent, and the sand tray is a useful medium to get them to act out and discuss their emotional problems.

Hoag *et al.* (1971) and Bemporad *et al.* (1971), in studies of 10 and 17 encopretic patients respectively, stressed that they were all boys and generally firstborn. The fathers tended to be passive, depressed and isolated individuals, who were intimidated by their dominating wives. Both groups of authors stress the importance of seeing the problem in its family setting, for successful therapy depends on modifying parental attitudes.

It can also have some physical associations and Coekin and Gairdner (1960), from a paediatric unit, investigated 69 patients with faecal incontinence. Forty-four were mechanical in origin due to constipation, 15 were psychogenic and in 10 'the somatic and psychic factors were so interwoven that neither could be ascribed a primary role'. In this series the psychogenic cases showed a sex ratio of 2 : 1 of males to females as against a 1 : 1 ratio in those of mechanical origin. In the latter, constipation was a common feature, but in the former it was generally absent. Even the 'mechanical' group of encopretics have been claimed as functional, the aetiology of the constipation being regarded as psychologically determined (Pinkerton, 1958, 1960).

EATING PROBLEMS

These constitute a major source of disordered behaviour in children. Vining (1952) summarizes the problem and those allied to it thus:

> Most of us are well acquainted with the food-forcing, bowel-forcing, sleep-forcing and obedience-forcing parents, to whom belong all those children who refuse to eat, to sleep, to have their bowels moved and to obey.

Refusal of Food

This is a marked feature of western civilization and can be considered the resultant of two forces: the urge for the parent to give and the need for the child to deny. It is therefore a manifestation of a variety of parent-child situations and as it is an obvious route for the child to express himself, it is a mechanism which is frequently invoked. Kanner (1960) defines three principal factors in a typical feeding problem: (1) culturally imposed mechanization and over-regulation of feeding; (2) obsessive and coercive maternal over-protection; and (3) infantile response to maternal attitudes. He quotes from Bossard (1943) who reported a breakfast scene between 5-year-old Martin and his mother. It is a model of its kind and illustrates admirably Kanner's three factors.

Over-eating

This too has an emotional aspect. Bruch (1940) has shown that it may be the only source of satisfaction for the child, for if it is insecure and unloved it may be unable to develop creative sources of satisfaction and takes to over-eating with resultant obesity. In addition to it providing some compensation for the lack of personal security, it is a means of gaining parental approval and may also be an indication of the mother's needs.

Treatment is directed to help the child to free himself from this form of dependence and become self-reliant and as Bruch says 'to make constructive use of his good physical and mental endowment, so that he can find more dynamic outlets for his creative drives than the static form of physical largeness'.

Other feeding difficulties are aerophagy (air-swallowing) and rumination (the habit of bringing up food without nausea or retching). These can prove to be very resistive to treatment as they are frequently a source of pleasure and are reluctantly relinquished. In the former instance, social pressure from the child's friends is more likely to cure the habit than the exhortations of the parents or for that matter, medical treatment. In the latter instance, severe dehydration and electrolyte loss may result and even simulate an aldosterone deficiency.

The most effective measure is strict supervision, for it is a similar problem to that of anorexia nervosa and unless the child is made aware that his conduct is observed and that his subterfuge is no longer successful, he may persist with consequent danger to life.

Anorexia Nervosa

In the child this problem is similar to that in the adolescent and may alternate with compulsive eating.

Pica (after the Latin for Magpie)

This is the name given to a craving for unnatural articles of food and is seen in pregnant women (p. 301) as well as in children. Infants put what is to hand in their mouths but this is not really pica, but an inability to differentiate normal articles of diet from the perverse. Kanner (1960) in 30 consecutive cases of pica admitted to the Harriet Lane Home found severe lead encephalopathy in 20 per cent, but the range of materials ingested included many substances other than those containing lead. Slightly more than half were severely retarded and all were below average intelligence. In only one instance did the child come from a satisfactory home. Recently the psychological factors in pica have been questioned and it has been postulated that the ingestion of earth and clay is an attempt by the child to supplement its iron stores. Landzkowsky (1959) showed that whereas wood, black soil and clay were occasionally eaten, the major predilection was for sand. Samples were analysed and were found to contain iron as Fe_2O_3 in proportions ranging from 0·38 per cent to 1·04 per cent and he successfully treated his patients with oral iron. This aspect had been reported previously by Carlander (1958) who found that all his cases of pica had sideropenia and that treatment with iron produced recovery in less than two weeks, which was earlier than the relief of the anaemia.

NEUROTIC ILLNESS

This should not be confused with neurotic reaction. It is relatively rare, because the child is still in a developmental phase and the effects of maturation are still operating. As adolescence approaches, neurotic illness tends to become more frequent, while neurotic reactions in childhood such as phobias concerning heights, open and closed spaces and animals, readily give way. Anxiety reactions precipitated by maternal deprivation or separation are common but usually resolve. Compulsions such as touching lamp posts, or concern over the health of members of the family or perseverative questioning are so common as to be normal and they too usually go with the approach of adolescence.

Conversion hysteria which is now a rare event in the adult is one of the commoner forms of neurotic illness in the child, and it can range over a wide field of symptomatology, but tends to group round abdominal complaints which may lead to hospital addmission and even laparotomy. A normal white cell count is a useful screening test, but porphyria must always be kept in mind. There is usually a readily accessible psychopathology which may be trivial but in some instances may present a major challenge to the psychotherapist.

PSYCHOSOMATIC DISORDERS

In childhood these have provided a satisfying field of operation for psychiatrists, paediatricians and family doctors and there is no dearth of reports of diagnostic and therapeutic successes. Unfortunately failures are not usually published so it is difficult to obtain a reliable account of the prognosis in these disorders. The psychiatrist who sees adults does meet patients who exhibited these disorders in childhood, but who did not meet these perceptive physicians. Their illnesses either recovered spontaneously or ran a recurrent course.

Apley (1959) gives these complementary aspects of psychosomatic diagnosis:

> First is *negative evidence* adequate to eliminate organic disease. The evidence should be adequate; but what William Penn called a 'wantonness in enquiry' is a sign of medical immaturity, is unnecessary, and may be harmful.
>
> Second is *positive evidence* of emotional disturbance. Often it is found, too, that symptoms recur when stress recurs.
>
> Third, treatment, not of the symptoms, but of the emotional disturbance or,

better still, of the stressful situation, which underlies them both, often improves or removes the symptom . . .

He lists the commoner disorders as recurrent abdominal pain or 'the little bellyacher', asthma, feeding problems and sphincter disturbances, but the commonest is 'the periodic syndrome' with recurrent abdominal, head or limb pains, vomiting and fever, which may occur singly as cyclic vomiting or a recurrent pyrexia or together. They masquerade under a variety of diagnostic labels such as 'grumbling appendicitis', 'mesenteric adenitis', 'abdominal epilepsy or migraine' which Apley quotes are 'names men use, to cheat despair'. He adds 'the more critically such supposed causes are examined, the less convincing they appear, with rare exceptions; but when we widen the scope of our enquiries the evidence for psychosomatic disorders becomes very convincing'.

CHILDHOOD PSYCHOSES

As in the adult these stem from a variety of causes including organic disease, especially of the central nervous system. Organic psychoses which do not completely remit usually result in intellectual impairment and these are dealt with in Chapter 16. Before this deterioration becomes apparent, psychotic features may present and these are primarily of the acute or chronic organic reaction pattern. Organic causes which should be borne in mind are brain infections such as encephalitis and meningitis, degenerative disorders such as Schilder's disease, cerebral tumours, hypertensive crises and chorea. Toxic states are notorious for precipitating psychotic reactions in children and those agencies which are most commonly implicated are lead, which may be ingested through pica, and belladonna, by eating the berries of the deadly night-shade. Febrile episodes, severe shock due to trauma or burns, septicaemia and over-dosage of drugs such as amphetamine, thyroid, or alcohol may all cause acute psychoses.

Functional psychoses are, as in the adult, divided into the manic-depressive and the schizophrenic varieties. The former are considered to be very rare in childhood but they do occur and not merely as responses to obvious situations, but as deep psychotic depressions which do not yield to environmental manipulation or antidepressant drugs. The author had a young boy with such a psychotic episode which was so severe that a course of E.C.T. was given with good results. Several years later his younger sister, then aged 9, had a similar condition which was associated with a severe anorexia. She, too, remitted with a course of E.C.T. and both have since remained well. One is quite prepared to see hysterical conversion as a mechanism in adult depression but hysterical features in the child are usually regarded as an unadulterated neurosis. It may be that a number of them are really depressive states.

Childhood Schizophrenia

This is a term which has been used by some to include all functional psychoses in childhood, but the above statement on depression would suggest that the term be reserved for those conditions which approximate to schizophrenia. It has naturally many of the features of the adult form, but as Potter (1933) said:

> Children cannot be expected to exhibit psychopathology with all the elaborations of the adult. It must be remembered that the level of intellectual development and the life experiences of the child are limited in comparison with those of the adult. Language developed to a degree of complexity is a product of a mature intelligence. Children, therefore, do not possess the faculty to verbalize fully their feelings, nor are they capable of complicated abstractions. Consequently, delusional formations seen in childhood are relatively simple and their symbolization is particularly naive . . . The outstanding symptomatology is found in the field of behaviour and a consistent lack of emotional rapport.

Aetiology. This is no more definite and no less varied than in the adult form.

1. *The biological concept* has been advocated by Bender (1953) who considered the primary symptom to be due to a biological difficulty with the secondary symptoms resulting from awareness of and attempts to master this difficulty. She postulated a lag in maturation with disturbance in body image, identity and orientation to impersonal objects and outside forces. One of her arguments in support of the biological view was the 'Whirling Test' which is based on the abnormal persistence of primitive postural and righting reflexes, expecially the tonic neck reflex in schizophrenic children. The child is asked to close his eyes and stand with his arms extended and parallel. The child's head is then rotated as far as possible without discomfort. In a positive response the child turns his body in the direction of the rotation of the head as long as the pressure is applied. The validity of the test has been assessed differently by different workers, *e.g.* Pollack and Krieger (1958) found it present in 27 per cent of a group of schizophrenic children, and Goldfarb (1961) found it in only 23 per cent of his schizophrenic group, but it was completely absent in his normal controls. They were uniformly inferior to the controls in the more complex behavioural functions,

such as in perceptual processes involving figure-ground discrimination and configurational closure, in conceptual functions requiring abstraction and categorization, and in psychomotor capacities. The question as to whether these deficiencies are organic or non-organic is not yet answered and Goldfarb comments:

> ... there is no question that perceptual and conceptual deficits can result from altered brain physiology ... It is also reasonable, however, to postulate that similar behavioural disturbances can result from environmental experiences which confuse rather than enhance the child's efforts to structure his world.

2. *Psycho-social factors* are implicit in the above comment and these seem to predominate in some schizophrenic children when the organic clues are not in evidence. Goldfarb continues:

> If the psychiatric classification 'childhood schizophrenia' includes a large proportion of brain-damaged children, it is reasonable to postulate that another universe of children, those initially diagnosed by neurologists as brain-damaged, include a sizeable percentage of children who cannot be differentiated from the childhood schizophrenics in terms of ego characteristics.

He claims that in both groups a psychodynamic appraisal is always essential to explain the specific symptomatology. Two elements in functional disturbance should be assayed in all cases:

> (1) The adequacy of the child's physiological basis for receiving impressions, evaluating them, conceptualizing and acting, and (2) the adequacy of the child's psycho-social environment, the family, particularly in terms of its ability to enhance the child's efforts to structure his experiences, to give meaning to them, and to improve his adaptive efficiency.

Clinical Features. These have been divided by Kanner (1960) into those with acute and those with insidious onset.

1. *Acute cases* are mainly found in older children with a previously adequate personality. Performance at school deteriorates, concentration is impaired and there may be an accompanying anxiety with the usual physical concomitants. Perplexity, restlessness, insomnia, bizarre hypochondriasis, in fact, most of the features seen in the adolescent, including auditory hallucinations, may appear. Precipitating factors are again those found in the adolescent group—severe emotional upsets, operations, and infections. The episode is usually short-lived and responds to treatment but it may drift into chronicity.

2. *Insidious* cases are difficult to recognize in the early stages. There is a gradual withdrawal and less tendency to engage in speech or communicate and they therefore approximate to the criteria of Potter (1933) who described the following:

1. A generalized retraction of interests from the environment.

2. Dereistic thinking, feeling and acting.
3. Disturbances of thought, manifested through blocking, symbolization, condensation, perseveration, incoherence and diminution, sometimes to the extent of mutism.
4. Defect in emotional rapport.
5. Diminution, rigidity, and distortion of affect.
6. Alterations of behaviour with either an increase of motility, leading to incessant activity, or a diminution of motility, leading to complete immobility or bizarre behaviour with a tendency to perseveration or stereotypy.

A working party was set up by the Hospital for Sick Children, Great Ormond Street, London, under the chairmanship of Dr Mildred Creak, to study 'psychotic' children and their findings were reported in the *Cerebral Palsy Bulletin* of April 1961. The following is a summary of the *British Medical Journal* (1961*c*) report on the memorandum.

The working party reviewed the varied terminology of schizophrenia-like states and opted for the term 'schizophrenic syndrome'. They defined nine points as diagnostic criteria, but emphasized that:

These nine points were not intended as absolute criteria in the sense that all, or any particular one, must be present; nor were they designed for use as a rating scale. While no attempt was made to arrange them in order of importance, it was found when they were 'tried out' by different members of the group 'on four samples totalling 68 children who had already been diagnosed as psychotic or schizophrenic' that the first point was present in every case except one. Many of us regarded the ninth point as a *sine qua non*.

THE NINE POINTS

1. *Gross and sustained impairment of emotional relationships* with people. This includes the more usual aloofness and the empty clinging (so-called symbiosis); also abnormal behaviour towards other people as persons, such as using them, or parts of them, impersonally. Difficulty in mixing and playing with other children is often outstanding and long-lasting.
2. *Apparent unawareness of his own personal identity* to a degree inappropriate to his age. This may be seen in abnormal behaviour towards himself, such as posturing or exploration and scrutiny of parts of his body. Repeated self-directed aggression, sometimes resulting in actual damage, may be another aspect of his lack of integration (see also point 5), as also the confusion of personal pronouns (see point 7).
3. *Pathological preoccupation with particular objects* or certain characteristics of them, without regard to their accepted functions.
4. *Sustained resistance to change in the environment* and a striving to maintain or restore sameness. In some instances behaviour appears to aim at producing a state of perceptual monotony.
5. *Abnormal perceptual experience* (in the absence of discernible organic abnormality) is implied by excessive, diminished, or unpredictable response to sensory stimuli—for example, visual and auditory avoidance (see also points 2 and 4), insensitivity to pain and temperature.

6. Acute, excessive, and seemingly illogical *anxiety* is a frequent phenomenon. This tends to be precipitated by change, whether in material environment or in routine, as well as by temporary interruption of a symbiotic attachment to persons or things (compare points 3 and 4, and also 1 and 2).

(Apparently commonplace phenomena or objects seem to become invested with terrifying qualities. On the other hand, an appropriate sense of fear in the face of real danger may be lacking.)

7. *Speech* may have been lost or never acquired, or may have failed to develop beyond a level appropriate to an earlier stage. There may be confusion of personal pronouns (see point 2), echolalia, or other mannerisms of use and diction. Though words or phrases may be uttered, they may convey no sense of ordinary communication.

8. *Distortion in motility patterns*—for example, (*a*) excess as in hyperkinesis, (*b*) immobility as in katatonia, (*c*) bizarre postures, or ritualistic mannerisms) such as rocking and spinning (themselves or objects).

9. *A background of serious retardation* in which islets of normal, near normal, or exceptional intellectual function or skill may appear.

Other workers have contributed their experiences to this diagnostic group and though there are some doubts as to whether the children they described were in fact schizophrenic, they did emphasize that what is generally regarded as childhood schizophrenia may be a collection of a variety of conditions and that to itemize them helps in the differential diagnosis.

INFANTILE AUTISM

Kanner (1943) described primary infantile autism which consists of a primary defect in ability to respond to the environment. Since this report, what was at one time regarded as a rare condition has now become a popular diagnosis. This may be in part due to Kanner's statement that the parents of his patients were mainly highly intelligent and from the professional classes. Initially the condition was equated with childhood schizophrenia and regarded as a functional psychosis, but this view is no longer generally held, though it is no doubt a comfort to a parent to be told that the child is suffering from an illness which can be successfully treated. Rutter (1970) concludes that:

1. Early childhood autism begins at birth or within the first three years of life.
2. It is not a form of schizophrenia.
3. The basic handicaps are produced by organic and not emotional pathology and are not caused by the personalities of the parents or their child-rearing practices.
4. Problems of comprehension and use of language are important aspects of the condition.

Kanner *et al.* (1972) followed up the 96 children who had been diagnosed as autistic at the Children's Psychiatric Clinic of the Johns Hopkins Hospital before 1953. Those selected for study were sufficiently integrated into society to be employable, able to move among people without obvious behaviour problems, and were acceptable to those around them. This well-adjusted group included 1 female and 10 male patients. Their occupations were: bank teller, laboratory technician, duplicating machine operator, accountant, blue collar worker, office worker, library page, 'bus boy, truck-loading supervisor, helper in drug store, and college student. As the parents were mainly professional people it is not difficult to see that some owed their jobs to their parents' positions rather than to their competitiveness in the labour market.

In comparing those employed with those who were not, the former used speech before the age of 5 years and showed a steady succession of stages in its development: (a) no initiative or response; (b) immediate parrotting; (c) delayed echolalia with pronominal reversals; (d) utterances related to obsessive preoccupation; (e) communicative dialogue with the proper use of personal pronouns; and (f) greater facility in the use of prepositions. None had at any time been resident in an institution for the mentally subnormal and while this may be seen by some as an argument for not sending autistic children to such institutions, there are other more pertinent explanations.

A recurrent theme which was regarded as specific for the well-adjusted group, in clear contrast with the non-emerging autistic children, was a chronicle of gradual changes of self-concept and reactions to them along the road of social adaptation. In their early teens the eleven children showed a remarkable change from the isolation and its corollaries which all the autistic children had shared. Unlike the others they became uneasily aware of their peculiarities and began to make a conscious effort to do something about them, and this increased with age.

It is not possible to deal with childhood autism in the usual systematic way under the headings of aetiology, signs and symptoms, treatment and prognosis for it is not a clinical entity in spite of the considerable propaganda to make it one. Post-mortems on such children have revealed a variety of clinical conditions such as tuberous sclerosis and the lipoidoses, and follow-up has shown that a disproportionate number develop epilepsy.

The partisan approach to childhood or infantile autism with its own society acting as a pressure group is an interesting social phenomenon which has repercussions in a Welfare State. These were pointed out by Sim (1970):

> Since Kanner in 1943 described the condition a considerable and disproportionate effort has been directed at this problem, both in the United States and in Britain, and in general the results have been disappointing.
>
> This does not mean that these children should be neglected. One would certainly not advocate that they be given less in the way of treatment and rehabilitation than other children with mental subnormality, but what is the case for giving them more? Is there any work to show that similar investment in children with other forms of mental subnormality would produce materially less improvement? Why has there been such a clamour for facilities for the autistic child at the expense of the less well-publicized needs of the more numerous mentally subnormal? What is behind the powerful lobby that is capable of promoting this disproportionate effort?
>
> One reason may be that these children usually do not look like other subnormal children and at times behave as if they had normal intelligence. Because of this their parents are reluctant to have them labelled mentally subnormal, and have used their group influence to ensure that they are regarded as a very special case. Yet in the field of adult dementia one does not confine the diagnosis to intellectual deterioration alone. Behavioural and emotional deterioration is regarded as no less important, and in child psychiatry social and emotional immaturity is a no less significant criterion for handicap.
>
> Another reason is that autistic children, or at least those diagnosed as such, tend to come from middle-class homes. Wing *et al.* (1967) found that 60 per cent of the fathers were in social classes I and II, compared with 18 per cent in the general population of England and Wales. It would appear that it is parental advocacy which has largely contributed to the greater concentration of resources on this problem and to its separation from other forms of mental subnormality, including, paradoxically, those recoverable patients who manifest with behaviour disorders or where the condition is based on early deprivation.
>
> I am not one who would interfere with the liberty of people to provide advantages for themselves or their offspring, be it in the field of education or medical treatment, provided that they pay for them. It need hardly be repeated that resources in the Health Service are scarce, and before one advocates further public expenditure on this problem there is a need for more critical assessment of the results already obtained, and how this investment compares with similar investment in other fields of mental subnormality.
>
> This is not the only instance where the intelligent and articulate, if given access to the resources of the Welfare State, take more than their share. It used to be argued that by giving them this access facilities would be improved for all. In fact it has exposed the poor and the inarticulate to unfair competition. The shocking conditions of hospitals at Ely and Coleshill are symptomatic of disproportionate investment not only *vis à vis* other branches of medicine but within the field of subnormality itself. It is disturbing to see a lobby agitate for even greater privileges for an already privileged class while those who cannot plead are even more deprived.

As autism is primarily a fault in communication and comprehension there has been more intensive research into these aspects, but to date nothing specific has emerged, and this is not surprising in a condition with multiple aetiology. The understanding of the problem will depend more on advances in paediatric neurology than on the studies of psychologists and ethologists, yet it is the latter that are primarily involved. They see the autistic child's tendency to ignore objects and people to the extent of running into them as a psychologically determined pattern of behaviour. A similar if not a sinister interpretation could be placed on a patient with a poorly compensated left-sided hemianopia who bumped into objects on the left.

Chess (1959) gives some useful hints for differential diagnosis, particularly from mental retardation, and stresses that the child's behaviour must be assessed in terms of its intellectual level and that if there is evidence of its functioning at or above the chronological age, then mental retardation is unlikely. She also mentions the dangers of using terms like autism, dissociation, perseveration, echolalia and echopraxia descriptively as these connote schizophrenia and one may be 'almost trapped into having made a diagnosis'. Contrary to the Working Party Report which regarded point nine as a *sine qua non,* she is emphatic that 'there is no pathognomonic symptom in schizophrenia'.

Psychopathic Personality

This aspect is dealt with in Chapter 10 and though primarily a problem in the adult, it is essentially a constitutional problem, accent now being placed on the early formative years of the patient. Institutional children and those from broken homes seem particularly vulnerable and if the potential psychopath can be detected, and if something constructive can be done to help him, then early diagnosis becomes of prime importance. There are, however, factors other than environment which affect the condition, one of which is maturation, though even this can be influenced by the environment. A child with an immature EEG pattern may stabilize both clinically and electro-encephalographically with psychotherapy or environmental manipulation.

Special Stress Situations

In adult life such situations spring readily to mind. They include bereavement, employment, housing, marriage and traumatic experiences such as battle, earthquake and flood. Children undergo stresses which may not in themselves be very specific, but which interfere with the normal processes of emotional and intellectual development. It should be stated at the outset that though there is some evidence of the influence of these factors on the child, it is not conclusive, and many children undergo similar experiences without any adverse effects, suggesting that other factors must be taken into consideration.

Physical Illness and Handicaps

These are frequently quoted as causative of emotional disturbances, and it is easy to convince parents of the relationship. The diabetic child who cannot tuck in to all the good things at a party; the cardiac child who is unable to join in at games; the polio victim who cannot walk or has to wear calipers, can all excite in the adult the capacity to project himself into the child's situation and 'understand' how the child must feel. But this does not tell us the effect these disabilities have on the child. A simple and useful way of appreciating these issues is to apply the Adlerian concept of organ inferiority and the compensatory mechanism used in the handling of it (p. 46). The parents may be more in need of help than the child, for they tend to over-protect and shelter and thus obstruct the usual processes which make for the child's independence. A common result of this over-protection is a tendency by the child to exploit the illness and to react similarly in future situations. There are, of course, differences between acute and chronic illness in that the former does not permit time for dependency situations to develop. In chronic illness, there is time and the way the child is handled may well influence his subsequent behaviour.

Battered Babies

Since Caffey (1957) described the periosteal changes and other injuries seen on X-ray films of children who had been swung fiercely by their ankles or wrists, there has been a spate of reports on what is now termed the 'Battered Baby Syndrome'.

The condition should be suspected if a child sustains an unusual or severe injury and the parents have delayed in seeking advice, or if they give unsatisfactory explanations of the 'accident'. There may be a sequence of minor injuries to one child which a parent would normally avoid by taking the necessary precautions to see that the burn or fall did not happen again. There may be a contrast between the attention to the child's clothes and cleanliness and its failure to gain weight. The parents may adopt an attitude of extreme defensive sensitivity to the doctor who may be unaware that he has touched on such an area (Isaacs, 1972).

In spite of these early clues, such is the reluctance of doctors to accept that parents could so treat a child, the diagnosis is frequently missed, or if made is met with denial mechanisms which is translated into giving the parents the benefit of the doubt or failing to take the appropriate action. Yet the situation does not permit delay or failure to act, for it tends to be repetitive, and even when one child has died as the result of its injuries other children may be at risk.

Isaacs (1972) sees the problem as a personality disorder in the parent or parents:

> It may evolve from their being reared in emotionally abusing situations themselves; situations which, like the disorder they later develop, are not confined to any social class. Unwanted, unloved, neglected, frequently moved from home to relatives or residential care, witnesses of parental quarrels and violence, sometimes even physically abused themselves, the parents remember these situations only partly consciously and try to forget, and overcome, by starting their own families young and with the intention of treating their own children better. These early situations have left the parents very unsure of their own worth, very vulnerable to the opinions of others, and unduly reliant on external proof that all is well—hence their tendency to clothe and feed their children particularly well and their susceptibility to disturbance when things go wrong, or appear to do so. Thus they may perceive the wetting or soiling of even a normal infant as a rejection and an accusation of failure, and other such events include illness or unhappiness in the child or just its inevitable childish failure to fulfil the role of loving child to the tragic parent who has never had consistent experience of such affection and care.

Dr Isaacs does not favour a register of 'batterers' and is very much against bringing in the police or amending the existing law. She claims that with adequate supervision much can be done to remedy the problem, though initially it may mean taking the child or children into care. The present Children and Young Person's Act (1969) permits this 'if his proper development is being avoidably prevented or neglected or his health is being avoidably impaired or neglected or he is being ill-treated'. There is also a clause which permits preventive action if one child in a family has already died in a similar situation.

There is much wisdom and experience in Dr Isaac's views, but there is also much that suggests special pleading. No doubt a large number of child batterers are included in her description, but more research into the background of many more instances is needed before her generalizations can be accepted entirely. The report by Skinner and Castle (1969) is a good start.

The Battering Child

Adelson (1972) reported on five infants, all less than a year old, who were killed by children aged 2½-8 years. All died from craniocerebral trauma, and in only two of the victims were other areas of the body affected. One assailant was mentally defective and another had a low I.Q., but all displayed a sense of rejection and rivalry with a sibling or resentment of the younger child. This real or fancied threat to the assailant's place or priority in the household provoked the lethal violence.

A battered baby may therefore not necessarily be the victim of a battering adult, for if in one County Coroner's Court there can be 5 lethal cases in 3½ years, the condition cannot be regarded as rare.

Burnt Children

Martin (1970) in a study which compared 50 children burned or scalded in accidents with 41 healthy children from families of similar size and matched for age, sex and social group found that there seems to have been an unconscious wish to injure the child with motives similar to those in the battered baby syndrome. There was a difference; battering parents expressed little guilt while the parents of burned children showed marked guilt. While parents of battered children abuse them again and again, burns did not recur during a year's follow-up.

Seligman *et al.* (1971) reported an intensive study of 56 children who sustained major burns and lists the following characteristic events in the history of the burnt child: (1) early bereavement of parents; (2) unconscious motivation; (3) possible significance of anniversary dates of parents' bereavements. In spite of the psychopathology, follow-up studies of the children who were discharged revealed an adjustment which was far more adequate than anticipated.

Admission to Hospital

This has received much publicity and has been equated with maternal deprivation (Bowlby, 1951). Personality development is said to be impaired and many Children's Hospitals now permit unrestricted visiting or make arrangements for the mother to be admitted with the child. The corollaries to these reforms are also being introduced, namely unrestricted visiting of adults by children and the admission of children with their mothers. The latter is of course not new in the case of patients with puerperal psychosis. MacCarthy *et al.* (1962) review the history of admitting mothers with children under 5 years of age to a paediatric unit. They point out that nursing by the mother was the principal aim of the late Sir James Spence when he founded the Babies Hospital in Newcastle-upon-Tyne in 1925; in 1953 they established their unit and in support they quote the film study by Robertson, *A Two-Year Old goes to Hospital* for its portrayal of the fretting child. Robertson (1958 *a & b*) who has written extensively about the problem advised MacCarthy *et al.* on their project, thus indirectly showing how the child psychiatrist can make a constructive contribution to child care. The results of the experiment are regarded by the authors as generally advantageous and it is adopted by many paediatric hospitals. Schaffer (1958) has pointed out that infants under 7 months do not exhibit fretting behaviour, and it is generally agreed that in children over 5 years, the need is not so great. On the other hand, a sick child tends to regress and chronological age may not indicate the emotional needs of the patient. The authors show that the usual objections of nursing obstruction, cross-infection, and difficult mothers are easily overcome and in fact indicate that the mother acts as an unpaid nurse for her child.

Now that the principle of unrestricted visiting and even residence of parents of children in hospital has been universally received, critical comments are now filtering through. A major attack on the principle of maternal deprivation has come from Bettelheim (1969), who studied children reared on a Kibbutz, which is a communal settlement in Israel. Here the children spend relatively little time with their parents, and were mainly in the care of an indifferent or cold attendant who could have been a burnt-out schizophrenic. These children do very well and eventually become the *élite* in the armed forces, the professions and the government service. The major factors in their development are: (1) the Kibbutz; (2) their peer groups and (3) their parents, in that order.

One cynic, on seeing the Robertson film where the child reacted catastrophically to the mother's departure, remarked: 'Any mother who could bring up a child to be so dependent should be barred from visiting'. The fashion is popular and has won government support. It will take many more objective studies to counter the propaganda of a film.

Khan (1971) has started to chip away at the universal application of unrestricted visiting with his paper on 'Mama's Boy Syndrome'. He treated 13 such children who had developed a critical social deficit as a result of an excessively prolonged mutually dependent relationship with the mother. After failure to respond to six months of out-patient treatment, each child was admitted and parental visiting was barred till the child had achieved an adequate degree of independence.

School

This is a universal experience of children in societies which have compulsory education. It has become so much part of the normal background that one is apt to forget the upheaval it can represent in the lives of some children. It signifies the first break with the home, the spending of a greater part of the day with strangers and being initiated into new relationships outside the family including children of the same age. Any difficulty the child may have in adjustment will probably be reflected in learning difficulties which in their turn lead to social and psychological problems. Chess (1959) distinguished between 'an emotional learning block in which the emotional problem is primary and the learning difficulty is symptomatic' and 'a primary learning difficulty caused by faulty brain functioning, which directly interferes with the learning process'. For the former a psychotherapeutic approach with the definition of the emotional factors concerned is necessary. Parental ambition with consequent resistance by the child or the child's need to remain dependent may block his capacity to learn.

Primary learning difficulties are generally reflected in the child's capacity for speech or for writing, and some are popularly regarded as problems in cerebral dominance with resulting crossed laterality. Orton (1937) who has written a standard work on the subject favours a physiological interpretation of what he called *congenital developmental alexia.* The habit of initiating the intricate motor responses required for speech and writing from one hemisphere begins in childhood and is associated with a preference for the right or left hand. Dominance is thus established and Orton holds that delays and defects of speech may be due to interference with the ability of the patient to ignore the impulses from the non-dominant hemisphere. Though much has been written about the neurophysiological basis of such defects, in remedial training emotional factors are probably more important. A good relationship between the teacher and the emotionally disturbed child is more likely to lead to improvement in a reading disability than a training programme which does not include such a relationship.

Adoption of Children

This includes several aspects which may involve the psychiatrist. A childless couple may consult a psychiatrist for an assessment of the part adoption may play in fulfilling their emotional needs; or they may wish to ascertain their suitability for the role of adoptive parents, particularly if one or both has had a history of mental breakdown and the adoption society has expressed its doubts. It is, however, the adopted child who is more frequently referred, for when things go wrong, the parents have a strong sense of guilt and readily seek the help of the psychiatrist. There is thus a danger that the psychiatrist may get a distorted view of the adopted child and its parents, for, as he is usually consulted when things have gone wrong, he is relatively ignorant of the large number of adopted children who are happily reared and give no trouble. Nevertheless, a fair number of problems do occur in children who are adopted and that fact must be considered, though it may not be the most important one. It can be argued that adoption is only an incidental factor and that had these parents reared their own children, an identical situation would have resulted. Adoption with its attendant formalities does place a legal obligation on the parents and they are more likely to be concerned with minor deviations in behaviour and wonder where they went wrong, or what is equally disturbing, what was wrong with the child's antecedents. Concealment of the true parentage and accidental discovery by the child can be traumatic, especially as these children frequently weave romantic tales about their true parents and cannot accept the fact that they were rejected. Generally, the child should be told at a relatively early age that he is adopted and his questions should be answered frankly and sympathetically. It is however a field of study which still awaits the searchlight of a patient and inspired investigator.

Lewis (1965) who had considerable experience of the problems involved, states that 87 per cent of adoptions are successful. In a sample year, 20 per cent of the children were legitimate and of the illegitimate, 25 per cent went to one or both parents. She lays great store on the type of home where the child goes. '*The character of the house* in which the child will develop (and not its economic class) strongly influences his ultimate intellectual functioning, whatever his genetic endowment.' She lists the following difficulties in adoption:

1. Temporary adjustment problems. These can be overcome by counselling.
2. Threatened breakdown of placement and rejection of the infant. This calls for a complete re-appraisal of the adoption.
3. Telling the child. (This has already been discussed.)

She affirms that difficulties and failures are few in proportion to the successes but these happy results could only be obtained by experienced workers.

Lewis advocates that the mother should always see her child which is contrary to some who feel that once the mother has seen her child she will never be able to relinquish it and assumes insuperable social handicaps. These objections are dismissed by Lewis and such is her experience and patently sensible approach to the problem that she is more likely to be right. She also advocates that the mother breast-feed the child for the first month.

Support for the above views has come from Gifford *et al.* (1969), who compared adopted children referred to a child psychiatric out-patient department with children referred who were living with their biological parents. No significant difference was found between the groups with respect to the severity of the illness. Seglow *et al.* (1972) studied 200 adopted children after seven years and compared them with children born in the same week who were living with their biological parents. Eighty-nine per cent of the adopted children were illegitimate. The authors conclude that the favourable environment enjoyed by most adopted children enabled them to achieve normal development despite their greater vulnerability at birth, and that the adoption procedure had proved to be a 'remarkable success'.

School Phobia

This was first described as a syndrome by Broadwin (1932) but the term was later coined by Johnson *et al.* (1941). It signifies a persistent refusal to attend school, the child remaining at home with the full knowledge of his parents, as opposed to *truanting,* where the child usually absents himself from home and school. Hersov (1960 *a* & *b*) has pointed out that school phobics are more intelligent, of higher social class, work and behave better at school, are more timid, have been less frequently separated from their mothers in early childhood, have mothers who are over-protective, and have a higher incidence of family neurosis. Burns (1959) has emphasized that it is the separation-anxiety rather than fear of school which is the main problem and Davidson (1961) has suggested they be called motherphiles rather than school-phobes. It is usually a symptom of neurotic disturbance, while truancy tends to be associated with delinquency.

The incidence is difficult to gauge; as with most recently described conditions, collectors become enthusiastic and a number of other conditions are re-named and included in the new syndrome. Some may have been previously regarded as truants or as suffering from other neurotic features, for many present with somatic complaints such as abdominal pain or nausea on school mornings.

Treatment is still a matter of empiricism as is shown in a summary of the problem in a leading article in the *Lancet* (1960*b*):

The treatment of early cases consists in firm support, and encouragement of mother and child towards a return to school. Attempts to force the child only generate greater panic. If this fails, psychotherapy, usually of both mother and child, may be required; but a compromise solution, such as allowing the mother to remain with the child at school, may bring about an early return. Change of school in itself is useless, for it is not there that the trouble lies; but such a change does provide a fresh start and, in combination with other methods, may help. Separation from the parents by residential schooling may be needed, but only after careful judgment and individual treatment; for in the obstinate case the child will immediately abscond. Half of Hersov's group of severe cases required in-patient treatment; but on the whole the outlook is good, especially for children below 11 years old of whom 89 per cent. attending one clinic were going to school regularly (Rodriguez *et al.*, 1959); over that age the figure dropped to 36 per cent. The 'hard core' cases were found to come from the most seriously disturbed families; in such cases the school refusal may well be a clinic refusal, and, later on, a work refusal. Clearly, the sooner treatment is started the better; and this requires efficient and rapid communication between parents, school, and many other agencies that may become involved.

In the older age groups, treatment should be as for phobic anxiety in adults (see p. 470) where the results are much better than the 36 per cent quoted above.

Children of Psychotic Parents

This subject is receiving increasing attention for different reasons. For some the psychotic process with its disruption of inter-personal relations presents as a ready-made experimental situation which should be reflected in the child's development, while for others who subscribe to the theory that neurotic and psychotic traits are inherited independently, the presence of neurotic features in the children of psychotic parents would indicate the environmental effects of a psychosis. Cowie (1961) surveyed 330 children of psychotic patients treated at the Bethlem Royal and Maudsley Hospitals and compared them with a similar number of control children of mentally healthy patients treated in general hospitals. The overall rating for neuroticism did not differ materially between proband and control groups though there was an excess of neurotic symptoms during the 2 years after the onset of the parental psychosis. The author took this to indicate the transience of environmentally precipitated childhood neuroses. A small number of obsessive-compulsive parents of either sex produced the highest proportion of disturbed children in that they were over-dependent, faddy and prone to tantrums, but generally not obsessional.

Other data which emerged showed that parental psychosis when the child was under 2, produced no excess of neurotic features but the incidence was higher but not significantly so in the 3–5 years group. The sex of the parent mattered most with schizophrenia, in that a schizophrenic father did little harm, but schizophrenic mothers were associated with adverse circumstances more than any other group studied. Too much importance should not be placed on the latter finding, for a diagnosis of schizophrenia does not indicate the effect the illness has on the child. Newman and San Martino (1971) have shown that the degree of psychosis in the parent has no correlation with the adverse effect on the child. It depends more on the nature of the disturbance and whether the child is incorporated or not. Landau *et al.* (1972), in a controlled study, do regard the child of psychotic parents as at risk, but this could be due more to the social and economic handicap than to the psychosis, though the psychosis itself could be a contributory factor to the family's social disadvantage.

A more important point is the response to treatment and the degree of supervision the family can be given. Where the patients are living literally on the door-step of a psychiatric clinic and where adequate social support is available, the author has been impressed with how the children of psychotic (mainly schizophrenic) mothers appear to thrive under what one would expect to be a severe handicap. Some social workers have reported that even in the mother's more disturbed phases, the children are not neglected, and maternity and child welfare services do not report adversely on the development of these children. In the course of 30 years of history-taking, the author has met very few instances indeed of psychotic, or for that matter neurotic patients who had schizophrenic mothers, thus reinforcing his opinion that such a parent need not constitute the handicap in the child's development that one has been led to expect.

PSYCHIATRIC PROBLEMS IN ADOLESCENCE

These do not include all the behaviour problems of the adolescent, even though they may be explained in psychosociological terms. The exploits of the gang, rebelliousness in the school and home and the general flouting of authority come within the province of preservers of law and order, rather than of the psychiatric clinic. This does not deter magistrates and others from constantly requesting psychiatric reports on every boy who is caught throwing a stone at a lamp post or defacing public property. In addition, intelligence testing is undertaken in the hope that in this age of repeated screening a mentally subnormal person may have been overlooked and some clinics must utilize a considerable proportion of the time of their professional staff in providing such a service to the Courts. If payment for these services was separately accounted, the Home Office or the Local Authority might eventually ask or be asked whether they are really worth the expenditure, and the Minister of Health might be more reluctant to divert staff, whose main function should be therapeutic, to provide many unnecessary and even useless reports for the Courts.

Adolescence, however, is for some a stress situation and mental disturbance may result. Some understanding of the stresses involved is therefore necessary.

Denial of Death–Longing for Immortality

Sarwer-Foner (1972) discusses the above factors in the terminal stage of adolescence, which act as impediments to becoming adult and accepting adult roles and responsibilities. Physical growth leads to bodily interest and pride and a feeling that this state of physical glory is eternal and unchangeable. Beneath these conscious feelings lie a yearning for and an insistence on immortality and indestructibility and a gross denial of death and dying. The non-medical use of drugs, dangerous behaviour and risk-taking are affirmations of one's capacities and prowess and also represent a challenge to one's elders.

For some adolescents the mystical attraction of the hallucinogens lies partly in the 'expansion of the mind' experience which offers hope of an enhanced present supra-corporal "destiny" under immediate control. The adolescent's fear of dying and nothingness, a fear rooted in the need to maintain his new-found glory, leads him to reject adulthood and its responsibilities as compromises and its implications of ageing as weakness and decrepitude. Such attitudes may be reinforced by the attitudes of those parents who share some of the existentialist anxiety and, succumbing in part to the adolescent's mood, adopt his appearance and more and more of his life-style. Many parents have lost at least some of their ability to accept death, and as a partial result have ceased to be a worthwhile stable force or a good identification model for maturity and ageing. The former valued role of elders with their acquired wisdom and experience is largely absent from the nuclear family in a culture dedicated to the nurturing of individuality. The adolescent then turns to his peer group to combat loneliness and existentialist anxiety.

Religion no longer plays its traditional role in the affirmation of the eternity of God, the immortality of man and the stability of his institutions. Thus the adolescent longs for and yet cannot intellectually believe in indestructibility and immortality. The assurance of continuity and a future has been shattered by nuclear armament, and by way of defence it is assumed that only the present exists. Anxiety and depressive feelings about change, decrepitude and fallibility are often transformed into hypochondriasis or into unrealistic salvation fantasies of the restorability of bodily beauty, strength and health, together with 'magical' attitudes about medicine and medicaments.

Puberty

This is a phase from which most boys and girls emerge unscathed, but by virtue of the wide age range (9-16 years in girls and 11-16 years in boys) early or late puberty can lead to difficulties. Because of the associated secondary sexual characteristics, there is usually considerable focus of interest on these phenomena and their early or late emergence will be noted by their peers and be remarked on. Failure to achieve an erection in a late developing boy can accentuate his organ inferiority, and similarly, failure for the voice to break may result in suggestions of homosexuality. In the girl, early puberty may result in sexual precocity, for she may try to emulate the older girls and yet not have the intellectual and emotional maturity to handle the situations to which her conduct exposes her. It is at this age that a more serious interest is taken in the opposite sex and the author had a schizophrenic patient who claimed his whole life was ruined because of his shyness which prevented him sitting next to a girl in class.

External Stresses

These are usually those of school and home. In the former, there may be conflict between the increasing demands of the curriculum and the instinctive urges of puberty. Super-ego demands tend to assert themselves; compulsive masturbation and expiation go hand in hand and a good deed for the day may be essential to resolve such conflicts. Increasing awareness of cultural and racial differences can at this age be contaminated with the prejudices of the adult and give rise to the ostracism and even cruelty which some young people manifest towards each other. It is not only those children at the receiving end who need protection but also those who pursue such activities. They either build up a load of guilt which they later are unable to handle or what is socially more dangerous, they acquire the habit of deriving a perverse pleasure in inflicting suffering on others and are constantly obsessed with the enemy in their midst, and create one where none exists.

As well as being a vulnerable phase in development, adolescence, as has already been said, can help to resolve a number of childhood neurotic problems. It supplies motivation to overcome those patterns which are patently childish, such as temper tantrums, undue dependence on the parents and hysterical invalidism. It provides one of the very few examples in psychiatry where hormones (though personally produced) can effect a cure. The commoner problems in adolescence are obsessional states, phobic anxiety (including school phobia), anorexia nervosa, schizophrenic disorders and depressive states. Treatment for these is as for the adult though this is more likely to be handicapped by parental influences and attitudes.

DELINQUENCY

In spite of the fact that delinquency often has no psychiatric significance, it is a problem which is commonly presented to the psychiatrist. Though most of the psychiatric aspects are dealt with under Psychopathic Personality (Chapter 10), one should also see delinquency as a problem in the differential diagnosis of childhood psychiatric illnesses and their treatment. Chess (1959) quotes H. B. Peck as saying:

> A child brought into court for having committed a delinquent act may be psychotic or neurotic, psychopathic or normal, intelligent or defective, physically healthy or manifesting behaviour chiefly derived from organic brain disease or an intolerable family or neighbourhood situation.

The definition of delinquency has legal limits and this introduces a number of variables such as different laws in different countries and states, the capacity of the parents to make restitution, the efficiency of those forces responsible for detection and apprehension, and the milieu of the child which may not inculcate that respect for law and order which society might wish. Even Tappan's (1949) definition, which reads: 'Any act, course or conduct, or situation which might be brought before a Court and adjudicated, whether in fact it comes to be treated there or by some other resource or indeed remains untreated', does not convey all the complexities of the problem. The mentally normal is by far the commonest perpetrator of delinquent acts and the psychiatrist should bear this in mind when he is asked by the Court to examine a child. Even if he finds some mental abnormality, he should consider whether this has any causal relation to the act.

There are however certain physical and psychological disturbances which have a direct bearing on conduct and these have already been described in relationship to their associated mental disturbances. They are:

1. *The brain-damaged child* who may lack the capacity to control his impulses has a handicap which may exclude him from more conformist groups, so that he drifts towards those which are likely to come into conflict with the law.

2. *Reactive behaviour disorders* which may become manifest in episodic outbursts of delinquency. These are usually of a minor nature and may be an expression of a venturesome spirit which has been stimulated by the need to resolve inner tensions. Stone-throwing, interference with and destruction of public property such as stealing light bulbs from railway carriages and being a general nuisance are examples of the types of reaction commonly found under this heading.

3. *The neurotic child* may indulge in behaviour which reflects his inner conflicts. Aggression and hostility may manifest as destructive tendencies, cruelty to animals or persistent stealing. The latter may be particularly significant when the child steals exclusively from one of its parents.

4. *The psychotic child* is relatively rare and the one with delinquent features is certainly uncommon. A schizophrenic process may result in disturbing behaviour such as pyromania or fetishism, though the latter may be associated with temporal lobe disturbances (Entwistle & Sim, 1961).

5. *The psychopathic child* does not differ markedly from the psychopathic adult, except that it is difficult to distinguish abnormal behaviour from childish behaviour. A particular group of 'affectless' children were described by Bowlby (1944) who showed that they suffered from early maternal deprivation.

6. *The mentally subnormal child* is described in Chapter 15 and his aberrant conduct is better understood against the background of his handicap.

Suicide and Suicidal Attempts in Children

Toolan (1962) states that 'contrary to popular opinion, suicide and suicidal attempts are not rare in childhood and adolescence'. He quotes vital statistics (U.S.A.) for 1959 as listing only 3 deaths from suicide under 10 years but in the 15-19 years group there are more deaths than those from nephritis, nephrosis, leukaemia, all forms of pneumonia, tuberculosis and poliomyelitis in a similar age group. Many 'accidents' which cause death may have been successful suicidal attempts, so the problem is a considerable one.

Among attempted suicides admitted to Bellevue Hospital more than a third came from broken homes. Diagnostic categories were:

Childhood schizophrenia	12
Schizophrenic reaction	33
Personality pattern disorder	10
Personality trait disorder	25
Transient situation reaction	2
Mental deficiency	4
Neurotic reaction	16

In his analysis of causes for the attempts Toolan suggests the following:

1. Anger at another which is internalized in the form of guilt and depression;
2. Attempts to manipulate another to gain love and affection, or to punish another;
3. A signal of distress;
4. Reactions to feelings of inner disintegration, as a response to hallucinatory commands, etc;
5. A desire to join a dead relative.

Connell (1965) emphasizes the severity of childhood stresses and the child's reactivity to them and the frequent history of 'depression' for some time before the suicidal threat or attempt but which was not understood or taken seriously by the parents.

EXAMINATION OF PATIENT

The examination is traditionally carried out at a clinic which is staffed by a team consisting of a psychiatrist, psychologist and social worker. A popular, though in the author's opinion, undesirable procedure, is for the social worker to take the history from the parents and present it to the psychiatrist who can then 'fill-in' with a brief interview of the parents and proceed to the examination of the child. There may be reasons for this, such as a previous home visit by the social worker, where she has obtained the case history in the natural setting of the child's home and as she may be expected to support the mother, an early relationship with her may be an advantage. Yet it pre-supposes that she will be responsible for the mother's support and this may prejudice the psychiatrist's assessment of the problem and his plans for dealing with it. A better arrangement is for the psychiatrist to regard the referral to the clinic as he would any referral to his out-patient department. He should, if possible, see the patient first and the parents afterwards, for in this way he approaches the problem with a fresh mind and is better able to assess the parents' statements. Even with very young children, it is usually possible to conduct the interview more profitably without the mother being there. A child who may have a reputation of being most refractory with strangers, may settle down quietly in the consulting room. A useful tip is not to be too outgoing initially but to motion the child to the sand-tray with its numerous objects, human and animal. If he feels he is not being watched he will begin to busy himself and after a few minutes be prepared to share his experiences with the benevolently neutral figure who has not tried to confront him.

TREATMENT

Play Therapy

Therapy with children is now a highly specialized subject with an extensive literature, and covers a wide range of techniques.

Play has already been referred to, but it need not be confined to the sand-tray. A number of specialized toys which are said to be of fundamental importance in treatment have been devised. These include dolls that can be fed with bottles and which wet their 'nappies' and require changing. It is alleged that the child can identify more readily with these toys and act out its own problems in relation to feeding and excretion as well as sibling rivalries. A model house which can be used by a few children permits the child to take part in a group situation and act out those problems which may be related to the home and which would otherwise not be introduced into the clinic. Water and mud excite childhood reactions to excreta, and their manipulation may tap earlier memories and patterns of behaviour which had hitherto been dormant. The sand-tray with its numerous contents—houses, farms, cows, sheep, lambs, fences, soldiers, parental figures and other children—permits the creation of an infinite variety of situations and the display of attitudes to meaningful situations in the child's background. Questions and interpretations while the child is at play help in uncovering for the child some of those aspects which had been incompletely repressed and were leading to symptom formation.

Projection tests have a therapeutic as well as a diagnostic value and Raven (1951) and Duss (1950) have used different techniques. The former gets the child to draw while he is responding to questions designed to tap the child's early experiences. The latter brings the child into a story-telling game in that he is asked to fill in his side to a story which is psycho-analytically structured. It is about the feeding of lambs by their mothers and another lamb is introduced to gauge the reaction of the child to the advent of a sibling.

Painting and drawing have both therapeutic and diagnostic uses as they permit the child free expression, or indicate his inhibitions and restrictions. They can be interpreted and as they form part of the child's own creations, their content is likely to be significant.

Psychoanalysis

This has now become established practice in the treatment of the neurotic and psychotic child, limited only by the scarcity of trained personnel, and as a research tool it has contributed much to the understanding of child development and the origin of neurotic and psychotic behaviour. Freud (1909*a*) published the celebrated case history of 'Little Hans' in his paper 'Phobia of a Five-year-old Boy' but did not actually treat the boy personally. He used the father as a vehicle for this purpose and believed that analysis of a child could only be satisfactorily achieved if the parent were to play the role of the analyst. This was later disproved by his own daughter, Anna (Freud, 1946), and by Klein (1932). Anna Freud was already developing a different approach to therapy by her emphasis on analysis of the ego and its unconscious defensive mechanisms (Freud, 1937). She pointed out that the ego tries to defend itself against three dangers; (1) the protests of the super-ego, (2) the dread of the strength of the instincts, and (3) objective anxiety from the environment, which in the young child is dominant before the super-ego is structured. She describes five defence mechanisms: (1) denial in phantasy (2) denial in word and act (3) restriction of the ego (4) identification with the aggressor (5) a form of altruism. Brown (1961) gives the following examples of these mechanisms:

Denial in Phantasy. A 7-year-old boy used to please himself with the phantasy that he owned a tame lion which terrorized others but loved him. It came at his call, made its bed in his room, and followed him like a dog wherever he went. This phantasy is interpreted as follows: the lion was a substitute for the father, who was hated and feared as a rival in relation to the mother. In his imagination the boy simply denied a painful fact and turned it into its pleasurable opposite. The anxiety-animal became his friend, and its strength, instead of being a source of terror, was at his service. Such stories for children as *Little Lord Fauntleroy* in which a small boy or girl is pictured as taming a bad-tempered old man are regarded as coming into this category. Denial in word and act is illustrated by the behaviour of the child when he tries to reassure himself in face of dread of the external world. 'I am as big as daddy' or 'I am as clever as mummy' or 'I *don't* dislike this medicine—I like it very much' are all examples of denials of reality which protect the child from a knowledge of his helplessness and dependence.

Restriction of the ego is illustrated by the case of a small girl of ten who went to her first dance full of pleasurable expectation. She admired her new dress and shoes and fell in love at first sight with the best-looking boy at the party. But although the boy had the same surname as herself, and she had already imagined in phantasy that there was some sort of secret bond between them, she was chided by him during their first dance together for her clumsiness. From that time onwards she avoided parties and took no trouble to learn to dance, although she liked watching others do so. Finally she compensated herself for this restriction of her ego by giving up feminine interests and setting up to excel intellectually, and by this roundabout means she later won the grudging respect of a number of boys of her own age.

Identification with the aggressor is a method of mastering anxiety by assuming the opponent's qualities through a process of introjection. Thus the little boy who has undergone dental treatment will play at being a dentist with his sister as patient.

A form of altruism describes the contrary mechanism of satisfying one's own desires through the lives of others, as in the case of a young governess who as a child was possessed by two desires: to have beautiful clothes and to have many children. In later life she was plain and unassuming, indifferent to her clothes and childless. But her childhood desires had not disappeared and manifested themselves in her interest in the lives of others. She took work looking after other people's children and was intensely concerned that her friends should have pretty clothes. As Anna Freud points out, the most detailed study of this altruistic surrender in literature is to be found in Edmond Rostand's play *Cyrano de Bergerac*—the French nobleman who, handicapped by an ugly nose, but the possessor of all the cultural graces, helps a suitor win the hand of a girl he himself loves by sending her poems allegedly by the suitor and defending his rival with his sword to keep all other rivals at a distance.

Melanie Klein claimed it was possible to psychoanalyse children from the age of 2 years and gain considerable knowledge of early mental phenomena. She was supported by a number of analysts who became known as the British or London School and included such prominent members as Susan Isaacs, Joan Riviere, D. W. Winnicott, R. E. Money-Kyrle and Ernest Jones, though her views were not accepted by all analysts and her findings have been questioned by those who accept orthodox Freudian theory. Brown (1961) usefully summarizes the difference between the two schools of thought thus:

In respect of theory:

A.

1. Anna Freud accepts the orthodox Freudian theory while attaching more significance to the ego and its defences than was formerly the case.

2. Accepting the orthodox theory, she therefore believes:

(*a*) that although unconscious and instinctual factors are of great importance, such environmental factors as the parent's attitude towards the child are equally important. To a considerable extent the child's problems change with a changing environment.

(*b*) that the superego arises during the fourth year or thereabouts.

(*c*) that the important drives are the sexual ones.

B.

1. Melanie Klein also accepts orthodox theory, but, as noted above, claims to have opened up a hitherto unexplored region in the pre-Oedipal stages.

2. Differing from the orthodox school in this respect, she therefore believes:

(*a*) that environmental factors are much less important than had previously been believed.

(*b*) that forerunners of the superego are demonstrable during the first two years of life.

(*c*) that for this reason any analysis which fails to reach back to the stage of infantile anxiety and aggressiveness in order to resolve them is necessarily incomplete.

(*d*) that the important drives are the aggressive ones.

In respect of practice:

A.

1. With the methods of Anna Freud, children from three years onwards may be analyzed.

2. The details of the method used depend upon the age of the child. In younger children (*i.e.* before the latency phase) relaxation upon a couch for free association cannot be expected, nor can it always be used in older children. The child, therefore, may walk about, talk, tell stories and dreams, or play games, and all these activities are used in interpretation which as in the adult is gradual.

3. There are two essential differences between the young child and the adult, so far as analysis is concerned:

(*a*) the young child's ego is undeveloped and his main problem is that of achieving control over his primitive instincts. This is the reason why, in the child as in the psychotic, caution is needed in analysis when interpretations are being made.

(*b*) the young child does not develop a typical transference neurosis; he is constantly reacting to the actual situation and does not reproduce the experiences of the past in his reaction to the analyst.

4. The co-operation of the parents is sought, both in sustaining the regularity of the child's visits to the analyst, and in giving information and reports on progress. The analyst makes no attempt, as was done in the earlier history of child-analysis and ordinarily today amongst non-analytic child-psychologists, to give advice or change the home situation. On the contrary, it is in the analyst's interest to maintain the home situation unchanged during treatment, since he wishes to discover how the child's symptoms and character have developed.

B.

1. Children as young as two years old are treated by Melanie Klein.

2. The method is centred around the phantasy life of the child as revealed in play. Interpretations are given directly and even the deepest interpretations may be given during the first meeting.

3. The co-operation of parents is not sought, firstly because their reports are likely to be distorted by their own unconscious conflicts and secondly because little significance is attached to the reality situation.

4. The material recovered (at any rate as interpreted) includes a wide range of sexual and aggressive phantasies from the first year of life, including Oedipal wishes, the wish to destroy the mother's body, and the desire to incorporate the father's penis. There is stated to exist even at this age an awareness of parental intercourse which is conceived as taking place orally by analogy with the nipple.

A main source of conflict between classical Freudians and Kleinians in respect of adult psychoanalysis is that, if the latter are right in ascribing these important phantasies to the earliest months of life, it follows that orthodox analysis has been seriously incomplete in failing to deal with aggression in its most primitive form and the baby's first attempts to handle the problems associated with it.

Superficial Psychotherapy

But not all psychotherapy with children is so heavily committed to psychoanalytic theory. Some forms are at a very superficial level and any beneficial results are not due to the unravelling of the child's problems, but to the introduction into the family of a benevolent figure who as a doctor or psychologist possesses prestige and unlike well-intentioned neighbours or spiritual guides is prepared to listen rather than assail the relatives with advice. Here the therapist acts as a stabilizer for a craft which is pitching alarmingly with a sea-sick child as passenger. Such treatment operates best when the problem is a situational one, and would be better conducted by the family doctor rather than at the Child Guidance Clinic. It would not be very helpful in the deeper-seated problems where full training in child analysis would be a necessary qualification, but fortunately these cases are much fewer and the time may come when the clinics will really specialize and the more general problems be treated by the family doctor.

As things are, not only is much time wasted with reports for the courts which in most cases do little more than provide a semblance of a humane and enlightened approach, but the wrong children are referred. The whole question of the manner of referral and location of the clinic is now being earnestly considered and it may be that the recent tendency for school authorities to multiply these services will be checked. The general practitioner should be given the facilities and be encouraged to deal with the vast majority of the situational problems and the others referred to child psychiatric departments run by the district hospital.

The Schizophrenic Child

The treatment of the schizophrenic child becomes increasingly important as the problem is increasingly recognized. In the early stages, this may well be ambulatory and the first objective is to establish affective contact with the patient. Mahler (1952) points a way: '. . . the autistic child is most *intolerant of direct human contact.* Hence he must be lured out of his autistic shell with all kinds of devices such as music, rhythmic activities and pleasurable stimulation of his sense organs'. Chess (1959) criticizes the pessimism of some psychiatrists towards treatment;

> Such an attitude, I believe, is not justified. Just as a scrutiny of the development of the psychopathic personality has led to important advances in preventive treatment, so a scrutiny of the development of the biologically deviant infant into the schizophrenic youngster may give clues to the prevention and cure of the frank schizophrenic picture.

She is also critical of the 'modified goal' which some therapists adopt for the schizophrenic child and she advocates a more optimistic approach. As she regards the basic elements of the condition to be 'the primary affect disturbance, reinforced by affectless parents, or the blunting in a potentially affect-normal infant of the capacity to develop normal affect', she utilizes techniques such as playroom activities to foster affective relationships. These children usually relate better to objects than to people and such objects are exploited to lead the child to express its feelings. She utilizes the child's 'intensification and prolongation of the usual modes of mastery—primary repetition, which we call perseverance, practice and imitation'. In the schizophrenic these are replaced by perseveration, compulsion, echolalia and echopraxia and she provides a repetitious and familiar background for her programme of rehabilitation. She describes in some detail her efforts with a 4-year-old girl (Jacqui) who had been diagnosed as schizophrenic. The technique demanded considerable patience and was based on the principles mentioned. Balloons were used to give the child experience of physical laws and how they operated. One was filled with water till it burst, one was blown up and punctured; the first splashed, the second did not, and the child became aware of the difference. Then building blocks were used and all the time an effort was made to show the child the essential differences between animate and inanimate objects. Later the child herself introduced people into her conversation and generally improved. Chess, while not discounting the influence of a warm relationship, attaches more importance to the feeling of mastery over her subject matter that the child was given. She summarizes her treatment approach thus:

> 1. One small segment of reality—such as Jacqui's balloons—is employed as a basis for activity.

2. The physical nature of this object is explored. It is compared with other objects and the laws governing its behaviour under varying circumstances are examined.

3. In the course of play, these laws which are discovered are stated and restated.

4. Differences between the object and the young patient are established in terms of the play activity being carried on.

5. One after another, new activities are introduced. As each one enters the treatment situation, the pattern of stating the laws which govern the activity is repeated, and the play is structured so as to necessitate examining, and defining what is being done.

6. People are brought into the discussion and the significance of human wishes and desires are explained in the same kind of terms which are applied to objects.

7. Rules of behaviour are discussed and demonstrated. These include: what is expected of one in a given set of circumstances; what are good manners; what is meant by sharing; or by contrast, what hurts others or makes them uncomfortable. If necessary, an issue is made of forbidding or of demanding certain forms of behaviour.

Behaviour Therapy

As one would expect, with the close identification of psychologists with child guidance clinics, behaviour therapy is being increasingly advocated in the treatment of childhood neuroses. The process is called the *reversal* of the learned maladaptive responses which constitute the neurotic behaviour pattern (Eysenck and Rachman, 1965). These authors who advocate operant conditioning methods to generate and/or sustain stable behaviour patterns list the following advantages:

1. Non-verbal operations
2. Strict control of variables
3. Quantification of operations
4. Exclusion of 'clinician-variables'
5. Single-case studies.

As disadvantages they list:

1. Operant methods usually demand special equipment and experimental rooms
2. They can be time-consuming.

But these are not regarded as unsurmountable, '. . . better equipment provides for more automatic control and saves time'.

One might expect such authoritative statements to be based on extensive clinical experience, but the authors conclude, 'What is needed above all, however, are clinical trials of operant methods.

With very few exceptions operant conditioning has not been used as a *clinical* procedure'. Many may consider the above approach entirely inappropriate for sick children.

Transitional Phenomena. This term was introduced by Winnicott (1953) and has come to include anything, behaviour or object, that habitually comforts the child, especially at bedtime or at times of loneliness, sadness or anxiety, with the exception of objects like the whole or part of the mother's or child's own body. Ekecrantz and Rudhe (1972) investigated 130 mothers each with 3 children, and of the 390 children 74 per cent used or had used some kinds of transitional phenomena. These phenomena were highly cathected, as 84·8 per cent had a clear-cut wish for them and 30·2 per cent had a strong demand for them. There was a significant relation between first use and the onset of spoon feeding. This finding supports Winnicott's suggestion that they symbolize the mother or part of her (the breast).

There was an association with oral activities in 32·1 per cent, and genital behaviour in only one child, which contradicts the hypothesis that they are fetish-equivalents. The similarity in ego status in children with and without transitional phenomena indicates that they are not a cause of or sign of disturbance in ego development, though long-standing use is significantly related to a low level of frustration tolerance.

CHAPTER 18

Psychopharmacology and Drug Therapy

GENERAL REVIEW

From time immemorial man has used plants and their products to give pleasure or relieve pain and suffering. Brewing infusions, chewing the bark and leaves of trees, and fermenting fruit or cereals are still popular in the habits of tea, coffee and cocoa drinking, indulgence in alcohol and the use of tobacco. In some countries, cocaine, opium and hashish have their enthusiasts, though these are now generally regarded as dangerous drugs of addiction and their production is controlled. Their active principles have now been identified and while their mode of action is not entirely understood, they have one thing in common in that all act on the central nervous system. For example, tea, coffee and cocoa owe their success as stimulants to their caffeine content, while hashish distorts perception to such a degree that phantasies assume a reality which excites and fascinates the addict. Alcohol in its many forms, including tinctures of otherwise innocuous substances, and tonic wines, is freely used the world over and achieves its effect, not by stimulation, but by inhibiting the higher control and permitting more primitive impulses to seek expression.

While naturally occurring substances have not yet been entirely exploited, the science of chemistry has, in recent years, made tremendous contributions to the variety and effectiveness of agents uses to influence the mind. Some, like bromides, chloral hydrate and paraldehyde, have been in use for many years and still enjoy a reputation for soothing the excited and restless, but it was the synthesis of barbital in 1903 by Fischer and von Mering which initiated the present flood of manufactured drugs. There are now many barbiturates, varying in their speed, duration and intensity of action, and their great popularity with patients and doctors is reflected in their high incidence as agents in attempted suicide and in drug addiction.

Psychopharmacology is not synonymous with drug therapy in psychiatric illness, but is a young science which has grown not only with the manufacture of different drugs that act on the central nervous system, but with increasing knowledge about the anatomy and physiology of that system and how drugs can affect it. Much of this knowledge derives from experimental work on animal preparations, though an increasing amount of information is being obtained from human volunteers and patients, who can be given drugs which have already established their worth in empirical trials or because of their chemical structure give reasonable prospect of being efficient.

Chemical mediators of nerve or brain action such as acetylcholine, sympathin and serotonin have been defined and their site and mode of action have been studied. The discovery by Berger that the activity of the brain can be recorded electrically has helped to initiate a number of neuropharmacological experiments with recordings from the cortex or through the stereotaxic implantation of needle electrodes to the deeper brain nuclei. Olds has compared this method with the rather diffuse search by the biochemist for biochemical pathology in mental disease. The latter he regards as looking for a needle in a haystack, but the former as looking for a haystack with a needle!

In 1943, Hofmann, who was working on the synthesis of d-lysergic acid diethylamide (LSD 25) accidentally got a speck of the drug in his mouth with unusual mental sequelae. He repeated the experiment with what he then regarded as a small dose (0·25 mg.) but with devastating results, and when he had recovered, he realized he had stumbled on the most potent hallucinogenic drug which could produce mental changes in man in a dose of as little as 1 μg. This drug has since been extensively used in neuropharmacological studies, for it can produce EEG changes which are neutralized by some of the tranquillizing agents. The first of these, chlorpromazine, was initially used by Laborit *et al.* (1952) as a potentiator of barbiturates in hibernation, but later Delay and his associates applied the drug to the treatment of mental disorders with considerable success. Since then, pharmaceutical firms have continued to turn out a large number of tranquillizers, the majority being phenothiazine derivatives.

Another tranquillizer of importance which is unconnected with the phenothiazines is reserpine, which is derived from *Rauwolfia serpentini* and is of benefit in the treatment of schizophrenia, but it is not only its therapeutic success which gives it prominence in psychopharmacology, for it also increases the excretion of serotonin which, as has already been stated, is one of the chemical mediators of brain action and in susceptible subjects reserpine can produce profound depression. That one of the brain enzymes, monoamine oxidase, is essential for the breakdown of serotonin, and that this enzyme can be inhibited by a group of drugs which are called the monoamine oxidase inhibitors (MAOI) and that these drugs are of value in the treatment of depression, has given rise to a very attractive theory. This explains in a fairly tight system of neuropharmacological and neurophysiological data, the major psychoses (schizophrenia and depression) and their treatment. The theory receives additional support in that hallucinogenic drugs like LSD 25 and mescaline produce EEG changes which are neutralized by resperine, but there are flaws in the argument, one of which is that the most effective of the antidepressants is not a monoamine oxidase inhibitor. The other defects in the theory are described in detail later.

In spite of the success of the tranquillizing and antidepressant drugs in the treatment of the psychoses, there is no conclusive evidence that they are of any value in the neuroses and there has no lack of clinical trials. Effective drug therapy in the neuroses is unfortunately still largely confined to drugs which are habit-forming though it could be argued that it is not the drugs which are habit-forming, but the neurotic processes within the patient. This problem is dealt with under Drug Addiction.

The great benefit psychopharmacology has brought to the treatment of patients and to the unravelling of modes of action of the nervous system has led to over-enthusiasm in some workers, though the more responsible are cautious. Most of the experimental work has been on animals, such as cats, rats, mice and fish, and it is unwise to predict, from data thus derived, the effects on man. For example, behavioural psychologists have studied the reactions of the goldfish, the guppy and the Mexican cave fish to stimulants, depressives and tranquillizers—and these creatures are presumably normal mentally! The essential nature of the neurotic process has not yet been taken into account in pharmacotherapeutic studies and Lawrence Kubie poses some very pertinent questions as to what the drugs do and do not (see below). Criticism has also come from neurophysiologists and Eccles has suggested that if conclusions are to be drawn from the experiments of drugs acting on the C.N.S. they should be coupled with studies on the single nerve cell.

Kubie (1958) levels the following criticisms at current psychopharmacological theory:

To try and correlate fluctuations in the neurotic processes as expressed by symptomatology, with the efficacy or otherwise of drugs used in their treatment may be misleading. Dreams may show fluctuations in their ideational content and affective tone without any real change in the dreamer. Such fluctuations would not be regarded as an indication of changes in the underlying personality or in the stream of the dynamic process, yet what is true of the dream is also true of the neurosis, as they both show superficial changes without the deeper aspects being materially changed. As the usual method of therapeutic trial is to see whether certain symptoms are increased or decreased by drugs, he puts forward the following points for consideration:

1. In psychotherapy, increases in symptoms may occur without indicating that the patient is deteriorating—they may actually indicate that the therapeutic process is effective.
2. Subjective descriptions are fallacious and even neutral observers can disagree on whether symptoms are present, aggravated or reduced.
3. Counting devices as a measurement of severity of illness can be misleading. Changes in the frequency of hand-washing may not be an index of the illness as it tells us little of the struggle the patient is putting up against his obsession or the amount of suffering caused by it, or how much the symptom may relieve the underlying problems which have motivated it.
4. Is there any way of telling whether drugs influence the severity of the neurosis or the secondary and tertiary consequences of it? *e.g.* an agoraphobe may not venture outside the house—another will, and suffer torture. Even if the drugs change the former to the latter, is the neurotic process fundamentally affected?
5. At what point does the drug exercise its influence on the neurotic process? Does it affect the inhibitory or facilitatory influences?
6. Breakdown is but one phase of a neurotic process. For years a person may compensate adequately and then circumstances change, *e.g.* (*a*) the compulsive benefactor who loses his appreciative beneficiaries; (*b*) the height phobic working on the flat plain who has to move to a mountainous region.

Having shown the difficulties in the evaluation of the effects of drugs on such processes, Kubie suggests the following areas for further study:

1. The repetition of behaviour patterns in neurosis.
2. The effect of drugs on regressive phenomena which are inherent in the neurotic process, in which there is a tendency to relieve sufferings and other unpleasant experiences—Do drugs increase or decrease this tendency or alter the tendency qualitatively?
3. The same drug can influence man in quite different ways and the same man differently on different occasions. (He quotes the example of alcohol.) How does one distinguish between a mere unmasking of a concealed affective state and a quantitative or qualitative change in its intensity?
4. The inner lives of men vary. One man may spend his life organizing a

central affective state of gentle euphoria; another in warding off and defending against a painful central emotional position. Drugs are unlikely to produce identical effects in such widely varying individuals.

5. The effect of drugs on neurotic illness cannot be divorced from the trigger mechanism. All affective states respond to trigger stimuli and the threshold of such individuals to these stimuli is an important factor for the drug may well be operating at that level.

6. The effects of drugs on the relative roles of conscious, preconscious and unconscious processes. (He suggests that Free Association and the Transference Situation would be suitable subjects for study.)

Comment

The points raised by Kubie even without the answers, provide an essential corrective to the mechanistic approach of psychopharmacology and emphasize that psychodynamic factors cannot be lightly dismissed in physical treatment and clinical trials.

BIOCHEMICAL AND NEUROPHYSIOLOGICAL BACKGROUND[1]

There is some basic information about the chemistry and neurophysiology of the brain which is essential to the understanding of psychopharmacology and the following is only a brief resumé. For fuller details the reader should consult one of the many textbooks or symposia which deal with the subject.

ENERGY AND THE BRAIN

The central nervous system derives its energy mainly from the metabolism of glucose and from oxygen. *Glucose depletion,* as was commonly practised in the form of insulin coma treatment for schizophrenia, produces easily recognizable physical signs and these can be reversed by giving carbohydrates. Similarly *oxygen deprivation* produces the classical picture of cerebral anoxia which if not prolonged can be reversed by giving oxygen. Glucose is oxidised to carbon dioxide and water and is readily usable, for like oxygen it passes the blood-brain barrier.

There are three phases whereby the body derives energy from foodstuffs.

1. Fats, carbohydrates and proteins are broken down to fatty acids, glycerol, hexoses and amino acids.
2. Each of these breakdown substances is converted into one of the three carboxylic acids, acetic acid, a -ketoglutaric acid or oxaloacetic acid and in this process one third of the total energy is produced.
3. These three acids are completely oxidised by what is known as the citric acid cycle during which the remaining two thirds of the energy is released.

The hydrogen atoms which become available during these procedures convert nicotinamide or flavoprotein coenzymes to their reduced forms which are

[1] I am very grateful to Roche Products Ltd. for permitting me to extract freely from their excellent monograph 'Neurophysiological and Pharmacological Aspects of Mental Illness'.

reoxidised by molecular oxygen through the respiratory chain of enzymes. During this procedure adenosine triphosphate (ATP) is produced from adenosine diphosphate (ADP). ATP may be regarded as the form in which energy derived from oxidation is stored, transferred or utilised in the living organism.

Glucose Metabolism

As the brain gets its energy mainly from glucose, one must consider its metabolism in greater detail. It enters directly into phase II of carbohydrate metabolism and is converted into two molecules of pyruvic acid by the reaction sequence called glycolysis (see Fig. 4). This can occur aerobically or anaerobically.

In the absence of oxygen the pyruvate is converted to lactic acid and further

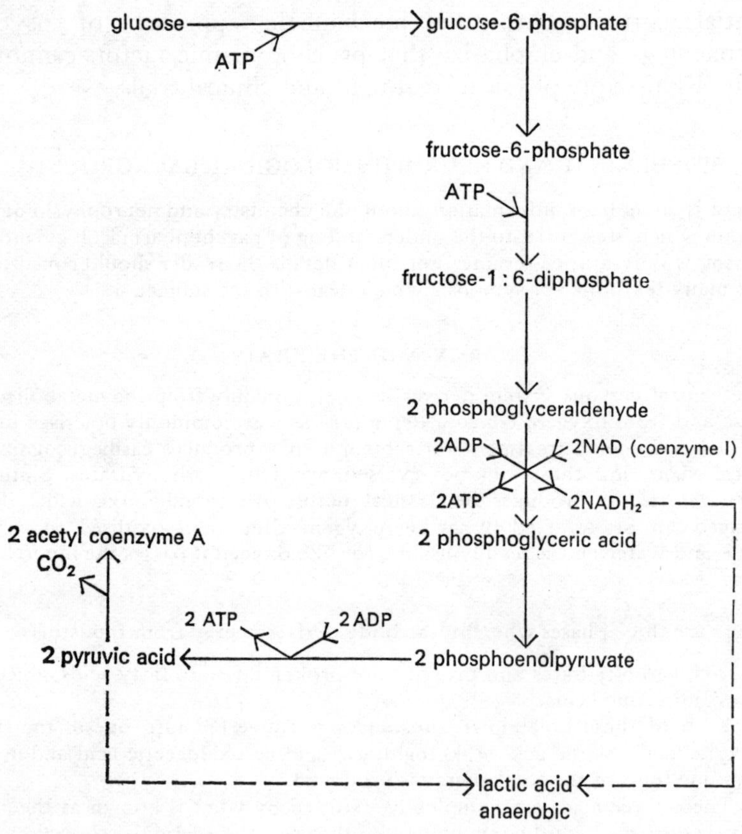

Fig. 4

metabolism does not occur. In such circumstances the breakdown of one molecule of glucose leads to the net synthesis of 2 molecules of ATP.

In the presence of oxygen pyruvic acid can be oxidatively decarboxylated to

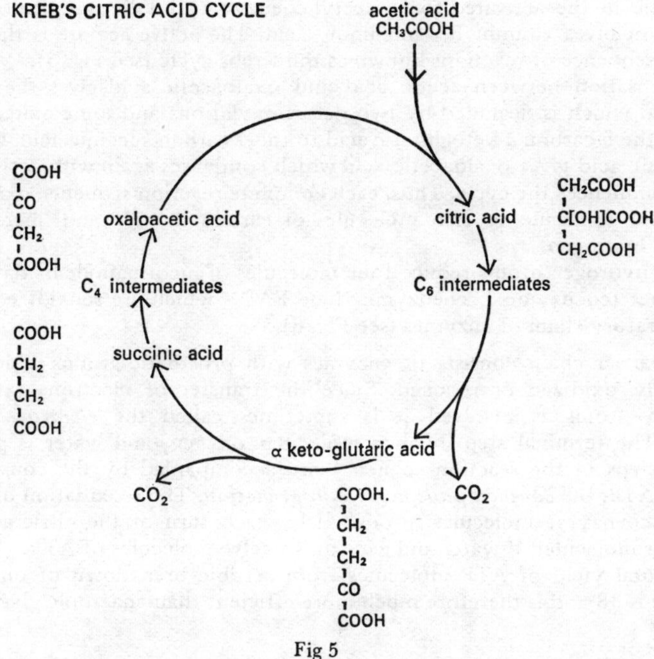
KREB'S CITRIC ACID CYCLE
acetic acid
CH_3COOH
COOH
CO
CH_2
COOH
oxaloacetic acid
citric acid
CH_2COOH
C[OH]COOH
CH_2COOH
C_4 intermediates
C_6 intermediates
COOH
CH_2
CH_2
COOH
succinic acid
α keto-glutaric acid
CO_2
COOH.
CH_2
CH_2
CO
COOH
CO_2

Fig 5

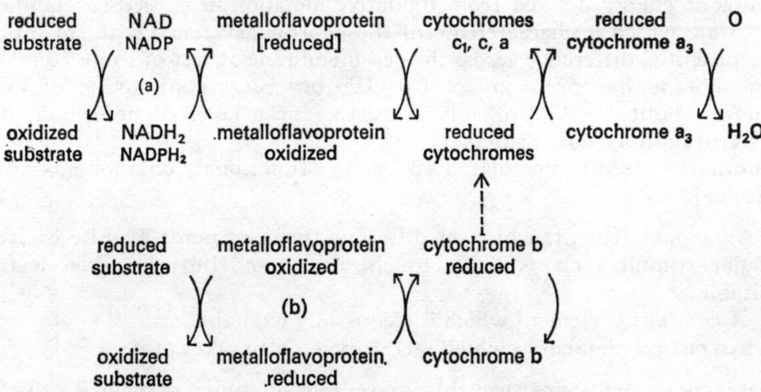
THE RESPIRATORY CHAIN OF ENZYMES
reduced substrate
NAD
NADP
metalloflavoprotein [reduced]
cytochromes
c_1, c, a
reduced cytochrome a_3
O
(a)
oxidized substrate
$NADH_2$
$NADPH_2$
metalloflavoprotein oxidized
reduced cytochromes
cytochrome a_3
H_2O
reduced substrate
metalloflavoprotein oxidized
cytochrome b reduced
(b)
oxidized substrate
metalloflavoprotein reduced
cytochrome b
Most substrates react with the nicotinamide coenzymes
as primary oxidants (a) but some systems, notably
succinic dehydrogenase, use a flavoprotein (b)

Fig 6

give acetic in the activated form, acetyl-coenzyme A. This complex enzymatic reaction involves vitamin B_1 and lipoic acid. The active acetate is then drawn into the sequence of reactions known as the Krebs cycle (see Fig. 5).

Condensation between acetic acid and oxaloacetic acid gives the 6-carbon citric acid which is degraded by two decarboxylations and some oxidative steps through the 5-carbon a-ketoglutaric acid to the 4-carbon succinic acid. Oxidation of succinic acid gives oxaloacetic acid which condenses again with active acetate and recommences the cycle. Thus, each complete reaction sequence oxidizes one acetic acid molecule to two molecules of carbon dioxide and liberates eight atoms of hydrogen.

These hydrogen atoms reduce four molecules of nicotinamide or flavoprotein coenzymes (coenzyme I, coenzyme II or FAD), which are reoxidized through the respiratory chain of enzymes (see Fig. 6).

This carrier chain consists of enzymes with prosthetic groups which can be alternately oxidized or reduced. Since the transfer of electrons rather than hydrogen atoms is involved it is sometimes called the *electron transport system*. The terminal step involves molecular oxygen, and water is produced. Certain steps in the reaction sequence are accompanied by the conversion of ADP to ATP, the *coupled phosphorylation reaction.* The reoxidation of the four reduced coenzyme molecules, produced by each turn of the citric acid cycle, gives four molecules of water and generates twelve molecules of ATP.

The total yield of ATP molecules from aerobic breakdown of one glucose molecule is 38 and is therefore much more efficient than anaerobic glycolysis.

ENERGY FOR MAINTENANCE

As a result of studies on peripheral nerves, the neuromuscular junction, the ganglia and autonomic innervation of the bodily organs, there is evidence that the bulk of energy derived from oxidative metabolism is used to maintain the *steady state* which is characteristic of the neuronal system, *i.e.* the maintenance of the potential difference across the cell membrane at rest of some 70 mV. This cell membrane has been shown by electron microscopy to be of uniform thickness (about 50 A) probably consisting of a layer of phospholipids and cholesterol supported by protein.

Grundfest (1959) postulated 3 main functional components of the membrane:

1. An *input* element, which in different types of nerve may be excited by particular stimuli such as light, touch, heat, etc., but which is electrically inexcitable.
2. A *conductile* element which is electrically excitable.
3. An *output* element at which secretory activity takes place.

These components are probably present in all types of neurone, including primary, receptor, final common path and synaptically excited neurones.

The system works in this way. The excitation aroused by the input component is converted to electrical activity which gives graded, summated and sustained potentials and may excite the conductile portion by generating a depolarising potential of sufficient magnitude to give rise to 'all or none' propagated impulses or 'spikes'. These are specially adapted to conduct the information acquired by the input.

The conduction of an impulse is therefore associated with the passage of an action potential along the axon.

The propagation of the impulse is effected by electrical current which flows between the active area of the nerve and the inactive region ahead.

The velocity of the impulse in an unmyelinated axon is much less than of a myelinated fibre of equal diameter which suggests that the mechanism of propagation may be different and has led to the hypothesis of *saltatory conduction* which is a process whereby the impulse leaps from node to node of Ranvier. Finally the output component is excited to release transmitter agents at the motor end-plate. Little is known of the interior of the neurone but it is postulated that there must be some correlation with the membrane because the presynaptic vesicles are concerned in the quantal emission of the transmitter compound, the membrane potential determining the rate of emission as in the production of acetylcholine (see below).

Ionic Composition

Between the two fluid compartments (outside and inside the neurone) there is a distinct difference in ionic composition of sodium concentration which internally is only 10–20 per cent of the external and the reverse is true of the potassium ion concentration. The cell membrane would appear to behave as if it were selectively permeable to potassium ions and impermeable to sodium and chloride ions.

If the system were permeable only to potassium ions the calculated potential difference would amount to −90 mV. The actual voltage is about −70 mV. The resting membrane potential can be altered by changes in either external or internal potassium concentrations and alterations in sodium concentration; *e.g.* an increase in external sodium ion concentration produces depolarization.

The Ionic Pump

It would appear that the cell membrane is also permeable to sodium ions and this view is supported by direct measurement with radioactive sodium. Sodium ions therefore enter the cell membrane but are forced out again at the same rate by some active process which has been called the 'ionic pump' and it differs from the passive diffusion down a concentration gradient. To expel sodium, the ions have to be pushed outwards against the concentration gradient and by a similar process potassium ions are prevented from passing down the gradient into the external fluid and are held within the membrane. This 'pumping' action is thought to be one of the major metabolic processes of the neurone and there is evidence that it is dependent on oxidative metabolism which provides the energy-rich phosphate compounds such as ATP.

During *anoxia* there is a decline in the potential difference across the membrane and a metabolic inhibitor such as cyanide markedly decreases the production of ATP and increases the proportion of inorganic phosphate in a nerve, simultaneously affecting the activity of the 'ionic pumps'. Conversely, direct injection of ATP into the axon during cyanide inhibition restores the 'pumping' function to a significant extent. Thus, a large part of the cellular energy generated within the neurone by oxidative metabolism of glucose is concerned in the maintenance of the active transport system or steady state of the neurone.

ENERGY FOR CONDUCTION OR COMMUNICATION

Acetylcholine (ACh)

The biogenesis of acetylcholine requires the presence of free choline and active acetate which can be derived from glucose metabolism but may also be provided, if necessary, by amino acids and fatty acids. The choline acetylase catalyzes the combination of acetate (as acetylcoenzyme A) with choline in the presence of energy as ATP.

It is generally supposed that the synthesis of acetylcholine takes place in the cell body of cholingeric neurones. It is then carried peripherally by the flow of the axoplasm. The acetylcholine is held, in an inactive or bound form, within small vesicles, about 300 A in diameter, which migrate towards, and concentrate at, the synaptic knob. It is thought that, whenever a vesicle makes an effective collision with the presynaptic membrane, a unit (some hundreds of thousands of molecules) of acetylcholine is released. Such collisions occur singly at random intervals even when the membrane is at rest, for spontaneous miniature end-plate potentials have been recorded in the absence of stimulation. When the membrane is depolarized by a nerve impulse, the collisions occur synchronously in large numbers. For a brief moment the acetylcholine released is free and crosses the synaptic gap. It presumably forms some sort of attachment to the receptor site, but is then eliminated by diffusion or destruction by the specific enzyme acetylcholinesterase.

Acetylcholinesterase (AChE)

It has been shown by Koelle (1961) that acetylcholinesterase is present throughout the entire length of cholinergic neurones, and he postulates two fractions which he has named 'reserve' and 'functional' AChE. The former he considers to be recently synthesized as part of the cell's protein turnover. From this reserve of enzyme, some is conveyed to the axonal and dendritic processes of the cell and incorporated into the membrane, and it is that AChE, which is directly involved in the hydrolysis of ACh in the course of synaptic or neuro-effector transmission. The membranes of both pre- and post-ganglionic cholinergic neurones are said to contain AChE, whereas in sympathetic ganglia, practically all the functional AChE is localized presynaptically.

Catechol Amines

Present knowledge of the biogenesis of the catechol amines originated with the discovery of dopa decarboxylase by Holtz *et al.* (1938). Blaschko (1957) proposed that the normal pathway for the synthesis of adrenaline is as shown in Fig. 7 and much recent work has established that this is the main biosynthetic route.

Blaschko has pointed out that noradrenaline is both a neurohormone and an intermediate in the formation of adrénaline. He has suggested that the same may apply to dopamine which may be a neurohormone as well as the precursor of noradrenaline. That it may have a functional role is suggested by its disappearance from brain tissue after resperine administration. The fact that dopamine in large amounts is found in the brain, in the adrenergic neurones and in the lungs, makes it necessary to consider the possibility that this third catechol amine is not simply a precursor.

Holtz (1959) has made the suggestion that the part played by dopa decarboxylase in the biogenesis of the catechol amines depends upon the organ in which the primary product of its action, *i.e.* dopamine, is formed. Thus, in the adrenal medulla, the biosynthesis proceeds via noradrenaline to the methylated end-product, adrenaline. Dopamine in this situation is a precursor. In nervous tissues, the biosynthesis stops at the noradrenaline level. Here, dopamine is the precursor of the transmitter, and probably also an effector substance. In lungs, liver and intestine, dopamine itself is the end-product of the biosynthesis. Here it may act as a local hormone.

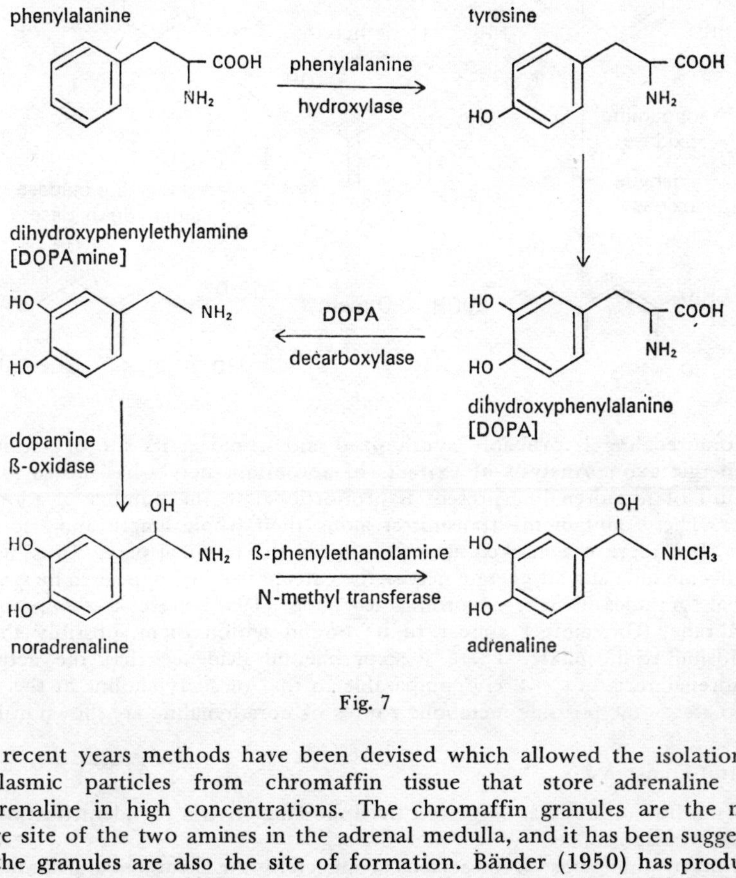

Fig. 7

In recent years methods have been devised which allowed the isolation of cytoplasmic particles from chromaffin tissue that store adrenaline and noradrenaline in high concentrations. The chromaffin granules are the main storage site of the two amines in the adrenal medulla, and it has been suggested that the granules are also the site of formation. Bänder (1950) has produced evidence to show that there are two types of cell in the medulla, which he called P and F because of their staining properties, and he suggested that the P cells synthesize adrenaline whilst F cells do not. Blaschko (1959) considers that, if the two cell types exist, it must be assumed that they differ, in that one of them is fitted with a mechanism for methylating noradrenaline, whereas the other is not.

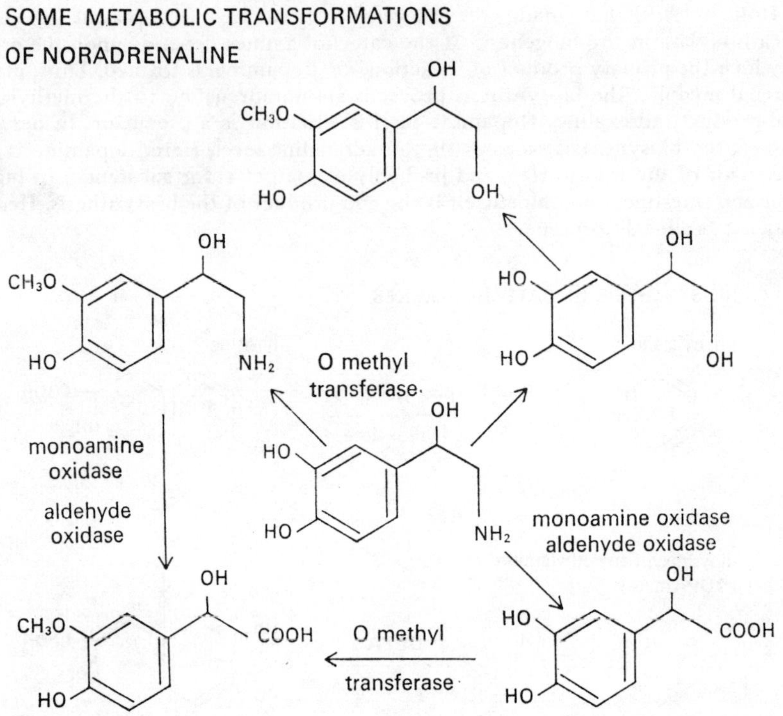

SOME METABOLIC TRANSFORMATIONS OF NORADRENALINE

Fig. 8

Noradrenaline is probably synthesized and stored at its site of action, the adrenergic axon. Analysis of extracts of autonomic nerves has shown that the amount of noradrenaline present is proportional to the number of adrenergic fibres. These contain the transmitter along their whole length and also in the soma, but there is a marked accumulation in the terminal parts. Thus, in both adrenal medulla and adrenergic nerves, the catechol amines appear to be stored in special granules which, according to Eade (1958) have a semipermeable membrane. The amines appear to be bound within them, possibly through adenosine triphosphate. There is experimental evidence that the action of noradrenaline is not entirely comparable to that of acetylcholine at the motor end-plate. Some possible metabolic routes of noradrenaline are shown in Fig. 8.

Central Transmission

Grundfest (1959) has suggested the following criteria for identification of a transmitter substance.

It must mimic closely the actions produced by the natural neural stimulus; its actions must be affected by the same drugs and in the same way as neural excitation: it must be a naturally occurring substance found in close proximity to the relevant synaptic structures and it is desirable to demonstrate that it is formed by an appropriate metabolic pathway, that it is released at the time, place and in the degree suitable to transmitter action, and that its accumulation to excess is prevented by another metabolic pathway.

Although it is generally conceded that acetylcholine and noradrenaline are transmitter compounds at the periphery and may well exert similar activity in the brain, the complexity of the problem is such that irrefutable evidence is not available concerning even these two substances.

Two other compounds which fulfil some of the criteria suggested by Grundfest are gamma-amino butyric acid (GABA) and serotonin. The evidence for their being transmitter substances is much more circumstantial than that pertaining to acetylcholine however. GABA has been shown to exist only in the brain and there is therefore no model of its possible mode of action to be investigated at peripheral situations. Serotonin, by contrast, is almost ubiquitous in its distribution and appears to have many functions.

Amino Acids

The predominant group of amino acids in the brain is that which includes glutamine, glutamic acid, γ-amino-butyric acid (GABA) and aspartic acid; these together account for some 75 per cent of free amino acids in the brain, their distribution being largely confined to grey matter. The only member of the group which passes the blood-brain barrier at all easily is glutamine, but the available evidence does not support the view that glutamine is the source of glutamic acid in the brain; its principal source is probably glucose, the glutamic acid being a product of the Krebs cycle when α-ketoglutaric acid is converted to L-glutamic acid. The reaction is important in ammonia and amino group metabolism. It can be summarized by the reversible reaction.

$$\alpha\text{-ketoglutaric acid} \underset{}{\overset{\pm NH_3}{\rightleftharpoons}} \text{L-glutamic acid.}$$

It takes place as two parallel reactions; one by the intervention of glutamic dehydrogenase, and the other by intervention of glutamic transaminase.

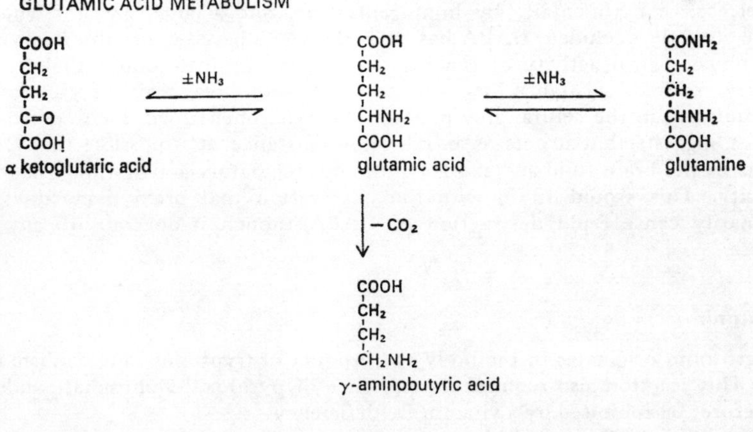

Fig. 9

Depending on the direction (which is reversible) the first reaction is known as reductive amination (α-ketoglutarate to glutamate) or as oxidative deamination (glutamate to α-ketoglutarate) and requires diphosphopyridine nucleotide (DPN) as coenzyme. The second reaction (transaminase) requires pyridoxal phosphate as coenzyme, and is one of the principal ways in which vitamin B_6 pyridoxine, enters into brain metabolism. This is one of several reactions concerned in amino acid metabolism involving the transfer of an amino group of an amino acid to the α-keto acid in which pyridoxal phosphate plays an important role.

At least two other important compounds may be synthesized from glucose. Glutamine can be formed by reaction of ammonia with glutamic acid, the energy being derived from ATP. This reaction can therefore also serve as a means of removing excess ammonia from the brain. By decarboxylation, glutamic acid is converted to γ-aminobutyric acid (GABA). This also is a reaction which is of great importance in brain metabolism and which is pyridoxine dependent (Fig. 9).

Gamma Aminobutyric Acid

Gamma aminobutyric acid (GABA) was identified by Ackermann and Kutscher (1910) who found that it was produced from glutamic acid by putrefied material. Since that time, its presence has been demonstrated in various bacteria, in yeast, in moulds, fungi and higher plant tissues. Its presence in the brain of mammals was discovered in 1950 by Roberts *el al.* (1950) and its identity proved by Udenfriend (1950). Brain tissue extracts have been shown to contain specific decarboxylases which catalyse the production of GABA from glutamic acid. After intravenous administration of labelled glutamate to mice there is rapid exchange with the glutamate of the brain; labelled glutamate, glutamine and, to a smaller extent, GABA, appear very quickly and thereafter slowly disappear.

A relationship seems to exist between the compound discovered by Florey (1953), which he named Factor 1, and GABA, and it has been suggested that they may, in fact, be identical. There is some evidence that GABA in the brain is divided into three kinds, a minimal amount which is truly free, a portion which is released experimentally by homogenization, and a larger amount which is more strongly occluded. GABA has been shown to have important effects upon the physiological activity of brain and there can be little doubt that it, or a closely related substance, is concerned in some way with regulation or transmission in the central grey matter. The experimental work with crustacean nerves suggests that it acts as an inhibitor substance. It is possible that GABA exists in the brain fluid and exerts continuous regulatory activity upon neuronal activity. This would fit in with the observation that brain tissue does not ordinarily cause rapid destruction of GABA though it does absorb any free excess.

Serotonin

Serotonin originates in the body as a product of tryptophan metabolism (Fig. 10). This reaction also requires the presence of pyridoxal-5-phosphate and will, therefore, be inhibited by a vitamin B_6 deficiency.

Distribution of serotonin is not confined to the central nervous system; it is present in many tissues. In mammals, the largest concentrations are found in the mucosa of the gastro-intestinal tract. Another storage site is the blood platelets which have a remarkable capacity for storing serotonin. There is much in the spleen, probably derived from breakdown of platelets. The absolute amount in the brain is small but this seems to have great importance.

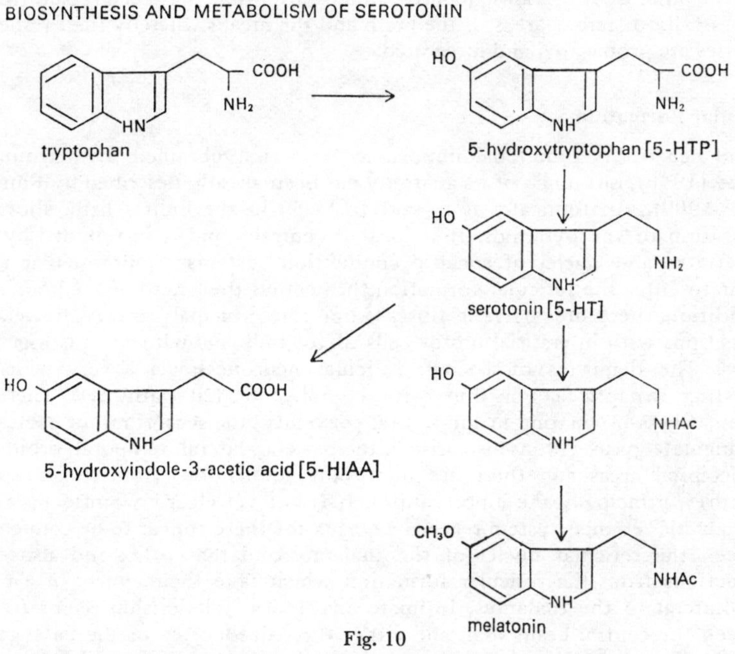

BIOSYNTHESIS AND METABOLISM OF SEROTONIN

tryptophan → 5-hydroxytryptophan [5-HTP] → serotonin [5-HT] → 5-hydroxyindole-3-acetic acid [5-HIAA]; serotonin → N-acetylserotonin → melatonin

Fig. 10

The administration of 5 HTP has been shown to increase the amounts of serotonin in most tissues, including brain. The amino acid penetrates into cells and is decarboxylated to serotonin wherever 5 HTP decarboxylase is present. By this means, prolonged, marked elevations of serotonin levels have been obtained in a number of animal species, and when sufficient is administered to increase the 5 HT level to twice or thrice normal, there occur somatic, autonomic and behavioural changes resembling those produced by lysergic acid diethylamide. For example, in dogs and cats, large doses produced excitement with loss of reflexes, blindness and disorientation.

Serotonin is rapidly oxidized by monoamine oxidase, first to aldehyde and then to 5-hydroxyindole acetic acid, (5 HIAA) and this is excreted in the urine (Fig. 7). This oxidative process may be only one of several metabolic pathways, however, for if an injection of 5HT be given, only about one third can be accounted for by increased urinary excretion of 5 HIAA and only traces of 5 HT are found. It would seem, therefore, that the evidence at present available is not sufficient to justify the assumption that either GABA or serotonin are true neural transmitter substances, and although the picture of acetylcholine action at the motor end-plate and at peripheral synaptic sites can be used to illustrate a possible mode of action of transmitter substances within the central nervous system, it can only be used with important modifications.

ROUTES OF COMMUNICATION

During recent decades many advances have been made in the anatomy and physiology of the brain and central nervous system by the use of new techniques, including microelectrodes, the electroencephalograph and the electron microscope. Consequently much attention has been paid to the anatomically different areas of the brain and the means whereby their respective activities are propagated and integrated.

Reticular Formation

Evidence of its functional importance was first obtained by Magoun and Rhines (1946), but much of its anatomy has been already described by Ramón y Cajal (1909). Anatomically it is said to begin in the bulb a little above the decussation of the pyramids. It is located centrally and is surrounded by long fibre tracts and nuclei of specific conduction systems. Spinoreticular axons appear to enter the reticular formation throughout the length of the brain stem. In addition there are afferent fibres from the principal sensory nuclei, and connections with interstitial motor cells of the bulb and with the quadrigeminal bodies. The dendrites of a single reticular neurone cover a very wide area suggesting synaptic connection with laterally located pathways. There are efferent fibres originating in the frontal convexity, the sensori motor cortex and the cingulate gyrus. Axons also arise in the parietal, lateral, temporal, orbital and paraoccipital areas and there are important connections from rhinencephalic structures, principally the hippocampus. It is not yet clear how influences from the thalamic reticular system reach the cortex for there appear to be connections between the reticular nuclei of the thalamus and the cortex and also direct connections from the reticular formation which take their course in a region ventrolateral to the thalamus. Intimate anatomical relationship seems to exist between the central brain stem and either the palaeocortex or the basal ganglia or both. There is, too, an important projection system of the reticular formation into the cerebellum.

Functionally the reticular system has been shown to consist of ascending and descending influences. Magoun and Rhines (1946) have shown that movement induced either by reflex action or by cortical stimulation can be *inhibited* by stimulation of the ventromedial part of the medullary reticular formation. They have also found that movement of the same kind can be *facilitated* by stimulation of the tegmentum of the mid-brain and the pons or of the hypothalamus and subthalamus. It appears that the descending reticular formation can inhibit or facilitate impulses to the spinal neurones through the extra-pyramidal projections of the spinal cord.

The reticular activating system consists of two parts, one located caudally and the other a rostral thalamic portion. Whilst EEG and behaviour studies appear to show that these are identical, the two portions show differences in their response to drugs and contrasting effects upon spinal structure. Much experimental use has been made of the discovery that lesions of the reticular formation in the mid-brain cause profound somnolence in chronic survival animals and that electrical stimulation of this area modifies the EEG, causing desynchronization. It would appear that sensory information to the thalamus and thence to the cortex is conveyed by ascending tracts in the reticular formation, thus maintaining wakefulness.

Most present concepts of the functions of the reticular formation are based upon electro-physiological studies. Demonstration that the process of arousal depends upon excitation of the central brain stem is due to Moruzzi and Magoun

(1949). More recently it has been shown that rapidly repetitive stimuli have the effect of arousal, but slow frequencies to the thalamic portion of the reticular system can induce sleep. In the arousal reaction all parts of the brain stem reticular system take part, but it has no capacity to induce or maintain wakefulness except by its action on higher structures.

Limbic System

The expression 'le grand lobe limbique' was coined by Broca (1878), who suggested that several different structural elements of the cingulate gyrus and the hippocampal gyrus bear a certain relationship to one another, forming a system which is placed around the mid-brain between the mid-brain and the neocortex. The structures associated with the limbic system had previously been regarded as essential parts of olfactory function, and consequently, were known as the rhinencephalon. Having observed the strongly developed fibre connections between certain parts of the rhinencephalon, namely the hippocampus, mamillary bodies, anterior thalamus and cingulate gyrus, Papez (1937) suggested the existence of a functional circuit largely concerned with emotion and its expression. Convincing evidence of the credibility of this theory was produced by Klüver and Bucy (1939). MacLean (1949) has brought forward electro-anatomical and physiological observations concerning the limbic system.

The limbic system may be divided into three essential elements. First are the cortical and subcortical grey regions of the limbic system to which belong the hippocampus, indusium griseum, area entorhinalis, cingulate gyrus, amygdaloid nucleus and the septal area. The second element consists of the intramural fibre layers and, finally, there are the extramural connections. The hippocampus, indusium griseum and area entorhinalis form part of the so-called palaeocortex. The cortex of the cingulate gyrus may represent the morphological transitional form between palaeocortex and neocortex. The amygdaloid nucleus and the septal region are subcortical nuclear areas in the basal fore-brain. There are also a few nuclei in the pre-optic region.

The intramural fibre layers which link the various parts of the limbic system together, include the cingulum, the striae longitudinales, the diagonal ligament and a fibre connection between area entorhinalis and hippocampus. There exists, therefore, a long- and short-fibred network which describes a curve round the corpus callosum. The subcortical nuclear areas, especially the septal area and the amygdaloid nuclei are connected by the strong fibre bundle of the diagonal ligament of Broca. Direct connections between the amygdaloid nuclei and the hippocampus have not been proved with certainty, but according to Klingler and Gloor (1960), certain fibres of the cingulum appear to project into the amygdaloid nucleus.

Its extramural connections connect the limbic system with certain nuclear areas of the diencephalon and mesencephalon. The grey areas of the limbic system are situated close to the medial hemispheres, and it seems as if the intermediate nuclei of the brain stem belong generally to the limbic system. Connections between the limbic system and the hypothalamus are established by the fornix, stria terminalis and the ventral amygdaloid nuclear radiation of Klingler and Gloor. Through these channels, the limbic system can influence the vegetative centres and the neurosecretory and neuroendocrine systems.

One part of the fornix leads from the hippocampus to the mamillary body, where the Vicq d'Azyr bundle (mamillo-thalamic tract) originates and projects towards the nuclei of the anterior thalamus. From this point, the connections fan out into the cingular cortex, to flow back again into the hippocampus via the cingulum. In this neuronal circuit, the mamillary body has a key-position in so far as important connections between the limbic system and the mid-brain also pass through it. Pathological increase of the processes of excitation leads to enormous discharges of affect, or even to the outbreak of the neurone discharge of an epileptiform type. In this connection, it should be remembered that the neocortex has direct efferent channels (pyramidal tract) through which agitation can run off to the skeleton muscles. On the other hand, excitation of the limbic system may finally be transmitted to the neurovegetative and neuroendocrine end-organs.

In the mid-brain, almost exactly arranged around the medial line, there is an area which is connected with the limbic system via the mamillary body, the Nauta loop. This limbic area of the mid-brain consists of discreet groups of nuclei (Gudden nuclei, Bechterew nuclei, etc.) and, owing to its situation, it is in direct relationship with important structures of the mid-brain. Beside these cross-connections within the mid-brain, there also exists a remarkable excitable loop which connects the limbic mid-brain area with the mamillary body, and this establishes connection with the Papez circuit. This circuit consists of mamillotegmental fibre layers leading in the dorsal direction into the area of the Gudden nuclei; the return takes place in the ventral direction via the mamillary peduncle.

The efferent connections between the hippocampus and the reticular formation pass through the fornix. In analogy to this, the 'medial fore-brain bundle' mediates between the amygdaloid nucleus, the septal area and the pre-optic region on one side, and the reticular formation on the other. Opposite both these ventral efferents, there is a dorsal conducting loop consisting of the stria medullaris and the Meynert bundle, with a site of communication in the nuclear complex of the habenula.

The afferent pathways between the reticular formation and the limbic system also pass via the 'medial fore-brain bundle' and, from the septal area, special ascending fornix fibres lead back into the hippocampus. These connections explain the physiologically established fact that signals from several sensory organs can be registered by the limbic system.

It is suggested that the limbic system, in addition to controlling motor patterns of affective behaviour may also be responsible for the subjective moods and feelings which we associate with such behaviour. This has been investigated by the so-called self-stimulation experiments of Olds and Milner (1954), in which electrodes are implanted in various places in the brain. By lever pressing or some similar action the animal can give itself a mild stimulus through the electrodes. According to the localization of the electrodes the animal may respond by stimulating itself almost continuously until it is exhausted, or avoid any possibility of further stimulus after the first time; in other instances the animal is indifferent to the effect. From this evidence it would appear that stimulation of certain brain structures brings about a pleasurable or rewarding experience whereas stimulation of other areas causes a feeling of pain or dislike. These experiments have been reproduced with consistent results for some years in a variety of animal species, and have been modified in a number of ways in attempts to assess the intensity of the desire for self-stimulation as compared with external affective stimulation such as that of eating or drinking. This experimental method has also been used to determine drug effects.

Therefore, in calling the limbic system the visceral brain, MacLean suggests that the functions of the limbic system are the interpretation of experience in terms of 'feeling' rather than in terms of 'intellectualized' symbols, the experience being obtained from all the body structures, both visceral and somatic. The 'visceral brain' is without doubt in an anatomically favourable position to integrate all forms of internal and external perception. In contrast to the neocortex it also has many connections with the hypothalamus by means of which it can discharge its impressions. Stimulation or destruction of any part of the limbic system will bring about widespread functional changes in the whole nervous system, including the cortex, which will be manifested by changes in emotional responsiveness and emotional behaviour. These, however, are greatly dependent upon the state of activity in the reticular formation.

Hypothalamus

The hypothalamus is an area containing more centres, or nuclei, with special functions than any other part of the brain and anatomically it may be divided into four principal regions, the preoptic, the supraoptic, tuberal and mamillary regions.

From the hypothalamus there are both afferent and efferent fibre connections. Thus there is a medial fore-brain bundle relaying impulses from the frontal lobe of the cerebral cortex; thalamo hypothalamic fibres which probably relay somatic and visceral sensory impulses to the hypothalamus and thus set up connections between the neopalaeal cortex and the hypothalamus; the fornix bundle which arises in the hippocampus and terminates in the mamillary bodies; the stria terminalis which arises from the amygdala and appears to have connections with the preoptic regions and others. The efferent connections include the mamillo-thalamic tract which in turn is connected with the cingulate gyrus and possibly relayed to the frontal cortex; diffuse descending connections extending as part of the medial fore-brain bundle which are thought to be important in conducting impulses from the hypothalamus towards lower anatomic centres; connections between hypothalamus and pituitary body; a diffuse projection system to the cortex which originates in the posterior portion of the hypothalamus and in the nearby reticular formation and is important in maintaining the waking state.

Perhaps the most important function of the hypothalamus is integrative. Although it is especially concerned with autonomic functions it ought not to be considered in isolation but as part of a system related to the fore-brain, the mid- and hind-brain which integrates sleep and waking phenomena, emotional, autonomic and behavioural activity.

Thus, the hypothalamus is intimately connected with control of body-temperature; its complete destruction allows the body-temperature to fluctuate with that of the environment; destruction of the anterior part abolishes the heat-loss mechanisms; heat production and conservation seem to be controlled by more caudal regions of the hypothalamus. By electrical stimulation of the hypothalamus, in experimental animals, autonomic activity including increased arterial pressure, cardiac acceleration, pupillary dilatation, sweating, piloerection, hyperglycaemia and cessation of peristalsis have been brought about. Especially in the anterior portions, essentially parasympathetic responses such as bladder contraction, peristalsis, cardiac depression and vasodilatation have also been obtained.

INTEGRATION

It would appear, therefore, that the brain stem reticular formation and other parts of the brain modify the composition of perceptive and projective neural patterns and help higher centres by diminishing or increasing the strength of signals according to their immediate significance. In other words, the brain exerts a certain freedom of choice regarding its awareness of the environment.

On the basis of present evidence there has been much speculation concerning the significance of the various parts of the central nervous system in the control of behaviour. Those special parts of the brain already described are considered to form a feedback mechanism or reverberating circuit. Though each member of the circuit makes a special contribution to the integrative process, the total effect on behaviour is modified by the reciprocal activity of all the other members.

Thus it is said that hypothalamic function is involved in the pattern of movement associated with strong emotion, the hypothalamus activating extrapyramidal discharges which may be reinforced by impulses from the cortex.

By means of the limbic system the reactions of the brain structures especially concerned in emotional activity reach consciousness. Such activity having reached consciousness, however, the cortex may then modify the reactions of the other parts of the limbic system and the hypothalamus. The limbic system may also affect, or be affected by, the amygdaloid complex, which can send signals to the hippocampus by way of the stria terminalis to the septum, the hypothalamus, the mid-brain tegmentum and the mid-brain reticular formation. In the reticular formation are nuclei which send fibres to the hypothalamus, the amygdala and the septal area and thence to the hippocampus.

By these means at least the fore-brain, the limbic system, the hypothalamus and the reticular formation are linked into one unifying system which can mobilize the complex activities required for self-preservation such as the acquisition and assimilation of food, sexual activities and the preservation of the species.

Obviously, all the parts and the functions of the various parts of the brain are not yet known. Until recently, the cortex was looked upon as the dominant influence in human activity. Some twenty years ago, it was suggested that possibly the reticular formation, with its complex system of reverberations and feed-back, might be of paramount importance. At present, great attention is being paid to the limbic system and its connection with emotion and drive. Doubtless, some other part of the CNS will become the focus of investigation before long.

AMINES AND ABNORMAL MOOD

Serotonin

Dewhurst (1969) critically assessed the relationship between amines and abnormal mood. He examined the hypothesis that serotonin deficiency is associated with depression. Although no cerebral effects occur after exogenous oral 5-hydroxytryptamine (5-HT) or in the usual carcinoid syndromes with hypersecretion of 5-HT, this does not mean that 5-HT has no cerebral effects but that it does not pass the Blood Brain Barrier (BBB). Because of this, the precursor of 5-HT, namely 5-hydroxytryptophan (5-HTP) has been tried in affective disorders because this passes the BBB and is decarboxylated in the brain to serotonin. Results have been disappointing, and although this has been attributed to inadequate dosage, carcinoid tumours secreting 5-HTP do not support the hypothesis.

Another type of evidence which is cited is the change produced in endogenous amines by various drugs which affect mood. The monoamine oxidase inhibitors (MAOI's) cause rises in cerebral 5-HT due to diminished destruction, and imipramine which is said to hinder access to the enzyme. On the other hand, reserpine, which is sometimes followed by depression, causes depletion of 5-HT from the cell and lithium possibly favours monoamine oxidase attack. The problem with this type of evidence is that other amines are also affected and it is difficult to separate the effects.

Furthermore the correlation between amine levels and a particular type of mental illness is not constant. For example, 5-hydroxyindoles may be low in depression but may also be low in schizophrenia as well as in mania. This would suggest that cerebral 5-HT changes are secondary and without causal significance as far as mood is concerned.

Catecholamines

In contrast to 5-HT, the case for catecholamine involvement is stronger. Schildkraut and Kety (1967) have hypothesized that some, if not all, depressions are due to catecholamine deficiency, particularly noradrenaline, while in mania, the converse holds. When scrutinizing evidence, it is important to bear in mind that what are effects are frequently paraded as causes.

Noradrenaline does not pass through the blood brain barrier, and for this reason, the amine acid precursor, dopa, which does, and is subsequently decarboxylated to form dopamine and other catecholamines, is used. It produces arousal but this is probably due to a direct amine acid effect as well as catecholamine formation in extracerebral tissues which causes altering via vascular responses (Dewhurst, 1969). As far as mood is concerned, studies to date have been negative.

Monoamine oxidase inhibitors are known to increase brain noradrenaline, but they also increase other amine levels. Imipramine is believed to protect noradrenaline from attack by monoamine oxidase and amphetamine may have a similar action; they would therefore liberate noradrenaline. Similarly the euphoriant action of tryptophan is attributed to noradrenaline release occasioned by 5-HTP, even though it has been shown that 5-HTP is ineffective in depression.

Reserpine and tetrabenazine administration may be followed by depression, and this is attributed to depletion of noradrenaline, although other amines are also affected. Nevertheless, reserpine combined with monoamine oxidase inhibitors or with imipramine alleviates depression supposedly by potentiation of noradrenaline release. Lithium too favours access of noradrenaline to monoamine oxidase, but again other amines may also be affected.

Urinary levels of noradrenaline excretion are raised where there is anger or increased activity, while adrenaline is only raised in states of uncertainty with anxiety and inactivity. Noradrenaline excretion is raised in mania but in depression the levels are equivocal. Bunney *et al.* (1967) have reported extremely high levels of noradrenaline in psychotic depression which they attribute to the massive and prolonged psychological distress in these patients. Yet brain noradrenaline in suicides who were depressed has been found to be within normal limits. Dewhurst (1967) summarizes thus:

. . . there is no clear evidence that cerebral actions of exogenous amines or precursors have an effect on *mood* nor that drugs which elevate or depress mood have significantly selective effects on noradrenaline rather than on other amines (indeed the reverse is the case). Because of blood brain barrier considerations urinary results must reflect peripheral activity and in the only brain study done noradrenaline was found to be normal. It is particularly important not to equate peripherally induced arousal with euphoria.

Dewhurst (1967) puts forward his own hypothesis:

Lowering of mood and some forms of depressive illness may be due to either deficiency of excitant (Type A) amines, or diminished responsiveness of the A receptor. Elevation of mood and some manic states may be caused by an excess of excitant (Type A) amines or increased A receptor sensitivity. Psychosocial factors are co-determinants of more complex behavioural features . . .

A number of amines acting on the A receptor such as amphetamine, phenmetrazine (Preludin), α-ethyl tryptamine (Monase) and tranylcypromine (Parnate), have euphoriant effects in man, and in the case of the last two these effects occur before inhibition of monoamine oxidase, i.e. they are due to direct action on the receptor and they all pass the blood brain barrier. Dewhurst favours tryptamine as the main agent even though it has been shown that tryptamine given intravenously is ineffective, but he attributes this to its instability in aqueous solution, particularly at pH 7.4. The amino acid precursor, tryptophan, on the other hand, has a well-established euphoriant action, though its effects are difficult to explain in terms of 5-HT because 5-HTP is ineffective.

His evidence for selecting tryptamine is based on the following experiment. Simultaneous measurements of the three main brain substrates of the enzyme in urine before and after an amino oxidase inhibitor (phenelzine) showed differential effects. Tryptamine was quadrupled, 5-HT was not quite trebled and meta– and normetanephrine showed less increase still. He explains:

The two substrates showing least change can also be metabolized by O-methylation, whereas tryptamine cannot, and hence is much more sensitive to interference with MAO . . . tryptamine, unlike the others, can pass the blood brain barrier so that not only is tryptamine the dominant physiological change in brain metabolism but the large amounts of tryptamine occurring in extracerebral tissues will also contribute to cerebral effects.

As to other anti-depressants, imipramine hinders access to MAO of various amines and it again follows that the amines mainly dependent on this route of catabolism will be affected most. The same is true for a combination of reserpine and MAO and reserpine and imipramine. The action of amphetamine is a direct one and this is why it acts after reserpination . . .

Correlation studies in affective states show that although urinary tryptamine is low in depression, it rises after successful treatment and may or may not be elevated in mania . . .these effects reflect the peripheral tissue activity associated with the different illnesses rather than the cerebral happenings.

Interactions between Sympathomimetic Amines and Anti-depressants in Man

As many patients, such as asthmatics, are treated with sympathomimetic drugs and there is the evidence that some anti-depressants interact with these drugs, it is important to gauge what the hazards of interaction are. Boakes *et al.* (1973) gave healthy human volunteers intravenous infusions of phenylephrine, noradrenaline, adrenaline and isoprenaline after they had been having phenelzine, tranylcypromine or imipramine for 5–7 days. Cardiovascular responses were compared with those observed under control conditions and the following observations were reported.

(1) With MAO Inhibitors, there was a 2–2½ times potentiation of the pressor effects of phenylephrine, but no clinically significant potentiation of the cardiovascular effects of noradrenaline, adrenaline or isoprenaline.

(2) With *imipramine,* there was potentiation of the pressor effects of phenylephrine (2–3 fold), noradrenaline (4–8 fold) and adrenaline (2–4 fold). There were dysrhythmias during adrenaline infusions but no noticeable or consistent changes in response to isoprenaline.

Noradrenaline and adrenaline in amounts contained in local anaesthesia used in dentistry are not likely to be MAO inhibitors. Hazardous potentiation of their cardiovascular effects might occur in patients receiving tricyclic anti-depressants. The authors conclude that their observations do not suggest that the hazards associated with isoprenaline inhalation by bronchial asthmatics would be increased by coincident therapy with a MAOI or tricyclic anti-depressant.

Catecholamines and Mania

As it has been suggested that functional levels of brain catecholamines are elevated in mania and decreased in depression, Brodie *et al.* (1971) tried the effect of alpha-methyl-para tyrosine (AMPT), which is the rate-limiting enzyme in catecholamine synthesis, in manic and depressive states. The work was conducted in metabolic research wards and the protocols of a controlled trial were rigidly observed.

They concluded that AMPT had a suppressant effect on manic symptomatology which could not be accounted for by its sedative effect, as those patients who improved showed definite changes in manic thinking and behaviour which were qualitatively different from the sedative effects of large doses of barbiturates and phenothiazines. *It was not as effective clinically as lithium carbonate* even though it did have a specific action on catecholamine metabolism, thus supporting the hypothesis that mania is linked to a functional excess of catecholamines in the brain.

TRANQUILLIZERS

Tranquillizers have a sedative effect without as a rule lowering the level of consciousness and though they are extensively prescribed for neuroses, their main action is with the psychoses. Although the clinical effects may be similar, their pharmacological actions may vary.

RESERPINE

This is one of the most potent alkaloids of *Rauwolfia serpentini Benth.* which is an Indian shrub whose extracts have for centuries been used in the treatment of a variety of diseases, including mental disease. The first report in modern medical literature was by Gupta *et al.* (1943), and Hakim (1953) gave the first scientific account of some of its pharmacological actions. After Hakim's report there were a number of clinical and pharmacological studies, including those of Kline (1954) which established its place in the treatment of schizophrenia. It has later been reported by Prince (1960) that another Rauwolfia plant has been used for many years in Western Nigeria for similar purposes.

Pharmacology

Reserpine, like serotonin, has an indole nucleus and although its effects can be long-lasting, it is rapidly broken down in the body, 50-60 per cent being excreted in three to four hours. Its prolonged action has been explained by its slow release from body fat. Vogt (1958) reported that its analogues interfere with the retention in brain tissues of such amines as 5-hydroxytryptamine, and the catechol amines, which include adrenaline, noradrenaline, and hydroxytryptamine, of which noradrenaline is the main representative in nervous tissue. As these substances are mainly concentrated in the hypothalamus, the tegmentum of the midbrain and in parts of the limbic system, they presumably play a role in the specialized functions of those regions. Vogt's paper is a highly informed corrective to the over-enthusiastic, as she deals mainly with the existing facts and points out the limits of our knowledge.

The biochemical action of reserpine is, however, not restricted to the brain for it causes 5-HT to disappear from platelets and intestine, noradrenaline from peripheral sympathetic neurones and occasionally from the adrenal medulla. She adds:

> We do not know whether the depleting action in brain is restricted to the

amines just listed: there may be others of even greater functional importance which are as yet unidentified and which are also lost . . . Altogether, the assessment of the relation between disturbance of function and state of the amines stored in special parts of the brain is at present entirely speculative. We do, however, know that in the peripheral nervous system, where conditions are less complex, the disappearance of noradrenaline from adrenergic neurones leads to failure of peripheral sympathetic activity. It is to be expected that, in prolonged treatment of psychiatric patients with large doses of reserpine, depletion must be such as to cause varying degrees of peripheral 'functional sympathectomy'. Analyses of urinary excretion of noradrenaline after administration of reserpine have confirmed this expectation by demonstrating a fall in the excretion of noradrenaline (Gaddum *et al.*, 1958). How far the disappearance of noradrenaline from the hypothalamus interferes with the activity of the sympathetic centres cannot at present be decided.

Removal of the cerebral cortex in animals produces a state of sham rage which is said to be due to removal of the inhibitory functions of the cortex on the diencephalic centres, and reserpine markedly but not completely antagonizes this action in the decorticated animal, but in the intact animal it intensifies the inhibitory effect of the cortex. Schneider *et al.* (1955) produced evidence that it could facilitate neuronal transmission by cholinergic predominance together with inhibition of afferent impulses. In contrast to barbiturates, it produces an alert EEG pattern in rabbits, probably by stimulating the mesodiencephalic activating system. By itself it does not produce sleep. In rhesus monkeys 'avoidance performing' and food rewarding situations are depressed (Weiskrantz & Wilson, 1955) and amygdalectomized animals show similar responses. It potentiates the action of metrazol, causing convulsions, while in the animal pre-medicated with phenobarbitone these are absent. It has a different but not antagonistic action to barbiturates—rather it competes with them by intensifying the inhibitory action of the cortex.

Relation to Serotonin

The principal action of reserpine is to change the cells of the brain so that they no longer maintain serotonin at a high concentration against a low extracellular concentration and it would appear that the cell-binding sites for serotonin are modified or filled by reserpine. When 5-hydroxytryptophane (a serotonin precursor) is fed to rabbits previously treated with reserpine, serotonin is formed in the usual way, but not bound by the cerebral cells (Brodie *et al.*, 1955). The action of reserpine may be mediated by the unbound serotonin, displaced from the cellular tissue sites prior to its conversion to 5-hydroxyindoleacetic acid by monoamine oxidase.

Clinical Uses

In psychiatry it is primarily used in the treatment of schizophrenia and has probably been used for this purpose for many centuries in India and Africa. In the former country, in Bihar and United Provinces, it has been called 'pagal-kawada' or insanity remedy. R. H. Hakim used it in India in 1953 and found it more valuable than E.C.T. and when combined with E.C.T. it gave even better results. The drug soon became popular in America, the U.K. and in Eire. In addition to its value in schizophrenia, it is useful in very disturbed and excited patients, including the senile, but has no place in the treatment of depression.

Dosage. This is geared to the degree and nature of the mental disturbance; 5 mg. is initially given intramuscularly but this may be exceeded if necessary. Oral therapy follows the settling of the excited patient; 2–8 mg./day is used, and it can be combined with E.C.T. Treatment (which is of course not confined to the administration of the drug) is continued for three to four months or even longer. Acute problems respond better.

Side-effects. *Depression.* This in susceptible subjects can be profound and present a serious suicidal risk, though in the 'pure' schizophrenic disorders this is unlikely. It can occur in schizo-affective psychoses but it is commonest in depression-prone individuals who are having reserpine for hypertension. Antidepressants such as imipramine have been combined with reserpine as a prophylactic against or treatment for depression. Withdrawal of the drug does not necessarily stop the depression and this after-effect has been attributed to its slow discharge from the body fat (see above).

Parkinsonism. This is found in up to 5 per cent of patients on treatment. It clears with antispasmodics or stopping the drug.

Oedema of Face and Feet. This may be transient and can frequently be controlled with antihistamine drugs.

Hypotension. This is found only in very susceptible subjects or where heroic doses are used.

Tremors of Limbs. These can occur in addition to the Parkinsonism.

With the exception of depression, all the other side-effects disappear rapidly on stopping or reducing the drug.

Deserpidine. An alkaloid from *Rauwolfia cenescens*. This is reputed to less toxic than reserpine and to enjoy a comparative freedom from depressive sequelae. Its therapeutic effects are very similar to reserpine and its dose is 2–3 mg./day.

THE PHENOTHIAZINES

The core of the molecular structure of the phenothiazine compounds is, of course, the phenothiazine nucleus This consists of two benzene rings connected by a sulphur atom and a nitrogen atom. The phenothiazines had already figured in chemotherapy, ever since Ehrlich showed that phenothiazine methylene blue had an anti-malarial action. Phenothiazine as a ring system was used in the production of antihistamine drugs, which frequently possessed anti-emetic, hypothermic and muscle-relaxant actions as well. A number of phenothiazine derivatives were therefore tried in efforts to reduce shock in surgical procedures, and it was found they could potentiate general depressants of the nervous system and assist in the production of artificial 'hibernation'. In this state, temperature and autonomic responses were lowered and these drugs proved a valuable aid to anaesthesia.

CHLORPROMAZINE

This was the first of the phenothiazines to have a useful action in the treatment of mental disorders. It has a chlorine atom attached to the phenothiazine nucleus in the 2-position, and a three-carbon 'side chain' attached to the nitrogen atom of the nucleus. The third carbon atom in the side chain is followed by another nitrogen atom, and the remaining valences of the nitrogen atom are filled by two methyl groups.

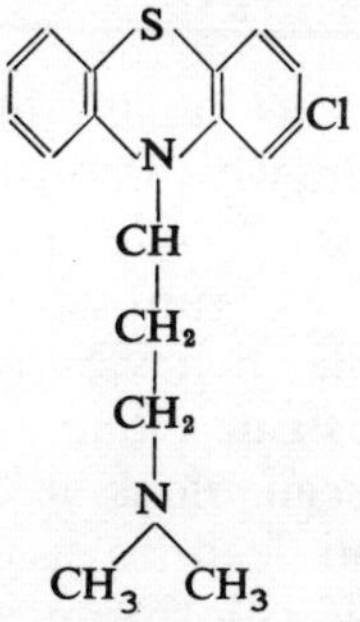

S
Cl
N
CH
CH_2
CH_2
N
CH_3 CH_3

Other phenothiazine derivatives have been developed since the introduction of chlorpromazine. Some have less than three carbon atoms in the side chain between the two nitrogen atoms; others have more than three carbon atoms in the side chain. But most of the phenothiazines which are useful in the treatment of mental illness like chlorpromazine, have three carbon atoms in the side chain. The main differences in these compounds are in the attachments made to the nucleus and to the end carbon on the side chain.

Laborit *et al.* (1952) considered that chlorpromazine would be worth trying in psychiatric patients as an aid to prolonged narcosis, and the phenothiazines had arrived in psychiatry. It was soon shown that their main function was not as a potentiator of barbiturates but as a 'tranquillizer', for Delay and Deniker (1952) reported their use of the drug in the treatment of psychoses.

Pharmacology

Himwich (1957) suggests that chlorpromazine depresses the hypothalamus where the centres for the control of basal metabolism, temperature, sleep, waking and blood pressure are located. This in turn impairs the function of the anterior pituitary which becomes less susceptible to stimulation, an effect similar to a lowered production of ovarian hormone, with consequent stimulation of lactation (see below). The depression of the hypothalamic functions would therefore cause a fall in basal metabolic rate, a lowering of body temperature, a fall in blood pressure and facilitation of sleep with potentiation of the action of barbiturates and other hypnotics. As the posterior hypothalamus contains sympathetic centres, there is also inhibition of emotional responsiveness. The hibernatory effect is explained by the drug's capacity to block the sympathetic ganglia with lowering of the blood pressure.

Neuro-electrical Findings

Chlorpromazine even in small doses can block the meso-diencephalic alerting system, which consists of the reticular formation (Moruzzi & Magoun, 1949) and the thalamic diffuse cortical projections (Jasper, 1949*a*). Stimulation of this system consists in behavioural arousal, while behavioural sleep occurs when it is depressed. A pain stimulus can evoke an arousal response, but small doses of chlorpromazine can block it, and so inhibit the inflow of stimuli to the cortex and lead to a diminution in affect responsiveness. Large doses of chlorpromazine, however, can, in the experimental animal, produce the reverse effect and cause an arousal reaction. The threshold to stimuli such as pain, electric currents, and injections of adrenaline is raised, and the responses shortened or even abolished (Hiebel *et al.,* 1954; Himwich, 1955; Bradley, 1957; Bovet *et al.,* 1957). Preston (1956) considers that the therapeutic effect of chlorpromazine is more closely linked with the electro-encephalographic changes in the limbic system, where high doses cause bursts of spikes which originate in the amygdala and can lead to generalized seizures. Vogt (1958) indicates her approval of Preston's work with the statement: 'The attractiveness of this view lies in the fact that it provides a common basis for the action of reserpine and chlorpromazine'.

The reticular formation and the reticulo-spinal tract carry the main motor outflow of the extrapyramidal system and it has been suggested that over-activity of the system may be responsible for the Parkinsonian tremor and that stimulation by chlorpromazine could produce such a picture just as well as by a lesion in the basal ganglia or substantia nigra. The alerting system here, too, may not be the only site of action; it has already been shown that synaptic transmission in the cord is facilitated, and if the cortex is similarly facilitated, this would augment the cortical inhibition exerted on the thalamus.

Olds *et al.* (1957) have demonstrated a third site of action of chlorpromazine. Olds had already discovered that animals with electrodes implanted in certain parts of their brain seemed to derive satisfaction from electrical stimulation of these parts. The technique is called 'self-stimulation', for when the animals have found that by treading on a lever they received an electric shock to their brain, they begin to operate the lever at frequent intervals. Rats given chlorpromazine no longer give themselves shocks when the stimulating electrodes are implanted in the posterior hypothalamus, but continue self-stimulation when the electrodes are placed in the anterior hypothalamus. These experiments would suggest that the drug acts on the posterior hypothalamus.

Neurochemical Findings

When chlorpromazine is injected into rats and the brain tissue analysed, there are no changes in the oxidation of the excised brain tissue, but there is an accumulation of adenosinetriphosphate (ATP) which could be due to increased production or slower utilization. The midbrain region of the rat containing the thalamus and hypothalamus showed the greatest increase of ATP. Unlike reserpine, chlorpromazine does not increase the excretion of 5-hydroxyindole-acetic acid (5 HIAA or 5-hydroxytryptamine) but in some respects acts like serotonin and is therefore serotonin-mimetic and competes for its receptors, thus reducing its effectiveness. Uterine contraction in the rat, produced by serotonin, is blocked by chlorpromazine but not to the same extent as by reserpine.

Vogt (1958), who reviews the pharmacology of chlorpromazine, not only fills in some of the gaps, but again underlines the limitations of our knowledge. She states:

> Chlorpromazine is known to be a potent inhibitor of many enzymatic processes, and its depressing action on the brain is likely to be related to this property. The turnover of phospholipids, so important in cerebral function, is among the processes affected; and the respiration of electrically stimulated slices of guinea-pig brain is inhibited by very low concentrations of chlorpromazine (Ansell & Dohmen, 1956; McIlwain & Greengard, 1957). In view of the general action of chlorpromazine on enzymes it is not surprising to find that its pharmacological actions are usually numerous (Courvoisier *et al.*, 1953). Many of these are undesirable side-effects from the point of view of the clinician; such are the depression of the bone marrow, the autonomic actions, the galactorrhoea, and the production of Parkinsonism, an effect chlorpromazine shares with reserpine.
>
> *Changes in Personality.* The use of these pharmacological observations for the explanation of the therapeutic action is limited by our lack of knowledge of cerebral function. If one assumes the therapeutic effect in psychoses to be due to an inhibition of overwhelming drives and irrepressible stimuli which are kept up by pathological processes in the brain, one can visualize these drugs as acting by inhibition of the metabolism in the offending regions of the brain. It is impossible to tell whether the limbic system is one of these offending regions and the spikes observed correspond to certain inhibitory phenomena occurring there, or whether the limbic system is stimulated by drugs and such stimulation leads to useful inhibitions of other parts of the brain. ... More striking still are the effects observed in animals, to which the drugs can be given more freely: previously aggressive animals become tame and easy to handle; they develop an indifference to unpleasant stimuli shown in the loss of conditioned avoidance responses. Rats and monkeys, for example, were trained to avoid an electric shock by leaving a particular area of their cage when an acoustic or visual signal heralded the coming of the shock. After an injection of chlorpromazine or reserpine they failed to heed the conditioning signal, though they were perfectly capable of performing the motor effort required to avoid the shock (Smith *et al.* 1957). Their behaviour had become inappropriate, and normal contact between animal and environment had been lost.

Bradley *et al.* (1966) consider that chlorpromazine has a selective action on the sensory inflow into the reticular formation from afferent pathways. Bradley and Wolstencroft (1965), by using micro-iontophoresis had already measured the effects of acetylcholine, noradrenaline, and 5-hydroxy-tryptamine on brain-stem neurones in the cat and found that all these compounds excited some neurones and inhibited others. In their later communication they compared the effects of these substances on the same neurone before and after the application of chlorpromazine. The only consistent findings were the reduction, abolition, and sometimes even replacement, by weak inhibitory effects, of the excitatory effects of noradrenaline, but the inhibitory effects were not antagonized. They conclude that the central actions of chlorpromazine are primarily related to those of noradrenaline and support their hypothesis by quoting other work which shows that chlorpromazine partially blocks the uptake of noradrenaline by nerve terminals.

If this effect occurred at sites in the brain where noradrenaline is released as an inhibitory transmitter, its local concentration at the receptor site would be increased and inhibition potentiated. If a similar effect occurred at sites where noradrenaline was an excitatory transmitter, the disappearance of an excitatory response would suggest that chlorpromazine may also selectively block the excitatory action of noradrenaline. They also showed that the effects of chlorpromazine on the neurones from the reticular formation which are concerned with arousal are mediated by these mechanisms resulting in an increased threshold for their activation.

Chlorpromazine and Plasma Levels

The estimation of the value of drugs by observing the effect on the patient is so customary as to make an estimation based on plasma levels appear almost revolutionary. In the majority of cases it is not necessary, but in some, such as anorexia nervosa it can be mandatory, for if the patient is secreting the drugs and is obviously not responding, larger doses may be given. If concurrently greater supervision is exercised, a dangerous situation may arise, for the patient would then receive and ingest a much larger dose than is necessary or safe. Though Marshall *et al.* (1970) advocate the regulation of dosage by plasma levels as a routine, it need only be reserved for situations of doubt.

THERAPEUTIC USES

Mental Illness

Schizophrenia. All forms respond, including schizo-affective reactions, paranoid schizophrenia and catatonic states. The rationale is that in schizophrenia there is an over-sensitivity to sensory stimulation which tends to disrupt personality structure and this is damped down by the drug and gives the patient a chance to settle. The effects in a catatonic state can be most dramatic and a wildly excited patient who is vividly hallucinated can be rendered calm and rational in less then 24 hours. Considerable dosage may be needed and though some recommend that the drug be built up slowly from say 25 mg. t.d.s. to the dose required, if the patient can be put to bed, large doses are well tolerated; 100 mg. t.d.s is not unusual and occasionally 1000 mg./day may be necessary. The maximum dose should be continued till the patient has completely settled which may be in three or four days and then gradually reduced, but a maintenance dose of 50 mg. t.d.s. for at least six months is advisable and if all goes well further reduction is possible. Some patients have been maintained on the drug for years, without untoward effects.

Mania. The same regimen is used as in schizophrenia, the dose depending on the severity of the case.

Agitation and Restlessness. These may be associated with melancholic states or occur in dementia and other forms of organic brain disease. Patients with organic dementia have a limited tolerance to the drug and dosage should not be heroic unless the circumstances are compelling. Normally 50 mg. t.d.s. should suffice, but it may be divided into a major dose for the evening to combat the nocturnal disturbance and a smaller dose during the day.

Post-operative Excitement or Confusional States. These psychotic episodes may also occur in medical conditions such as recovering from heart failure and anoxic states. The treatment of the physical condition such as electrolyte imbalance may not be enough and chlorpromazine is a useful supplement.

Post-leucotomy Behaviour Disorders and Aggressive Tendencies. These constitute a limited but important group. They are seen especially in those who have had the operation for severe compulsive neurosis and, with the general freeing of the patient's mental energies, there can result a state of uncooperation and resistance to even ordinary nursing care. The drug has proved useful as a prophylactic in such cases, the patient being given 50 mg. t.d.s. for several days prior to the operation and the dose thereafter continued and if necessary increased.

Mixed Psychotic Reactions. The drug can be prescribed in combination with a number of other drugs, such as antidepressants, and is useful in the schizo-affective reactions, or in paranoid states with depressive features.

Other Uses

(*a*) Nausea and vomiting.
(*b*) Acute alcoholism.
(*c*) Withdrawal of drugs in drug addiction.
(*d*) Relief of pain from various causes including inoperable cancer.
(*e*) Potentiation of effect of hypnotics and analgesics.
(*f*) Treatment of porphyria. Reported by Melby *et al.* (1956) who

consider it to be most effective. Confirmatory reports are still awaited.

Therapeutic Misuses

Neurotic Reactions. Numerous therapeutic trials have been carried out on these states and some claims made for the drug, but it is still very doubtful if it has any place in their treatment and the points raised by Kubie (p. 820) should be borne in mind. In clinical trials where chlorpromazine and other tranquillizers have been compared with barbiturates for their capacity to relieve neurotic symptoms, the latter have led the field and the former have not performed better than placebos.

Depression without Agitation. Though chlorpromazine has not got the reputation of reserpine in precipitating or aggravating existing depression there is considerable evidence that, at least, it does not help and is better avoided.

Mental Changes Associated with Toxaemia of Pregnancy. The liver in this condition is highly sensitive to the drug and permanent damage has occurred. Surprisingly the damaged liver of the alcoholic is less vulnerable.

Small Doses where Large Doses are Essential. These may fail to control the illness and earn the drug a reputation for failure which it does not deserve.

Toxic Effects

It is to be expected that with a drug that is freely prescribed, nearly every possible toxic effect will have been noted. This has had disadvantages for chlorpromazine, for it conveys the impression that it is a dangerous drug, and as a result other drugs in the field that are not as freely prescribed have earned a reputation for greater safety which they may not deserve. In fact it is possible for such a drug to be even more toxic than chlorpromazine and yet be regarded as less toxic.

The toxic effects of chlorpromazine are:

Jaundice. This was reported by Lehmann and Hanrahan (1954) as a complication of chlorpromazine therapy and the clinical features were well described by Cohen and Archer (1955). It is generally agreed that the jaundice is of an obstructive type due to a cholangiolstatic hepatitis which is regarded as due to drug sensitivity. Incidence is estimated at approximately 1·5 per cent of those receiving the drug, though for some unexplained reason, there seems to be less of it now than in the earlier days of the drug. The jaundice does not depend on dosage for it may follow very shortly after a relatively small dose, and it must therefore single out susceptible patients. Graham (1957), working in a general hospital, stressed the importance of keeping the diagnosis in mind as it is possible for such patients who do not declare that they have been having the drug, to be subjected to laparotomy. Out of 65 jaundiced patients investigated over a 12-month period he found that in seven, the jaundice was due to chlorpromazine. It is frequently associated with fever and may resemble an attack of hepatitis. Liver function tests show an obstructive type of jaundice with a high serum alkaline phosphatase and the mechanism of the jaundice is initially a stasis of bile in the canaliculi with lymphocytic infiltration. It usually clears spontaneously and further medication does not produce relapse but in a number of patients the sensitivity persists. A few develop permanent liver damage with atrophy and cirrhosis and Whitfield (1955) has reported such a case. Special treatment, other than withdrawing the drug, is not usually indicated though some favour corticoids and special diets. Patients have continued with the drug and yet recovered from the jaundice completely so there are no clear indications as to what to do but, generally, stopping the drug is desirable.

Sensitivity to Chlorpromazine in Patients with Hepatic Disease. Read *et al.* (1969) compared the effects of chlorpromazine on patients with liver cirrhosis with normals and showed that the former had a greater variability in EEG response with some becoming unduly drowsy. They conclude that such patients are extremely sensitive to chlorpromazine and that it should be used cautiously in such patients especially if there is evidence of delirium tremens, for it may be, in fact, hepatic delirium.

Dermatitis and Urticaria. This is more commonly found in those handling the drug, such as nursing staff and dispensers. Protective gloves should be worn. In the patient the rash can be generalized but is more often on the face and associated with gross oedema which may resemble an angioneurotic oedema. Treatment with antihistamines such as promethazine, 25 mg. t.d.s., is usually effective.

Leucopaenia. This can creep up insidiously and give rise to agranulocytosis with fatal results. It is wise to do regular blood counts on patients on prolonged therapy and should a sore throat develop, the drug should be discontinued, antibiotics started and the blood re-examined.

Parkinsonism. This tends to be related to dosage and is usually found in patients on prolonged treatment. The characteristic facies and tremor is unmistakable but it is not a permanent change and disappears when the drug is withdrawn or reduced. Oculogyric crises can also occur and these may in susceptible subjects follow relatively small doses of the drug.

Dystonic (Dyskinesic) Reactions. These may occur at the commencement of treatment and are frequently bizarre. A usual feature is involuntary movements of the face, jaw and tongue and the author had a hysterically prone patient who insisted that her tongue kept sticking out of her mouth and just would not go back. To the uninitiated this can appear quite ridiculous and almost wilful. Stopping or reducing the drug, or adding an anti-Parkinsonian drug should suffice to control the situation, but there have now been reports of irreversible dyskinesias affecting the face, mouth and jaw, which developed insidiously after prolonged medication. Hunter *et al.* (1964) found 5 per cent with such features out of 450 chronic mental hospital patients. They were all female, and had evidence of brain damage and were aged from 56 to 84. Six had undergone leucotomy and others had had up to 212 E.C.T.'s. The most striking feature was the continual grimacing and writhing movements of mouth, tongue and jaw. In some patients protrusion and withdrawal of the tongue was so severe as to interfere with eating and drinking and there were also choreiform movements of all four limbs. Stopping the drug, even for 8–13 months, failed to stop the movements.

TARDIVE DYSKINESIA

Relationship to Neuroleptic and Antiparkinson Drugs

Turek *et al.* (1972) set out to clarify the relationship of the abnormal movements to the cessation of neuroleptic medication, increases in dosage levels and the use of antiparkinson agents. The sample consisted of 56 chronic schizophrenics with tardive dyskinesia and was divided into those who received no neuroleptic drugs (8 patients); those who did (32 patients): and those who received a neuroleptic drug in combination with the antiparkinson drug, Trihexyphenidyl. All were processed through four treatment phases totalling 44 weeks. Throughout the entire study period, the original drug-free group served as a control and were not given any neuroleptics. The remaining protocols were of a good standard.

Mean scores indicated that dyskinetic symptoms were less when neuroleptic drugs (mainly phenothiazines) were given than when they were not, and that the antiparkinson agent was of little value in controlling the type of dyskinetic activity under study. Mean changes associated with dosage manipulation were minimal. Thus in five of the six instances where neuroleptic drugs were discontinued there was a significant rise in dyskinetic symptomatology during the drug-free period, while in the sixth instance there was a similar tendency. In two of the five instances in which neuroleptic drugs were reinstated, there was a significant drop in symptomatology for the subsequent medication period. Patients were also rated by film studies and these provided further evidence of the inverse relationship between dyskinetic symptom severity and the administration of neuroleptic drugs.

Treatment with Dopamine-Depleting and Dopamine-Blocking Agents

Kazamatsuri *et al.* (1972 *a, b*) used the dopamine-depleting agent, tetrabenazine, and the dopamine-blocking agents, haloperidol and thiopropazate, in the treatment of tardive dyskinesia. The results in the former supported the hypothesis that reducing brain dopamine suppresses the abnormal movements. In the latter, their results supported the hypothesis that the symptoms of tardive dyskinesia are caused by over-stimulation of dopaminergic synapsis. Haloperidol had a more striking effect on oral dyskinesia than did thiopropazate, though both drugs caused a significant increase in extrapyramidal symptoms. The inverse relationship of reversible extrapyramidal symptomatology during haloperidol medication suggests that the antidyskinetic effect of the drug may be due to increased rigidity or akinesia. The authors are cautious in recommending these drugs for long-term therapy as some patients show a tendency to aggravation of oral dyskinesia on a stable or increasing dose of antipsychotic agent.

Extrapyramidal Disorders and Prolonged Phenothiazine Therapy. Kennedy *et al.* (1971) describe five types of phenomena in 63 patients who had been on trifluoperazine for 3–13 years: (1) static tremor; (2) muscular rigidity; (3) dystonic spasms; (4) choreiform dyskinesia; and (5) restlessness and akathisia. Factor analysis defined 3 types:

1. Restlessness of trunk and all four limbs (32·5 per cent of variance)
2. Tremor of upper limbs with rigidity at wrists and elbows and facial immobility (19·1 per cent of variance)
3. Choreiform dyskinesia of tongue, lips and jaw is negatively correlated with tremor of tongue, lips and jaw (13·0 per cent of the variance).

Persistent Oral Dyskinesia and Brain Damage. Edwards (1970) reported on 34 elderly women with chronic psychiatric illness and persistent oral dyskinesia who were compared with matched controls on similar dosage of phenothiazines and found in the former a high incidence of brain damage (28 out of 34). The criteria of brain damage were: focal cerebral attacks; confusional episodes; incontinence; character change; neurological signs; perplexity; atypical psychiatric syndromes; grossly abnormal EEG; and inability to learn the meaning of 6 out of 10 new words after 6 trials (Modified Word-Learning Test of Walton).

Thiopropazate Hydrochloride in Persistent Dyskinesia. Thiopropazate was found to be significantly more effective than a placebo in relieving dyskinesia in 23 psychotic patients who had been on prolonged phenothiazine therapy (Singer & Cheng, 1971). The trial was placebo-controlled and each patient had the dyskinesia for at least one month and was treated for three weeks with either the placebo or thiopropazate. When the latter was given psychotic behaviour also improved.

Photosensitivity. Patients on high doses or who are particularly sensitive should be protected from sunlight or ultra-violet light. Some alarming skin reactions on the exposed parts can result but this is a variable condition and many can expose themselves to sunlight with impunity. As with skin sensitivity, antihistamine drugs are of value. Some have attributed a bluish skin discolouration of the face (*un visage mauve*) to prolonged high dosage and it has been linked with the diffuse melanodermia sometimes seen in endocrine disorders.

Lactation. The breasts may engorge and lactate and unless this action of the drug is explained, the patient may worry unnecessarily, particularly as a positive Aschheim-Zondek has also been reported following administration of the drug.

Pyrexia. This may occur without the presence of jaundice and can be associated with general malaise. Reducing or stopping the drug is all that is necessary. Large doses of phenothiazines given in hot and humid weather may contribute to heat stroke.

Hypotensive Effects. Some people, particularly the old and demented, are susceptible, but others may feel 'light-headed' and 'faint'. Reducing the drug or nursing the patient in bed is the answer and the condition frequently settles.

Barraclough and Sharpey-Schafer (1963) demonstrated acute loss of circulatory reflexes in poisoning due to phenothiazines, barbiturates and monoamine oxidase inhibitors. These are particularly dangerous in chronic problems, such as alcoholic and diabetic neuritis as well as tabes dorsalis, for reversal of the process even by increasing the blood volume with a plasma expander may be unsuccessful. In the acute cases, this is the method of choice once the diagnosis has been made. The condition is not sufficiently recognized for the mechanism is rarely appreciated.

Phenothiazines interfere with orthostasis by inhibiting centrally mediated pressor reflexes and by peripheral alpha-adrenergic blocking action. Jefferson (1972) has stressed the importance of distinguishing the drowsiness occasionally seen with postural hypotension, for, if it is regarded as sleep, the appropriate corrective measures of laying the person down and encouraging the pumping action of the leg muscles may be omitted. Otherwise a potentially fatal situation may arise. It is the present writer's practice when giving large doses of chlorpromazine to monitor the patient for postural hypotension (standing and lying) till stability has been reached. It has the added advantage in that as some patients complain of symptoms suggestive of postural hypotension, these can be correctly assessed.

Sudden Death. Moore and Book (1970) reviewed 12 cases who died suddenly and unexpectedly under phenothiazine therapy. No morphological changes in the brain were found, and the authors postulate that it could be due to chemical interference with the neural mechanisms affecting cardiac rhythm and leading to ventricular fibrillation or cardiac arrest, or asphyxia due to depression of the cough reflex.

Other Phenothiazines

Since the advent of chlorpromazine, there has been a spate of similar drugs which have been alleged to be less toxic or more specific in action. It is doubtful if any are more effective and the sheet anchor tranquillizer is still chlorpromazine, which in the acutely disturbed patient, has a certainty of action which the others cannot match; in fact their efficacy is frequently measured against the original drug. Some, however, are useful in cases of chlorpromazine sensitivity or resistance. While emphasizing the present supremacy of chlorpromazine, it would be wrong to suggest that it could not be supplanted by an equally or more efficient drug with fewer side-effects, and an open but critical mind should be kept on all new claims.

Promazine Hydrochloride. The chlorine atom on the phenothiazine nucleus has been replaced by the hydrogen one and this manoeuvre has been claimed to make it less toxic, but it is generally less effective. It has also been responsible for agranulocytosis and increased tendency to epileptic fits but is reported to be less liable to cause jaundice. Dosage is about equal to chlorpromazine.

Piperazine Side-chain

Prochlorperazine. This is an analogue of chlorpromazine and the chlorine atom is retained. It is not as effective in psychotic states and is more useful in the treatment of nausea and vomiting. It is more liable to cause somnolence and, in large doses, Parkinsonism. Liver damage is negligible. Dose is 15–30 mg. daily.

Perphenazine. This, too, has retained the chlorine atom and its action is very similar to chlorpromazine but is said to be six times stronger. Some have claimed success for it in the milder disorders but those who have tried using it with a large number of patients showing a variety of disorders, found it effective mainly in the acutely disturbed (Ayd, 1957). Dose is 2–4 mg. t.d.s. and it is rare to exceed 16 mg./day.

Trifluoperazine. This is alleged to be less toxic to the liver than chlorpromazine and is probably as effective as chlorpromazine. It does, however, induce Parkinsonism more readily and oculogyric crises are not infrequently seen. It has the capacity of inducing a dystonia of mouth and tongue with torsion spasms and myoclonic jerkings to a greater extent than one meets with chlorpromazine. The drug is a useful substitute for chlorpromazine in resistant cases, or where it produces somnolence. Dose is 2–4 mg. t.d.s.

Thiopropazate. This has retained the chlorine atom, and it has no real advantage over chlorpromazine. It causes hypotension, blurred vision and Parkinsonism, as well as jaundice and skin rashes. Dose is 5–30 mg. t.d.s.

Piperidine Side-chain

Mepazine. The action of mepazine is similar to chlorpromazine but it has an even more formidable list of side-effects including visual disturbances, paralytic ileus, jaundice, agranulocytosis, atonia of the bladder and postural hypotension. Ayd (1957) regards its clinical use as hazardous and though it is reputed to be twice as strong as chlorpromazine it has no real advantage.

Thioridazine. This was initially alleged to be less toxic than chlorpromazine, but with increasing use, undesirable effects are being reported, including retinal damage when given in large doses. It can produce breast enlargement but jaundice and extrapyramidal effects have not been reported. Dosage is 100–200 mg. t.d.s.

Fluphenazine Enanthate. The enanthate ester of fluphenazine gives promise of controlling schizophrenic symptoms with one injection of 25 mg. for 10–28 days. This has obvious advantages, for the greatest single cause of relapse in a schizophrenic illness which has been brought under control is failure by the patient to take the prescribed drugs. The drug has marked Parkinsonian side effects, so it should be coupled with benzhexol and a small dose should be given initially in case of hypersensitivity. It is still being evaluated and apart from the Parkinsonian and dystonic features, reports are encouraging. The enanthate has now been superseded by the decanoate, and the drug has now a firm place in long-term treatment of schizophrenia.

Phenothiazine Maintenance Therapy in Schizophrenia

Leff and Wing (1971) tried to determine the value of such maintenance therapy in an out-patient population who had recently recovered from an acute episode of schizophrenia. Those in the trial (treated and placebo controls) amounted to 20 and 15 respectively and the trial lasted for one year. Of 12 who completed the placebo trial, 10 (83 per cent) relapsed and 2 remained well; of the 18 who completed the trial on the active drug, 6 relapsed. Eighty-one patients were not included in the trial because the prognosis was considered favourable in any case or they were too precarious to be given a placebo. Their overall relapse rate was 56·9 per cent compared with a relapse rate of 53·3 per cent in both the trial patients (drug and placebo groups combined).

The follow-up showed that a patient who was given a good prognosis did well without drugs and the authors conclude that in a first episode of illness with acute onset with features of a psychotic depression and a good pre-morbid personality, maintenance therapy does not appear necessary.

Hirsch *et al.* (1973) were able to demonstrate the advantages of this form of medication in out-patient maintenance treatment of schizophrenics using a double-blind placebo trial (see under Schizophrenia, Chapter 13).

Depression Following Slow-release Fluphenazine Therapy

Alarcon and Carney (1969) reported 16 patients in whom schizophrenia was initially diagnosed and who developed severe depression after being treated with long-acting fluphenazine. In five patients suicide occurred. It is debatable if the total could be entirely due to the fluphenazine. It presupposes that an affective component was absent prior to treatment but this is unlikely as it may have been masked. Furthermore, many schizophrenics have depressive features and do commit suicide with or without phenothiazines. Nevertheless the authors' caution that patients on long-acting fluphenazine be carefully supervised should be heeded.

Mutism induced by Phenothiazines

Behrman (1972) reported a syndrome of mutism in 11 patients treated with phenothiazines in average doses referred to one physician in one year. In the majority, speech loss was almost complete, but unlike aphasics, they could respond to repeated questioning by simple utterances, usually in a whisper; occasionally they could speak appropriately and normally. About half showed one or more neurological toxic signs, e.g. akathisia, buccal dyskinesias, dystonias, tremor and Parkinsonism.

The condition followed a similar course in each patient, usually starting within several weeks of treatment though in a few it occurred 18 months later. Disturbances of speech with aphonia and impaired articulation were frequently the first signs to occur and later the whisper developed with slurring of syllables and a tendency for sentences to end in an unintelligible mutter and then complete loss of vocalization supervened. Disintegration of mental functions rapidly followed, the patient becoming increasingly more inert, and eventually lapsing into akinetic mutism.

In six patients the mutism gradually remitted when phenothiazines were stopped; in one patient who developed it after a week, it remitted within a week of stopping the treatment, but progress was much slower in the remaining cases. The author suggests that such features should alert the doctor to an idiosyncratic response to the drug.

FLUPENTHIXOL

This drug belongs to the thiaxanthenes which resemble in many respects the phenothiazine derivatives to which they are

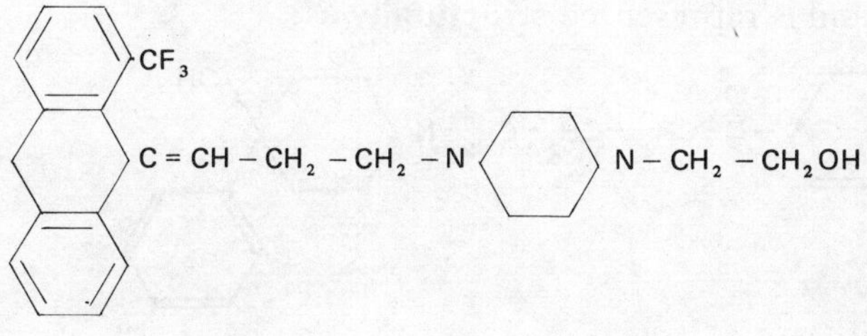

CF_3

$C = CH - CH_2 - CH_2 - N \quad N - CH_2 - CH_2OH$

related. It has gained a reputation, particularly in Scandinavia, as an effective antipsychotic agent and possessing, in addition, a fairly marked alerting action, so that it has been found useful in the apathetic or anergic types of schizophrenia. It is unsuitable for patients in whom agitation or restlessness predominates. Onset of action is more rapid than with analogous phenothiazine derivatives, and effect is shorter.

Gottfries (1971) reported a double-blind controlled trial, comparing its efficacy with trifluoperazine and found it to be roughly comparable. Like fluphenazine, it has been put up as a decanoate with a long action and is thus the second preparation to cater for the problem of the schizophrenic patient who neglects to take his medication. It has a greater tendency to produce striatal side-effects, but is beginning to gain a reputation as an anti-depressant agent (Reiter, 1969) which may be useful, as some patients report severe depression when on fluphenazine decanoate.

It is given by deep intramuscular injection in doses of 20–40 mg. (1–2 ml.) at intervals of 2–4 weeks depending on response. Fresh patients should start with a test dose of 20 mg. (1 ml.) and patient response and appearance of extrapyramidal symptoms should be carefully assessed over the following 5–10 days. If there is no over-reaction the dose may be repeated or increased. Those transferred from phenothiazine depot dosage should start with 20–40 mg. of flupenthixol, and, if necessary, antiparkinson agents should be used. As with all oily preparations, it is important to ensure by aspiration prior to injection that inadvertent intravascular injection does not occur.

It is still too early to decide whether the claims that it is superior to fluphenazine decanoate are substantiated, but it is being increasingly used as an alternative.

THE BUTYROPHENONES

These are a group of drugs whose chemical structure is related to γ-amino butyric acid (GABA) which is a product of normal brain metabolism. The one which is now established in clinical practice is haloperidol and is represented structurally as:

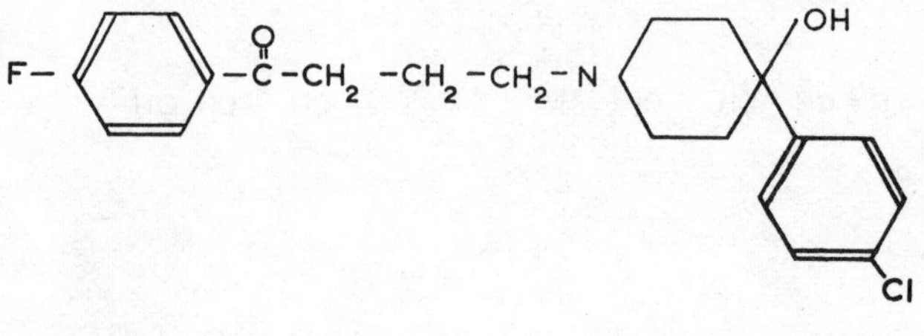

$$F-C_6H_4-\overset{O}{\overset{\|}{C}}-CH_2-CH_2-CH_2-N\langle\text{(piperidine, OH)}\rangle-C_6H_4-Cl$$

The influence of haloperidol on the brain content of GABA and other amino acids has been studied in rats and though it can produce significant changes in the amino acid content in respect to a number of different compounds there is no evidence of a selective effect on GABA or monoamine oxidase.

Historically, haloperidol derived from studies of substituted piperidine compounds. Some of these belong to the class of narcotic analgesics such as meperidine (pethidine) and substituted meperidine derivatives with side chain lengths up to 3-carbon atoms which may have analgesic properties depending on other structural features. The compounds with a 4-carbon side chain, including haloperidol and other related butyrophenones are completely lacking in the analgesic properties of the narcotic drugs. In monkeys, haloperidol fails to suppress morphine abstinence signs and it induces no opiate-like physical dependence.

Action

This is similar to the more potent phenothiazines except that it has negligible adrenolytic activity and no significant effect on blood pressure.

Clinical Uses

The author has not regarded haloperidol as a first choice in those conditions which traditionally respond to chlorpromazine, such as schizophrenic disorders, paranoid reactions and in the treatment of drug addiction. It has proved valuable in acute mania and has the edge on large doses of chlorpromazine. It was so frequently resorted to as a second choice that it has now become a first choice for that condition, either alone or supported with chlorpromazine. Persistent delirium tremens which is resistant to phenothiazines particularly when hallucinosis has supervened, also responds quickly.

Dosage

Haloperidol (Serenace) is put up in tablets of 1·5 mg. and 3–4 tablets/day is a minimum dose for the severely disturbed. Generally 3 mg. t.d.s. or even more is required and in an emergency 6 mg. t.d.s. can be used coupled with chlorpromazine 100 mg. t.d.s. After the condition has been brought under control the dose can be reduced gradually but a maintenance dose of not less than 1·5 mg. t.d.s. for some months is needed in manic patients.

Side - effects

Extrapyramidal. These are similar to those described as a result of phenothiazine treatment and are usually found after high dosage and resemble the excitomotor dystonic syndrome seen with the more potent phenothiazines rather than Parkinsonian rigidity. They consist of painful muscular spasms involving most commonly the face, neck and eyes and when severe, may resemble oculogyric crises. More rarely, dysarthria and dysphagia may appear. These reactions occur early in treatment, are not related to total dosage and are seldom seen if a small dose is given initially and gradually increased. They are easily controlled if the drug is temporarily discontinued or, rather surprisingly, if the patient is given 50 mg. of chlorpromazine (i.m.i.). Antiparkinson treatment by benzhexol, either orally or parenterally, controls the painful muscular spasms and it may be possible to continue with haloperidol at the same dose the following day without recurrence of dystonic reactions. It is usual with high dosage to give benzhexol (Artane) 2 mg. t.d.s. concurrently.

Pseudo-Parkinsonism. This occurs later in treatment and is more commonly restricted to muscular rigidity and fixed facies, the other features such as tremor, ataxia, festinant gait and increased salivation being more rare.

Motor Restlessness. This is a minor form of excitomotor reaction and consists of an uncontrolled restlessness with continual changing of position by sitting, standing or walking about.

Other Side-effects. These are uncommon and consist of drowsiness, increased salivation, hyperpyrexia and skin reactions.

Precautions

The drug should be used with caution in patients with lesions of the basal ganglia, including spastic cerebral syndromes of arteriosclerotic origin, as some of these patients may have occult basal ganglia damage. It has no anticonvulsant effect so if given to epileptics, the anticonvulsant drugs will also be required.

Droperidol

Droperidol is another butyrophenone which Neff *et al.* (1972) reported as useful in the rapid control of agitation. Doses of 1–4 ml. (2·5–10 mg.) were given intramuscularly, and after 30 minutes 75 per cent were showing evidence of reduction in agitation and in 60 minutes 85 per cent were responding. Out of 32 patients, 2 showed extrapyramidal symptoms which resolved with standard anti-parkinson agents without recurrence. The authors claim that it has an extremely high therapeutic/toxic ratio compared to chlorpromazine. It remains to be seen whether this drug has advantages over the other butyrophenones, haloperidol and triperidol.

Benperidol

This drug, which is a synthetic neuroleptic of the butyrophenone series has the following chemical structure:

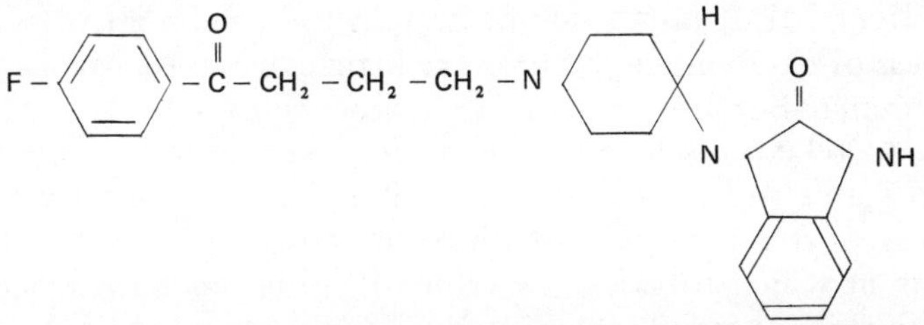

It is regarded as a useful agent for inhibiting sexual desire and it has therefore been tried on sexual offenders (Field, 1973). He treated 28 male patients who had been convicted of offences against children, 14 of whom were serving prison sentences and 14 were discharged and attending out-patient departments as a condition of probation. After 18 months' treatment with benperidol they all reported that the drug had effectively controlled their abnormal sex drive and none was charged with a further sexual offence.

Antiparkinson Drugs and the Major Tranquillizers

Because of the tendency for the major tranquillizers, phenothiazines or butyrophenones, to produce extrapyramidal signs (EPS) it is customary to cover this contingency with antiparkinson drugs. It has not been accurately established at what dose level this should be done and if the patient is under constant supervision it has been customary to wait and see and treat such side-effects when they occurred.

Pecknold *et al.* (1971) tried to define the indications for the use of antiparkinson drugs by suddenly withdrawing such medication in 77 in-patients who were also on neuroleptic drugs. There was no recurrence or first occurrence of EPS in 64, while 13 did have a recurrence and had to go back on the drug. The authors concluded that prophylactic antiparkinson therapy should not be given routinely. They also showed that patients with lesser dosage of neuroleptics developed EPS more frequently, and that recurrence was not related to high levels of neuroleptic medication.

OTHER PREPARATIONS

The following are some of the preparations which have enjoyed and may still enjoy some reputation in the treatment of neurotic states:

Meprobamate. This is chemically related to the muscle relaxant mephenesin, and has similar properties in addition to its tranquillizing effects. It is not a potent drug in the treatment of acute mental illness or excitement and has very little place in the treatment of schizophrenia. Because of its relative absence of side-effects and its capacity to relax muscle it has been used extensively for anxiety and tension states and minor psychiatric illness and there have been enthusiastic reports. This field of illness is, however, a notoriously difficult one in which to assess the value of a drug, since the placebo reactor is lurking behind every bush, which, coupled with the fluctuating nature of these conditions, defy the most carefully prepared therapeutic trials.

Tablets contain 400 mg. Dose, 1–6 tabs. per day.

Side-effects are rare, the commonest being drowsiness which is counteracted by giving *d*-amphetamine sulphate. Addiction is not uncommon and this may lead to overdosage, while withdrawal can lead to a state of tension and craving.

Benzodiazepines. These constitute a group of drugs which have become extremely popular as minor tranquillizers, though they have other actions.

Chlordiazepoxide. This is marketed as an *anxiolytic* drug and has the following structural formula:

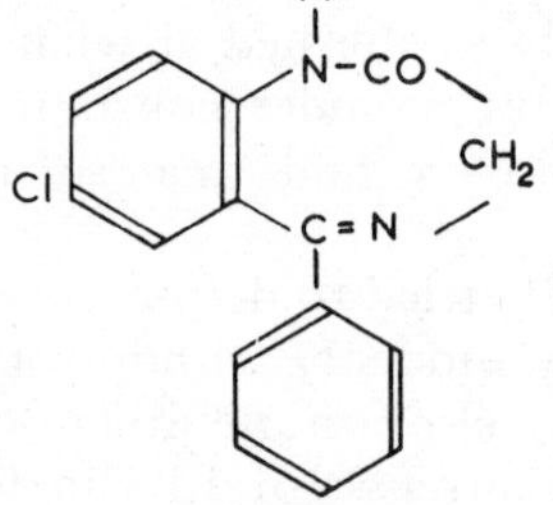

It has gained a vogue as a minor tranquillizer in the treatment of anxiety and tension states and no doubt, like many of its predecessors, satisfies some of the minor problems found in general practice. In the more severe problems it has no special use and in addition it tends to be addictive. It is difficult for the hospital psychiatrist or physician to evaluate such drugs, for the type of patient who apparently benefits rarely comes his way. It has been gaining a reputation in the treatment of delirium tremens, and if this proves to be so it will have earned its place in hospital treatment. Dosage is 50 mg./day for delirium tremens.

Diazepam. This is another anxiolytic drug and is chemically related to chlordiazepoxide. It has the following structural formula:

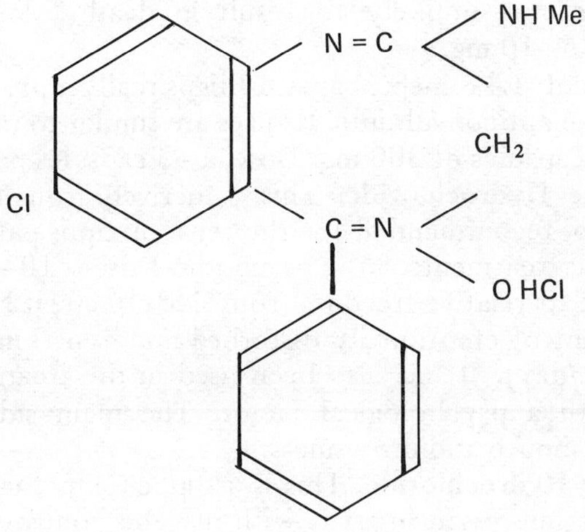

NH Me
N = C
CH_2
Cl
C = N
O HCl

It is reckoned to be more potent than chlordiazepoxide and has earned a reputation as a muscle relaxant, particularly in the treatment of the interesting condition called the Stiff Person Syndrome. It enjoys considerable popularity in general practice in the treatment of milder disorders, but is ineffective with greater degrees of morbidity seen in hospital practice. Dosage is 20 mg./day.

It has also been used in dental 'anaesthesia'. It is given intravenously (20 mg.) and the patient is not only fully relaxed and free of pain but has little memory for the event in spite of being conscious. Some psychiatrists have been using intravenous injections to decondition phobic anxiety states with varying success. As with intravenous barbiturates there is a tendency for patients to become dependent. It is of real value in the treatment of status epilepticus.

Nitrazepam.

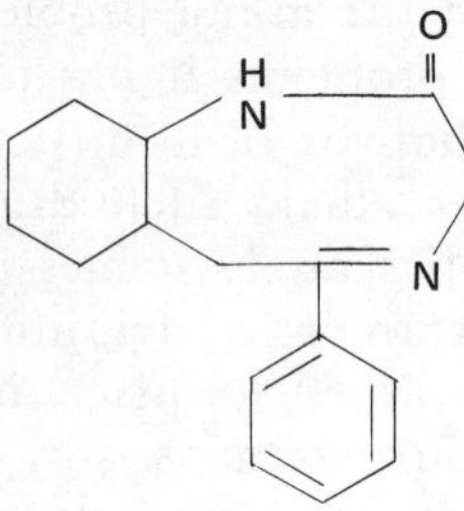

This bids fair to be the best hypnotic of the century. It is effective and strongly counters excess of paradoxical (REM) sleep. It has very little in the way of side-effects and is very safe. Even a large overdose is unlikely to result in death (Matthew *et al.*, 1969). Dose is 5–10 mg.

Phenaglycodol. Like meprobamate this is really a propanediol and is related to the anticonvulsants. Its uses are similar to meprobamate. It is put up in capsules of 300 mg. Dose, 1–3 capsules per day.

Hydroxyzine Hydrochloride. This is derived from the diphenyl methane group, recommended for the tense anxious patient, but has no place in the treatment of the psychoses. Dose is 10–50 mg. t.d.s. and because of its relative freedom from side-effects, it has been used in the treatment of emotionally disturbed and hyperkinetic children (200–300 mg./day). It has also been used in the treatment of skin conditions with a psychological factor. The main side-effects are dryness of the mouth and drowsiness.

Benactyzine Hydrochloride. This is a diphenyl methane derivative which has not impressed in trials with placebo controls. Dose, 1–3 mg./day.

Ectylurea. This is an ureide derivative which is used chiefly for daytime sedation. Dose, 150 mg. four-hourly–450 mg. nocte.

Azacyclonol. This is an isomer of piperadol hydrochloride but with a different effect. It is capable of obliterating model psychoses induced by LSD 25 or mescaline. It has been used for hallucinated schizophrenics though it is not constant in its action, but it is relatively free from side-effects and is alleged to enhance the efficiency of chlorpromazine and reserpine.

Methaqualone and Diphenhydramine Hydrochloride (Mandrax). Hypnotics are commonly prescribed, and while they have their place they also have their dangers. Barbiturates have had a long spell of popularity, but their addictive properties, their serious withdrawal effects and above all, their use as an agent for suicide attempts have made their prescription less popular. Newer hypnotics have been produced, and one which is still popular is a combination of methaqualone, 250 mg. and diphenhydramine hydrochloride 25 mg., marketed as Mandrax. It is effective as a hypnotic but is unfortunately a very effective poison and as such has replaced barbiturates.

Matthew *et al.* (1968) reported on 116 patients who were admitted to the Edinburgh Royal Infirmary during the 18 months ending 31st December 1967. They strongly advise against forced diuresis which may aggravate the tendency to pulmonary oedema and myocardial damage, and at the same time is quite ineffective in eliminating methaqualone or its metabolites. Another danger is that many patients take the drug prior to going to bed, run their bath, and get in. It is then that the drug is at its most potent, and some have been overwhelmed with a deep sleep while in the bath and have drowned. The author no longer uses it, preferring nitrazepam (5–10 mg.), which does not have this dangerous action and is not a dangerous suicidal agent.

BARBITURATES

These derive from barbital, which was first synthesized by Fischer and von Mering in 1903, and were, until recently, the most popular hypnotics; once a patient had been prescribed them, he was unlikely to be satisfied with a substitute. Unfortunately, because of their popularity and widespread distribution, they were the commonest vehicle for attempting suicide, though second to carbon monoxide in successful suicide.

Chemistry

Cumming (1961) summarizes the chemistry:

> Barbituric acid results from the condensation of malonic acid and urea.

```
                          O
      H                   ‖                     H
      N—H          HO—C                  N—C      H
     /                     \                 /       \    /
O=C                      CH₂  ——→  O=C          C
     \                     /                 \       /    \
      N—H          HO—C                  N—C      H
      H                   ‖                     H
                          O
```

the pyrimidine nucleus

Table of common barbiturates

B.P. Name	Common Name	R_1	R_2	Dose (mg.)
Group I. Short acting (3–6 hours duration)				
Quinalbarbitone (Na)	Seconal	Allyl	1. Methyl-butyl	50–200
Cyclobarbitone	Phanodorm	Ethyl	Cyclo-hexenyl	200–400
Group II. Medium acting (4–8 hours duration)				
Pentobarbitone (Na)	Nembutal	Ethyl	1. Methyl-butyl	100–200
Butobarbitone	Soneryl	Ethyl	Sec-butyl	100–200
Amylobarbitone	Amytal	Ethyl	Iso-amyl	100–200
Group III. Long acting (8–16 hours duration)				
Phenobarbitone	Luminal	Ethyl	Phenyl	30–120
Phenobarbitone (Na)	Soluble luminal	Ethyl	Phenyl	30–120
Barbitone (Na)	Veronal	Ethyl	Ethyl	300–600

Therapeutic Indications

These are primarily to induce sleep, though they may be prescribed during the day for acute anxiety states following a traumatic experience. They should not be prescribed for chronic anxiety or tension states as they can readily become drugs of addiction and the resulting addiction may prove a more serious problem in therapy than the original psychiatric condition. Some firms market preparations where the short- and long-acting barbiturates are combined in order to cope with the individual disturbance of the sleep rhythm. This has its danger for it treats insomnia as the disease itself, rather than as a symptom. For example, the early morning waking may be the main evidence of an underlying depression and to deal with this aspect in isolation may mean leaving the patient without effective treatment for an illness which carries a serious risk of suicide.

Action on the Central Nervous System

This is summarized thus by Cumming (1961):

> All degrees of central depression from mild sedation to deep anaesthesia may be achieved with barbiturates, dependent only upon dose of drug, method of administration and the previous level of reflex excitability. The method of action on the central nervous system has been a matter for debate, but it is now generally agreed that attempts to localize such action to any particular anatomical structure are probably misguided, and that the drug acts at all levels in greater or lesser degree. With an adequate oral dose of barbiturates, sleep

ensues within 20–60 minutes and closely simulates normal sleep, both with respect to subjective response and to EEG investigation. With sufficient dosage surgical anaesthesia may be induced in a similar manner to the volatile anaesthetics but having some differences, for instance in the relative ratio of muscle relaxation and respiratory depression. The barbiturates produce a more marked respiratory depression. The analgesic actions of barbiturates are small, and pain sensation remains substantially unimpaired when the patient is almost asleep, having taken a therapeutic dose. The psychic response to the experience of pain is, however, modified. In adequate dose all the commonly used barbiturates exert an anticonvulsive action and will control convulsions initiated by strychnine, tetanus or epilepsy. Phenobarbitone has a selectively anti-convulsant activity which is unrelated to its narcotic effects since these may be counteracted with amphetamine without abolishing the anticonvulsant action.

Removal of the drug is by destruction in the tissues and excretion in the urine. Cumming (1961) writes:

The liver is the chief organ of detoxication, and the process is effected principally by oxidation of the side chains to alcohols, ketones and carboxylic acid derivatives. These compounds may then be conjugated with glucuronic acid or excreted unchanged in the urine. The residual ring structure possesses little pharmacological activity as a narcotic, and is rarely disrupted by hydrolysis into urea and malonic acid, only traces being excreted.

The medium-acting compounds amylobarbitone, pentobarbitone and quin-albarbitone are mainly degraded by the liver, whilst butobarbitone and cyclobarbitone are degraded by the liver and also excreted by the kidneys. The long-acting barbiturates phenobarbitone and barbitone are mainly excreted by the kidneys without modification. The very short acting barbiturates like thiopentone are deposited rapidly in body fat, then slowly detoxicated by the liver and excreted by the kidney.

Renal elimination occurs slowly, and this may explain the long action of the two drugs which depend in large measure on this route. Renal clearance of barbiturate occurs in the same way as that for urea. This fact is of some significance, since it implies that renal clearance during an osmotic diuresis is greatly increased. Fifty to sixty per cent of filtered barbitone is excreted as compared with only 10 per cent during water diuresis.

The respective dependence of the two long-acting compounds on the renal route of excretion is exemplified by the fact that 80 per cent of barbitone and 25 per cent of phenobarbitone may be recovered unchanged in the urine. Since excretion is slow, this creates the conditions for the cumulative toxicity seen in repeated dosage of barbiturates. Only 20 per cent of a therapeutic dose of barbitone is excreted in 24 hours. When these and other barbiturates dependent on renal excrction are administered in the presence of renal insufficiency, severe poisoning may occur from rapid cumulation. Before this group of barbiturates is adminstered, information on renal function should be sought.

Barbiturate Poisoning

In Britain this is second only to coal-gas (carbon monoxide) as a cause of death from poisoning. Cumming (1961) cites the following figures for different countries showing that geographical and cultural factors influence incidence:

United Kingdom. From 1954 to 1958, approximately 14 per cent of deaths due to poisoning were from barbiturates (total 600–700) compared with 74 per cent resulting from carbon monoxide (total 3000–4000). Barbiturates were, however, the commonest cause for hospital admission.

Denmark, because it has centralized treatment for poisoning, has more reliable figures. From 1953 to 1957, 75 per cent of their admissions resulted from barbiturate overdosage.

United States has about 1500 deaths per year from barbiturate overdosage.

Cumming estimates that in England and Wales there are probably 3000 cases per year requiring admission and 6000 cases per year requiring treatment in the casualty department.

Symptoms and Signs

These vary according to whether the poisoning is mild or severe.

Mild cases display slurred speech, drowsiness, ataxia, nystagmus and hypotonia in the presence of normal respiration, blood pressure and skin colour. Corneal and gag reflexes are present and the patient is readily rousable. This does not mean that the condition will not deteriorate to a severe case of poisoning, for symptomatology depends on the amount of drug taken and its rate of absorption and removal and a severe case may go through a mild phase in the initial stages.

Severe cases are stuporose with difficulty in being roused, though they may respond to noxious stimuli. Reflexes may become impaired and blood pressure and ventilation are affected. From this stage, coma may develop and the patient is deeply unconscious and does not respond to noxious stimuli. Absent knee and ankle jerks indicate a severe degree of intoxication. Cumming (1961), whose approach to poisoning and its management differs from the traditional, does not see it as a problem of a poison and its antidote, but of disturbed physiology and its restoration. He therefore stresses the effect of the resulting arterial hypotension in reducing the renal blood flow and the potentiating of this handicap by the antidiuretic properties of barbiturates. This may result in oliguric renal failure and as the kidneys play an important part in eliminating one type of barbiturate, dialyzing, by means of an artificial kidney, may be the most rational form of treatment and it is now being commonly practised with success.

Serum barbiturate levels are, of course, diagnostic and Locket (1957) gives the following figures which are consistent with stupor and coma.

	(mg./100 ml. in blood)			
	Stupor	*Average*	*Coma*	*Average*
Amylobarbitone	0.3 - 3.1	0.8	0·3 - 6·5	1·8
Butobarbitone	0·5 - 1·8	1·4	0·8 - 3·5	2·1
Pentobarbitone	0·25- 1·1	–	0·45- 1·8	–
Quinalbarbitone	0·3 - 1·5	1·0	0·7 - 2·0	–
Phenobarbitone	2·4 -10·4	4·3	4·0 -15·2	8·0
Barbitone	5·2 -10·0	6·8	11·0 -17·0	13·4

The resuscitation of a severe case of barbiturate poisoning requires a well-equipped unit with full laboratory facilities, mechanical respirators, artificial kidney and medical team trained for the job. Although the mortality rate has been reduced to 1·7 per cent, with better facilities this figure could be improved.

Barbiturate Antagonists

Because of the frequency in the use of barbiturates in attempts at suicide, there has for long been a search for an antagonist which if combined with barbiturates would render the risks of overdosage less dangerous. Bemegride, which is an analeptic, has been advocated for such a role and there have been favourable reports. In the author's department this claim was investigated (Orwin, Sim & Waterhouse, 1964) by using the sedation threshold test (Shagass, 1954). The patient was given an intravenous injection of amylobarbitone sodium and the sedation threshold defined clinically and with EEG monitoring. A few days later bemegride was added to the barbiturate in the same proportion as in the tablets recommended, and the sedation threshold again charted for the same patient. Although in the 50 patients studied there was a statistically significant shift upwards in the sedation threshold with the bemegrated barbiturate, the clinical significance was that a dose of 2·1 g. of barbiturate required to produce sedation would have to be increased to 2·2 g. to produce the same effect. This is clinically insignificant, but in addition it illustrated that statistical analysis may be entirely at variance with clinical assessment.

Drug Overdose and Brain Recovery. It has been assumed that after a patient who had taken an overdose recovered consciousness the brain had reverted to normal function. Haider and Oswald (1970) question this assumption. In a study of 10 patients who had taken overdoses, abnormal sleep features, particularly raised paradoxical (REM) sleep persisted for up to two months. There were, in some, withdrawal symptoms, including epileptic phenomena and delirium as late as three weeks after the overdose.

ANTI–DEPRESSANTS

MONOAMINE OXIDASE INHIBITORS

These have been used extensively in the treatment of depression and though there are still doubts as to their relative efficacy, the psychiatrist should be familiar with the chemical background of their development and the theory of their action.

Monoamine oxidase is an enzyme which is widely distributed in the body and its known action is oxidatively to deaminate amines to pharmacologically inactive acidic derivatives (Davison, 1958). It probably provides the main route by which 5-hydroxytryptamine is inactivated to 5-hydroxyindoleacetic acid, which is a normal constituent of the urine. The most widely-studied inhibitors of monoamine oxidase are the hydrazine derivatives of nicotinic acid or phenylethylamine of which the best known is *iproniazid* (1-isonicotinyl-2-isopropyl hydrazine), originally developed from isoniazid (isonicotinyl hydrazine) which is used in the treatment of tuberculosis, and whose monoamine oxidase inhibitor effect *in vitro* was described by Zeller *et al.* (1952). Not only does isoniazid inhibit the growth of the tubercle bacillus, but it also produces euphoria and mental alertness, and this led to the drug being used for depression. Iproniazid, while not as bacteriostatic as isoniazid, has a more marked euphoriant effect. Schayer *et al.* (1954) showed that iproniazid inhibited monoamine oxidase *in vivo* and conclusions were drawn by others that the euphoriant effect of the drug was related to this inhibition. As iproniazid was toxic, particularly to the liver, a search was started for monoamine oxidase inhibitors which were less toxic and more effective, hoping thereby to produce a better antidepressant drug, and phenelzine (β-phenylethyl hydrazine) and nialamide (1- 2-(benzylcarbamyl)ethyl 2-isonicotinyl hydrazine) among others have undergone clinical trials with varying degrees of success as far as their antidepressant action is concerned, though they have less side-effects than iproniazid. In a leader in the *British Medical Journal* (1959*a*) the problem is reviewed thus:

The postulated relation between therapeutic action and monoamine inhibition forms an attractive, if tentative, hypothesis for which there is considerable experimental evidence. For example, in a study of a series of monoamine oxidase inhibitors some degree of correlation was found between capacity to inhibit monoamine oxidase and therapeutic effectiveness (Pletscher, 1959). But there are other observations which suggest a more complex picture. Thus isoniazid, structurally closely related to iproniazid, is also a central stimulant and has been used in the treatment of depression (Salzer, 1953), yet as a monoamine oxidase inhibitor it is inactive (Zeller *et al.*, 1952). Conversely, the compound 1-benzyl-2methyl-5-methoxytryptamine is an effective monoamine oxidase inhibitor in man, but has tranquillizing and sedative rather than stimulating properties (Feldstein *et al.*, 1959). Furthermore, the observation that the major route of metabolism of adrenaline and noradrenaline involves methylation to give the pharmacologically inactive 3-methoxy derivatives, and that this occurs before oxidative deamination by monoamine oxidase (La Brosse *et al.*, 1958), makes it difficult to relate the central action of the monoamine oxidase inhibitor to an effect on the rate of inactivation of the catechol amines. It is perhaps pertinent to recall that the theory of monoamine oxidase inhibition of the pharmacological actions of ephedrine and amphetamine receives little support today (Goodman & Gilman, 1955). At all events it is clear that, until we know more about the normal physiological functions of amines in the body, only tentative interpretations are possible.

The first of the monoamine oxidase inhibitors (iproniazid) was alleged to cause fatal jaundice in up to 1 in 250 patients treated, but with the advent of phenelzine, nialamide, phenylisopropyl hydrazide and isocarboxazid, the physician has a wide range of these drugs which are less toxic to the liver, but unfortunately not entirely devoid of undesirable and occasionally dangerous side-effects.

Sargant and Dally (1962) have used the monoamine oxidase inhibitors, phenelzine, isocarboxazid, phenoxypropazine and iproniazid in the treatment of anxiety states, or what some would call neurotic depression. They report favourable results and receive support from Hare *et al.* (1962) who claim that phenelzine owes its therapeutic effect in depression to a sedative action, which relieves the anxiety, rather than to any specific antidepressant effect. The main therapeutic effect of these drugs is in psychotic depression, provided it is not too severe. To claim that because a depressive illness responds to a monoamine oxidase inhibitor it belongs to the neurotic group, and that if it fails to do so, it belongs to the psychotic group is really mistaking severity of a reaction for its nature. Pare *et al.* (1962) have gone further and postulated that there are two genetically determined specific types of depression which can be distinguished by their response to monoamine oxidase inhibitors or imipramine respectively, and that there is therefore a different biochemical basis for these reactions. Reliable evidence in support has not been produced.

Those still in common use are:
phenelzine, iproniazid, isocarboxazid, and tranylcypromine and while there are many psychiatrists who prefer to use them, there is now a considerable body of evidence that they are not as effective in the treatment of depression (psychotic) as other antidepressants or E.C.T., and that they are responsible for many dangerous and even fatal side-effects.

The Medical Research Council (1965) compared the treatment of depression by E.C.T., imipramine, phenelzine and a placebo. The enquiry was based on 250 patients from various parts of the country and results were estimated on a short and long term basis. E.C.T. and imipramine (see below) came out best and phenelzine did no better then the placebo.

Side-effects

Drugs of doubtful value have been used in the practice of medicine for centuries, and many patients, and doctors too, have sworn as to their efficacy. When drugs have dangerous side-effects and more effective treatments are available and are safer, one must have compelling reasons for continuing to use the more dangerous drugs, especially now that the mechanisms involved in these side-effects are understood.

Pressor (hypertensive) attacks. The first description of such attacks was by Ogilvie (1955) who reported severe headaches associated with palpitations, flushes, sweats and raised blood-pressure in 4 out of 42 patients receiving iproniazid but not in 47 patients receiving isoniazid which is not a monoamine oxidase inhibitor. The cause was unexplained until Blackwell (1963) incriminated cheese as a precipitating factor and Astoor *et al.* (1963) provided evidence that tyramine which is present in cheese was the active pharmacological agent. In normal subjects the ingestion of cheese is followed by the excretion of large amounts of the harmless phenolic acid ρ-hydroxyphenylacetic acid which is formed from tyramine by oxidative deamination and is an intermediary metabolite. In patients treated with monoamine oxidase inhibitors, tyramine remains unoxidized and being a pressor amine it produces severe clinical effects.

Horwitz *et al.* (1964) found that all types of cheese examined except cream and cottage cheese contained considerable amounts of tyramine, New York State Cheddar having the highest (1416 μg./g.). Beers and wines contained rather small amounts except Chianti (24 μg,/ml.). As little as 20 g. of Cheddar cheese could initiate a pressor response in a patient treated with the monoamine oxidase inhibitor, pargyline, and it could be controlled by injecting phentolamine, thus confirming what was already known, viz. that tyramine produced its effects mainly by releasing adrenaline and noradrenaline.

Although Chianti contained less tyramine, when more was drunk compared with cheese eaten, it was shown that between one-tenth to one-hundredth of the amount of tyramine was required during monoamine oxidase inhibition to produce the pressor effect compared with control periods. Cheese samples vary in their content and this may explain why some people can eat cheese while on these drugs with impunity, while others suffer.

Other foodstuffs have been incriminated such as broad beans which contain DOPA. Yeast extract prepared by autolysis and subsequent fermentation contained as much as Cheddar cheese, *i.e.* 1·5 mg./g. Yeast extract also contains histamine which can further aggravate the reaction.

Tranylcypromine has been the greatest offender of the MAOI group in this respect and there have been numerous reports of subarachnoid haemorrhage with fatal results, though sudden severe headaches with flushing are much commoner.

Other Side-effects As if some hypertensive crises were not enough, these drugs are dangerous when combined with pethidine or with other anti-depressants such as imipramine or with amphetamine which has certain affinities with the MAOI group. This can prove difficult in treatment, for in order to change over to a more effective and safer anti-depressant like imipramine, the patient must cease taking the MAOI for not less than 2 weeks.

Hypotension of a persistent nature can occur and the author had one such patient where the condition persisted in severe form for six months.

Liver Damage. Iproniazid, which was the first of the MAOI drugs to be generally used was alleged to cause *fatal* jaundice in up to 1 in 250 patients treated. Those in common use now are less lethal but severe liver damage is still reported.

Allergic Reactions. They may aggravate asthma or eczema.

Retrobulbar Neuritis. Fortunately recovery is almost complete when the MAOI is discontinued.

Combining the Anti-depressant Drugs. Some psychiatrists advocate a form of 'cocktail' by combining an MAOI drug with a tricyclic compound such as imipramine should the patient prove refractory to either. The risks are of two sorts:

1. A synergism between the milder side-effects shared by both types of drugs.

2. An acute syndrome of hyperpyrexia, excitability, coma and fluctuations in blood pressure which can lead to death.

That some doctors have used these combinations without serious sequelae does not invalidate the accumulating reports of the dangers of this practice. The main defence against accusations that MAOI drugs cause liver damage is that it is not possible to distinguish the hepatoxic effects from viral hepatitis, a case or two of which can usually be found in the area. Popper (1965) states: 'as long as there are no aetiological tests for viral hepatitis, and experimental readministration of the drugs remains absolutely contraindicated, this reaction will not be differentiated with certainty from viral hepatitis'. The doctor who prescribes such drugs can therefore feel reasonably secure that a court of law could not at present prove that he was responsible for his patient's death or severe disability. This is not the type of defence behind which a responsible doctor should shelter.

It has already been stated that antidepressant action and monoamine oxidase inhibition are not synonymous and this artificial distinction of antidepressants may be dropped without disadvantage. It would be more helpful if these drugs could be classified according to their efficacy, speed of action, toxicity and side-effects.

THE TRICYCLIC ANTI-DEPRESSANTS

IMIPRAMINE HYDROCHLORIDE

The chemical structure of imipramine resembles that of chlorpromazine

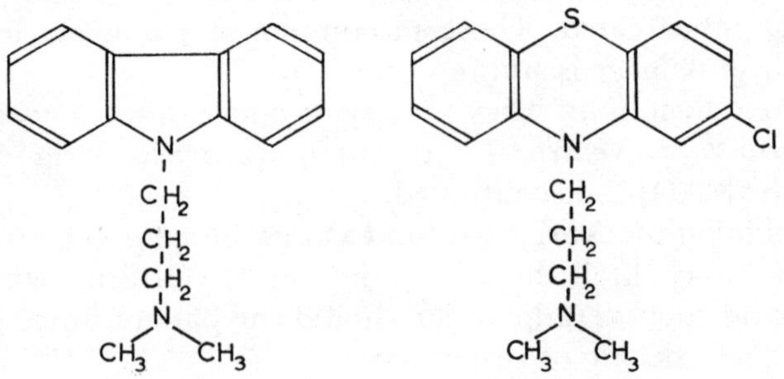

Imipramine Chlorpromazine

It is surprising that a drug with some of the sedative properties of a tranquillizer should be a most effective anti-depressant. Kühn (1957) tried out the drug in an unbiased manner and reported on its anti-depressant properties. It belongs to a group called the Tricyclic Compounds of which amytriptyline, desimipramine and trimipramine are also commonly used and it is not a monoamine oxidase inhibitor. It does not affect levels of brain amines or interfere with the release of amine by reserpine but when given together with the drug that rapidly releases brain catecholamines it can produce excitation and therefore can potentiate the action of amphetamine.

Since its introduction in 1957, numerous trials have been carried out and the general consensus is that it is the most effective and safest of the anti-depressant drugs and is the treatment of choice in those depressive states which are not severe enough to warrant a course of E.C.T.

Dosage. The patient should be started on 25 mg. t.d.s., increasing by 25 mg. daily to 50 mg. t.d.s. and all the side-effects explained as well as the delayed response. A patient may find it easier to tolerate these inconveniences if told about them beforehand. It has to be taken for 10–14 days before an adequate response is obtained and provided that the patient has reached an effective dose. As the condition is liable to persist if inadequately treated, a minimum period of eight weeks' dosage is necessary, but it may have to be continued longer. Reduction of dose should be gradual, and 25 mg./day at weekly intervals is safe, but if there is any evidence of relapse, the dose may have to be increased. Some patients may have to be maintained on imipramine for very long periods, two years or more, and therefore serious consideration should be given to the desirability of substituting a course of E.C.T. if the response is either initially unsatisfactory or chequered. It had been claimed that imipramine like other anti-depressants was useful in maintaining progress after E.C.T. or in reducing the number of treatments. The author has been unable to substantiate these claims. It does not appear to cause addiction or even habituation.

Side-effects In this waiting phase, a number of side-effects are liable to occur which to depressed patients can be very distressing and convince them that the drug is making them worse. These are: giddiness, dryness of mouth, constipation, increased sweating, skin rashes, difficulty in accommodation, urinary retention (particularly in the male), trembling and occasionally muscular jerkings. Their incidence is variable, but most complain of dryness of the mouth. The sweating and flushing in the female may lead her to attribute them to the menopause.

Cardiovascular changes occur in the form of palpitations, tachycardia, hypotension, and after exercise the ECG may show inversion of T waves in leads 1 and 2, and this finding has also been reported in cases of over-dosage. Galactorrhoea which recovered after withdrawal has been reported in a 34-year-old woman.

It is just possible that some of these side-effects may be due to other drugs which have been concurrently prescribed. Whatever else may be given with imipramine, and chlorpromazine is frequently and justifiably used, it must never be combined with a MAOI. In view of its mydriatic effect, it should not be given to patients suffering from glaucoma.

The author, who after 32 years' extensive experience with E.C.T. has had no fatality directly caused by the treatment, in his early use of imipramine had two elderly female patients who fell and fractured femurs and died. This is an important consideration in deciding whether it should be given in preference to E.C.T., for it may in old people prove more dangerous, exposing them to the risk of suicidal attempt, as well as prolonging their agony with inadequate anti-depressive measures.

Adult Poisoning from Tricyclic Antidepressants

Noble and Mathews (1969) from their vast experience report the clinical features of overdosage with tricyclic anti-depressants. There is restlessness, agitation and twitching movements with both pyramidal and extra-pyramidal signs. Some of the features resemble atropine poisoning with persistent tachycardia. Of 100 consecutive cases, 51 were in coma and it was of interest that there were no severe cases of coma with imipramine. Most patients (68 out of 100) had taken amitriptyline. There were no cardiac arrhythmias but 3 had conduction defects. All recovered eventually, but this does not reflect the gravity of overdosage by amitriptyline, which is steadily gaining a reputation as a cause of death. Sedal *et al.* (1972) stress the gravity of such over-dosage and the dangerous cardiac complications.

Combination of Tricyclics and Monoamine Oxidase Inhibitors

Theoretically such combinations are regarded as hazardous, yet Schukit *et al.* (1971) in their review of 350 out-patients, a survey of the records of 50 in-patients and a drug trial with 10 patients could find no evidence of this. They were unable to report that the combination was more effective than tricyclics alone.

Imipramine and Pregnancy.

Sim (1972) had treated 81 pregnant women who were depressed with imipramine (50 mg. t.d.s.). Forty-five received the drug throughout the pregnancy and in fact the 45 were on the drug while they became pregnant. All proceeded to term and in no instance did the child show any congenital abnormality. In a large series of puerperal psychosis (280) there were nine babies suffering from congenital defects and in no instance had the mother received imipramine during her pregnancy. This is not conclusive evidence that imipramine cannot produce congenital malformation, but it does suggest that the risk, if any, is very slight.

Imipramine in Organic Emotionalism

The author has for many years used imipramine for the treatment of depression occurring in multiple sclerosis with gratifying results. Lawson and MacLeod (1969) report its use in pseudobulbar states with organic emotionalism resulting from cerebrovascular disease. They found these conditions to be particularly responsive after a controlled double-blind trial. These findings on a small series cannot be accepted as valid for the whole population of such patients. The present writer has used imipramine in such cases with varying results. All one can say is that it is worth trying.

CLOMIPRAMINE HYDROCHLORIDE

This is a dibenzazepine derivative, 3-chloro-5-(3-dimethylaminopropyl)-10, -11-dihydro-5-H-dibenz-[b.f.]-azepine (clomipramine) hydrochloride.

$CH_2 - CH_2$

Cl

N

$CH_2 - CH_2 - CH_2 - N\langle^{CH_3}_{CH_3} \cdot HCl$

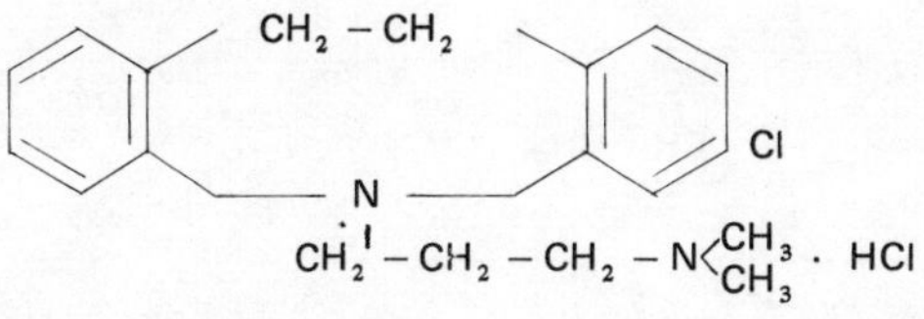

It potentiates the effect of adrenaline and noradrenaline on the blood pressure and on the contraction of the nictitating membrane of the anaesthetized cat and inhibits the pressor effect of tyramine. Its anticholinergic effect is similar to that of related tricyclic substances and investigations of its pharmacological properties suggest that is occupies an intermediary position between imipramine and amitriptyline. It has the same hypotensive drawbacks of imipramine so it should be used cautiously in elderly patients.

Contraindications and Precautions

(1) It should not be given in conjunction with or within 14 days of treatment with a monoamine oxidase inhibitor.

(2) It is contraindicated in patients with existing liver damage.

(3) ECG studies suggest it would be unwise to prescribe it in the presence of pronounced cardiac or circulatory failure, recent myocardial infarction or ischaemic heart disease, because of its hypotensive action.

(4) It may precipitate or aggravate glaucoma and retention of urine.

(5) It may cause convulsions so its use in epileptics would be undesirable.

(6) Overdosage can be very dangerous so a large supply should not be given to the suicidal patient.

Side-effects are similar to those of imipramine.

Generally the drug is not as effective an antidepressant as imipramine though it has been used by some psychiatrists intravenously for severe depression and a rapid response has been reported. It was at one time thought that it may be a substitute for E.C.T. but the early promises have not been fulfilled.

AMITRIPTYLINE

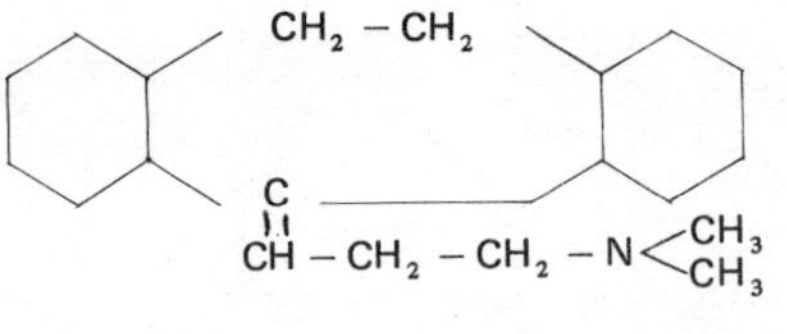

$CH_2 - CH_2$

C

$CH - CH_2 - CH_2 - N{<}^{CH_3}_{CH_3}$

This tricyclic anti-depressant has become very popular in general practice becuase it has fewer side-effects than imipramine, but is not quite as effective in the more severe depressions. It has a soporific side-effect which can be troublesome, and it has a bad record for inducing cardiac irregularities, particularly in the predisposed; it is also hepatotoxic. Dosage is 25–50 mg. t.d.s.

Epileptic Fits and Amitriptyline

Betts *et al.* (1968) described 7 patients encountered in one year where it was reasonably certain that amitriptyline in normal doses precipitated epileptic seizures. With one exception where there was a previous history of grand mal in childhood, the fits occurred within a few days of either commencing medication or changing to a higher dose. The authors suggest that patients with low convulsive thresholds, i.e. with a history of brain damage, past or present or family history of epilepsy, should be given amitriptyline only under close supervision, ideally in hospital.

Dothiepin

This is a thio analogue of amitriptyline with the formula 11-(3-dimethylaminopropylidene)-6 H-dibenz (b,c) thiepin. In clinical trials conducted by the author it is almost as effective as imipramine but has fewer undesirable side-effects, and should therefore be a suitable anti-depressant for general practice. Dosage is 50 mg. t.d.s, though one should start the patient off with 25 mg. t.d.s. and increase by 25 mg./day.

Cinanserin (2'- 3- dimethylamino-propylthio cinnamanilide Hydrochloride) in Manic and Schizophrenic Patients

Turan *et al.* (1971) conducted clinical trials on cinanserin which is

$$\begin{array}{c} O \\ \| \\ -NH-C-CH=CH- \\ S-(CH_2)_3-N(CH_3)2 \end{array}$$

Cinanserin Hydrochloride

an anti-serotonin compound, on the hypothesis that certain psychotic states were associated with a disturbance of indole metabolism, particularly 5-hydroxytryptamine (serotonin). Patients with classical manic symptoms showed dramatic global improvement within 12–24 hours after being given 300–500 mg. of cinanserin. Schizophrenic patients after three days on the drug became markedly agitated and had to be given tranquillizers. The authors concluded that cinanserin was useful in the treatment of mania, controlling the symptoms without altering the level of consciousness, but it was ineffective in schizophrenic symptoms unless these were linked with a manic state. In view of the specific nature of the drug, they suggest that the disease processes underlying mania and schizophrenia are different.

THE AMPHETAMINES

These belong to the sympathomimetic amines and are related to adrenaline (epinephrine) and ephedrine, and amphetamine was included by Barger and Dale (1910) in their survey of sympathomimetic agents. Initially used as a vasoconstrictor, its stimulant action was noted and it was tried in the treatment of narcolepsy (Prinzmetal & Bloomberg, 1935). Excessive dosage was found to maintain the waking state and Bonhoff and Lewrenz (1954) called the group Weck-(Wake)amines. They described how Africans, to increase endurance used the leaves of *Khat,* a local shrub, whose active principle, d-nor*iso*ephedrine, is a close relative of the amphetamines. In the 1930's it began to supplant caffeine as the student's favourite cerebral stimulant and its use was unfortunately not confined to the cause of learning but was (and probably still is) a popular stimulant of 'the party spirit'.

EEG Studies

Animals. In the intact conscious cat it produces desynchronization coupled with behavioural 'arousal'. In the 'encephale isolé' the intermittent electro-cortical activity was abolished but restored with midbrain section, after which further doses were without effect (Elkes *et al,,* 1954). These findings suggest that the effect on the EEG is through the mesencephalon.

Man. It produces a shift to faster frequencies with increase in total voltage level, similar to caffeine and adrenaline (epinephrine). These changes are found when dosage is high but in ordinary therapeutic doses the changes are slight and are mainly an increase in the frequency of parietal and occipital *alpha* rhythms as found in hyperkinetic and disturbed children (Cutts & Jasper, 1939), although there was a marked improvement in behaviour. A 'fatigued' EEG is restored to regular rhythm, and the classical barbiturate (fast) record is neutralized.

Physiological Effects. Vasopressor, cardiac accelerator, respiratory stimulator.

Psychological Effects. In animals, large doses increase the number of errors in rats running through a maze, previously learned.

Biochemical Studies. *In vitro,* low concentration has no effect on oxygen uptake of brain slices in a glucose medium, but it inhibits cerebral respiration at higher concentrations. Low concentrations could diminish or prevent the inhibition of respiration produced by the addition of tyramine, *beta*-indole-thylamine or iso-amylamine to the glucose medium. This action is based on three factors:

1. These amines plus tryptamine and adrenaline 'compete' for amine oxidase and are destroyed by it.
2. Amphetamine is not destroyed by amine-oxidase.
3. It is not the amines *per se* which inhibit cerebral respiration but aldehyde breakdown products and ammonia produced with the help of amine oxidase.

Mann and Quastel (1939, 1940) have suggested that the drug's efficacy in fatigue and narcolepsy may be due to these states being a result of amine metabolism. Wikler (1951) has speculated that toxic psychoses produced by large amounts of amphetamine may be related to derangement in the metabolism of amines through its inhibitory action on amine oxidase.

Clinical Uses

Amphetamine sulphate, dextroamphetamine sulphate and methyl amphetamine sulphate have similar effects, but there are individual susceptibilities. Their clinical uses are now very much less, and in some countries doctors have imposed on themselves a voluntary ban. This is not because the drugs are in themselves dangerous but because they have become popular drugs of addiction, especially with the young. Restriction in prescribing is designed to prevent the drug from leaking into the 'black market' and to remove the temptation to break into chemists' shops where they may be stored. Because of a social problem, patients are deprived of a drug which, though of limited use, has still some advantages.

Behaviour Disorders in Childhood and Adolescence (including Hyperkinesis).

Abreaction. Methyl amphetamine sulphate is usually used either by itself or combined with Pentothal. For details see under narcoanalysis (Chapter 20).

Epilepsy with Disturbed Behaviour. Not infrequently anti-convulsant drugs (particularly barbiturates) aggravate or even initiate the behaviour disturbance and a combination with amphetamine may counteract this. It has also been recommended together with Mysoline in temporal lobe seizures which progress to twilight states. Dose is 2·5 mg. morning and noon.

Depression in the Old. Some elderly patients who would react with severe hypotension to tricyclic anti-depressants, frequently benefit from amphetamines.

Toxic Effects

1. Hypomanic excitement, accompanied by giggling and inappropriate behaviour, with garrulousness.
2. Erratic behaviour, with failure in judgement.
3. Acute psychotic states, including delirium.
4. Insomnia.
5. Tremors.
6. Cardiovascular changes—palpitation and rapid pulse.

Antidote. Chlorpromazine 50 mg. four-hourly if necessary.

Caution. In order to diminish the somatic effects and the restlessness and wakefulness of the drug, it has been combined with a barbiturate. This can lead to the patient becoming addicted to the barbiturate—masked addiction. The patients most likely to show this somatic intolerance to amphetamine are the anxiety-prone, and barbiturate, particularly amylobarbitone, is liable to produce addiction in these patients. The author has known some patients obtain over a gramme of amylobarbitone per day in this way, yet these patients were referred as amphetamine addicts.

Addiction. As the drug was originally obtainable without prescription it rapidly became a popular drug of addiction, but legislation which in the United Kingdom has placed it on Schedule IV (only obtainable on prescription by a registered medical practitioner) has reduced its prevalence. A common source for the addict was the Benzedrine Inhaler with contains 300 mg. of the drug. In Japan it has become a widespread addiction among teenagers and it is, and is likely to remain for some time, a serious social problem. (See under Drug Addiction, Chapter 8).

LITHIUM

Chemistry

Lithium (χίθος = stone) is a metal which belongs to Group 1A which contains the alkali metals, having an atomic weight of 6·94 (sodium 22·99: potassium 39·10). Immediately preceding each alkali metal in atomic numbers in the periodic tables is an inert gas element. In passing from Group 0 to Group 1A, i.e. from unreactive non-metal to highly reactive metal, there is the most abrupt change of chemical type in the whole of the periodic classification. In the outermost shell of each alkali metal atom there is only one electron, and the loss of this electron converts the atom into a unipositive ion which has the same electronic configuration as the insert gas, which immediately precedes it in the periodic classification.

Clinically the alkali metals provide an example of extreme metallic behaviour; thus, their electrode potentials are among the highest of all, with a powerful affinity for oxygen and the capacity to displace hydrogen from cold water. As they have a very low ionization energy their electronegativities are also among the very lowest. Thus their compounds are of an extreme ionic type and show the characteristic properties associated with ionic binding, particularly as one descends the group. The lithium ion being the smallest of the group, differentiates the behaviour of its compounds from the other elements in the group.

Clinical Applications

Because of its resemblance to sodium, it was at one time regarded as a sodium or salt substitute in patients with heart failure. It was Cade (1949) in Australia who first reported the successful treatment of manic states with lithium carbonate. The monitoring of such treatment by frequent estimates of serum levels meant that its systematic application had to wait till such facilities were readily available and it was Schou *et al.* (1954) from Denmark who first submitted lithium carbonate to a double-blind experiment of a placebo-controlled design. They concluded that 'lithium treatment of mania represents a very welcome addition to the therapeutic measures against a disease that is very resistant to most types of treatment or in which the improvement after treatment is short-lived'. It was later used for the treatment of recurring depressive states, particularly those associated with the bipolar form of manic-depressive psychoses, and then as a prophylactic agent (Baastrup *et al.*, 1967). This latter claim was severely attacked by Blackwell and Shepherd (1968), and Lader (1968), mainly on the methodology of the trial, but the original authors came back with more rigorous trials (Baastrup *et al.*, 1970; Angst *et al.*, 1970) and vindicated their earlier claims.

It is now generally accepted that lithium carbonate is an effective drug in the treatment of mania and of recurrent depressive reactions in manic-depressive (or bipolar) depression though its use as a prophylactic while demonstrated clinically should be used with considerable reserve because of the prolonged commitment to a drug with a number of undesirable features.

Therapeutic Uses

(1) **Manic States.** Schou *et al.* (1971) state that the drug in fully developed mania only begins to work after 2 days and generally after 7 days. It is therefore advisable to start treatment with one of the neuroleptics to allow time for lithium to act. The manic features disappear with lithium treatment without the appearance of lethargy, though some patients who felt 'liberated' during the manic phase may complain that they feel 'curbed'. It is better than neuroleptics in the treatment of hypomanic states where the improvement can be observed in a few days.

(2) **Depression.** In unipolar depression it is of no value but it can be very useful in the recurrent forms of bipolar depression (Goodwin *et al.*, 1972).

(3) **Prophylaxis.** It was first recommended as a prophylactic for recurring attacks of mania and later (Baastrup *et al.* 1967) for preventing recurrence of depression. As Schou *et al.* (1971) remark:

> The idea of a drug capable of exerting a prophylactic action in preventing attacks of depression yet with little therapeutic effect on an established attack was something new, and it gave rise to much questioning of the findings and their interpretation. However, further studies, under double-blind conditions with matched partners randomly given either lithium or a placebo, provided evidence in support of the view that lithium indeed had the postulated prophylactic action in patients suffering from recurrent endogenous depression as well as in patients with recurrent manic-depressive disorders.

The effect is independent of the patient's age and sex and duration of illness and Schou *et al.* (1971) state that: 'Patients whose attacks have been many and frequent may be able to lead stable and happy lives for the first time under the influence of continuous lithium treatment. The effect may be immediate, but in some instances depressive episodes may occur for up to 12 months though these tend to be less severe and peter out progressively. This should be explained to the patient, otherwise he may abandon an effective answer to his problem. Should depressive episodes occur, these may be treated with anti-depressants or ECT but the lithium treatment should be kept up throughout'.

Dosage

An average starting dose is 20–25 mEq./day (or 140–175mg.) which may be reduced to 10 mEq./day should side-effects be troublesome. In patients with known renal or circulatory disease one should start with 10 mEq./day. If after the 7th day the blood level is below 0·7 mEq./l. or above 1·3 mEq./l., proportionate increase or decrease of the dose is necessary. On the 14th day a second estimate is made to assess the need for further adjustment, and it may be reasonably assumed that once the optimum level has been found this will remain satisfactory, though it is common practice to assess levels at regular intervals, once per week for four weeks and once per month for 12 months, to see whether the patient is taking the dosage as instructed and for general supervision.

Further checks of serum lithium levels should be made when: (1) signs of poisoning appear; (2) signs of manic or depressive episode occur; (3) dosage has been changed (i.e. after 7 days); (4) intercurrent disease, apart from trivial ailments, develops; (5) there has been a significant change in the intake of sodium; (6) diuretic treatment is administered; (7) pregnancy occurs. In the presence of acute kidney disease lithium should be stopped forthwith.

Estimations are done on 10 ml. venous blood collected in a plain tube. Results should be immediately available.

Schou *et al.* (1973*c*) recommend two doses per day, a smaller one in the morning and a larger one at bedtime and sustained release preparations have been recommended so that a single dose per day can be given. One of the drawbacks of sustained release lithium is the difficulty in producing rapid elimination should this be desired. In patients who are at high risk for overdosage this is a material consideration. It is still not possible to decide when treatment should be discontinued. Some patients who have been maintained on lithium for 2 years or more have relapsed when it has been discontinued.

Administration and Action

The concentration of lithium in blood serum can be rapidly and accurately determined by flame photometry. Dosage is frequently calculated in milliequivalents (mEq.) and concentrations in milli-equivalents per litre (mEq./l.); one milliequivalent of lithium is equal to 6·9 mg. of lithium. It is administered by mouth, the ion being readily absorbed, and the serum level is maximum in 1–2 hours until passage to tissues and urine causes the level to fall. Because of this it may be desirable to delay estimating samples for about a week, though in hypertensive patients where renal damage is suspect even if not demonstrated, more frequent estimates are necessary. Generally, blood samples should be taken not less than 10 hours after the last dose and every attempt should be made to keep the interval between the last dose and the taking of the blood sample as constant as possible for each patient, and the author has made it a rule that patients omit the first dose of the day until the sample has been taken.

As lithium is excreted mainly in the urine and as renal clearance varies individually, so should dosage be determined individually. There is some relationship between the excretion rate of sodium and lithium so patients who are on sodium restriction require less. As some manic patients have an appetite for salt, they may require more.

Toxic Effects

The authors provide the following table:

Side Effects	Initial, harmless	Persistent, harmless	Prodromal signs of intoxication
Nausea, loose stools	+	–	–
Vomiting, diarrhoea	–	–	+
Fine tremor of the hands	+	+	–
Coarse tremor of the hands	–	–	+
Polyuria and polydipsia	+	+	+
Weight gain	–	+	–
Oedema	–	+	–
Sluggishness, sleepiness	–	–	+
Vertigo	–	–	+
Dysarthria	–	–	+

Precautions

Urine should be tested for protein, glucose and cells. Renal or heart disease increases the risk but this should be weighed against the physical hazards of prolonged spells of manic-depressive psychosis but if one embarks, frequent monitoring is essential.

Mild side-effects are common in the early weeks of treatment but usually disappear. The hand tremor is fine and does not respond to anti-parkinson drugs. Excessive urinary output should not be treated by fluid restriction, but rather the reverse. Of the many other side effects that are attributed to lithium, the authors concede acne, allergic skin reactions, transient impairment of muscle tone and epileptiform seizures. There may also be reversible non-specific changes in the EEG and flattening of T_1 and T_2 in the ECG may be observed. They state that lithium does not cause addiction or tolerance and withdrawal symptoms are unknown and they base these observations on many patients who have been treated with lithium for more than 15 years.

Lithium Retention and Response

Serry (1969) emphasized the importance of the Lithium Excretion Test which consists of the following: (1) void urine; (2) put to bed and tranquillize with phenothiazines; (3) loading given of 1200 mg. lithium carbonate (4 tablets) orally and time noted; (4) liberal fluids for 4 hours as excretion of 100 ml. is needed for valid result; (5) take blood after 2 hours to make sure tablets have been taken; (6) collect all urine till end of 4 hours; (7) estimate specific gravity and total lithium content (using flame photometry).

His findings were:

1. 24 of 30 manic patients excreted 11 mgm. lithium in 4 hours and these he labelled lithium retainers.
2. Two patients excreted 11·1–20 mg. lithium (intermediate group).
3. Four patients excreted 20 + mg. lithium (lithium excretors) and they failed to respond to 1800 mgm./day for 12–14 days.
4. Five out of 21 depressives were lithium retainers.
5. Six out of 11 schizo-affectives were lithium retainers.

All this looks very convincing and gives a pointer to those who may benefit but Stokes *et al.* (1972) tested the hypothesis and did not find the test valid and regarded it as useless as a screening test as it would exclude many who would benefit. They suggest that Serry's high percentage of retainers may be an artefact due to delayed absorption of the lithium carbonate preparation and recommend that in future studies the rate of absorption will need to be monitored and controlled.

Patient Rejection of Lithium Prophylaxis

Polatin and Fieve (1971) report that highly creative individuals who suffer from recurring manic-depressive episodes may depend on their hypomanic drive and creativity to earn their living and find lithium robs them of their ability to express themselves and diminishes their drive and incentive. They may also enjoy their hypomanic state so that treating it with lithium robs them of the enjoyment of life. The authors wisely counsel that before starting treatment each patient should be assessed individually and if his lifelong adaptation to his chronic recurrent illness results in high productivity with success and well-being without serious annoyance to anybody, it may not be in the patient's best interests to prescribe lithium carbonate.

Lithium compared with Chlorpromazine in Excited Schizo-Affective States

Prien *et al.* (1972) selected 83 schizo-affectives and randomly assigned them to a treatment programme of either lithium carbonate or chlorpromazine after dividing them into moderately active (41 patients) and highly active (42 patients). In the highly active group chlorpromazine was significantly superior to lithium in all symptom areas while in the moderately active group there was very little to choose.

Lithium and Thyroid Function

Sedvall *et al.* (1969) reported that in Scandinavia some patients treated for several months with lithium developed diffuse goitres or even symptoms of hypothyroidism. They found that there was only a moderate alteration of thyroid function and in most patients was of no practical importance in treatment, but should the patient be suffering from latent hypothyroidism further impairment of function could be deleterious. This point was emphasized by Rogers and Whybrow (1971) who recommend that the evaluation of any individual for lithium treatment should include thyroid function. They base this on studies of five patients whose thyroid function was profoundly depressed following lithium therapy, all but one had either a compromised thyroid function prior to treatment or a strong family history of thyroid disorder, suggesting that lithium was only contributory rather than the main causal factor. Family and personal histories of thyroid disorder should therefore be checked.

Lithium Treatment and Goitre

Schou *et al.* (1968) reported on 330 patients given lithium for manic-depressive illness of whom 12 developed goitre after treatment periods of 5 months to 2 years. All patients remained clinically euthyroid though pressure symptoms led to subtotal thyroidectomy in 2 patients. In 9 out of 10 patients with goitre and in 2 out of 7 without goitre, radioactive iodine studies showed abnormal findings in iodine metabolism. When lithium was stopped, the goitres disappeared and thyroid metabolism returned to normal. Thyroxine or desiccated thyroid produced shrinkage of the gland in spite of lithium medication.

Lithium Treatment in Bipolar Depression

Though it has made a significant contribution to the treatment of mania it is also gaining a reputation in the treatment of bipolar depressions. Goodwin *et al.* (1972) evaluated its anti-depressant effect in 52 hospitalized depressed patients, 40 bipolar and 12 unipolar. Of the bipolar, 80 per cent showed some improvement compared with 33 per cent of the unipolar. The 4 unipolar who improved had histories of more frequent and more regular depressive episodes than those who did not and the authors suggest that the degree of cyclicity which is independent of polarity may also be relevant to the anti-depressant action of lithium.

Lithium-induced Diabetes Insipidus

Polyuria and polydipsia have been reported in man and experimental animals. For example, rats given toxic doses of lithium passed dilute urine, and the kidneys did not succeed in concentrating the urine despite the administration of vasopressin. Later the animals died in oliguric renal failure and these effects were more easily produced if the animals were salt-deficient. These findings suggest that lithium may interfere with the action of vasopressin on the nephron, resulting in an acquired form of nephrogenic diabetes insipidus such as may also be associated with hypercalcaemia and hypokalaemia.

Some patients may develop a disturbing degree of polyuria and polydipsia on conventional doses even when there is no previous evidence of renal disease or electrolyte imbalance (Ramsey *et al.*, 1972). Such patients failed to concentrate their urine or reduce the flow normally during water deprivation tests or after being given hypertonic saline stimulus, in spite of haemoconcentration and loss of weight, indicating a diagnosis of diabetes insipidus. As the urine did not become concentrated after the giving of vasopressin either, it would appear that the patients had acquired nephrogenic diabetes insipidus, but fortunately the condition is generally reversible when the drug is stopped.

Pregnancy

Schou *et al.* (1973*a*) collected information about 118 children born to mothers who were given lithium treatment in the first trimester of pregnancy. The data showed that the teratogenic effects were lower than one might have expected from some of the animal studies on rats and mice. Two of the four authors were so impressed by the findings that they have ceased to collect information on lithium babies.

In a second study (Schou *et al.*, 1973*b*) the authors found that the renal lithium clearance of a manic depressive woman rose when she became pregnant and fell to the pre-pregnancy level when she gave birth, emphasizing the need for frequent determinations of the serum lithium concentration and dosage adjustments during pregnancy and delivery.

Lithium Intake and Mental Hospital Admission

Dawson *et al.* (1972) studied mental hospital admissions in Texas and found that there was an increase from those countries where there was a lower level of lithium in the drinking water. They suggest that a community should derive a prophylactic benefit from lithium ingestion, depending on the quantity, as far as the four major mental illnesses are concerned and also for those with homicidal tendencies. It had no effect on those admitted for drug abuse, alcoholism or mental retardation, the first two being more dependent on population density.

DRUG TOXICITY

Agranulocytosis and Psychotropic Drugs

As agranulocytosis has a mortality rate of 20–50 per cent even after treatment, it is important to determine the onset of leucopaenia in patients who are having psychotropic drugs. Litvak and Kaelbling (1971) investigated 54 patients whose leucopaenia was associated with psychotropic drugs. Their definition of agranulocytosis was a combination of a white blood count below 3,700/cu.mm. with a decrease in neutrophils to less than one third of their normal percentage, and with secondary symptoms resulting from the lowered resistance to infection, such as ulceration of the mucous membrane and fever.

The authors found that routine white blood counts were not helpful in the early detection of agranulocytosis and in the very few cases that were discovered, other symptoms appeared 2–5 days earlier. They suggest that routine white blood counts have fostered complacency and the frequent finding of innocuous leucopaenia with routine white cell counts has made some physicians less vigilant. They urge that physicians and nurses be cautioned to remain alert to the appearance of general malaise, mucosal ulcers, sore throat, fever, or other evidence of infection. A white blood count could return to normal despite continued treatment with the suspect drug and it is suggested that cyclic leucopaenia may occur without relation to drugs, so that not every white blood count below 3,700/cu.mm. is a proper cause for abandoning a helpful drug.

Drug Induced Jaundice

Although a number of psychotropic drugs induce jaundice, it is salutary to look at the whole scene to gauge the extent of the problem. This was done by Maxwell and Williams (1973) who present the following table (abridged) from a report to the Committee on Safety of Medicines (1964–1971) from hospitals and general practitioners.

Drug	Number of Reports	Number of Deaths	Type of Reaction	G.P. Prescriptions in 1970
Monoamine oxidase inhibitors				
Phenelzine	26	16	Hepatitis	17,000
Iproniazid	7	4		10,000
Isocarboxazid	3	–		50,000
Phenothiazines				
Chlorpromazine	213	60	Cholestasis and hepatitis	1,540,000
Other Phenothiazines	58	14		4,800,000
Tricyclic anti-depressants				
Amitriptyline	55	20	Cholestasis and hepatitis	3,420,000
Imipramine	31	8		1,400,000
Iprindole	46	2		240,000
Anxiolytics				
Chlordiazepoxide	50	14	Cholestasis and hepatitis	6,400,000
Diazepam	24	9		5,450,000

As such reports are not mandatory the numbers are probably much larger. It should also be appreciated that patients may have been on more than one drug and many, like alcoholics, may have had pre-existing liver damage. Nevertheless, it is a disturbing thought that drugs prescribed as mild tranquillizers may cause serious illness and even death.

NEW DRUGS

The introduction of new drugs places a very heavy responsibility on the psychiatrist. Should he be first in the field with every drug that is placed on the market and give his patients the benefits of the new cures or should he be cautious and wait till more extensive trials have been conducted and a better appraisal of their efficacy is available? Precipitate use can be harmful, for drugs are no longer vehicles for transferring the doctor's affection to the patient, but dangerous instruments either in their toxic effects or in producing addiction. Psychiatric problems, especially neurotic ones, are particularly difficult to assess and no doubt because of an honest attempt to relieve humanity of their prevalence, drug houses keep pouring out new agents for their treatment, and the doctor is presented with more dilemmas. Inspired by this widespread application of new drugs, such as antidepressants for neurotic disorders, the *British Medical Journal* (1962*b*) in a leader pointed out that:

> Anxiety is one of the commonest of human afflictions and it is no wonder that much energy and ingenuity have been spent in attempting to treat it. Long before the term psychopharmacology became fashionable the drug treatment of anxiety was well established, and its history is one of somewhat transient victories which seem to follow one another at an increasing rate. The era of alcoholic nerve tonics, of valerian and asafetida, and of the bromides is over. Only the barbiturates have kept a fair reputation over the years, perhaps because no one suggests that they provide more than partial symptomatic relief. . . . The major neuroleptics such as reserpine and members of the phenothiazine family have in turn been claimed as effective in controlling anxiety. Their value is perhaps best indicated by the rapidity with which each is discarded when something new is introduced.
>
> Experimental evidence suggested that the tranquillo-sedative drugs would be beneficial, but their careers have on the whole been short. Mephenesin, benactyzine, meprobamate—there have been many disappointments. Such effects as they exert are slight and often evanescent and the few strictly controlled and comparative trials to which these substances have been subjected have shown that they are generally of less value than amylobarbitone (Raymond *et al.*, 1957). . . .
>
> Why should this pattern of uncontrolled enthusiasm and subsequent disappointment be repeated over and over again? . . . .

THERAPEUTIC TRIALS

The above question brings us to the core of the problem of therapeutic trials, particularly for psychiatric illness, namely, the *placebo reactor.* Whitehead (1938) had shown that when work conditions were varied with a view to increasing production in a factory, each change was beneficial, including the final one which was a reversion to the original conditions. Weatherall (1962), commenting on this, states that it is just as well to remember that the administration of any drug whatever is likely to benefit symptoms, provided the dose is not excessive. To circumvent the problem of the placebo reactor a number of devices have been elaborated, including the *'double-blind therapeutic trial'.* In it, neither the patient nor the physician knows what is being prescribed. Usually an inert substance is compared with a drug which is intended to have a beneficial effect, or two active agents may be compared for their efficiency, but to compensate for the placebo reactor a third inert substance is thrown into the trial, which is usually conducted in a 'controlled random order'. It is generally held that in any such therapeutic trial, at least 30 per cent of patients will be placebo reactors. The controlled double-blind therapeutic trial does not, however, supply the complete answer for testing new drugs. Apart from technical imperfections, such as tablets when crushed tasting differently, the drug having distinguishable side-effects which are absent from the placebo, or the patient (particularly, though not exclusively, an out-patient) not taking his tablets or capsules as directed, the double-blind trial can convey a false sense of security. This point was emphasized by White and Sim (1959) who in their attempt to subject imipramine to a severe test on patients with a high degree of morbidity, rejected the double-blind method as it would have meant introducing an inert substance in the treatment of a patient who was severely depressed, and also because of the defects in pharmacological knowledge which the double-blind trial assumes to be present. They say:

> The clinical assessment of drugs in the treatment of depression is notoriously difficult. The illness frequently fluctuates diurnally and/or over long periods, and the changes can be quite marked. Diagnosis, too, may be difficult, for the condition may be adulterated with obsessional, anxiety, paranoid or schizophrenic features which may or may not yield to specific treatment for the depression. It has become fashionable to use the double-blind trial which in some quarters carries the hall-mark of objectivity and is regarded as the method most likely to reveal the true action of a drug. But this can give a false sense of security. It does not exclude the pitfalls of diagnosis, selection, delayed response, assessment of results, and what is probably the most serious criticism, it compares the responses of different people to different agents. Even the

self-controlled and self-recorded trial (Hogben & Sim, 1953) has drawbacks, for it presupposes a knowledge of the pharmacology of a drug which we may not possess. For example: does it work immediately, or is its action delayed? Does its action cease to work as soon as it is withheld? Does it set in motion a train of events which will make the subsequent introduction of an inert substance quite meaningless and cause us to attribute to the latter some of the effects of the drug? Are we able in the early trials of a drug to decide on the individual variations in terms of effective dose and total reaction?

Another method devised by Hogben and Sim (1953) is the Self-Controlled and Self-Recorded Clinical Trial which uses the patient as his own control. This has considerable limitations for it places a heavy responsibility on the patient who must be able to record objectively, and in neurotic disorders where symptoms may be protean, this can prove a serious handicap. It also presupposes a knowledge of the drugs and their side-effects which in new drug trials may be completely lacking, and it demands that the condition lend itself to quantitative estimation of its progress, an aspect which at best is fraught with difficulties but is frequently impossible. It is more likely to be of value in organic states such as spasmodic torticollis where the patient is considerably handicapped and objective tests can be devised. The author was able to conduct such a trial in a patient by using a series of tests, such as threading beads (which could be counted), pouring water into a glass jar (the height of which could be measured) and the time taken to read a column of a newspaper. The drugs were administered 'double-blind' and the patient co-operated well, but the effective drug did not do better than the placebo; yet when its dose was doubled there was a dramatic improvement and the patient was returned to work and has coped satisfactorily since, which illustrated the difficulty that individual responses to drugs can produce.

Hogben and Sim (1953) in the same paper discuss the place of statistical analysis in these trials and point out their limitations. In support of their arguments they quote Claude Bernard (1865) and the lesson that pioneer in experimental method laid down is just as appropriate today as when he first wrote it:

By destroying the biological character of phenomena, the use of *averages* in physiology and medicine usually gives only apparent accuracy to the results. From our point of view, we may distinguish between several kinds of averages; physical averages, chemical averages, and physiological and pathological averages. If, for instance, we observe the number of pulsations and the degree of blood pressure by means of the oscillations of a manometer throughout one day, and if we take the average of all our figures to get the true average blood pressure and to learn the true or average number of pulsations, we shall simply have wrong numbers. In fact, the pulse decreases in number and intensity when we are fasting and increases during digestion or under different influences of movement and rest; all the biological characteristics of the phenomena disappear in the average. Chemical averages are also often used. If we collect a man's urine to analyse the average, we get an analysis of a urine which simply does not exist; for urine, when fasting, is different from urine during digestion. A startling instance of this kind was invented by a physiologist who took urine from a railroad station urinal where people of all nations passed, and who believed he could thus present an analysis of *average* European urine! Aside from physical and chemical, there are physiological averages, or what we might call average descriptions of phenomena, which are even more false. Let me assume that a physician collects a great many individual observations of a disease and that he makes an average description of symptoms observed in the individual cases; he will thus have a description that will never be matched in nature. So in physiology, we must never make average descriptions of experiments, because the true relations of phenomena disappear in the average; when dealing with complex and variable experiments, we must study their various circumstances, and then present our most perfect experiments as a type, which, however, still stands for true facts. In the cases just considered, averages must therefore be rejected, because they confuse while aiming to unify, and distort while aiming to simplify. Averages are applicable only to reducing very slightly varying numerical data about clearly defined and *absolutely simple cases*. . . . I acknowledge my inability to understand why results taken from statistics are called *laws;* for in my opinion scientific law can be based only on certainty, on absolute determinism, not on probability. . . . In every science, we must recognize two classes of phenomena: first, those whose cause is already defined; next, those whose cause is still undefined. With phenomena whose cause is defined, statistics have nothing to do; they would even be absurd. As soon as the circumstances of an experiment are well known, we stop gathering statistics; we should not gather cases to learn how often water is made of oxygen and hydrogen; or when cutting the sciatic nerve, to learn how often the muscle to which it leads will be paralysed. The effect will occur always without exception because the cause of the phenomena is accurately defined. . . . Certain experimenters, as we shall later see, have published experiments by which they found that the anterior spinal roots are insensitive; other experimenters have published experiments by which they found that the same roots were sensitive. These cases seemed as comparable as possible; here was the same operation done by the same method on the same spinal roots. Should we therefore have counted the positive and negative cases and said: the law is that anterior roots are sensitive, for instance, 25 times out of a 100? Or should we have admitted, according to the theory called the law of large numbers, that in an immense number of experiments we should find the roots equally often sensitive and insensitive? Such statistics would be ridiculous, for there is a reason for the roots being insensitive and another reason for their being sensitive; this reason had to be defined; I looked for it, and I found it; so that we can now say: the spinal roots are always sensitive in given conditions, and always insensitive in other equally definite conditions.

This illustrates another fallacy in therapeutic trials. Drug 'A' is tested against Drug 'B' and the latter is successful in 70 per cent of the group and the former in 30 per cent. One might conclude that the 30 per cent were placebo reactors and the 70 per cent were responding to the effective drug. Yet the 30 per cent may have been hard-core who were resistant to Drug 'B' and a valuable remedy may have been unjustifiably discarded. Another fallacy is to assume that because a drug is effective in say 70 per cent of cases, these are genuine reactions to the drug and that all the placebo reactors are in the other group. The reverse is just as likely and therefore a 70 per cent recovery rate may well include a 30 per cent placebo response. If placebo reactors were constant in their behaviour, one might be able to isolate them and identify the genuine response, but this is still not possible. Not only may a placebo reactor respond to a pharmacologically inert substance, but he may fail to respond to an active one. Wolff (1948) has shown that if the subject is hostile to the investigator he may respond paradoxically to a physiological drug like acetylcholine, and Joyce (1959) pointed out that patients could develop symptoms with dummy preparations. Patients are very prone to attribute their most recent symptoms to the most recently prescribed drug, a common human failing when logic is denied and the *post hoc, propter hoc* argument is substituted. This is more likely to happen with those suffering from neurotic symptoms, for the neurotic process itself predisposes to false logic and the need to rationalize, and in therapeutic trials with such patients, even greater care is needed in interpreting results.

A Placebo Test

Shapiro *et al.* (1968) reviewed the methodological problems involved in studies of the placebo effect and put forward their own methodology. Twenty-seven subjects were instructed that they were to receive a test drug that was a non-specific autonomic nervous system stimulant which was not harmful or dangerous. The patients were to record changes in any symptoms, such as increase, decrease, no effect or the occurrence of new symptoms. The 'drug' was given with a glass of water and recordings were made every 15 minutes. Contrary to previous reports, the authors predicted, correctly, that positive and negative reactions to the placebo would be unrelated to old age, female sex, lower intelligence, lower social class, authoritarianism, short duration of illness, or a diagnosis of neurosis or psychosis. They predicted, correctly, that anxiety and depression would be significantly correlated with positive and negative reactions and that absence of anxiety and depression would be associated with neutral response.

They arrived at the following conclusions:

(1) Inferences made about placebo effects vary with methods of

scoring: (2) The placebo effect occurs in a group of non-reactors without regard to positive or negative direction; (3) The reactive group is subdivided into predominantly positive or negative groups and therefore to compare positive reactors with a combined group of non-reactors and negative reactors, obscures important differences among groups; (4) Patients with positive reactions to placebo tend to improve more rapidly and have a better prognosis than patients with neutral and negative reactions; (5) Patients with absent and negative responses may respond to treatment eventually but not as predictably as positive reactors.

They claimed with some justification that their placebo test combined the best features of a simple, standardized, quantitative and reliable laboratory test of suggestibility with the clinical relevance and validity of the placebo effect.

Factors Contributing to the Placebo Effect

Lowinger and Dobie (1969) on the basis of four double-blind placebo-controlled trials concluded that the milieu in which drugs and placebo are administered may exert a considerable effect on the patient's chance for improvement in a variety of contributory psychiatric illnesses. A study in which large doses of the active drug are in use is a more impressive therapeutic endeavour, even to the doctor who does not know whether he is giving a particular patient the active drug or a placebo. He is more enthusiastic about this double-blind study, more alert to toxicity and somehow conveys this to the patient. The doctor participating in a double-blind study in which he knows the drugs are milder or used in low dosage is perhaps less optimistic about the patient's progress and less concerned about toxicity. A study which requires frequent tests offers an extended emotional relationship with the clinic and the patient gains additional support from identification with the research personnel.

MEDICAL ETHICS AND CONTROLLED TRIALS

Hill (1963) poses the following six questions which are applicable to clinical trials.

1. Is the proposed treatment safe, or in other words, is it unlikely to do harm to the patient?

Hill argues a practical and ethical advantage of the controlled trial, which is, that by its exact comparisons it may more rapidly pinpoint the unsuspected undesirable side-effects of a treatment, therefore even harm can be justified, but the circumstances would have to be most exceptional.

2. Can a new treatment ethically be withheld from any patients in the doctor's care?

The true question is not, can the doctor withhold the new, but can he withhold the established in favour of what is still quite unproved? Only the actual circumstances involved for each case can provide the answer.

3. What patients may be brought into a controlled trial and allocated randomly to different treatments?

The doctor is ethically in a stronger position if he 'rings the changes' of treatment *within* patients rather than *between* patients. It must be *necessary* to 'ring' these changes, for, as with the law, 'where it is not necessary to change it is necessary not to change' (MacMillan, 1937). Here, too, much will depend on the individual circumstances, such as pregnant women, the old and infirm and the very young where special hazards may be present. The ethical obligation always and entirely outweighs the experimental and should the patient's condition deteriorate, any measure which can help should be used even though the trials be nullified.

4. Is it necessary to obtain the patient's consent to his inclusion in a controlled trial?

Hill states: 'Having made up your mind that you are not in any way subjecting either patient to a recognized and unjustifiable danger, pain, or discomfort, can anything be gained ethically by endeavouring to explain to them your own state of ignorance and to describe the attempts you are making to remove it; and what is true of 2 patients is equally true of 20 or 200'. This argument is not acceptable. Doctors generally take their patients into their confidence in regard to therapy as well as to diagnosis. In the latter, many procedures are undertaken just because the doctor is ignorant and whether it is examination of a urine specimen or a cerebral biopsy, these are explained to the patient as being necessary because the doctor is still ignorant of the nature of his condition. Patients should be told even if this interferes with the clinical trial, but it need not.

5. Is it ethical to use a placebo, or dummy treatment?

If there is already an orthodox treatment which is reasonably effective it would be unethical to substitute a placebo for it. If there is no effective and established treatment then it should be acceptable to devise means to create one. One group in a trial need not *always* be a mirror image of the other and Hill points out that during the M.R.C. trial of streptomycin in the treatment of pulmonary tuberculosis, they did not think it necessary to mimic the injections. The argument as to whether it is less ethical knowingly to administer a placebo than to do so unknowingly is a complex one and it will again depend on the special circumstances of the case.

6. Is it proper for the doctor not to know the treatment being administered to his patient?

This question arises out of the 'double-blind' procedure in a controlled trial. It required that neither patient nor doctor should know the nature of the treatment being given in the individual case. It is not enough to say that it is all right as long as no harm comes to the patient. There should be no detriment compared to active treatment by existing methods. There must also be the firm understanding that if things are not going well, the code of the trial must be broken.

James (1969) poses a relevant question:'Where will we obtain our new medical knowledge if our present generation will not volunteer?'. He puts forward two options for man:

1. He who offers the best in ultimate hope through prevention and research.
2. He who demands the total allocation of our major resources in the futile struggle against the insatiable demand of the population for medical care, using our present ineffective armamentarium against today's killers and disablers.

He adds: 'We must dedicate our programmes to the citizens of tomorrow even though they cause inconvenience, pain and great cost to the citizens of today'

This view is becoming prevalent, yet it may be questioned whether it may not in itself contribute to the 'insatiable demand of the population for medical care'. At the same conference Fr.T.J. O'Donnell, S.J., while agreeing it would be immoral to deny future generations their birthright of improved medical care, believed that it would be more immoral to deny human rights in experimentation, for this would be depriving those future generations of a greater value while handing over to them something of a lesser value.

The present writer remains cynical over arguments re the 'birthright' of future generations put forward by people who are usually in the van of those who would deny future generations the right to birth through their advocacy of abortion as a legitimate aid to population control. Another contributor to the conference, Dr F. Ayd, also questioned the experimenter's philosophy: 'Too many of them are impatient with moral restraint. They want everyone to march to the beat of the scientific and technological drummer. The biological achievements of amoral researchers may lead only to spiritual decay'.

CHAPTER 19

The Psychotherapies

If one could assume that the minds of men the world over were subject to identical influences and that their functional disturbances were also similar, then psychological treatment or psychotherapy should be constant and based on a uniform theory of causation in mental illness. But the mind varies from culture to culture, between members of the same family and at times in the same individual. It is this complexity which defies a universally valid psychopathological theory though some theories have come close to general application. Protagonists of such theories are usually more concerned in emphasizing the differences that divide them, while the common ground tends to be overlooked, and we now have a bewildering variety of psychotherapeutic techniques, some based on well-formulated theories and others based on no theory at all. It is therefore inaccurate to talk of psychotherapy as a specific form of treatment and the generic term 'the psychotherapies' should be used with, if possible, further definition.

Because of the dominance of the Freudian (psychoanalytic) school, many equate psychotherapy with psychoanalysis, but the following accounts of a number of other therapies should help to correct this impression. Neither are all therapies neo-Freudian, for some have their origins in Oriental religions like Zen Buddhism, while others are based on modern philosophies like Existentialism. The theory of cybernetics which is largely based on the principles of electronic computers, has now invaded the field of psychiatry and a number of distinguished workers have developed what was initially regarded as an attractive analogy into a whole system of brain function. Pavlovian psychology with its strong emphasis on the conditioned reflex has always enjoyed a high reputation among psychiatrists in the Soviet Union and it is now being freely adapted elsewhere and has given rise to what is called Behaviour Therapy.

An immediate reaction to this formidable array of theories and therapies is that they cannot all be valid. A valid theory should be based on a careful study of the disease process and its aetiology and be generally applicable to mental illness in its protean manifestations, *but it need not be equated with successful treatment.* In fact a less valid theory may be more successful when applied to treatment and the most dramatic results may be based on no theory at all, but on the enthusiasm and confidence of the practitioner, who may believe he has a divine gift. Successful treatment may in itself be open to different interpretations. To some, and particularly to patients, it may mean the removal of symptoms, while to others it should mean the greater understanding of mental mechanisms and the early experiences of life which have made the patient more vulnerable. Some illnesses will respond to the first criterion, but there are others which are so closely linked with the patient's personality development, that only a careful analytical approach will give any hope of relief.

Some theories have been elaborated in opposition to existing ones without regard to their intrinsic merit, and such is the enthusiasm of their protagonists that disputes over percentages of cures are now no longer confined to the pages of reputable scientific journals, but have flowed over to the mass media of communication: radio, television and press. Such disputes are not only unseemly, in that they are reminiscent of the competing claims of the market place, but are unscientific, since no serious attempt is made, or for that matter can be made, to match adequately the selection of patients and criteria in response. Yet the public are asked to adjudicate in controversy which calls for the most expert assessment of all the factors, not the least being that of the protagonists.

There are, however, other difficulties. Psychotherapy in its many forms has attracted a host of workers, medical and non-medical, professional and amateur, and each claiming to have mastered some technique. Unorthodox and even unqualified practitioners may practise medicine, but it is generally accepted that a sound medical training is an important if not essential qualification. When it comes to psychiatric treatment, people are less scrupulous. Diagnosis is either disregarded or is dismissed with the comment 'my guess is as good as yours' and treatment is regarded as the province of anybody who can spare the time. Of course, the medical practitioner is immediately dismissed as being too busy and an army of willing helpers including psychologists, social workers, welfare officers, parsons, teachers, marriage guidance counsellors, hypnotists and evangelists have entered the field. They are backed by even greater numbers of enthusiastic amateurs whose need for a person in distress overcomes any inhibition their lack of training and experience may give them. They may be successful, with their particular clientele, and no amount of argument about the advantages of a medical education or the dangers of the layman practising what is essentially a branch of medicine is likely to curb their activities. Doctors are of course prejudiced for a variety of reasons and the one which instantly springs to mind is that a number of patients with serious mental disturbances have been treated by such practitioners with apparent ill-effects. There are other reasons which are less closely related to the patient's welfare. But this is not an issue on which the doctor should be violently partisan. His duty is clear and it is to try and gain as much understanding as he can of healers and their art and to equip himself with a knowledge and experience of the psychotherapies so that society will be in no doubt as to who is the most highly trained practitioner; just as it gives the doctor first place in diseases affecting the body, so it will give him first place in matters affecting the mind. His medical training and ready access to the most private affairs of his patient give him a tremendous advantage. The rest is a matter of training and study.

PSYCHOANALYSIS

This derives from Freud's treatment of hysteria by hypnosis and its later replacement by Free-Association, the techniques of which were laid down in Freud's earliers papers (Freud, 1910 *a* & *b*, 1912 *a, b* & *c,* 1913*a* & *b,* 1914, 1915*a,* 1919). Although these papers are models of clarity and pregnant with clinical expertize, the beginner must not expect to *learn* the technique merely by reading. As Freud himself states (Freud, 1913*b*):

> He who wishes to learn the fine art of the game of chess from books will soon discover that only the opening and closing moves of the game admit of exhaustive systematic description, and that the endless variety of moves which develop from the opening defies description; the gap left in the instructions can only be filled in by the zealous study of games fought out by master-hands. The rules which can be laid down for the practical application of psychoanalysis in treatment are subject to similar limitations.

Selection of the Patient

Before starting treatment there is the problem of selection of the patient. For successful analysis three criteria are regarded as essential and these have been listed by Gitelson (1951) as: (1) *the ego-functioning,* which is the degree of contact, the capacity for reality testing, appropriate affect, the general adequacy of ego-defences, or if decompensation is evident, its degree and rate of development; (2) *motivation,* which should be strong and should spring from within the patient and not from external pressure; and (3) *the capacity of the patient for psychological work.* As regards this last point, some patients are just incapable of appreciating psychological causes in their illness and seeing the relationships. A fourth point which is just as essential as the other three is the patient's or his family's capacity to pay, for a prolonged and intensive analysis is a costly business. It is not fair to expect the therapist to treat even colleagues and their families *gratis.* A person who is engaged full-time in psychotherapy can have only about eight patients and if he takes on one *gratis,* he is sacrificing one-eighth of his total income; with two such patients, a quarter is sacrificed. This economic aspect has other implications, particularly in a National Health Service which is being financed by the taxpayer. To refer for, or to undertake psychotherapy, is a decision which should be made with the greatest circumspection and should be given no less consideration than the selection of the patient for pre-frontal leucotomy. The questions to be answered are: (1) can this patient be helped by any other treatment? and (2) if not, what are the chances of psychotherapy doing good or harm?

The treatment sessions should be long enough to give the patient a chance to settle down and get over the preliminary resistances and leave time for resistances to be overcome for these may include relatively long periods of silence. A time of 50 minutes is generally accepted as adequate. Frequency of visits varies among different therapists, but five times a week is general, though Freud saw his patients six days a week and even then had some difficulty in breaking through the 'Monday crust'. Perhaps the five-day week is more symptomatic of the psychotherapist's adoption of modern labour conditions than evidence of greater efficiency.

In practice, the number of patients who must have this intensive psychoanalysis are not many, compared to the large numbers who do very well with other speedier and less costly treatments. But there are still some who do require this psychoanalytic approach, which also has a place in the shorter forms of psychotherapy.

In order to assess the original motivation of patients Sifneos (1968) lays down the following criteria: (1) an ability to recognize that the symptoms are psychological in nature; (2) a tendency to be introspective and give an honest and truthful account of emotional difficulties; (3) willingness to participate actively in the treatment situation; (4) curiosity and willingness to understand oneself; (5) willingness to change, explore and experiment; (6) expectations of the results of psychotherapy; (7) willingness to make reasonable sacrifices.

These factors constituted *'the motivational process'* and patients who fulfilled all seven criteria had the best prognosis in both anxiety-provoking or dynamic psychotherapy and anxiety–suppressive or supportive psychotherapy.

Free Association

This is the technique employed to get the patient to communicate with the therapist and also with himself, for awareness of the underlying motives is important for both. All censorship of items of thought must be removed and whatever emerges should be declared without regard to shame or offending the therapist. This is based on the principle that the unconscious factors in the neurosis are seeking expression but are concealed by the neurosis, and by allowing the mind to associate freely, they will emerge in verbal form and ultimately declare themselves. Orthodox analysts use a couch in a semi-darkened room to encourage a feeling of relaxation and freedom from distraction and the analyst sits behind the patient. allegedly for this purpose, though Freud admitted that it was because he could not bear to be gazed at by his patients for eight hours a day! He did however add that as his own unconscious processes were working, he did not wish to distract the patient by letting him see them through his facial expression.

The treatment situation has been likened to a battle with two opposing forces: (1) those on the side of the analyst, and (2) those which oppose him. The former include the conscious rational ego of the patient who is motivated to seek help through psychoanalysis; the positive transference which motivates the patient towards cooperation, the *id* and the repressed which are seeking conscious expression; and super-ego factors which motivate the patient to do the right thing. The latter include those aspects of the ego which are irrational and unconsciously motivated to preserve the neurotic defences in order to suppress painful memories; conscious though irrational ego-attitudes which are designed to avoid social embarrassment; the negative transference which may try to defeat the objective of the analyst; the patient's masochism which may deprive him of his motivation towards recovery; and secondary gain from the illness which is preferable to recovery. Greenson (1959) states:

> The reasonable ego of our patient is our main ally. This portion of the ego seeks our help, is willing to risk once more facing the old, formerly overwhelming, unconscious impulses and their derivatives, is willing to endure and to wait and to attempt to understand.

The Psychological Meaning of Silence

Reik (1968) critically assessed the significance of silence in the analytic situation, its emotional evaluation by the patient, and its latent meaning. In the beginning of analysis, when used by the analyst it usually has a beneficial and calming effect on the patient. It gives him confidence, encourages him to express himself freely, and helps to establish communication. The patient reacts to the analyst's silence by speaking. It indicates to him that the analyst is willing to listen but may later indicate that he is unwilling to speak and this can be interpreted as a threatened loss of love or even punishment. This can engender a hostile reaction in the patient with accusations of the analyst's lack of feeling but it can also uncover his guilt feelings.

Silence can therefore take on contradictory meanings such as sympathy or hostility. It is therefore a form of speech and is not mere muteness; it is rather pregnant with unsaid words.

Resistance

This includes all those conscious and unconscious factors which interfere with a rational recovery-motivated ego and will therefore consist of all those factors which are mobilized against the therapist. It need not be confined to the negative transference, for a very strong positive transference may prompt the patient to seek substitute love from the therapist rather than experience painful uncovering and understanding of unconscious guilt processes. In the days before psychoanalysis, psychotherapy would deliberately avoid the resistances of the patient, but orthodox analysis attempts to uncover and analyze these resistances for it is only then that a fully rational cooperative ego can be prepared for further treatment. Resistance can assume many forms, such as turning up late for the appointment, long periods of silence, rudeness and irrelevant and irreverent remarks. The author had a patient who was a meteorological instructor in the Royal Air Force and who with each therapeutic session recited a lecture on meteorology. The 'course' consisted of ten lectures and it was only when they had all been delivered that this facet of resistance ended. This is, of course, an extreme example.

Freud (1914) gives the following advice in dealing with resistances:

> Now it seems that beginners in analytic practice are inclined to look upon this [recognizing and pointing out the resistance] as the end of the work. I have often been asked to advise upon cases in which the physician complained that he had pointed out his resistance to the patient, and that all the same no change

had set in; in fact, the resistance had only then become really pronounced and the whole situation had become more obscure than ever . . . only the analyst had forgotten that naming the resistance could not result in its immediate suspension. One must allow the patient time to get to know this resistance of which he is ignorant, to 'work through' it, to overcome it, by continuing the work according to the analytic rule in defiance of it. Only when it has come to its height can one, with the patient's co-operation, discover the repressed instinctual trends which are feeding the resistance; and only by living them through in this way will the patient be convinced of their existence and their power. The physician has nothing more to do than to wait and let things take their course, a course which cannot be avoided nor always be hastened. If he holds fast to this principle, he will often be spared the disappointment of failure in cases where all the time he had conducted the treatment quite correctly.

Transference

Though generally referred to as positive feelings the patient has towards the analyst, it includes all feelings, positive and negative, which derive from earlier emotional relationships with other figures and which have been transferred to the analyst. They originate from the earliest infantile experiences and are therefore connected with parents, siblings and other household figures such as domestics and relatives. They may be associated with people in the more recent past, but just as in the transference situation with the therapist, these experiences, too, can be linked with the earlier childhood ones.

The transference situation may be strongly positive and from the patient's standpoint represent a falling in love with the analyst. Freud (1915*a*) regards the resistance as an *agent provocateur* of the transference-love which is frequently irrational and infantile but can nevertheless be very disturbing. He states:

> The analytic psychotherapist thus has a threefold battle to wage—in his own mind against the forces which would draw him down below the level of analysis; outside analysis against the opponents who dispute the importance he attaches to the sexual instinctual forces and hinder him from making use of them in his scientific method; and in the analysis against his patients who at first behave like his critics but later on disclose the over-estimation of sexual life which has them in thrall, and who try to take him captive in the net of their socially ungovernable passions.

There therefore rests a heavy responsibility on the analyst who though dealing with the most intimate details of his patients' experiences must refrain from psychological familiarity.

The transference situation, like the resistance, must be analysed and interpreted and is a crucial aspect of treatment for it is a replica of the patient's infantile attitudes to the key figures in his life, from which the neurotic pattern may have originated. *Transference neurosis* is the term for the neurotic and other inappropriate attitudes towards the analyst and as these include later patterns of neurotic behaviour it helps the analyst to gain some insight into the patient's character structure. As the therapist can represent to the patient parental figures of either sex, the earlier intense emotional attitudes of love and hate will be directed towards him and do not depend on his physical or mental equipment, or for that matter, his sex. The 'couch' method favours this process for the patient is not confronted by the incongruity of some of his unconscious drives. Similarly, negative transference does not depend on the analyst's lack of social grace, but on an expression of infantile attitudes towards the therapist who represents to the patient earlier objects of his hostility. Absence of transference, positive or negative, can be a serious obstacle to therapy. It is seen in withdrawn patients who are deficient in a rational well-motivated ego structure such as incipient schizophrenics or severe obsessive-compulsive states where the patient's thoughts are overwhelmingly pre-occupied with the obsession and the mind cannot be freed to develop the necessary relationships for the therapeutic situation.

The analyst should not neglect the clinical approach in his therapy and Freud (1913*b*) gives two interesting examples.

> The first symptoms or drama actions of the patient, like the first resistance, have a special interest and will betray one of the governing complexes of the neurosis. A clever young philosopher, with leanings towards aesthetic exquisiteness, hastens to twitch the crease of his trousers into place before lying down for the first session; he reveals himself as an erstwhile coprophiliac of the highest refinement, as was to be expected of the developed aesthete. A young girl on the same occasion hurriedly pulls the hem of her skirt over her exposed ankle; she has betrayed the kernel of what analysis will discover later, her narcissistic pride in her bodily beauty and her tendencies to exhibitionism.

While many of these observations may be valid, there should always be the reservation that a false interpretation may be placed on them, for observable phenomena may not always be what they seem. Experienced clinicians with an intimate knowledge of abnormal gait occasionally may be mistaken in their spot diagnoses and most medical students can recount episodes when they 'fooled' the physician or surgeon by getting the patient to parade features which were at variance with the diagnosis.

Interpretation

This should not start till a dependable transference and rapport has been established and certainly should not be initiated as soon as the therapist himself perceives the meaning of the patient's symptoms. As Freud (1913*b*) states:

> . . . but what a measure of self-complacency and thoughtlessness must exist in one who can upon the shortest acquaintance inform a stranger, who is entirely ignorant of analytical doctrines, that he is bound by an incestuous love of his mother, that he harbours wishes for the death of the wife he appears to love, that he conceals within himself the intention to deceive his chief, and so forth! . . . Such conduct brings both the man and the treatment into discredit and arouses the most violent opposition, whether the interpretations be correct or not; yes, and the truer they are actually the more violent is the resistance they arouse.

Generally, interpretation must take into consideration the reasonable ego of the patient and what may be accessible to it, and therefore proceeds from conscious to pre-conscious and unconscious material. The patient himself may dictate the interpretation through repetition of material, either spontaneously during analysis or by relating a recurring theme in his dreams. Then interpretation is called for, but again the therapist must be sure that the patient is close to him in understanding, for otherwise interpretation may shock, frighten or even terminate the treatment. It means therefore that defences take precedence over the instinctual forces in interpretation as they are more likely to be nearer to consciousness, though one aspect of behaviour may be a manifestation of both, such as prolonged silence which can be evidence of resistance and/or hostility towards the analyst. The amount of interpretation which a patient can absorb at one session is, of course, limited and the analyst can only gauge this through his empathy with his patient and this, too, varies. If in doubt, err on the side of caution, for in this way least harm will be done. On the other hand, interpretations which do not 'click' with the patient because they are too inadequate or superficial may increase the resistance.

Manifest Dream Content during Analysis

Jones (1971) stresses the importance of manifest dream content as an aid to communication during analysis. The patient should be encouraged to participate in interpretation, thus creating a therapeutic alliance. The author lists five specific uses:

1. Direct exposure on the less-disguised affect-laden content.
2. A vocabulary of a unique and specific character with its catalogue of reference points.
3. Facilitation of memory for significant achievements in the analysis.

4. Resolution of conflict and sequestration of neurotic problems expressed in manifest dream content.

5. A reference point for analysis of counter transference.

Counter-transference

This is a transference reaction of the analyst to the patient and is one of the most formidable obstacles to treatment if it gets out of control. There are naturally likes and dislikes in everybody, and most patients will excite a positive or negative reaction in the analyst. It is only when these reactions are based, like the patient's transference on the early neurotic conflicts of the analyst, that the term 'counter-transference' is justified. It interferes with the conduct of the analysis by impairing judgement, inducing anxiety in the therapist and may even lead him into conduct which is inappropriate. Self-analysis may help the therapist to see his reaction more clearly and deal with it, but he should not hesitate to consult a colleague and get his help for he may be just as much in need of it as the patient.

Working Through. This is the constant repetition of interpretation which had previously sufficed to give the patient insight into his neurotic conflicts. The old resistances which have been dealt with may return either in similar or different guise and demand further interpretation. There is a repetition-compulsion about the neurosis which will not yield to the single interpretation of an episode, but must have it recurrently interpreted so that the understanding eventually permeates. Freud's (1914) explanation of 'working through' has already been given (p. 906).

Termination of treatment can be a difficult decision. Frequently it is made by the patient who, after having gained considerable insight and been relieved of pathological anxiety, feels confident that he can cope satisfactorily without further help, and it is obvious to the therapist that this new confidence is genuine and not a form of resistance. It is however frequently the therapist's task to terminate treatment and prepare the patient for it. It should be introduced to the patient several months before it becomes effective and its implications discussed. The patient will have to adjust to separation from his analyst and a period of acclimatization is necessary to avoid an abrupt break with consequent separation-anxiety. It gives the patient time to introduce unfinished business and feel that everything has been dealt with and it also permits a running down of the sessions which can become less frequent and even shorter. If the analyst is satisfied that the infantile neurosis and transference neurosis have been resolved and that the ego has consequently been strengthened in its handling of the problems derived from the super-ego and the id, then he can confidently terminate the analysis. Greenson (1958) summarizes the whole problem thus:

> Psychoanalysis is that method of treatment of emotional disorders in which the relationship between the patient and the therapist is so structured that it facilitates the maximal development of a transference neurosis. The analyst's interpretations are the decisive and ultimate instruments, used in an atmosphere of compassionate neutrality, which enable the patient, communicating via free association, to recapitulate his infantile neurosis. The analyst's goal is to provide insight to the patient so that he may himself resolve his neurotic conflict, thus effecting permanent changes in his ego, id and super-ego, and thereby extending the power and the sovereignty of his ego.

Just as Freud was prepared to modify his earlier views, *e.g.* giving up hypnosis for free-association and not elaborating his final technique till he had over 20 years' experience with psychoanalysis, so other workers have modified his views. Reference has already been made to the theoretical differences of Sullivan, Horney, Fromm and Rank, as well as those of Jung and Adler, but there were others.

Ferenczi and Rank (1925) reacted against what they called the over-intellectualized procedures of many analysts who overlooked the dynamic handling of resistances and transference. They believed that after dealing with the transference neurosis there was no need to continue to probe the infantile memories as they considered insight could be gained solely through the different transference experiences. They argued that much of the child's repressed material was not verbalized in any case and could therefore not reach consciousness. Their theories, if correct, would have considerably shortened the analysis as the need for 'working through' would be eliminated. The extension of this approach was to ignore more and more the infantile experiences and concentrate on the life situation. Rank was the main practitioner of this method, for Ferenczi soon abandoned it, as he found it of little therapeutic value, and instead concentrated on the abreaction factor, that is the discharge emotion which is associated with buried memories (Ferenczi, 1926*a*). It could be argued, however, that this discharge of emotion consequent on the ego's ability to recall buried memories, may in fact be evidence of the ego's increased capacity to face psychological content and is evidence of improvement, rather than the cause of it.

Reich (1933) held similar views, and hoped that by concentrating on the analyses of the resistances, he would permit the discharge of highly emotional experiences and he linked this objective with his orgone theory which laid great stress on orgastic potency. The energy released by psychotherapy, he believed, was that which was bound up in neurotic symptoms and character trends and it could be transformed into orgastic genitality. While many do not accept his theory, his contributions to technique have been widely recognized. He laid great stress on the less overt manifestations of resistance, such as pseudo-cooperativeness, over-conventional or over-correct behaviour. He paid more attention to resistance interpretation than to content interpretation and emphasized the value of 'layer' analysis, which depended on typical emotional sequences such as early oral receptivity, when deprived, leading to sadistic revenge, guilt and self-punishment and finally to regression to a dependent level. Alexander (1957), while accepting the concept of layer analysis, points out that it is not new and is well known to experienced analysts, and that there are inherent dangers in approaching material with a preconceived idea of stratification, for it may vary from patient to patient. He states:

> Though certain general phases in the individual's development succeed others with universal regularity, the different emotional attitudes do not necessarily appear during the treatment in the same chronological order as they developed in the patient's past history. Moreover, the pathogenetic fixations occur at different phases in different cases, and the fixation points determine what is the deepest layer in any given case. Often we find an early period of sadism leading to anxiety and covered consecutively by a layer of passivity, inferiority feelings, and a secondary outbreak of aggression . . . it is not uncommon for a patient, in the course of the first two or three interviews, to reveal in his behaviour and associations a sequence of emotional reactions belonging to different phases of his development.

Yet Reich's work contributed to the newer trend in technique which has been called *Ego Analysis*. Freud himself stimulated it by his publication *The Ego and the Id* (Freud, 1927) and Alexander (1929) backed it up by explaining that the complex symptomatology of compulsion neurosis was an attempt of the total personality to reconcile ego alien tendencies with the demands of the super-ego, in a fashion rather like the dream work. The task of the ego was becoming more apparent, as that of harmonizing the instinctual needs with each other and with the environment. Nunberg (1931) emphasized that the process whereby unconscious content became conscious was an integrating act of the ego and that every neurotic symptom and even most psychotic symptoms were synthetic products. It is only by appreciating the ego's task of integrating the emergent unconscious material that the process of 'working through' can be adequately understood. The therapist by his interpretations assists the ego in its work of integration and thus helps to resolve the actual life situation.

With the increasing popularity of psychoanalytic therapy, there has been an increasing concern with the length of treatment. The short-cut methods of Ferenczi and Rank were frowned on, rapid cures were attributed to the transference and that without a systematic 'working through', relapse was certain. Poor results with prolonged treatment were attributed to the patient's weak ego-structure and consequent inability to resolve conflict. Alexander *et al.* (1946) challenged these and other views with a series of questions. They asked: is it true (1) that the depth of therapy is necessarily proportionate to the length of treatment and the frequency of the interviews? (2) that therapeutic results achieved by a relatively small number of interviews are necessarily superficial and temporary, while therapeutic results achieved by prolonged treatment are necessarily more stable and more profound? and (3) that extreme prolongation of an analysis is justified on the grounds that the patient's resistance will be eventually overcome and the desired therapeutic result achieved? They introduced the *principle of flexibility* in the application of the different therapeutic factors to different types of patients and this raised another question as to whether one can draw a sharp line between psychoanalysis proper and other analytically oriented forms of psychotherapy. Alexander (1957) tries to steer a middle course and states:

> The question whether or not in certain individual cases a 'personal psychotherapy' can be substituted for 'personal analysis' is an open one which for lack of experience cannot be answered in a dogmatic fashion . . . The view is slowly gaining acceptance that these procedures represent a continuum in which the two extremes are radically different but are connected by borderline procedures which blend into one another gradually . . . profound changes in personality occur sometimes not only through therapy but spontaneously under the influence of life's experiences. They often do occur, but not always, after penetrating prolonged psychoanalysis and they also occur frequently after so-called transference cures. They also occur under the influence of psychotherapeutic procedures which, quantitatively at least, differ from standard psychoanalysis . . . For evaluating the different forms of dynamic psychotherapy, treatments must be carefully recorded and observed by several trained persons before these controversial questions can be satisfactorily answered.

He points out the dangers of 'wild analysis' which is the unsound application of partial or vague knowledge and supports the view that psychoanalytic concepts in psychotherapy should preferably be taught in psychoanalytic institutes, but need not necessarily be restricted to them. He considers that the institutes of psychoanalysis with their exclusive interest in the standard technique do not give their students such an advantage in the application of new and experimental methods of treatment which must be designed to meet our changing social structure.

Psychoanalysis proper, which is the most extensively practised, like other depth therapies, cannot be learned out of a book, but requires personal experience with supervision, though Alexander (1957) has proposed a form of analytically oriented psychotherapy which may be practised by the less intensively trained psychiatrist and there is no doubt that such a technique based on an adequate theoretical knowledge can considerably extend the range of usefulness of the non-analytically trained psychotherapist.

It is apparent that in the vast welter of psychotherapeutic problems, most can be helped by superficial therapy, a large number by analytically orientated psychotherapy, but that the more intractable problems require an intensive analytical approach, with at least five sessions per week and continuing for three years or more.

Berg (1948) gives a simplified account of psychoanalytical technique and defines four general principles:

1. *Passivity*. This must be 'utter and complete and sustained' by the analyst. This may mean the enduring of long periods of intolerable silence, perhaps as intolerable for the psychiatrist as it is for the patient.

2. *Free-association of Thought*. This applies to the patient. He is asked to relax and just say what he wants to say or whatever enters his mind.

3. *Daily Sessions of* 50 *Minutes each with a Minimum of Five Sessions a Week*. This principle is the one which has aroused great controversy on account of expense and inconvenience to the patient, and thc necessary restriction of such treatment to those few who can afford it. Short-cut methods are constantly being introduced and though there are undoubtedly instances where the long-term and intensive approach is essential, there are many patients who can be helped to recovery with less intensive treatment. It is, however, on occasions difficult to gauge the patient's requirements till information derived from intensive treatment is available.

4. *The Recumbent Position*. This, too, has given rise to controversy, for some object to its regressive implications which they claim heighten suggestibility and that this element should not be introduced into a situation where theoretically it has no place. It does, however, help to cast the psychiatrist in a less personal and obtrusive role.

The process of psychoanalysis he divides into the following stages:

1. *The Pre-transference Stage*. This he states is the one which most psychiatrists even without analytical training manage successfully, provided they are passive.

2. *The Transference Neurosis*. This includes the 'displacement of

affect, positive and negative, from one person (usually the parent) on to another person, *e.g.* the analyst, or . . . a projection on to the analyst of affects originally experienced towards the parents during the period of infantile amnesia'. It may manifest with improvement in the patient and a general reduction of symptoms.

3. *Transference Analysis.* This is a highly skilled process requiring analysis of the patient's resistances, the uncovering of early infantile attitudes and the judicious use of interpretation.

4. *The Terminal Stage.* This can be as difficult as the preceding stage for many patients are content to remain in the transference stage. Berg describes the process as 'libidinal weaning' and 'ego education', 'the patient's ego being encouraged to take over the direct control of his instinctual life in place of the previous directors of this life'. These directors were in turn the super-ego and the analyst.

The factors which interfere with the ordinary progress of analysis are:

1. *Defence-resistance.* This interferes with free-association and Freud defined five aspects: (*a*) ego resistance; (*b*) transference resistance, which should be interpreted by the analyst; (*c*) gain resistance, which is an attempt by the illness to achieve advantage: (*d*) super-ego resistances, which though they disappear usually in the early stages may have to be completely uncovered in the transference analysis; (*e*) id resistances, which consist of an urge to be repetitive as is seen in obsessional neurosis and may prolong the analysis.

2. *Counter-transference and Counter-resistance.* These may consist of the patient's tendency to project his own insecurities on to the analyst. Some of the patient's accusations may contain a modicum of truth and upset the analyst who may as Berg points out,

> have to do some analytical toilet of his own so that these, often very stimulating accusations will no longer arouse his own emotional tendency to revulsion, however determinedly suppressed. He must never retaliate either actively or passively. For instance, he must beware of excessive interpretation emotionally motivated, as this may prove on the unconscious levels to be the equivalent of counter-attack or of sexual assault, if not of positive sadism. Conversely, excessive silence when help should be given, may be an outlet for the analyst's revenge tendency, or a reaction-formation against sadistic trends in himself.

The above points in analytical technique illustrate the difficulties and complexities of the treatment and the reader should not consider that even an intimate knowledge of psychopathology is adequate to start practising this technique on patients. He should seek training either individually or in a group situation so that neither he nor his patients suffer from his untutored efforts.

There are many who deny the specificity of psychoanalytical treatment and attribute any good results to suggestion or 'brain washing'. Others have tried to explain psychoanalysis in terms of a behaviourist model and have gone back to Pavlov (1921) for their inspiration, for in certain circumstances his experimental animals developed behaviour patterns which resembled neurotic behaviour in man. As these patterns could be induced under controlled laboratory conditions, Pavlov considered that these experiments could be used to assist in the understanding of the aetiology, nature and treatment of mental illness. Masserman (1943) following in this path, but with a psychoanalytical background, trained cats to obtain their food when hungry by approaching and lifting the lid of a food box. After this response was established, the approach to the food was interrupted by air blast or electric shock with striking changes in the animal's behaviour:

> . . . somatic manifestations of anxiety in or out of the apparatus, hyperaesthetic startle reactions, consistent 'phobic' responses to the feeding signal, to space constriction, or to other meaningful configurations previously associated with the conflict situation, typical 'compulsion' and 'fixation' patterns of hiding or escape, 'narcissistic' or regressive manifestations such as excessive licking and preening, and even protracted food-avoidance and self-starvation to the point of extreme cachexia.

Other workers have reported similar findings. Maier (1949) observed persistent fixation in rats when the conflict involved two incompatible tendencies, while Gantt (1944) reported severe behaviour disturbances in dogs which continued for as long as 10 years after induction, in and out of the laboratory. Many experiments have since been conducted on goats, sheep, pigs, rabbits, monkeys and chimpanzees. Physiological changes were recorded in the heart rate, respiration rate, sexual function, and frequency of urination and defaecation, while there were wide individual differences between the species and between animals of the same species.

The danger of drawing conclusions from such experiments has been pointed out by Anderson and Liddell (1935) who attributed the results to the confinement of the animals, for they found that unconfined animals did not develop abnormal symptoms. Even with confined animals, not all developed behaviour disturbances and individual differences have been attributed to genetic or constitutional factors. Hall (1938) showed that by selective breeding, rats may within filial generations be divided into two groups, one very 'emotional' and the other very 'unemotional' in situations of conflict. As with many models, there has been considerable anthropomorphism introduced into the descriptive language, *e.g.* Masserman has reported varying degrees of success, by decreasing the intensity of one of the conflictual drives; by petting and gentle hand-feeding the animal ('transference') during a retraining period; by altering the environment and forcing the animal at the height of its hunger drive into the vicinity of the conflict situation; by 'irritation' of a 'non-neurotic' animal in the conflict situation; and by training the animal to control the essential features of the environment, thus learning to 'work through' its conflict.

The above attractive analogy has given theoretical support to Behaviour Therapy (p. 918) and by implication has been used as an argument against the tenets of psychoanalysis, though some workers have claimed the reverse. For example, Hunt (1941) obtained results which indicated that frustration in the feeding of the infant rat leads to abnormal hoarding of food in the adult animal and Levy (1934) has shown that artificially nourished puppies and calves which are not permitted to indulge in nipple-sucking to the point of satiation develop abnormal behaviour patterns, licking their paws or other objects to a degree dangerous to their health.

The quotation by Walshe (1965) of Sir James Paget's views on clinical science is most appropriate to these animal studies:

> within our range of study that done is true which is proved clinically and that which is clinically proved needs no other evidence . . . a failure to obtain similar observations in cat, dog or monkey, leaves their validity untouched. Conversely the obtaining of data in animals identical with those found in man in similar circumstances does not lend confirmation to the clinical observation, it merely establishes a homology, and the establishment of a homology between the phenomena of clinical observation in man and those of experiment in animals rests upon an accurate knowledge of both so that their assemblances, and their differences, if any, may be evaluated.

Psychotherapy is still the big enigma in therapeutics and, in spite of much theory and experimentation, we are still very far from knowing what makes the patient better. Apart from spontaneous remission, about which nothing is known, there are a host of procedures which can result in cure. These are listed by Meares (1962) thus:

> Many patients lose their nervous symptoms after such vastly different forms of treatment as a quiet talk with the family physician, simple sedation, ataractic drugs, superficial psychotherapy, abreaction, conditioning, waking suggestion, hypnotic suggestion, hypnoanalysis, narco-analysis, autogenic training, psychoanalysis, Adlerian analysis, and Jungian analysis. The psychopathology of the condition is not a reliable guide to how it will respond to different forms of treatment.
>
> Many patients lose their nervous symptoms after such non-medical procedures as Christian prayer, yoga meditation, Zen practices, self-taught autohypnosis, or just a good holiday.

Meares would be less than human if he did not postulate his own theory of the process of recovery and he calls it *'atavistic regression'*, which he defines as 'the process by which the mind ceases to function at a logical critical level, and reverts to a biologically more primitive mode of functioning'. He believes that this process takes place in every procedure which is able to make the patient better and he bases his theory on his experiments with hypnosis (Meares, 1960).

It would be giving a wrong impression to suggest that one type of treatment is as good as another or that it didn't really matter what you did to the patient, as long as you did something. Patients and their illnesses vary and there is no doubt that some will respond to a relatively simple approach, while others will require a more prolonged and deeper one. What is required will depend on a careful assessment of all the factors based on a full and intimate knowledge of the patient and his problems and to gain this, psychoanalytical insight may be necessary. An untutored charlatan may in a percentage of instances produce dramatic results, but if one is to understand the psychological processes that are operating, and be able to help the patient in the greatest possible number of instances and not do the patient harm, then a detached knowledge of psychopathology and instruction in psychotherapy is essential.

Common Features of Psychotherapy

Frank (1972), in an overview of Western psychotherapy since Freud, emphasizes two points: (1) the dominant psychotherapeutic approach of an era reflects the cultural attitudes of its time and place; and (2) the same psychotherapeutic techniques keep recurring under different guises, suggesting that despite their superficial differences, they all may be variations on a few underlying themes.

He mentions six features common to all which contribute to their effectiveness:

1. An intense, emotionally charged, confiding relationship with a helping person.
2. A rationale or myth which includes an explanation of the cause of the person's distress and a method for relieving it. To be effective, the therapeutic myth must be compatible with the cultural world-view shared by the patient and therapist. The supplying of a conceptual scheme, for what seems to the patient to be a group of nonsensical symptoms, provides powerful reassurance to him. It is the function of the rationale and technique rather than their specific content and form which really count.

3. Provision of new information concerning the nature and sources of the patient's problems and alternative ways of dealing with them.
4. Strengthening the patient's expectations of help through the personal qualities of the therapist, enhanced by his status in society and the setting in which he works.
5. Provision of the experience of successful mastery over symptoms which heighten the patient's hopes.
6. Facilitation of emotional arousal, a prerequisite of attitudinal and behavioural changes.

He distinguishes four groups of Americans who seek psychotherapy:

1. Those struggling with modern problems of identity and alienation, who, instead of requiring psychotherapy, may receive help from groups or religious sects who can restore meaning to life.
2. Essentially sound individuals who are overwhelmed by a crisis and can be helped by non-professionals offering brief, empathic support.
3. Individuals with constitutional weaknesses so deeply ingrained that they cannot be undone by psychological means, and though medication may help, non-professionals can provide the psychological support.
4. Those who respond differentially to different approaches because their symptoms seem to be related primarily to specific learning defects or traumatic experiences in early life, and they may require professional psychotherapy. The author suggests that this last group be categorized so that the most appropriate therapy be selected.

This thoughtful contribution may prove unpalatable to some but it does highlight the large number of patients who receive but do not need skilled psychotherapy.

BEHAVIOUR THERAPY

This is a relatively new term for something which is as old as man himself, in fact older, for some of its methods are used by the lower animals. At the human level, wherever fear (or anxiety) had to be overcome, or where bad habits had to be eliminated, re-education was tried and the pill either sweetened or made more bitter to achieve the desired result. Long before Pavlov had described his experimental work on conditional reflexes, human society had evolved such proverbs as 'burnt bairns dread the fire' and 'spare the rod and spoil the child'. For centuries teachers and parents have used techniques in the training of the young which were not dissimilar to some used by Pavlov in the training of his dogs, and no doubt drill sergeants who served with Alexander could show a thing or two to modern practitioners of behaviour therapy. It is also likely that these methods were in ancient times not confined to the training of the young but were also applied to the treatment of the mentally ill and certainly to the mentally subnormal. It is literally only a few steps from the anxiety and fear associated with diving into the water from a modest height to have a general fear of heights; fears of riding a bicycle can readily deteriorate to a general nervousness in traffic. Such fears are usually overcome by what is regarded as the ordinary educative processes of life and we can all remember our own insecurities and how 'treatment' of a de-conditioning nature was employed. In this scientific age when analogies are freely borrowed from experimental work in order to explain the workings of the mind, it is not surprising that a system of therapy has been developed which is based on the theoretical aspects of conditioned reflexes and the more recent advances of learning theory.

In its formal and present-day sense, behaviour therapy has been used for at least 40 years. Dunlap (1932) described a method where the patient actively and consciously practised the undesired habits in order to get rid of them and Goresky (1948) reported the technique he used in general practice. More recently, Goresky (1961) has redefined his aims, saying that he is mainly concerned with the amelioration of symptoms and these he attributes to conditional responses to environmental stress. The patient is encouraged to examine his problem by reviewing past unpleasant experiences and in this way to learn to respond normally to present stresses. If this cannot be achieved, 'situational adjustment' is used. The patient is taught to ask three questions:

1. What is happening that upsets me?
2. What is my emotional reaction and what are its disadvantages?
3. What should be the right reaction to keep me out of trouble with my conscience in the light of my duty to my family and other people?

When reviewing his past experiences, similar questions are posed and the patient is taught to use this technique by himself, at first for several times a day and less often as the need diminishes.

The most comprehensive account of this 'new' therapy is by

Eysenck (1960). He is a non-medical psychologist who has established himself as the major protagonist of the treatment, yet as Stengel (1961) remarks 'there is no evidence that Professor Eysenck has ever carried out a treatment himself'. Hull's theory, which expresses in mathematical terms the factors determining the formation and extinction of conditioned reflexes, gives the treatment a scientific basis which its exponents declare is absent from psychoanalysis and in fact a considerable amount of space is devoted to dismissing many of the latter's accepted tenets. Methods of treatment are by reciprocal inhibition, negative practice, aversion therapy and positive conditioning, and as with most new measures whether by drugs or even in surgical procedures and especially in psychotherapy, early results are most encouraging but many reports are of successful treatment in a single case. Wolpe (1958), who is a major contributor to the literature, has claimed 90 per cent recovery in a large series. This is a very substantial claim, and it remains to be seen whether it will be confirmed by the large number of workers in the field.

Neurosis, which has already been proven to the satisfaction of the 'school' as a statistical factor, is not regarded as a disease, but a collection of symptoms acquired as conditioned reflexes. People develop these conditioned responses at different speeds and in different degrees. A third aspect is the tenacity with which these symptoms are held, but all three depend on the individual's personality. The conditioned reactions are regarded as surplus in dysthymics and as deficient in hysterics and psychopaths. Underlying anxiety is regarded as the basis of all symptoms and motor activity such as tics and compulsive movements are said to be anxiety reducing. The unconscious is given scant recognition, and is in fact ignored in treatment and the patient is 'cured' when symptoms and anxiety are removed, for neurotic symptoms are regarded merely as learned patterns of behaviour which for some reason or other are unadaptive, there being no underlying disorder. Psychotic illness has to date escaped serious attention, but no doubt some intrepid spirits are preparing to attack this field.

Among the variety of conditions treated are phobic states and there have been reports of individual cases including one of cat phobia (Freeman & Kendrick, 1960) where the patient was gradually deconditioned by placing pictures of cats round the house so that she would be confronted unexpectedly with the appearance of the animal. Later this was supplemented with stroking a piece of fur and so on till the fear of cats was resolved. Other clinical states treated in a similar way are transvestism, fetishism, alcoholism and homosexuality. In a case of transvestism reported by Barker *et al.* (1961) colour transparencies of the patient in female attire were taken and a tape-recording was made of his description of the process of dressing up. Aversion therapy was employed by means of apomorphine hydrochloride, but this was later replaced by emetine hydrochloride because of the establishment of tolerance to the apomorphine. Each injection was followed by presentation of the slides and the tape recording, with subsequent recovery. After three months the patient had not relapsed but the authors criticize its apparent therapeutic efficiency.

> It is time-consuming and expensive, and is extremely unpleasant for the patient. It is clumsy, for using emetic drugs creates great difficulties in timing the introduction and cessation of the conditioned stimulus (slides and tape recording) for optimal conditioning, and possibly in some trials the stimulus preceded pleasant rather than unpleasant drug responses owing to fluctuations in the degree of nausea as reported by the patient. Also apomorphine, which has central depressant properties, reduces the value of the conditioned stimulus at the time of presentation and tolerance develops rapidly to this drug which had to be administered in increasing doses to produce any effects. . . .

They conclude their refreshingly frank report thus:

> Because of these numerous difficulties it is clearly misleading to regard this procedure as straightforward deconditioning, and at present we are unable to demonstrate the precise mechanisms which alleviated symptoms in our patient.

These authors are not alone in questioning the theoretical basis of behaviour therapy.

The subject is at present on a wave of enthusiasm and has a distinct appeal to the 'directive and organic' type of psychiatrist; it has therefore already achieved considerable prominence in British psychiatry and is now beginning to make an impact on the American scene. Carefully controlled work on the treatment of phobic anxiety states by behaviour therapy has been carried out by Marks and Gelder (1966) and they report that the method *in this condition* is superior to traditional psychotherapy (see Chapter 11). Others are using the treatment for compulsive gambling, smoking, drug-addiction and thrustful car drivers, but unlike Marks and Gelder, the method employed is that of aversion therapy, by means of electric shocks. While it is too early to pass judgement, it is possible to state some of the arguments in its favour as well as those against.

For

1. It is bringing the concept of psychotherapy to a group of psychiatrists who to date have had great difficulty in accepting the

value of psychotherapy and were almost exclusively organic in their approach. This new superficial approach may eventually lead to an appreciation of depth psychology.

2. It had underlined the fact that treatment of symptoms can help some patients towards a working adjustment and that full analysis in these cases would be unnecessary and uneconomic.

3. By its attack on psychoanalysts, it has stimulated the latter to a re-appraisal of their tenets and to seek experimental proof, and though much of the criticism is ignorant, it has made the more serious psychoanalysts think of how they can reconcile their researches with modern scientific criteria. This process was already in evidence but there is no doubt that it will now be accelerated.

4. As it is based mainly on psychological theories, it provides a link between the psychologist and the clinician, introducing the latter to the former's techniques of research and validation and it may prove a useful medium for teaching general psychology to medical students.

Against

1. By ignoring underlying causes, behaviour therapy offends the cardinal rule of clinical practice, to seek out the cause of the disease and then eradicate it. To regard a thinking and feeling human being as a variety of conditioned reflexes resulting in symptoms and to treat these by some form of deconditioning can only be a retrograde step and is reminiscent of those happily bygone days when medical practice consisted of three mixtures labelled 'head', 'stomach' and 'the rest' and a bottle of the appropriate mixture was dispensed entirely on the basis of the patient's complaint. Even hypnotherapy, which till recently was the most symptomatic form of treatment, allows for the unconscious and handles its material by hypnoanalysis.

2. Some of the clinical concepts on which the theories are founded are not generally accepted and even though complicated arithmetic may apparently prove that neuroticism and psychoticism are clear-cut entities, psychiatrists know that mixed states occur. For example, obsessional states can decompensate and give way to either severe depression or even schizophrenic reactions. Diagnostic labels such as hysteria and schizophrenia are freely used but it is obvious that while the psychologist has made an impact by his factor analysis and learning theories on his psychiatric colleagues, the latter have not yet influenced the psychologist, whose knowledge of psychiatry is too limited to permit the generalizations he uses.

3. Conditions treated are predominatly monosymptomatic and

include tics, stammering, bedwetting and writer's cramp, but these constitute only a fraction of neurotic illness and may on closer inquiry extend into other symptoms which presumably have been overlooked by the behaviour therapist.

4. Aversion therapy has its own dynamic significance for both patient and therapist and while the latter may choose to ignore the unconscious of the patient he should be fully cognizant of his own. The use of violent emetics, electric shocks and other brutal forms of therapy can encourage his own sadistic drives and instead of a patient he may have found a masochistic partner.

5. The overt hostility to all things psychoanalytic is most unfortunate for it makes the motivation of the school suspect. An objective appraisal of psychoanalytic concepts is one thing, though one might argue it could be better undertaken by those with some real knowledge and experience of the subject and what is perhaps even more important, a thorough knowledge of clinical psychiatry. Much of the work of behaviour therapists and theorists, though highly critical of the unscientific methods of the analysts, falls far short of the criteria of clinical science. Sophisticated statistics can never invalidate sound clinical observation and it would be a sad day for medicine if they did. It is on the clinical rock that spurious theories from whatever source will founder.

6. Although behaviour therapy is put forward as a 'scientific' treatment and free of the dynamic contaminants of psychoanalysis such as transference and resistance, Rhoads and Feather (1972) report a study of five patients where the phenomena interfered significantly with treatment. They used a therapist-observer method, with one psychiatrist continuing to see the patient as observer while the other carried out the behaviour therapy. In one instance the patient developed an intense dislike of the therapist and his 'authoritarian ways' and she refused to co-operate. Another female patient's treatment foundered on the resistance of the patient to facing an unresolved Oedipus complex, complicated by an erotic transference to the therapist.

The authors illustrate that failure to deal with the resistance and transference phenomena in these cases through rigid application of the behaviour model prejudiced successful treatment. This point needs emphasis, for many behaviour therapists are unaware of the dynamic factors in all such treatments.

Aversion Therapy and Behaviour Disorders

There has been criticism enough of the dynamic components and theoretical constructs of behaviour therapy from those who are prejudiced against the treatment. It is refreshing to read valid criticisms from those who were at one time enthusiastic advocates but are now more circumspect. Rachman and Teasdale (1969) state: 'Although there is strong evidence that aversion therapy is frequently effective in terminating alcoholism, it is not definitive. In particular, we require conclusive demonstrations that aversion therapy contributes more to the therapeutic process than the non-specific factors involved in general treatment and rehabilitation procedure'. They refer to the notable absence of control studies in the treatment of sexual disorders, with the possible exception of homosexuality, and the 'punishment training' for alcoholism and obesity. This is all to the good and should help to modify the earlier exaggerated claims.

Suxemethonium Chloride in Aversion Therapy. Suxemethonium chloride is a muscle relaxant used in anaesthesia for electroconvulsant therapy. It induces muscular paralysis with apnoea and this is used to decondition heroin addicts who indulge in self-injection, and for alcoholics. Thomson and Rathod (1968) describe the verbal accompaniment in the heroin addict. They say: 'This is how "stuff" can kill you, you may suffocate to death'. After minor cyanosis has developed oxygen is given. It is not surprising that three patients abandoned treatment after one or two sessions and two absconded.

GROUP PSYCHOTHERAPY

The present fashion of working with groups has given a stimulus to the use of group psychotherapy, though the psychotherapy may in many instances be quite unstructured and not directed towards any goal, other than a general desire to make people feel better. Man is born into a group and his earliest relationships are with a group; it is not surprising therefore that he derives considerable support from group acceptance. In pre-historic times, the group must have organized such support for those in need, and throughout history there are examples of groups of men and women who banded themselves together for their own emotional well-being and/or the glory of God. The Essenes, on the west shore of the Dead Sea, the monasteries, convents, colleges, Secret and Friendly Societies, clubs, fraternities and sororities, all testify to the need of individuals to belong to a group and the more exclusive the better. It may represent a need to recreate the original family group which is the most exclusive group of all, and the prefix 'brother' and 'sister' which these groups frequently employ is suggestive.

Modern group psychotherapy as a branch of psychological medicine is a relatively recent innovation. This is not surprising, as it had to wait for the formulation of group dynamics, which were inspired by the two-body relationship of individual psychotherapy. Freud (1922) in his *Group Psychology and the Analysis of the Ego*, summarized some of the basic mechanisms of group behaviour, stressing the group mind, suggestion, identification, and the herd instinct. It is doubtful however, whether he has group psychotherapy in mind. Moreno's psychodrama (p. 940) is probably one of the earliest examples of a group technique but the main impact came with the Second World War. In Great Britain, the War Office sponsored resettlement units for repatriated prisoners of war in an effort to reintegrate them into the community. It had been learned that after the First World War, the repatriated prisoner of war proved a very difficult social problem. He carried within him a certain load of guilt at having been taken prisoner and tried to project it on to society. Many of them had anxiety features and their group psychotherapy consisted of explanatory talks on the physical concomitants of anxiety, and the operation of some mental mechanisms. These talks together with the other measures, which included a marked reduction in formality and military discipline, helped to settle many of these men, some of whom were very disturbed, in a relatively short time. Visits were arranged to local industries and the Ministry of Labour played its part; overall, it was probably one of the smoothest and most successful exercises of the war. Such a simple approach is probably adequate for a homogeneous group with identical problems.

The practice has spread and there are now numerous forms of group psychotherapy, some with a theoretical basis and a well-formulated order of procedure, while others are just 'groups'. Slavson (1950) is credited by some with having introduced psychoanalytical concepts into the practice, which he used originally with disturbed children, but Foulkes (1948) had been using these methods with the British Army during the Second World War. This permissive or analytically oriented method was also used by Maxwell Jones at Belmont with psychopathic personalities and there have since been many reports of the technique and its results.

Theoretical Considerations

In addition to Freudian psychopathology, group psychotherapy makes use (as did Freud) of Le Bon's concept of the 'Group Mind'. Freud (1922) quotes:

The most striking peculiarity presented by a psychological group is the following. Whoever be the individuals that compose it, however like or unlike their mode of life, their occupations, their character, or their intelligence, the fact that they have been transformed into a group puts them in possession of a sort of collective mind which makes them feel, think and act in a manner quite different from that in which each individual of them would feel, think, and act were he in a state of isolation. There are certain ideas and feelings which do not come into being, or do not transform themselves into acts except in the case of individuals forming a group. The psychological group is a provisional being formed of heterogeneous elements, which for a moment are combined, exactly as the cells which constitute a living body form by their reunion a new being which displays characteristics very different from those possessed by each of the cells singly.

It is easy to prove how much the individual forming part of a group differs from the isolated individual, but it is less easy to discover the causes of this difference.

The first is that the individual forming part of a group acquires, solely from numerical considerations, a sentiment of invincible power which allows him to yield to instincts which had he been alone, he would perforce have kept under restraint. He will be the less disposed to check himself from the consideration that, a group being anonymous, and in consequence irresponsible, the sentiment of responsibility which always controls individuals disappears entirely.

The second cause, which is contagion, also intervenes to determine the manifestation in groups of their special characteristics, and at the same time the trend they are to take. Contagion is a phenomenon of which it is easy to establish the presence, but that is is not easy to explain. It must be classed among those phenomena of a hypnotic order, which we shall shortly study. In a group every sentiment and act is contagious, and contagious to such a degree that an individual readily sacrifices his personal interest to the collective interest. This is an aptitude very contrary to his nature, and of which a man is scarcely capable, except when he makes part of a group.

A third cause, and by far the most important, determines in the individuals of a group special characteristics which are quite contrary at times to those presented by the isolated individual. I allude to that suggestibility of which, moreover, the contagion mentioned above is only an effect.

Groups are classified as Didactic or Leaderless.

Didactic or Directive

These have a leader who should be familiar with the individual patients and their problems and who can steer the discussion and bring into it those who may be otherwise too inhibited. It is a useful medium for elaborating on a common problem like that of anxiety in repatriated prisoners of war, or phobic anxiety in housebound housewives. Some psychiatrists, particularly psychoanalysts, are unsympathetic to the didactic group because it offends their training and they argue that is creates a dependence on the leader which is unhealthy. While theoretically this may be a valid argument, the same could be said of any lecturer or even tutor, and the realities of the situation suggest that didactic methods have their uses, not only with neurotic patients, but with psychotic patients, particularly schizophrenics.

Leaderless or Non-directive

These are usually run on psychoanalytical lines and as has been said is the method favoured by Slavson and Foulkes and also by the Tavistock Clinic, which at one time was almost group-committed. The optimum number is usually eight persons though it can contract to six or extend to ten. In addition to the psychiatrist, there is often a psychiatric social worker, and some have argued that these two especially if of opposite sexes, help to recreate the family situation and permit the easier development of transferences and resistances and their expression.

The selection of patients is most important and it has been found that hypomanic patients are particularly disruptive in that they monopolize conversation and never give the others a chance, yet their efforts do not relieve their own problems. Psychopathic personalities have also been regarded as disruptive in that they may lack the essential factor of conscious honesty. Psychotherapy can deal with the distortion of the unconscious but conscious deceit is a different matter. This difficulty with psychopaths is not yet proven and some have claimed good results with them either singly or comprising the whole group.

The arrangement of the group may also be important, in that a retiring and sensitive person on the fringe may be extruded. The seats should be arranged so that the less assertive are brought into the centre or put between a couple who tend to talk it out between themselves. The group in a leaderless situation will generally 'elect' the psychiatrist as their leader and all he can do is refrain from being didactic, so in fact a leaderless group is really a nondidactic one. Interpretation is usually given and the essence of the group is the feeding-in of information, as in individual psychotherapy. Membership is usually decided by the group and they may exclude a member of the medical staff of the hospital or a visiting psychiatrist who wishes to learn techniques. This can be a nuisance, but it is the patients' confidences on which the group functions, and they are entitled to decide who shall share them.

The range of groups that are in being must now include every conceivable grouping of people, both spontaneous and artificial.

Some do group therapy with entire families, alcoholics, drug-addicts, prisoners, schizophrenics, phobic anxiety states, psychopaths, chronic hospitalized psychotics, disturbed children, business executives, and religious sects, to mention a few. It is debatable whether a patient in group therapy should also attend for individual therapy. If the psychiatrist is responsible for the overall treatment of, say a schizophrenic patient, it would be quite in order to see the patient individually and allow him to attend the group with another psychiatrist. It is a different matter if the group psychiatrist sees the patient individually and should this be so, the group should be informed and the situation explained to them; even then it can give rise to difficulties.

Semrad and Arsenian (1951) used group psychotherapy as a medium for training in group dynamics and Balint (1957) had a group of general practitioners with an interest in psychotherapy attending the Tavistock Clinic, who by learning of their own problems, were better able to handle those of their patients.

The challenge of a group situation is apparently less than the two-body one in individual psychotherapy and it is therefore easier for psychiatrists in training to integrate themselves in such activities. The author has found it a valuable medium for helping the registrar, with a hitherto directive and organic background and training, to overcome his resistances to dynamic psychiatry and to learn to appreciate, at first hand, mental mechanisms. Just as group therapy is often an expedient and successful measure in the treatment of a larger number of patients than can be handled in individual therapy, so it is now proving a successful and economic method in the training of psychiatrists.

Termination in Group Psychotherapy

When the therapist is one of a leaderless group, one may ask how therapy is terminated. McGee *et al.* (1972) discuss the problem as it concerns patients. Termination may take the form of a 'phone call or letter to the therapist or failure to attend. It may follow a 'flight into health', represent an unwillingness to advance further or be announced in advance and carefully worked through. They recommend that the individual contemplating termination should be encouraged to announce his intentions openly in the group, at a time sufficiently in advance to permit adequate discussion and when it does occur it should be regarded as irrevocable. On the question as to how the therapist can terminate treatment or leave the group himself, the authors are silent. Presumably, as long as people are prepared to attend they must be in need. It would be interesting to test the validity of such an assumption.

Group Psychotherapy. A Patient's View

It is as well to try and see this treatment through the eyes of a patient, though it must be admitted the following quotation may not be typical. The patient was admitted for this treatment to his local mental hospital and writes (Cox, 1965):

> In the unit I was introduced to the Alice-in-Wonderland world of group psychotherapy. The discussion groups usually occupied three or four hours a day, but, in our desperation to be cured, informal groups often met until the small hours of the morning. This practice was well known to the psychiatrists and staff and, I suspect, approved by them, since no measures were taken to stop or curtail these cock-crow debates. Some of the official groups were held in the enigmatic, and usually silent, presence of a psychiatrist. Other groups were under the supervision of nurses, or more often occupational therapists, perhaps 20 or so years old.
>
> We were encouraged to express our feelings about anything in general, including personal interreactions with each other. Heaven knows how many millions of words were expended, to such apparently small purpose. At times the groups were sullen and uncommunicative. At other times a patient would dramatically express or confess feelings of, say, anger, hatred, or lust. This reaction was what the psychiatrists wanted; but, when the tears or fuss had died down, there was no apparent result.
>
> The unit developed a jargon and language of its own. The insistence on feelings led us to preface almost any statement or opinion with the words 'I feel'. Another well-aired verb was to 'escape'. This covered a multitude of situations. For example, most evenings I left the unit for a beer or two (which was officially permissible), and often I was then accused of 'escaping'. Indeed, the insinuation of 'escape' could apply to almost any situation, including oversleeping, reading in a quiet corner, or visiting the cinema.
>
> I sometimes felt like a goldfish, swimming endlessly and hopelessly with its fellows around a glass bowl, under the eyes of psychiatrists and staff. The groups went on and on. Discussion followed discussion. We squeezed our memories and feelings like a sponge and awaited the cure. Every month or so, an evening group was held, to which ex-patients were invited. Very few attended, and it was only too apparent that most of those who did were far from well, or whistling in the dark.
>
> More than half of the patients in the unit were women, aged from 22 to 55. I know of two illegitimate children conceived during the 'treatment', many broken marriages, and some suicides by discharged patients. These casualties might be considered as unhappy but necessary side-effects of psychotherapy; but the lamentable truth is that the treatment was far from beneficial.
>
> Many dismal features confronted the new patient. For example, some patients had been in hospital for three years or more, and had been readmitted several times. Despite these obvious facts, the new entrants were told briskly that a cure was usually obtained in 4 to 6 months. My own treatment lasted about 10 months. I finally left the unit more in a sense of desperation than of confidence. I was given outpatient treatment for almost another year with weekly individual psychotherapy.

Though I was now back at my job, I was without interest or confidence. In fact, I had developed what I can only describe as an obsession about neurosis. I sought opportunities to discuss nervous breakdowns with anybody and everybody—my friends, family and casual acquaintances.

This patient later responded to anti-depressant drugs. It does illustrate that even when group psychotherapy is undertaken there should be a constant review of the patient's clinical state, preferably outside the group situation. It should again be emphasized that many patients do benefit from group therapy and write equally informative reports to that effect.

T-Group and Acute Psychosis

A T-group is a relatively unstructured group in which individuals participate as learners, the learning data being the transactions among members. Thus each individual may learn about his own motives, feelings and strategies in dealing with other persons, and about the reactions he produces in others. These groups, particularly in the United States, are sponsored by industry, universities, social service agencies, and non-profit groups, but little has been said of their possible harmful effects.

Jaffe and Scherl (1969) describe two patients who suffered an acute transient psychosis precipitated by an intensive T-group experience. They suggest that participation in these groups be voluntary and informed, that participants are screened and that there are clear limits regarding acceptable behaviour as well as individual follow-up. Their main criticism is that the T-group is a social setting that encourages openness, intimacy and closeness, but has little structure for handling the anxiety that is provoked.

EXISTENTIAL PSYCHIATRY

A period of intellectual snobbery, whether in religious practice or in philosophy, brings its reaction. Thus the 'sensible' Anglican attitude generated the Shakers and the Wesleyan movement. Rabbinical and Talmudical supremacy led to Hassidism, and the rationalism of Hegel led to Kierkegaard's insistence that truth could be found only in existence. Perhaps more significant was his feverish agitation against the theology and practice of the state church, on the ground that religion was for the individual soul and should be separated from the state and the world. His philosophy was a reaction against speculative thinkers and was based on the absolute dualism of Faith and Knowledge.

It is not surprising therefore that the rationalism and objectivity of the psychoanalytic movement should produce among its reactions existential psychiatry, that this relative newcomer to the psychiatric field should find its inspiration in Kierkegaard and that one of its greatest protagonists and theorists should be Martin Buber, who had already distinguished himself as the apostle of Neo-Hassidism. It has already attracted a number of well-known psychiatrists, including psychoanalysts and has claimed its philosophers (Buber, Kierkegaard, Nietzsche, Sartre and Schopenhauer), its authors (Dostoevski, Kafka and Rilke) and painters (Cézanne, van Gogh and Picasso), and runs a quarterly journal. It will doubtless appeal to a large number of psychiatrists who like Binswanger protest against 'the subject-object cleavage of the world'.

Its adherents insist that it is not just another splinter group of analytical psychiatry, but that it is concerned with the concept of man, the basis of psychotherapy and the reality of human beings under stress. They claim that it has the character of a pure rather than an applied science, that the trained existential psychiatrist can see reality without adulterating it with preformed concepts and that all value judgements are excluded. He may even try to exclude the distinction of subject and object and thus gain a clearer picture of total phenomena. Minkowski (May, 1959) lived with and studied a schizophrenic patient for 24 hours per day for two months, and learned that the patient could not experience time in continuity and had no appreciation of or even hope for the future. His delusion was that his execution was imminent. It is alleged that the traditional psychiatrists would say that the patient could not relate to the future because of his delusion, whereas Minkowski suggests that the delusion itself was a result of the patient's inability to relate to the future.

The author is indebted to Dr Israel Sussman,* formerly Isaac Wolfson Travelling Fellow in the Department of Psychological Medicine of the United Birmingham Hospitals for the following account of 'Psychiatry and Existentialism': *(Masra Hospital near Acco, Israel).

Existentialism, like psychoanalysis, has introduced an entirely new aspect into psychology as it too deals more with motivation than with appearances. They both share an antipathy towards traditional and conventional theories, are products of our modern age and gain momentum with time, but here the analogy ends, for in their fundamentals they are really antagonistic.

Mind and Matter has been and still is the main 'problem' of philosophy, and the past 3000 years of history have thrown up many varieties of idealism, materialism and dualism to deal with it. The impact of the exact sciences has raised hopes that the 'essence' of Man might be defined in terms of mathematical formulae (cybernetics). Existentialism, on the other hand, seeks to characterize Man through its 'dynamic' formulations rather than through its 'essence'. This dynamic has been called **existence.**

Historical Note

With the advent of a bourgeois society, new ideas were introduced which led to Protestantism in religion and disintegration of aristocracy in the social system, which were tantamount to the dissolution of Divine Authority. The new laws were man-made and were accepted by the mass of the people as 'humanistic'. Destruction of idols is potentially dangerous, for one can never be certain that one has righted the real wrong, or one may have done too little or too much, probably the latter. Even if one were successful, the act of breaking down is likely to encourage more destruction by others with a resulting snowballing effect. To use another analogy, such a process can be compared with low and high pressure atmospheric regions with their resulting currents leading to instability and insecurity. One cannot accuse Protestantism of deliberate cynicism, but neither can one refrain from the conclusion that a mercantile society, in order to develop, must accumulate wealth with consequent decentralization in order to cut down the outflow of treasure to the Royal Court, or to a religious centre like the Vatican. Protestantism, therefore, though it is based on a spiritual ideology, served well the cause of the bourgeoisie. One might at this stage digress to discuss the origins of the bourgeois society, but we can summarize the situation thus: there is a relationship between the rebellion against the Divine hierarchy by Protestantism, and the insecurity resulting from such iconoclasm.

The ideology of Protestantism can also be compacted into one sentence: Man does not need an intermediary between himself and God for this relationship is an individual one; an **'I–Thou'** relationship. Is this assumption correct? The answer would appear to be in the negative, when one does not speak of Man, but of 'men' or 'people'. It seems that the new religion could be said to exist only where a rigid social rule was imposed on communities by the Presbyters, or, in other words, by the establishment of smaller, but once again, theocratic states. Elsewhere this 'I–Thou' relationship became the prerogative of the very few.

In parenthesis, one could follow the same process of idolization of other gods, like 'nationalism', 'communism', and 'capitalism' and observe the shifting centres of pressure with their resulting currents and insecurities, but here we are concerned only with Protestantism, which gave birth to Existentialism, for it was there that Man was left alone with his God, or as some would have it, where Man lost his God.

Psychiatrists need not be concerned with the academic study of this new school of philosophy, except to appreciate that in common with other disciplines, philosophy has its own language, history and rules for discussion. Psychiatrists should however be familiar with the conclusions of the Existential school about the nature of Man in order to gauge their relevance in their practice.

The first point that existentialism makes (a direct result of the loss of God), is the voidness or nothingness that faces and surrounds Man. As voidness breeds insecurity and insecurity is anxiety, Man becomes inseparable from anxiety, and this is a natural process common to all exposed to these influences and not an accidental or chance finding. The second point posed by existentialism is a question. Is Man himself 'something' in the midst of nothing? The answer given, is that each of us belongs to the human race and shares with other human beings certain characteristics which can be described in terms of the physical world. We also share some facts that are not 'matter' but can be labelled 'historical' because they apply to events which have happened such as in the process of natural development. This physical and historical information which is common to all men has been defined by philosophers as the 'essence' of *homo sapiens.* Existentialists feel that this knowledge describes some aspects which they call 'non-authentic' but that these do not help us to know or identify a man or Mr X. The authentic Mr X, or a man cannot be studied by these common phenomena in his present or past, but only from his future. Mr X exists only in terms of a projection of his intentions. He does not 'exist' in what he was because that is already dead, or colloquially 'simply vegetative'. Playing on the double meaning of 'exist' in its authentic and non-authentic senses, Sartre states: 'What exists does not exist, but what does not exist, exists'. He also states that the position of man in the world is that of 'a projection of nothingness to nothingness'. One cannot express anxiety in more dramatic terms and this definition also provides an answer to the eternal question: 'Is man something?'

There are two ways whereby anxiety can be overcome; firstly, to secure the nothingness or in other words to make something from nothing, which is a God-like action; secondly, to cease to exist and relinquish being human. The latter attitude is criticized as being really self-deception or 'acting in bad faith', it being explained that to 'act in good faith' is to be conscious of nothingness and to permit anxiety to continue or to project freely into anxiety, as consciousness and free will mean responsibility of the self. This implies moral responsibility and being conscious of other 'existences' as well, in contrast to psychoanalysis with its accent on the unconscious and pre-determinism.

There is a considerable difference in attitude to these problems if one assumes the existence or non-existence of God, which is not the same as believing or not believing in God. If there is God, and many Existentialists believe He does exist, then human existence is facilitated by the 'God–I' relationship which can make the individual feel truly God-like. For Martin Buber, who is one of the more prominent existentialist philosophers, the experience of God is rooted in Jewish Hassidism which is an emotional feeling of the universal existence of God. As very few people could experience God directly, the members of the Hassidic sect would foregather in the courts of their 'rabbis' (the equivalent of saints) and through their holiness, the ordinary person could share their religious experience. The same is true for other religious groups who believe in Divine revelation through intermediaries, and for that matter those who overcome anxiety or become lost through religious substitutes where a few dedicated 'ists' take the place of the priests. For atheistic existentialists like Sartre, any interposition of God or a God-like substitute in the nothingness, must be a form of acting in bad faith. Sartre's purpose is a heroic one, but he offers little help in terms of support or instruction on how to act in good faith. Furthermore very few can remain so independent and alone, for most people wish to assert their existence by being something or by searching for something which will be eternal and ever-lasting.

By inspired observation one can occasionally appreciate the singleness of purpose of a man and his life project by which he hopes to assert himself as eternal or 'existing' in the authentic and non-authentic senses simultaneously. This type of observation Sartre calls 'existential psychoanalysis' and he adds that the Freud of this kind of analysis has not yet been born. Sartre's purpose is to reduce all human phenomena into one of three modes of eternity: being someone, making something or someone, and having something or someone. It is significant for psychiatrists that whenever Sartre describes a person with singleness of purpose, one recognizes a psychotic or very pathological personality. As far as psychiatry is concerned, existentialism is still restricted to diagnosis and is not a method of treatment. History continues to create and shatter ideals, with the existentialist as an anxious observer, unable to help.

To summarize, existentialism is the philosophy of being nothing in the nothingness. It was born from the ashes of iconoclasts of all times. For a few, it supplies the strength to live virtuously in the midst of despair; for a few more it is the way back to God or a substitute; but for the mass of the people, it is a pessimistic diagnosis of our time. Some have misinterpreted it as a false prophet who justifies vice.

In order to explore the contribution of existentialism to psychiatry, one is tempted to compare it with psychoanalysis and some have tried to do this. But existentialism does not challenge psychoanalysis as long as the latter does not become a philosophy and the former in its true sense does not suggest any method of psychological treatment, though a number of psychiatrists have elaborated a treatment which has borrowed some of its concepts and have labelled it existential psychiatry.

It is generally agreed that the symptomatology of the schizophrenic is not meaningless and that the psychosis is a form of reaction by the extremely handicapped both mentally and organically. 'Mental' symptoms like paranoid delusions, euphoria or stupor are in themselves not enough to make a diagnosis of schizophrenia, for they may also present in organic states and similarly schizophrenics may exhibit a severe dementia which may closely resemble an organic state. Goldstein (1939) has pointed out that the greater defect there is in one's personality, the more rigid and less numerous are the patterns of reaction that remain, and with the narrowing of personality there is an accompanying increase of anxiety. An alternative way of putting it would be: the greater the defect, the greater the anxiety and the narrower the reaction.

Behind the symptomatology of schizophrenia there is usually one basic problem which was recognized by Sullivan who based his theories on their singleness of purpose which was their acceptability by other human beings as an equal. The schizophrenic loses his mind because he failed to belong, the alternatives being homicide or suicide. In the course of therapy, schizophrenics explain that their own weak and tender selves are not suitable for the human society of the natural, strong, domineering and amoral man. Either the schizophrenic is right and society is a herd with whom he cannot associate, or his view of society is wrong and he can be treated and brought back into society. Unlike the neurotic, the schizophrenic takes up an extreme position; either he feels able to identify with society or he denies himself a place entirely. Borderline or established cases frequently have this alarming insight and do not deceive themselves as to their place in society. There is another difference between the neurotic and the schizophrenic in that the former profits from treatment by reducing his personal responsibility by means of a deterministic theory. This does not apply to the schizophrenic, and many therapeutic failures have resulted from efforts to try and remove from the psychotic patient his sense of responsibility, for his guilt feelings do not resolve like those of the neurotic.

The amount of anxiety which the schizophrenic carries, his singlemindedness concerning the nature or constitution of the world, his insight, his lack of self-deception and his sense of responsibility are all reminiscent of existentialism. This has raised the question as to whether existentialist philosophers are schizophrenics, or schizophrenics are existentialist philosophers. It is not possible to give a categorical answer, except that schizophrenics have been more intensively studied and are better understood, and a 'pathological' outlook on life does not necessarily mean that the individual is psychotic. Furthermore existentialists tend to associate because they are capable of doing so and realize that their feelings of anxiety and nothingness are not abnormal in themselves.

What is apparent from a study of existentialism is that it affords a vehicle for bringing to the schizophrenic the world on his own terms and it may be that it does give some hope of helping him on a psychotherapeutic basis.

DEFINITIONS

Like most psychiatric movements, it has developed its own jargon, and the following are some of the terms and concepts used:

Dasein. This is used to describe the human **being** (*sein*=being, *da*=there). It is claimed that it is concerned with ontology or the science of being and that *dasein* is used to describe the patient before the therapist. It is primarily a verb form and includes an awareness of self or of being. It is an *ur* phenomenon, *i.e.* original and not derived and is a level of experience prior to the dichotomy of subject and object, or differentiation of the ego.

Daseinanalyse. The process of therapy which considers that man not only has a position in place but has a 'there' which includes a position in time and is aware of his own existence.

Instantaneous Encounter. The moment when we experience the *dasein* of another person. It yields direct knowledge and not knowledge about the person such as one would derive from case records and it is this aspect which completes the picture. The therapist's capacity to handle the encounter will determine the degree of understanding of the patient, and spatial proximity, while not essential, is regarded as an advantage.

Anxiety. This is regarded as an ontological characteristic of man and rooted in his existence and therefore differs from other affects. It is something people *are* rather than *have,* and is the inward state of becoming aware that existence can be lost. As such it is closer to the German *angst* than the English *anxiety*; it differs from *fear* and can only be understood as a threat to the individual's *dasein.*

Guilt. This, too, is regarded as ontological and is not to be confused with guilt feelings which depend largely on external influences.

World. A dynamic pattern in which the individual plays a part. May (1959) states:

> My world is not something static which I accept or fight against or adjust to . . . I am in the process of forming and designing. It includes the deterministic influences of the past which condition my existence, but it is these as I relate to them, am aware of them, carry them with me—moulding, forming, building them in every instant of relating.

(*a*) **Umwelt** (world-around). The biological world or environment to which one adapts and adjusts.

(*b*) **Mitwelt** (with-world). The world of interpersonal relationships with *encounter* between people, the experience changing the participants.

(*c*) **Eigenwelt** (own-world). The personal relating and interpretation of the real world by the individual and therefore the basis on which he accepts reality.

These three worlds are simultaneously experienced and classical psychoanalysis is criticized for over-emphasizing the Umwelt at the expense of the Mitwelt and certainly the Eigenwelt.

Transcendence. This does not have a religious significance, but is seen in Goldstein's sense of the capacity of the individual to abstract himself from the concrete situation. Man has the capacity of speech and reason and can modify his own world; he can therefore transcend the immediate situation. It may be that the pre-occupation among certain groups with psychodelic drugs in order to obtain a 'transcendental experience' is an expression of the existentialist philosophy which pervades them.

Time. It is not merely a quantitative measure, but is related to *dasein* which is able to relate the very old and even the future to the present. The term 'having been' is preferred to 'past', and the present also includes the individual's moving into the future as well as his emergence of what has been. The future is regarded as the most important of the three modes of time and everybody whose *dasein* is not overwhelmed by anxiety or depression is constantly engaged in planning it.

Therapy

Adherents of different schools employ existential concepts in therapy and a full *daseinanalyse* has not yet been produced. Technique is regarded as of less importance than understanding the patient as a 'being in his world'.

Presence. The relationship of therapist to patient is one where the former is preoccupied with the *existence* and is part of the field of relationship of the latter. He must enter this field for successful therapy and May (1959) quotes Binswanger as saying that when therapy fails the fault may be the therapist's, not necessarily in any technical sense:

> . . . but the far more fundamental failure that consists of an impotence to wake or rekindle that divine 'spark' in the patient which only true communication from existence to existence can bring forth, and which alone possesses, with its light and warmth, the fundamental power that makes any therapy work—the power to liberate a person from blind isolation . . . and to ready him for a life of genuine community.

Anything which interferes with full presence in the therapist may require some form of analysis to increase self-awareness so that he can participate in the encounter and not diminish the existential aspect of the relationship.

Cure. Existentialists do not subscribe to conventional cures which imply the successful adjustment of the individual to the culture. This may result in relief of symptoms but *dasein* is forfeited and the therapist has become the agent of the culture which may possess greater defects than the patient. The aim of therapy is for the patient to be able to realize his *dasein* fully, but awareness is only part of the process and it must be supplemented by action to enable the individual to achieve his full potential.

The Unconscious. this concept is not held in high esteem by the existentialists. May quotes Straus: 'The unconscious ideas of the patient are more often than not the conscious theories of the therapist'. As they are committed to an indivisible human being, there is a reluctance to accept divisions of the mind, even though these are recognized as artificial and are used merely as a means of classification.

Existential Psychiatry and Schizophrenia

Laing (1960) who is regarded by the New Left as the reflection of the true image of psychiatry, first attracted serious attention with his book, *An Existential Study in Sanity and Madness.* Schizophrenia was not really an illness and schizophrenics were not really sick. It was society that was sick and it used the schizophrenic as its scapegoat. This approach accorded well with the philosophy of those who regarded our 'bourgeois' society as the epitome of all that was bad in the world, and the schizophrenic, whose ego-disintegration was regarded as a true revolt against the super-ego forces, was the complete man. The family, with its emphasis on basic morality, starting with incest taboo, was the source of all the trouble and it must be discredited.

A permissive or rather a regressive therapeutic community was established at Kingsley Hall and individual cases became book titles. For example, Barnes and Berke (1971) *Mary Barnes: Two Accounts of a Journey Through Madness,* relate the story of a female aged 42, who, after previous breakdowns, moved into the permissive therapeutic community of Kingsley Hall where regressive behaviour, including nudity and smearing with faeces, was tolerated with eventual benefit. Dr Berke quotes:

> . . . the reason why most psychiatrists are unable to communicate with people who have entered the deeper levels of depression is that they do not utilize their own enormous reservoirs of primitive emotion to make contact with such individuals. To try and force the other to speak in rational modalities long after he or she has decided to declaim an 'irrational' tongue. And by 'irrational' I do not mean 'unintelligible'. I am referring to the language of the infant, the melodies of primary feeling, which are, in themselves, quite comprehensible.

The above attitude is not new in psychiatry and many psychiatrists before and since Laing have used regressive techniques to assist the schizophrenic to a better level of functioning. It is the accent on the 'scapegoat' theory whereby the families of schizophrenics exploit their weaker relative, that has attracted considerable attention and comment. The 'double-bind' factor in the genesis of schizophrenia had already been evolved by Bateson *et al.* (1956) and Lidz and Lidz (1949) had defined the schizophrenogenic parent. Laing and Esterson (1964) went much further, and Esterson (1970) on the basis of a single case history devotes a book to the theme. His approach is Marxist and he dismisses the time factor or even failure in treatment as irrelevant, using as his analogy the success of the Russian Revolution 1917 which he claims was made possible by the failed attempt of 1905. Whether this is historically accurate is another issue, but if it were, and it could be shown that it was sound revolutionary strategy, it would be bad medicine. It is of interest that a Marxist psychiatrist should labour the theme of the 'scapegoat' and attack society for attributing insanity to its dissenting members, yet this behaviour has been recently highlighted in the society of the Marxist heirs of the Russian Revolution.

The original impulse to analyse the role of the family in the genesis of the patient's difficulty has deteriorated into a cult with much of the associated mysticism. For example, Laing (1972) puts forward this gem:

> . . . if thoughts cannot be thought; and among the thoughts that cannot be thought is the thought that there are certain thoughts that cannot be thought, including the aforementioned thought, then he who has complied with this calculus of antithought will not be aware he is not aware that he is obeying a rule not to think that he is obeying a rule not to think about X . . .

There are plenty more passages like the above.

Comment. In psychiatry one is used to all manners of theories and practices, which is not surprising in a subject dealing with the mentally ill. Existential psychiatry, especially of the type advocated by Laing and his colleagues, is just another example, though in this instance it is allied to a powerful and vociferous political creed with a strong fascination for the young, who, in their adolescent identity crisis, feel they have much in common with the schizophrenic patient. To make common ground is laudable: to obstruct effective treatment is deplorable.

Remarks

This is a powerful, new impulse in psychiatry which because of its intellectual support in the profession itself and outside, is already making useful contributions. It is no doubt a timely corrective to the over-intellectualized analytical movement, but its historical setting must be appreciated and it should be borne in mind that one of its progenitors, *Hassidism,* soon became adulterated with *Cabbalah* and the miracle-working *Zaddik.* While Wesley and Baal Shem (the founder of Hassidism) kept within the bounds of a religious ethic and liberated their followers for religious zeal and prayer, the world has also recently had the horrible experience of a mass movement nourished on similar philosophies without religious and ethical controls. It can be heady wine with an appeal to many with little head for it.

PSYCHODRAMA

This method of therapy is probably very old and indeed Moreno (1959), its modern founder, quotes instances when it was used by priests in primitive tribes to cure hysterical and anxiety symptoms. His first experiment was directed to solving the domestic problems of a young married couple who acted in his *Stegreiftheater* (Theatre of

Spontaneity) founded in 1921, and by 1925 a method had evolved and was already being applied elsewhere. The ingredients are (1) the protagonist or subject, (2) the director or chief therapist, (3) the auxiliary egos, and (4) the group.

Technique

This varies according to the theoretical bias of the therapist and the resistances of the subject which may be (1) private, (2) social, (3) ethnic, or (4) symbolic.

A number of methods are used to overcome resistance, such as:

(*a*) creating a situation which is superficially far removed from the patient's problems;

(*b*) using an auxiliary ego (another patient) to play the role of the patient so that he can see his own problem mirrored and obtain help by identification;

(*c*) using group rivalries as material for the drama;

(*d*) caricaturizing serious problems;

(*e*) replacing the therapist by an auxiliary to meet the needs of the patient.

Technical Terms

Psychodrama has developed its own language and the following are some of the commoner terms used.

Acting Out. This is the bringing to the surface of important inner experiences giving the therapist and the patient the opportunity to evaluate the situation, the latter being called *action insight,* of which Moreno defines two types:

1. *Irrational and incalculable,* which is found in the ordinary life situation and disturbs the patient's relationships and indirectly himself.
2. *Therapeutic and controlled.*

Tele (Distance) Relations. A feeling of people into each other such as patient to therapist and to other members of the group and *vice versa.* 'The telic relationships between protagonist, therapist, auxiliary egos and the significant dramatis personnae of the world which they portray are crucial for the therapeutic progress' (Moreno, 1959). This definition is very close to the existentialist concept of the *encounter.*

The Cultural Conserve. 'The accumulation and preservation of creative moments such as books, musical compositions, etc.' The need for this definition arose out of the belief that the concept of the moment is the most important in human thinking and that it is responsible for being, living and creating. This concept is however intangible and some more concrete and definable term was needed. Seen against the background of the tangible cultural conserve, the concept of the moment is given greater clarity.

Spontaneity. This retains its orthodox meaning, but is extended to include the response of the protagonist to a new situation or a variation of the old one. Spontaneity is regarded as an essential element of the healing process but is not the whole process though it is most important as the mainspring of creativity. All creations of the human mind are however not necessarily healthy and some are in fact grossly pathological.

A number of terms such as *free association* and *catharsis* have been borrowed from other psychotherapies though their meanings have been bent to the theory and purpose of psychodrama. Catharsis in psychodrama is intended to be a primary phenomenon for the benefit of the actor and not in the sense of the classical Greek Theatre as a secondary one for the benefit of the spectators.

In the production of a psychodrama the patient is expected to provide the director or therapist with clues as to the behaviour and positioning of the auxiliary egos and these have to enter into their parts as if they were in fact the patient's parents or sibs. All this can place a tremendous responsibility on the therapist who can have a group acting out the most emotionally charged material and must maintain control over the situation, yet Moreno insists that a cold detached attitude is undesirable and describes techniques for 'warming up' the group.

The patient may be asked to soliloquize, portraying either his own life or that of a relative or other person with whom he is or has been in contact. He can be given a few helpers and if necessary put his hallucinations and delusions to a reality test. A conflict can be presented in both forms with the help of an auxiliary ego, or the patient may fractionate himself into several auxiliary egos and deal with several facets of himself at the same time.

The Mirror Technique. This permits the patient to see someone else take his place and how another experiences him, and this if caricaturized may stimulate a patient to change his role from spectator to actor. Roles can be reversed and the patient takes on the therapist or another patient and there are no limits to the phantasies or even dreams that can be enacted—in fact a whole world can be created which need not have any relation to facts. The '*therapeutic community technique*' permits disputes between patients to be settled 'under the rule of therapy instead of the rule of law'.

Modifications

Hypnodrama. This was introduced by Moreno himself. The patient is hypnotized on the stage and the drama proceeds as usual with the advantage that inhibitions are freed more quickly and unconscious factors can more readily emerge.

Direct Analysis. Rosen (1953) confronts the patient with a factual challenge to his hallucinations and delusions. The method has been criticized as too traumatic by Moreno, but no doubt the personality of the therapist may help the patient to overcome situations which some therapists would shrink from creating.

Accessory Drug Therapy. Stimulants such as caffeine, lysergic acid, methedrine or depressants like alcohol are used to aid the acting out process of selected episodes or for more general effect. The dangers of drug addiction should constantly be borne in mind.

Didactic Psychodrama. Members of staff—medical and nursing—may play the part of the patient and his relatives so that he can see and accept an interpretation to which he was hitherto inaccessible.

Rehearsed Psychodrama. This method was used by Maxwell Jones at Belmont. The patient writes his play and other patients and staff rehearse their parts and it is in the rehearsing that catharsis and improvization with occasional revelation occur.

Conditioned Psychodrama. This is based on Pavlovian principles. A traumatic situation which has resulted in a distressing symptom is re-enacted till the symptom no longer occurs. It is a limited approach to the patient's problems, but in highly selected cases with a specific disability it may have a place.

A number of modifications have been used in the treatment of children. These make use of symbolic material and the language of children and are not far removed from the games that children have played from the beginning of time, except that the groups are therapeutically designed and the therapist usually participates.

Psychodrama as originally propounded by Moreno and in its subsequent modifications is of value as a group psychotherapeutic agent, and the author has seen good results in a military neurosis centre and in civilian day hospitals. Much of its success depends on the enthusiasm and skill of the therapist and it is not given to everyone to handle a group on the stage. A compromise could be made by having a member of the team skilled in stage direction, the psychotherapist playing his role through the medium of his producer.

The above summary is based on Moreno's contribution to the

American Handbook of Psychiatry, 1959, which describes the theoretical basis and techniques of psychodrama lucidly, informatively and of course, authoritatively, and also contains a useful bibliography. No summary can adequately interpret his classical account, and it is highly recommended reading for the student who wishes to be more fully informed about the subject.

Psychodrama combined with Videotape Playback

Gonen (1971) distinguishes psychodrama from role-playing. The former is the staging of an actual or fantasied event, emotionally charged for the person involved and never worked through, while the latter is the staging of situations which could happen and for which practice can serve as a good preparation. An act which starts as role-playing can become psychodrama if it evokes a sense of intense personal relevance and becomes highly charged emotionally for one or more participants.

He uses psychodrama and role-playing for short-term inpatient treatment. The session lasts for one hour per week and is videotaped and exhibited four hours later. This treatment involves the audience intellectually and emotionally while in the theatre, which is a safe setting. Insight is promoted, so that the observer develops an observing or reflecting ego, thus strengthening ego boundaries. The playback sessions served as valuable tension relievers and the author found it could reach patients more strongly than therapists.

HYPNOSIS

Historical

It is probable that the phenomenon of hypnosis was used by man in the earliest stages of civilization and the deliberate induction of states identical with, or closely allied to, hypnosis has been practised by primitive people, mainly for ceremonial purposes. The sound of drums, monotonous songs and movements were used to induce a trance-like state in which the individual was highly suggestible and could be made to perform feats which were almost super-human such as walking on live coals, being buried in a state of almost suspended animation and the like. Western medicine did not appear to be seriously interested till the sixteenth century when Paracelsus described the 'sympathetic system', according to which the stars and other bodies, especially magnets, influence man by means of a subtle emanation of fluid that pervades all space. J. B. van Helmont extended this doctrine by saying that a similar magnetic field radiates from men, and that it can be guided by their wills to influence directly the minds and bodies of others. In the seventeenth century there were already people in Western Europe who claimed they could cure diseases by stroking with the hand, and an Irishman, Valentine Greatrakes, claimed he could cure scrofula, and scientists, including Robert Boyle, confirmed some of these cures.

It was F. A. Mesmer (1733–1815), a graduate in medicine from the University of Vienna, who further publicized the theory of *animal magnetism.* He met a priest John Joseph Gassner who was renowned for his cures of nervous complaints and who claimed they were a spiritual act. Mesmer, who had hitherto regarded his own cures as due to his use of magnets, noted that the priest effected his by manipulation alone, so he discarded his magnets and claimed that he possessed a special force which could influence others. He moved to Paris and invaded the salons with his demonstrations of 'mesmerism' and he soon excited the hostility of the medical faculty who regarded him as a charlatan. He certainly exploited the sensational for he practised in a dimly lit room, hung with mirrors, with occasional strains of music breaking the prolonged silences. The patients sat around a kind of vat where chemical ingredients were concocted. Mesmer, dressed as a magician, glided among them, touching one, looking into the eyes of another and making 'passes' with his hands over a third. The Academy of Sciences appointed a commission to investigate these phenomena and it included such distinguished scientists as A. L. Lavoisier and Benjamin Franklin. They found that many of the facts were genuine, though they disputed Mesmer's theory of animal magnetism. An interesting by-product of mesmerism is that Mary Baker Eddy, the founder of the Christian Science movement, developed her interest in healing through an association with a mesmerist, Phineas Quimby.

In England, as elsewhere, there was much charlatanism associated with mesmerism and in an attempt to counter it John Elliotson, a leading London physician, founded and edited a professional journal, the *Zoist.* It is said that Elliotson had to resign his hospital appointment because of his interest, but James Esdaile, a surgeon in a hospital in Calcutta, so impressed the East India Company by his ability to perform operations painlessly, including amputations and removal of large scrotal tumours due to filariasis, that it built him a new hospital. This new flowering of mesmerism was due to a greater expertize in medical diagnosis, the extension of surgery and the *absence of efficient anaesthesia.* In 1841, James Braid, a Manchester doctor of high repute, enhanced the practice, coined the term 'hypnotism' and placed it on a more rational and ethical basis. It then looked as if hypnotism would become a popular and orthodox part of medical practice, but in 1848 Simpson discovered chloroform and about that time modern spiritualism started to spread and many equated the practice of hypnotism with the activities of a number of very questionable spiritualists.

J. M. Charcot (1825–93), who dominated neurology in the latter part of the nineteenth century, taught at the Salpêtrière in Paris that hypnosis was a symptom of hysteria, but Freud who studied there saw it as evidence of unconscious mental processes. Bernheim, who was professor of medicine at Nancy and had been influenced by a general practitioner A. A. Liébeault, published in 1884 his book, *De la Suggestion,* and gave a factual and clinical account of the phenomenon.

In 1892, a committee of the British Medical Association reported favourably on hypnotism, after a searching investigation, and again gave it the cloak of respectability, but it fell into disuse as a medical treatment till the First World War, when it was found to be of value in the rapid removal of hysterical symptoms. It again lost favour but in the Second World War it was revived largely for the same purposes as in the First World War, though the incidence of these disorders was not as great. Lay hypnotists have constantly disturbed the medical profession. The dangers of public exhibitions of hypnotism were regarded as harmful and legislation has been introduced banning them in England.

The present position is that hypnosis is practised by doctors and others, and that many extravagant claims are made which tend to bring treatment into disrepute. It lost ground with the introduction of anaesthesia; it also lost ground as an abreactive agent with the introduction of pharmacological aids. It still has its adherents among the medical and dental professions, the latter using it for painless extractions and other dental surgery, while among the former are enthusiasts who regard it as a panacea for most human ills and as a substitute for an extensive training in psychiatry.

The Technique

The author was once asked to write an article for the lay press on hypnotism and he then stated: 'If trade unions were to rate the practice of hypnotism, it would not rate higher than semi-skilled labour'. The vast majority of people can be hypnotized, probably not less than 90 per cent, and there is no evidence that it is easier to hypnotize hysterics or other unstable people; the author in demonstrating the technique to medical students, prefers to select the more stable. What is needed in any subject is confidence in the therapist and good motivation. The consciously resistant person is likely to prove difficult. Some prefer to have the patient lying down on a couch; others prefer him to sit in a comfortable chair. A variety of methods are used, the commonest being the use of a 'fixation object'. The patient is asked to gaze fixedly on a pencil, or a coin or a spot on the wall or ceiling and the therapist makes monotonous suggestions of relaxation and sleep. He tells the patient that his eyes are getting more and more tired, that he is feeling drowsier and drowsier and that the eyes are closing and he is getting sleepy. This suggestion goes on till the patient's eyes flicker, lower and close and the breathing takes on the characteristics of a sleeping rhythm. The patient, however, is not asleep and can hear what is being said and can answer questions and obey instructions.

Effects of Hypnosis

In the above somnambulistic state, suggestions can be made which can influence the patient's mental or physical state, such as easing of breathing in asthmatics and loss of irritation of skin in appropriate cases. Anaesthesia can be suggested and this can be localized to one limb, or one eye, memories can be reactivated, regression can be induced and the patient brought to experience again events in his earlier life which had been repressed. This abreactive aspect is used extensively by those who practise hypnotherapy (p. 949).

The senses can be rendered hyperacute and a subject may hear from the back of a room the hypnotist whisper, while those in the front may not hear. Similarly, time can be counted with an accuracy which in the unhypnotized person would not be possible. Hallucinatory experiences either of a positive or negative nature may be induced, such as telling the subject something is present when it is not, and *vice versa.*

Post-hypnotic Effects. After the subject has been brought out of the somnambulist state, suggestions which were given during it can still operate and this phenomenon is exploited in treatment.

Antebi (1963) enunciates the following seven principles in the practice of hypnotherapy which are useful in overcoming resistances. These are effected by suggestion.

1. Distortion of the time concept.
2. Distortion of the space concept.
3. Dissociation of the personality.

4. Links are forged in the dissociation process.
5. Induced changes in the emotional state.
6. Reinforcement of the process of concretization of the object in the patient's thought process. This is a form of regression therapy.
7. Distortion of the body image.

These manoeuvres can only be attempted with patients whose ego-structure is sufficiently well-integrated. They would be highly dangerous otherwise.

THE PRACTICE OF HYPNOSIS

This is a very different matter from the technique. No one should undertake the hypnosis of a patient without having made a careful medical and psychiatric appraisal. The patient who comes asking to be hypnotized for some condition should first be interviewed in the same manner as any other patient, for there are certain categories where hypnosis may be harmful.

Contra-indications

The Hysterical Character (p. 478). The patient is usually female with a superficially bright personality but there is a histrionic streak which is easily recognized. Unless a careful medical history is taken the diagnosis may be missed and the hysterical behaviour, which to the patient is a way of life, attaches itself to the hypnotic session and beyond. These patients may be responsible for the so-called irreversible hypnotic states, false accusations against the hypnotist, litigation and other difficulties. They are really very disturbed people and the relatively superficial help that hypnosis has to offer does not improve, but may even reinforce their basic instability.

The Schizophrenic. An obvious schizophrenic disorder is unlikely to suggest hypnotic treatment, but the pseudo-neurotic types with their somatic pre-occupations may be mistaken for a conversion syndrome or an anxiety state and it is therefore essential that an experienced psychiatric opinion be sought before embarking, for the ego is barely holding together and a dissociative phenomenon like hypnosis may accelerate breakdown.

Paranoid States. Like schizophrenics, these patients may present with hypochondriasis or a ruminative disorder and seek help to get the disturbing thoughts out of their minds. Hypnosis is not only unlikely to be successful, but may substitute for the more concrete delusions of persecution, those involving telepathic influences, with the hypnotist incorporated in the system.

Psychotic Depression. The origins of this state are relatively inaccessible to suggestion and the risk of aggravation with suicide would strongly urge the application of the much more effective treatments that are available.

Obsessional States. Just as these patients prove formidable in psychotherapy, so with hypnosis. They lack the capacity to dissociate and indeed their whole problem is held with such tenacity that the hypnotic suggestion is most unlikely to break this down. When exacerbation occurs as a result of anxiety, it is possible that the relaxation induced by the therapist may lighten the condition.

Indications

Hysterical Symptoms. These have been the traditional objectives of hypnotic treatment. They should be seen in their true setting and symptomatic treatment undertaken only when the full clinical picture is understood.

Psychosomatic Disorders. A number of these states which are associated with tension like asthma, eczema, ulcerative colitis, peptic ulceration, can be helped with the relaxation induced by hypnosis.

Tics and Habit Spasms including Stammering. If these are functionally determined they are usually aggravated by anxiety-provoking situations and hypnosis may remove them, though in the case of stammering the suggestion may have to be repeatedly reinforced.

Anaesthesia. In patients who are very apprehensive of an anaesthetic or whose physical state makes the administration of one unduly hazardous, deep hypnosis may be able to induce a state of surgical anaesthesia. One of the difficulties is that the results are uncertain and frequent rehearsal may be needed, which would preclude emergency procedures.

Pregnancy and Labour. These not only involve anaesthesia, but also include relaxation, and hypnosis may be particularly useful in those mothers who are very apprehensive and may therefore have a prolonged third stage, with consequent danger to the foetus. The variety of other techniques which are concerned with relaxation in pregnancy are probably hypnotic equivalents.

Hypnotherapy. In the hands of a well-trained psychiatrist who is perceptive of resistances and can handle them and who can also deal with the material that may result from the accompanying abreaction, hypnotherapy can be of benefit in selected cases. It can also be used to recover lost memories, though the indications for doing so must be very few.

Children's Functional Disorders. These include stammering, tics, nocturnal enuresis, and phobias. Children are generally very good subjects for hypnosis.

Dermatology. In addition to those skin disorders which are psychologically determined, a number of skin conditions which have not got an obvious psychological origin may respond to hypnosis. Among the commonest are warts, but there have also been reports of successful treatment of psoriasis, congenital ichthyosis and urticaria.

Mode of Action

This is still one of the mysteries of life. Even though a variety of physical conditions can be produced or removed by hypnosis, practically nothing is known of how it works. Yet many autonomic changes have been reported following hypnosis, including slowing of pulse rate, lowering of blood pressure and increase or diminution of gastric secretions. Barber (1962) who has contributed extensively to the subject concludes that trance induction is not necessary to elicit post-hypnotic suggestion. This has been recognized by a number of workers, and White (1961) in his treatment of asthmatics noted that symptomatic relief did not depend on the depth of hypnosis. It is probably true that the induction of trance is not essential, but it helps. Some have gone as far as saying that the trance state is simulated, but there is ample evidence from many sources that it is a valid phenomenon and one hopes there need be no more commissions to decide whether hypnosis works; what is needed now are enquiries as to how it works.

Quantitative EEG Analysis during Hypnosis

The development of electronic frequency analysis of the EEG has made it possible to study afresh EEG responses in situations which had hitherto failed to reveal EEG changes. Ulett *et al.* (1972) selected the 10 best and the 10 poorest hypnotic subjects and took a 10-minute resting (eyes closed) EEG recording before the hypnotic session followed by a 10-minute recording during trance induction and an 8-minute record during the trance testing period.

Statistical evaluation demonstrated significant changes between groups in the trance induction period, with a decrease of slow and an increase of alpha and beta waves accompanied by an increase in amplitude and decrease in amplitude variability in the best hypnotic subjects. The changes in the poor subjects were in almost the opposite direction; a similar situation was found during the hypnotic trance period. This increase in alpha activity in the best hypnotic subjects has been observed during different behavioural techniques such as Yoga, Zen meditation, and autogenic training, suggesting that hypnosis has something in common with these states.

SUPERFICIAL PSYCHOTHERAPY

This term covers a multitude of approaches, some of which have a theoretical basis, while others are purely *ad hoc* practices and range from a 'pat on the back to a kick in the pants'. Most are based on that doctor-patient relationship which invests the doctor with healing powers and ascribes to him an authority which has a powerful influence on the patient. Suggestion is therefore facilitated, positive advice is accepted, and placebos are given the force of potent drugs, while if the patient is allowed to talk about himself, tensions may be eased and anxiety relieved. If the doctor is gentle and passive, he may fill the patient's need for a comforting maternal figure; if he is positive and authoritarian, the patient may accept him as a father figure. This latter role can be the more difficult for the doctor, for even though it may fit in with his personal inclination, it is liable to excite in the patient negative reactions with at times resentment and hostility. According to the rules the doctor should be able to recognize these as part of a negative transference and deal with them accordingly, but even if he does not, it can still have the therapeutic effect of psychodrama (p. 940).

The analytically trained psychiatrist frequently either frowns on superficial psychotherapy, or adopts a patronizing attitude, yet there must be a greater number of patients who receive considerable benefit from such attentions, and many of them may be better off with a superficial than with a depth approach.

Structured forms of such therapies may, like those of Dubois (1949), consist of persuasion, in an attempt to encourage the patient to yield his symptoms, or supportive therapy, with insight therapy during times of crisis. Some are based on a full appraisal of the individual's life history, and an attempt to correlate the illness with past events and environmental influences. Others are goal-directed and approach the problem as the behaviour therapists do (see above).

Meditation

Gellhorn and Kiely (1972) define: (1) the *ergotropic syndrome* as associated with an increase in sympathetic discharges and in skeletal muscle tone together with a diffuse cortical excitation (desynchronization of EEG potentials) as in awakening and (2) the *trophotropic syndrome* as associated with an increase in parasympathetic discharges, relaxation of skeletal muscles and lessening of cortical excitation (increased synchrony as in sleep). The physiological changes which accompany meditation are a shift in the balance to the trophotropic side. Alpha potentials are found in stage I; they increase in amplitude in stage II; they decline in frequency in stage III; theta potentials appear in stage IV.

The authors used the systematic practice of meditation in the treatment of formerly drug-dependent adolescents and young adults with benefit. The patients reported a heightened sense of inner-directed self-control in contrast to the anxiety-provoking loss-of-control affects of psychedelic and other drugs. There was also much improved clarity in cognitive function and in emotional-behavioural integration. They consider the technique an easy one to learn in contrast to the rigorous training involved in Zen and Yoga exercises. They also propose its use in psychosomatic disorders.

Crisis Therapy

A crisis may be defined as a transitional period which presents an individual with either an opportunity for personality growth and maturation or the risk of adverse effect with increased vulnerability to subsequent stress. Past maladaptive patterns of problem solving may be repeated since old memories are characteristically revived during crisis.

Brandon (1970) reviews crisis theory as evolved by Caplan (1964):

Phase I. When a threatening situation is perceived and habitual coping mechanisms prove unsuccessful within the time span of expected success.

Phase II. Rising tension and increasing disorganization will result in some interference with functioning. Feelings of anxiety, fear, guilt or shame are accompanied by a feeling of helplessness and ineffectuality in the face of the apparently insoluble problem. During this phase the individual is more suggestible.

Phase III. Rising tension leads to a mobilization of internal and external resources when emergency problem-solving techniques are called up and novel solutions may be attempted. A solution which may terminate discomfort and disorganization may still be neurotic or maladaptive and ultimately harmful.

Phase IV. If normal resolution is not achieved, major disorganization results.

The most effective intervention will be during the period of disorganization (Phase II) in the form of early and frequent support with encouragement of dependency needs together with stress on the reality situation as well as discouraging denial and evasion. The author recommends intervention on the basis of crisis theory as a short-term eclectic therapy.

Brief Psychotherapy

This should be distinguished from superficial psychotherapy in that it uses interpretation and exploits the transference relationship. Malan (1963) describes 21 patients so treated, the duration varying from 10–40 sessions. Results after long follow-up showed that 50 per cent improved and the conclusions drawn were that prognosis was best when patient and therapist were prepared to become seriously involved and bear the tensions that invariably ensued. The hoped-for changes in psychodynamic terms were listed before treatment began so that follow-up could be assessed according to changes effected, scored on a rating scale and not on clinical impressions. The book made quite an impact for it showed that psychodynamic theories are susceptible to the formal ordering and analysis of statistical method and that brief psychotherapy in selected cases could be as successful as more prolonged treatment.

Although it is generally accepted that well-motivated patients carry the best prognosis, the poorly motivated patient may present the greater challenge. Brill and Storrow (1963) emphasize that poor motivation should be regarded as a symptom to be treated, not an irritation to be avoided. The author would add 'in the presence of material disability'.

Evaluation of Psychotherapy

Cawley (1971) poses the following series of questions:

1. Do patients chosen for psychotherapy fare better than they would if treated differently?
2. What components of the treatment determine its effectiveness?
3. What proportion of patients with defined disabilities are suitable for one or another kind of dynamic psychotherapy and how can they be identified?
4. For how many patients is this treatment available?
5. When dynamic psychotheraphy is freely available to a community, will suitability and responsiveness remain stable factors, or are they subject to subcultural influences such as fashion and other psychosocial variables?

Oriental Psychotherapy

Modern systems of psychotherapy are based on Western standards and cultures and it would appear reasonable to suppose that they may not be as relevant in oriental cultures. Kishimoto (1962) puts forward the hypothesis that psychotherapy based on orientalism should be more effective for Japanese. He explains that both Zen (which means meditation, *i.e.* the placing of the body and soul in good order) and psychoanalysis aim at surpassing ethics and both claim to be independent of all authority. The aim of Zen is to set one free from self-tenacity and is not so much a therapy for neurosis as a way to well-being through accomplishing unity with the world.

Another philosophy is that of Vasubandho (Idealism) which explains that we view things incorrectly because of overtenacity of the ego to things. What is really true does not issue from antagonism between existence and non-existence, but in between. Improvement would involve an understanding of causes and conditions, practice of austerities, acquiring discriminating knowledge and application of wisdom.

The above brief statement does not convey one fraction of the complexity of Zen and its associates but it does indicate the tremendous difference between oriental and Western requirements. Cultures do change and it may be that the mass media will produce an amalgam of cultures though if history is a guide, there is a stubbornness in these things which will defy uniformity.

Japanese Psychotherapy (Morita)

Nishizono (1969) suggests that the main reason why Freudian psychoanalysis did not become a major force in Japan was because it was not congruous with Japanese culture. Westernization influenced industry, commerce, the fighting services and the universities but made no impact on Japan's traditional family system. A person's livelihood and mental stability were guaranteed as long as he remained within the framework of the family and obeyed its patriarchal authority. Such a system was not limited to the family but formed the basic structure of Japanese society. Emotional problems were dealt with by the family and psychoanalysis, which aimed at establishing individual freedom and independence, was generally inacceptable.

Professor Morita of Tokyo Jukei Medical College developed a uniquely Japanese psychotherapy, which, though linked with Zen Buddhism, is far from religious. It attaches great importance to perfectionism as an inherent aspect of man's nature. A person thus heavily endowed would be over-preoccupied with even trivial signs that are not basically morbid and neurotic features may supervene since he strives to get rid of these trivia. The purpose of Morita-psychotherapy is to help the patient to acquire a mental state which enables him to get on with the business of life though still aware of the irritations.

Technique. The patient is completely isolated and put to bed all day for about a week. During this period he is barred from reading and talking and therefore forced to face up to his anxiety. He is then assigned light work and then graduated to normal social relationships, and during this time he is exposed to persuasion and advice on how to cope. The treatment is designed to establish the patient's proper mental attitude towards life rather than focussing on the unconscious. The patient's role is that of a seeker after truth.

The author admits that the situation is changing and Morita psychotherapy is being challenged, and he compared the behaviour of patients and the results of Morita psychotherapy and psychoanalysis. Results were similar but the attitude to the therapist was very different, being excessively dependent in the psychoanalytic group. He considers that while psychoanalysis fosters a parent-child relationship in therapy, Morita psychotherapy gives rise to a master-disciple relationship. The demand for the psychoanalytical approach in Japan is growing at a time when people in the West are growing disenchanted with it and as a substitute are turning to Oriental mysticism.

The Repertory Grid in Therapy

Ryle and Lunghi (1971) used a modification of the repertory grid, which they called the 'dyad grid test' as an aid to psychotherapy. They say:

> A neurotic patient is like a traveller in unfamiliar country forced to rely upon a deficient and systematically falsified map. The joint exploration undertaken with the therapist can enable the patient to revise this map. One condition which must be met for this to occur is for the therapist to recognize clearly how the patient sees his relationships with others, including the therapist.

When patient and therapist had completed the dyad grid, the therapist having predicted the patient's response, there was substantial agreement but also an important misconstruction on the part of the therapist. It is possible that this method will gain in popularity, particularly among non-medical practitioners. Reading tea-cups and crystal gazing have always had their fascination; a scientific variation is sure to attract its adherents.

Peer Group Psychotherapies

These have arisen because orthodox psychotherapies and counselling have failed to meet the needs or preferably the requirements of certain groups such as young people, often university students who are antipathetic to orthodoxy and wish to talk to 'their own kind'. Others are 'unattached' and lack the formal machinery of referral, while some, who may feel isolated and depressed, wish immediate access which is generally not available. These therapies are anti- or atheoretical, relatively unstructured, the training of the therapist being informal, and they rely more on 'doing' than on 'thinking'. They are found in coffee bars, the university campus and basic encounter (T) groups

Crown (1973) defines the basic factors in the patient which are considered essential for successful psychotherapy. These are summarized in the word YAVIS–Young, Attractive, Verbal, Intelligent, Successful, whereas the therapist should have accurate empathy, non-possessive warmth and genuineness. *A treatment alliance* is the relationship therapist and patient develop during the initial assessment interviews and when arrangements are being made for treatment.

Conditioning Factors

Cognitive Control. Cognitive factors can influence autonomic functioning including autonomic conditioning and these are likely to operate in the treatment alliance and subsequent psychotherapy.

Verbal Conditioning. This operates in both behaviour and dynamic psychotherapy. The basic experimental demonstration is that if certain forms of speech such as personal pronouns are verbally reinforced by the experimenter with the word good, subjects will produce more of the rewarded class of words as a form of operant conditioning (Verplanck, 1955).

Modelling. Learning theorists have emphasized the role of social learning in psychotherapeutic change. Modelling is a social learning technique when, for example, a child who is unafraid of dogs 'models' for a child who has a dog phobia. Other forms of social learning, for example, imitation or identification, whereby the patient takes into his or her personality certain aspects of the therapist's personality, appearance, behaviour and attitudes, probably occur during psychotherapeutic interaction.

ASSESSMENT OF RESULTS

This is now becoming a major concern not only of psychotherapists but of the taxpayer. As long as psychotherapy was a private arrangement between the individual and the doctor the financial aspect was not questioned. Now that psychotherapy in all its forms is being provided by the State Health Service, the results must, sooner or later, be correlated with the cost. The emphasis on psychotherapy which derives to some extent from the distinction of its clientele has, in an affluent Welfare State, become an objective for those members of the public who lay great store on these things. It is evident that the clamour will come from the middle class who, in this particular instance, see themselves as tailor-made for the treatment, and being articulate, are most likely to get it.

Does it do any good? To whom? For how long? What would happen if the person had a different type of treatment or no treatment? These questions were the concern of a joint enquiry between the Maudsley Hospital, a general psychiatric unit, and the Tavistock Clinic, which is predominantly devoted to psychotherapy. They circulated 85 psychiatrists in London who would be likely to treat patients suitable for psychotherapy. They referred 113 patients, but when the particulars were subjected to the scrutinizing panel only 8 were accepted as suitable and of these 2 dropped out. It was intended to expose matched groups to varying forms of psychotherapy, intensive, brief and supportive, and to assess the results, but with such a small residue it was impossible to complete the experiment in its intended form (Candy *et al.* 1972).

Nevertheless, the experiment has important lessons. Even when a validation experiment is contemplated, many experienced psychiatrists selected many patients who are eventually regarded as unsuitable or unpromising material for psychotherapy according to a panel interested in comparing results. This means that many, probably too many, are receiving all forms of psychotherapy without being really in need or likely to benefit. The completion of such an experiment is absolutely essential before services are expanded. It may also be coupled with a study in the redeployment of a number of psychotherapists.

In a sequel to the paper by Candy *et al.* (1972), the same authors (Cawley *et al.,* 1973) describe what happened to the 8 patients who were accepted. Two refused the vacancies offered and one showed motivation only for support and encouragement, causing psychotherapy to be abandoned after 22 sessions. Of the 6 patients who were judged to be the most suitable after those selected, but were not included in the trial, all found alternative psychotherapy. One immediately regressed to a state of child-like dependence, showing motivation only for support, while the other 5 all broke off prematurely, apparently as soon as their main problems were touched on.

One explanation for this poor showing of psychotherapy was that the most suitable patients, and those felt to be most in need, were referred directly to psychotherapy, while the less suitable were referred to the trial, where they were known to have a one-third chance of not receiving psychotherapy. This sounds like and probably is a rationalization. It does not counter the logical inference that many unsuitable patients are taken on for various forms of psychotherapy and that more rigid selection is indicated. It would be of interest to scrutinize those patients who are regarded as well-motivated, taking into account their background, disability and the results of psychotherapy. This evidence is essential if any credence is to be given to the above argument.

Psychotherapy in a Changing World: a Fresh Look

Crown (1973) said:

> Psychotherapy, more than any other treatment in psychiatry, reflects the sociocultural and economic climate of a country and a period . . . Young people, who form the majority of patients of psychotherapists of all approaches, have a sceptical attitude towards the supposedly mind-bending propensities of both dynamic and behavioural psychotherapies. Psychotherapists have to be prepared to state clearly to a potential patient what they have to offer, to say something of their own background and attitudes and why they think their treatment might be more effective or 'relevant' than someone else's. Other social factors include economic pressures in the private sector, the influence of Eastern religious ideas and, with those influenced by the Women's Liberation Movement, a suspicion that orthodox psychotherapies of all types attempt to mould them into the middle-class wife-and-mother image.

Counselling

Though this has developed outside the medical, psychoanalytical and behaviourist traditions, it is a rapidly developing field, particularly in the universities, but is also sponsored by local authorities in Marriage Guidance Clinics, Citizens Advice Centres, Samaritans, Open Door Centres for Young People and the like. Much of it is based on the client-centred therapy of Rogers (1951) whose thesis was that 'the individual has within himself the capacity and the tendency, latent if not evident, to move forward toward maturity'. The approach is non-directive, and though the theoretical basis is weak, it has 'caught on' largely because it is used by non-medical practitioners in a milieu where spontaneous maturation of the individual is likely to occur, so that results are bound to be good. It usually operates with an adequate medical 'back-up' so that in the few instances where it fails and is doing harm the counsellor and his client are protected.

All this may seem innocent enough, but it is not a question of an expensive medical approach to a situation as against one which costs nothing. It *is* costly and with its expansion is becoming increasingly so. Neither does it save the medical expense, for it breeds its own medical requirements in terms of supervision and salvage. It could even be argued that it creates a demand where none was previously justified. The issue is becoming a major one and the author has been asked by professional bodies with responsibility for training whether they should appoint qualified counsellors. In a society where tutors are sympathetic and experienced, and medical, including psychiatric, advice is readily available, it should not be necessary to create a large corps of professional counsellors. Much of their expertise is based on a theory and practice which in any case is being seriously questioned as far as its universal application is concerned.

CHAPTER 20

Other Treatments

At one time it was possible to distinguish between physical treatment and psychological treatment in psychiatry even though all physical treatment involves psychological factors in terms of doctor-patient relationship and the powerful suggestion that some of these treatments convey. Now the situation is more confused, as some physical treatments are used for their psychological influence rather than for the production of a physical change in the patient. For example, Behaviour Therapy, which is reckoned by its practitioners to be a form of psychological treatment, and indeed most are non-medical psychologists, makes use of physical techniques such as electric shocks. There are still some treatments where the intention is to induce a physical change which is in itself beneficial and the following is an account of those in common use.

PSYCHOSURGERY

The term 'Psychosurgery', like psychosomatic medicine excites in some, considerable resistance. A few surgeons develop scruples about it and rationalize that as there is no anatomical location for the 'psyche', there can be no such regional surgery. Others who are more aware of the origin of their resistance maintain that specialized neurosurgery has its own fields and are reluctant to enter into the field of mental illness. There are, however, some who have devoted themselves energetically to improving and modifying techniques and it can now be said that it has a secure place in psychiatric treatment.

The present era of psychosurgery was ushered in by a paper by Jacobsen (1936) which was read at the Second International Neurological Congress in London. He reported the absence of frustrational behaviour in chimpanzees following bifrontal lobectomy, and it is said that the Portuguese neurologist Egas Moniz who attended the Congress saw the possibilities of such surgery in the treatment of mental illness. He enlisted the support of his surgical colleague, Almeida Lima and published the results of the operation on the first 20 patients (Egas Moniz, 1936) with approximately a third recovered, a third improved and a third unimproved.

It had been reported a century before that damage to the frontal lobes could cause personality changes in man, for in 1848, Phineas Gage while working on the railway had a crowbar driven through his frontal lobes and he changed from being a conscientious foreman who commanded the respect of his labourers, to a careless, uninhibited person who was no longer suited for the responsible job he had previously done so well. Brickner (1936) had already shown that extensive bilateral frontal lobectomy could be undergone for cerebral tumours without impairment of memory or intelligence, though with social deterioration. Freeman and Watts (1941) extended the work of Egas Moniz and noted that although the operation did not remove the abnormal thoughts from the patient, there was a marked change in the patient's attitude to his psychosis. He was less anxious, tense and pre-occupied, and these authors suggested that there was a bleaching of the affect as a result of the operation. They also studied the effects of the operation on intractable pain (Freeman & Watts, 1946) and found that though the pain could still be felt, its effects on the patient were reduced and there was less need for drugs.

The Anatomical Rationale of the Operation

This was defined by studies on patients who had been operated on, and who at necropsy showed retrograde degeneration in the dorsomedial nucleus of the thalamus, with insignificant cortical changes (Freeman & Watts, 1947; Meyer & Beck, 1954), indicating the interdependence of the frontal region with the thalamus, hypothalamus and the rhinencephalic centres. The operation therefore severs fronto-thalamic fibres, which form a rather diffuse projection on to the cortex. Experimental attacks on other areas, including the occipital, parietal and temporal, were carried out with little benefit, and it was obvious that if substantial improvement was to take place the fronto-thalamic fibres must be severed *on both sides.* This could be done by attacking the dorso-medial nucleus of the thalamus, or the fibres in their course either from above, from the side or from below, or by under-cutting selected areas of the cortex, or by topectomy, which is the excision of portions of the frontal cortex (Pool, 1949; LeBeau, 1954). Scoville's (1949) method of cortical undercutting is considered to give the same advantages as topectomy, while preserving the cortical blood supply and thus reducing the risk of post-operative epilepsy.

The Standard Operation

This was described by McKissock (1943) and had a considerable vogue. It has largely given way, however, to more selective operations but where a more extensive procedure is indicated, it still has a place. McKissock used the following technique: A point 3 cm. behind the lateral margin of the orbit and 5–6 cm. above the zygoma is selected as the centre of the skin incision. A 1-cm. burr hole is made in the dura. After first locating the anterior horn of the lateral ventricle, the brain needle is directed in front of it and pushed to a depth just short of the grey matter of the medial aspect of the frontal lobe. The needle is made to take an upward sweep, being pushed deeper to ensure that the line of the section runs parallel with the falx. When it has come close to the superior convexity, it is withdrawn and reintroduced along the original line to sever the fibres running from the lower part of the frontal lobe, again taking care to see that the needle travels parallel with the falx, only on this occasion, it is progressively withdrawn to avoid damage to the grey matter of the orbital surface of the frontal pole. The procedure is then repeated on the other side.

Objections have been raised on account of the extent of the damage, the risk that the cut may be more posterior than is desired, and the possibility that not enough may be done, for it has been shown that in some cases the leucotome has merely rotated instead of cut and there was virtually no mass severing of the white fibres. Posterior cuts can produce severe and even fatal complications (McLardy, 1950). These are mainly inanition leading to wasting and death from starvation, the patient being reduced to a 'cabbage-like' existence with resulting trophic lesions, uraemia and delayed post-operative death.

The number of operations and other procedures designed to interfere with frontal lobe function, continues to grow and while it is not necessary to know them all, the psychiatrist should not be merely a referring agency to the neurosurgeon, but an active partner in deciding the best type of procedure for his patient's needs. Operations favoured by neurosurgeons are those which can be performed under direct vision through trephine openings, some of which have been described by Paul *et al.* (1956) and Poppen (1948), while a **transorbital leucotomy** has been described by Freeman

(1949). This last procedure which was reputed to be performed by psychiatrists in the United States of America in their offices, consists of thrusting a sharp instrument (legend declares it is an ice-pick) through the orbital plate, 3 cm. from the midline and severing the fronto-thalamic fibres in the inframedial quadrant. Anaesthesia can be produced by 'stunning' the patient with E.C.T. previously and after doing the one side, a second 'stun' is used for the other. While this procedure has been condemned by most neurosurgeons, Freeman (1954) considers that it gives a higher proportion of good results than operations on the convexity or frontal poles.

Coagulation by chemicals or electric current of fronto-thalamic fibres or of the dorso-medial nucleus of the thalamus has been tried either by inserting electrodes under X-ray control or by **stereotaxic methods.** The relevant white matter has also been injected with novocaine in order to produce a temporary result to gauge the effectiveness of surgery. Lindstrom (1954) used **ultra-sonic sound** in patients who were suffering mainly from inoperable cancer with intractable pain, and claimed good results. His apparatus could be handled conveniently and was no bigger than many instruments used by surgeons; he christened it 'the bazooka'.

SIDE EFFECTS OF THE OPERATION

Before selecting a patient for leucotomy, it is not enough for the psychiatrist to be familiar with the clinical conditions which are likely to benefit from the operation, but he should also be aware of the results, desirable and otherwise, of the operation, for it may be those which concern the patient and his relatives most. Mention has already been made of the case of Phineas Gage, which was reported by Harlow (1869) though the relationship between the brain lesion and the personality changes were not pointed out, the object of the report being the equally remarkable recovery of the patient. Welt (1887–8) saw the connection very clearly and entitled his paper: 'Concerning changes in character in man following lesions of the forebrain' and to him must be given the credit for being the first to see the relationship between the anatomical lesion and the disturbed behaviour. Oppenheim (1890, 1891) introduced the term *Witzelsucht*, which is the cracking of feeble jokes, a phenomenon which has since been regarded as an essential feature of the frontal-lobe syndrome, though it is in fact not particularly common.

It was the development of neurosurgery and the plethora of head injuries in both World Wars, which contributed most to our knowledge of frontal lobe deficit, a notable contribution to the psychological implications of frontal lobectomy being that of Rylander (1939). There is little general agreement on what constitutes the frontal-lobe syndrome, and Bleuler (1951) stated: 'The so-called frontal syndrome is not characteristic of a frontal lesion but occurs also in most other brain lesions if they are localized'. Jarvie (1954, 1958) reported on the mental changes of 71 men with wounds of the brain, of whom 46 had damage to the frontal lobes, and he found clear evidence that certain permanent changes in behaviour took place only when the frontal lobes were involved, but it was severe in only nine cases. The changes noted, though not present in all the nine cases, were restlessness, increased drive, stereotyped actions, increased sexual activity, talkativeness, inappropriate talk, impulsive and foolhardy behaviour, emotional blunting and loss of anger in response to provocation. Jarvie did not subscribe to the views of Meyer (1950) that the degree of change was proportional to the amount of damage and states that similar changes occurred in one patient when only one frontal lobe was damaged, a phenomenon which had already been noted by Margolis *et al.* (1952).

Personality Changes

These do not occur in more than a small proportion of cases with frontal lobe damage and Jarvie noted them in only 25 per cent of his patients who had sustained severe damage, and suggests that this may be due to previous personality, rather than to anatomical factors. Those with changes had a background of being model children and were generally more inhibited than the average person and it would appear that the frontal lobe damage in them released behaviour which had previously been kept under control. This accords with the author's experience, for the most disturbing post-operative behaviour changes occur in patients with severe obsessional neuroses. Fortunately this type of behaviour can be controlled readily with adequate doses of chlorpromazine and tends to settle within a period of three months.

The answer to the patient or his relatives about the adverse personality effects following leucotomy would be, that they occur in only a minority of cases and that most of them settle with appropriate treatment in less than three months. But the type of operation cannot be entirely ignored.

THE SELECTION OF THE PATIENT

This is the most important aspect of the whole business of

leucotomy. In the early days, the operation was used as an instrument of therapeutic despair on patients who had not been helped by other forms of treatment and whose illness carried a hopeless prognosis, and it therefore tended to be recommended too freely for chronic psychotics whose behaviour made their management in a mental hospital a serious nursing problem. The surprising thing is that with such unpromising material there was any improvement at all. Yet, early reports with the standard operation yielded as many as a third of recoveries, including schizophrenic patients who had failed to respond to deep insulin shock therapy, which was then considered a specific remedy.

Indications for Leucotomy

Indications are varied and the operation has been tried for recurrent depression, obsessional states, tension states, depersonalization syndrome (Shorvon, 1947) psychosomatic disorders, with tension, such as eczema, asthma, anorexia nervosa (Sargant, 1951), hypertension (Tibbetts, 1949) and intractable pain (Freeman & Watts, 1946). That the patient should be suffering from one of the above conditions, is not enough. A leucotomy does not add anything to a patient, it can only take away and therefore the more a patient is endowed with intelligence and with a good pre-morbid personality, the better the results of the leucotomy are likely to be. Even though measurements of intellectual deterioration do not reveal any deficit after operation, there is sure to be some deficit which is more likely to be recognizable in the less well-favoured subjects. This does not mean that leucotomy will produce a marked reduction in capacity, for the author has had patients who have gone back to their previous jobs such as accountant, garage proprietor, senior business executive, and performed very well, for these patients had the reserves and could compensate for their deficit. An effective pre-morbid personality is probably the most important criterion for selection and as this assessment must be based on several years of stability and satisfactory employment, it is preferable not to choose too young a subject, for the instability which manifests may well be the precursor of schizophrenic breakdown, and there is no evidence that leucotomy may be of prophylactic value. Tension and obsessional features are also regarded as favourable, though the former may be difficult to assess. Neurotic depressives can create a façade of tension as part of the hysterical accompaniment which can superficially be indistinguishable from a genuine tension state or in fact appear to be in excess of it, and it is this aspect which frequently helps in the differential diagnosis.

The choosing of a surgeon is probably just as important a matter for the psychiatrist and his patient as it is, for example, for the physician and his patient with ulcerative colitis. The surgeon should have a feeling for the psychiatric problems which will come his way, be able to appreciate and enter into the discussion of a pre-leucotomy conference, interview patient and relatives and balance the conflicting views that will undoubtedly be expressed. He will also share the responsibility for the early post-operative phase which is most important in the patient's rehabilitation. In the team approach which has evolved at the United Birmingham Hospitals, the neurosurgeon's views on the patient's psychiatric state are highly valued and his contribution to the pre-leucotomy conference is as important as his role as surgeon. It is a convenient way of introducing him to the patient and relatives and ensuring that his part in the subsequent management is likely to be in accord with the views of his psychiatric colleagues.

THE PRE-LEUCOTOMY CONFERENCE

It has been the custom, in the author's department, for all cases for consideration for leucotomy to be submitted to a pre-leucotomy conference, at which the patient, relative(s), family doctor, neurosurgeon, psychiatric colleagues, nursing staff, social workers, occupational therapist—in fact all who have or will have experience of the patient—attend. The presenting psychiatrist reports the essential features of the problem as regards history of illness and its treatment to date, the pre-morbid personality, the family and home background and its capacity for rehabilitation as well as other relevant factors. Gaps are filled in by question and answer and then the patient is introduced and if necessary can be asked about specific aspects of the history or symptoms. The relative is then interviewed and after further discussion, with questions to the family doctor by the neurosurgeon and some 'devil's advocacy' by psychiatric colleagues, those present record individually their assessment of the problem, the case for or against operation and its type, and the result expected from the operation. The most important question on the form is 'What will happen if there is no operation?' and the recommendation will largely depend on its answer. Results are graded:

I = satisfactory with relief of symptoms.
II*a* = improved but not symptom-free.
II*b* = improved but with residual personality changes due to the operation.
III = unsatisfactory.

The patient retires and recommendations are then discussed; if there are suggestions which are generally accepted as offering the patient a reasonable prospect of recovery without operation, these are given an extended trial depending on the patient's capacity to continue without effective treatment. If there is general agreement that operation is desirable, the neurosurgeon can discuss the type of operation and get the psychiatrists' views at a live meeting where all statements can be critically tested. Although the discussion is most democratic, the decision to operate is not based on a vote, for it would not be in the patient's interest to go ahead say, on the casting vote of a junior medical officer with little experience of the patient or psychiatry. It is the neurosurgeon's decision alone and it is up to the presenting psychiatrist to make his case.

THE POST-LEUCOTOMY CONFERENCE

Post-leucotomy conferences at intervals up to six years have been held on approximately 100 of these patients and the results, which will be discussed later, have been gratifying. The recommendations of the pre-leucotomy conference are then reviewed and the opinions expressed compared with the actual result which is assessed independently by an assessor who was not present at the pre-leucotomy conference. It has been shown that the best predictions are those of the presenting psychiatrist, and the question has been raised: 'Is all this fuss of the pre-leucotomy conference necessary?' The author and his colleagues are in no doubt that it is, for there is a great deal of difference between a private talk with the neurosurgeon and having to make one's case in open court. The criteria of selection are sharpened and the surgeon is in a position to evaluate all the evidence, while the patient, relatives and family doctor are able to appreciate the care which is taken over these matters and a general feeling of confidence is inspired.

RESULTS OF LEUCOTOMY

There have been many studies of the results of leucotomy, and it can be said at the outset that those of the larger series are likely to yield the least helpful information, if only because of the diffuseness of the population and the varying standards of selection, surgery, post-operative care and rehabilitation. The Board of Control (1947) reported the results of 1000 cases of pre-frontal leucotomy, the patients being by definition inmates of mental hospitals and mainly psychotic. Yet in the relatively few obsessional patients operated on,

55 per cent were living outside the mental hospital after operation compared with 40 per cent manic-depressives and 16 per cent schizophrenics, who comprised more than 50 per cent of the total. Tooth and Newton (1961) surveyed 10,365 patients who had the operation in its various forms between 1942 and 1954. Of all cases, 41 per cent were regarded as total or social recoveries or greatly improved. Thirteen per cent were classed 'family burden and social defect'. Results were better for affective disorders than for schizophrenia. Twenty-five per cent were unchanged, 2 per cent were worse, 4 per cent were dead, the death being wholly or partly attributable to the operation, and 21 per cent who improved subsequently relapsed. Partridge (1950) personally followed up 300 patients who all had the same operation, by the same surgeon and described results which in general were in accord with those of the larger series. It is of interest that his carefully investigated smaller group can be used as corroborative evidence of some of the findings of the much larger but less intensively studied groups.

In spite of improvements in the operation, the numbers selected are diminishing year by year, but this need not mean that it is generally falling into disrepute, though it is a procedure which engenders violent reactions among the public as well as in the medical profession. In Russia, the operation has been banned, presumably because it conflicts with Pavlovian theory and practice. Freeman (1959) reports that Pope Pius XII (1952) gave guarded approval on the principle that it is licit to sacrifice a portion for the preservation of the whole. In this country Winnicott (1951) has been a persistent antagonist while in France, Baruk (1956), has attacked it on moral grounds. The correspondence columns of the *British Medical Journal* have at times borne the most heated arguments on the subject, and it must be conceded some of the objections may well have been justified by faulty selection in the early stages and perhaps by operations which did not suit the particular needs of the patient.

TYPES OF OPERATION

Much has been written of the various types of operation and their indications suggesting that some produce better results in some cases than in others. McKissock (1951) reviewing his results with the blind Freeman-Watts technique regarded it as still the operation of choice in most cases of mental illness requiring surgical treatment and claimed that its results were probably as good as those of topectomy, coagulation of the thalamic dorso-medial nucleus or selective cortical undercutting. He did, however, put forward another operation which he called 'rostral leucotomy' which is essentially the same as Scoville's (1949) undercutting of areas 9 and 10. McKissock recommends it as a limited operation when it is desired to preserve as much of the personality as possible but adds that it would be no bar to a more complete operation at a later date, if necessary.

Among the modified operations, that of the bilaterial infero-medial quandrant cut would appear to be theoretically the least damaging to the higher functions, as it spares the superior convexities and therefore the 'isocortex' and is mainly confined to the more primitive or 'allocortex' (MacLean, 1949, 1955). This operation like transorbital leucotomy has given very good results in recurrent depressions where E.C.T. has been producing diminishing results but has, however, proved disappointing in severe obsessional states. In the author's experience, the operation which has given consistently good results in both depression and obsessional states is the undercutting of areas 9 and 10 which as has been said approximates to McKissock's rostral leucotomy, and this is in spite of the theoretical objections mentioned above. It is always wise to recommend, in the first place, a modified operation, for if that is not enough, a second or even a third may be performed. This approach has much to commend it, for there is nothing so irremediable and disturbing as a patient who has been 'over-leucotomized'. The author had referred to him such a patient, who had previously been a conscientious member of the nursing profession and who, following her operation, had deteriorated to an almost unemployable level. Pippard (1955) has reported 27 cases who had a second leucotomy, with indifferent results, but these may have been due to the selection of patients rather than the second operation. Cingulectomy was introduced by Cairns for the treatment of obsessional and tension states as it was considered to have least effect on intelligence. The rationale may be valid, but the results in the author's experience have been disappointing. A number of the patients who had the cingulectomy which consisted of a bilateral removal of the rostral 5 cm. of the cingulate gyrus, had to have a second operation (undercutting of areas 9 and 10) which fortunately proved successful.

Knight (1965), who has favoured restricted orbital undercutting, regarded the area of the substantia innominata as crucial for the success of the operation. To make the lesion more localized he implanted radioactive yttrium-90 seeds with a stereotactic device under radiological control and he has reported on 90 patients so tested. Patients suffering from intractable depression did well. It is too early to say whether this method is superior to others, for this form of depression does well with the surgical techniques already described. What may prove to be its best indication are the elderly patients with cerebro-vascular disease and intractable depression. These constitute a higher risk group for traditional surgery and Knight's method may provide the only safe answer to their problem.

POST-LEUCOTOMY MANAGEMENT

Most candidates for leucotomy have contained their aggression and indeed have turned it relentlessly on themselves. The sudden release of this aggression can make post-operative care difficult and the author has, in suitable cases, prescribed chlorpromazine as a prophylactic. Dosage of 50 mg. t.d.s. is usually sufficient to ensure a quiet convalescence and render the patient suitable for early rehabilitation.

All patients after operation should be considered as candidates for rehabilitation, which is a standard procedure in hospital, and consists of early stimulation by nursing staff and occupational therapist. The social worker is also available to enter into a new relationship with the patient, whom she had already met. She has had to assess the family background for its tolerance to a changed patient, who is no longer helpless and dependent, proclaiming her unworthiness or tortured by her obsessions, for this object of pity may have given way to a rather boisterous over-confident person who is outspoken and tactless and no longer expresses gratitude. Some relatives who have been so used to their role of martyrdom have great difficulty in relinquishing it and may unconsciously try to recreate the old problem in the patient in order to cater for their own needs.

The early post-operative problems of lying abed, turning up late for appointments, and difficulty in getting to work, may tax the tolerance of the household and instead of constant stimulation, the patient may be permitted to drift. If the home is far removed from the hospital, prolonged stay in hospital with consequent delay in integrating the patient into the community may result. Ideally the patient should reside near the hospital so that early discharge with attendance at the Day Hospital should take place. It also permits more frequent visiting by the social worker and easier attendance for follow-up at the out-patient department as well as attendance at the out-patient social club. An industrial rehabilitation unit in the vicinity may be another advantage, for residential training lacks many of the advantages the patient has when he lives at home. The above points indicate how important rehabilitation is in the treatment of the leucotomized patient and it is no exaggeration to say that a suitable subject, expertly operated on, may fail to obtain maximum benefit, if the rehabilitation services are inadequate, or if the home background is unsatisfactory.

To summarize, the criteria for successful results are: (1) good selection; (2) good surgery; and (3) good rehabilitation. If any one of these ingredients is deficient, the result may be prejudiced. As published data on the operation rarely include the more detailed criteria of selection or all the essential features of rehabilitation, it is difficult to draw conclusions from one set of figures or to consider that results in a similarly operated group of patients would be similar; they may be better, or worse.

PROGNOSIS

Schizophrenia is not a good indication, although in chronic schizo-affective patients who remit on 'maintenance' E.C.T., some useful recoveries may be expected. Generally, about one-third show some improvement, though Kalinowsky and Hoch (1952) claim better results in pseudoneurotic forms of schizophrenia; some independent observers, however, may doubt the validity of classifying all these patients as schizophrenics.

Freeman (1972) reported on 415 patients with schizophrenic reactions who were followed up from 4–30 years (average 14·3 years) and who were operated on within 12 months of hospitalization and compared with the 300 patients whose operations were done after one year or more in hospital. Of those 415 operated on early, 97 had prefrontal leucotomies and 45 per cent of their total years since operation were gainfully or constructively employed, 28 per cent of their years were spent in idle dependency at home or in a sheltered environment, and 27 per cent of their years were spent in state or private psychiatric hospitals. The corresponding percentages for the 318 patients with transorbital leucotomies were 65 per cent, 22 per cent and 13 per cent, indicating a well-marked difference between the long-range results of the two types of operation, in favour of the transorbital.

When these results were compared with the long-stay patients the latter showed very little improvement, and the author concluded that in a disease like schizophrenia it may be better to operate than to wait. An important factor in rehabilitation was the ability and willingness of the families to provide a home life. A factor which favoured a poor prognosis was the preponderance of prefrontal leucotomy as opposed to transorbital in the long-stay patients. The advent of the tranquillizers made it easier to manage patients at home so that instead of leucotomy being a final heroic remedy it could mark the turning point in effective therapy.

Affective disturbances which do well are primarily psychotic depression, mainly of the involutional period. These patients usually have a good pre-morbid personality and it should be possible in these states to give a very good prognosis, which may approximate to that given for a course of E.C.T. Manic-depressive swings are much less common and there are therefore relatively few reports on the results of leucotomy in these patients. Stevenson and McCausland (1953) have reported suppression of cyclic depression, in that 18 out of 22 patients were able to leave hospital after leucotomy. Sargant and Slater (1954) do not consider that patients who are liable to attacks of both excitement and depression and are of pyknic build should be considered for psychosurgery unless the prognosis otherwise would appear to be hopless; they suggest that in these severe cases a more posterior cut is justified. Some consider that should these patients relapse after such a leucotomy, they are rendered more receptive to further courses of E.C.T.

The commonest psychoneurotic state which benefits from leucotomy is the **obsessional neurosis**. It is important to assess the problem carefully and make sure that decompensation with some schizophrenic features has not set in, for this would adversely affect what should otherwise be an excellent prognosis. An accompanying depression with perhaps suicidal preoccupation should enhance the prognosis, if only because it makes the possibility of schizophrenic deterioration less likely, and also because these features in themselves are good indications for the operation. In the obsessionals operated on for the author, the results have been most gratifying and in one particular case, even remarkable. A young married woman with obsessional features of a checking and germ-avoidance nature had for years disrupted her home life with her conduct and had incorporated her husband in her rituals so that neither could get to bed till 2 or 3 A.M. She had a history of what was considered primary amenorrhoea and had had prolonged courses of hormone therapy since she was 16 years to initiate normal menstruation, but without success. It was even suggested that the constant checking of dates and rectal temperature might have reinforced the obsessional features. Following the operation, she lost her obsessional features and promptly became pregnant, giving birth to a normal child. She has continued well, menstruated regularly till she again became pregnant and this time gave birth to twins.

As has been mentioned in Chapter 11 (p. 449) obsessional states pose a unique problem in the violence of the post-leucotomy response and it has now become standard practice in the author's department to place these patients immediately on adequate chlorpromazine dosage, which may mean 100 mg. thrice daily, maintaining them on this dose for periods of up to a month or more and then gradually reducing to zero. **Anxiety states** either free and floating, with somatic dysfunction, or phobic, may occasionally be considered for the operation, but are not promising subjects unless there is much accompanying tension. Occasionally a patient with a very severe degree of anxiety may be referred for consideration for leucotomy, but on careful inquiry, the patient may be having large quantities of barbiturates and may be already addicted. This addiction is usually based on phobic anxiety and the proper course is to admit the patient to hospital for treatment of the barbiturate addiction and then treat the phobic anxiety which is usually amenable to less drastic measures than leucotomy. **Hysteria** as a conversion symptom is unlikely to yield to leucotomy, and as a manifestation of the hysterical character is a direct contraindication. **Psychopathic states** are also contraindications as the little control the patient may be abe to exercise over her conduct may be removed.

Intractable pain which has defied other neurosurgical procedures such as tractotomy, sympathectomy, ganglion block or root section, may be referred for consideration. The operation had gained some favour in the earlier years after its introduction for intractable pain by Freeman and Watts (1946), particularly for the pain of inoperable cancer (Otenasek, 1948; Dynes & Poppen, 1949), where the former author reported good results in all 11 cases and the latter authors reported good results in 11 out of 18 cases. As inoperable cancer has a short expectation of life, a good result need not last very long. It is, however, a very different matter when the pain is long-standing and the patient has a high expectation of life. Elithorn *et al.* (1958) reported on 25 patients with pain mainly of 'neuralgic' type. Nine had extensive leucotomy operations, and the rest were modified ones, being unilateral. Elithorn *et al.* (1955) had previously demonstrated that leucotomy does not affect the actual perception of pain, nor is there any selective interference with the perception of autonomic or visceral pain. The operation alters the reaction of the patient to anticipated pain, which is really the psychological reaction rather than the pain itself. The authors used a rating scale to assess the patients' social behaviour after operation, which included the patient's and his family's reactions to the persisting symptoms. Only one-third of the patients said their pain was better, though three-quarters seemed improved as far as their social adaptation was concerned. Standard leucotomy was more successful than modified operations in the patient's estimation, but rating scales which were compiled with the help of the relatives, suggested that the latter was in fact better. Other authors (Botterell *et al.*, 1954; Fischer-Williams, 1956) had already demonstrated the relative inefficacy of the operation in intractable pain and Elithorn and his colleagues emphasized the importance of a correct assessment of the psychiatric picture, yet it is still very difficult to decide who will benefit and who will not. Where depression is a major component, there would appear to be a better prospect of recovery, for the operation relieves suffering rather than pain.

Complications of the Operation

These are not many and will depend to some extent on the physical state of the patient. As **haemorrhage** is the commonest complication, if there is marked cerebral arteriosclerosis, the risks are increased. **Incontinence of urine** may occur and can be troublesome, but it usually settles, though rigorous training may be necessary to help it on its way. **Obesity** is common as appetite is increased and the patient may not seem to be aware that he has had enough to eat and will continue to gorge. **Epilepsy** with the standard operation was not uncommon, but it is rarely seen now. Some surgeons if operating on the superior convexity place the patient on phenobarbitone, 60 mg. twice daily for a period of up to two years to prevent the occurrence of fits. The type of operation also influences complications and Freeman (1953) found the frontal lobe syndrome 20 times as frequent after the standard operation as after the transorbital one.

Psychological Effects

These are confined mainly to the immediate post-operative period and Ashby and Bassett (1949) demonstrated this most effectively by getting the patient to draw from still life in the pre-and post-operative phases. In the latter there was frequently complete distortion of form and colour, with the patient showing no evidence of awareness of the deficient response. This effect tended to wear off. Tow (1955) studied 36 patients before and after operation and found that they lost significantly in tests for accuracy, Raven's progressive matrices, persistence, and the ability to handle abstract. When the patient is given a structured situation, he performs quite well, but in an unstructured test, such as writing an autobiography, deterioration in performance could be gross. Yet most patients emerge from this phase and perform quite well in everyday life, including business, which contains a large number of unstructured situations.

OTHER BRAIN OPERATIONS

Stereotactic Hypothalamotomy for Behaviour Disorders

Schvarcz *et al.* (1972) reported on 11 patients with aggressive behaviour which had failed to respond to extensive psychiatric treatment. They all had exhibited severe episodes of hetero-and/or auto-aggressiveness, usually with violent, destructive behaviour. One patient was schizophrenic, 2 were aggressive psychopaths and 8 were epileptics, of whom 5 were mental defectives.

With the exception of one patient who had a unilateral lesion, all had bilateral lesions under general anaesthesia with an average interval of 10 days between lesions. The method was fractionated electrocoagulation and lesions were 3–4 mm. in diameter, the target point being 3 mm. perpendicularly below the mid-point of the inter-commissural line and 2 mm. from the lateral wall of the third ventricle which corresponds to the medial part of the posterior hypothalmic area. The ventro-medial nucleus, the lateral hypothalmic area and the mamillothalamic tract were all carefully avoided and electrical stimulation was done in all cases for physiological corroboration before electro-coagulation. The stimulus produced an arousal reaction with opening of the eyelids and vocalization as well as the autonomic responses of midriasis, marked hypertension and tachycardia, but these effects disappeared after two minutes. There were also somatic responses, with convergent strabismus and/or downward deviation of gaze, and the lesions were made at the site of strongest symptomatic responses.

At follow-up between 6–48 months, 7 showed marked improvement, 3 improved with the addition of drugs and one failed to improve. Best results were obtained in patients with normal intelligence while those who were oligophrenic and hyperkinetic were least satisfactory, again illustrating the point that any form of leucotomy gives nothing to a patient; it merely takes away, in some instances, that little which he hath.

Stereotactic Lesions in the Knee of Corpus Callosum

Laitinen (1972) reported 46 patients with intractable anxiety who had small stereotactic lesions in the rostral cingulum, anteroventrally to the genu of the corpus callosum (GCC). Good responses were observed in 25 patients, 12 showed some improvement, while 9 did not benefit. During the series the author on experimental evidence of bipolar low intensity stimulation produced in the patient a sudden strong feeling of inner well-being and relaxation. Lesions of 6 x

6 mm. in diameter were produced with high frequency electro-coagulation 6 mm. to the right and left of the midline, followed by bilateral pea-sized cingulate lesions. In this patient, all anxiety, fears, and obsessions disappeared and drug therapy was stopped. Cognition, memory and psychomotor function improved and there were no signs of emotional blunting, disorientation or euphoria. A subsequent 11 patients with anxiety had equally good results but 3 patients with melancholia did not respond either to the stimulation or to the lesions.

LEUCOTOMY AND SOCIAL RESPONSIBILITY

There is a primitive fear in man that interfering with the brain, such as in leucotomy will render the patient completely indifferent to the social customs and even to the morality of his culture. In the immediate post-operative phase, this could happen, though in modified operations it is very rare. Crimes have been committed by leucotomized patients, though they frequently have been criminal before operation. The author had a patient who after a leucotomy for a severe tension state, found his wife was having an affair with a business associate. He wrote him a blackmailing letter asking him to deposit money at a certain time in a public place. The police were informed and saw the patient loitering near the spot, went to his home and found traced on the blotter an imprint of the letter he had written with a ball-point pen. They were impressed with this evidence and he was charged. It is very doubtful if leucotomy made him a criminal, though it may have contributed to his crude attempt at blackmail and the trail of clues which assisted the work of the police.

It could be responsible for minor peccadilloes and one patient was very careless in his dress to the extent that he offended and frightened his teenage daughter. Most of the aggressive behaviour following leucotomy can be controlled with chlorpromazine and occasionally the aggression is replaced by a general negativism and lack of pliability; this state too will yield to phenothiazine.

The operation still has a place in the treatment of mental illness but where once it was a last despairing effort to influence a hopeless problem, it is now reserved for patients with good pre-morbid personalities who have a good prognosis with the operation. Paradoxically, it is best in the very patients one may fear to operate on, because one does not think they are sufficiently deteriorated to risk the operation. The number of leucotomies performed has dropped considerably, and this is probably due to more efficient treatment by more conservative measures. The more frequent use of lithium carbonate is also playing a part in reclaiming some of the 'hard-core' manic-depressives.

INSULIN SHOCK TREATMENT

Insulin shock treatment was introduced in 1932 by Manfred Sakel in Vienna following his empirical observation that accidental hypoglycaemia improved the mental state of schizophrenia. It rapidly gained recognition as the only effective treatment of early schizophrenia and most mental hospitals organized their insulin units.

This treatment is now rarely used and most psychiatrists feel, with justification, that they can obtain better results in schizophrenia without it. Social factors which can be manipulated and the advent of the phenothiazines, rauwolfia preparations and the butyrophenones have made this treatment unnecessary. Some clinics which have built their management of the schizophrenic round insulin coma induction have felt unable to renounce it but they are a diminishing group and it is unlikely that there will be a resurgence of interest in its use. For this reason, it is not proposed, in this edition of the 'Guide', to give all the details of the technique. For those who are interested, these can be found in the first edition (Sim, 1963). For those who may feel this attitude is too cavalier, the following criticisms of insulin coma treatment are offered.

Criticisms of the Treatment

A number of psychiatrists had for long wondered whether insulin coma therapy was a specific treatment and found it difficult to isolate its therapeutic effects from all the other accompanying features of the treatment. These included special dieting; the controlled games and exercises; the little bag of sweets that the patient carried around to cope with delayed insulin reaction; the group morale of the insulin ward; the fuss and nursing attention associated with the coma treatment; the glucose drinks after termination; and the rub down with a warm dry towel to mop up the excessive perspiration. It seemed that these measures in themselves when applied to a schizophrenic patient together with the time the treatment lasted, might conceivably have contributed to remission in a group which, as has been said, tends to remit in any case.

Bourne (1953) crystallized these views in his provocative paper 'The Insulin Myth'. He stated that treatment for schizophrenia may be evaluated by its immediate and remote effects on: (1) early cases, in which spontaneous remissions make it very difficult to assess the value of any treatment; (2) dilapidated chronic cases in which spontaneous remission is unlikely so that good results in even a few cases might be significant; and (3), individual cases observed over long periods with repeated courses of treatment. He pointed out the fallacies of drawing conclusions from the treatment of early cases. Some of these cases were diagnosed on flimsy evidence such as a clinical suspicion reinforced by a Rorschach test. Schizophrenic reactions seemed to be more benign than previously, or were being increasingly recognized and Bourne quotes from his study of 376 schizophrenic soldiers, 84 per cent of whom were discharged within nine months as recovered or sufficiently improved not to require further hospital care. He adds: 'The influences of nuances of environment on the course of schizophrenia involves so many imponderables which cannot be isolated or controlled that to compare results at different times and different places may be quite invalid'. Environment has been known for long to influence the course of a schizophrenic psychosis and Bourne points out that this was early evident in the contrasting effects of the neglect of the chronic schizophrenic in the backward institution with those of enlightened hospitals which promote freedom and social life. Bourne's paper critically analyses previous controlled trials with insulin as against another or no treatment and concludes that when these are statistically reliable and properly planned, such as that of Penrose and Marr (1943), insulin therapy is of no real value. His conclusions are that the evidence for the value of insulin treatment is unconvincing and that in the early case, the chronic case, and in individual case studies, there is no proof that insulin has a specific therapeutic effect or that it influences the long-term prognosis.

As one would expect, this challenge from one who was then a young and very junior medical officer in a mental deficiency institution, produced a barrage of letters to the editor from a number of senior psychiatrists, but unfortunately as Bourne later illustrated in his replies, there was little convincing argument in them, and some were really attacks on his lack of experience. The matter could not now rest and 'The Insulin Myth' became a popular topic for discussion. Medical superintendents felt that to abandon their insulin units would be bad for staff morale, as much of the therapeutic effect in the form of traditional medical and nursing sense was centred on these units. They feared that without them their staff would lose interest and there would be a return to the therapeutic nihilism which had for years been associated with schizophrenia.

Ackner *et al.* (1957) carried out a carefully controlled trial where young schizophrenic patients were matched for age and sex, and one group given insulin comas, while the other was given barbiturate anaesthesia, each patient having the same number of injections. They found no significantly greater improvement in the insulin-treated group. Boardman *et al.* (1956) followed this up by comparing insulin and chlorpromazine in the treatment of 100 previously untreated schizophrenics. The results were slightly more favourable in the chlorpromazine-treated group and they concluded that chlorpromazine was the first treatment of choice in schizophrenia.

Since then, other workers have reported even more enthusiastically on the value of chlorpromazine, and insulin has gradually declined in popularity. Many units have been closed, although regions try to maintain at least one unit, so that the treatment should still be available. It is now about 20 years since Bourne delivered his attack, and it appears that the years have vindicated him.

Modified Insulin Therapy

This is the term used for subcoma treatment and was introduced by Sargant and Craske (1941) who, on the basis of the Weir Mitchell technique (Mitchell, 1881), used insulin to produce a state of relaxation and sopor and to stimulate the appetite in the treatment of war neuroses. The patients were generally suffering from severe anxiety states with insomnia and anorexia, following prolonged exposure to stress. The technique consists of putting the patient to bed and fasting him from 8 P.M. At 7 A.M. the following morning, 20 units of soluble insulin are injected intramuscularly and the dose increased by 10 units daily till 100 units is reached, or less if coma threatens on a smaller dose. Complete rest is imposed and as soon as the patient becomes soporific, he is propped up and encouraged to take a sweetened drink; this is followed by a meal. If there is no emergency, three hours are allowed to elapse from the time of the injection before a meal is given. The effect of the hypoglycaemia is to stimulate the appetite and large amounts of food, particularly buttered toast and jam, may be consumed at this time. The patient then gets up, has a shower to wash off the perspiration, makes his bed and is occupied in ward duties. In the afternoon he is free to take exercise or play games, and he is given some sweets to counteract any delayed hypoglycaemic effects; he should be under loose supervision. Treatment is continued till he has regained his previous weight.

Good results have been claimed, particularly in battle neurosis but as with deep insulin coma, it is very difficult, perhaps even more difficult, to assess whether improvement is due to the effects of the insulin or the other factors. Sargant and Slater state that during the time he is gaining weight, the patient is amenable to suggestion and can be encouraged to relinquish many of his symptoms. Acute stress reactions are considered to yield the best results, while chronic hysterical problems are unsatisfactory indications. There are so many factors at work that it is virtually impossible to define accurately the role of the insulin, but there is no doubt that in some patients it provides a vehicle for recovery from an acute neurotic reaction which is far more economical of effort and medical man hours than intensive psychotherapy. It has gained a reputation as a stimulator of appetite, and many cases of anorexia nervosa have been treated by modified insulin, but the results are generally disappointing, for it is not the appetite which is impaired in these states, but rather a wilful refusal to eat.

CONVULSION THERAPY

Convulsion therapy was introduced for the treatment of mental illness by Meduna, who in 1933 recommended the intramuscular injection of 25 per cent camphor in oil for the treatment of schizophrenia. At about this time there was much interest in the physical illnesses of patients in mental hospitals, and in defining symbiotic and antagonistic illnesses, a certain degree of symbiosis was noted in that tuberculosis was rife in schizophrenics. There was also evidence of disease antagonism, in that schizophrenia and epilepsy rarely occurred together. Legend has it that someone had tried to treat epilepsy with the serum of schizophrenics, but was unsuccessful, and Meduna saw the possibilities of the reverse procedure, namely treating schizophrenia with epilepsy and published his findings (Meduna, 1936). Cardiazol (Metrazol) and other chemical convulsants replaced camphor, and Cerletti and Bini (1938) replaced the pharmacological agents with electric current; this method has now almost entirely supplanted any other form of convulsant therapy. Chemical convulsants are, however, of some value, especially in areas where electricity is not available or should the current fail, and details of the technique are as follows.

TECHNIQUES

Cardiazol is injected intravenously in a 10 per cent aqueous solution, the dilution being necessary to avoid venous thrombosis at the site of the injection. Speed is essential in order to cut down the time between the prodromal phase and the convulsion which can last several seconds, during which time the patient is conscious and is aware that he is about to lose consciousness. The feeling has been described as one of impending death and some schizophrenics who were extremely apprehensive of the treatment would claim improvement and make heroic efforts to demonstrate this in order to avoid further injections. Cardiazol, 10 ml., is loaded in the syringe and an initial dose of 5 ml. is given rapidly to test for undue sensitivity, for some with an epileptic diathesis will convulse with as little as 4 ml. If there is no convulsion, after a minute a further 2–3 ml. may be given. On subsequent occasions 7–8 ml. can be shot in quickly and this usually suffices to produce a convulsion. As the drug is broken down fairly rapidly, too much delay during the injection would render it ineffective. A close watch should be kept on the patient's face and limbs, for there is usually a 'march' of clonic movements prior to the generalized convulsion. It is this phase which gives the therapist time to remove the needle from the vein before the arm goes into spasm. The usual precautions for an epileptic fit should be taken.

Electric convulsant therapy or electroplexy, as it is now being called, consists of the passage of an electric current through the forehead of the patient, the two electrodes being applied to either temple. In the earlier days of the treatment, machines were very complicated, with dials to measure resistance, voltage, and time switches which could be set to a variety of readings. A 'phantom' could also be introduced to test that the machine was in working order and voltages and resistances would be juggled with till satisfactory readings were obtained. Machines are now much simpler and the author has for many years used the 'Ectron' stimulator (Ectron, No. 543) which delivers a steady current.

Preparation of the Patient

The patient should have had no food or drink for three and a half hours, and just before the treatment should be asked to empty the bladder. A physical check should be made before initiating treatment, and even with subsequent treatments the patient should be asked about his health, for otherwise an incipient chest infection may not be declared, with the possibility of risk to the patient. Dentures are removed and the skin of the temples is wiped with an electrolytic solution or with electrojelly such as is used for contact in electrocardiography.

Treatment may be given either 'straight' or 'modified'. In 'straight' treatment, the patient will experience a full major convulsion with spasm of jaw muscles and violent jerkings of the limbs, and various measures have been suggested to avoid damage to teeth, tongue and skeletal system. A number of different mouth gags are available, some shaped like horse-shoes, others like mouth-organs with holes in them to permit the patient to breathe and saliva to escape. Rubber dog's bones are also used to guard an awkward part of the mouth where irregular dentition makes the use of the horse-shoe bite impracticable. The author has found a rubber ring pessary of the greatest value in patients with occasional dental pegs. The ring can be placed round these and thus protect the teeth and the mouth from harm. These appliances should naturally be sterilized before re-use. There is still some doubt as to the value of **restraint** when the treatment is given. Some insist on hard, padded couches, restraining sheets and a band of attendants who pounce on the patient in an attempt to prevent movements of the limbs and trunk in order to avoid fractures. The author has never been convinced of the efficacy of these measures and in a very long and plentiful experience with no restraints, has not found that his patients were more liable to fractures than those of his colleagues who practised restraint. There was the not inconsiderable advantage that fewer staff were required to administer the treatment.

Of greater importance is the provision of reliable suction and adequate oxygen supplies which can be delivered at a controlled pressure, such as by the Oxford inflator.

Fractures are not infrequent with 'straight' E.C.T., though they may be confined to a minute chip off a transverse process of a vertebra. The author took part in a study of the incidence of bony injury in 100 young servicemen following E.C.T. Patients' vertebral columns and pelves were X-rayed before and after the course of treatment and nearly 50 per cent revealed some bony injury though, in most instances, it was very slight. The usual fracture is one of compression in the region of the dorsal kyphosis (D. 5, 6 or 7) and though the radiological lesions appear gross, it must be very rare indeed for neurological involvement to occur; the author has never seen such a case. If long term adverse results occurred, there would have been a spate of reports from orthopaedic clinics, but apart from a few accounts of the radiological changes, these have not appeared. The author had a female patient in her late 60's who was suffering from severe depressive delusions and had attempted suicide. She was started on E.C.T. and was responding dramatically till her fourth treatment when she complained of pain in her back. X-ray showed marked compression of the 6th thoracic vertebra. Treatment was stopped and the family informed. She began to relapse and the family who were very loyal to their mother asked what would be the risk if treatment were continued. On being told that it might aggravate the spinal injury, they unanimously decided that they would rather have their mother as they used to know her and with an injured back than in her present pathetic mental state. Treatment was therefore continued and the patient's mental state improved, the pain in the back disappeared and everybody was pleased, but the X-ray still showed the compression fracture. This experience has since been confirmed in a number of patients and the question arises as to whether these compression fractures are radiological diseases rather than clinical states. As one cynical colleague remarked: 'I never see the spinal fractures—I don't X-ray my patients'.

Other injuries are fracture-dislocation of the shoulder joint, dislocation of the jaw, fracture of the pelvis due to the head of the femur being driven through the acetabulum with resulting rupture of the bladder, and a rather strange event, haemorrhage from the ear due to rupture of the tensor tympani (Hodgson & Sim, 1959). These are all very rare and the most serious complication of the treatment is cardiovascular failure.

Apart from the complications and hazards, 'straight' E.C.T. is a most inelegant procedure. The patient utters a loud cry due to the sudden expiratory phase and this is followed by the strong tonic phase with cracking of joints and possible fractures and then the prolonged clonic phase during which the patient becomes more and more cyanosed followed by stertorous breathing. In large clinics, patients would hear and perhaps even see others being treated and one can imagine their horror.

Modified E.C.T.

A modification of the method was needed and attempts to achieve this were soon made. Palmer (1939) reported the use of the muscle relaxant, *d*-tubocurarine chloride, an alkaloid obtained from crude curare, but had to interrupt his work because of the war. Bennett (1940) has since been credited with propagating this form of treatment though in his earliest paper he used the crude curare. Though this modification prevented fractures, it was still hazardous, for curare and *d*-tubocurarine had a rather prolonged action with resultant apnoea which had to be counteracted with oxygen delivered at positive pressure. Hobson and Prescott (1947) who had used *d*-tubocurarine with E.C.T. were concerned with patients' complaints 'of the terrifying feeling of suffocation and extreme weakness' and that some refused further treatment on account of this. They first tried to produce unconsciousness with a sub-convulsive shock immediately after injecting the *d*-tubocurarine, but they found it impossible to gauge the dose required for the sub-convulsion and they were also fearful of the risk of cardiac arrest which might result (Kalinowsky & Hoch, 1952). They used preliminary anaesthetization with intravenous thiopentone and found that this provided an adequate suppression of undesirable sensations and any memory of them. It also permitted the treatment to be given to patients with a variety of physical states which would have made straight E.C.T. either hazardous or impossible. These included elderly patients, hypertensives, recent fractures, pregnant women, and one who had had a haematemesis from a peptic ulcer following unmodified E.C.T. A more humane and safer method had been evolved.

Relaxants were improved, *d*-tubocurarine chloride was replaced by decamethonium iodide which was shorter in its action, and in 1952, Bovet introduced *succinylcholine* which, though it has no antidote like curare which has prostigmine, is very brief in its action, the muscular paralysis lasting only two to three minutes. An even shorter-acting relaxant, suxethonium bromide, has also been introduced, but in electroplexy has no real advantage over succinylcholine which is said to act by depolarizing the muscle-nerve endings like acetylcholine. There was at one time a suggestion that modified E.C.T. did not have the same therapeutic effect as the 'straight', but there is no reliable evidence to support this.

Technique of the Treatment

The following is a description of the technique now used in the author's clinic, on both out-patients and in-patients. The patient is thoroughly examined physically, but physical diseases are not necessarily contra-indications. For example, a number of severe hypertensives who have become acutely depressed and suicidal after the administration of rauwolfia or other hypotensive agents, may be given the treatment. Occasionally, after consultation with a cardiologist, patients with a recent history of coronary occlusion may be given the treatment, though these high risk patients should be treated, initially at least, as in-patients.

As with 'straight' E.C.T., the patient has nothing to eat or drink for three and a half hours prior to the treatment and the bladder is voided, artificial teeth are removed, tight clothing is loosened and the patient is given a single intravenous injection containing 0·2 g. thiopentone and 0·6 mg. of atropine sulphate. The latter helps to reduce salivation and bronchial secretions and thus is a useful prophylactic against respiratory difficulties (Hargreaves, 1962). Gahagan (1962) criticizes this dose of atropine and recommends 1·2 mg. 'to prevent the undesirable cholinergic effects which are otherwise induced by E.C.T. The chief aim in premedication with atropine is the prevention of cardiac arrhythmias of vagal (*i.e.* cholinergic) origin. The lessening of secretions is an important secondary gain'.

Clement (1962) supported this view. He premedicated 100 patients with 1 mg. of atropine intravenously 75 seconds before treatment. In the subcutaneous group, 22 patients exhibited circulatory disturbance, while in the intravenous group, one patient developed complete disappearance of pulse and heart sounds for four seconds. In this instance the shock was given inadvertently 45 seconds after the administration of atropine and not after the required 75 seconds.

Methohexital Premedication. Thiopentone has been the most popular anaesthetic for E.C.T. but Woodruff *et al.* (1968) reported a systematic study comparing methohexitone with thiopentone which showed that the latter was associated with a greater frequency of five types of ECG abnormalities: atrial premature contractions, ventricular premature contractions, multifocal ventricular premature contractions, T wave changes, and ST segment changes. These occurred more frequently between the end of seizure activity and the resumption of spontaneous breathing, particularly with thiopentone. The authors did not find pre-oxygenation an advantage but they do not indicate whether the patients were in oxygen debt prior to treatment.

Succinylcholine 40–70 mg. according to the weight and muscularity of the patient is then given through the same needle, and after about 15 seconds the fasciculation of the muscles, due to depolarization, begins. This twitching can be quite violent at times and may almost simulate voluntary movement, but it peters out after a minute and the electrodes can be applied. These, which are soaked in electrolyte (sodium bicarbonate solution, 1 tablespoonful to a pint), are applied to the temples, which have been cleaned with the same electrolyte solution. The patient who is now apnoeic is given oxygen at positive pressure by the Oxford inflator. This is a very important aspect of this form of treatment and gives it a distinct advantage over the 'straight' form, for the patient is never in oxygen debt and consequently the risks are lessened. The gag or airway is placed in position, the electrodes and the current applied for about one second and the electrodes removed. The patient may show only the slightest flicker of the muscles or a modest degree of movement, depending on the degree of relaxation achieved. Oxygen is again given and the patient kept a good colour, care being taken not to overdo the oxygenation. When the swallowing reflex has returned the airway can be removed and the patient turned on his side and made comfortable.

After a short time, he will regain consciousness and it is important that he be not disturbed, for his memory is defective and he may misinterpret any movement made towards him. A smile from the nurse is generally reassuring, but the psychiatrist should not be too outgoing and the author has found his neutral back less disturbing to patients than his friendly face. If the patient is restless, it is tempting to try and restrain his movements, but the author finds that sitting on the edge of the bed with his back to the patient to prevent him from falling out is less likely to lead to trouble, for one should understand that the patient is confused and may misinterpret any approach as a hostile one. If he is sleeping peacefully, he should not be disturbed; if the bed is to be wheeled back to the ward he should be told what is happening and if he has not properly received the message, he should be left a little longer, for an excited patient trying to get out of bed is a formidable problem in a hospital corridor. When he has fully recovered, he can be given a drink of tea or coffee, followed by some food. As an out-patient he should be able to go home by ordinary transport within two hours of the first injection.

Out-patient electroplexy has brought a treatment, at one time reserved for in-patients, to many people who might otherwise have had to enter a mental hospital (Hodgson & Sim, 1959), and the results are no less gratifying than with those treated as in-patients. In the author's department, which is a general hospital unit with, to date, inadequate facilities in the in-patient department for the disturbing patient, it is not uncommon for him to tell the relatives: 'We can treat the patient as an out-patient, if you will undertake to keep a close eye on him at home and bring him regularly for treatment, for he is really too ill to be admitted'. It is most encouraging to see how often relatives will shoulder these responsibilities and when the patient begins to improve, the benefit spills over to the relatives who are overjoyed to see their efforts crowned with success.

E.C.T. in Delirium Tremens

This treatment has been recommended for some time, and as prognosis in delirium tremens worsens with the persistence of delirium and hyperkinesis, Dudley and Williams (1972) decided to subject it to a controlled trial against patients who received the standard treatment of sodium diphenylhydantoin and phenobarbitone in diminishing doses. Ten patients who had received E.C.T. on the first or second day in hospital were matched for age and sex against 10 controls.

Mean length of delirium was 0·85 days for the E.C.T. group as against 2·8 days for the controls. In 7 out of 10 of the E.C.T. group, the delirium stopped on the day E.C.T. was given. In all cases, one treatment produced sedation with a clearing of the sensorium and termination of hallucinations within 24 hours. Combative patients began to take oral fluids and food readily in contrast to an average of 72 hours in the control group.

Other Forms of Electroplexy

These have been used to reduce the severity of the convulsion, either by using different forms of current or by altering their wave form (Liberson & Wilcox, 1945; Wilcox, 1946; Liberson, 1947). A machine which is alleged to give all the benefits of convulsion therapy without the convulsion is the Reiter apparatus which gives modulated brief spiked impulses (Wilcox, 1948). Milligan (1951) who reviewed these development concluded that: '. . . it was possible to produce a smooth convulsion in which the clonic stage is completely masked'. Heath and Norman (1946) had suggested that a convulsion was not essential in order to gain benefit from electric therapy and that the benefits derived were due to hypothalamic stimulation.

A large variety of techniques using electricity in the treatment of mental illness have been elaborated, some of them based on experimental work. Russell *et al.* (1953) described 'intensified E.C.T.' which was later called interrupted fused-dosage (I.F.D.) and in 1956, Russell devised the 'ectonus' technique, which is the continuous application of a current of varying voltage for a period of 30–60 seconds. A control knob permits the therapist to alter the voltage so that clonic movements can be reduced to a slight twitching which acts as a useful index of the duration of the stimulation. Its sponsors have claimed that it is safer and more effective than ordinary E.C.T. and reduces the memory disturbance. MacDougall (1958) coupled the 'ectonus' treatment with promazine (EPT) and claimed excellent results in the treatment of schizophrenia. Jacoby (1958) described 'regressive shock therapy', where the patient is given daily treatment until a severe but temporary confusional state is induced and this method has been used in the treatment of maniacal states. By varying the type of current a 'glissando' effect is obtained which cuts out the sharp stimulus produced by the ordinary machine and a smoother convulsion is achieved. Some of these methods have found favour in a few clinics as they permit the psychiatrist to administer a type of modified E.C.T. without the risks of anaesthesia and eliminate the sometimes very real difficulty of getting anaesthetist assistance. Generally, these methods have not become popular and E.C.T. modified with thiopentone and succinylcholine is the one most generally used. Some clinics omit the thiopentone, claiming that the patients do not remember the effects of the relaxant, but the author has had referred to him quite a number of patients who have had this type of treatment and they give graphic and accurate descriptions of their experiences. There is so much in favour of giving the treatment modified with thiopentone and succinylcholine that there should be very strong reasons for using an alternative.

Unilateral E.C.T.

Post-E.C.T. confusion with memory loss is a universal accompaniment of the treatment; some have proposed that it is an essential part of the treatment. Yet, in some patients the degree of disturbance can be more than is tolerable and in efforts to minimize these side-effects, unilateral E.C.T., applied to the non-dominant hemisphere, has been used. The main problem is how to assess the results. Patients who confuse most are elderly and often vitamin-depleted; they are notoriously unreliable subjects for formal testing and the vitamin deficiency can be so variable as to invalidate conclusions. Memory deficit is often a subjective experience, the obsessional patient with little memory loss making more complaint than others with greater loss.

This has not deterred a large number of investigators from trying to decide the advantages of unilateral E.C.T. over bilateral E.C.T. One of the more carefully controlled studies was by Cronin *et al.* (1970) who concluded that unilateral, non-dominant E.C.T. was less likely to lead to confusion than unilateral dominant or bilateral E.C.T. It was not as rapid in its anti-depressant action and this could be a material consideration in the treatment of a patient whose depression exposes him to danger. This point was emphasized by Abrams *et al.* (1972). It was only on two auditory verbal tasks that those receiving bilateral E.C.T. showed greater decrements than those receiving unilateral treatment, and where it is important to minimize auditory verbal memory impairment and *where severity of illness and rapidity of treatment response is not overriding*, non-dominant unilateral E.C.T. may be indicated. In older, more deeply depressed patients, bilateral E.C.T. may be used despite the associated greater memory impairment.

A technique for placing the electrodes has been suggested by Man and Bolin (1969). A line is drawn from the lateral angle of the orbit horizontally to the external auditory meatus and from the midpoint of this line a perpendicular is drawn 1½ inches upwards. This is the site for the first electrode. One inch away from the midpoint, towards the ear, another perpendicular line of 4½ inches is drawn, and this is the site for the second electrode.

Pratt *et al.* (1971) were sufficiently confident of the difference in memory following unilateral E.C.T. to the non-dominant hemisphere as opposed to the dominant one, that they recommended a couple of such treatments with subsequent testing before continuing with the full course. They regarded this method as less hazardous and unpleasant than intracarotid sodium amylobarbitone in other situations where language laterality had to be established. Naming of objects from verbal description at 7 minutes proved to be the best discriminant between the hemispheres in right-handers in 11 out of 12 patients.

Multiple E.C.T.

Abrams and Fink (1972) found M.E.C.T. useful in patients with schizophrenia, mania and involutional paranoid psychosis but not in depression; in fact, no depressed patient recovered after a single session of M.E.C.T. x 4 or x 6. Hallucinations and delusions were most responsive. As with ordinary E.C.T. they found that memory disturbance was worse after bilateral applications.

The role of the anaesthetist in the giving of the treatment is still a controversial one. It is unwise for one doctor to carry out the whole treatment on his own, for in an emergency, he has no qualified colleague at hand and this may prove disastrous if resuscitation like external cardiac massage has to be organized, and as another medical colleague is essential, he should preferably be one who is expert at dealing with the unconscious patient, namely an anaesthetist. This is often impossible to arrange and in that case, the psychiatrist giving the treatment should have received instruction from an anaesthetist in the correct administration of the drugs, their hazards, and methods of resuscitation. After six practical tutorials, the psychiatrist should have achieved a reasonable standard of proficiency and could be entrusted to treat low-risk patients. High-risk patients should always have an anaesthetist in attendance.

The number of treatments and their spacing can only be decided by regular, careful assessments of the patient. It is the responsibility of the psychiatrist in charge of the case and requires considerable experience, not only in the examination of the patient, but in eliciting reliable information from relatives. Treatment should never become a routine matter of once or twice a week till an arbitrary total has been reached, but should be individually prescribed, depending on the patient's response. It may have to be more intensive, such as once daily for three or four days or spaced to twice or once weekly. Generally the treatment can be given twice weekly for the first five or six treatments and thereafter spaced at weekly intervals. Most patients show some response after even the first treatment, if only in that they have slept better or that the depression is not quite so severe. After two or three treatments, there is usually considerable progress with marked lightening of the depression and a return to the pre-morbid personality. It used to be said that if a patient shows no response by the third or fourth treatment, it should be abandoned; but there have been many instances, in the author's experience, when such a policy would have been disastrous. Some may not begin to respond till the seventh or even eighth treatment and the proper way to deal with a suggestion that the treatment be given up, is to re-assess the problem; if the clinical decision to have started on a course of E.C.T. is still the right one, then it should be pressed to its conclusion, which is usually recovery. Sargant and Slater (1954) consider that the treatment may fail if it is given at the wrong time, and that the correct phase of the illness should be selected. It is difficult to assess this advice. Firstly, the patient who is regarded as being in need of the treatment is so distressed and even unreliable, that delay may be dangerous. Secondly, in the author's experience, if the patient is well selected, the chances of recovery are not less than 90 per cent and this without any special attention to the most favourable time to initiate treatment. It seems as if it must, as in other branches of medicine, depend on the clinical assessment of the patient. Hodgson and Sim (1959) discuss the optimum number of treatments and though they appreciate that a fixed number would be too arbitrary, their two years' follow-up study of 364 patients treated as out-patients with E.C.T. showed that those who had seven treatments had a higher relapse rate than those who had eight treatments. As those patients who were given seven treatments generally had better pre-morbid personalities, responded more rapidly to treatment and were thought to have a more favourable prognosis, they conclude that eight treatments should constitute a minimum course to give the patient the greatest insurance against relapse.

Confusion of a mild nature is almost normal after treatment, but in some instances it can be severe and associated with paranoid reactions. This may be due to arteriosclerotic changes, but also to vitamin depletion and is seen most commonly in elderly people who because of their disordered mental state have been indiscreet with their diet. It is useful to prescribe a vitamin quota as a prophylactic in these cases.

E.C.T. and Brain Damage

The situation may arise when a patient with severe and recent brain damage requires E.C.T., and the author was recently faced with such a problem. A 52-year-old man was knocked off his bicycle and suffered a severe head injury with rupture of the right middle meningeal artery. After emergency surgery he was left with severe dysphasia, a left-sided hemiplegia and a marked dysmnesic syndrome. After a spell at a rehabilitation centre there was considerable reduction of hemiplegia, though the dysphasia and the dysmnesic syndrome persisted and in addition there was a severe psychotic depression with strong suicidal risk. What to do? The EEG, brain scan and cerebral angiography showed no evidence of further brain involvement and mentally he was a classical indication for E.C.T. What effect would this have on his dysphasia and the dysmnesic syndrome? It was not possible to say and neither was there time to experiment with unilateral E.C.T. for it was important that the depression be cleared quickly.

A course of E.C.T. x 8 suitably modified with methahexetone and succinylcholine produced a dramatic recovery as far as the depression was concerned. This released his considerable ability and capacity to concentrate with resulting improvement in the dysphasia which is now hardly in evidence. The dysmnesic syndrome was aggravated initially with post-E.C.T. confusion but when this cleared the dysmnesic syndrome gradually lifted and 10 months after the head injury his memory is functioning well and he has returned to skilled engineering work.

Another patient had a severe head injury in the First World War with the insertion of a metal plate to replace the bony defect in the skull. A severe depression in later life required a course of E.C.T. and one was concerned over applying an electrode near a metal area covering the brain. As frequently happens, these fears were unfounded and there were no adverse sequelae.

Risk of Treatment

The treatment is not without risk, though in the ordinary case the major hazard is no more than that of the short-acting anaesthetic and is therefore minimal. Barker and Baker (1959) investigated, out of a group of 55 hospitals, the cause of death in nine patients who had died following E.C.T. The fatality rate worked out at one death per 28,000 treatments and the cause was predominantly cardiovascular. Pilling *et al.* (1962) have given the treatment successfully to a patient with complete heart block. They do stress that with a high risk cardiac patient full resuscitation measures, including defibrillator and pace maker should be available, though in their case, these were not required in spite of a ventricular asystole lasting 8 seconds. Barker (1958) in the same enquiry found that muscle relaxants were used at 85 per cent of the hospitals; 60 per cent used E.C.T. modified with thiopentone and succinylcholine, 15 per cent used E.C.T. modified with thiopentone and suxethonium and 6 per cent used the ectonus technique without relaxants. These figures refer to male patients only. Barker and May (1959) reported three cases with prolonged apnoea following suxethonium-modified E.C.T. without a general anaesthetic and suggested that P.A.M. (pyridine-2-aldoxine methiodide) which successfully reverses some of the symptoms of alkyl-phosphate (Parathion) poisoning instantaneously, and restores the serum-pseudocholinesterase to normal levels, might act as a specific antidote for these cases.

The author experienced a most unusual complication recently. The patient, a 36-year-old woman with a puerperal depression after her fourth baby was having her first treatment. She was pre-medicated with intravenous atropine and the treatment was modified with 0·2 g. of pentobarbitone and 40 mg. of succinylcholine. The convulsion was minimal but it did not completely settle and she continued to have convulsions which became stronger as the muscle relaxant wore off. She had in fact developed *status epilepticus* and was eventually controlled with 10 ml. of intramuscular paraldehyde. All physical investigations before and after treatment were negative and the only significant aspect of her history was one of childhood asthma and skin sensitivity. As many such patients have had E.C.T. without this sequel, there was probably another reason. The only one that might be relevant was that the pads over the electrodes had been changed and only one layer of thin gauze was used. Whether this was a factor may never be known. The author has no desire to experiment! Subsequent mental progress apart from the prolonged amnesia was satisfactory, which is not surprising as she had had the equivalent of a full course of E.C.T. at one go.

Physical Concomitants of E.C.T.

A large number of physical and physiological investigations have been made during the administration of E.C.T., particularly on blood pressure which is usually raised during the 'straight' treatment, but may be lowered with thiopentone induction. Cardiac irregularities have been demonstrated electrocardiographically and these have been attributed to vagal stimulation and anoxia, two factors which are counteracted with atropine and oxygen inflation prior to the stimulus as in the modified treatment described above. Urinary corticoids are increased, weight is gained and sleep is restored, but whether these are primary endocrinological changes or are results of the increased well-being of the patient is still debated, though the latter explanation would appear more likely. Funkenstein *et al.* (1950) studied the responses of patients treated with E.C.T. to adrenaline (epinephrine) and mecholyl chloride and claimed that the differences in response were of prognostic significance in the patient's reaction to E.C.T.

The Funkenstein Test

These studies have now been called the *Funkenstein Test* and consist of the following:

1. Normally, a small intravenous dose of adrenaline (epinephrine) causes a rise in blood pressure and the authors found that best clinical results with E.C.T. were obtained in patients with a pre-shock adrenaline (epinephrine) response of 60–80 mm. Hg and after shock with a response of 15–25 mm. Hg.
2. After intramuscular injection of mecholyl chloride most patients show a decrease of 20–40 mm. Hg and best results with E.C.T. were obtained in patients with a pre-shock decrease of more than 10 mm. Hg and a decrease of more than 20 mm. Hg after shock.
3. Intramuscular injection of mecholyl chloride after successful treatment no longer produced the shock and anxiety which was evident following a similar injection prior to the treatment.
4. If a patient showed anxiety after an injection of adrenaline (epinephrine) he was unlikely to improve with E.C.T.

These findings were initially received with enthusiasm for they seemed to indicate that physiological tests could be substituted for clinical diagnosis, but they have not supplanted clinical assessment, which is still a finer and more reliable indicator of prognosis. Furthermore, as many psychiatric states are mixed in their symptomatology, such as in schizo-affective psychosis, it is possible to treat the depressive aspect successfully with E.C.T. and there is more to be gained for clinical psychiatry in psychiatrists sharpening their end-points of diagnosis than in placing too much reliance on physical tests. In fact, clinical selection of patients can in experienced hands be so successful that it can be used as a standard to measure laboratory tests.

Complications of Treatment

The course of the treatment and its sequelae can produce a range of complications which may concern the patient, relatives and even the family doctor. The commonest of these is *memory disturbance,* which is variable, but in some patients it may be gross or the patient may be so obsessed by it that it assumes a greater importance than the facts warrant. It is normal for the patient to forget after treatment. This amnesia may extend to some events just before and after treatment and may cause embarrassment to patients in hospital who write letters of thanks for flowers or gifts on more than one occasion to the same person. On returning home they may have difficulty in recalling how and when some of their previously familiar household objects were acquired and keep asking questions; on return to work they may have forgotten the names of their employees or associates. Friends and acquaintances usually make allowances and are happy to see the patient back at work. The patient, however, may be particularly sensitive and equate losing his memory with losing his reason and become considerably upset though he may be afraid even to mention it. The patient and the relatives should be told about this but as the patient may forget, the author has made a habit of getting him to write down on a card, which will not be easily lost, the following: 'While I am having this treatment, my memory will become muzzy. This is temporary and will clear when the treatment stops'. When the assurances of relatives fail, a glance at the card helps to convince the patient.

Occasionally one sees acute confusional episodes, which if not due to vitamin deficiency, may be due to minor vascular changes and are alleged to be more common in patients with cerebral arteriosclerosis. A rather rare condition which is occasionally found after E.C.T. is the *Gerstmann syndrome* (1940) which usually manifests as finger agnosia, disorientation for right and left, agraphia and acalculia and is considered to be due to interference with the angular gyrus. The syndrome which can also be caused by more serious pathology, is reversible after E.C.T.

The practice of psychiatry in a general hospital has brought to the author large numbers of patients suffering from a variety of physical disorders, who underwent a course of E.C.T. without mishap. These included recent coronary occlusion, severe hypertension, hemiplegia, parkinsonism, mitral stenosis, recent fracture, post-operative states including mitral valvotomy, diabetes, resuscitated cases of barbiturate, aspirin and carbon monoxide poisoning, cancer in various organs (but excluding cerebral primary and secondary growths), pulmonary tuberculosis, severe anorexia, and ulcerative colitis. Pregnancy in all its stages is not a contraindication.

Contraindications

After such a formidable list which is by no means complete one may justifiably enquire into the contraindications. In the author's experience the most consistently adverse results were obtained in patients with cerebral organic disease which had masqueraded as depressive illness. Sim (1947) reported instances where dementia paralytica and demyelinizing states have been aggravated or declared by a course of E.C.T., while brain tumours are notoriously aggravated by the treatment. In some patients who have been carefully screened by a neurologist, E.C.T. may result in the first physical signs and the establishment of the diagnosis. A patient with cerebral arteriosclerosis may show marked confusion after the treatment, yet the depression for which the treatment was given may clear.

Psychiatric Contraindications. Although the treatment was initially given for schizophrenia, it was soon found that these patients did not generally respond favourably, and unless there is a marked affective or catatonic component associated with the schizophrenia it is rarely of benefit. It has been claimed that a very disturbed schizophrenic can be made more amenable to social influence after E.C.T. and it used therefore to be common for many schizophrenic patients to have a 'maintenance' dose of the treatment at about weekly intervals. With the advent of phenothiazines; 'maintenance E.C.T.' or E.C.T. for tranquillizing purposes is rarely used.

Anxiety states of all types do not respond to E.C.T. and obsessional states are frequently made worse. Their pre-occupation with the memory loss usurps their other symptoms and the whole clinical pitcure is therefore blamed on the E.C.T. As depression of a psychotic pattern is probably the only strong indication for E.C.T. it can be said that any functional state which does not contain an appreciable psychotic depressive element, apart from catatonic states, is a contraindication. Neurotic depression, on the other hand, should not be regarded under any guise as an indication.

Other uses of Electricity

In conventional E.C.T. approximately 100 volts is applied to the head and a current above 200 milliamps is produced, depending on tissue resistance, and the convulsion rather than the current produces the therapeutic effect. In sub-convulsive strengths below 200mA, an electric current produces psychological and physiological effects which vary according to current strength, duration of flow, wave form and of course the personality of the patient and his type of illness. Effects aimed at are electronarcosis, electrical sleep and electrical abreaction. Although convulsions do not occur, pain frequently does and intravenous anaesthesia may be required.

Weaker currents have been used on conscious patients. Techniques have varied and unidirectional currents from a scalp electrode to a peripheral point have been applied using lower intensities, *e.g.* 1mA. It has been claimed that selective effects may be obtained by varying the position of the electrodes in order to focus current on a particular part of the brain. It is not certain whether the effects of such treatment are due to cerebral stimulation, for some patients derive similar benefits when both electrodes are applied to the arm, leg or lumbo-sacral region.

A greater significance has been attached to the polarity of the stimulating electrodes and the direction of current flow and it is claimed by Lippold and Redfearn (1964) that when current flows between a peripheral electrode and a positive scalp electrode, mood elevation results. When the scalp electrode is negative, current flowing in the reverse direction produces quietness and withdrawal. Costain *et al.* (1964) evaluated the treatment in 24 depressed patients using a double-blind crossover trial but the results were not conclusive. It is of interest that workers are searching for variations in technique even with a well-tried treatment like E.C.T. This is because there is still a hard core of patients who, though initially responsive to E.C.T., relapse readily and yield diminishing returns. These patients have eventually had to have leucotomies and even though these operations in well-selected cases are successful, a modification of E.C.T. if it worked would be preferable. Some of these machines are intriguing. The patient literally dials his treatment as on a telephone, but, to date, 'H' for Happiness has no more than a 30 per cent chance of coming through. As has already been stated, leucotomies are much less frequently performed and many of the 'hard-core' problems who failed to respond to E.C.T. are being reclaimed with lithium carbonate.

'Electrosleep' Therapy

Electrical machines which are alleged to induce sleep are being sold in large numbers to the general public. Achté *et al.* (1968) subjected such a machine to a clinical trial on 24 patients. All were suffering from severe insomnia, and half were abusers of narcotics or sedatives with addictive tendencies. Most had a variety of psychiatric treatment for years with no benefit.

During treatment, each subject lay in bed with eyes closed. The electrodes of one pole were placed over the orbits and those of the other pole on the neck. In each case the strength of the current and the impulse frequencies were chosen exclusively on the basis of the patient's skin sensations, the criterion being that the patient should feel the current as pleasurable. Duration of application varied from half to two hours and the number of treatments from 6 to 29 per patient. The currents were too weak to induce convulsions.

Six patients (25 per cent) fell asleep under the treatment, and the rest were relaxed. At the end of the trial, 20 patients (83 per cent) reported favourable results and this accorded with medical and nursing observations. The authors concluded that it was possible to reduce the intake of drugs, the effect of the electrosleep being chiefly suggestion, depending on the sleep-producing influence of monotonous sensory stimuli and the conditioned reflex. It should not be used for agitated or very anxious patients, or for those suffering from schizophrenia or melancholia.

Auditory Feedback Training

Many machines are being marketed to decondition anxiety, depending on auditory feedback converted from either the psychogalvanic response (PGR) dependent on finger-tip sweating or from an electromyographic (EMG) recording of the frontalis muscle or of the forearm extensor, just below the elbow. The subject is instructed to keep the auditory tone low by relaxing the relevant muscle group in the latter experiment or by general relaxation in the former. Many physiological readings can be influenced in this way, including heart rate, blood pressure, bowel and stomach movement and skin conditions. Wickramasekera (1972) reported on a successful EMG experiment with auditory feedback in the treatment of tension headaches. By varying the sensitivity readings, *i.e.* low, medium and high, the response could be made increasingly difficult with resultant greater degree of relaxation. Initial results have been encouraging and it remains to be seen whether these methods will supplant other treatments for anxiety symptoms.

CHAPTER 21

Legal Aspects of Psychiatry

Most societies have had to take cognizance of their mentally ill and pass laws dealing with their social and criminal responsibilities, their capacity to testify, their ability to handle their affairs and their involuntary detention. Legislation such as the introduction of a National Health Service, a Criminal Justice Act or a new Divorce Act is continually being amended to deal with new situations, and the psychiatrist should be familiar with the law as it affects or may affect his patients. The special concern of the law with *mens rea* gives the lawyer a particular interest in the mental state of his client, and so the two professions of law and medicine have common ground in the mental state of man, the former using a language and an attitude which is heavily coloured with words like 'intent', 'sound mind', 'defect of reason', 'partial delusion', while the latter talks in terms of 'motivation', 'compulsion', 'altered state of consciousness' and 'character disorder'. This must surely lead to difficulties and it does. The legal profession, quite rightly, are very jealous of their privilege of administering the law and resent psychiatrists telling them how to do it. Some psychiatrists, exasperated by what they consider to be 'outmoded' notions of the disturbed mind entertained by the law, campaign perhaps a little too enthusiastically and injudiciously, and engender some of the reactions which they most resent.

Yet man in society must live and abide by the law and reform is a never-ending process though it is probable that some of the resistance to change may in fact be emotionally rather than rationally determined. There is, however, a much more fundamental aspect, in that the whole essence of the law regarding the conduct of man depends on *mens rea,* which till recent times had not been seriously challenged. The law has gradually accepted defect of reason, diminished responsibility and irresistible impulse, but it will not and cannot accept determinism, for it must attribute to man, free will, so that in the main, he can be held accountable for his actions. The most psychiatrists can expect from the law is that it be just and not that it subscribe to the latest in psychiatric theory and practice. The controversies within psychiatry must make it very difficult for the law to appreciate what is well-established practice and this may account for the law in some situations appearing so reactionary.

Some very important steps forward have been made in recent years, and psychiatrists should not forget that the law has reformers among its own ranks who in the long run are probably more effective, though that should not deter sober and constructive comment.

In this chapter, legal procedures in countries other than those of the United Kingdom are mentioned, not only for the benefit of those residing in those countries, but also to instruct the inhabitants of these islands in what is happening elsewhere. We have much to learn from each other and what today, like the Durham decision, may be regarded purely of domestic interest to the United States of America, can tomorrow be the prototype of new legislation in other countries including our own. Similarly, the Mental Health Act (1959) designed for the British National Health Service may provide a prototype for medical care elsewhere.

PSYCHIATRIC REPORTS AND THE PSYCHIATRIST IN COURT

At one time, a chapter on the legal aspects of psychiatry would start with the administrative and legal arrangements for the admission, detention and discharge of patients in mental hospitals. This time-honoured practice is being forsaken, for circumstances have changed. The infrequency of formal detention in mental hospitals, the de-designation of mental hospitals and the development of out-patient and community services for the mentally ill have meant that appraisal of patients by psychiatrists for legal purposes is more likely to be undertaken outside rather than inside an institution.

As has been indicated the psychiatrist may be associated with legal procedures in criminal and civil actions as well as having to provide statutory reports. Henderson (1956) gives very sound advice on the compilation of these reports and on giving evidence:

> Never hesitate to request permission to make several examinations; one may be quite insufficient. Your aim will be to obtain a comprehensive accurate clinical picture of the individual in relation to all the surrounding circumstances,

and therefore in addition to your examination of the patient you may find it essential to seek information from relatives, friends, business associates, doctors, ministers, teachers, social workers, or any other persons. All of them are nearly always willing to be most cooperative.

The extent of your enquiries will be some indication of your thoroughness, and of your anxiety not to leave anything to chance. At all times and on all occasions maintain high professional standards, and in your examinations do not depend too much on the help of others. There is a certain sting in the tail of that remark, because I am disturbed by the knowledge that the art of good history-taking—an art which has been developed by the psychiatrist—is passing out of his hands into those of the social worker . . . I believe the doctor should carry out all examinations and the interviewing of relatives and others by himself. . . . Your prepared report should seek to do justice to all the relevant facts, which no doubt you will have grouped in an orderly way and expressed positively. You should be ready to explain and elaborate your report whenever called upon to do so. Be as concise and free of ambiguity as possible.

. . . Write your report in language which is easily understood and when technical terms are introduced, it is advisable to define them at once. It is surprising, for instance, how perceptions and beliefs so different as illusions, hallucinations, delusions, and obsessions are referred to as if they were synonymous. We know that each has its own peculiar significance, which may affect prognosis, diagnosis, and treatment, and with a little care they can all be defined easily enough and made understandable. The same sort of difficulty applies to the interpretation of schizophrenia, hysteria, psychopathic personality and more so to the language of the psycho-analyst involving such terms as the super-ego and the id, and such mechanistic phenomena as sublimation, projection, displacement of affect, introjection, dissociation and so on. . . .

. . . In framing your report you should state at whose instance you are acting, and where and when you carried out your examination. If information—for example, police reports, a history from lawyers or relatives—has been supplied to you, you should state so before giving the details of your own observations. . . . In case there may be any doubt in the examinee's mind you should always explain who you are, and what is the purpose of your examination. There must be no element of subterfuge, no attempt to cloak your identity.

. . . In your final summing-up the relevant points will be grouped and emphasized, and a particular clinical entity will be described which will be correlated with the family history, the personality type, and the environmental circumstances. In certain instances it may be both wise and necessary to suggest a diagnosis and even to consider the prognosis and probable effect of treatment. You may even in the most humble and tentative way venture to suggest to the court how the case might be disposed of. . . .

If there is any doubt in your mind you should not be afraid to express it, but at the same time you must realize that it is quite reasonable to talk in terms of probability rather than of certainty.

When you enter the witness-box you must be prepared to testify to the truth of your report, to maintain your opinion, to answer all questions in an unequivocal manner, and to speak in a clear confident voice so that the judge and jury know what you are saying. If you have told the truth, and nothing but the truth, and if you know your work, and can vouch for what you have said, then you need not be disturbed by your examination-in-chief, by your cross-examination, or by any special questions which the judge may ask you. It is the cross-examination which so many witnesses fear. An astute and clever counsel may make you uncomfortable by querying your opinion, by pointing out flaws and inconsistencies in your argument, by criticizing the form of your examination, the extent of your enquiries from outside sources, and the actual time you have been engaged on the case. Do not become either irritated or flustered—the cooler you are the better—and never try to score off counsel, for he is usually a good deal more nimble-witted than you are. Never mind if you have to concede a point here and there, but never allow your opinion of the main issue to be disturbed. Above all, you will be wise to avoid being patronizing or presumptuous so that no one can accuse you of trying to ape the Almighty.

If you are asked questions which you are unable to answer, admit your ignorance, and if you don't know your work you had better keep out of the witness-box altogether. If, on the other hand, you don't understand the questions asked, appeal to the judge, who is always ready to clarify the question and to advise and direct counsel. It is important, no matter how strongly one feels, not to overstress the situation, not to overplay your hand, but to strike a reasonable balance between sense and sentimentality; the one is, to a certain extent, complementary to the other. If you have been so indiscreet as to write papers and text books you must be prepared to have them quoted against you. It may be advisable to ask that the passage referred to should be shown to you, as a statement may often be taken from its context. You can always counter the suggestion made by saying that opinions previously expressed are always susceptible to change and modification. And certainly you need never hesitate to state, when a medical colleague's opinion is quoted against yours, that he is entitled to his opinion, but that you are perfectly satisfied with, and indeed prefer, your own. . . .

CRIMINAL RESPONSIBILITY

Prediction of Dangerous Behaviour in Mentally Ill Criminals

Society expresses confidence in the notion that a psychiatrist can predict dangerous behaviour in a patient though there is no supporting evidence. Time after time a mentally disordered criminal is released on the advice of a psychiatrist, with often disastrous results. On the other hand many mentally ill criminals are not released on psychiatric advice, who, given their freedom, would behave responsibly. Rubin (1972) reckons that even with the most careful and lengthy clinical approach to the problem, false positives may be at a minimum of 60-70 per cent. What is needed is the design of morbidity-experience-prediction tables which can be systematically tested to determine the possibilities of dangerous behaviour in various sub-populations.

The question still remains as to what should be done pending the accumulation of such data. It is probably easier to say what should not be done. In a recent case, a young man was released from a top security mental institution with a history of having murdered his mother and with a strong interest in poisoning. He was released on the recommendation of the psychiatrist in charge of his case and made immediately for London where he was to contact a social worker and a psychiatric clinic. It was not long before he was indulging in mass poisoning while engaged in the kitchen of a works canteen. This case illustrates certain points:

1. There should be no 'private deal' between the psychiatrist and the authorities about such a patient's discharge. The psychiatrist's case for discharge should be made 'in open court' with all informed and interested parties present. As in the case of a recommendation for a prefrontal leucotomy the doctor who puts it forward is usually in close touch with the patient and for a variety of reasons, some of which are not based on objective evidence, he wishes to press the matter. Open discussion permits the opposite point of view to be mobilized and stated. It permits weaknesses in the argument to be spotted and alternative suggestions to be made. It is much easier to turn the recommendation down.

2. A tribunal, faced with such a decision should interview, not only those who had the patient under their care, but those who will be responsible for his supervision and treatment on discharge. The social worker and the psychiatrist of the reception area should be present and be confronted with the degree of responsibility they are expected to shoulder and be asked to state whether they are able and willing to do so. It is a very different matter being informed that Patient A has been discharged from a top security hospital and is now in your area for supervision and treatment, and having to be part of the decision-making process of discharge. It may provide information on the level of competence of the social services in this field and whether a different model for rehabilitation and supervision is needed.

3. For various reasons, it appeared that less serious cases were rehabilitated gradually. They were first given work outside the hospital and later allowed to live outside the hospital, yet the serious problem mentioned was allowed to go immediately to London where many an innocent and normal lad would get himself into trouble. It may be that the reputation of the hospital with the neighbourhood discouraged rehabilitation of such patients on the doorstep, but if so, he was decidedly not suitable for London.

4. The degree of incompetence in this field of psychiatrists, psychologists and social workers is not a matter to be concealed or denied. It must be honestly and freely admitted so that serious efforts may be made to evaluate it and remedy it.

The law at one time took no notice of madness except to punish it, frequently by burning or hanging, and considerations for the criminal responsibility of lunatics did not exist. In 1723 an English court declared that for an accused to escape punishment, he must 'not know what he is doing, no more than . . . a wild beast'. To escape execution the accused had to show a '*total* want of reason'. A lunatic made an attempt on the life of George III and this led to the passing of the Criminal Lunatics Act of 1800, which recognized that an accused could be 'under the influence of insanity'. Eighty years later an attempt was made on the life of Queen Victoria and the assailant was found to be 'Not guilty, being under the influence of insanity'. The Sovereign is reported to have retorted, 'Insane he may be, but guilty he most certainly is'. The following year the Trial of Lunatics Act, 1883, gave official status to the somewhat paradoxical verdict of 'guilty but insane'. This situation persisted till the passing of the Criminal Procedure (Insanity) Act, 1964 which substituted for the illogical verdict of 'guilty but insane' the special verdict of 'not guilty by reason of insanity'. The treatment of persons on whom such a verdict is passed and of persons found unfit to plead is now brought within the ambit of the provisions of the Mental Health Act, 1959 (see p. 1033).

THE McNAUGHTON RULES

The spelling of McNaughton has aroused considerable controversy largely because the man himself was said to have spelt it in different ways. Morton (1956) produced convincing evidence that it was spelt 'McNaughton' but his scholarly paper has not had the influence it deserves.

In 1843 Daniel McNaughton was tried for the wilful murder of Edward Drummond, the private secretary to Sir Robert Peel. McNaughton had for years had delusions of persecution and had tried on several occasions to escape from them, had complained to public authorities, and eventually tried to right his imagined wrongs. (He was one of the first patients to be admitted to the new Criminal Lunatic Asylum, Broadmoor.) His case caused a great sensation, and a discussion in the House of Lords proposed five questions to the 15 judges of England regarding the law of insanity. The answers of the judges can be reduced to two rules, now referred to as the McNaughton Rules. The first is the one most commonly invoked and reads:

> To establish a defence on the ground of insanity it must be clearly proved that, at the time of committing the act, the party accused was labouring under such a defect of reason, from disease of the mind, as not to know the nature and

quality of the act he was doing, or if he did know it, he did not know he was doing what was wrong.

The second rule was a reply to the question as to whether a person, labouring under an insane delusion as to existing facts, commits an offence in consequence thereof, should thereby be excused. The judges replied that a great deal would depend on the nature of the delusion, though they stressed that if it were only a partial delusion, and that otherwise the individual were not insane, he should be considered responsible for his act. Should the delusion cause him to believe that somebody was attempting to take his life and he killed that person in what he supposed was self-defence, he should be exempt from punishment.

Some cynic, commenting on the rules, remarked that there could not be anybody that mad, and there is considerable support for this attitude, for the vast majority of certified (mental) patients in this country would not qualify. There has been considerable dissatisfaction expressed, as well as movements for reform but with no success, and in 1922 the Lord Chancellor appointed a committee to consider and report on what changes, if any, were desirable in the existing law, practice and procedure relating to criminal trials in which the plea of insanity as a defence was raised. The McNaughton Rules were again approved and it was recommended they may be maintained.

Other countries have not been so conservative. Although America adopted the McNaughton Rules and they are still valid in many States, the Supreme Court of New Hampshire in 1869 handed down an opinion sweeping them aside. The court recognized simply that an accused person is not criminally responsible if his unlawful act was the result of mental disease or mental defect. Under this decision, insanity is no longer defined as a matter of law; instead it is made a question of fact to be determined by the jury like any other fact. This determination rests upon the testimony of the psychiatric expert respecting the latest knowledge of human behaviour and his interpretation of such knowledge in terms of his observations of the accused. If the accused has a mental disease and if the criminal act is the product of it, he is found not guilty by reason of insanity.

In 1953, this view was put before the Royal Commission on Capital Punishment by an American, Justice Felix Frankfurter, who stated:

> The McNaughton Rules were rules which the judges, in response to questions by the House of Lords, formulated in the light of the then existing psychological knowledge. . . . I do not see why the rules of law should be arrested at the state of psychological knowledge at the time when they were formulated.

In 1954, in the case of Durham *v.* United States, the Court of Appeal for the District of Columbia Circuit handed down a decision adopting in substance the same rule as the New Hampshire one. The appeal court ruled that the trial court was in error in declaring Durham sane on an obsolete test of responsibility. They said:

> We find that as an exclusive criterion the right-wrong test is inadequate in that (*a*) it does not take sufficient account of psychic realities and scientific knowledge, and (*b*) it is based upon the symptom and so cannot validly be applied to all circumstances. We find that the 'irresistible impulse' test is also inadequate in that it gives no recognition to mental illness characterized by brooding and reflection and so relegates acts caused by such illness to the application of the right-wrong test. We conclude that a broader test should be adopted. . . .
>
> The rule we now hold . . . is not unlike that followed by the New Hampshire court since 1870. It is simply that an accused is not criminally responsible if his unlawful act was the product of mental disease or mental defect.

English law has moved a little recently in that the Homicide Act of 1957 recognizes diminished responsibility, but there still exists in our legal system an undeclared conflict between psychiatrists and the law as it stands today. Yet the law turns to psychiatry for assistance for a variety of services. The court can order a psychiatric examination to determine whether a prisoner is fit to plead. A psychiatrist may be called by the defence to assist in what may be the accused's only possible defence. The prosecution may call a psychiatrist to refute the claims of the defence. The Home Secretary may ask for independent psychiatric assessment of a prisoner who, though found guilty and sane at the time of the crime, may since the crime be suffering from mental illness. Some may argue that it is unlikely therefore that a person who is insane will hang, but all crimes are not murders and there have been many instances where people who would have been held not responsible according to the Durham case, were dealt with as common criminals.

The author had such a case. A young man of hitherto unblemished character was arrested because of Post Office frauds. He was reluctant to yield his previous history and would not permit his counsel to use it in his defence. He had a steady skilled job, but had been worried about his face, because girls had refused to dance with him, probably because of his strange manner. He tried to get a plastic operation but was told (rightly) it was not necessary and so he decided to have it done privately, and to get the money he gave up his job and embarked on his life of crime. He was markedly schizophrenic and in need of treatment but he was sent to prison for four years. There was apparently no machinery whereby his mental state could be brought to the notice of the court. He was, in fact, anxious to go to jail and told the author he hoped for 10 years.

Even in capital charges there are anomalies and attitudes which do not encourage psychiatrists to take part in proceedings which are not designed to relieve sickness but to satisfy legal requirements. During a session of the Royal Commission on Capital Punishment in 1949, Lord Goddard, then Lord Chief Justice, was asked in the course of the evidence: 'Do you agree with the general view, that it is wrong to hang those who are insane in the medical sense?" He replied 'I think it very largely depends on what one means by "in the medical sense"', again emphasizing that mental disorder can be defined legally. In March 1947 a man (T. J. Ley of the chalk-pit murder) was tried and committed before him and sentenced to death. A statutory enquiry under the Criminal Lunatics Act, 1884, Section 2 (4), was held on Ley six weeks later and he was found to be insane and reprieved. In less than three months he died in Broadmoor from a brain haemorrhage. Lord Goddard said, 'I had no doubt he was insane; his whole conduct including his demeanour and evidence at the trial showed a typical case of paranoia. But he refused to allow his counsel to raise the defence of insanity.' Later Lord Goddard was asked: 'I suppose you would not think it proper that he should hang?' He replied: 'I should have thought it was very proper that he should have been hanged'. When it was put to him that 'the medical point of view would be that the disease had altered his (Ley's) personality so as to make such wickedness possible', Lord Goddard replied: 'If that is the medical point of view, I am afraid, frankly, that it does not appeal to me at all. If that was the case, I think it is one of the reasons why he should be put out of the way'.

Further Criticisms of the McNaughton Rules

Slater (1954) puts forward the following criticisms of the method of administration of the Rules:

1. They are inequitable as between case and case, for they may be applied loosely, or not at all.
2. They are inequitable as between judge and witness, for the judge need not be bound by them, but he can tie the witness down to them.
3. The judge rather than the jury can be the arbiter of what should be a matter of fact by being able to decide whether to apply the Rules in directing the jury.
4. 'The Rules are not applied candidly.' If the judge were to give the jury a full briefing, he would point out that very few of the certified insane come within the definition of the rules.

5. Slater leaves to the end what he considers the worst effect of the Rules. It is that they prevent the court from hearing and adjudicating the essential psychiatric aspects of the case, for the court is committed to an evaluation of the problem within the framework of the McNaughton Rules. He illustrates this most aptly with the judge's summing up in the Straffen case. Straffen was a feeble-minded youth who, on the occasion of a previous murder, had been found unfit to plead because of mental deficiency. Some years later he escaped from Broadmoor and in a few hours of liberty committed another murder. This time he was found fit to plead and the court had to decide whether he was responsible in law. Slater quotes from Mr Justice Cassels' address to the jury:

> Ask yourselves whether you are satisfied by the defence that at the time when he did that murder he was insane within the meaning of the criminal law; not that he was feeble-minded; not that he had a lack of moral sense; not that he had no feeling for his victim or her relatives; not that he had no remorse; not that he may be weak in his judgment; not that he fails to appreciate the consequences of his act; but was he insane through a defect of reason caused by disease of the mind, so that either he did not know the nature and quality of his act, or if he did know it, he did not know that it was wrong.

Psychiatry is a branch of medicine which, like others, is constantly tackling and solving problems in human behaviour and it has been shown that much of what has been regarded as criminal conduct is overt evidence of disease. Studies on epilepsy, biochemical and structural changes in the brain, and psychological influences may provide just as reliable evidence of disease as a solid lung does of pneumonia. But it may not be quite so easy to explain these things to a jury who tend to choose the testimony they can best understand and which corresponds to their own sentiments. The explanation of a crime to a jury by a competent psychiatrist may be too complex both intellectually and emotionally for a jury trial to understand or act on.

Wiseman (1961) describes a case which occurred in Boston, U.S.A., which illustrates these difficulties. A young man was engaged to a girl who was constantly threatening to break it off. He asked for his ring back but she kept making excuses. He felt, probably rightly, that she was just playing with him and that he would like to shoot her. He went to her house; she opened the door; he took out the gun but couldn't pull the trigger; she shut the door and he then fired repeatedly through the door. He gave himself up and had the greatest difficulty in persuading a policeman he had shot a girl. After four hours of argument they made enquiries and he was charged. The court was bound by the McNaughton rules and the defence psychiatrist had written in his report that 'At no time did the accused express regret that her life had been interrupted'. The State's attorney reasoned that if Cooper did show regret then he would know that this act was 'wrong' and therefore knew the difference between 'right' and 'wrong'. He proceeded this way:

Q. So, I ask you, sir, in your opinion . . . was he or did he indicate in any way that he was sorry that he killed this girl?
A. He did not say he was sorry he had killed this girl and he was expecting the electric chair.
Q. Doctor. Can't you answer that question—yes or No?
A. I can only answer it on the basis of what I observed. I observed that . . .
Q. What is your opinion, doctor? Was he or was he not sorry that he killed the girl?
A. . . . .

and so it went on.

It became even more involved when the attorney asked for a definition of a personality disorder and was given two. When he asked which applied to the accused he was given an intermediate definition. The attorney then confused behaviour which was consistent with the accused's personality, with normal behaviour.

The accused's father had lost his life by trying to help the boy who was in difficulties on a frozen lake and guilt feelings were being discussed.

Q. On what theory do you base that, doctor?
A. This is based on the common psychiatric technique of explaining a pattern of activity, or a pattern of thought in the person's life by the type of events to which they were subjected, the types of stress, actual and traumatic events to which they were subjected in their younger years

A psychologist who had tested the accused with personality tests talked of his feelings and phantasies in a frank way which would have been meaningful to a case conference but not to a lay jury. When the attorney begins to ask her how the Rorschach Test (a projection personality test) is scored, the situation becomes ludicrous. Reference to cars and guns as power or phallic symbols was also questioned. His fear of impotence which was manifest in promiscuity in order to prove his masculinity brought an interruption from the court.

The Judge (who had got it wrongly): 'You mean the way to prove you are inadequate sexually is to keep having sexual intercourse?'
The Witness: No. In order to keep proving that he is not inadequate to himself is to continue having sexual relations because . . .
Judge: Don't you think that would satisfy him that he was adequate?

The Witness: Well, unfortunately these things don't happen that way, that if the feeling is very deep within a person . . .

Judge: Have you had any personal experience?

The judge's reaction was only one of a number of possibilities, some of which must have occurred to the jury. Some of them may have a passion for guns or big cars and they might fear a psychologist's similar verdict about them. They might feel that because it couldn't be true of them, it couldn't be true of the accused. A jury is no more prepared to accept or understand deeper psychological interpretations than any other unprepared individual or group, including the judge.

Yet we go on in our old-fashioned way. But the law has long recognized that certain items are better settled by experts and there are special divisions such as the Admiralty Division, where it is appreciated that the technicalities of a ship are more likely to be understood by the experts than by a jury. The vagaries of the human mind and body are so well known, however, that any 12 jurors can understand them. It often makes one wonder why we have medical schools.

There is one redeeming feature. The law can be changed and with the passing of the Homicide Act of 1957 and the reduction of the chances of hanging, one now rarely meets those wrangles over the McNaughton Rules. The truth has come out. It was not the McNaughton Rules that were really being debated. It was hanging.

The law will one day appreciate that psychiatry is a rapidly developing branch of medicine with an increasing understanding of aberrant, including criminal, behaviour and that if it wants the best psychiatric advice it will have to constitute itself differently. At present there is great reluctance on the part of many, if not most, reputable psychiatrists to take part in a game whose rules offend their whole experience and training.

Psychiatrists themselves have not been blameless and a number have regaled the courts with 'expert' evidence which must have done more to confuse than clarify. Baroness Wootton (1963) in her Winchester Address stresses this point in her quotation from Szasz (1957).

> It is unlikely that toxicologists would be tolerated in courts of law if one would assert that he found a large quantity of arsenic in the body fluids of a deceased person, and another would state that he found, by the allegedly same operation none. Yet this sorry spectacle is commonplace in regard to psychiatric findings.

She adds her comments:

> Certainly, the eminent medical woman who once remarked that what Lady Wootton does not understand is that a mental abnormality is a definite condition like a broken leg, must admit that this deficiency is shared by many of her own professional colleagues.

There is now a considerable body of opinion in legal, sociological and medical circles which would ask the court to decide on the factual guilt of the prisoner, *i.e.* did he or did he not commit the crime? The sentence or 'treatment' they would leave to a more experienced agency. It has also been suggested that court decisions be followed up to see how successful they are; there is a corollary to this in that those who treat rather than punish should also publish their results. At present there is an overwhelming argument for change; there is an equally strong case for collecting the facts.

One last word: it is illegal to break the law; it may be our duty to criticize and change it.

A Psychiatric Classification of Homicide

Tanay (1971) on the basis of an evaluation of 100 homicide offenders proposed the following classification:

1. *Ego-syntonic.* This is where the act was committed without disruption in ego-functioning in that it was rational, goal-directed, and committed for the purpose of fulfilling a consciously acceptable wish.
2. *Ego-dystonic.* The killing occurs against the conscious wishes of the perpetrator and is frequently carried out in an altered state of consciousness, akin to a dissociative state. The following factors are usually present: (*a*) an overcontrolling superego in the perpetrator; (*b*) a sadomasochistic relationship between victim and perpetrator; (*c*) the occurrence of an altered state of consciousness; and (*d*) the presence of a weapon. The author claims that this is the commonest form.
3. *Psychotic.* These are rare.

The author regards punitive measures as appropriate for the ego-syntonic group but not for the ego-dystonic group. For them, the most easily manipulated variable in the process is the availability of a weapon and therefore the possession of firearms exposes the owner to the risk of committing 'dissociative homicide' through inability to contain aggression.

Abolition of Capital Punishment

The abolition of capital punishment is now regarded as one of the hallmarks of a civilized society and the legislation which made it effective is rarely questioned. Sparrow (1969) posed the question. He stated:

What was it that really determined the votes of the majority in either house upon this issue? The decisive factor was not the statistical evidence (which they did not wait to see completed), or any other evidence, about the effectiveness of the death-penalty as a deterrent; it was a deep conviction, based not upon reason but upon emotion, that the gallows—or any other machinery for judicial execution—is an anachronism and a horror, and should have no place in a civilized society in the twentieth century even if it provides the most effective means of deterring the potential murderer. A society which dispenses with the death-penalty and has a murder-rate of x per annum is *pro tanto* a healthier and more civilized society than one which reduces its annual murder-rate below x by maintaining the machinery of capital punishment: better a few more murders in the year than the possibility of even a single judicial execution.

This humanitarian view invites two comments: (1) it is held by only a small minority of the public, and (2) most of those who hold it belong to categories, e.g. peers, M.P.'s, bishops, academics, from which the murderer does not usually draw his victims; the people who are murdered are 'ordinary' people—bank-clerks, post-mistresses, policemen, prostitutes. It is natural that the enlightened minority should pay more heed to the outrage inflicted on their own sensibilities by the existence of the gallows than they pay to the risk of murder run by the mass of ordinary people and the loss of a few 'unimportant' lives.

But is it right, one may ask, that they should make this preference a basis for legislation? Will it not increase the sense of alienation, not only from the Government, but from Parliament itself, that is even now becoming widespread among the electorate? This, after all, is not an issue with which the enlightened are more concerned, or one (like, say, the Common Market) on which they are better able to judge, than is the man in the street.

This is only half the story. The humanitarian feeling thus dominant among the 'enlightened' minority extends beyond the death-penalty to alternative punishments for murder, and to punishments for other crimes. Already *The Observer* has declared that, 'Since some murderers may have to be detained for much longer than the so-called 'average' of nine years in custody, conditions in our prisons must be made tolerable for them.

This far-reaching suggestion—for it could hardly be intended that conditions should be made more tolerable for murderers than for those convicted of less serious offences reveals clearly where we are being led by the trend of feeling responsible for the abolition of the death penalty; the goal is the removal from judicial penalties of every harsh or painful or humiliating element. Is there not a danger that if you remove these elements from judicial penalties you will also remove their efficiency as deterrents? To the extent that you make the penalty imposed upon X for an offence a 'tolerable' one you diminish the likelihood that it will deter Y from committing a similar offence. *The Observer* was aware of this dilemma, but could offer no solution of it.

Parliament, it seems, has taken its first step along the road to Erewhon and

Utopia—a desirable road, no doubt, but one along which it is possible to move too fast. The time has not arrived, at any rate in this country, when crime can be prevented by treating criminals as mental patients, or single contract debtors to the state, and hoping that this will serve as a sufficient warning to the thug, the cheat and the crook.

It is, no doubt, the function of Parliament to give a lead to the country at large in matters such as this; but it is useless, surely, to talk of 'leading', along this or any other road, if Parliament is so far out of touch with the mass of its constituents that they are not prepared to follow. But at least it is desirable that they should be made aware of where it is that their representatives are set to take them.

The situation became even more complicated in that more police are being armed and make more use of their arms. A bank robber may be and in fact has been shot dead, but a convicted murderer who killed in the furtherance of crime is given a prison sentence. Already more people have been 'executed' by the police since abolition than were executed judicially in the equivalent years before abolition.

Homicide and the Lunar Cycle

The moon and insanity have long been associated with intermittent insanity, hence the term lunatic, and the author once tried to test the hypothesis when working in an acute psychotic ward during the Second World War. Full moon was associated with a greater and recordable degree of disturbance because of the need to prescribe more sedation during this phase, but as the hospital was on the edge of the Sinai Desert and curtains were an unknown luxury, the moon shone brightly through the windows and must have impaired, if not disturbed sleep. Furthermore, one patient if excited could unsettle the whole ward, so the index of drugs prescribed could be fallacious.

Lieber *et al.* (1972) tried to test the following hypotheses: (1) a relationship exists between the lunar synodic cycle and human emotional disturbance; and (2) any measurable disturbance would be directly proportional to the magnitude of gravitudinal force exerted upon the earth at that point in time. Homicides were used as a quantifiable reflection of massive emotional upheavals. If a lunar effect on homicides does exist, it was postulated it would resemble a tidal periodicity, with greatest frequency around full and new moon. If gravity were the main determinant of such an effect, it should occur at times of maximum tidal force, *i.e.* coincidence of new moon and/or full moon with lunar perigee (that point of the orbit at which it is nearest the earth.) Data on all homicides occurring in Dade County, Florida during a 15-year period (1949 cases) were compared with similar data from Cuyahoga County, Ohio (2033 cases).

Homicides in Dade County plotted for lunar phase intervals showed an apparent lunar periodicity; they peaked at full moon and showed a trough leading to a new moon followed by a secondary peak just after the new moon and showed statistically significant groupings around full moon and new moon. The number of cases within the 24 hours before and after full moon over the 15-year period was also significantly greater than expected values. Starting 24 hours after the new moon, the homicides committed in the next 24-hour period showed a significant increase. Cases occurring around apogee (that point in the orbit of the moon at which it is farthest from the earth) and perigee differed significantly from expected values.

In the Cuyahoga sample, homicides peaked at two intervals after full moon: (1) starting 24 hours after new moon, the cases in the next 24-hour period approached significance; (2) starting 48 hours after full moon, the cases in the next 24 hours also approached significance. As in the Dade sample, there was no significant increase in the frequency of homicides relative to the apogee-perigee cycle.

These findings suggest that a lunar influence on the frequency of homicides may exist. The fact that lunar periodicity for homicides occurring in Dade County was statistically significant, while a similar periodicity was found in the Cuyahoga sample, although the peak was shifted to the right and did not quite reach significance, could be interpreted that the geographic location may be a significant variable, just as it frequently operates for geophysical and meteorological phenomena.

Fitness to Plead

It is a cardinal principle of English law that no man should be tried unless he is in a mental condition to defend himself. If the accused is charged with an indictable offence and is dealt with in a higher court, such as an Assize Court, counsel may claim that his client is unfit to plead either at the beginning of the trial (on arraignment), or during the trial itself. It is then for the jury to decide whether the prisoner is fit to plead and certain criteria of fitness are laid down:

1. The prisoner should be able to instruct his counsel.
2. He should appreciate the significance of pleading 'guilty' or 'not guilty'.
3. He should be able to challenge a juror.
4. He should be able to examine witnesses.
5. He should be able to understand and follow the evidence placed before the court and court procedure.

Such prisoners are usually in custody before trial, so the court has the benefit of the prison medical officer's report. Mental deficiency is the commonest cause of 'unfitness to plead', though schizophrenic and paranoid states may also qualify.

The prisoner's fitness to plead may be questioned when he is called on to plead guilty or not guilty. He may stand mute and then the court must determine whether he is *'mute of malice'*, or *'mute by visitation of God'*; the latter meaning that he is deaf or dumb. A judge said (R. *v.* Sharp, 1957, 41, Criminal Appeal Reports 197), that if the defendant is unable to communicate with his legal advisers, he is unfit to plead as a matter of law. Though he be mute, if he can communicate by reading and writing or by signs, he may be considered sane.

Even if the accused is capable of answering to the charge, the question of his fitness to stand trial may be raised either by the prosecution or the defence. If he is found unfit to plead, he will be committed 'until Her Majesty's pleasure shall become known', probably to Broadmoor. If he should return to sanity and be discharged, he may again be brought to trial. This rarely happens, but there was such a case in 1958, when a man confessed to a murder, was charged, found unfit to plead and sent to Broadmoor. While there he responded well to treatment and was discharged after a few months as sane. He was brought to trial again and found not guilty. His confession was based on hallucinations and delusions.

The above arrangements for the prisoner who is considered unfit to plead, though still valid, are becoming obsolete. The terms of the Mental Health Act and the Criminal Justice Act (see below) are more commonly invoked, especially for lesser offences.

The Insane Person as a Witness. Insanity does not bar a person from being admitted as a witness if the court find he is capable of giving evidence. An idiot is not admissible, though a feeble-minded person or an imbecile may be admissible at the discretion of the judge. (The Mental Health Act, 1959, uses different terms for these categories of mental disorder.) An affidavit (written evidence) is admissible under similar conditions. The issue is however not entirely agreed. It was pointed out in relation to the above case, that a less fortunate person may have to wait years before he could be discharged from Broadmoor as sane, yet would be still liable for trial. By this time defence witnesses may no longer be available, while the prosecution would hold the depositions of its witnesses. Another criticism is that, in spite of the accused's inability to take sufficient interest in the proceedings, defence counsel may consider there is a good chance of an acquittal and therefore not immediately raise the issue of fitness to plead, leaving the matter to be raised at a later stage if necessary. The right of counsel to do this has produced conflicting judicial decisions. In R. *v.* Roberts (1953), Mr Justice Devlin supported defending counsel; firstly on the grounds that when the charge is one of murder, it would be intolerable that counsel should have to gamble his client's life in order to obtain an acquittal; and secondly, that if the accused were incarcerated in Broadmoor without a trial, the real murderer might still be at large. In R. *v.* Benyon (1957) Mr Justice Byrne regarded the decision in the previous case as incompatible with the principle that no man should be tried unless he is in a mental condition to defend himself. With the suspension of hanging, counsel need no longer gamble with his client's life.

Hysterical Amnesia as a Psychiatric Defence. A precedent was created in the English courts on 24th September 1959, when the defendant, one Podola, appeared at the Central Criminal Court charged with the capital murder of a policeman. He claimed amnesia for the whole event and his fitness to plead was raised by his counsel. The judge ruled it was for the defence to establish that the defendant was insane so as to be unfit to plead to thc indictment and that the burden of proof would be sufficiently discharged if they could show on the balance of probabilities that he was unfit to stand trial. He was tried and found guilty and though he did not appeal, a petition was submitted to the Home Secretary who referred the whole case to the Court of Criminal Appeal. The defendant had relied solely on a hysterical amnesia preventing him from remembering events during the whole of the period relevant to the crime. The Court found that hysterical amnesia did not amount to insanity and the appeal was dismissed.

Contracts

A person of unsound mind can make valid contracts involving 'necessaries' which include food and clothing and whatever other articles the court may decide. Otherwise an insane person is regarded as incapable of entering into a valid contract, though if it were during a 'lucid' interval, it would be binding. Even if the patient is formally detained because of mental disorder, he may execute a will provided that his responsible medical officer testifies that the patient has a 'sound disposing mind' (see below). Should mental disorder supervene after the person has entered into a contract, it is still binding, though there is now an exception in the marriage contract (see below).

Torts are wrongs done to a person, his reputation or estate which are dealt with by the civil law. A person of unsound mind is considered liable to tort if his insanity did not prevent him from understanding the nature and probable consequences of the act. The more common torts involved are libel, slander, trespass and adultery.

Marriage

If either party at the time of marriage was incapable of understanding the nature of the contract, its duties and responsibilities, or of taking care of himself or his property, then this contract, as with any other, is void. The situation is now governed by the *Matrimonial Causes Act,* 1965 (England and Wales) with its corresponding Scottish Act. The relevant section is: that the respondent is incurably of unsound mind and has been continuously under care and treatment for a period of at least five years preceding the presentation of the petition (which is generally not less than three years since the date of marriage). To qualify as 'incurably of unsound mind', the person should have been under care and treatment (until 1958) within the terms of the Lunacy Act of 1890 and the Mental Treatment Act, 1930.

This emphasis on detention was removed, however, by the Divorce (Insanity and Desertion) Act, 1958, by which a person was deemed to be under care and treatment at any time when he was receiving treatment for mental illness as a resident in an approved hospital. For example, the transfer of a mental patient for more than 28 days to a tuberculosis hospital, where no treatment for mental illness was given, would be regarded as sufficient interruption of the continuity of treatment and make it necessary to start counting the five-year period from the date of re-entry to the mental hospital.

Mr Justice Phillimore laid down some important criteria in the leading case of Whysall *v.* Whysall, 1959, which was upheld by the Court of Appeal in Webb *v.* Webb, 1962. They stressed that 'unsoundness of mind' and 'incurability' were not medical terms and that each term was a matter of degree. A man is of unsound mind in the context of the term used in the Matrimonial Causes Act, 1965, if he is incapable of managing his affairs without undue protection from the incidents and problems of life. 'Incurable' was also given a broad construction, and a man was not incurable merely because he needed to continue with drugs. The Court of Appeal added that the husband's capacity to lead a normal life must be related to a wife who would receive him as a husband. The Legal Correspondent of the *British Medical Journal* adds:

. . . medical witnesses should be asked to direct their minds to two questions in addition to those arising out of the decision on Whysall *v.* Whysall:

1. If in the opinion of the witness the respondent is at the date of the trial 'of unsound mind', is his state of mind such that he is capable of dissembling and concealing the particular unsoundness when he wishes?

2. Is the particular unsoundness such that the respondent could not surmount it with the assistance of a loving spouse without being unduly shielded by that spouse from the difficulties of the world? *(British Medical Journal, 1962a.)*

This may be good law, but it can lead to a mockery of medical treatment. The author has known of cases where the patient's family have kept taking the patient in and out of hospital in order to avoid the 'qualifying period' in their efforts to prevent the spouse from obtaining a divorce. The marriage is already broken and yet divorce in thse instances can be obtained only on grounds of cruelty, though the patient is medically, though not legally of unsound mind. This is another unfortunate example of a law which was designed to take a person's mental state into consideration, but where the legal implications are generally at variance with medical opinion and gives the former precedence. Neither does the law take into consideration other aspects of treatment such as out-patient and day hospital, and the present trend to keep mental patients in the community. In other countries, like the U.S.A., most States allow divorce if a spouse has been three or five years in a mental hospital and is certified by two doctors as 'incurably insane'.

A recent case (Woolley *v.* Woolley, 1966) has highlighted another difficulty in divorce law. A patient who had been detained for 16 years (well over the statutory period) under the Lunacy and Mental Treatment Act was later considered by the consultant in charge to be suffering not from insanity (chronic schizophrenia) but from severe subnormality with a secondary diagnosis of epilepsy. The judge accepted the change of diagnosis and interpreted the Act as not applying to mental defectives.

Testamentary Capacity

This is the capacity of a person to make a will and it traditionally rests on the following criteria: (1) that he knows he is making a will and what such an act implies; (2) that he knows the nature and extent of his property; (3) that he knows the persons who have claims on his bounty; and (4) that his judgment and will are so unclouded that he is able to determine the relative strengths of these claims, which means he should know the members of his family and close friends. It is also said that the testator should have a 'sound disposing mind' which does not necessarily mean that he must not be suffering from mental illness, for even gross forms of mental disorder are compatible with making a perfectly valid will. If, however, the patient suffers from delusions which are directed at a member of the family and that person who would normally have a claim on the patient's bounty is excluded, then it would be invalid as the patient would not have a 'sound disposing mind'. If the patient suffers from delusions which have not influenced the will, then even if detained formally in an institution he may be capable of making a perfectly valid will. It is not enough, therefore, to say that the patient was insane at the time; he had to be insane in the preparation of his will.

Though the influence of a delusion in the making of a will may fascinate the psychiatrist, the commonest problem in testamentary capacity is that of the senile patient, who may or may not have delusions in association with the dementia. In ordinary senility there is disturbance of memory but not to the extent which is associated with senile dementia, though naturally there are some border-line instances in which it may prove difficult if not impossible to decide. The task is rendered no easier by the fact that the testator may have already died and a psychiatric opinion may have to depend on a history of the patient's health and previous documents prepared by him, with particular reference to writing, spelling and contents. Many elderly dements are particularly suggestible and can be easily influenced, particularly by those with whom they are living, and whom they may even misidentify, *e.g.* a housekeeper may be regarded as a daughter or her husband as a son.

Though undoubtedly many wills have been changed by undue influence while the testator was not really of sound disposing mind, it may be difficult for the family doctor, who may be asked to witness it, to assess the degree of dementia present. The patient's vocabulary may be relatively well preserved and in ordinary conversation on a superficial plane, create a favourable impression.

The doctor may be reluctant to expose his ageing patient to strict questioning and he may not wish to offend the good people who are looking after him by appearing unduly suspicious. He may therefore be tempted to be less careful than he should. In order to avoid later embarrassment he should insist on conducting his examination of the patient in private and ascertaining whether the patient can fulfil the criteria already mentioned. It is not enough to get the patient's assent to leading questions, for one may only demonstrate suggestibility rather than testamentary capacity. If the housekeeper is to be a major beneficiary he should be asked her name, how long she has been with him, what exactly he intends to leave her and what proportion this is of his estate. If the doctor knows of any close relatives who have been excluded he should make sure that this is a deliberate and rational act of the testator and not due to a lapse of memory or to a delusion.

The best way of avoiding such problems is to appoint a *receiver* or, in Scotland, *curator bonis* so that the patient is protected during his life, as well as ensuring that valid wills are not cancelled and disputable ones substituted. The importance of this measure cannot be too strongly emphasized and it should be initiated by the family doctor who is probably the only person in contact with the patient with the necessary training and experience to note the signs of intellectual deterioration. If in doubt he should obtain psychiatric advice and the family should be told of the possible implications of not taking action. It is surprising how often an elderly person with money and property is regarded by complete strangers as a pebble on the beach ready to be picked up. They disregard the claims of relatives and in some instances deny the patient his own comforts and in a short time may have usurped the whole estate. There is of course another side, in that devoted servants may be excluded from benefits which should normally have been theirs and a Receiver would ensure that they are not forgotten.

Another source of dispute is the patient with a stroke and residual aphasia or dysphasia with perhaps a hemiparesis. Superficially he may appear to be incapable of making his wishes understood, but usually the 'way in' is unimpaired and he can be made to understand what is wanted and give perfectly valid instructions in the drawing up of the will, though some members of the family who have been unable to communicate with the patient and are not beneficiaries may remain sceptical.

COMPENSATION CLAIMS

These are matters which frequently come to court and the psychiatrist may be asked to report on the mental state of the patient and express an opinion as to whether the injury caused the disability or aggravated an underlying instability, to assess the prognosis and the probable effects of treatment. The advice given by Henderson (see above) in preparing reports holds for compensation cases too and a strict objectivity is essential, for identification or resentment may lead to the inclusion of doubtful data or the suppression of facts which are vital to the patient's claim. From the psychiatrist's point of view many of these cases are very disturbing, for what was originally a minor disability which would have yielded readily to treatment has become a major issue, and desire for retribution has replaced that for recovery. It is true that the patient should not be deprived of his just compensation, but when that depends on his demonstrating a disability, it is often futile for the psychiatrist to try and treat the patient while litigation is pending and attempts to remove the patient's disability may be resisted.

Frequently the disability has been present for some time and enquiry should be made into what treatment has been prescribed and what degree of cooperation the patient has shown, for persistence with a most ineffective form of treatment and refusal to accept more positive help may be a crucial aspect of the history. Gross memory disturbance may be a symptom, but it is inadvisable to start immediately to test the degree of this handicap with the usual tests. A full anamnesis is as good a general test of memory as there is and it can later be supplemented with a more specific examination of memory. Usually, what the patient considers memory loss, is an inability to concentrate or make the effort to register or recall an experience, and though this may be no less a handicap than true organic impairment of memory, it is just as well to get the record clear for the sake of accurate diagnosis and the bearing this has on prognosis. Formal testing takes time and one should not hesitate to see the patient again. This is not only because a second interview may be more productive, but also to obviate the element of fatigue in both the patient and in the examiner. Of greatest importance is a complete record of the patient's pre- and post-accident medical history, for this frequently gives a clue to the patient's capacity and stability and creates a better perspective. (See also under Compensation Neurosis, p. 494.)

ABORTION AND THE PSYCHIATRIST

The medico-legal aspects of abortion in England are still governed by the Criminal Abortion Act of 1861. It is an offence to procure or attempt to procure an abortion and anyone doing so is guilty of a felony. The law regarding therapeutic abortion is not so clear. In other European countries the situation is no less equivocal, and Bleuler (1924) states:

> . . .In the Protestant part of Switzerland the sensibilities of the people demand an attitude that is more favourable to abortion and I should let social considerations count with the legal. Plain legal determinations exist nowhere: one has to fall back on local and customary interpretations. . . .

In Sweden the situation is more clearly defined in that five grounds for termination are listed (Ekblad, 1955). These are: (1) medical; (2) medico-social; (3) socio-medical; (4) humanitarian; and

(5) eugenic. Yet the strict medical indications are no more positive than in England and the impression is gained that the law in Sweden merely gives the doctor a wider field in which to manoeuvre.

Until 1938 most reputable doctors would not abort on therapeutic grounds unless they felt sure that the continuation of the pregnancy was a serious threat to the mother's life. Mental state was also considered and the dangers of suicide and severe and intractable mental illness were regarded as indications though they had not been tested in the courts. In 1938 the celebrated case of Rex *v.* Bourne moved the law towards a more liberal interpretation by allowing that an abortion was lawful if performed in the interests of the mother's health. The actual term used by the judge was 'to prevent the mother becoming a physical or mental wreck' but in actual practice the interpretation of a wreck could cause dismay to, and elicit violent protests from an underwriter at Lloyds.

The main issue facing the psychiatrist is whether the mother is likely to develop a puerperal psychosis and the effects of such a psychosis on her future health. Some psychiatrists concern themselves with minor grades of morbidity, others with the effect of the unborn child on existing children, but the ultimate decision to terminate is the responsibility of the gynaecologist and most would not operate unless they were advised that the mother would almost certainly suffer permanent mental damage of a serious nature or would commit suicide.

The Foetus as a Personality

Although attitudes to abortion are frequently emotional and irrational, much of the argument hangs on the foetus and its disposability. Is it human? When does it become human? The answers to these questions are not in themselves difficult. The fertilized human ovum is human after about the 5th day of conception and can become nothing other than a human being unless somebody interferes with it or there is a spontaneous abortion. The Abortion Act, 1967, was got through Parliament with the help of a bit of smart showmanship. One of the sponsors of the Bill held aloft a test tube containing what he claimed was a human foetus measuring a few centimetres. Humanity was being defined by centimetres. It is as well to know what the foetus is.

Liley (1972) points out that far from being an inert passenger in a pregnant mother, the foetus is very much in command of the pregnancy. It is the foetus who guarantees the endocrine success of the pregnancy and induces all manner of changes in maternal physiology to make her a suitable host. After 25 weeks it will respond to sudden noise in a quiet room. Development of human form is rapid, with discernible limbs after several weeks, and it is this aspect which has disturbed nursing personnel who have to work in operating theatres where abortions are done. As somebody has pointed out, only a lunatic could have devised a law for the destruction of the unborn child and then asked doctors and nurses to implement it.

Before such an Act is passed, there is much propaganda that doctors and nurses are queueing up to perform abortions on willing subjects, but the cruel State has not made it legal. In the United Kingdom, we now know that this is not so. A very large number of abortions are performed in the private sector and doctors are not queueing up; if they were, the considerable fortunes to be made would be drastically reduced by competition.

Abortion on psychiatric grounds is increasing, especially when compared with abortion for organic disease. Calderone (1958) from a large series (1309 abortions between 1951 and 1953), reports 37·8 per cent on psychiatric grounds compared with 13·1 per cent on similar grounds out of 3046 therapeutic abortions between 1943 and 1947. It is unlikely that this increase could have been due to the greater incidence of strict psychiatric indications, or to any new information which might suggest a more grave prognosis in puerperal psychosis; and one suspects that socio-economic factors were probably the main consideration. These figures pale into insignificance compared with those now available since the Abortion Act, 1967, when in 1973 out of a total of nearly 150,000 therapeutic abortions, over 90 per cent were performed on psychiatric grounds.

Serious doubts have been expressed as to whether these factors come within the province of the psychiatrist and Donnelly (1958) makes the following statement in the Calderone (1958) symposium:

> . . . As medical men, I believe we should definitely confine our indications for therapeutic abortion to strictly medical reasons. . . , We should be doctors of medicine, not socio-economic prophets. How many students in medical school today who were born in the depths of a depression in 1932 were good socio-economic risks at the time of their birth? If we could go back three or four generations in any of our families and eliminate all the poor economic risks among our antecedents, this conference today might never have been convened.

Abortion as a Method of Population Control

Though protagonists for abortion reform frequently deny that more freely available abortion is intended as a method of population control, it has been used as such in Japan (Gordon, 1973). In the 1940's, with a birth rate of 34·3 per thousand steps were taken to limit population growth. By 1957, using abortion as the chief weapon, a 50 per cent decline in birth rate to 17·2 per 1000 was achieved. This may have called for congratulations, but by 1969 Premier Sato publicly advocated an increase in the birth rate, for, in spite of overcrowding, there were new problems of a declining labour force and an ageing population. With legal abortions in the United Kingdom now running at about 150,000 per year, these problems are no longer confined to the Japanese.

The Unwanted Child

This term is commonly paraded as adequate grounds for abortion. Apart from the extremely doubtful argument that the unwanted child is at social and psychiatric risk (Forssmann & Howe, 1966) there are other objections. There are unplanned and unwanted pregnancies in plenty, but rarely an unwanted child. Most doctors before the 1967 Act had personal experience of patients, married and unmarried, who initially rejected their pregnancy, but after the 3rd and 4th month accepted it and when the child was born there was not a hint of rejection at the time or in its subsequent development. Even the *unwanted pregnancy* requires scrutiny, for in the author's experience it is important to ask: 'Who doesn't want?' If the patient is unmarried, it is the parents or the boy friend who doesn't want; if she is married it is generally the husband. The author, when discussing the problem with the patient, on her own, has been given the reply which is almost a stereotyped one: 'Doctor, if it were left to me, I would have the baby; it's my husband who is upset'.

Indications for Termination

In any other aspect of medicine, be it renal disease, heart disease, diabetes or neurological disorder, the physician when confronted by the problem of termination asks himself the question: 'Can this patient be delivered safely?' If the answer is 'Yes' there is no further argument. In psychiatry, the question of abortion is usually raised not because of any hazard from the pregnancy, but because the pregnancy is unwanted. If the baby is wanted, the most adverse social factors are discounted; if the baby is unwanted, remediable social problems are paraded as unsurmountable and abortion is recommended. The issue of not wanting the child should be viewed with caution, for in the author's clinic where a number of such patients are referred, 'not wanting' has proved to be a state of mind which is generally short-lived and many happy mothers have subsequently written appreciatively of the decision not to terminate. Ekblad (1955) found that out of 479 women aborted on psychiatric grounds, 25 per cent regretted the operation. It is likely that this figure is conservative, for a woman who had persuaded a tribunal to grant her an abortion is unlikely to turn round on them later and say she regretted it, if only because it would prejudice her future chances of an abortion (156 out of 427 non-sterilized were pregnant again between the time of the abortion and the follow-up). It can therefore be accepted that 'not wanting' in a substantial proportion of Ekblad's patients was not a true reflection of their permanent attitude. In an affluent society with highly developed social services, it should be possible to cope with social factors; abortion only diverts the attention of society from what may be its legitimate objectives, and it is a very final decision.

Psychiatric indications for termination should not be based on sentimental guesses, but on a strong body of facts. The following questions should be carefully considered by the psychiatrist:

1. Is a puerperal psychosis likely to develop?
2. What would be its outcome?
3. What are the chances of avoiding it by termination of the pregnancy?
4. What would happen if patients, who according to present-day practice would be aborted, were left alone?
5. What are the risks to the mother's mental health of a therapeutic abortion?

PUERPERAL PSYCHOSES

Some psychiatrists have criticized the criteria of suicide or irrecoverable puerperal psychosis as being too rigid, yet these conditions are the ones which are generally quoted by psychiatrists in their reports to gynaecologists. The author has seen many of these reports as patients have been referred to him by gynaecologists who have doubted (rightly) the grave prognostications. Other psychiatrists have talked of the impact on the family and the impairment of the quality of human life, yet no factual evidence for these criteria has been produced.

The answers to the above questions are intimately associated with the problem of the puerperal psychoses and it would be appropriate to deal with the subject here.

Studies on substantial numbers of patients with puerperal psychoses have been reported by Ellery (1927), Zilboorg (1928, 1929, 1931), Solomons (1931), Anderson (1933), Cruikshank (1940), Skottowe (1942), Hemphill (1952), Tetlow (1955), Polonio and Figueiredo (1955), White *et al.* (1957), Schneider (1957) and Martin (1958). Although there are some differences in the conclusions drawn by these authors, there is also a wide measure of agreement, particularly over symptomatology. Anderson (1933) in a carefully controlled clinical study found nothing significant in the pre-morbid personality structure of his patients with puerperal psychoses, compared with a matched group of patients suffering from psychoses not associated with childbirth. Others have stressed the similarity of the symptomatology and insisted that apart from the delusional content which may be concerned with the child, there is nothing to distinguish these states from other acute psychotic breakdown, such as post-operative states.

Prognosis in Puerperal Psychosis

This varies according to the efficiency of the treatment. In an early paper, Ellery (1927) reported 49 per cent of recoveries in his most favourable prognostic group; Hemphill (1952) in his unselected total of 116 cases, had an 80 per cent recovery, and these included 19 schizophrenic reactions, of whom only one recovered. Martin (1958) had an 86 per cent recovery in her group of 75 cases, which included 15 schizophrenic reactions, thus suggesting that the prognosis in schizophrenia has been considerably modified by developments in treatment. It has also been suggested that the condition is not so malignant as it used to be but this may be due to the elimination of organic factors such as haemorrhage and infection. The author (Sim, 1963) reported on 213 patients with puerperal psychosis and found that in no instance was the patient's ultimate mental state worse than it was before her pregnancy and in many instances, it was better. This series included a number of mothers who were suffering from schizophrenia.

Post-abortive Psychoses

It is an axiom in medicine that a measure designed to avert a situation should not in itself precipitate such a situation. Ekblad (1955) found that in a series where psychiatric morbidity was not generally gross, 11 per cent of those aborted had undesirable sequelae and concludes:

The psychiatrically abnormal find it more difficult than the psychiatrically normal to stand the stress implied in a legal abortion. This means that the greater the psychiatric indications for a legal abortion are, the greater will be the risk of unfavourable psychic sequelae after the operation.

Ekblad (1961) came to an exactly similar conclusion over the problem of sterilization.

Siegfried (1951) found 59 per cent of guilt reactions in his series of *therapeutic* abortions, while Polonio and Figueiredo (1955) found that out of 244 puerperal psychoses, 20 per cent occurred after *spontaneous* abortion.

In post-abortive psychoses (some of whom were 'therapeutic'), which the author had referred to him, the psychosis proved more stubborn than in the puerperal states. A post-abortive psychosis may therefore be a real and severe hazard of termination, especially in the conscientious type of person who may be stirred by guilt feelings.

The author in a paper (Sim, 1962) reported eight patients with post-abortive psychoses and then raised the issue whether a measure which can precipitate a psychotic reaction could be legitimately used to prevent one. In a more recent analysis of data (Sim, 1972) the total of post-abortive psychoses had risen to 34. Out of a total of 280 with a puerperal psychosis, only 4 (1·4 per cent) had a prognosis which was unsatisfactory; out of the 34 post-abortive psychoses, 16 (47 per cent) had an unsatisfactory prognosis. The paradoxical situation has evolved that patients who may have a conceivable claim to an abortion on psychiatric grounds, are those who should not have an abortion, for their psychiatric hazard would be greater.

The role of the psychiatrist is therefore not to recommend an abortion on psychiatric grounds for this rarely, if ever, is justified, but to use his clinical judgment to recommend that an abortion does not take place on psychiatric grounds, and thus spare the patient much suffering and the gynaecologist much embarrassment. The author has personal experience of four patients for whom he refused to recommend abortion on psychiatric grounds who got an abortion elsewhere and who developed severe post-abortive psychoses. If these patients had not been aborted but had gone to term the chances of a puerperal psychosis were not high and the prognosis would have been excellent.

Suicide and Pregnancy

It is frequently suggested that a puerperal psychosis or instability in pregnancy greatly increases the risk of suicide and that this factor should be given due consideration. Lindberg (1948) reported on 304 women who were refused legal abortion and of whom 62 indicated they would commit suicide; none did. It is not known, however, how many (if any) of the 62 had criminal abortions. Dahlgren (1945), in a study on 'Suicide and Attempted Suicide', found that 3·7 per cent of the women were pregnant which would suggest that a pregnant woman may attempt suicide, though the incidence of suicide is very low. The author approached the Coroner of the City of Birmingham for information concerning suicide in pregnant women and received the following reply:

> . . . I can now tell you that my staff have gone through the 119 cases of suicide of females up to the age of 50, 22 of whom were unmarried. They date from January 1950 up to today, 8th November 1956.
>
> I can now summarize our research as follows:
>
> In no case has pregnancy been established as a factor in bringing about the suicide. In two cases the woman thought she might be pregnant, but it was certainly not confirmed by medical examination or post-mortem examination. We have no record of any woman known to be pregnant having committed suicide. . . .

In a subsequent six-year study, the same coroner reported one death in a pregnant woman. This patient was married, had two children and was attending a psychiatric clinic for a depression which was not associated with her unwanted pregnancy. In her case, abortion would not have cured her psychosis; she was in need of more active treatment. If the question of suicide in pregnancy is raised, the answer is that a pregnant woman is less likely to commit suicide than one who is non-pregnant.

The Unmarried Mother

It is frequently claimed that the unmarried mother is more vulnerable to mental disturbance, yet in the author's series of 213 cases of puerperal psychosis, there were no unmarried mothers, apart from one who was not psychotic but really an acute hysterical reaction which required no special treatment. In an attempt to broaden the enquiry, a survey of admissions of puerperal psychoses to five mental hospitals was undertaken. Out of 119 cases, two were unmarried, and in one of these the reaction was a hysterical one and the other was schizophrenic prior to her pregnancy. With an increasing illegitimacy rate (6–8 per cent) these figures are significant, and would suggest that the unmarried mother carries a high degree of immunity to puerperal psychosis.

The Unpredictability of Puerperal Psychosis

As the condition occurs in approximately 1 per 1000 live births, it would be a bold person who would predict its occurrence. Even where there is a family history or a previous history of breakdown, either puerperal or from other causes, the chances are not increased by more than 20 per cent. The author had a patient who had four puerperal psychoses, one with attempted suicide and all requiring electroplexy, and who became pregnant with number five. She was then 43 years old and this baby was not planned. Although she always recovered well from her breakdowns, it was a dilemma. It was put to her that most psychiatrists would advise termination but that in view of her conscientious nature, therapeutic abortion carried its own hazard. She elected to go to term and had no puerperal psychosis. There have been other instances and the author has no hesitation in advising another pregnancy in these patients.

Treatment

This is as for other psychiatric disorders. Most of the clinical pictures are depressive, schizo-affective or schizophrenic, and as they are usually acute reactions in otherwise good personalities the results are excellent. The author does not reckon that a patient even if psychotic during pregnancy should deteriorate after her pregnancy; in fact, a number have improved, as the necessary psychiatric treatment is applied to a condition which might have been allowed to pass unnoticed. Some have justified their recommendation for termination on psychiatric grounds, not on severe mental sequelae or suicide but on neurotic handicap. Adequate evidence for this attitude has not yet been forthcoming. Gencrally, it can be accepted that a woman will come to no psychiatric harm if she continues with her pregnancy.

Conclusions

There are no psychiatric grounds for termination of pregnancy. Pressure may be brought to bear on the psychiatrist to recommend termination. He may be told the patient is threatening suicide or be regaled with the dreadful social consequences. The answer is still not to recommend termination, which indeed may be harmful, but to nurse the patient through her unstable phase. There is a parallel here between the present legal grounds for termination and the law in relation to murder. There is a move afoot in society to make abortion easier, which resembles in some ways the campaign against hanging. In the latter instance, the psychiatrist became involved in unseemly wrangles over the McNaughton Rules, but now that diminished responsibility is accepted, the psychiatrist is no longer asked to defend an untenable position. Similarly with abortion, the problem is certainly not one of preventing mental illness, for abortion is not a prophylactic against psychosis, but rather a precipitant. It is a socio-economic problem and the psychiatrist should stick to clinical facts in his practice of medicine. Whether at other times he campaigns for reform in the law relating to abortion is his own private business, but he should not distort medical facts to serve other ends As Taylor (1958) in the Calderone symposium puts it: 'If you are going to find medical reasons for aborting 750,000 per year in the U.S.A., there is a medical reason for aborting anybody'.

Abortion Act, 1967

This act breaks new and controversial ground in that its provisions have not been subject to judicial interpretation and neither is it derived from an exhaustive enquiry into the social and medical facts concerning pregnancy and its sequelae. It therefore does not represent the results of responsible legal and medical enquiry but reflects a climate of opinion which was formed without the benefit of all the facts already available and with no serious attempt to provide answers to relevant questions.

The Act *is permissive only,* for abortion remains a criminal offence. The Offences Against the Person Act, 1861, Sections 58 and 59, which consolidated the law relating to offences against the person, from murder to simple assault, remains in force. The Abortion Act creates exceptions by providing that a person shall not be guilty of an offence when a pregnancy is terminated in certain circumstances, and by a registered medical practitioner, not necessarily by a consultant or specialist. Case law relating to therapeutic abortion laid down in R. v. Bourne (1939, 1, K.B. 689) and other decisions no longer apply.

The circumstances in which an abortion may be carried out are:

1. Two registered medical practitioners must form in good faith the opinion set out in the next succeeding paragraph and certify it in accordance with the regulations made under Section 2 of the Act.

2. The opinion must be to one or more of the following effects:

(*a*) that the continuance of the pregnancy would involve risk to the life of the pregnant woman greater than if the pregnancy were terminated; or (*b*) that it would involve risk of injury to the physical or mental health of the pregnant woman greater than if the pregnancy were terminated; or

(*c*) that it would involve risk of injury to the physical or mental health of any existing children of the pregnant woman's family greater than if the pregnancy were terminated; or

(*d*) that there is substantial risk that if the child were born it would suffer such physical or mental abnormalities as to be seriously handicapped.

Any treatment for the termination of pregnancy must be carried out in a National Health Service hospital or in a place approved for the purpose by the Minister of Health or by the Secretary of State for Scotland. The fact of the termination must be notified in a prescribed form to the Chief Medical Officer of the Ministry of Health or to the Chief Medical Officer of the Scottish Home and Health Department.

There are two exceptions to the normal rules.

1. *Emergencies.* An abortion may be performed by a practitioner who is of the opinion, formed in good faith, that the termination is immediately necessary to save life or to prevent grave permanent injury to the physical or mental health of the pregnant woman. In such a case a second medical opinion is not required by law nor is there any restriction on the place where the operation may be performed. The regulations regarding certification and notification apply.

2. *Visiting Forces.* The Act is applied with modifications if the pregnant woman is associated with a body within the purview of the Visiting Forces Act, 1952, or the International Headquarters and Defence Organisation Act, 1964, provided that the abortion is performed in a hospital controlled by such a body, and is carried out by a registered medical practitioner or an official medical practitioner of that body.

Certification and Notification

An opinion given by a practitioner that an abortion is lawful must be certified in accordance with regulations made by the Minister of Health or the Secretary of State in Scotland.

The practitioner who terminates a pregnancy must give notice of the termination and such other information relating to the termination as is provided by the regulations to the relevant Chief Medical Officer.

Conscientious Objection

The Act lays down that no person shall be under any legal duty to participate in any treatment authorized by the Act to which he has a conscientious objection unless the treatment is necessary to save the life or prevent grave permanent injury to the physical or mental health of a pregnant woman. Should there be lawful grounds for abortion and he feels that were it not for his conscience she should have an abortion under the afore-mentioned circumstances, he should refer the patient to a colleague who would not expose the patient or her children to what would presumably be material risks.

Abortion on Demand. It was stated repeatedly by the sponsors of the Bill before it became law that it was not intended to make abortion available on demand and the Act though it makes abortion lawful on certain grounds does not make it available on demand. Quite independently of his rights under the conscience clause, which are personal to him alone, a doctor is not compelled to abort even when presented with certificates from two registered practitioners. Indeed, if in good faith, he is of the opinion that abortion is not indicated, he would be in the wrong if he collaborated. Any practitioner who recommends abortion when it is contra-indicated, and there are many contra-indications, would also be in the wrong as he would not be acting in good faith.

The term 'good faith' does not mean being obliging or yielding to pressures, but forming an opinion based on the complete facts and taking into account the clinical realities. That the law was passed without due inquiry does not exonerate those who do or do not perform or recommend abortions from informing themselves of the risks to which they consider their patient may be exposed through abortion or refusing abortion. An up-to-date knowledge of the literature of the subject is an important aspect of acting 'in good faith' whether it is over the question of abortion or any other part of medical practice.

It is still too early to assess the effects of this Act. Immediate results have been tremendous pressures on clinics and doctors who had declared a liberal attitude to abortion with a reaction against this pressure in the forms of rationing of available appointments and operating theatre time. Some have publicly protested; others have tried to involve their more conservative colleagues with appeals for help. Most of the promised social benefits have not yet materialized. The poor are at the end of a longer queue. Private practitioners are finding new patients in increasing numbers from abroad and by making abortion more legal for the doctor, it has not made it less attractive but even more attractive to the unqualified practitioner. The pressures are now building up for a full enquiry such as a Royal Commission, which was rejected by Parliament and the medical profession before the law was passed.

The Homosexual Act, 1967

This permits homosexual practices in private between two consenting adults over the age of 21 years. The passage of this Act was much less controversial than the Abortion Act, 1968, presumably because the medical and legal professions and the public were well informed by a Royal Commission prior to the law being passed.

THE MENTAL HEALTH ACT (1959)

Not all patients are cooperative, but that does not mean that they should be compelled to have treatment they do not wish. It is only when their illness is of such a nature that they may be a danger to themselves or others or are so disturbing to the community that measures are taken to ensure that they are given the appropriate treatment. The factors leading to the recent changes in the law dealing with the certification and detention of persons of unsound mind are many, and while some are obvious, others can only be inferred. The climate of opinion in the country, in Parliament and in the medical profession was ready for a change and when the Bill was presented to Parliament it received an enthusiastic welcome from both sides of the House and was probably the least controversial piece of legislation in the post-war years. Everyone agreed that a change was due for the Lunacy Acts of 1890 and the Mental Deficiency Act of 1913 were considered to be outmoded. It may be that people were more disturbed by the names of these Acts rather than their contents, for the new Act at once abolished the terms 'lunatic' and 'mental defective' and replaced them by the terms 'mental disorder', 'subnormal' and 'severely subnormal'. The old Acts were designed for an age when patients were sent to hospital for custody; the idea of detaining someone suffering from mental disorder formally in an ordinary ward of a general hospital had not yet been considered. The new Act de-designated mental hospitals and put them on the same footing as general hospitals and though not creating new units in general hospitals, implied that such units would be developed, for the only way the mental hospital could treat its patients like those in the general hospital was either to become a general hospital or to merge its work into one. Accent was also put on the community care of the mentally ill with the Local Authority responsible for the 'prophylaxis' and 'after-care' of mental illness, though these functions were not made mandatory.

Definitions of persons liable to be dealt with under the Act differ from the old Acts and are laid down in Section 4, as follows:

1. *'Mental disorder'* means mental illness, arrested or incomplete development of mind, psychopathic disorder, and any other disorder or disability of mind; and 'mentally disordered' shall be construed accordingly.

2. *'Severe subnormality'* means a state of arrested or incomplete development of mind which includes subnormality of intelligence and is of such a nature or degree that the patient is incapable of living an independent life, or of guarding himself against serious exploitation, or will be so incapable when of an age to do so.

3. *'Subnormality'* means a state of arrested or incomplete development of mind (not amounting to severe subnormality) which includes subnormality of intelligence and is of a nature or degree which requires or is susceptible to medical treatment or other special care or training of the patient.

4. *'Psychopathic disorder'* means a persistent disorder or disability of mind (whether or not including subnormality of intelligence) which results in abnormally aggressive or seriously irresponsible conduct on the part of the patient and requires or is susceptible to treatment.

It will be noted that *'mental disorder'* is used as a generic term which includes 'mental illness, arrested or incomplete development of mind, psychopathic disorder, and any other disorder or disability of mind' but there is no definition of 'mental illness' while the other two are defined. This has led to confusion. Under Section 60, the nature of the mental disorder has to be stated and some doctors because of the manner in which the Act is drafted, put *'mental disorder'* instead of *'mental illness'*, which is wrong. A redrafting of the Act would appear necessary, though an attempt to define mental illness could conceivably give rise to even greater difficulty than that produced by the definition of psychopathic personality.

The following paragraph is inserted not as a definition but for guidance:

5. 'Nothing in this section shall be construed as implying that a person may be dealt with under this Act as suffering from mental disorder described in this section, by reason only of promiscuity or other immoral conduct.'

This paragraph is an interesting one and while one can see that promiscuity or other immoral conduct may not be evidence of mental disorder, neither are a number of other socially undesirable forms of behaviour and it strikes one as odd that vice should be specifically given this protection. The Act makes is more difficult to deal with a dull girl who is engaged in prostitution, and is probably spreading disease, than with a dull girl who is failing in her social duties, such as being unable to maintain herself in more virtuous employment. One of the commonest forms of behaviour which leads dull girls into vice rackets and crime is no longer considered a reason for ensuring their rehabilitation and treatment. Yet there is no compensatory legislation to ensure their welfare. A vice 'lobby' could not have achieved more sympathetic treatment.

The term 'certification' has been abolished and instead there are 'applications for admission' which is a euphemism for compulsory detention, provided that the application is successful. Prior to the present Act a judicial authority could order the detention of a patient but now there must be an application for admission and there is always the possibility of refusal on the ground that the medical superintendent does not regard the patient as suitable. This change was introduced to take the legal and lay side out of the Order and also to give mental hospital doctors the same rights to refuse admission as those possessed by doctors in general hospitals. It is not a very convincing argument either way, for though much has been said of the disadvantages of lay magistrates taking the responsibility of ordering a patient's detention, such as his lack of psychiatric knowledge and his occasional over-ruling of the medical opinions expressed, it was an excellent rule that the individual's freedom should be in the hands of magistrates rather than of doctors. Refusal to admit has never been regarded as a privilege by those doctors working in general hospitals, but rather a matter for regret. Refusal has never been used as an instrument of policy to deny admission to patients on grounds that they are unsuitable or that they can be just as well looked after elsewhere, but because there just was no accommodation available.

Though the word 'asylum' has become debased, it is a matter for regret that the principle is being allowed to lapse. For centuries people with mental affliction have been able to seek asylum in order to be sheltered from the stresses of life which they could no longer endure. First the Church provided them with this service and later the State. The Mental Health Act (1959) has swept it aside and a patient must pass a scrutiny test before he is admitted formally or informally and the right to refuse him admission is regarded as a privilege. It diminishes somewhat claims that the new Act is a patient's charter. Some of it reads like the mental hospital doctor's charter, for not only has he the right to refuse admission, but he can sign medical recommendations for admission into his own hospital, a power that was specifically denied him under the old Lunacy Act. That changes were due, in order to meet the new developments in psychiatry, is accepted, but all changes are not necessarily for the good and an Act which had unanimous support because of its allegedly better safeguards for the patient's liberty does not, in fact, measure up to these requirements and in some respects is less concerned with these safeguards.

Formal Admission

This can be arranged under two procedures (*a*) for observation and (*b*) for treatment. As no hospital is compelled to admit, it is advisable to enquire first from the hospital if they are prepared to admit. In practice there has been no detectable tendency for hospitals to refuse admission but should they do so, the Regional Hospital Board can exercise some influence.

Application for a patient can be made either by the nearest relative or a mental welfare officer who is usually a local government official. A number of forms are available for this purpose and are as follows:

Form 1. Application for admission for observation (Section 25).

Form 2. Emergency application for admission for observation (Section 29).

Form 4A. Application by nearest relative for admission for treatment (Section 26).

Form 4B. Application by mental welfare officer (Section 26).

If the nearest relative has notified the mental welfare officer or the local health authority that he objects to the application being made, then it should be deferred till the mental welfare officer has consulted with the objecting relative, provided delay would not be prejudicial to the patient or society.

Grounds for Application for Observation

(*a*) That the patient is suffering from mental disorder of a nature or degree which warrants the detention of the patient in a hospital under observation (with or without medical treatment) for at least a limited period.

(*b*) That the patient ought to be so detained in the interests of his own health or safety or with a view to the protection of other persons.

Grounds for Application for Treatment

(*a*) That the patient is suffering from mental disorder, being—

(i) in the case of a patient of any age, mental illness or severe subnormality.

(ii) in the case of a patient under the age of 21 years, psychopathic disorder or subnormality and that the said disorder is of a nature or degree which warrants the detention of the patient in a hospital for medical treatment.

(*b*) That it is necessary in the interests of the patient's health or safety or for the protection of other persons that the patient should be so detained.

Medical Recommendations

These must be signed on or before the date of application by medical practitioners who have personally examined the patient either together or at an interval of not more than seven days. One must be completed by a doctor approved for the purposes of Section 28, by a local health authority as having special experience in the diagnosis or treatment of mental disorder. One medical recommendation should be completed by the doctor who is normally attending the patient and has previous knowledge of him. One of the recommendations may be completed by a doctor on the staff of the hospital to which the patient is being admitted, provided that the accommodation is not Section 5 of the National Health Service, *i.e.* private accommodation. A number of forms are available as follows:

Form 3A. Medical recommendation for admission for observation (Sections 25 or 29).

Form 3B. Joint medical recommendation for admission for observation (Sections 25 or 29).

Form 5A. Medical recommendation for admission for treatment (Section 26).

Form 5B. Joint medical recommendation for admission for treatment (Section 26).

This is useful when both doctors see the patient together.

Certain people are excluded from signing a medical recommendation for admission to hospital or for guardianship. These are:

(*a*) the applicant;

(*b*) a partner of the applicant or of a practitioner who may be making the other medical recommendation;

(*c*) a person employed as an assistant by the applicant or by the practitioner making the other medical recommendation;

(*d*) a person who receives or has an interest in the receipt of any payments made on account of the maintenance of the patient;

(*e*) if one medical recommendation is already signed by a member of the staff of the hospital to which the patient is to be admitted, no other medical officer on the staff is eligible.

As has already been stated, if the patient is to be a private patient, no medical member of the staff of that hospital can sign the recommendation and neither can the husband, wife, father, father-in-law, mother, mother-in-law, son, son-in-law, daughter, daughter-in-law, brother, brother-in-law, sister or sister-in-law of the patient or of any of the other people excluded or of a practitioner who is signing the other medical recommendation.

An application for admission for observation under Section 25 authorizes the removal of the patient to the hospital within 14 days, beginning with the date on which the patient was last examined by a medical practitioner before making his medical recommendation. The patient may then be detained for a period not exceeding 28 days from the day of admission and cannot be detained after that unless a subsequent application or order is made. This can be extended for a further 7 days under Section 52 (4) if there is pending an application to the county court to deprive the nearest relative of his rights on the ground that he has exercised his power to discharge the patient without due regard to the welfare of the patient or the interests of the public, or is likely to do so.

Emergency Admissions

In case of urgent necessity, an 'emergency application' for admission for observation can be made either by a mental welfare officer or by any relative of the patient, and includes a statement that it is of urgent necessity for the patient to be admitted and detained and that compliance with the ordinary procedure would involve undesirable delay. Such an application may be founded on one medical recommendation, signed preferably by a doctor with previous knowledge of the patient and who is not disqualified (see above). A second medical recommendation must be obtained within 72 hours of admission and the two together must fulfil the requirements of the ordinary procedure for admission. An emergency application authorizes the transfer of the patient to hospital within three days beginning with the date the patient was examined by the doctor or the date of the application, whichever is earlier. If the second medical recommendation is received by the managers of the hospital within 72 hours of the patient's admission, the period of authorized detention will be the same as for any other admission for observation.

Abuse of Section 29. This section of the Act was designed to be used only in real emergencies where action must be taken before there is time to obtain the two medical recommendations. In practice, it is being increasingly used as the routine method of formal admission and in some areas it accounts for over 90 per cent of mental hospital admissions (Enoch & Barker, 1965). This confirms the fears the author expressed in the First Edition of the 'Guide'. that many of these patients (quoted as one-third) became informal within 3 days does not minimize the serious threat to individual liberty that this common practice implies. In the 1890 Lunacy Act which the 1959 Act replaced, such cavalier disposal was reserved for pauper lunatics or lunatics wandering at large, but it was still the responsibility of a magistrate to scrutinize the doctor's certificate. We claim that our society has outgrown the concept of 'pauper' and 'lunatic'. This abuse of Section 29 gives one serious cause for doubt.

Emergency Provisions

These are to help to remove a person to hospital as a matter of urgency and permit the use of the police to help the mental welfare officer. The information is laid before a magistrate on oath by the mental welfare officer that he has reasonable cause to suspect that a person believed to be suffering from mental disorder:

(*a*) has been, or is being, ill-treated, neglected or kept otherwise than under proper control, or
(*b*) is unable to care for himself, and is living alone.

The magistrate may issue a warrant authorizing any constable to enter, if need be by force, any premises specified in the warrant where the patient is believed to be, and if the constable thought fit, to remove him to a place of safety with a view to making an application for his admission to hospital. The constable executing the warrant *must* be accompanied by a mental welfare officer and by a medical practitioner, and it is not necessary to name the patient on the constable's warrant. Such a patient may be detained for 72 hours which allows time for an application to hospital to be made.

A constable may find a person who appears to him to be in immediate need of care or control, and if he thinks fit, he may in the interests of the patient or for the protection of others remove that person to a place of safety, where he may be detained for 72 hours, permitting him to be examined by a doctor and a mental welfare officer. In this instance no magistrate's warrant is necessary.

A Place of Safety. This is defined as a police station, a mental nursing home or residential home for mentally disordered persons or any other suitable place, the occupier of which is willing temporarily to receive the patient.

Application for Guardianship

This can be made on the grounds:

(*a*) that a person is suffering from mental disorder being—

(i) in the case of a patient of any age, mental illness or severe subnormality;

(ii) in the case of a patient under 21 years, psychopathic disorder or subnormality;

and that the disorder is of a nature or degree which warrants the reception of the patient into guardianship and that it is necessary in the interests of the patient and for the protection of others. Two medical recommendations must accompany the application and the rules pertaining to them are similar to those for treatment and observation.

The patient may be kept under guardianship for a period of not more than one year from the day the application was accepted. A further period requires a renewal of guardianship which in the first instance is for another year and successive renewals will be at intervals of two years, except that a psychopathic or subnormal patient ceases to be subject to guardianship on attaining the age of 25 years.

Appeals

With the introduction of the National Health Service Act (1946), the Board of Control, which had exercised a statutory role as 'protector' of patients in institutions, was merged with the Ministry of Health, and with the new Mental Health Act (1959), the Board of Control was abolished entirely and some of its functions replaced by Mental Health Review Tribunals. These consist of legal members appointed by the Lord Chancellor and medical members appointed by the Lord Chancellor after consultation with the Minister of Health, as well as a number of persons with experience in administration or knowledge of social services or other suitable experience. One of the legal members of each tribunal is appointed by the Lord Chancellor to act as chairman. Membership of the tribunal is barred to Members of Parliament.

The tribunal has the power to discharge a patient from hospital if they are satisfied that he is not then suffering from the condition for which he was detained; that it is no longer in the patient's or public interest that he should continue to be detained; that the patient if released would not act in a manner dangerous to himself or to others. Similar conditions are applicable to patients under guardianship. It is possible for a private medical examination to be made on behalf of the patient to advise whether an appeal to the tribunal should be made.

Appeals to tribunals can be made within a period of six months of admission and the variety of patients and conditions which can be dealt with by tribunals are very wide indeed and include subnormal or psychopathic patients detained over the age of 25 years, challenges to a barring report, when a nearest relative's request for a patient's discharge has been refused, reclassification of patients on attaining the age of 16 years, special referrals by the Minister, persons ordered to be kept in custody during Her Majesty's pleasure, and persons serving sentences who have been removed to hospital.

Applications to be considered by a Mental Health Review Tribunal are made on an appropriate form—Form 1 when completed by the patient and Form 2 when completed by the nearest or displaced relative. The numbers of the forms indicate the priority in the minds of the legislators of the Act and the procedure laid down is such that every consideration is given to spare the patient embarrassment. For example, should the applicant request a formal hearing, the tribunal, if of the opinion that such a hearing would be detrimental to the patient's health, can ignore the request and determine an informal hearing. Though the patient may appear personally before the tribunal, medical examination is in private by the medical member and the medical records can be examined. The tribunal may interview the patient at his request, but the essential evidence of the medical member is obtained privately and the patient or applicant is not in a position to contest it. This is obviously meant to spare the patient, but it again yields considerable power to the medical member and, as cases appearing before tribunals are likely to have been in hospital for at least six months, the issue is not usually one of waiting for the results of short-term treatment, but of long-term custody and the reasons for detention would be largely behavioural and not dissimilar from those which are dealt with by courts of law. It is merely another example where for 'medical considerations' traditional legal safeguards of liberty are shelved.

For those who desire a lucid account of the complete Mental

Health Act, 1959, Speller (1961) has produced an excellent review of the subject.

THE LAW IN SCOTLAND

This is in most respects similar to that of England. In criminal proceedings, if the accused is insane, he will be found so on arraignment so that the psychiatric wrangles which till the passing of the Homicide Act, 1957, were so common in English courts, hardly occur. Diminished responsibility has been a feature of Scottish law relating to murder for many years.

Mental Health Act (1960) Scotland

This follows very closely the pattern set by the Mental Health Act (1959). Among the main differences are:

1. The Mental Health Act abolished the Board of Control and put the administration of mental health in England and Wales into the hands of the Ministry of Health. The Scottish Act dissolves the Scottish Board of Control and replaces it by an independent central body called the Mental Welfare Board which will consist of not fewer than five or more than seven commissioners, of whom at least two must be medical.
2. It will exercise general protective functions over those who are mentally disabled.
3. It will have wide powers including complete supervision of the conditions under which mental treatment is carried out in Scotland, inquiry into cases of improper detention, and the right to discharge a patient at any time, and in certain circumstances a duty to do so.
4. It will be able to delegate its powers by appointing committees to carry out specific tasks.
5. The Mental Health Review Tribunals of the English Act are not introduced into the Scottish one. There is less machinery for investigating alleged wrongful detention. The patient or his nearest relative has the right to appeal to a sheriff against refusal to discharge, and it appears as though the Mental Health Review Tribunal's functions will be carried out by the Mental Welfare Board, who may accord a private interview to patients on request. The Board has power to enquire into conditions of treatment. The machinery for dealing with complaints would appear to be less cumbersome than the English system.
6. Compulsory admission is dealt with by application by a relative

or mental health officer supported by the opinion of two medical practitioners, one having special psychiatric knowledge, which is similar to the English, except that in Scotland they have retained the lay person in the form of the sheriff who must approve all applications before they become effective.

7. Compulsory admission to hospital of convicted persons suffering from mental illness by means of a Court Hospital Order is almost identical with the English provisions.

8. In the Scottish Act all forms of abnormality are described simply as 'mental disorder', but a more exact definition is required in certain of the clauses, which contrasts with the English subdivision of severe subnormality, subnormality and psychopathic disorder.

A commentator on both Acts stated that there would be very little difference in practice as the intentions of both are basically the same. This could be said of legislation for mental illness the world over, but unfortunately the intentions of the legislator and everyday practice based on such legislation may be very different. The time has surely come when these matters can be discussed at international level so that new legislation may benefit from practices in other lands.

The Court of Protection

The function of the court is to manage the property and affairs of persons who, by reason of mental disorder, are unable to do so themselves (Jennings, 1962). It is therefore only concerned with their property and not their persons and it cannot direct where a patient shall live or that he shall enter or leave hospital, though by its control over the patient's property, it can exercise some influence over these matters. It acts by appointing a *receiver* who has authority from the court to act on behalf of the patient as a form of statutory agent. Occasionally, there will be no need for a receiver and the court will instruct that a legacy or policy to which a patient in hospital has become entitled should be paid to the hospital on the patient's behalf. The court generally exercises its jurisdiction only after scrutinizing medical evidence under Section 101 of the Mental Health Act, 1959. This section applies to a person who is incapable, by reason of mental disorder, of managing and administrating his property and affairs. 'Mental disorder' is defined in Section 4 of the Act (see above).

The Degree of Disorder. This is less than that usually required for compulsory detention under Section 25 and 26 and the majority of patients are not in hospital, but are usually suffering from mental confusion accompanying old age with difficulty in distinguishing past from present and forgetfulness leading to unpaid bills and uncashed cheques, or in danger of being imposed on by a scheming so-called friend. Jennings (1962) states:

> In all these cases, and indeed in all cases of mental infirmity, protection is given, and can only be given, by the Court of Protection, and the appointment of a receiver will often relieve the family doctor from an embarrassing position.

He also stresses the fallacy of trying to compromise with *power of attorney*.

> If a power of attorney is said to be required in the context of a failing intellect this is cogent evidence that in fact the patient is incapable of managing his affairs . . . any power of attorney will, with few exceptions, be void *ab initio* or voided by the subsequent incapability.

The Lord Chancellor's Visitors. There are at present four Visitors, appointed by the Lord Chancellor, a Queen's Counsel and three physicians, specially qualified in psychological medicine. They visit patients who are, or who are thought to be, incapable of managing their affairs and report to the court. They have the statutory right of requiring the production of any medical record relating to the patient and interference in the carrying out of their duties is an offence punishable by imprisonment. The family doctor who wishes to obtain for his patient the protection of the court should consult his solicitor or write directly to the Chief Clerk, Court of Protection, Store Street, London, W.C.1.

Detention of Criminals in Mental Hospitals

Section 60 of the Mental Health Act, 1959, permits a court (assize, quarter sessions and magistrates) under certain circumstances to transfer a convicted person to a mental hospital. The relevant conditions are:

(*a*) The court is satisfied on written or oral evidence of two medical practitioners that the offender is suffering from mental illness, psychopathic disorder, subnormality or severe subnormality and that the mental disorder is of a nature or degree which warrants the detention of the patient in a hospital for medical treatment, or his reception into guardianship under the Act;

(*b*) The court is of opinion, having regard to all the circumstances including the nature of the offence and the character and antecedents of the offender, and to the other available methods of dealing with him, that the most suitable method of disposing of the case is by means of an order under the Act.

This order is called a *hospital order* and can only be made if the court is satisfied that arrangements have been made for the patient's reception into hospital within 28 days beginning with the date of the making of the order. The form of mental disorder should be specified.

Section 61 carries the implication of Section 60, but applies to children or young persons who are found to be in need of care or protection or beyond control.

Section 65 is used for a hospital order with special restrictions concerning discharge, but to be effective, at least one of the medical practitioners whose evidence is taken into account by the court under Section 60, should have given evidence orally before the court. These orders have already given rise to difficulties and the case of R. *v.* Higginbotham, 1961, illustrates some of these. Mr. Justice Glyn-Jones delivering a judgment of the Court of Criminal Appeal made the following observation:

> It was unsafe for courts to assume that the making of a hospital order coupled with a restriction order under Section 65 was sufficient by itself to ensure that the convicted person would be kept in custody. The only way to ensure this was for the court to ascertain before making the order, which mental hospital hospital could receive the man: this must be done. Further the court must find out whether the hospital had facilities for keeping the patients in safe custody, so they would not have the opportunity to walk out and commit a crime. If there were no such vacancy it should be remembered that the power to make a hospital order was permissive and not mandatory. If there was no such vacancy in a secure hospital and the protection of the public demanded that the accused be incarcerated, he should be sent to prison and his treatment left to the prison medical officer.

The Legal Correspondent of the *British Medical Journal* states: '. . . the difficulty of finding places in secure hospitals will no doubt result in an increasing number of prisoners being sentenced to prison, although the court would wish them to receive treatment' (*British Medical Journal*, 1961d).

That the difficulties are not confined to the court has been amply demonstrated by Rollin (1966) who stresses the incompatibility between the modern mental hospital with its 'open door' and permissive regime, and the security conditions required for the dangerous criminal. In two years 66 men on hospital orders, including 10 with restrictions on discharge (sections 65 and 72) absconded from his hospital 188 times. There is obviously room for more consultation between judges and doctors about these patients and also the Act could be improved in this respect.

Transfer of Prisoners to a Mental Hospital. If the Home Secretary is satisfied by reports from at least two medical practitioners that the person is suffering from mental illness, psychopathic disorder, subnormality or severe subnormality and that the mental disorder is of a nature or degree which warrants the detention of the patient in hospital for medical treatment, he (the Home Secretary) may direct that the patient be transferred to such a hospital. Mental nursing homes are specifically excluded. Sections 72-78 of the Mental Health Act are those which deal specifically with the subject.

The Criminal Justice Act (1948)

This provides the court with power to order psychiatric treatment as well as punishment. At the magistrates' court level, it frequently means that the convicted person is required to submit himself for out-patient treatment as a condition of his probation. Prior to the Mental Health Act, 1959, an English court could not order a person to undergo treatment in a Scottish hospital, but this has now been remedied. A new Criminal Justice Act (1961) deals mainly with offenders under 21, and it does not alter the arrangements for treatment in the 1948 Act.

The Homicide Act (1957)

In addition to accepting the principle of diminished responsibility in certain types of murder, it reduces the offence of the survivor in a suicide pact to manslaughter. Section 2 of the Act provides for a verdict of manslaughter instead of murder where it is shown that the accused 'was suffering from such abnormality of the mind . . . *as substantially* impaired his mental responsibility for his acts or omissions in doing or being party to the killing'. The word 'substantial' has already given rise to difficulties in that it does not indicate whether it excludes minor or trivial impairment of responsibility or whether it means a high degree of impairment. Although it does not mean to equate diminished responsibility with irresistible impulse, in Rex *v.* Simcox, 1964, the Court of Criminal Appeal quoted the opinion of one of the defence doctors that the accused could control himself if he wanted to. It is certainly no easier to give a jury (who have to decide) clear guidance on the matter. It may be that was the intention of the Act in that it gives the judge considerable room for manoeuvre and he can therefore direct differently according to the nature of the case.

The Suicide Act (1961)

Throughout the centuries suicide in England (though not in Scotland) has been a criminal offence as well as an ecclesiastical sin. Attempted suicide has been a crime since 1845 and though the police seldom used their powers, the climate of public opinion, including that of the Church of England, felt that these people required treatment rather than punishment. In practice the Act makes very little difference, for nearly all cases of attempted suicide admitted to hospital received the appropriate psychiatric treatment. In fact, the legal implications could on occasion prove a useful lever to persuade the patient to cooperate, while with the present Act an uncooperative patient has to be dealt with formally, which may mean transfer to a mental hospital. It also provides a penalty for members of suicide pacts who survive, in that they can be accused of aiding, abetting, counselling, or procuring the suicide of another or an attempt by another to commit suicide.

The Psychiatrist as Witness and Professional Confidence

Professional confidence between patient and doctor was given a rude jolt in a divorce suit (Nuttall *v.* Nuttall and Twyman, 1964). Counsel for the husband called as a witness a psychiatrist who had been consulted by the wife and the co-respondent. The psychiatrist said he did not wish to give evidence. The Judge informed him that according to the law he must. The doctor replied: 'These parties consulted me professionally in my consulting-room. They entrusted their confidence to me and I accepted their confidence on the basis that everything said between us was privileged'.

The Judge: It is not privileged.

The Witness: If you order me to give this evidence it will really strike at the roots of my profession. How can people consult a psychiatrist if they cannot feel sure their confidence will be protected from disclosure?

The Judge: I cannot alter the law. You must go to your M.P. to do that . . . The alternative before you is either to give evidence or to go to prison.

The witness protested but gave evidence.

The correspondence in the medical journals that followed this case left no doubt that there is a very strong body of support for a change in the law. In many other countries such confidences are privileged. The case for the legal and ethical right of privacy in medical practice has been well put by Cass and Curran (1965). They accept that there are instances when information should be revealed such as the reporting of contagious disease to a public health official, but they stress that physicians are bound by a code of ethics to act at all times in the best interests of those they serve.

Medical records should be given the same respect as verbal communications and the present tendency to forward such documents to government departments even with the patient's consent may lead to unforeseen trouble. The author had one such experience when a relative of a paranoid patient had given information concerning him which was duly recorded in the notes. He was a war pensioner and was appealing against his award and had given written consent for his notes to be made available. The custom is for an extract of these notes to be given by the Ministry to the appellant. Although the author was assured that nothing which would disturb the patient would be disclosed to him, the risk of violent behaviour towards the relative precluded the taking of any chances and instead of the case records, a prepared summary was forwarded. This was acceptable to the Ministry.

PHYSICAL DISABILITY AND CRIME

There are conflicting views on the causal relationship between physical abnormality and crime. Goring (1913) concluded: 'On statistical evidence, one assertion can be dogmatically made: it is that the criminal is differentiated by inferior stature, by defective intelligence, and . . . by his antisocial proclivities'. The first two are now no longer regarded as peculiar to the criminal and East (1942) who thought they were, urged caution in determining any association. Healy (1915) who saw the problem in terms of treatment, made the impassioned plea: 'It ought to be generally realized in all common sense, that any physical peculiarities, defects, or diseases of the offender which stand in the way of social success should be as efficiently treated as possible'. Ogden (1959) working in Portland Borstal Institution corrected cosmetic disfigurements as well as using remedial surgery for varicose veins, hernia and congential heart disease. He deliberately exploited the psychological potentials of the treatment by encouraging the prisoner to earn the recommendation for treatment, trusting him with responsibility, altering the environment and giving supportive psychotherapy. Attitudes improved not only in response to facial operations but to removal of varicose veins.

Lewison (1965) submitted 450 male prisoners to plastic surgery for the correction of misshapen noses, ears, and chins and for the removal of scars. The offenders were selected because of good (criminological) prognosis and youth, but like Ogden he had no control groups and results were favourable. Similar work has been done at the new psychiatric prison at Grendon Underwood and elsewhere and while improvement has been recorded while in prison, follow-up is important, for a scarred or mutilated face which is made attractive can merely shift the nature of the crime from, say, larceny to confidence tricks. It has already been reported that some prisoners were looking forward to improving their position in the criminal world with their new-found charms. At present these methods must be considered experimental and while no criminal should be deprived of surgical facilities which are available to the general public, the case for priority has not yet been made.

Frequency of Concussion and Types of Criminality

Lidberg (1971) investigated the frequency of concussion in a sample of individuals sent by the court for forensic examination to the department of psychiatry at the Karolinksa Institute. There was a statistically significant higher frequency among those previously committed for crimes of violence compared with crimes of forgery and theft. Those with no previous convictions had the lowest frequency. The severity of the concussion did not seem to influence the type of criminality, and of the 10 in the sample who had suffered open brain damage with symptoms of neurologic defect, none had committed crimes of violence after the head injury. Thus severe brain damage by itself does not necessarily imply a greater degree of criminal violence.

Malingering after Injuries to Brain and Spinal Cord

The psychiatrist is frequently asked to decide whether a claimed disability is 'genuinely hysterical' or malingering. Miller and Cartlidge (1972) use the term 'malingering' to encompass all forms of fraud relating to matters of health which included: (1) the simulation of disease or disability which is not present; (2) the gross exaggeration of minor disability and the conscious and deliberate attribution of a disability to an accident that did not in fact cause it, for personal advantage. The major criterion of distinction was the context, since medical simulation occurs only where it is hoped it will yield personal, economic or social gain.

Malingering is most common in the following conditions: post-concussion syndrome and its variants; blackouts; abnormal gait; varied visual complaints, the most prominent being asthenopia;

speech disturbances; and anosmia. The commonest forms of malingering are subjective psychiatric complaints, and here the distinction between malingering and neurosis or psychosis will depend on the credibility of the witness and objective clinical evidence.

Simulation is most conspicuous in middle-aged men for whom job advancement is bleak. The examiner's suspicions may be aroused:

(*a*) when the claimant's hope of financial gain is implicit in the context of the disability;
(*b*) when severe, continued and disproportionate disablement is claimed to follow trivial injury;
(*c*) when the disability is one that can be simulated;
(*d*) when the simulated complaint follows no organic pattern.

The authors state that it is exceptional to be able to prove malingering but that such a conclusion may be reached on the 'balance of probabilities'.

SHOPLIFTING

With the proliferation of supermarkets and the increased accessibility of goods on display, it is not surprising that there has been an increase in shoplifting. Most instances are of no great concern to the psychiatrist, but there are examples where the act is intimately associated with mental illness. In a general survey of shoplifting in the London area, Gibbens (1962) found that a third of the women were foreign visitors—students, *au pair* girls and visitors' wives. These figures would obviously not apply to the provinces and indicate the importance of not generalizing from the London scene. In the provinces the problem tends to divide between those who do it out of greed and those who are in a disturbed mental state.

The latter are usually middle-aged women in a depressive state who get the impulse and almost welcome detection as part of their expiation for unconscious guilt. Some have behaved in this way under the influence of drugs like amphetamine. The author had a patient who had a cyclothymic personality and was in a depressed state. She took some amphetamine and felt a gay abandon and decided to 'challenge' the store because it had the audacity to tempt people with such desirable goods. She literally stuffed her bag to overflowing and stated she felt most exhilarated at the time. Another patient succumbed following a pre-frontal leucotomy; a middle-aged woman with hypertension had an automatism when she went back twice for the same goods and was unaware that she had done so; one patient had a temporal lobe tumour. Some have a complicated psychopathology which includes self-punishment with vengeance as is frequently found in suicide or attempted suicide.

These are only a few of the conditions the author has met in a general psychiatric practice, so medical factors are not uncommon. It is another matter trying to convince a court that such factors are material.

Victim and Offender Relationship

Schultz (1968) described the results of pre-sentence investigations and pointed out that there are many offences where the victim invited, initiated and worked diligently towards the success of the offence. Obvious examples were criminal abortion and prostitution but less obvious were 'con' games where the victim's larcenous impulse is exploited by the criminal A victim can contribute to the crime by provoking a hostile reaction, by direct incitement, by omitting preventive measures and by unconsciously inviting the offence through his psychopathology.

The author recommended that in crimes of violence and sex offences, the victim's police record should be checked as routine. In sex, the victim may be collaborative, participating or seductive in a large percentage of cases. In assault and homicide the terms aggressor and victim are sometimes interchangeable. Provocation may be so great that the victim may be using the killer as an instrument of suicide. Victims should be encouraged to express their feelings about the trauma, lest a deeper significance go unrecognized. Not uncommonly the quest for compensation or restitution may be pursued to a degree which prejudices rehabilitation and the security of the family.

LSD and Manslaughter

Williams (1969) discussed the case of a defendant aged 37 who was charged with the murder of a girl of 18 years. He had taken LSD and experienced a 'trip' in which he claimed he had the illusion of descending to the centre of the earth and being attacked by snakes which he fought. He claimed no knowledge of the crime and denied intention to harm. He was found guilty of manslaughter because it was proved that 'he must have realized, before he got himself into the condition he did by taking drugs, that acts such as those he subsequently performed and which resulted in death were dangerous'. He appealed on the grounds that even in cases of manslaughter a degree of *mens rea* was essential. Lord Justice Widgery saw no reason to distinguish between the effects of drugs voluntarily taken and of drink voluntarily taken: 'When killing resulted from an unlawful act of the defendant, no specific intent had to be proved to convict of manslaughter and self-induced intoxication accordingly was no defence'.

GUILT AND THE LAW

Some consider that guilt is a personal matter and that we should all be better off .without it and that a legitimate objective of psychiatric treatment and/or social reform would be its removal. Lord Devlin in his Ernest Jones lecture to the British Psycho-Analytical Society (Devlin, 1964) took a different view. He considered that the function of the Law was to maintain order and no system of penalties could be a sufficient deterrent unless there was almost 100 per cent likelihood of detection. The sense of guilt, in his opinion, played a greater part in the maintenance of law and order than any legal deterrent. Because of this he felt that the imposition of the penalties imposed by the criminal law should be reinforced by the judge's moral observations. If the existence of a moral law, by affecting the conscience of the average citizen, was essential to the functioning of the criminal law, then those who spread rational and philosophical criticism of traditional morality had a grave responsibility, unless they were prepared to supply something else to support the maintenance of law and order.

These views are today controversial but they should be seriously considered by psychiatrists, who more than any other section of the medical profession are involved in reforms which fundamentally affect the foundations of our culture.

CHAPTER 22

Legal Aspects of Psychiatry in the United States

by John Donnelly, M.D., F.R.C. Psych. (G.B.), F.A.C.P., F.A.P.A.
Psychiatrist-in-chief, Institute of Living, Hartford, Connecticut, U.S.A.

INTRODUCTION

Most societies have recognized mentally ill persons as being different from other members of the group and as requiring different treatment in respect to responsibility, behaviour and management of their affairs. Statutes have been enacted to protect other members of the society and the individual himself. With increasing knowledge concerning mental illness and with social and legal attitudes towards the ordinary individual and his rights constantly in a state of change, the laws and procedures relative to the mentally ill person are also in a continuing state of change.

In the United States, special difficulties arise out of the fact that there are so many different jurisdictions. The Federal jurisdiction extends over all areas in which the constitutional rights of the individual are concerned. The fifty States each have constitutional jurisdiction over all matters within their individual boundaries, subject to conformity with the Constitution of the United States. The Federal jurisdiction extends to all matters involving inter-State matters, while the laws of each State are binding only within the geographical borders of that State.

As a consequence, the laws pertaining to the mentally ill present a patchwork quilt across the nation. Certain principles are uniform but from State to State the variations are innumerable. Each physician, and especially each psychiatrist, should become aware of the laws which govern in the State or States in which he practises. Contiguous States often have quite different statutes on, for example, the commitment of patients.

Until recently, the primary drive for modification of the law with respect to deviant members of society has come from psychiatrists and prominent jurists whose orientation has been a humanistic one. In recent years the influence of psychiatry has become secondary to that of the strong libertarian movement. The orientation of this is essentially a legalistic one which, in the eyes of psychiatrists, often sacrifices right to treatment in favour of the civil right of non-deprivation of liberty. The consequences of this shift have had profound effects on the practice of psychiatry and the training of psychiatrists and have resulted in an emergence of a new emphasis on protecting the patient from the established patterns of care. In contrast to the recent past, there has been developing a movement hostile to psychiatry and the behavioral sciences in general, not only in the basic sciences but also in some segments of the public.

The processes available to effect change are two in number: the first through enactment of statutes in the various legislatures of the States; and the second by pursuit of issues in individual cases through the legal system to the ultimate decision by the Supreme Court of the United States. Both avenues have been constantly used. The legislative process has often been the mode for emotionally involved lay persons, resulting in a tremendous range of methods with which patients are dealt. The legal route, on the other hand, establishes, when completed, a uniform approach throughout the country.

Starting with a primary focus on the civil rights of minorities and of accused and convicted persons, the civil rights movement spread to the constitutional rights of the mentally ill, including due process with respect to his involuntary confinement in a psychiatric hospital, abrogation of civil rights by prolonged confinement of a defendant incompetent to stand trial, the issue of 'informed consent' of a patient to submit to any medical, surgical or psychiatric procedure, and a host of related problems.

Whereas the societal position had been that justice and humanity demanded that mentally ill persons be provided with protection and treatment, there has developed a powerful movement to deal legally with the mentally ill person in the same way as if he were fully competent to take care of himself. The advocates of this approach include not only social activists, but also the far-right, politically conservative group loosely known as the John Birch Society and, in the field of psychiatry, those most prominently represented by Thomas Szasz, a psychoanalyst, who philosophically believes in the Kantian categorical imperative. This philosophy, enunciated prior to recognition of the 'unconscious' element of the human psychical structure, appeals strongly to physical scientists and lawyers, the two groups which, with the political conservatives, are the strong and powerful advocates of this approach to the mentally ill. Szasz's position that mental illness is a myth has, curiously enough, a strong appeal to a number of young psychiatrists and especially those whose orientation is toward 'social psychiatry'.

In contrast, those on the liberal left are concerned primarily with the constitutional right to freedom of the individual and hold the extreme position that no person should be involuntarily deprived of his freedom unless there is demonstrated evidence that he is dangerous to himself or others. Accordingly, if he is not, no matter how mentally ill he may be, he has the right to choose whether or not he wishes to seek treatment.

This chapter endeavours to outline some of the basic principles and laws which are of especial importance to the psychiatrist and his potential patient.

CRIMINAL RESPONSIBILITY

It has long been accepted that an individual suffering from insanity, a legal term, should not be held responsible for his criminal acts. Underlying this principle lies the philosophy that an individual exercises free will in the execution of his actions and a criminal act is the result of premeditated malice. The 'insane' person suffers from impairment of the exercise of free will and from impairment of objective reasoning and is, therefore, not capable of criminal intent and is not to be held responsible for acts which otherwise in a normal person would be judged to be criminal in nature.

The methods of establishing criminal responsibility, *i.e.* the legal tests or rules, have been phrased in language which set up the test in terms of lack of criminal responsibility. Though this would appear a simple procedural matter, there are important principles and practices underlying the establishment of responsibility. *First,* a person is presumed innocent until proven guilty. *Second,* at trial a person is presumed sane or responsible until the issue of irresponsibility due to mental illness or defect is raised by either of the adversaries. *Third,* when the issue of insanity as a defense has been raised by a defendant *and* some evidence of insanity has been introduced, the burden is imposed on the prosecution to provc sanity beyond reasonable doubt. The final decision is as always for the triers of fact, that is, the jury or the judge sitting without a jury. *Fourth,* the jury may accept lay testimony with regard to insanity as well as expert opinions and may reject the latter provided it does not do so arbitrarily.

The problem of establishing criminal responsibility and of formulating an adequate and just test has long occupied the minds of eminent psychiatrists and jurists. In the United States, the established test in the vast majority of jurisdictions has, until recently, been the so-called McNaughton Rule laid down in 1843 by the Law Lords of the House of Lords.

Although referred to as the McNaughton Rule, it is to be noted that this test was not established in the McNaughton case itself. The origin of the term commences with the assassination of Edward Drummond, Secretary to Sir Robert Peel, Prime Minister of England, by Daniel McNaughton who believed mistakenly he was shooting the Prime Minister. At that trial, evidence clearly established that McNaughton was insane, that he suffered from a paranoid disease, and that he believed he was saving England by assassinating the Prime Minister. All the medical testimony supported this conclusion and McNaughton was found not guilty be reason of insanity and ordered to be confined during Her Majesty's Pleasure (the customary procedure in England).

The verdict aroused much public outcry. The country was, at that time, torn by strong political dissension, while the Queen and the press were disturbed by threats against the lives of prominent persons. As a result, a series of questions was placed before the fifteen Law Lords of the House of Lords (comparable to the U.S. Supreme Court). Their answers to the questions became the basis of the test for criminal responsibility in the English speaking world. While these questions and answers were intended to cover a wider field of criminal responsibility than the case of Daniel McNaughton, it is obvious that they were posed in the narrow context of this crime and verdict.

In response to the question about the instructions to be delivered by the presiding judge to the jury, fourteen of the fifteen justices agreed to this formulation of the charge which ought to be made:

> . . . the jurors ought to be told . . . that to establish a defence on the ground of insanity, it must be clearly proved that, at the time of the committing of the act, the party accused was labouring under such a defect of reason, from disease of the mind, as not to know the nature and quality of the act he was doing or, if he did know it, that he did not know he was doing what was wrong.
>
> If the accused was conscious that the act was one which he ought not to do, and if that act was at the same time contrary to the law of the land, he is punishable. . .[1]

From the time the rules were enunciated, there has been discontent with them, voiced by medical and legal authorities. The criticisms have been made on a number of grounds. The questions and answers were clearly influenced by the type of McNaughton's illness, namely, a paranoid one. They were greatly influenced by the then concurrent concepts of psychology, but especially by the traditional legal doctrines formulated by Lord Hale more than a century before. The current psychology of the day compartmentalized the faculties and functions of the mind, believing them to be separate entities and operating independently of each other. The judges ignored the concepts of Isaac Ray, M.D., author of *A Treatise on the Medical Jurisprudence of Insanity*,[2] published in 1838, whose views were extensively presented at the trial itself.[3]

Another criticism has been the vagueness of the language. Although the phraseology gives an impression of precision, the key phrases have presented significant problems. What, for example, does 'the nature and quality of the act' really mean?

Equally ambiguous is the meaning of the word 'wrong'. Is 'wrong' to be interpreted in the moral or legal context? The formulations by the judges appear to be contradictory and there appears to be an implicit identification of legal wrong with moral wrong. Yet a person suffering from delusions and hallucinations may commit an act which he knows to be legally wrong but believes to be morally right, for example, an act carried out in response to an auditory hallucination of a command of God.

The greatest objection to the McNaughton Rule is that the test of legal sanity is founded on the very narrow basis of the presence or absence of abnormality in a single aspect of mental functioning, namely, the 'knowledge' of the accused, while excluding other, and often more significant, symptoms which determine the diagnosis of mental illness.

From the medical viewpoint, the fundamental criticism is the failure of the test to take into account accumulated knowledge concerning the human personality. The vast majority of psychiatrists maintain that the McNaughton test prevents them from presenting all about the accused which ought to be known by the jury. Many psychiatrists have protested that they are obliged to testify in a way which they believe to be morally wrong.

The application of the Rule has become inconsistent, and in many jurisdictions in the United States it has been ignored, giving rise to inequitable justice. The Honorable Simon E. Sobeloff[4] has stated: 'All seem to be agreed that McNaughton is obsolete.' And again: 'Why should we maintain a Rule that must be breached in order to make it work?'

The general position of psychiatrists is well summarized in the Report of the Royal Commission on Capital Punishment:[5]

> The McNaughton test is based on an entirely obsolete and misleading conception of the nature of insanity, since insanity does not only, or primarily, affect the cognitive or intellectual faculties, but affects the whole personality of

the patient, including both the will and the emotions. An insane person may therefore often know the nature and quality of his act and that it is wrong and forbidden by law, and yet commit it as the result of the mental disease. . . . In our view the test of criminal responsibility contained in the McNaughton rules cannot be defended in the light of modern medical knowledge and modern penal views.

THE IRRESISTIBLE IMPULSE

One attempt to overcome some of the problems inherent in McNaughton was the introduction of the concept of an irresistible impulse as an acceptable defence. The leading decision adopting this was delivered in 1886 in the Alabama Supreme Court.[6] Since responsibility implies the use of free will, an uncontrollable impulse, resulting in a criminal act, is a competent defense. Although the irresistible impulse concept has been accepted in a few jurisdictions, there have been considerable objections to it. First, there is the question as to whether there is a truly irresistible impulse; second, several States had already established McNaughton as the crucial test; third, it is difficult, if not impossible, to prove; fourth, it cannot exist without concurrent impairment of the capacity to know right and wrong; and, fifth, it is unlikely to occur except in conditions of organic aetiology, when other symptoms of mental illness would be found.

The term 'irresistible impulse' usually is interpreted to denote a sudden overwhelming urge of very brief duration and its usefulness is, therefore, extremely limited. Yet certain individuals do experience impulses of an extremely powerful nature, the control of which is possible when environmental pressures reinforce internal forces. Removal of these external pressures may result in expression of the impulse, for example, in kleptomania, exhibitionism and pyromania. There would appear to be a spectrum of such personalities, at one end of which is the individual with complete internal control of impulses and, at the other, the person who is able to repress the impulses when the superego is reinforced by strong external controls, such as a deterrent in the form of the presence of a policeman. In practice, the doctrine of the irresistible impulse is rarely invoked because the legal penalty for the crime, where its use would be appropriate, is usually preferred to the finding of insanity and confinement to a mental hospital.

THE NEW HAMPSHIRE RULE

With one exception, all the jurisdictions of the United States adopted the McNaughton Rule as the test of criminal responsibility. The exception was New Hampshire. In the Pike[7] and Jones[8] cases in 1869 and 1871, Justice Doe of the New Hampshire State Supreme Court enunciated the *Product Rule:*

The legal principle, however much it may formerly have been obscured by pathological darkness and confusion of law and fact, is that a product of mental disease is not a contract, a will, or a crime. It is often difficult to ascertain whether an individual had a mental disease, and whether an act was the product of that disease; but these difficulties arise from the nature of the facts to be investigated, and not from the law; they are practical difficulties to be solved by the jury, and not legal difficulties for the Court. [9]

Justice Doe was greatly influenced by Isaac Ray, the foremost American forensic psychiatrist of his day, with whom he corresponded frequently about mental illness and its medico-legal implications. Dr. Ray, extensively quoted at McNaughton's trial, appears to have had no influence on the English Law Lords; but in New Hampshire, and more recently in a number of United States jurisdictions, the changes he advocated have been introduced in the application of justice for the mentally ill criminal.

THE DURHAM RULE

In 1954, the Court of Appeals for the District of Columbia, in the Durham case, rejected the McNaughton Rule and the irresistible impulse formulation as the test for criminal responsibility. Judge Bazelon wrote in this decision:

The rule we now hold must be applied on the retrial of this case and in future cases is not unlike that followed by the New Hampshire Court since 1870. It is simply that an accused is not criminally responsible if his unlawful act was the product of mental disease or mental defect.[10]

Many jurists and a few psychiatrists expressed alarm concerning the administration of justice and the possible abuses under the Durham Rule. Most psychiatrists and some jurists regarded the Durham decision as a major breakthrough because it removed the right-and-wrong test and permitted the psychiatrist to testify as to his findings in his own language without artificial restrictions. The Rule was deliberately written in such a way that it could be applied in accordance with the principles of current psychiatric knowledge and of scientific data which would become available in the future.

The Durham test was subjected to a number of criticisms.[11, 12] Thus it was claimed that acceptance of the Durham Rule made the legal test of criminal insanity the same as the medical test of mental disease and placed the decision as to guilt in the hands of the psychiatrists.

The test has been held to be vague and variable in application. There was no clear definition of mental disease or mental defect and, because of the differences between psychiatrists, it generates uncertainty and inequality in the administration of the criminal law. There was initially the criticism that some psychiatrists regard all who commit criminal acts as mentally ill persons. Special difficulties were quickly foreseen in the category of offenders known as psychopaths or sociopaths who are diagnosed by psychiatrists as character disorders, a class of mental illness different from psychosis and neurosis. At the same time, the statutes on civil commitment are usually applicable only in the case of the psychotic individual.

In the years following, later decisions of the Court of Appeals for the District of Columbia attempted to deal with the specific criticisms. For example, the fact that lay, as well as medical, testimony was acceptable at trial controverted, at least in theory, the criticism that the psychiatrist makes the decision and not the jury. The Court subsequently clarified and defined the language of the Durham Rule. Of special interest is the case of United States *v.* Leach.[13] Leach, a sociopath in 'pure form', pleaded mental illness, was found not guilty by reason of insanity under the Durham test, and was committed to a Federal mental hospital. Shortly afterwards, he filed a petition for a writ of habeas corpus alleging he was of sound mind. Seven psychiatrists testified that, though not psychotic, he would, if released, be a danger to the community. In spite of this, the District Court (the Court lower than the Court of Appeals) ordered his release. On appeal by the Superintendent,[14] the Court of Appeals reversed the District Court on the grounds that Leach was one of a special group of persons, who had been found not guilty by reason of insanity, and for whom the standards of the statute regarding civil commitment of the mentally ill person did not apply. Eligibility for release must include 'freedom from such abnormal mental condition as would make the individual dangerous to himself or the community in the reasonably forseeable future'.

This decision appeared to produce the same effect as the English verdict of preventive detention but in a mental hospital. At the same time, the legal philosophy is strongly opposed to loss of freedom without due process.

Another important criticism of the Durham test was the problem of demonstrating the causal connection between the illness and the criminal act. The Court in a later decision, Carter *v.* United States,[15] defined this relationship as follows:

When we say the defense of insanity requires that the act be a 'product of' a disease, we mean that the facts on the record are such that the trier of the facts is enabled to draw a reasonable inference that the accused would not have committed the act he did commit if he had not been diseased as he was. There must be a relationship between the disease and the act, and that relationship, whatever it may be in degree, must be as we have already said, critical in its effect in respect to the act. By 'critical' we mean decisive, determinative, causal; we mean to convey the idea inherent in the phrases 'because of', 'except for', 'without which', 'but for', 'effect of', 'result of', 'causative factor'; the disease made the effective or decisive difference between doing and not doing the act.

THE AMERICAN LAW INSTITUTE MODEL TEST

Despite the continuing controversy regarding the Product Rule, a number of States adopted it, some by passing statutes because of the reluctance of their individual Appellate Courts to act. Delay in more extensive adoption of the Durham decision was probably influenced by the fact that the American Law Institute, the research arm of the American Bar Association, developed a Model Penal Code and recommended a new test. The Institute suggested:[16]

A person is not responsible for criminal conduct if at the time of such conduct as a result of mental disease or defect he lacks substantial capacity either to appreciate the criminality of his conduct or to conform his conduct to the requirements of law.

The terms 'mental disease or defect' do not include an abnormality manifested only by repeated criminal or otherwise anti-social conduct.

In 1961, Chief Justice Biggs of the U.S. Court of Appeals for the Third District in the Currens case[17] formulated the following test:

The jury must be satisfied that at the time of committing the prohibited act the defendant, as a result of mental disease or defect, lacked substantial capacity to conform his conduct to the requirements of the law which he is alleged to have violated.

It will be noted that the specific reference in the Durham decision to the unlawful act being the product of mental disease was eliminated, while the phrase, 'either to appreciate the criminality of his conduct or', was removed from the American Law Institute's recommended test.

The American Law Institute's recommendation, like the Durham Rule, has been subject to extensive and intensive criticism. The Law Institute's test in effect adheres to the McNaughton Rule to the degree that the criterion 'know right from wrong' has been replaced by the test 'to appreciate the criminality of his conduct'. There has been substantial criticism that this phrase is equally indefinite and vague and difficult to establish in an offender. The Currens test has also been criticized because there is no definition of what is meant by 'substantial capacity to conform his conduct . . .'

Nevertheless, until recently, it became abundantly clear that the McNaughton test for criminal responsibility was being rapidly replaced by either the Durham, Currens or the American Law Institute test. Of the ten U.S. Courts of Appeals, other than for the District of Columbia, the majority adopted the American Law Institute test and it now appears that this test will in time become the rule throughout all Federal and State jurisdictions.

Indeed, the Durham Rule received in June, 1972, a mortal wound by a decision of the U.S. Court of Appeals for the District of Columbia, the jurisdiction in which it was first enunciated. Dissatisfaction with this test grew greater and greater as the appellate reasoning in individual cases required more and more detailed instructions to the jury. The intent of the promulgator of the Durham Rule, Judge David Bazelon, had been to provide psychiatrists with the opportunity to present psychiatric evidence on behalf of the defendant, detailing his life history and indicating the influence of past experiences in bringing him to his current personality and situation. In time, Judge Bazelon became disillusioned with psychiatric evidence and, in thc case of Washington *v.* United States,[18] he laid down specific instructions as to how the psychiatrist should testify and prohibiting psychiatric opinion on the issue of productivity.

Final disillusionment with the Durham Rule was reached in the case of Archie Brawner *v.* United States.[19] In this case, the U.S. Court of Appeals for the District of Columbia decided to have a full hearing *en banc* on the issue. *Amicus Curiae* briefs were solicited from the major national organizations whose members participated in trials in which the accused pleaded the insanity defence, including the American Bar Association, the American Psychiatric and Psychological Associations, the American Medical Association, the American Civil Liberties Union and other national associations, representing groups such as public defenders.

As a result of this full examination of all opinions, the Court eliminated the Durham Rule and enunciated a new test close to that of the American Law Institute. Under the new test, an individual is considered not responsible for criminal conduct if 'at the time of such conduct as a result of a mental disease or defect he lacks substantial capacity to appreciate the wrongfulness of his conduct or to conform his conduct to the requirements of the law.' The Court retained the existing definition of mental disease or defect of *Durham-McDonald,*[20] namely,

A mental disease or defect includes any abnormal condition of the mind which substantially affects mental or emotional processes and substantially affects behavior controls.

Philosophically, the death of the Durham Rule represents a significant change not only within the legal confines of the District of Columbia, but also in the tenor of thinking regarding the mentally ill defendant. Indeed, it is symbolic of the passing of an era in which 'humanistic' as opposed to 'legalistic' or 'intellectual' concern has held dominance. It is representative of the changing attitudes in the administration of the law.

Although the insanity defence is usually invoked in major crimes, the influence of psychiatry has resulted in its increasingly frequent use in other offences.

DRUG ABUSE

Symbolic of the change in social attitudes, especially toward the established order, there was in the nineteen sixties, in the United States as elsewhere, an epidemic of drug abuse, especially amongst adolescents and young adults.

Historically, Federal and State drug abuse legislation, enacted in the nineteen-twenties and thirties to cope with increasing use of opiates, specified severe criminal penalties for the use of narcotic drugs and included under this umbrella drugs of the cannabis type. Many judges, with reactionary attitudes arising out of a general ignorance and fear, imposed harsh and unjustifiable penalties. For example, adolescents apprehended in a police raid, which netted a single possessor of marijuana, might be sentenced to a period of years in prison, even though they did not themselves possess or use any prohibited drugs. Because of the harshness of the penalties, plus the changing social attitudes in the more educated segments of American society, new laws were passed in many States reducing the use of marijuana to a misdemeanor, with correspondingly less punitive penalties. As the social turmoil has subsided, new legislation has tended to be very punitive towards the seller, with mandatory sentences up to 25 years and, in some States, life imprisonment.

One of the consequences of the extensive use of drugs was the attention paid to the chronic alcoholic. In practically every State public drunkenness has been a criminal offence, resulting in large numbers of individuals going through the circle of arrest, release and rearrest, often many times a year. Arising out of the civil rights issue and out of the humanistic motives of those interested in helping persons addicted to drugs or alcohol, several lawsuits were initiated.

In a landmark case, Robinson *v.* California,[21] the vital distinction was made that simple narcotic addiction was an illness and not a crime. The application of this principle to public drunkenness was raised in several important cases. In the cases of Easter *v.* District of Columbia[22] and Driver *v.* North Carolina,[23] the respective Appellate Courts ruled that a *chronic* alcoholic charged with public drunkenness could not be punished or jailed as a criminal because such a person had lost self-control in the use of intoxicating beverages and to do so was 'cruel and unusual punishment in branding him a criminal'.

However, in a parallel case, Powell *v.* Texas,[24] which reached the U.S. Supreme Court, the Court divided 5 to 4 in ruling that the criminal conviction for public drunkenness must stand in those States in which the statutes define public drunkenness as a crime. This decision was reached despite 'the widespread recognition today that "alcoholism" is a "disease" for the simple reason that the medical profession has concluded that it should attempt to treat those who have drinking problems. There the agreement stops. Debate rages within the medical profession as to whether "alcoholism" is a separate "disease" in a meaningful biochemical, physiological or psychological sense or whether it respresents one peculiar manifestation in some individuals of underlying psychiatric disorders'.

Fortunately, modifications of the statutes have already been made in many State legislatures, and introduced in others, to remove chronic alcoholism, essentially public drunkenness without other unlawful behaviour, from the criminal statutes. While this has resulted in a substantial increase in the number of arrests for creating a 'public nuisance' in some jurisdictions, there has been a definite trend toward developing special treatment facilities for such persons as alternatives to jail.

ABOLITION OF THE INSANITY DEFENCE?

Despite the long-standing philosophical reasoning that 'an insane person' should not be held criminally responsible for acts arising out of mental disease or defect, the unsatisfactory nature of psychiatric testimony has led an increasing number of legal scholars and psychiatrists to question the usefulness of this concept.[25] Too often the expert witness appears to lose the objectivity required of his role and to become an advocate not only of the party who pays him but often of his own theoretical concepts and philosophy.

Because of a few highly publicized cases, the belief has grown widespread that attorneys in many cases appear to use this defence where it is not, in fact, appropriate. This has also been criticized as a manifestation of the general permissiveness developing in all areas of the social order.

In the past four years, as a result of an alarming increase in crimes of violence, there has emerged a powerful law and order sentiment in large segments of the public, with demands for stronger action by the courts to protect the law-abiding person. This popular movement has provided the public support for the theoretical position mentioned above.

The President of the United States has recently submitted to Congress proposals for extensive revisions of the Federal criminal statutes, with severe restrictions on the use of insanity as a defence because present law has led to 'unconscionable abuse by defendants'. In this revision, insanity would be a defence only if the crime requires an element of intent and the defendant's mind was so beclouded that he could not form such intent. Mental disease or defect would not otherwise constitute a defence.

MENTAL COMPETENCY TO STAND TRIAL

It has long been a constitutional right that an individual accused of a crime shall be given a fair trial with the assistance of legal counsel. If, because of mental illness or defect, the accused person is unable to comprehend the nature of the trial or to assist counsel in his defence, he is held to be unfit to plead and the trial must be postponed until the individual becomes mentally competent.

It is to be emphasized that the question of mental competency to stand trial is quite different from that of criminal responsibility. Lack of understanding of this important distinction is to be observed in psychiatrists, attorneys and judges. Capacity to stand trial may be present in a frankly psychotic person. If an accused person is determined by the Court to be incompetent to stand trial, he is committed to hospital until such time as he becomes competent. Psychiatrists and lawyers should understand that, with the recovery of competency, even while the individual remains psychotic, the accused should be brought to trial in the interests of justice for the accused. Otherwise, he will continue confined without due process and under the continued stress of a trial pending in the future.

The criteria to be utilized in evaluating mental incompetency relate to (*a*) comprehension of the proceedings and (*b*) the ability to advise counsel in the preparation and execution of his defence. With respect to his capacity for comprehension, the individual should be aware of the purposes of the trial, the nature of the proceedings, the possible decisions and the penalties which may be imposed in certain eventualities. He must be aware that it is he who is being tried; he should be cognizant of his legal rights and of the crime with which he is accused. With respect to the level of intellectual capacity, there is no firm rule, for intelligence quotients, while helpful, do not completely define in every case the capacity of the individual to understand the nature of the proceedings.

In order to conduct a fair and competent defence, an attorney must have the full co-operation of his client who must be able and willing to give him the relevant facts. This requires an ability to communicate rationally with the attorney, even if there are distortions of facts due to emotional reasons. He must be able to understand the questions which the lawyer puts to him. He must be able to agree with counsel on the nature of his plea. He must be able to understand the testimony rendered by other witnesses and be able to advise his lawyer with regard to the accuracy of such evidence. He must be able to give testimony in his defence if this is deemed advisable.

The examining psychiatrist must, as mentioned above, be fully aware of the reason and purposes of his examination. He must know the charges against the accused, their levels of seriousness and the complexities of the case. The psychiatrist must fully evaluate any existing mental disease, but it is unnecessary for him to form an opinion as to criminal responsibility at the time of the crime because this is not relevant to the evaluation. The latter issue can arise only after the Court has decided that the accused is presently mentally competent for the trial to proceed. Because a trial is a source of considerable stress, an important aspect of the evaluation of incompetency is the probable ability of the individual to tolerate the stresses which will be generated during the course of the trial.

The psychiatrist testifies at the hearing on mental competency as an expert witness and his evidence should, therefore, include his detailed observations of the accused on which he bases his opinion. The judge, of course, decides the question.

The areas of functioning to which special attention should be paid are in the cognitive, emotional and behavioral field. The person should be interviewed to establish the presence or absence of disorders of cerebral function, such as gross defects in memory, disorientation as to time, place or person; instability in time relationships, inability to comprehend and elaborate on necessary information and gross impairment of judgment. The presence of delusions or hallucinations does not render a person incompetent, unless they directly interfere with his capacity to understand the nature of the proceedings or to advise counsel in his defence.

In the affective sphere, the presence of severe depression may be sufficient to cause mental incompetency if, for example, he has ideas of guilt and worthlessness and believes he should be punished. Similarly, marked emotional instability with fluctuating mood and behaviour may interfere with his competency.

While there has been considerable debate about the use or abuse of the insanity defence, the actual number of cases involved are remarkably few. What should be of much greater concern are the consequences of the determination of incompetency to stand trial. Two important issues are involved: the deprivation of liberty without due process and the degrading conditions and total lack of treatment in many hospitals to which these persons are sent.

A number of studies have revealed that the number of persons confined in mental hospitals because of incompetency to stand trial exceeds by many times those institutionalized because of the finding of not guilty by reason of insanity.[26, 27] A related group of patients are persons who have been convicted but later develop overt psychiatric illness and are transferred to the maximum security sections of mental hospitals, there to remain long after the time when the period of their sentence has expired. One study reported more than half of those found incompetent to stand trial would spend the rest of their lives in the hospital.[28]

Following the decision in the case of Baxstrom *v.* New York, the confinement of hundreds of such patients at Matteawan State Hospital for the criminally insane was declared unconstitutional and almost half of the patients there were transferred on civil commitment to other mental hospitals, many to be discharged soon after.

Just as there have been questions raised about the insanity defence, so now are questions being raised about the miscarriage of justice which so often follows a finding of incompetency to stand trial.[30] Many persons in the legal and psychiatric professions are now advocating that a person found incompetent to stand trial should be confined to a hospital for a limited period of time, for example six months, during which he would receive adequate treatment. Should he become competent to stand trial, he would be returned to the Court. If, after treatment for six months, he remains incompetent to stand trial, a further period of six months of treatment would be required. If still incompetent, criminal charges should be dropped and he would be subject to civil commitment procedures where the issue of his dangerousness would be assessed. In those cases in which he is found not to be dangerous, the decision should be made as to whether he requires involuntary confinement or whether he could be treated on an outpatient basis. Those patients found to be dangerous would be confined and treated in a maximum security institution.

Alternatively, persons who, after a period of twelve months, remain incompetent to stand trial should be returned to trial or be confined under civil commitment.

It is recognized that some criminal defendants charged with grave offences might attempt to malinger for the period of six or twelve months with the expectation of escaping a trial. This type of defendant would require special consideration but, of course, the diagnosis of malingering can be very difficult to establish in a sophisticated individual in a way that is convincing to the judge.

SEXUAL PSYCHOPATH LAWS

In no other area of deviant human behaviour are the changes in attitudes towards psychiatry more apparent than in dealing with aberrant sexual offences. The criminal statutes with respect to sexual activity vary from jurisdiction to jurisdiction. They reflect local public attitudes, public morality and public fear of the 'dangerous'. The prescribed penalties in each State vary for each offence, from mild to extremely harsh, but the consequence of the very punitiveness of the laws has been that in many cases they are not enforced. Distinction is often not made as to the dangerousness of the offender to other members of society and not infrequently the evaluation of dangerousness appears to be related to the existing code of public morality, even where this is clearly at variance with the general private morality.

Since 1938, legislation has been enacted in over half the individual States to deal with sexual offenders under 'Sexual Psychopath' laws. Usually passed after sexual crimes of violence which have received widespread publicity, these statutes provide for the confinement of offenders on indeterminate sentences, ranging from a day to life, with the final decision made by the psychiatric expert. Offenders under these laws are not regarded as ordinary criminals nor are they legally insane. They are theoretically confined for treatment of their personality disorder.

Many persons have been declared sexual psychopaths for single offences, including exhibitionism. The procedures for commitment under these laws vary widely and often there is no protection of the individual's constitutional rights. Under some laws, only a person convicted of a sexual crime is subject to commitment, while in other jurisdictions those who have only been indicted are subject. Only the District Attorney or Attorney General of a State may initiate commitment proceedings. Jury trials are mandatory in some States but not in others. In some jurisdictions, the proceedings are held in private and in others a jury trial may be demanded by the accused. In still other States, the judge has discretionary powers.

It is the consensus that these statutes have been ineffective. Treatment programmes, presuming treatment is effective, are by and large non-existent. The offenders are usually incarcerated in overcrowded, understaffed mental hospitals. They are generally viewed as untreatable by hospital authorities who advocate that they be managed in correctional facilities. The authorities of these institutions in turn see them as mentally ill persons and whom they are not qualified to treat. The non-dangerous offender goes his way unnoticed and forgotten in the institution.

The attention paid to the civil rights of involuntarily confined persons has resulted in studies in greater depth of the sexual offender. The courts are becoming less punitive in the administration of the laws. Exhibitionism, for example, has come to be seen in many jurisdictions as not only not a dangerous offence but not even 'harmful' in this day and age and not warranting confinement. In some jurisdictions, psychiatric examination is ordered prior to a Court decision and judicial disposition is determined on the basis of such testimony. In other jurisdictions, the disposition is made prior to examination by a psychiatrist.

After two decades in which seemingly magical powers have often been attributed by many to the psychiatrist as having the ability to effect beneficial personality change, the lack of interest of psychiatrists in such problems has forced re-evaluation of these laws. Moreover this re-evaluation has extended to the limitations of psychiatry as an agent of change. There is increasing recognition that only a few such offenders suffer from definitive mental illness and that the greatest number belong in a group that is untreatable by either medical or criminal law measures.

The truth of the matter is that society, through its legislative and judicial systems, makes use of psychiatrists to avoid proper assumption of responsibility for more adequate procedures to deal with these persons. With the current emphasis on the constitutional rights of the individual, the Courts are being confronted with issues of disposition which will protect society from the dangerous sex offender and of new approaches for dealing with the non-dangerous offender. Other issues that are emerging include the right of protection of the law-abiding members of society and synthesis of rapidly changing public and private moralities.

HOSPITALIZATION OF PSYCHIATRIC PATIENTS

In the United States, hospitalization of the mentally ill person as a national institution dates from the middle of the eighteenth century with the establishment of 'asylums', usually for the poor. In legal matters, except for the intermission of a few years rapidly ending, the criminal and the mentally ill have been dealt with in similar fashion. This parallelism has its origin in the early statutes which were intended to provide for the custody of the dangerously insane. The statutes and procedures of the criminal trial were followed in dealing with them and the stigma of criminality has continued ever since, though evidence of change has been forthcoming recently. The statutes, the language and procedures relating to the hospitalization of psychiatric patients were based upon the corresponding criminal laws. Thus in varying jurisdictions, the mentally ill person may be arrested by a sheriff or policeman, charged before a judge, detained in jail, tried in open court before a jury, and committed and transported to a mental hospital by a representative of the law.

The widespread use of the jury in involuntary hospitalization arose in part from the Packard case in Illinois in 1860. Mrs E.P.W. Packard, wife of a minister who disagreed strongly with her husband on religious matters, was hospitalized involuntarily on the signature of her spouse. After her discharge, she claimed that she had been unjustly placed in the hospital and, as a result of her arousal of the public, the right to a jury trial was established in the State of Illinois. Later, Miss Dorothea Lynde Dix, in her crusade for improved care of the mentally ill, led a widely supported movement, resulting in the enactment of new statutes and/or the revision of the old statutes on commitment. Many of the statutes were designed to guard against wrongful detention rather than with adequate treatment and rehabilitation.

In the last two decades there has been a strong movement concerned more with effective therapy than with detention and custody. Increasing psychiatric knowledge and increasing acceptance of psychiatric illness as a disease process have led to a further revision of old statutes and the enactment of new ones in many jurisdictions. The first statute, providing for voluntary admission, was enacted in Massachusetts in 1881. By 1924, twenty-eight statutes provided for voluntary admission and by 1955 all States except Alabama permitted voluntary hospitalization. In the past decade many State legislatures have attempted to revise their legal codes in respect to hospitalization of the mentally ill and this process is very active in many States today. There is no consistent pattern, however, with regard to the statutes, the procedures, or the methods by which the mentally ill are admitted to hospital.

INFORMAL ADMISSION

A few States have enacted statutes permitting informal admission to a psychiatric hospital in the same manner as admission to a general hospital. The patient is admitted at the discretion of the superintendent, without requirement of a written request, and he may leave at any time he wishes. Some hospitals in these jurisdictions have attempted to secure some control over discharge by having the patient sign, at the time of admission, an agreement to abide by the rules of the hospital, including discharge at reasonable hours of the day.

VOLUNTARY ADMISSION

All States except Alabama provide for the voluntary admission on written application by the patient. More than thirty of the fifty States provide that the application may be made by the parent or guardian of a minor or the guardian of an incompetent.

Some five States specifically require that the patient be mentally competent to make application for his voluntary admission. There has been considerable discussion about the validity of the voluntary admission of an incompetent person but no test cases have arisen. The most usual opinion holds that a psychotically ill individual should not be denied the opportunity of treatment on a voluntary basis.

Most statutes dealing with voluntary admission provide that the patient be discharged within a definite number of days after he has requested it. In six States, the release is to take place 'forthwith' and in the other States, the period ranges from two to thirty days. In five States, the voluntary patient admits himself for a minimum period of time, thus yielding the right to be discharged before the end of the period.

INVOLUNTARY HOSPITALIZATION

It is very difficult to classify the procedures and statutes in the various jurisdictions. The classification in *The Mentally Disabled and the Law,* prepared by the American Bar Foundation,[31] divides these admission procedures into emergency, short-term (or observational) and extended term. In all three types, the statutory authority to confine may be judicial or nonjudicial, the latter being of two types, administrative and by medical certification.

Judicial hospitalization procedures are those in which the

determination of the need for hospitalization is made by a judge or jury. Administrative hospitalization is that in which the determination is made by a board on which may serve doctors, attorneys, and others. The procedures of such boards vary considerably, some having the power to conduct their own hearings, while other boards must present their findings to a judge.

Involuntary hospitalization by medical certification is the procedure in which a person is hospitalized on the basis of the certificate of one or more physicians. In some States, specific physicians are appointed as authorized examiners. In some jurisdictions, the certificates have to be verified by a judge as to signatures and qualifications of the certifiers.

Where a patient may be committed by medical certification, there are two different categories. In some jurisdictions, the confinement is compulsory even though the patient protests, while in eight States medical certification can be used only if the patient does not protest admission. In these States, a protesting patient must have a judicial hearing prior to confinement.

In many States, statutes providing for involuntary hospitalization authorize indeterminate detention while the illness persists, though there is an increasing trend to eliminate this kind of confinement.

There is no consistent pattern with regard to the statutory provisions relating to the formal application and who makes it, the pre-hearing medical examinations, the qualifications of the physician, the necessity for the patient to be notified of the hearing and conditions under which he will or may be present. The right to a trial by jury, the provision of legal counsel, and the notification to the patient of the determination also vary from jurisdiction to jurisdiction.

TEMPORARY HOSPITALIZATION

This method of hospitalization provides for the admission to hospital for observation and diagnosis for a specified period of time, after which the patient must be discharged or other methods of detention sought. The vast majority of the States now provide for this type of admission. The period during which the patient may be hospitalized under the order ranges as high as six months but there have been a number of suits, some successfully claiming that such deprivation of liberty without due process, that is, judicial determination, is unlawful and unconstitutional. As a consequence many State laws have been revised to reduce greatly the period of detention.

EMERGENCY DETENTION

All except thirteen States have statutory provision for the emergency detention of mentally ill persons who are dangerous to themselves or others. In some States, judicial approval is required; in others, the approval by the county commissioners; and in sixteen States, medical certification is sufficient. The minimum qualifications of physicians who may act under the above statutes are usually clearly laid down in order to protect the patient.

RECENT DEVELOPMENTS

In the United States there has been a strong movement towards emptying governmental hospitals of the hundreds of thousands of long-term patients. The emphasis has been on treatment 'in the community' with the drive to provide psychiatric and social services in the local area. The concept of the hospitalization of even the most disturbed patient is anathema to a few social psychiatrists and others of similar orientation but, generally, the developing attitudes with respect to psychiatric patients fall into two main categories. The first is that hospitalization in and of itself is wrong and justifiable only in very limited circumstances, with emphasis on 'dangerousness'. One aspect of this approach is that the civil rights of a patient must receive absolute priority as illustrated by a recent decision of the United States Court of Appeals for the District of Columbia. The Court ruled that formerly (that is, in that jurisdiction) juries were instructed in civil commitment proceedings that a person should be involuntarily committed if, 'by a preponderance of the evidence', the jury determined that person to be mentally ill and likely to be a danger to himself and/or others. The new ruling enunciated by the Court is that judges and juries must use the same 'beyond a reasonable doubt' standard as is applied in criminal proceedings.

The appellant in this case, Ballay *v.* United States,[32] was a man who approached the policemen at the United States Capitol and at the White House on three occasions, claiming *inter alia* to be a Senator from the State of Illinois and, on a latter occasion, to be President Nixon's son-in-law.

The Court held that the issues of the protection of society and the freedom of the individual were identical in civil commitment and criminal cases.

It is ironic that the reason the Court gave for this finding was that the stigma still attached to a person found mentally ill was equal to that of being a criminal. Since the stigma in the greatest degree arose in the first place because the mentally ill person was dealt with socially and legally as a criminal, one must ask whether society, as represented by the judges in this case in the very Court which promulgated the Durham Rule, has, indeed, turned a full circle. This is the Court which threw out the Durham Rule and established the standard of the American Law Institute Model Test which returned in large measure to McNaughton.

Increasing advocacy of the concept of treatment in the patient's local community, rather than in a mental hospital, has had a number of consequences, some far from desirable from the humanistic viewpoint. Politicians and administrators in governmental service have seized on this therapeutic principle to promote rapid evacuation of state mental hospitals by discharging thousands of long-term patients, many of whom, if not the vast majority, have lost all contact not only with their former local communities, but also with their relatives.

Under the guise of treating them in the community, thousands, especially those from the dehumanized large cities, such as New York and Chicago, are being placed—deposited is a better word—in single rooms in old and dilapidated hotels taken over by municipal authorities. There they remain completely withdrawn and neglected, without therapeutic supervision but having their civil rights to hallucinate all day without interference, and without the basic physical necessities which were at least provided when they were institutionalized mental hospital patients. Their miserable condition equals that which an aroused public about a hundred years ago tried to improve by building a network of hospitals.

But many public-minded individuals are becoming aware of the deplorable conditions in which the 'liberated' patients exist.

Of increasing public concern in a number of communities is the problem of premature discharge of dangerous patients who have subsequently committed criminal offences. It is to be anticipated that the reactions of citizens to this development will lead to a closer study of community psychiatry in practice as opposed to community psychiatry in theory.

THE COMPREHENSIVE COMMUNITY MENTAL HEALTH CENTER

In the past decade the major trends in the treatment of psychiatric patients have been in the direction of avoidance of hospitalization, management in the local community and emphasis on the solution of social and environmental problems confronting the patient as the principal curative and preventive approaches. Short-term hospitalization, where necessary, and the revolving door principle have been accepted by most persons in the field.

The community mental health center concept was originally embraced by President John F. Kennedy and the United States Congress which enacted Federal legislation to provide matching funds for the construction and staffing of such centers by local authorities. The long-term objective was to build a network of such centers covering the entire country. Each center was to have the capability of serving all persons in its catchment area, with an approximate limitation of 200,000 population per center.

Each center was to provide a minimum of five essential services: inpatient, outpatient, partial hospitalization, including day and night care, emergency services, and consultation to community agencies. Several other services were deemed desirable, including diagnostic, rehabilitative, pre-and post-hospital care, including foster home placement, home visiting, training, research and evaluation.

The Federal funds provided for construction must be matched by locally derived money, while staffing grants are on a declining basis over a ten-year period. 'Consumer' involvement in the establishment and in the operating of the center is essential in order to qualify. Over two hundred, and perhaps nearly three hundred, centers are in operation, while another two hundred are in various stages of development. But already disillusionment with the effectiveness of this large scale programme has set in. The provision of services has varied markedly from center to center. In many, there are few, if any, psychiatrists involved in providing services. Patients may pass through a center without even being seen by a physician. There has been strong criticism of the cost per unit of service. Many centers have developed into primarily social service organizations.

The Executive Branch of the Federal Government recently moved to cut off funding for new centers and the programme has become a political and, indeed, a constitutional issue in the Congress. While some centers are, indeed, operating at an acceptable level of effectiveness, many others are not. In fact, this programme is one which is involved in a constitutional dispute between the President and Congress which may be resolved only by the United States Supreme Court.

The future of many, if not the majority, of community mental health centers is in doubt because the financial resources necessary to make up for the scheduled declining Federal support call for local funding, a far from popular proposal.

The original concept of these centers was based on the philosophy that communities would support local services which were essentially psychiatrically, *i.e.* medically, oriented. The directions in which so many of these facilities have proceeded, together with the lack of community economic support for them and the impact of the emptying of the State hospitals, raise serious questions regarding the future provision of psychiatric services for very large segments of the population.

THE RIGHT TO TREATMENT

The resurgence of public and political interest in the condition of the mentally ill during the past twenty-five years demonstrated a concern comparable to that which abounded in the last half of the nineteenth century. At that time, the public was aroused about the degrading conditions endured by the mentally ill, especially the indigent, in the community. As a result, the majority of the States built and staffed public mental hospitals to provide both humane care and treatment.

Over the years, however, and in part as an offshoot of the waves of immigration into the United States near the end of the last century, these hospitals were increased in number and size but not proportionately to the need to provide adequate treatment. As happens with all popular movements, public interest gradually waned, especially as more and more tax moneys were required to maintain them. Consequently, with the exception of a few facilities, the typical public mental hospital became a grossly overcrowded, inadequately staffed and, usually, deteriorated institution.

Immediately after World War II, a group of psychiatrists, as a result of their experience in the Armed Forces, started a movement to alert the profession and the country to the inadequacies of medical treatment and facilities for the mentally ill. Forming a new association, the Group for the Advancement of Psychiatry,[33] they aroused the interest of the public and politicians on the State and Federal levels. The National Institute of Mental Health was brought into being by Congress in 1947. Citizen groups developed across the nation and became politically influential. At first, attention was addressed to improving the mental hospitals. But even greatly increased expenditures could do little to rapidly ameliorate the deplorable conditions.

Political action proving inadequate, the next approach was through the legal system. Suits were initiated against a number of States on the basis that involuntary commitment without the provision of adequate treatment was in fact a deprivation of liberty without due process. A constitutional right to treatment was claimed for patients committed to governmental institutions. This 'right' was first advocated in 1960 by Dr Morton Birnbaum, a lawyer-physician, though not himself a psychiatrist.

The earlier suits were on an individual-by-individual basis, usually on a writ of habeas corpus. More recently, these suits are 'class actions' in which a legal action is taken on behalf of one individual and the class of all other persons who suffer similarly to him. Originally class action suits were used on behalf of persons with legitimate but small financial claims who lacked the economic resources to pursue their rights, unless several individual suits were merged into one action. The class action suit has become a major legal tool of civil rights and 'public interest' organizations in the field of mental health.

The first important decision with respect to the right to treatment was Rouse *v.* Cameron[34] in which the Court of Appeals for the District of Columbia, in a split decision, ruled that a person judged not guilty by reason of insanity could not be incarcerated without adequate treatment being provided. The Court declared that 'the purpose of involuntary hospitalization is treatment, not punishment'. In the absence of the former, such confinement was held to amount to punishment.

Whereas this case applied to one individual in one type of situation, the first class action with respect to the right to treatment was that of Wyatt *v.* Stickney (1971),[35] on behalf of patients committed under civil statutes to the State hospitals in Alabama, which was taken to the United States District Court of Appeals. The judge ruled that patients involuntarily hospitalized in Alabama were being deprived of a constitutional right to adequate treatment and gave the State government a period of time to effect improvements. After failure of the State of Alabama to institute these, the judge himself set forth standards for minimal staffing patterns, physical facilities and the provision of adequate care.

In the second case, Burnham *v.* Georgia (1972),[36] identical to the Alabama case in all respects, that Court reached the opposite conclusion, namely that such a constitutional (that is, Federally protected) right did not exist, despite a 'right to treatment' statute enacted by the 1969 Georgia General Assembly. Both cases are being appealed and will doubtlessly go to the United States Supreme Court. Though confined at present to two of the fifty States, a decision by the Supreme Court in favour of a constitititutional right to adequate treatment would have far-reaching consequences, not only on the practices in governmental hospitals throughout the country but also on the financial resources of poverty-stricken States such as Alabama and Mississippi.

Right to treatment actions have been instituted with respect to four classes of patients involuntarily confined in governmental institutions: those committed as mentally ill under civil statutes, those found 'not guilty by reason of insanity', those confined by reason or 'not competent to stand trial' and the mentally retarded. Significant improvements have already been effected in those jurisdictions where the class actions have been successful.

CIVIL RIGHTS OF THE PATIENT

Because those citizens who are interested in the mental health field tend to be drawn from the segments of society concerned with humanity and the rights of the individual, it is inevitable that there has been great activity in the halls of the Courts and of the State legislatures. In most States, there is statutory provision for patients to contest their commitment, often with the automatic appointment of a *guardian ad litem.* In some, the patient may request a jury trial which may be held at the discretion of the judge, while in others the patient's request makes mandatory such a trial.

Under the Constitution of the United States, all persons, including patients, have the right to petition at any time for a writ of habeas corpus, though, in actual practice, this has been rarely sought. As noted above, there is a trend to view the commitment of a mentally ill person as exactly comparable to the incarceration of a criminal. In many States, patients have had few rights but the tenor of the times has led to the enactment of statutes delineating very specifically the individual rights of a patient. These include visitation by an attorney, clergyman, physician or friend of the patient's choice. In some States, the patient is now guaranteed the use of a public telephone. Censorship of mail is prohibited. Laws have been passed guaranteeing the patient the right to privacy, to wear his own clothing, to have his own money and property and to transact business while confined.

Some States have enacted laws which permit patients, hospitalized either voluntarily or involuntarily, to refuse treatment whether by mouth, by injection, or by other somatic procedures. In the case of involuntary patients, authorization for such treatment must be obtained from the nearest of kin, the committing judge or legally appointed guardian. Limitations have been placed on the seclusion and isolation of patients, with documentation and submission of such reports to the State mental health authority required. Some statutes are so written that in order to deal with disturbed, dangerous and assaultive patients, even the minimal measures would be strictly against statutory law, though, in practice, they can be managed under common law principles. While there has been some distress amongst the personnel of many State hospitals, nevertheless, the enactment of these rights of patients has undoubtedly led to far better care and treatment.

This emphasis on the rights of patients is to be seen in a recent document produced by the American Hospital Association, the vast majority of whose members are general hospitals serving the medical and surgical needs of their communities. In this document is laid down the responsibility of the institution, affirming the rights of patients to respectful care and to complete current information concerning his diagnosis, treatment and prognosis in terms he can be reasonably expected to understand.

This latest 'right', and most troublesome from the viewpoint of the physician, which has been afforded to patients by court decision, is that of 'informed consent'.

INFORMED CONSENT

A major cause for distress among physicians and hospitals has been the increasing number of malpractice suits and the sizes of awards made, some over one million dollars. So troublesome has this problem become that many insurance companies have withdrawn from offering this form of coverage; even Lloyds of London, which will insure against bad weather, has become cautious in accepting medical risks in the United States.

While the psychiatrist's exposure to malpractice suits has dropped significantly with the great reduction in the use of electroshock, he does suffer in that, as a physician, he is included in the actuarial calculations. Even though the use of electroshock has fallen off, there has been increasing exposure as the use of psychopharmacological agents has grown and, more particularly, as the long-term side effects, such as tardive dyskinesia, have become evident.

One effect of the drive on the civil rights' front for the protection of the individual has been the emphasis on the 'informed consent' of the patient to accept treatment recommended or prescribed by his physician. As the result of experience, for example, no wise surgeon would venture into the operating room without first having explained the possible risks, denied a guarantee of success and having the patient attest his consent in writing.

For psychiatrists the most common circumstances are the administration of electroshock treatment and the prescription of potent medication. The Federal Government requires pharmaceutical manufacturers to detail on package inserts all the possible undesirable side-effects which the drug may provoke. The psychiatrist, when prescribing, must alert the patient, already emotionally distressed, to these possible consequences and is faced with the problem of how much to tell.

In an attempt to set forth guidelines, the Supreme Court of California, in a landmark decision[37] on the question of informed consent, attempted to define the duty of the physician to inform the patient of the available alternatives in treatment and the dangers involved, both in the absence of therapy and with each alternative. The Court ruled that by 'reasonable disclosure' a physician must tell the patient everything that he needs to know in order to make an intelligent decision. Until recently, the general medical criterion throughout the country has been the standards of practice in the local community. This is no longer applicable. One clause in the guidelines is particularly ambiguous; a physician could not be held liable if he 'can prove by a preponderance of the evidence that he relied upon facts which would demonstrate to a reasonable man the disclosure would have so seriously upset the patient that the patient would not have been able dispassionately to weigh the risks of refusing to undergo the recommended treatment'. Because of the subjectivity of individual judgment, this standard may be impossible to meet.

In one particular area of psychiatry there has been widespread public debate in the news media, including papers, radio and television. This is the use of psychosurgery. While probably only about 500 to 600 such procedures are performed a year, the outcry against such treatment by a few vocal opponents has aroused considerable discussion, all based on underlying fears of the uses to which psychosurgery might be put.

Minority groups such as Negroes are fearful that lobotomy may be used as a political weapon of social control. The extreme civil libertarians see the procedure as irreversibly changing the person. The ordinary man identifies his very essence as residing in the brain and reacts in response to his fears of loss of himself. Parallels with the experimentation by the Germans in the nineteen-forties are drawn by some.

Underlying fears in the American culture become obvious by analysis of the presentations by the media. No distinction is made between ethical research and irresponsible experimentation on humans. The emotional distress about such procedures reflects the recent opposition to, or at least questioning of, the established order but probably has its origin in the basic history and traditions of the United States, namely, that the nation was founded on the overthrow of an authoritarian and controlling government.

The present fear of psychosurgery as a form of social control is also intensified by the publicity given to new technology now available. Some neurosurgeons have been conducting research by creating lesions in the amygdala to obviate or control violent behaviour in patients with uncontrolled impulses. Considerable media coverage has also been given to behaviour control as advocated by B. F. Skinner[38] and to behaviour modification as a psychiatric and psychological procedure. These factors, together with the emphasis on the rights of the individual, have combined to keep the controversy alive. In fact, legislation to prohibit psychosurgery has been introduced in the U.S. Congress.

In a recent landmark decision,[39] a Michigan Court of Appeals has ruled that a person, involuntarily confined under civil or criminal statutes, is incapable of giving valid informed consent to submit to a high-risk, low-benefit psychosurgical procedure because of the not-so-intangible factor of coercive influence. While the narrowness of the circumstances to which the legal decision applies has been lost in the nationwide coverage of it in the media, it almost certainly eliminates future research, using committed patients or prisoners as subjects.

CONFIDENTIALITY AND PRIVILEGE

A physician who examines and treats a patient thereby enters into a legal contract with him. In addition to the ethics of his profession he is under a legal obligation to maintain the confidentiality of the transactions between the parties. A breach of this right of privacy may constitute a tort, and certainly a lawsuit, if the patient believes he has been injured by such disclosure.

Because of the social attitudes towards emotional illness and mentally ill persons, the psychiatrist is in an especially vulnerable situation if he, without authorization, discloses information. There has been one action in which a psychiatrist was held liable through the act of sending his unpaid accounts to a collection agency. It has been held that a psychiatrist cannot, without authorization, provide information regarding a patient's illness to anyone, including an insurance company which is processing a claim by the patient.

It is now a cardinal rule that written authorization for the release of information or records be obtained from a patient, present or past, before any information is supplied to third parties.

In legal and court proceedings, both criminal and civil, a psychiatrist may be subpoenaed and forced to testify concerning a patient involved in litigation. This common law principle still rules in England, whence it came, and in many jurisdictions, State and Federal, in the United States. Only the lawyer-client relationship is privileged under common law and extension of this privilege to other relationships, such as priest-penitent or doctor-patient, must be enacted by the State legislatures and by the U.S. Congress in Federal jurisdictions.

In a number of States the importance of the confidential relationship between physician and patient has been recognized by the passage of special legislation, giving to the patient the privilege of preventing a physician who has treated him being forced to testify against the patient's wishes. The principle under which privilege is enacted is that a greater public good accrues when mentally ill persons are encouraged to seek treatment which would not be sought if privilege did not exist, than the public good which would be achieved if a psychiatrist could be compelled to reveal information conveyed to him in the therapeutic relationship.

This privilege, where it exists, belongs to the patient, not the physician. The physician has no right to refuse to testify if the patient waives his privilege. But, once a patient waives his privilege, the physician is obliged to testify as to all knowledge he has acquired in the patient-doctor relationship. The doctor may not edit his evidence.

When a patient introduces in Court the question of his own mental state he automatically waives privilege (if it exists under the laws of that State). Although privilege exists for the patients of all physicians in a few States and although great opposition to this privilege has been interposed by special interests, such as lawyers and insurance companies, a number of State legislature have enacted statutes giving privilege to patients of psychiatrists, though not other physicians. The right of privilege has been extended to patients of psychotherapists in a number of these States which have enacted laws licensing psychologists to treat patients by psychotherapy. One State has extended privilege to patients of psychologists but not psychiatrists, on the premise presumably that only psychologists treat patients by psychotherapy. The statutes in each particular State (where privilege exists) vary so widely that it is necessary to be alert to the exact situation in a particular jurisdiction. Some statutes give complete privilege, while in other States varying exceptions are included.

Almost universally, however, when a person charged with a crime is sent by a Court to a mental hospital for psychiatric examination, such examinations are not privileged, but the psychiatrist may not testify regarding communications which bear on the the alleged crime itself. This issue has become a sensitive one with some attorneys of defendants demanding the right to be present during the psychiatric examination. Even when the Court so orders, the psychiatrist who agrees to co-operate is a rarity.

A vast majority of the citizens of the United States probably believe, erroneously, that confidential communications by a patient to a psychiatrist are always privileged. Even in those jurisdictions where privilege has been enacted, only confidential information given in a diagnostic or therapeutic relationship is so privileged. Information given during a psychiatric examination for other purposes may not be protected.

A growing segment of psychiatrists in the United States have argued in favour of the privilege being given to the psychiatrist rather than, or as well as, to the patient. They argue that the patient when waiving his privilege cannot possibly know how damaging to his case might be the testimony of the psychiatrist.

These conflicting views are at issue at the present time. In a recent case in California,[40] a psychiatrist claimed the privilege for himself. Although the patient, who was involved in civil legal proceedings, had authorized the psychiatrist who had treated him years before to testify, the physician refused to do so. The case was appealed to the California Supreme Court which ruled against the psychiatrist but laid down guidelines with respect to the psychiatric evidence that a psychiatrist might be forced to give.

There is also another important arena in which there is controversy on this issue. The Rules of Evidence in Federal Courts are enacted by Congress which has requested the U.S. Supreme Court to make recommendations for revisions. Among the recommendations is one to abolish the current privilege for patients of all physicians, which is limited by a number of exceptions. Of interest is the recommendation that privilege be extended to 'psychotherapists' who are not psychiatrists. But, for the first time, appears the recommendation that psychotherapists be given the right to claim privilege on behalf of the patient. This would represent a very substantive change in the law.

On the other hand, the Sub-committee of Congress, also studying revisions of the Rules, is advocating complete abolition of all privilege in criminal cases, except as provided by common law, *i.e.* in the attorney-client relationship, and in civil cases granting privilege as enacted by the State in which the civil action originates.

THE PSYCHIATRIST AS A WITNESS

A psychiatrist may be called upon to testify in two capacities: the first as a witness of fact and the second as an expert expressing his professional opinion.

The psychiatrist is a witness of fact when he functions in the capacity of an ordinary citizen. He may, for example, have been an observer of an automobile accident and his testimony is similar to that of any other observer—recounting what he saw. He may also be called to testify with respect to medical facts relating to a patient whom he has examined or treated. In this role, he does not give, nor can he be forced in most States to give, an opinion or interpretation based on his examination.

The second role is as an expert who, by his training, knowledge and experience, is qualified to express a professional opinion. A psychiatrist or other expert cannot be compelled, in most jurisdictions, to express an opinion if he is called, by subpoena, to testify as to facts. In jurisdictions in which the patient does not possess the right of privileged communication the psychiatrist may be compelled to disclose all he knows, *i.e.* 'facts' about the patient, including those learned in the therapeutic relationship.

When a psychiatrist testifies as an expert he is entitled to a full professional fee; when he is a witness of fact he is entitled only to the ordinary witness fee. Financial arrangements should be clearly made prior to appearance in Court. In the event of conflict about fees when subpoenaed, the expert should advise the Court that he has been called as a witness of fact and not as an expert witness. It is important that the matter of fees be clearly established for another pressing reason. An expert expresses his professional opinion as an objective evaluation; he does not appear as a protagonist for either side. Thus a psychiatrist should never agree to be a witness paid on a contingency fee basis. In personal injury actions, it is wise to have fees agreed upon in advance of the trial. All reputable attorneys are willing to engage the services of an expert of this basis.

The psychiatrist as an expert witness is paid for his time, including that devoted to the study of documents or medical books, conferences prior to the court proceedings, as well as that devoted to his examination and writing of the report. He also includes time spent in Court on a portal-to-portal basis. His fee is calculated on the basis of his customary fee.

When requested to conduct a psychiatric examination the physician should obtain as much information as possible about the clinical condition of the individual. He should devote enough time to obtain a complete clinical picture and should be prepared to have as many interviews as are required. Interviews with other persons who know the individual may be appropriate.

The report should be comprehensive, detailing all pertinent findings, and phrased in clear language intelligible to the educated layman. Diagnosis and conclusions arrived at should be concisely expressed. As a witness the psychiatrist should be ready to elaborate on his findings and opinion, using language which can be understood by the jury.

In civil actions, including will contests and personal injury suits, the psychiatrist may be asked to give an opinion in respect to an individual whom he has never examined. In this situation, he is presented with the so-called 'hypothetical question'. In some jurisdictions even if he has examined and/or *treated* the individual, he may be obliged to give his opinion on the basis of information presented to him, on the witness stand, in the form of the hypothetical question. This question commences with the phrase, 'Assuming that. . .' and then contains all the pertinent information (selected by the attorney) which has already been introduced into evidence and on which the psychiatrist may base an opinion. After hearing the information the psychiatrist is asked, 'Do you have an opinion?'. On answering in the affirmative he then presents his opinion—based on only the information in the question—and is examined by the counsel calling him and cross-examined by counsel for the opposing party.

Since the attorneys on each side choose to include only information favourable to their cases, it is readily apparent that differing opinions may be reached by psychiatrists appearing on the opposite sides.

The hypothetical question is framed by the attorney who, prior to the trial, obtains the necessary data from the psychiatrist and tries to ensure that the necessary information is introduced into evidence. Opposing attorneys may attempt, on cross-examination, to unsettle expert witnesses, such as psychiatrists, by asking questions implying prior collusional conferences with the attorney who asked the hypothetical question. It should be emphasized that such conferences by an attorney with a witness prior to testimony are part of the ordinary and proper preparation of the witness.

One of the most unedifying aspects of forensic psychiatry is the so-called 'battle of the experts' in which are seen two or more psychiatrists, on opposing sides, presenting testimony which appears to be biased to the side by which the expert has been called. Sometimes these contradictions arise from the application of the Rules of Evidence, for example, pertaining to the formulation of the hypothetical question, which encourage the development of adversary positions. Often, however, the differences appear to arise from conscious or unconscious identification on the part of the psychiatrist with the party which 'employs' him. The expert should be alert to this natural tendency and must always realize that his role is that of an impartial expert, presenting objective opinions and conclusions, irrespective of the party for whom he appears. The psychiatrist is under an obligation to inform the attorney who calls him of the nature of the testimony he will present.

BRIGGS LAW

A number of solutions have been proposed to eliminate this conflict. Usually the solutions are different versions of the proposal that the Court itself appoint independent and neutral experts who report to the Court. Lawyers voice strong objections to this procedure, the strongest being that an accused is entitled to present all the evidence which will favour him. One attempt of considerable merit, which has achieved noteworthy success, is the Briggs Law in Massachusetts.

Passed in 1921, the Briggs Law provides that, when a person is indicted for a capital offence, or has been previously convicted of a felony, or has been indicted for any offence on two or more occasions, the Department of Mental Health must be notified. The Department than appoints psychiatrists to examine the accused to determine whether there is 'any mental disease or defect which would affect his criminal responsibility'. Copies of the reports are forwarded to the Court and to the prosecuting and defence counsels. The psychiatrists may be called by either side to testify in respect to their examinations and opinions. This procedure has been successful in no small part because a psychiatrist called by one side only will appear to be biased.

A few attempts have been made in other jurisdictions to establish panels of 'neutral' psychiatrists who volunteer to examine referred litigants, but utilization of such experts depends on agreement between opposing counsel.

TESTAMENTARY CAPACITY

The mental competency of a testator is not infrequently a

question which arises in contests involving wills. In most will contests, the deceased had not been examined by a psychiatrist, either as a patient or as part of the process in drawing up the will. Consequently, a psychiatrist may be called upon to give an expert opinion without having had thc opportunity of making direct professional observations. His conclusions must be reached on the basis of indirect evidence. The legal test of the validity of a will revolves on the following issues:

1. The individual must know the nature and extent of his property.
2. He must be cognizant of the persons who have a natural claim on his bounty.
3. His judgment and will must be so unclouded and free as to enable him to evaluate the relative strengths of these claims.
4. The testator must appreciate the nature and effect of his act.
5. He must be of full age and of sound disposing mind.
6. The will must be executed in due form.

Having a sound disposing mind is the same as possessing testamentary capacity, and the first four parts of the test provide the key questions to be answered by the psychiatrist.

The degree of knowledge of the testator is not a fixed criterion of competency. It is not necessary that the testator be able to enumerate in detail all his property. With regard to the degree of recall necessary, a large and diverse estate would require less detailed knowledge compared with one involving only a small amount of property. It is sufficient that the individual be aware of the nature and extent of the majority of his possessions. Moreover, the individual may not know the exact value of some of his assets. For example, an elderly person who has for many years owned real estate in a metropolitan area may not be aware that its value may have appreciated many times its original cost, yet he may be able to define the property accurately. Further, it is not expected that an individual should be able to recall without assistance the nature and extent of all his property. Similarly, the elderly person with memory deficits may not be able to enumerate all those who are the natural objects of his bounty. It is sufficient if, with prompting, he recognizes them as potential recipients. The testator must be aware of what he is doing and of the fact that he is determining the distribution of his estate, on his death, to particular persons.

The nature of the will may raise important questions with regard to the testator's mental state, especially when one or more of the objects of his bounty is excluded completely or is given a disproportionately small inheritance in comparison with others. Evaluation of his judgment, the clarity of his sensorium and the validity of his reasons become deciding factors.

In evaluating testamentary capacity it is wise to review the whole life of the individual, noting his lifelong patterns and any changes which have occurred in recent years, with special attention to the period in which the will was drawn. The psychiatrist should attempt to obtain as much information as possible from family members, business associates, friends and others who have had opportunities to observe him; for example, his personal physician. Information regarding alterations in attention to his affairs, to his personal care and in his interpersonal relationships should be sought. Lifelong eccentricity often has no significance whatsoever in relation to his business capacity.

Additional information may be obtained from samples of handwriting, letters, etc., and the will itself. The writing, evidence of tremors, spelling errors inconsistent with prior standards and syntactical structure may be significant. The complexity of the will may be of importance, since an individual requires a lesser degree of capacity to make a simple will compared with a complicated one.

The psychiatrist should be particularly concerned with the presence or absence of delusions, especially those of a paranoid nature directed against anyone who has a moral claim on the estate. Sometimes pathological antagonism and resentment do not reach obvious psychotic proportions and, superficially, good reasons may have seemed to justify the hostility. Very careful evaluation of the factual basis of these ideas should be made. Common delusions include those in which particular relatives have been waiting for him to die in order to obtain his money or have been actually plotting against him. When the sole or major beneficiary is an unusual one, an underlying delusion may have existed.

In the case of persons who have lived with one relative or other close person, the question of 'undue influence' may arise. The senile individual, for example, may in his dependency become quite suggestible, yielding to the wishes of those whom he feels have devoted themselves to him, or he may be easily deceived by false stories about others who are natural objects of his bounty, or he may yield to the wishes of a dominant relative or to the flattery of others.

Irrespective of apparent unfairness, the Courts are most reluctant to interfere with a will unless it can be shown that it is frivolous, fickle or malicious. If it can be shown to be the real intent of the testator, it is valid. The criteria with regard to delusions were well expressed in 1870 by Lord Chief Justice Cockburn (who had defended Daniel McNaughton):

> No disorder of the mind shall poison the affections, pervert his sense of right, nor prevent the exercise of his natural faculties; that no insane delusion shall influence his will in disposing of his property and bring about a disposal of it which, if the mind had been sound, would not have been made.

It is an interesting observation that McNaughton held sway where life and death were at stake but the Product Rule reigned when property was involved.

CONTRACTS

The question of mental capacity to enter into a contract is sometimes raised in litigation. The law requires that a person entering into a contract shall do so with full knowledge of the meaning of the contract and with due deliberation of the terms of the agreement. The consent of both parties shall be free and complete.

Problems may also arise when one of the parties subsequently is unable or unwilling to fulfill the contract, especially when an overt mental illness develops. A contract made by an incompetent mentally ill person is void and non-enforceable. A contract made by a person who subsequently becomes mentally ill, and who is unable thereby to fulfill the terms, may be voidable. However, a full restitution of any loss suffered by the other party must be made. Just as a person cannot legally gain by a criminal act, a mentally ill person may not benefit by his act.

The abrogation or the enforcement of the terms of a contract often is dependent on how easily the original position of the aggrieved complainant can be restored without any loss or sacrifice on his part.

A mentally ill person, including one who has been committed to a psychiatric hospital, may be capable of executing documents and entering into legal contracts, such as the sale or the transfer of property. As a precaution, it is advisable that a psychiatrist be requested to examine the person to evaluate, and certify to, his competency to conduct the transaction. The criteria to be used are that the patient understand the nature and effect of the act, the nature and extent of his property, be of clear mind and reason with respect to the proposed act, and that he be not motivated in the transaction by delusional ideas or by irrational emotions which are symptomatic of his illness.

A contract entered into by an incompetent mentally ill person is, nevertheless, enforceable on him in the case of 'necessaries'. These include those objects such as food, clothing and housing which have been supplied to the individual and which constitute necessities appropriate to his particular station in society. The Court must decide what constitutes 'necessaries' which include expenses incurred in taking care of the patient.

Problems may also arise in the case of persons who recover from an attack of mental illness and subsequently relapse. The legal rule is that a contract entered into in a lucid period or interval is a valid instrument, enforceable unless the illness renders the patient unable to fulfill it.

TORTS

A tort is an action resulting in injury to another person, whether physical or economic, or to his reputation, for which redress may be obtained by a legal civil suit. A mentally ill person, including the committed patient, or, in the case of a declared incompetent, the estate, may be liable for torts to other persons. Even if the patient were incapable of criminal intent he may still be subject to a civil action. In some cases, however, the lack of capacity, arising out of mental illness, may be a partial defence, especially when no great damage has resulted from the wrongful act.

In certain situations the responsible relative, for example the father, may be held financially liable for the tort of a mentally ill person.

GUARDIANSHIP AND INCOMPETENCY

A person who develops a mental illness may become unable to care adequately for himself or his property. As indicated above, a psychotic person may be able to negotiate legal instruments, effect transfer of property, etc., even when committed to a psychiatric hospital. Such an individual may be able to manage his affairs competently. When, however, he becomes unable to perform these obligations, the laws provide for the appointment of others to assume such responsibilities. Such persons are named variously: guardians, conservators or committees. The particular term used varies according to the legal terminology in the different State statutes.

There are two different types of guardianship. A guardian, conservator or committee of the estate is a person appointed by the appropriate Court to be responsible for the management of the individual's business and financial affairs. A corporation, such as a bank, may be appointed guardian of the estate. A guardian, conservator or committee of the person is charged with the duty of looking after the incompetent's person or making suitable arrangements for someone to do this. A guardian must submit to the Court, usually annually, an accounting of his stewardship. Major financial transactions require direct authorization by the Court.

Most modern psychiatric thinking supports strongly the position that Court hearings in regard to commitment to hospital and to the appointment of a guardian of the estate should be separated. Unfortunately, in a number of States such hearings are combined, while in others commitment automatically is a declaration of incompetency, resulting in unnecessary distress, diminution of personal dignity and subsequent difficulties when the patient recovers.

When a patient who has been declared incompetent recovers from the mental illness and wishes to be restored to full control of his property, it is necessary for him to apply to the Court for termination of the guardianship. Procedures are similar to those for the adjudication of incompetency. One, or more, psychiatrist is required to examine the individual in order to determine his opinion as to the competency of the individual. The same criteria are utilized as in the prior examination. The statement by the psychiatrist is sometimes referred to as a 'certificate of sanity'.

MARRIAGE AND DIVORCE

Marriage is, in the eyes of the law, a form of contract and the same considerations are applicable. A marriage by an incompetent mentally ill person is null and void. The criteria to be used in forming an opinion are the capacity of the individual to appreciate the nature of the marriage contract, to understand the obligations imposed under it and the ability to carry them out. The degree of understanding necessary for competency to enter into a valid marriage is probably the least demanding of all contracts.

In the vast majority of States mental illness is not grounds for divorce and, indeed, is a barrier to it. Normally, the usual grounds for divorce, such as desertion, cruelty or adultery, are not sufficient reasons if committed by a psychotic spouse.

In a few jurisdictions mental illness to the degree of psychosis is a basis for divorce with a variety of attached conditions. A duration of insanity for a minimum period of years, usually three to five, is required, together with medical evidence that the insane spouse is suffering from an incurable mental disease. In States where mental illness is cause for divorce, it is usually not a necessary condition that the ill spouse be hospitalized the full period.

In practice, psychiatrists are faced with two types of problems. The first is to swear that the person is incurable. With the increasing knowledge of the life history of mental illnesses and with the effectiveness of new forms of therapy, many have reluctance to make such declarations. The best guide is the use of the criterion: on the basis of present knowledge and of the failure of the treatment of the patient hitherto, is it reasonably certain that this particular patient is incurable?

The other problem for psychiatrists arises when the spouse develops an overt psychotic illness after divorce proceedings have been started. If the actions of the defendant spouse were symptoms of the incipient illness, technically the grounds for divorce may disappear.

While a mentally ill committed person often loses the civil right to sue for divorce, others may act for and on his behalf.

A new development in some States is the enactment of laws which remove many or all the conditions which hitherto have constituted the basis for divorce. In their place is the simple condition that the marriage has irretrievably broken down. In most of these laws, there is a stipulation that a sincere attempt be first made to mend the ruptured marital relationship through consultation with mental health professionals.

Nevertheless, the position of the psychiatrist in divorce and custody actions is often a difficult one in many jurisdictions, especially when the issue of divorce has not arisen until after the patient has started treatment. Unless the State statutes provide the patient with privilege, the psychiatrist perforce must often testify in a way damaging to his patient's case.

ABORTION

In January, 1973, the United States Supreme Court handed down a landmark decision in two cases, Roe *v.* Wade, Texas,[41] and Doe *v.* Bolton, Georgia,[42] in which was contested the right of a State to prohibit an abortion except as a life-saving measure. The Court held that the concept of personal liberty in the Fourteenth Amendment of the Constitution of the United States covered a woman's 'right to privacy' and her decision to terminate her pregnancy.

However, the Court upheld the legitimate interests of a State in safeguarding the health of the pregnant woman and in protecting the potentiality of human life. Thus, at some point in the pregnancy each of these interests becomes sufficiently 'compelling' to sustain State regulation of the factors governing the decision for abortion.

Accordingly, the Court decided that this point occurred at the end of the first trimester. Up to this time, the State may make no regulation except to provide that the abortion be performed by a physician. From the end of the first trimester until commencement of the 'viability' of the foetus, *i.e.* from the 24th to the 28th week, the State may regulate the procedures to the extent of protecting maternal health but may not prohibit the abortion. In the period of viability the State may fully regulate and prohibit abortion except when necessary to preserve the life or health of the mother.

Moreover, a State requirement of approval of abortion by a hospital committee or by two or more concurring physicians was declared unconstitutional. Removal of this requirement, which previously had resulted in psychiatrists participating in most abortion decisions, has relieved such physicians of the responsibility to legitimatize the procedure. In the future the psychiatrist will be as much concerned with the decision as to whether abortion is not indicated as he will be in recommending it. Since the psychiatric indications and contraindications with respect to abortion have long been unresolved, such decisions will continue to be made more by the personal orientation of the psychiatrist than by his scientific knowledge. In order to respect the religious convictions of those opposed to abortion, State statutes regulating this procedure now specifically include a conscience clause which protects hospitals which prohibit this procedure and hospital employees who refuse to participate in it or in the care of the patient.

The medical attitude to intervention has moved rapidly towards a more liberal approach. Psychiatrists as a group, more than other specialists, are apt to take a humanitarian attitude and to recommend termination more readily. The general indications for abortion on psychiatric grounds include the presence of a serious mental illness attributable to the pregnancy, the continuation of which would maintain or intensify the illness. Consideration is given to the probability that continuation of the pregnancy would result in the irreversibility of the mental illness or to the development of a post-partum psychosis. Some psychiatrists also take into consideration the potential injury to a child who would be reared by a grossly pathological mother. One of the considerations which arises is whether a post-abortion psychosis might occur should interruption of the pregnancy be therapeutically induced.

The incidence of psychosis due to such intervention is uncertain. The statistical studies which have been published are inconclusive.[43,44] Some psychiatrists still hold that patients who would react with strong guilt feelings are liable to develop mental illnesses following abortion, while others assert that the few women who do so are extremely vulnerable to any severe stress. They maintain that the continuation of pregnancy would in all probability have precipitated the mental illness or that psychosis would have ensued following normal parturition.

The evidence available suggests that women who develop puerperal psychosis tend to have unstable personalities and are subject to the precipitation of a mental illness with any comparable stress.[45] There is frequently some evidence of extreme dependency of the husband and ambivalence to the unborn child with fear of inability to take on maternal responsibilities. One study has shown that there are no apparent differences between psychoses associated with pregnancy and those not so associated, with the exception that the symptomatic content in the former may relate to the pregnancy. The interpretations of these findings vary. On the one hand they are taken to imply that the pregnancy has little to do with the aetiology of the illness, and on the other that the mental content of the symptomatology of the illness indicates that the pregnancy plays a significant role in the causation of the condition.

The prognosis regarding psychosis during pregnancy varies, depending on the author, and ranges from 50 per cent to 86 per cent favourable. There is some evidence that patients suffering from schizophrenia have a less favourable outlook than those who exhibit other forms of psychiatric disorders. A previous history of post-partum psychosis does not necessarily indicate the development of a subsequent one. An early study has led one author to the conclusion that there are no definite psychiatric indications for a therapeutic abortion,[46] while more recent investigations report low or no incidence of psychosis in series of women who had been aborted.

The threat of suicide raises considerable concern but is, in fact, a very unreliable diagnostic indicator. For obvious reasons the thought of suicide as an escape from an intolerable situation is a frequent accompaniment of an unwanted pregnancy. Few women, however, convert this thought into action. Severe depressive reactions may occur during pregnancy with suicidal attempts. On rare occasions, a severe schizophrenic reaction occurs, with attempts to injure the foetus as well as the mother herself. Threats of suicide, however, are rarely carried into action before or after the birth of the child.

At the present stage of knowledge it is difficult to take a scientifically strong position about the medical merits or demerits of the psychiatric indications for the termination of pregnancy. The underlying personal attitudes and beliefs of the psychiatrist are as likely to influence his decision as much as the clear-cut medical indications. Therapeutic abortion is becoming more and more a reflection of social trends, especially within the educated segments of the population, and it behoves the physician to be clear in his own mind about the real motivations in arriving at recommendations.

STERILIZATION

The issue of performing sterilization at the same time that a therapeutic abortion is carried out has arisen in a number of cases which have received considerable notoriety. Most of these cases have involved young women who are mentally retarded or who are regarded as social liabilities, having a history of promiscuity, multiple pregnancies by different fathers, and being maintained on the public welfare roles. As in most medico-legal situations today, the issues are far more related to constitutional and legal rights than to the medical aspects of the patient. With recent changes in statutes, the majority of States now have a provision for eugenic sterilization. The statutes vary from permitting sterilization for convenience to expressly prohibiting it for this reason. It is interesting to note that the sterilization of the male is not prohibited in any State. The biggest problems confronting medical decisions with regard to sterilization arise out of the question of informed consent.

SUMMARY

The past few years have seen a significant change in the directions in which the therapeutic and legal aspects of psychiatry in the United States are developing. Often there are massive contradictions inherent in these developments. Thus, the drive for the protection of the patient with respect to the right to treatment, his civil rights, including the right to refuse treatment, informed consent and other issues places increasing importance on the individual. The concept of treating the patient in the community, while theoretically emphasizing the welfare of the individual, is being prostituted to justify emptying governmental hospitals, thereby saving governmental expenditures. In the meantime, many discharged patients linger on, neglected and forlorn, in often deplorable conditions far worse than those in most hospitals.

In the courts of law, the credibility of psychiatry is increasingly questioned and its influence diminished proportionately. There is evidence in the courts of a beginning trend towards a return to using the same legal principles in dealing with the mentally ill offender and the criminal. All these changes are themselves symptomatic of the turmoil which the nation is experiencing.

REFERENCES

1. McNaughton's Case, 10 Clarke and Finelly, House of Lords 200, 1843.
2. Ray, I. (1838) *A Treatise on the Medical Jurispurdence of Insanity*. Boston: Little Brown.
3. Diamond, B. L. (1956) Isaac Ray and the Trial of Daniel McNaughton. *American Journal of Psychiatry*, **112**, 651.
4. Sobeloff, S. E. (1958) From McNaughton to Durham and Beyond. In *Crime and Insanity*, ed. Nice, R. W. New York Philosophical Library.
5. Report of the Royal Commission on Capital Punishment, Cmd 8932, (1953). **80**, 103, London: H.M.S.O.
6. Parsons *v.* State, 2 Southern **854**, 1886.
7. State *v.* Pike, 49 N. H. **399**, 1869.
8. State *v.* Jones, 50 N. H. **369**, 1871.
9. Justice Doe, Pike Case Decision, *Supra*, Quoted by Douglas, William O., in *Law and Psychiatry*, an address to the William Alanson White Institute of Psychiatry, 1956.
10. Durham *v.* United States, 214 F. 2d 874, 1954.
11. Krash, A., and Levine, S. M. (1959) Memorandum of Dissent, Bar Association of thc District of Columbia, Committee on Criminal Responsibility.
12. Watson, A. S. (1959) Durham Plus Five Years: Development of the Law of the District of Columbia. *American Journal of Psychiatry*, **116**, 289.
13. United States *v.* Leach Cr. No. 450-57, 1958.
14 Overholser *v.* Leach, 257 F. 2d **667**, 1958.
15. Carter *v.* United States, 252 F. 2d **608**, **617**, 1957.
16. American Law Institute, Model Penal Code Section 4.01, 1962.
17. United States *v.* Currens, 290 F. 2d **751**, **774**, 1961.
18. Washington *v.* United States, 390 F. 2d **444**, 1967.
19. United States *v.* Brawner, 471 F. 2d **969** (en banc), 1972.
20. MacDonald *v.* United States, 312 F. 2d **847** (cn banc), 1962.
21. Robinson *v.* California, 370 U.S. **660**, 1962.
22. Easter *v.* United States, 361 F. 2d **50**, 1966.
23. Driver *v.* Hinnant, 356 F. 2d **761**, 1966.
24. Powell *v.* Texas, 392 U.S. **514**, 1967.
25 Goldstein, J., & Katz, J. (1963) Abolish the 'Insanity Defence'—Why Not? *Yale Law Journal*, 72, 853,
26. Morris, G. (1968-69) The Confusion of Confinement Syndrome Extended: The Treatment of Mentally Ill 'Non-Criminal Criminals' in New York. *Buffalo Law Review*, **18**, 393.
27. Acher, J.P., Guzman, R., & Levin, T.H. (1967) *Psychiatric Evaluation in Criminal Cases.* Michigan Department of Mental Health.
28. McGarry, A.L. (1971) The Fate of Psychotic Offenders Returned to Trial. *American Journal of Psychiatry*, **127**, 1181.
29. Baxstrom *v.* Herold, 383 U.S. **107**, 1966.
30. Group for the Advancement of Psychiatry, *Misuse of Psychiatry in the Criminal Courts: Competency to Stand Trial* (1974) Report No. 89. New York, GAP.

31. American Bar Foundation (1971) *The Mentally Disabled and the Law*, 2nd edn. Chicago: University Press.
32. Ballay *v.* United States, 422 F. 2d 648, 1973.
33. Deutsch, A. (1959) *The Story of GAP*. New York: Group for the Advancement of Psychiatry.
34. Rouse *v.* Cameron, 373 F. 2d 451, 1966.
35. Wyatt *et al. v.* Stickney *et al.* 344 Supp. 373 MD Ala., 1972.
36. Burnham *et al. v.* Georgia, 349 F. Supp. 1335 ND Ga., 1972.
37. Cobbs *v.* Grant, 502 P. 2d 1, Calif., 1972.
38. Skinner, B.F. (1972) *Beyond Freedom and Dignity*. New York: Knopf.
39. John Doe *et al. v.* Department of Mental Health, Michigan *et al.* Civil Action No. 73-19434-AW, 1973.
40. In re Lifschultz: 2 Cal. 3d 415, 85 Cal. Rptr. 829, Sup. Ct. Cal., 1970.
41. Roe *v.* Wade, 93 S. Cr. 705 (U.S. Sup. Ct. Docket No. 70-18) 1973.
42. Doe *v.* Bolton, 93 S. Cr. 739 (U.S. Sup. Ct. Docket No. 70-40) 1973.
43. Patt, S.L., Rappaport, R.G., & Barglow, P. (1969) Follow-up of Therapeutic Abortion. *Archives of General Psychiatry*, 20, 408.
44. Jansson, B. (1965) Mental Disorders after Abortion. *Acta Psychiatrica Scandinavica*, 41, 87.
45. Protheroe, C. (1969) Puerperal Psychoses: A Long Term Study 1927-1961. *British Journal of Psychiatry*, 115, 9-30. *Brit. J. Psychiat.*, 115: 9-30, 1969.
46. Sim, M. (1963) Abortion and the Psychiatrist. *British Medical Journal*, ii, 145.

CHAPTER 23

Symptomatology and Examination of the Patient

Examination of the patient for psychiatric purposes should not differ materially from a general medical examination. The medical student who fails to elicit that his patient has had a previous nervous breakdown and excuses himself on the grounds that he had not taken a 'psychiatric history' condemns himself for having failed to take an adequate medical history. One cannot arbitrarily divide the patient's history into medical and psychiatric components for these are so intertwined that they are in essence one. Can a mutilating injury be divorced from the sensitivities resulting from it? Can admission to hospital in childhood for an organic disease be seen without the separation anxiety experienced? Similarly the prolongation, aggravation and even motivation of organic disease by psychological factors is too common to be ignored. There is no way round this problem. If the medical student or doctor is to understand the patient and his illness, he must be competent to assess the psychiatric factors pertaining to the illness and the psychological make-up of the patient. Less than this can be fraught with at least the same risks as those run by the psychiatrist who fails to take into account his patient's medical history and physical state.

It is customary in text books of psychiatry to describe 'symptomatology' and 'Examination of the Patient' at the beginning of the book, before 'Psychopathology' and the descriptions of the major clinical conditions. This can be defended on the grounds that such a procedure is relevant for a textbook of medicine, but it should be realized that medicine is based on disturbed physiology of which the student has already an intimate knowledge, and that he is also familiar with anatomy and pathology. In psychiatry, normal or general psychology has very little bearing on mental pathology. The pathology of mental illness can best be understood after a thorough grounding in psychopathology and the patient can only be expertly examined after the student has become familiar with the clinical conditions from which the patient may be suffering. One may legitimately enquire whether, in that case, it is necessary to devote a chapter to 'Symptomatology' and 'Examination of the Patient', if most of the information has already been given under other headings. The answer is, that it is still necessary, but it becomes more meaningful after acquiring a knowledge of psychopathology and clinical psychiatry. It helps to systematize the information obtained from the preceding chapters and revises the 'jargon' or language of psychiatry, so that the reader is able to study, assess and describe his patient in a language which is meaningful and generally accepted. The least one can do, is to encourage the student to use terms as accurately as possible so that not only will others understand his communications, but that he too will give a constant interpretation to the terms he uses. Loose descriptions and inappropriate terms have done as much as any other factor to bedevil psychiatric progress. Even those terms in current use and 'officially' approved are not faultless, but generally they provide a reasonable frame-work of reference.

SYMPTOMATOLOGY OR THE LANGUAGE OF PSYCHIATRY

Psychiatry is likely to be the last branch of medicine to lend itself to electronic computer diagnosis, for its symptomatology, in itself, cannot yield a reliable answer. It must be taken into consideration with the whole life history of the patient. A delusion, tension, ideas of reference, a hysterical symptom or euphoria can be quite meaningless unless seen as part of a whole and the whole should include confrontation with personal examination of the patient. Heart murmurs may be transient, but their disappearance is not nearly so confusing as the variability of symptomatology in psychiatric illness. Symptoms must be seen in the conscious setting, but they must also be related to unconscious mechanisms, so that they are based not only on a factual case history, but on the dynamic forces and trends in the patient's life history. A hysterical reaction may exploit a variety of symptoms for ego defence in one setting, while in another setting an entirely different picture may result. The process may be more important than the symptoms. A young man who is charged by the police for an offence may portray a degree of anxiety which could be related to his immediate predicament or may have existed previously and be intimately associated with the aberrant behaviour which brought him into conflict with the law.

Motor Disturbances

These can be studied by observation alone, and the capacity to see and describe them accurately can at times provide valuable information about a patient's mental state. Nursing staff and house doctors (interns) should be thoroughly familiar with the terms used to describe these phenomena, for it is frequently on their observations that a diagnosis may be reached or a fruitful line of enquiry initiated. The physician (internist) depends to a considerable extent on laboratory investigation, such as X-rays and haematological, biochemical and bacteriological findings, but the psychiatrist wants to know how his patients behave not merely for the relatively short time he is with them, but during the day and night and he therefore depends largely on the observations of others for reliable reports on the patient's behaviour. It is important that these are presented in a language which is unambiguous and generally approved, and one of the first things a psychiatrist in charge of in-patients should do, is to see that his nursing and medical staff are well-grounded in psychiatric terminology, otherwise communication can be very difficult or frankly misleading.

Overactivity can be general and may be referred to as a 'push' or 'pressure' such as is seen in manic states. The patient is continually on the go with marked restlessness, and bodily movements frequently involve the larger joints.

Partial overactivity is the term used when the increased movements are localized such as in tics and habit spasms. This type of movement may prove to be organic in origin, for it is not uncommonly seen in striatal conditions such as torsion spasm, spasmodic torticollis, Huntington's chorea or that interesting condition called ballismus or hemiballismus which is alleged to be due to a lesion in the sub-thalamic body (body of Luys).

Stereotypy is the repetition of an action or movements and is seen in chronic schizophrenic states. Occasionally it is highly organized and approximates to a ritualistic act.

Mannerisms are seen in normal people, are not as persistent as stereotyped behaviour and are more in keeping with the individual's personality. They are more frequently in evidence when the individual is under some stress, such as making a speech or meeting strangers. They assume many forms such as shoulder shrugging, repeated clearing of the throat, blinking, frank blepharospasm, or more general affectations and in this last instance approach the level of eccentricity.

Decreased activity as a pathological phenomenon is frequently overlooked, particularly in the general wards of a hospital, where the patient who is quiet and 'well-behaved' attracts little attention. Yet this may be the prodromal phase of an acute outburst of maniacal excitement. It can also be evidence of the psychomotor retardation found in depressive states or a phase of a schizophrenic psychosis, when the patient may lie in bed, completely immobile.

Negativism. This can manifest in a variety of ways. Generally it consists of a refusal or active resistance to do what is suggested. An example is the patient who has got out of bed and is staring out of a window. The nurse asks him to get back to bed, but he is heedless of her request and when she attempts to guide him, he stiffens under her hand, and the message is clear that he has no intention of complying. It may also be seen as refusal of food and drink as well as refusal to void urine, or defaecate, swallow saliva, or cough up bronchial secretions. Severe urinary retention and oral infections can result, and the author has seen patients who refused to cough almost drown in their bronchial secretions and have to be bronchoscoped and aspirated to save their lives.

Automatic obedience is in its appearance the reverse of negativism in that the patient shows a pathological degree of compliance. This is most dramatically evidenced in *flexibilitas cerea* or waxy flexibility, where the patient's joints can be moulded like wax, and the limbs and digits will retain their positions in a statuesque manner. It is found in schizophrenic patients, particularly in catatonic states and is a relatively rare phenomenon, but such is its dramatic impact that teachers of psychiatry rarely refrain from demonstrating it to medical students, who even when they forget most of the important psychiatry they ever learned, rarely forget *flexibilitas cerea.* There is no doubt a moral here for medical educators.

Other forms of automatic obedience are *echolalia* and *echopraxia* which are the tendency to repeat or mimic the words and actions of others in a stereotyped way. They are generally regarded as schizophrenic features, though they may be part of a post-encephalitic picture and the most florid example of echolalia the author has seen was in a patient who contracted trypanosomiasis in West Africa and showed other postencephalitic signs.

Other pathological movements are *automatic movements or automatisms,* which may be highly systematized and appear purposeful, though they lack the full conscious control of the patient and are usually associated with epilepsy. The disturbance of consciousness may not be recognized by the observer and a number of these patients are regarded as hysterical. The author had one such patient who, during interview, got up, walked over to the window, looked for a second or two and then left the room without saying a word. It was this lapse of manners which made one realize that she was behaving in a way which was contrary to her normal code even though she had been sentenced on more than one occasion for shoplifting. An EEG revealed a left temporal lobe lesion and surgical exploration confirmed the presence of a tumour in that region. Automatisms can include behaviour which is much more serious than shoplifting or being rude to the psychiatrist, and there are records of capital crimes being committed in these states.

Compulsive movements are the result of an irresistible urge to perform a certain act, which to the outsider may appear quite meaningless if not peculiar. They are very common and presumably normal in children, who among other things may insist on touching lamp-posts or not walking on the cracks of the pavement. In the adult it can take many forms some of which are described under 'Obsessional Neurosis' (p. 501).

Speech

This is usually seen as a compound of form and content. It is occasionally possible to gain some information about a patient's mental state by observing the form of the speech without a clear understanding of the content, as for example in manic states, when the speech may be voluble. It is said to be *circumstantial* if the patient never gets to the point, but just keeps talking round and round the topic. *Flight of ideas* is the term used for a tendency for the patient to start talking on one subject and then rapidly switch to another and another, with very little connection between them. In his speech the patient may show an extreme *distractibility* which leaves the listener quite unable to follow what the patient is saying. Someone entering the ward, another patient's movement—any incident, no matter how trivial and irrelevant, may be enough to set the patient off on another theme. Speech may be heavily contaminated with *rhymes* and *puns,* usually of a standard which is more likely to pain, than delight the listener. The rhymes may deteriorate in the grosser manic states to a mere *clang association* of words, such as 'ding-a-ling, sing, ring' the patient being so uncritical of his efforts that he may preen himself on what he considers to be creative art of a high order. The above features are seen in cases of mania.

Speech may be *slowed* to a degree that several seconds may elapse between words. This is seen in very retarded depressive states, the patient's answers to questions being almost unobtainable, though if enough time is allowed, they eventually come through. *Blocking* of speech is when the patient stops in his tracks in the middle of a sentence and gives the impression that there has been a breakdown on the line and he may return to the beginning of his sentence, only to halt again at the same place. This is a not uncommon feature in schizophrenia, particularly of the hebephrenic type.

Speech may be *relevant* or *irrelevant* depending on whether it applies itself to the topic under discussion. Irrelevant speech may be evidence of schizophrenia, the patient's thoughts being distorted by other influences. *Disconnected speech* is also seen in schizophrenia and may deteriorate to the stage when all the rules of syntax are forsaken and a *'word-salad'* results. The patient may even invent his own language and use new words which have an apparent meaning, but on further analysis appear strange and meaningless. These words are called *neologisms.*

Emotional Responses

These can be the most difficult to gauge, if only because people generally tend to conceal their true emotions, or if they declare them, may under—or over-emphasize them. The technical term for the emotional tone of the patient is *'affect'* and disturbance of affect may be the dominant feature in some, if not in the majority of mental diseases. Affects are composed of temperamental and developmental factors, and unconscious mental processes. It is still debatable which of these plays the dominant role, but with the introduction and success of the thymoleptic drugs, there is now considerable support for biochemical determinants, though there is equally no doubt as to the importance of psychological factors in their aetiology.

To some people, just as the unduly quiet patient in the ward is not considered abnormal, so the unduly cheerful or *euphoric* person is not regarded as being in need of psychiatric assessment or treatment. Cultural attitudes are also relevant in estimating the degree of euphoria, for during the Second World War, the boisterous and overtly cheerful were considered the norm in some army messes, while the aloof and less euphoric were frequently labelled schizoid. Euphoria can progress to *elation, exaltation* and *ecstasy,* which even though manifestly pathological, can under certain circumstances, such as intense religious experience, be accepted as normal behaviour. An interesting example which has been pointed out by Sim (1956) is that of Hannah, the mother of Samuel (I. Samuel, ii. 1).

Although the term *affect* which has given rise to the affective psychoses, is treated as a discrete aspect of mental life, it is very intimately connected with thought processes and even with levels of consciousness, for in profound depression there may be a reduction of awareness. The classical and in our culture by far the commonest affective state, is that of *depression* which can range from a variation in mood which is within normal limits to the deepest psychotic state, where the patient feels he has reached 'the bottom of the pit' and that life holds nothing more for him. Even this state can be further qualified in that it need not be pathological unless it is unwarranted by the circumstances or is disporportionate to them.

Depression is usually classified as *'reactive'* and *'endogenous'* though these descriptions can be very misleading, and *'neurotic'* and *'psychotic'*, though terms which have given rise to a great deal of controversy, are more reliable distinctions. 'Reactive' and 'endogenous' are essentially aetiological terms, yet it is virtually impossible to classify depression in this way. Firstly, it is a diagnostic conceit to use the term 'reactive', for it implies that the clinician is so expert at eliciting his history that if there are aetiological factors, he will find them. Secondly, 'endogenous' becomes a diagnosis by exclusion and not through any special criteria, but the clinical facts do not support these distinctions. Many of the most severe depressions follow a bereavement, an infection like influenza, an operation, moving into a new house and so on. Yet these may not be referred to as 'reactive', which really means a disporportionate display of depression following a relatively minor precipitating factor. It is the quality of reaction therefore, which is really being described in 'endogenous' depression, for it is equated with profound feelings of guilt and unworthiness and with other expressions of super-ego hypertrophy. As we are not yet at a stage where a diagnostic classification can be based on aetiological factors, it would seem more reasonable to base it entirely on the nature of the response, and as this is what is really being attempted with the inappropriate terms 'reactive' and 'endogenous', the argument for using 'neurotic' and 'psychotic' in their place is a strong one. It is certainly much less confusing for medical students, who in one statement are told that a depressive state is 'endogenous' and later, when the history is unfolded it transpires that it followed on a specific incident, but is still not 'reactive'.

Anxiety is basically manifest by the physical concomitants of tremor, tachycardia, hyperhidrosis and symptoms related to muscular tension such as headache, or pain in the back and neck. There is also a facial expression which is referred to as 'anxious' which can be present in psychiatric or even physical states where pathological anxiety is not the dominant feature. Clinical anxiety as described under 'Psychoneuroses' (p. 452) though presenting with the same symptoms as 'normal' anxiety or fear, is based on some neurotic conflict and is either *'free-floating' 'organ-fixated'* or *'phobic'*.

Apprehension like anxiety need not be a pathological process, but it can be a part of neurotic anxiety, psychotic depression or schizophrenia.

Diminution of affect or emotional blunting or apathy is the manifestation of an inadequate emotional response to life's experiences. Rapport is difficult to establish and the 'warmer' human emotions are rarely expressed. It varies in degree from the 'cold fish' individual with little 'heart' to the psychotic state where the apathy is so pathological that it is impossible to make contact with the patient. But things are not always what they seem, and the apparently detached, withdrawn individual may have marked hyperhidrosis and be hypersensitive to his surroundings.

Disharmony between mood and thought or *inappropriate affect* is common in schizophrenia and is not the incongruous phenomenon it was previously thought to be but really a futile attempt on the patient's part to make contact with the outside world from a background which is very much pre-occupied with inner problems, hence the presence of inappropriate laughter or giggling.

Emotional lability is the rapid change in emotional tone to tears or laughter with slight or even no provocation. It is found in functional and organic states such as manic-depressive reactions, schizophrenia, cerebral arteriosclerosis and disseminated sclerosis.

Emotional deterioration presupposes emotional growth or *maturity* and also *immaturity*. It need not be correlated with intellectual growth and it is not uncommon to see highly intelligent people, that is as far as educational attainment is concerned, behaving childishly, while less favoured people comport themselves with a maturity which inspires admiration and respect. This is not unimportant in everyday life, for one is likely to see maturity of judgment and behaviour in public matters among ordinary people, while those who should know better often behave in a highly prejudiced way or assume poses like temperamental prima donnas. Unfortunately, criteria for emotional maturity among the intelligent are most difficult to assess, though there are tests for grading the unintelligent, particularly in social maturity. Schizophrenics and hysterics are usually regarded as emotionally immature which may be due to a failure of emotional development or to *emotional regression*. Deterioration (which includes regression) is seen not only in schizophrenics, but in organic states, particularly in the senile and presenile psychoses. The second childhood of old age is a classical example, while in the schizophrenic it may show in speech, manner and even dress. The patient may appear childish and easily suggestible or present a facile expression.

Thought Processes

These, like affects, are not as discrete an aspect of mental life as was at one time believed, but are closely dependent on the affective state of the patient. A number of disturbances are described.

(a) *Autistic thinking* is that state where phantasy assumes large proportions and is over-indulged. *Phantasy* is a normal experience and can give pleasure or act as the spur to ambition and action, but in autistic thinking the phantasies are rarely corrected by reality and little if any positive action results. The patient may not discuss his phantasies but a fleeting smile may betray his mental state.

(b) *Obsessional thoughts* like compulsive acts are a form of rumination which the patient is unable to control and may pervade his whole consciousness.

(c) *Autochthonous ideas* are a passive form of thinking. Although the patient realises he has some responsibility for his thoughts, he may consider that they have been put there by an external agency, such as telepathy, thought control or some other phantastic source.

(d) *Ideas of reference* are a near-normal phenomenon. Many people under certain circumstances are sensitive and may feel that other people are taking notice of them, but this feeling can assume pathological proportions and be with the patient at all times and in situations which the ordinary person would not find embarrassing. The symptoms vary from a vague feeling of discomfort, to definite accusations that people are talking about them and even quoting what they are saying, which is approximating to a hallucinatory and delusional experience. The ideas need not always be of a derogatory nature, for in some schizophrenic states the patient may believe he is an exalted person and that people are referring to him by his delusional title.

(e) *Katathymic thinking* is emotionally-toned and the emotional aspect is sufficiently strong to twist the logical argument to fit the patient's emotional attitude. It is frequently at the root of prejudiced arguments.

(f) *Ambivalence* is really an attitude, though it does involve thought processes. It implies a dual attitude to a person or object, the attitudes being opposite in character such as love and hate. Such ambivalence is derived from unconscious conflict and paradoxical attitudes ensue.

Disturbances of Thought Content

Delusions are beliefs which are false or not true to fact, cannot be corrected by an appeal to the reason of the individual and are out of harmony with his educational and cultural background. Each of these qualifications is very important, for the term is now being loosely used even in hospitals, and it is the doctor's duty to satisfy himself that the patient is indeed suffering from delusions. The facts should be carefully checked and it is surprising how often the 'delusion' disappears under this scrutiny. The author was once presenting a patient who had a particular delusion that he had been everywhere before (*déjà vu*) and the case had added interest in that he had a temporal lobe disturbance. The medical registrar who acted as the convener of the meeting informed the author that his patient had arrived a little early for the conference and that he had a few words with him. 'He seemed quite certain that he knew me and had seen me before'. The registrar was told in a patronizing way that that was the main interest of the case and that he would know a little more when it was presented. 'But he does know me', was the reply, 'He and I were at school together'. A person may entertain a belief which is not true to fact, but when the position is carefully and sympathetically explained, the falsity of the belief is appreciated and it is no longer held. The cultural factor can be equally important, for the world over, there are cultures that hold beliefs which not only are not held by other cultures, but may be flatly contradicted; it would be a most prejudiced person, however, who regarded these beliefs as delusional. Frequently, in clinical practice, the reverse problem presents, in that the patient parades an argument which appears to be so logical and convincing, yet is entirely delusional.

Delusions may assume a variety of forms which have been described as those of grandeur, persecution, sin, poverty and nihilistic.

(a) *Delusions of grandeur* are not nearly as common as the music hall would have us believe. They may of course be more commonly maintained than expressed and it is possible that there are a number of people with these delusions, as with others, who do not come to the psychiatrist. It would be easier for the person with grandiose delusions to keep his problem to himself than the person with delusions of persecution and sin. A feeling of grandeur can be very satisfying and unless the patient is unduly elated over his exalted station, he may bear his honours like a true aristocrat, condescending, with a superior or patronizing smile and perhaps with some affectation, but not necessarily declaring them openly. Paranoid, manic and some organic states like dementia paralytica are usually found in people with such delusions.

(b) *Delusions of persecution* are among the commonest and are found in both paranoid and depressed patients. In the latter, they may be indicative of some guilt and the fancied persecutors, like the police, are frequently on the side of law and order, and the patient may amplify the situation by declaring the crime he believes he has committed. In such a setting, these delusions can be of grave significance as far as the risk of suicide is concerned. In paraphrenic disorders, the patient may be most vociferous in his protests about the persecution, writing letters to the Prime Minister, the Chief Constable and others in authority.

(c) *Delusions of sin* are almost always associated with depression and are accompanied by self-accusatory statements. The sin may be incorporated in a delusion about disease such as syphilis, the patient insisting he has contracted it, though the likelihood is that he has never exposed himself to the infection. Diseases with a social stigma, or associated with terrible suffering, are those which the patient strenuously believes he has contracted.

(d) *Delusions of poverty* are also depressive in origin and are usually entertained by people of substance. They feel they are ruined, cannot possibly afford the physician's fee and that they are a burden to their family.

(e) *Nihilistic delusions* are not commonly seen and are regarded by some authorities to be exclusive to involutional melancholia, though they may also be voiced by schizophrenics, but not with the same emotional intensity. The patient believes that nothing exists either inside or outside himself and this gives rise to bizarre delusions such as not having any blood, brain or bowel. The patient may use his delusions as excuses for refusing food and become severely anorexic.

Insight is the capacity of the patient to appreciate that his abnormal thoughts or delusions are in fact abnormal. At one time, it was regarded as being of good prognostic significance but this view is not so widely held and there can be instances where the patient may have too great a degree of insight, and the prognosis is accordingly less favourable. A psychiatrist once cynically defined insight as the patient's capacity to accept the psychiatrist's interpretation of his illness.

Systematization is the elaboration of a delusion in a logical manner. The patient may develop a whole scheme of explanations, facts and what he interprets as the attitudes of others and weave them into a composite picture. It is usually based on a false premise although the subsequent elaboration may seem reasonable enough. The degree of systematization is determined by the ego-integration of the patient and it may be referred to as 'well-systematized' or 'poorly-systematized'. In the latter, the patient may be intellectually inferior or the paranoid picture may have schizophrenic features.

Hypochondriacal delusions are usually referred to as *hypochondriasis* and patients who voice them are frequently seen initially by physicians and surgeons, and only later referred to the psychiatrist, or sometimes, not at all. They are generally found in older patients who may keep attending their doctors with complaints about their bowels or some other organ. Physical examination is negative and medicine is prescribed. Later the patient may have committed suicide, and at the inquest, the doctor can truthfully say that at no time did the patient complain of depression. What does not usually emerge is that the old man had a cancerophobia and that he took his life to forestall what he thought was the relentless progress of the disease that was destroying him. Hypochondriasis may also be present in paranoid and schizophrenic states. The complaints may then be rather bizarre either in their nature or in the language used to express them. In the schizophrenic, the appropriate emotional component of a distressing complaint may be lacking, or there may be frank disharmony between mood and thought. These delusions can in certain instances be difficult to distinguish from hysterical complaints and in fact some schizophrenics are so labelled because their complaints are entirely somatic, though quite irrational. If they complained about their neighbours or about telepathic influences with the same persistence, there would be no doubt about their mental disturbance, but because they stick to somatic symptomatology, their illness assumes a mantle of medical respectability and they are, for years, regarded by physicians and surgeons as legitimate objects for investigation, and even treatment.

Ideas of unreality or *derealization* are often associated with *depersonalization,* although the two conditions may exist independently. In the former, streets, houses, people and personal possessions like tables and chairs look unreal. In the latter the patient has a disturbance of appreciation of himself. He looks in the mirror and although he recognizes that the face is similar to his own, it lacks the personal qualities he had hitherto associated with himself. He may also have difficulty in recognizing his own voice.

DISORDERS OF PERCEPTION

Illusions

This is a perceptual distortion which need not be associated with a disturbed mental state and is frequently a normal phenomenon. Experts in camouflage, fashion designers, interior decorators and experimental psychologists go out of their way to create illusions whereby to deceive normal members of the community. Visual and auditory illusions, which can result in the misinterpretation of visual and auditory stimuli may, however, be part of a delirious process, the patient misidentifying his surroundings. These false perceptions are frequently coloured by the mental state of the person and an excellent example of such a delirious illusionary state is described in Goethe's ballad *der Erlkönig,* where the father riding with his delirious child, in each verse explains to the child the factual origin of his illusions. In depressed, paranoid and manic patients, illusions may be incorporated in their delusional symptoms.

Hallucination

It is important to distinguish between a hallucination and an illusion, though in delirious states both phenomena may coexist. A hallucination is usually defined as a mental impression of sensory vividness without external stimulus and it may be auditory, visual, olfactory or tactile. This sensory vividness is a very important diagnostic factor, for occasionally patients and even nursing staff report auditory hallucinations, which on closer enquiry are not the unequivocal auditory experience associated with a true hallucination. The patient may say she is 'hearing things' or has 'noises' but an auditory hallucination should sound as clearly in the patient's ear as the examiner's voice.

The content of the hallucination is usually related to the patient's mental state and the voices may be accusatory or laudatory. They may appear to know all the intimate details of the patient's life, accusing him of abnormal sexual practices, or in elderly spinsters, of normal ones. The mechanism of projection is usually very obvious and their super-ego quality may also be apparent. In some patients, an auditory hallucination may occur in an otherwise clear setting, almost like a 'primary delusion', but usually they are associated with more protracted mental disturbance. They may be very distressing to the patient who will seek refuge from them, or he may establish a *modus vivendi* with his 'familiars', occasionally indulging in conversation or calm disputation, but, at times, in argument.

The commonest 'functional' hallucinations are auditory, and are generally associated with all schizophrenic states, but occasionally they may be sexual and give rise to delusions of interference with the genitalia. Visual hallucinations are generally organic in origin, due to either a localized cerebral lesion or toxic state. Hallucinations of smell are also found in schizophrenics, the patient complaining about his own smell which he insists is offensive and will not be persuaded otherwise, but they may also be evidence of a temporal lobe lesion.

Hypnagogic Hallucinations. These occur in the state between waking and sleeping, or *vice versa.* They are associated with a dream-state and the patient recognizes their hallucinatory quality.

Oneiroid States. These usually contain vivid hallucinations, both auditory and visual, and are akin to dream-like states such as the twilight states of epilepsy. The condition was described in 1924 by Mayer-Gross and it may be that electroencephalography would now demonstrate some cerebral dysrhythmia. They are alleged to persist on occasions for months on end, the patient having vivid hallucinatory experiences usually of a visual nature.

Memory Disorders

Amnesia. This is absence or loss of memory and though allegedly common, in clinical practice, genuine cases are very rare indeed. The patient may complain of a partial loss, such as of his recent whereabouts, or a total loss. The latter is extremely suspect and is more likely to be malingering. In the former, there may be some obvious motivating factor, which may be no more complicated than a desire for a bed for the night in hospital. When associated with the 'fugue state' in the middle-aged, it may have more serious implications and be evidence of a severe depression or suicidal 'equivalent'.

Paramnesia. This is a distortion of memory and approximates to dysmnesia and the dysmnesic syndrome or Korsakoff state with confabulation.

Hypermnesia. This is a marked accuracy of memory, particularly for detail and is seen in pathological states like mania and paranoia. The patient is extremely sensitive to his environment and registers events acutely. In the paranoiac it is strongly motivated, while in the manic, it is part of the psychomotor hyperactivity.

Déjà vu. This is the feeling that something has been experienced before and is quite normal. It becomes pathological when it persists and it can be very distressing. It may be evidence of a temporal lobe lesion.

Disorders of Orientation

These are usually seen in organic states, especially in those associated with dementia such as the cortical atrophies or Korsakoff states. It is usually tested by asking the patient where he is, how long he has been in the place and what kind of people are working there, or in other words, orientation for place, time and person.

EXAMINATION OF THE PATIENT

THE PSYCHIATRIC INTERVIEW

The doctor who is asked to see a patient with an established or suspected organic disease has a fairly clear pattern to follow. He lists the patient's complaints and their duration, elicits a family and personal history, the history of the present illness and then continues with a physical examination, paying particular attention to those aspects indicated by the complaints and history. This system of examination has stood the test of at least a century and is usually adequate to establish the presence or absence of organic disease, within the limits of a clinical examination. It is to a certain extent based on the belief that the patient attends the doctor with one end in view, namely to cooperate as far as possible so that the doctor will be in possession of all the facts and arrive at the correct diagnosis.

In psychiatry, things are different. One cannot assume that the patient is cooperative. He may be overtly uncooperative and resist any attempt at examination, or he may appear to be cooperative, yet his unconscious resistances may distort, deny or conceal information. Furthermore, the psychiatrist knows that should treatment be necessary, this will depend on his relationship with the patient, and that an attitude which is too forensic may destroy this relationship. Psychiatric examination used to pattern itself closely on that used for organic disease, but with the accent on personality evaluation, which was usually based on current theories of personality organization and disorganization. This led to the recording of data, some relevant, some irrelevant, but which rapidly dated, and instead of a meaningful appraisal of the patient, there were lists of observations and conclusions which reflected the orientation of the examiner. It failed to initiate the therapeutic relationship and made the patient feel he was an object for scrutiny, rather than a person who required help.

Powdermaker (1948) in her paper on 'The techniques of the initial interview and methods of teaching them', stresses that 'the development of methods of conducting the initial interview are of strategic importance in the treatment of the patient. This includes the effect of the reactions of the doctor on his techniques and on the patient'. She recommends the seminar method of teaching students so that they can discover their needs and weaknesses and is critical of the obsessive and mechanical use of a guide, though she appreciates the importance of fact-gathering. It is when the patient senses that the doctor is a therapist rather than a fact-gatherer, that there is a greater understanding and some reduction in resistance, which in itself makes the interview more meaningful. It has been suggested that it is rarely possible to get a full history in the first interview and that subsequent ones may be essential, and if the aim of the consultation is psychotherapy, this may well be the case.

There are, however, a large number of patients referred to a psychiatrist for an opinion, from the family doctor, the courts, pension boards and insurance companies, and some formulation of the patient's problem is expected after the initial interview. In practice, it is not common to have to see the patient a second time to arrive at a conclusion as to what needs to be done, especially if the patient is accompanied by a relative or friend who can be interviewed independently. One should then be able to decide on the degree of morbidity and how urgent treatment is. In character disorders, which may require prolonged analysis, it may not be so important to initiate effective treatment after the first interview and several weeks may be allowed to elapse before a final formulation is made. But with depressive illness, phobic anxiety and schizophrenic disorders, the referral to the psychiatrist is frequently the end of a number of unsuccessful attempts to help the patient and the psychotherapeutic relationship which the patient may develop with the psychiatrist would be of secondary importance to initiating a course of E.C.T. in a depressed patient with suicidal preoccupation or prescribing tranquillizers to a disturbed schizophrenic.

It is, however, not possible to generalize. Much will depend on the type of psychiatric practice, which in turn will depend on the type of psychiatrist. A psychotherapist practising in an 'over-doctored' area has very little appreciation of the degree and incidence of morbidity that is referred to his colleagues working in a state or local authority service. In the latter, psychotic depression and schizophrenia abound, alcoholism frequently presents as delirium tremens, attempted suicides with their range of psychiatric problems are commonplace, dementia in all its varieties is not a rare condition, and puerperal psychoses can be referred at the rate of 25 in one year. There need be no apology for not adopting leisurely, six to seven initial interviews in these cases, for in fact, it would be medically wrong to do so. It is important therefore when discussing initial interviews to know what type of patient one is seeing and for what purpose. There is no one counsel of perfection which will cater for all types.

A certain minimum of facts must be gathered at the initial interview, otherwise one will not be in a position to say what should happen to the patient next, and in many instances, this would be a tragedy for the patient, either through suicide in the depressive, the onset of chronicity in the schizophrenic, or the prolongation of needless suffering. It should be possible to arrive at a compromise, in which the initial interview provides the doctor with the essential information, helps towards a therapeutic relationship and in addition permits the patient to get to know his doctor. This last aspect is frequently overlooked, but it is just as important that the patient has a good idea of the type of person who is going to treat him as it is for the doctor to get to know the patient. It can be very disturbing to the patient if one creates an initial impression of complete passivity and allows him to feel that his every whim will be countenanced, when after the first or subsequent interviews a decision has to be taken which presents a very different image.

The most important communication the psychiatrist can impart to the patient is one of *sincerity*. Anything which may detract from this must be avoided. It is not fair to one's colleagues to create an initial impression of interest, sympathy and trust and then to transfer the patient, sometimes against his will to another psychiatrist who not only has to take a more positive line, but has also to combat the distrust the patient has developed for doctors. So with all the permissiveness and passivity which is essential for the psychotherapeutic relationship, the psychiatrist should always bear in mind how the patient will react, if eventually he is to be rejected. This danger, and it is not an uncommon one, provides further cause for trying to decide as soon as possible what treatment the patient needs most. It is no disgrace to admit initially that the problem is beyond one's resources and should go elsewhere; it may be that only a period of observation in hospital can really decide and if so, one should say so. In a modern society there is no reason why one should offer a patient a less effective treatment, and social considerations though of some importance should not take precedence over the patient's medical needs.

Determinants of Psychological Reactions

Practical hints are useful but it is just as important to recognize that there is a systematic approach to the problem of patient evaluation. A psychological reaction can have a number of determinants. These have been itemized by Lipowski (1974) as:

1. *Intrapersonal,* which include biological variables such as age,

sex and constitution as well as psychological variables based on the personality all of which influence the patient's attitude to his illness.

2. *Interpersonal,* which includes the patient's relationships with other people, especially family and those involved in the therapeutic relationship. Bereavement may therefore be a common precipitating factor and family relationships are being increasingly recognized as a major factor in the presentation of some illnesses, particularly schizophrenia.

3. *Pathology-related,* which include those physical aspects which impair the integrity of the body and its functions. These may give rise to distortion of perceptions, thoughts, feelings and actions and therefore contribute to mental symptomatology.

4. *Sociocultural and economic,* which influence values, beliefs, and attitudes to disease in general.

5. *Non-human environmental,* which include the physical environment of the sick person, such as home and hospital.

The Language of Disease

This has socio-cultural determinants. Certain people dramatize their symptoms; others behave with a 'stiff upper lip'. Pain may be borne stoically (another cultural term) or be fussed over; some may convert it to psychological symptoms, others to somatic symptoms. Lipowski (1974) refers to *coping styles* and strategies; the former referring to enduring dispositions to act in a certain manner while strategies refer to the actual techniques employed. He lists three styles:

1. *Tackling.* This is the adoption of an active attitude to illness with 'fighting' as the order of the day. Therapeutic alliance is assured, for the patient wishes to be rid of his handicap as soon as possible.

2. *Capitulation.* This is the adoption of a passive or dependent attitude. Cooperation is poor and excessive demands for support are made with little or no attempt to achieve independence.

3. *Avoiding.* This is shown by those who cannot accept illness, hospitals or treatment and is therefore manifest by considerable denial.

Lipowski's 'Law'. In discussing the personal meanings of illness, Lipowski (1974) puts forward this 'law':

A patient's overall response to illness and disability and his motivation to get well, are related to the subjectively experienced losses and/or gains derived from the illness.

TAKING THE HISTORY

Treat the patient as a human being and do not neglect to comment on the weather or whatever national topic of conversation is appropriate.

The Patient's Appearance

This will frequently give one a clue as to how one should open the proceedings. If furtive and suspicious, then there will be little place for preliminaries for they may well be misunderstood. If the manner is open and friendly, one should not go to the other extreme and get involved in time-consuming irrelevant conversation. A marked depressive appearance or agitation should not be met by heartiness, but by a sympathetic approach, for the patient is probably undergoing the 'tortures of the damned' and good fellowship is more likely to aggravate the problem than help it.

Although a case history is apparently a matter of question and answer, there are undertones and overtones which will be missed unless the examiner is listening as Reik puts it 'with the third ear'. He should also be observing closely with the clinical eye, or he will miss essential clues to both the patient's mental and physical state. The face may show tremors around the lips which are more marked when an emotionally charged subject is being discussed. Grimacing and pursing of the lips may betray a schizophrenic process. Hands may be clasped tightly together in a state of tension and the patient may be constantly wringing them or just fidgeting. It is important to decide whether these latter movements are voluntary or involuntary, for on them may rest an early diagnosis of Huntington's chorea. Sweating, tremors and nail-biting may be pointing to anxiety. Levels of consciousness may fluctuate and what might pass for transient obtuseness may be evidence of intracranial disease. Facial symmetry, eye movements and the presence or absence of strabismus will be observed in the apparently casual process of the interview so that a mental note is made of what must be specifically looked for in the physical examination which is to follow.

The history can be dealt with under the usual headings of complaints, family history, personal history (including school and employment records), and history of present and previous illnesses, but there should be considerable flexibility, on occasions leaving a topic to return to it later. It should not be forgotten that a full and reliable case history is available only through the courtesy of the patient and nothing should be said or done which would hamper the process.

Date of Examination

This is a small but very important point which can cause considerable irritation when overlooked. It should invariably be recorded, and it is surprising how often this little item is later required. Medical students are instructed as to the importance of it in ordinary clinical examination, but some tend to think that *laisser-faire* and psychiatric case histories are synonymous and get careless.

Complaints

The Patient has no Complaints. This may well be the case and the patient is referred because of over-anxiety in a parent or spouse, or he may have engineered the interview himself so that his wife as the patient's nearest relative could be examined. This is not uncommon in paranoid reactions, where the patient insists she is normal and that her husband should see a psychiatrist. It may also occur in a paranoid patient who insists he is well and considers that his conduct, which has disturbed the family, is perfectly justified. It is most frequently seen in offenders who have been referred for psychiatric opinion by the courts to assess their degree of psychopathy. They often deny any psychiatric disability and regard the whole situation with whimsical humour.

The Patient cannot Ventilate his Complaints. In societies where verbal facility is low, the patient may have real difficulty in saying what is troubling him. 'I can't explain it to you doctor' is a common remark and there is no point in insisting that he completes his examination in the approved manner by listing his complaints; he needs help and the questions should be put in several ways if necessary—such as 'How do you differ now from when you were well?' or 'Just tell me about your illness as you would talk to your wife about it'. The blocking may be mental rather than cultural and this is seen in the thought-blocking of schizophrenics, who just stop in their tracks and do not proceed. It can also be found in depressive stupor where the statements may be so retarded that it is hardly possible to make sense of them. Speech defects of an organic nature such as dysarthria and dysphasia are obvious examples while stammering can be so gross that the prospect of going through a whole case history may terrify the examiner as much as it does the patient.

The Patient has too many Complaints. He may be verbose, and go on describing one thing after another and apart from recognizing that he must be very hypochondriacal, very little real information emerges. It is as well to listen attentively for he will become repetitive and he can then be interrupted by saying 'You've already told me about that', and then the torrent subsides. It is usually found in people who fear they will not have a chance to tell 'everything' and try to get it out all at once.

The history may be written down on a piece of paper, or what is more alarming, arrive in a parcel before the interview. The author recently had a 10 page letter and a large notebook with 167 pages of the patient's complaints in her own handwriting which was not particularly legible. It is not necessary to read it all. A cursory glance will give one the gist of the contents, which are usually repetitive, and the delusions are unlikely to be repressed during the interview in any case. The manic patient may also be extremely garrulous and though generally one should encourage the patient to talk, in a manic state this rule should be suspended, as the content of his talk is for the time being of less diagnostic importance than the form.

Family History

This can be a delicate subject and one should not immediately rush in with questions like 'Is there insanity in the family?' It is useful to start with the parents. Are they alive? Are they in good health? If not, what is wrong? If dead, what did they die from? At what age? When?; and so on. These questions may not only give helpful information about anxieties over the parents' health, dates of bereavements and their possible impact on the patient, but may also reveal family suicides which otherwise might not have been admitted. It is also the beginning of a test of the patient's memory and it is with such matters as parents' ages and dates of deaths that dementia may be suspected. The patient should preferably be seen alone and a relative interviwed later for otherwise one may be left with an excellent record of the relative's memory, and the patient may be reluctant to disclose family skeletons in the relative's presence.

One may then enquire whether any of the family suffered from 'nerves', where they were treated, and if possible the nature of the illness. It is as well to go back to grandparents, and sideways to uncles, aunts, cousins, brothers and sisters. This history may be the only opportunity for oneself or another research worker to get a full account of the family and it should not be missed. It also gives the patient an opportunity to talk about his family and become prepared for the next set of questions which relate to his early experiences.

Personal History

The date of birth should not be omitted. Apart from giving the patient's exact age, it is useful in coding information and plays an essential part in an identification number. The latter has its uses for registration and for transfer to punch card.

How many brothers and sisters did you have? Where did you come? Did you get on well with each other? Did you have a favourite? Were you generally accepted by the others or were you the odd man out? Place of birth? If it is a large city the district may be worth recording for it may indicate social mobility which is frequently associated with instability. Father's occupation? This gives some idea of his social class and whether he has moved up or down. How did you get on with your parents? With whom did you get on better? Did they get on well with each other? This question may be followed by a silence, the patient feeling it disloyal to criticize his parents. It should be explained to him that domestic disturbances may lead to insecurity, that it is his background that one would like to know about, and that to pretend things were otherwise would make it more difficult to assess his problem and help him. He may then talk of father's alcoholism and the rows and scenes and his fears of them. He may say 'I used to dread Friday nights when he came home drunk–I would sit at the top of the stairs outside my bedroom and pray he would not beat mother'. Did either of them ever leave home? What happened to you? . . . and so on.

Enquiries about neurotic traits in childhood can then be put. The commoner ones are bed-wetting, sleep-walking, sleep-talking, fears of the dark and undue shyness. Physical illness should also be enquired into, particularly as to admission to hospital.

School. Age at starting school and whether he liked it or not. Was he a good, average or poor scholar? What was he good at? What was he poor at? Particular enquiry should be made about arithmetic (or mathematics as it is now called), for this subject, of all educational attainments, has the highest correlation with general intelligence. In appropriate cases, he may be asked if he learned to read and write. Did he play truant? Did he attend a Special School? If he was above average, his place in the school and distinctions should be noted. Was he interested in games? If not, was he on the timid side? Did he mix with his school-mates and have friends or was he a poor mixer and tend to be solitary. Age at leaving school.

A rough guide to intelligence level and school attainment is the following:

Grammar school–I.Q. 120 +. Technical School–I.Q. 110 +.

Secondary Modern School–I.Q. 70 + (this low score would qualify for what was called the 'C' stream). Special School for the Educationally Subnormal–I.Q. 50 +. Occupation Centre–I.Q. 50 or below.

With the growth of Comprehensive Schools the first three criteria may become dated, but the type of class should become a good guide. It will not be long before the earlier distinctions of school will be transferred to classes.

Work. Number of jobs and their nature should be recorded. To assess stability in employment, the longest spell in one job should be noted. Occasionally a person may start off steadily and as the psychotic (schizophrenic) process develops, so the employment record becomes more erratic, with deterioration in performance.

Service Record. Thirty years ago most able-bodied young men were in the Armed Services, the Merchant Navy or in the mines and if not, the reason should be found, as it may well have been medical. If he did not serve his full time, the reason for discharge should also be noted. Overseas service and combat experience may give some indication as to his capacity to stand up to such stresses. Rank too may indicate how he fared in a competitive society. The unit he served in may also be of interest, as some were in the nature of labour battalions and the other ranks were of limited intelligence and not regarded as suitable for infantry or corps training. Psychiatric illness in the Forces offers the opportunity for perusing adequate documentation of his medical state at the time as well as the results of intelligence and aptitude tests. The patient's permission in writing should be obtained and the appropriate Service approached. It cannot be too strongly emphasized that previous information (especially documentary) about the patient's medical history is invaluable. The author has had occasion to 'lecture' house physicians (interns) who would order expensive laboratory investigations on a patently functional problem, yet fail to obtain from the War Office the much more relevant patient's medical history for the expenditure of a postage stamp.

Marriage. Age, children and their sex and ages. Husband's occupation. Marital relations. This can be a delicate subject with some patients and the phrasing of the questions may have to be altered to suit the situation. It should always be a neutral question, such as: How do you and your husband get on? Have you many interests in common? The responses may indicate reservations and the subject can then be followed up. Sexual relations can be enquired into, by asking whether there has been any difficulty in that respect.

Has he been able to perform as he used to, or has there been any falling off recently? Is she relaxed or does she tend to tighten up? Has she any particular fears about it? Would she regard herself as frigid? How does it affect her relationship with her husband? In appropriate instances these details may be further elaborated.

Sex. With the spread of formal sex education, one would think that ignorance on these matters no longer exists. Unfortunately this is not so, largely due to 'education' which today is biased heavily on the side of 'equal rights for women', Female sexual experience is treated as a legitimate cause for suffragettes and not as a biological function, which must differ from that of the male. We now have a generation of orgasm-directed women, who feel they are deprived if they do not experience orgasm with each intercourse. That biologically their role is receptive and passive, that psychologically it carries maternal overtones, seems now to be ignored and a number of sex problems present to the psychiatrist, which are really an artefact of our civilization. It extends to men who because they too are indoctrinated with magazine articles on female orgasm, feel inferior if they are unable to produce this reaction. Instead of it being a maternally satisfying biological experience, it becomes a charade, the man trying to create the orgasm in the woman, and she having to pretend she is experiencing one when she is not, in order to satisfy him. Another contribution from 'Women's Lib' is the aggressively sexual female who is basically a latent homosexual. Like her male counterpart, the 'Pub Casanova', she too boasts of her orgastic prowess. It is therefore important not to see sexual problems where they do not exist. In our culture, especially among the conscientious who require the help of a psychiatrist, some degree of frigidity in the female and indifferent sexual appetite in the male, particularly in middle age, is very common.

Specific sexual problems such as impotence and perversions are dealt with in Chapter 9. Psycho-sexual development may be enquired into though it does not lend itself readily to the question and answer of the initial examination.

Previous Breakdown

This may be easily elicited, the patient volunteering that he had a severe depression several years before, which required a course of E.C.T., or that he was invalided from the Forces on psychiatric grounds. Sometimes the information is not so readily forthcoming, the patient preferring to withhold the information, or disguise it with a euphemism. Gaps in the history may direct enquiries to a certain period: leaving a job which he had held for many years, changing from indoor to outdoor work 'to get into the fresh air', giving up work with higher pay in a more hazardous occupation like mining or steel-erecting, for one which pays less and is safer, are all pointers to a nervous reaction. Occasionally the change of work is more subtle and caters for the patient's unconscious needs, such as joining the fire-brigade, the police force or the regular army, and many re-enlisted 'regulars' were unable to settle down in civilian life and re-enlisted in an attempt (frequently futile) to solve their personal problems.

Previous Personality

This can prove a very difficult question for the patient to answer and it may have to be put in several ways before a satisfactory one can be obtained. What kind of a person are you when you're well? How would your friends describe you? Specific enquiries as to whether the patient is generally withdrawn, over-sensitive, suspicious, given to swings of mood, methodical or fussy, rigid or slap-dash, self-confident, sociable, dependable or unreliable, over-dependent or independent, are among a number that may be made. The patient's special interests should be recorded, such as club membership, holding of public office, religious belief and practice, and unusual interests in politics, religion or philosophy.

Examination

Although this is traditionally placed under a separate heading, the process starts with the patient entering the consulting room and continues throughout the case-history taking.

The appearance should be noted: facial expression, manner of dress, whether meticulous or untidy, perseverative movements and stereotyped behaviour, may all help towards the diagnosis.

Talk. Voluble, punning, circumstantial, ponderous, abrupt, retarded, thought-blocking, neologisms, incoherent.

Mood. Depressed or elated, boastful, irritable, apathetic, confused, or perplexed. Enquire as to diurnal variation or whether it depends on environmental factors.

Thought Content. Misinterpretations, over-weighted ideas, delusions, ideas of reference or of influence, ideas of unreality, excessive day-dreaming and phantasies. When discussing the patient's sexual orientation, masturbatory phantasies may give a clue. They may be homosexual in the patients who are heterosexual in practice, or may reveal sadistic and masochistic tendencies.

Obsessional Features. These may be ruminations or actions and some patients are reluctant to discuss them, for they may recognize the incongruity of their behaviour and fear that if they mention it, they may be considered insane. The extent of the problem should be gauged in terms of the amount of time it occupies, and whether the patient has incorporated other members of the family in his obsessions.

Phobic Features. These are frequently concealed by the patient on the same grounds as the obsessional features. They realize the illogicality of their conduct and fear that if they declare it, people will regard them as insane. They may therefore mention the accompanying depression only and because of this, receive a course of E.C.T. which clears the depression and leaves the phobic anxiety unaffected. They should be specifically asked: Have you lost confidence? Are you able to go out on your own? Can you do your shopping by yourself? Can you travel on a bus? The patient frequently believes that nobody else could be afflicted in this way and these questions reassure him that the problem is familiar to the psychiatrist and that he is no longer alone. These few questions can help to establish a good rapport.

Orientation. If the patient is disorientated, it is likely to be apparent before any specific questions are directed to this end, but they may be asked if they know where they are, the date, and if they can recognize persons.

Insight. This was at one time regarded as of great prognostic significance in delusional states. If the patient realized that some of his ideas were phantastic, he was considered to have insight and it could be a pointer to the recession of a psychotic process. One should enquire: What do you think of these things now?

Memory. This is a complex phenomenon and depends on attention, retention and recall and, if deficient, one or more of the ingredients may be responsible. During the history-taking, memory defect will become apparent in the failure to remember dates, names of members of the family, and periods in employment. It is likely, if the patient has been able to give a reliable and up-to-date history, that the memory is unimpaired.

If there is organic deterioration, memory for recent events tends to go first, the patient being unable to recall incidents that happened that day, but able to give in great detail accounts of events of long ago. In Korsakoff psychosis, or the dysmnesic syndrome, memory impairment may, initially, be less apparent, for the patient's confabulations can for a time conceal the deficit.

Testing of memory may then be undertaken. One gives the patient a personal name and an address, or names like that of a flower, a song, and an animal, and 10 minutes later asks for them to be repeated. Korsakoff states have a singular difficulty in learning new things and a strange sentence like the Babcock sentence may be put to the patient. He is asked to repeat: *The one thing a nation must have to be rich and great is a large secure supply of wood.* The average person gets it word perfect after two or three tries, but the patient with Korsakoff psychosis has much greater difficulty and shows an inability to learn with repeated tries. In cortical atrophies and arteriosclerotic dementia, the initial peformance is probably the best one and they deteriorate with subsequent tries and may eventually become 'catastrophic'. In some brain lesions, the patient may learn the sentence except for one word, but has a 'scotoma' for the error and numerous tries fail to correct it.

Digits forward and backward are traditional tests, but it is difficult to know what is being tested in the latter, and in the former rote memory is not a particularly good test.

Serial 7's. Take 7 from 100 and keep taking 7 from the answer. This is usually poorly performed in cortical dementias, but with Korsakoff states the faculty of handling numbers may be unimpaired. One should have assessed the patient's scholastic attainment before drawing conclusions from the test.

General Knowledge. The name of the sovereign, the prime minister and the leading items of news give some idea of the degree of contact the patient has. In some cases of dementia the name of the soveriegn or prime minister may be given as that of 20 years ago or more. The patient may also be asked to name capitals of countries or the names of animals, birds or fish.

Proverbs. In schizophrenic patients, the difficulty in handling abstracts may not be apparent during the ordinary case history and they should be asked specifically to interpret proverbs, such as: 'A bird in the hand is worth two in the bush'; 'People in glass houses shouldn't throw stones'. The schizophrenic tends to repeat the words used in the proverb and is handicapped in translating metaphor. Patients with organic deterioration are equally handicapped in handling abstracts. Some present the patient with a short story containing a moral and ask him to explain the point of the story.

EXAMINATION OF NON-COOPERATIVE OR STUPOROSE PATIENTS

Kirby (1921) described a scheme for such an examination which included:

General Reaction and Posture. Tests for flexibilitas cerea, the presence of voluntary movements, reaction to noxious stimuli such as a pin prick, attitude to staff such as resistive or cooperative.

Facial Expression. Evidence of emotional expression, such as depression or perplexity, may assist in differentiating a depressive psychosis from a schizophrenic one.

Eyes. The patient may or may not be taking note of his surroundings. If the eyes are closed an attempt should be made to open them and if he resists, it could be evidence of schizophrenic negativism, though some hysterical reactions may behave similarly. Blinking or corneal anaesthesia may help to distinguish the hysterical reaction.

Reaction to Verbal Instructions. These may elicit either a negative response or automatic obedience. Asking the patient to stick out his tongue to have a pin stuck in it may be confirmatory of the latter, but it is a crude test and there are more refined ways of arriving at the diagnosis. Echopraxia and echolalia may be elicited.

Muscular Reactions. Flexibilitas cerea may be recognized or the muscles may be rigid and tense when one tries to move them as in schizophrenic negativism.

Emotional Reactivity. The patient may respond when emotionally charged topics are introduced or when a particular person approaches. The eyes may fill with tears or there may be acceleration of the pulse rate.

Speech. The patient may be seen trying to talk and a whisper may emanate. Mutterings with turning of the head in an attitude of listening may suggest auditory hallucinations.

Writing. Some patients who will not communicate in speech, may write if presented with a pencil and paper.

EXAMINATION OF THE ORGANIC CEREBRAL CASE

Mayer-Gross and Guttmann (1937) designed a scheme for this type of examination which includes tests for mood disturbance (such as lability), attention and adaptability, memory, use of numbers, speech, and visual and related functions. Klein and Mayer-Gross (1957) have elaborated on this scheme in a comprehensive monograph. Dysphasia resulting from a vascular accident with the associated 'jargon' may convince the relatives that the patient is mentally ill and that psychiatric opinion is required. A rarer but more difficult problem is the differentiation of akinetic mutism from catatonic schizophrenia. Sours (1962) considers that in the former the patient has no memory for the event, while in the latter, the intravenous injection of amylobarbitone sodium frequently clears the catatonic state with an accompanying emotional release.

Comments

The above pointers to examination of the patient do not include the relationship which the psychiatrist establishes with the patient, the tone of voice, the inflection, the recognition of emotionally charged material, the meaning of silences, and the interpretation of words implying reservations on the patient's part. It cannot be emphasized too strongly that the worst system of examination is to go through a list like the above, ticking off the items. It should be conducted as an interview, and questions should flow naturally from one topic to the other. Intimate points should be introduced with great delicacy, the patient being told that he need not answer if he doesn't wish to, and this approach is more likely to produce the answer than a blunt attack. There should be no betrayal of curiosity on the doctor's part, for the patient will at once sense it and lose respect for the doctor. Some patients may even cater for curiosity by throwing out hints—'I don't think I should really tell you; it's too dreadful'. The doctor's role is to tell the patient that if it would distress him unduly to do so, he needn't. It may then be difficult to stop the patient from talking about it.

Frankness and scrupulous honesty are essential factors in any doctor-patient relationship. Should the patient ask a question it should be answered honestly and without trying to cover up. He will notice such a manoeuvre in any case and his suspicions would only be heightened. If honestly answered, he will feel that he is with somebody, who even if he has unpleasant news for him, will not deceive him. The author has on occasions been faced with a suspicious and hostile patient who asked, 'You don't think I'm mad?' One should tell the patient that his doctor and family are concerned about his mental state and have called in a specialist to see what can be done to help him. One should add that their anxieties may not be unfounded; that he may not be well mentally but that with his cooperation quite a lot can be done to get him better. Relations and sometimes family doctors who had tried to deceive the patient into believing that the specialist was a friend or a visitor, are appalled by this frankness, but the patient's response usually is, 'Fair enough' and rapport is established.

It is not possible to quote the thousand and one aspects of a psychiatric examination. Most develop out of personal experience and the doctor who knows his subject well will rapidly gain an expertise which his less well indoctrinated colleagues will lack. An attention to detail, an ability to recognize features which are out of the usual run of presentation, the enthusiasm to keep abreast of current literature and read up what has already been said on the subject, will not only equip the doctor well for diagnosis and treatment, but place him favourably to make a useful contribution to psychiatry from his own observations.

PSYCHIATRIC DIAGNOSIS

Over the years there has been considerable, if not undue, preoccupation with psychiatric diagnosis. Medical students always want to know the diagnosis of a patient and one feels like replying after the fashion attributed to Adolf Meyer: 'We don't label our patients in this clinic, we try to understand them'. Mental illness can be defined as the *total* reaction of a *total* person to his *total* environment, yet people insist on labelling such a reaction.

Psychiatric assessment carries a major handicap in that there is still considerable disagreement over diagnosis or the labelling of a patient with a psychiatric illness. Such labelling can only place a patient in a convenient pigeon hole and is unrealistic, for the illness itself, in contradistinction to other medical conditions, does not lend itself to such a manoeuvre. To overcome this difficulty psychiatrists have adopted two main approaches: (1) the descriptive; (2) the dynamic.

Descriptive Psychiatry

This is entirely committed to phenomenology. By meticulous attention to detail and defining criteria, it is believed that essential truth will be distilled and that all ambiguity will disappear. Hence the first-rank symptoms of schizophrenia as defined by Schneider (1925), the detailed analysis of symptoms by Jaspers (1963), the multivirate analysis techniques applied to the diagnosis of depression by Kendell (1968). Factor analysis has also been used to extract the ultimate from the patient's symptoms by Hamilton & White (1959) who analysed a correlation matrix derived from 17 symptoms on 3 to 5 point scales in patients with depression and defined Factor I–the retarded depression, Factor II the agitated depression, Factor III a depression with a specific response to treatment and Factor IV a psychopathic depression. This was later elaborated into a rating scale for depression (Hamilton, 1960), Kiloh and Garside (1963) extracted two factors in depression, a general one based on clinical features and a bipolar factor differentiating neurotic from psychotic types.

The list of classifiers is endless and their conflicts have taken up a disproportionate share of psychiatric journals, but factor analysis does not substitute for clinical observation and for an understanding of the problems involved. It has led to cross-national investigations where London psychiatrists were compared in their diagnostic criteria with their counterparts in New York (Cooper *et al.*, 1972) and it was found that the Americans were more prone to diagnose schizophrenia and less prone to diagnose depression in the same patients as recorded on videotape. Differences in usage of diagnostic labels were also found between psychiatrists in the British Isles, with Glasgow psychiatrists being the most "un-American" in their criteria (Copeland *et al.*, 1971).

What seems to have been overlooked is that a diagnosis is not a fact but an inference which is, or should be, based on observed facts or phenomena. It is in the recognition of phenomena and even the definition of phenomena that there is still considerable controversy and until this aspect is resolved there will always be controversy over diagnosis.

Dynamic Psychiatry

This tries to see mental illness as a process with the erection of ego-defences, their compensation and decompensation, and the way whereby these activities influence symptomatology. It is not independent of phenomenology but tries to explain it in dynamic terms so that the exercise is not to produce a shopping list of symptoms, give them loadings, extract factors and then group them under diagnostic labels, but to ask the simple question: 'What is going on here'. This implies that full appreciation of the individual patient is even more important than his symptomatology.

It would be a simple matter to retreat from systematic assessment and it could be argued that the individual patient would not suffer unduly, but there are many calls for systematic assessment and the collection of data. Therapeutic trials depend on some form of recording and its analysis; a simple form of documentation which is reproducible would make for a tidier form of hospital record, both in-patient and out-patient and permit conclusions to be drawn in terms of morbidity, recovery and the inter-relation between the patient's background and his illness.

PSYCHIATRIC ASSESSMENT AND RECORDING

The author has for long been interested in devising a system which will take into account many of the points mentioned above and after considerable trial and error evolved a system (Sim, 1971) which is simple, valid and reliable and has now been tried in over 500 patients and is also capable, with suitably indoctrinated psychiatrists, of being used in multicentre trials and other research projects.

Psychiatric Data

Psychiatric data tend to divide into two main groups: (1) those that are public, objective or 'hard' and (2) those that are private, subjective or 'soft'.

In the former, there is generally no disagreement between investigators or clinicians. The group includes basic information about the patient such as age, sex, family history, personal history including school and employment records, marital state, previous breakdown and the like. Though such data are not generally regarded by psychiatrists as being as important as the 'soft' data obtained in the relationship established in the first and subsequent interviews, their value should not be underestimated. Many commercial firms base production lines of consumer goods on much less 'hard' data than are obtained in even a brief psychiatric interview. These data do give useful clues to the patient's social and economic achievements and in themselves may provide a check on the reliability of the subjective assessment. For example, if one had a patient with stable school and employment records, an absence of any suggestion of delinquency and who was aged 40, one would be most reluctant to conclude that he was a psychopathic personality, no matter how sociopathic his recent behaviour may have been. Factors other than those commonly found in personality disorders would have to be considered in the aetiology and an entirely different diagnosis would probably be made.

Manifest Problems and Diagnostic Areas. 'Soft' data have to be evaluated and interpreted and it is over this subjective aspect that controversy arises. This is complicated further in that descriptions of the disability tend to be in two fields: *(a)* as a manifest problem or problems and *(b)* as a diagnostic area or areas.

The manifest problems in psychiatry have some parallels in general medicine except that in the latter they are no longer generally regarded as of diagnostic equivalence. Advances in pathology and physiology have made it possible to base most diagnoses on an aetiological or pathological process and therefore major manifest problems like jaundice, hepatomegaly, pyrexia or cyanosis are no longer equated with diagnosis. This is not yet the case in psychiatry and many manifest problems are given the status of diagnosis even though it is generally agreed that conditions such as mood disturbance, anorexia, obesity, drug addiction, alcoholism and insomnia can be symptomatic of a variety of underlying psychiatric disorders. Furthermore, the patient may manifest more than one problem, e.g., hypochondriasis, anorexia and insomnia, and these are also capable of quantitative estimation.

There is still some disagreement over a minority of diagnostic labels in psychiatry, such as schizoaffective psychosis and pseudo-neurotic schizophrenia, but it is generally agreed that most diagnoses have clinical validity, *i.e.* they represent an identifiable constellation of symptoms. As with manifest problems, it is common and indeed usual for the same patient to present in more than one diagnostic area, so that any valid assessment should take into account all the diagnostic areas. Such an orientation has the following advantages:

1. It ensures that the patient is assessed overall and avoids the error of ignoring relevant diagnostic areas because there is striking evidence of a reaction in one or two areas.
2. Improvement or deterioration in the patient's mental state is not confined to assessment of one or two areas but of all areas. This permits the recognition of new developments which may otherwise go unheeded.
3. In assessing response to treatment, recession in one area with no change in the others gives a useful clue as to the manner in which the treatment is helping the patient. For example, a patient may have depressive as well as phobic anxiety features. In some instances these conditions are interdependent and both may respond to the same treatment. In other instances they may be entirely independent.

Degree of Handicap. Although symptomatology, whether as manifest problems or as diagnostic areas, is of clinical interest, the main purpose of treatment is to remove disability or handicap . A person may have psychotic features of a paranoid nature and function well in employment and to some extent socially. On the other hand, a person who has a minor degree of sickness as measured quantitatively in terms of manifest problems or diagnostic areas may be considerably handicapped in his social functioning or even in his employment. Handicap should therefore be measured in terms of employment, social competence and personality deterioration for these give some estimate of the patient's functioning in society. It is apparent that these measures can only be crude but they have an important bearing on the results of treatment and these or similar criteria are going to become increasingly necessary in a public and expensive service where accountancy is likely to extend from the cost of treatment to the benefits derived.

Quantitative Estimation. Scales for quantitative assessment consist of an arbitrary number of divisions. It might be considered that the finer the scale the more accurate the assessment, but in practice, quantifying clinical components in psychiatry becomes extremely inconsistent between two trained observers when more than a five-point scale is used. In this project, it was decided to reduce this to a four-point scale, including zero. The scale would then be in accord with the traditional clinical assessments of mild, moderate, severe and absent. Though there would be some overlap between these grades, they are sufficiently distinct to reduce this to a minimum while at the same time offering sufficient range to draw valid comparisons in terms of improvement or relapse.

The Pro-Formas

(*a*) *The Public Data.* In a psychiatric interview a mass of public data is elicited but in the preparation of the pro-formas (Figs. 11, 12) these were reduced to a minimum. It is appreciated that these pro-formas could be modified for more specific enquiries but they should preferably not be enlarged. As they stand, they are easy to complete and do not interfere with the interview. Earlier samples included questions about twin status, hereditary disease, illegitimacy and many others but after a number of trials these were eliminated, though they could be reintroduced for specific enquiries. What has been retained is the minimum information consistent with providing a basic background of the patient. Although these pro-formas are the end result of several previous attempts and they could no doubt be further improved, in their present form they sufficed.

In all hospital records, the patient's hospital number is invariably included, though not his National Health Service number. The author found in a recent survey of schizophrenic illness treated in a general hospital that at follow-up many patients had drifted out of the area or left their previous domicile. The hospital number was then of no help in tracing them but the N.H.S. number when available was the most useful clue. As personal identity numbers are no longer used, the N.H.S. number is the best means of identification outside the hospital and was therefore included in the Public Data.

(*b*) *Manifest Problems* (Fig. 13). These include only the commoner problems and all headings have been selected because they can be symptomatic of a variety of psychiatric conditions. The review periods are listed in weeks as this reflects the short stay of patients in the department. It is also relevant to clinical trials where review and monitoring of laboratory data are initially at weekly intervals and thereafter four to six weeks from the commencement of the trial.

(*c*) *Diagnostic Areas* (Fig. 14). These are the diagnostic labels in general use, but again, they are restricted to a minimum. The terms neurotic and psychotic depression are preferred to reactive and endogenous for obvious reasons. There is in some instances a tendency for a diagnostic area to approximate to a manifest problem but generally there is a recognizable distinction. It is conceded that there could be further useful modifications in these pro-formas but for practical purposes they were adequate.

Analysis of Data

The public data are similar to those usually collected in patient studies. From these data, distributions of the patients with respect to age and sex, social class, duration of illness, etc. can be obtained.

The patients with a particular manifest problem, or who fall into a given diagnostic area, or who have a certain handicap, can be analysed in the following stages:

1. The progress of a patient with an individual manifest problem can, of course, be assessed serially by reference to the pro-forma which gives scores of the degree of severity at the initial assessment and after the first, second and sixth weeks of treatment. When a reasonable number of patients in a series present with a given problem, and if they are all scored on each successive occasion during treatment or observation, the progress of the group can be summarized by calculating the mean score at each assessment.

2. The speed of response is an essential piece of information in assessing treatment, for it is not enough to know whether it is successful but how quickly it succeeds. An index of the rate of response of a group of patients with a given problem can be calculated at each subsequent assessment by calculating the ratio of the mean score one week after treatment is started to the mean at the initial assessment, and similarly for later assessments.

3. Another method which will be used is to calculate for those patients with initial scores of 2 or 3 on a given problem (diagnostic area of handicap) the proportion who score 0 or 1 on subsequent assessments. Such a proportion can be a useful index of progress of the group, especially in the comparison of one treatment with another.

It should be mentioned at this point that a group of patients with a greater degree of severity at the outset might be expected to present a more formidable therapeutic challenge, but this is not necessarily so in clinical practice. Indeed the more florid the symptomatology in psychiatry the more readily does the condition respond to treatment; and it is frequently those with less florid symptoms who prove more refractory to treatment.

Any system of psychiatric assessment and recording, no matter what its theoretical basis, is only as good as it is useful. The above system has now been scored by a number of investigators in four double-blind clinical trials involving approximately 500 patients and it is both workable and informative. It is possible to assess and record changes in the patient's mental state, quantify these findings and compare the relative efficacy of drugs including their speed of action. Although the record cards are designed for economy of investigators' time, there is still much unused information which can be stored and analysed. This could provide details of the distribution of manifest problems and diagnostic areas in mental illness and those aspects which are or are not amenable to treatment. In patients who come in for observation rather than treatment, some information may be obtained of the process of spontaneous remission. The storage of the present data, scant though it may appear, can therefore be useful in general psychiatric assessments, independently of clinical trials.

With further experience and in the light of criticism, the above system will no doubt be improved, but even in its present form, it illustrates that a modern orientation of psychiatric diagnosis with the formulation rather than the label as the objective, is capable of being recorded simply and economically. The derived data are in a form which can be stored and analysed either by modern computer techniques or by simple arithmetic .

Fig. 11. Pro-forma to psychiatric interview (1)

Hospital..

Patient No. in Survey [| | | | | |]   Sex [ ] (M or F)

Surname..

Forenames 1st.. 2nd..

Date of Birth Day [ ] Month [ ] Year [ ]   Age [|]

Date Examined Day [ ] Month [ ] Year [ ]   Patient's Hospital No. [| | | | |]

Family Doctor Name..   Patient's N.H.S. No.

Address..   ....

....

Marital Status

Single	Married	Widowed	Divorced	Separated	Div. & Remar.	Wid. & Remar.
1	2	3	4	5	6	7

Cohabiting		
No	Permanent	Casual
0	1	2

Occupation (housewife — husband's/partner's occupation)

specify..

G.R.O. Social Classes				
I	II	III	IV	V
1	2	3	4	5

Employed	Unemployed	Unemployable	Other
1	2	3	4

Religion at present

None 0

C of E	Other non-Con.	R. Cath.	Other
Practising 1	Practising 3	Practising 5	Practising 7
Non-pract. 2	Non-pract. 4	Non-pract. 6	Non-pract. 8

Patient's complaints

Nil	Psychological only	Somatic only	Social only
0	1	2	3
	Psychological and somatic	Psychological and social	Somatic and social
	4	5	6
	Psychological, somatic and social		
	7		

Nature of complaints

Not applicable	Steady	Fluctuating
0	1	2

[|]

Duration of symptoms in months (e.g. 5 months code as 05)

Less than 1 month, code 00 and specify..

More than 99 months, code 99 and specify..

Fig. 12. Pro-forma to psychiatric interview (II)

FAMILY HISTORY

Father History of mental illness

No	Yes	N/K
0	1	9

Mother History of mental illness

No	Yes	N/K
0	1	9

PERSONAL HISTORY

Number of children in family

Only child	2-4 surviving children	More than 4 surviving children
1	2	3

Home Background

Secure	Insecure	Broken	N/K
1	2	3	9

Separated from parents in childhood

No	Yes	N/K
0	1	9

Psychological illness in childhood

No	Yes	N/K
0	1	9

School

Attendance		
Reg.	Irreg.	N/K
1	2	9

Educational Attainment			
Below aver.	Aver.	Above aver.	N/K
1	2	3	9

ADOLESCENCE

Social activities

Adequate	Restricted	N/K
1	2	9

Work record

	None		
	0		
Skilled	Steady	Erratic	N/K
	1	2	3
Semi-skilled	Steady	Erratic	N/K
	4	5	6
Unskilled	Steady	Erratic	N/K
	7	8	9

Delinquency

No	Yes	N/K
0	1	9

Sexual Development

Physical	
Mature	Immature
1	2

Mental		
Mature	Immature	Deviant
1	2	3

PREVIOUS BREAKDOWNS

No	Yes	N/K
0	1	9

PREVIOUS PERSONALITY

Interests			
None	Social	Other	Soc. & Other
0	1	2	3

Degree of Interest			
Obsess	Erratic	Normal	N/K
1	2	3	9

PRECIPITATING FACTORS

Precipitating Factors				
None elicited	Physical	Psychological	Phys. & Psychol.	N/K
0	1	2	3	9

AGGRAVATING FACTORS

Aggravating Factors				
None elicited	Physical	Psychological	Phys. & Psychol.	N/K
0	1	2	3	9

Fig. 13. Psychiatric survey of manifest problems

Patient's Reference No. in Survey.../..

MANIFEST PROBLEMS		Week 0 Date			Week 1 Date			Week 2 Date			Follow-up Date		
		Mild	Mod.	Sev.	Mild	Mod.	Sev.	Mild	Mod.	Sev.	Mild	Mod.	Sev.
Alcoholism		0 1	2	3	0 1	2	3	0 1	2	3	0 1	2	3
Drug Addiction		0 1	2	3	0 1	2	3	0 1	2	3	0 1	2	3
Behaviour Disorders	Neurotic	0 1	2	3	0 1	2	3	0 1	2	3	0 1	2	3
	Sociopathic	0 1	2	3	0 1	2	3	0 1	2	3	0 1	2	3
	Psychotic	0 1	2	3	0 1	2	3	0 1	2	3	0 1	2	3
	Organic	0 1	2	3	0 1	2	3	0 1	2	3	0 1	2	3
Mood Disturbances		0 1	2	3	0 1	2	3	0 1	2	3	0 1	2	3
Sleep	Insomnia	0 1	2	3	0 1	2	3	0 1	2	3	0 1	2	3
	Hypersomnia	0 4	5	6	0 4	5	6	0 4	5	6	0 4	5	6
Eating Disorder	Anorexia	0 1	2	3	0 1	2	3	0 1	2	3	0 1	2	3
	Obesity	0 1	2	3	0 1	2	3	0 1	2	3	0 1	2	3
	Pica	0 1	2	3	0 1	2	3	0 1	2	3	0 1	2	3
	Polydipsia	0 1	2	3	0 1	2	3	0 1	2	3	0 1	2	3
Psycho-somatic	Respiratory	0 1	2	3	0 1	2	3	0 1	2	3	0 1	2	3
	Cardio-vasc.	0 1	2	3	0 1	2	3	0 1	2	3	0 1	2	3
	Gastro-int.	0 1	2	3	0 1	2	3	0 1	2	3	0 1	2	3
	Skin	0 1	2	3	0 1	2	3	0 1	2	3	0 1	2	3
	Other	0 1	2	3	0 1	2	3	0 1	2	3	0 1	2	3
Hypochondriasis		0 1	2	3	0 1	2	3	0 1	2	3	0 1	2	3
Psychotic symptoms	Hallucinations	0 1	2	3	0 1	2	3	0 1	2	3	0 1	2	3
	Delusions	0 1	2	3	0 1	2	3	0 1	2	3	0 1	2	3
Personality deterioration		0 1	2	3	0 1	2	3	0 1	2	3	0 1	2	3
Depersonalization		0 1	2	3	0 1	2	3	0 1	2	3	0 1	2	3
Fits		0 1	2	3	0 1	2	3	0 1	2	3	0 1	2	3
Other episodic phenom.		0 1	2	3	0 1	2	3	0 1	2	3	0 1	2	3
Suicide attempt		0 1	2	3	0 1	2	3	0 1	2	3	0 1	2	3
Other problems		0 1	2	3	0 1	2	3	0 1	2	3	0 1	2	3

Remarks:

Fig. 14. Diagnostic classifications

DIAGNOSTIC AREAS		Week 0 Date			Week 1 Date			Week 2 Date			Follow-up Date		
		Mild	Mod.	Sev.	Mild	Mod.	Sev.	Mild	Mod.	Sev.	Mild	Mod.	Sev.
Anxiety	Somatic	0 1	2	3	0 1	2	3	0 1	2	3	0 1	2	3
	Phobic	0 1	2	3	0 1	2	3	0 1	2	3	0 1	2	3
	Free-floating	0 1	2	3	0 1	2	3	0 1	2	3	0 1	2	3
Depression	Psychotic	0 1	2	3	0 1	2	3	0 1	2	3	0 1	2	3
	Neurotic	0 1	2	3	0 1	2	3	0 1	2	3	0 1	2	3
Mania		0 1	2	3	0 1	2	3	0 1	2	3	0 1	2	3
Obsessional	Personality	0 1	2	3	0 1	2	3	0 1	2	3	0 1	2	3
	Colouring of illness	0 4	5	6	0 4	5	6	0 4	5	6	0 4	5	6
	Neurosis	0 7	8	9	0 7	8	9	0 7	8	9	0 7	8	9
Hysterical	Personality	0 1	2	3	0 1	2	3	0 1	2	3	0 1	2	3
	Adulteration	0 4	5	6	0 4	5	6	0 4	5	6	0 4	5	6
	Conversion	0 7	8	9	0 7	8	9	0 7	8	9	0 7	8	9
Schizophrenic	Simple	0 1	2	3	0 1	2	3	0 1	2	3	0 1	2	3
	Hebephrenic	0 1	2	3	0 1	2	3	0 1	2	3	0 1	2	3
	Paranoid	0 1	2	3	0 1	2	3	0 1	2	3	0 1	2	3
	Catatonic	0 1	2	3	0 1	2	3	0 1	2	3	0 1	2	3
	Pseudo-neurotic	0 1	2	3	0 1	2	3	0 1	2	3	0 1	2	3
Subnormality		0 1	2	3	0 1	2	3	0 1	2	3	0 1	2	3
Charact. disorder	Psychopathic	0 1	2	3	0 1	2	3	0 1	2	3	0 1	2	3
	Sexual dev.	0 1	2	3	0 1	2	3	0 1	2	3	0 1	2	3
Paranoid	Personality	0 1	2	3	0 1	2	3	0 1	2	3	0 1	2	3
	Adulteration	0 4	5	6	0 4	5	6	0 4	5	6	0 4	5	6
	Reaction	0 7	8	9	0 7	8	9	0 7	8	9	0 7	8	9
	Psychosis	A	B	C	A	B	C	A	B	C	A	B	C
Organic reaction	Acute (delirium)	0 1	2	3	0 1	2	3	0 1	2	3	0 1	2	3
	Sub-acute	0 4	5	6	0 4	5	6	0 4	5	6	0 4	5	6
	Chronic (dementia)	0 7	8	9	0 7	8	9	0 7	8	9	0 7	8	9
	Other	A	B	C	A	B	C	A	B	C	A	B	C
Physical Illness (specify if yes)		No (0)	Yes (1)	Mult. (2)	No (0)	Yes (1)	Mult. (2)	No (0)	Yes (1)	Mult. (2)	No (0)	Yes (1)	Mult. (2)
Course of illness		Steady 1	Fluct. 2		Steady 1	Fluct. 2		Steady 1	Fluct. 2		Steady 1	Fluct. 2	
		Mild	Mod.	Sev.	Mild	Mod.	Sev.	Mild	Mod.	Sev.	Mild	Mod.	Sev.
Nature of Handicap	Social	0 1	2	3	0 1	2	3	0 1	2	3	0 1	2	3
	Employment	0 1	2	3	0 1	2	3	0 1	2	3	0 1	2	3
	Personality	0 1	2	3	0 1	2	3	0 1	2	3	0 1	2	3

References

Abraham, K. (1912). Notes on the psychoanalytical investigation and treatment of manic-depressive insanity and allied conditions. *Selected Papers* (1927). London: Institute of Psychoanalysis and Hogarth Press.

Abraham, K. (1916). The first pregenital stage of the libido. *Selected Papers* (1927). London: Institute of Psychoanalysis and Hogarth Press.

Abrams, R., & Fink, M. (1972). Clinical experiences with multiple electroconvulsive treatment. *Compr. Psychiat.* **13**, 115–121.

Abrams, R., Fink, M., Dornbush, R. L., Feldstein, S., Volavka, J., & Roubicek, J. (1972). Unilateral and bilateral electroconvulsive therapy. *Arch. gen. Psychiat.* **27**, 88–91.

Abse, D. W. (1950). *The Diagnosis of Hysteria.* Bristol: Wright.

Achté; K. A., Kaoko, K., & Seppálá, K. (1968). On 'electrosleep' therapy. *Psychiat. Quart.* **42**, 17–27.

Ackermann, D. & Kutscher, F. (1910). Uber die Aporrhegmen. *Z. Physiol. Chem.* **69**, 265.

Ackner, B. (1954). Depersonalization: 1. aetiology and phenomenology. *J. ment. Sci.* **100**, 838.

Ackner, B., Cooper, J. E. Gray, C. H., Kelly, M. & Nicholson, D. C. (1961). Excretion of porphobilinogen and β-amino laevulinic acid in acute porphyria. *Lancet,* i, 1256.

Ackner, B., Harris, A. & Oldham, A. J. (1957). Insulin treatment of schizophrenia: a controlled study. *Lancet,* i, 607.

Adams, R. D., Fisher, C. M., Hakim, S. Ojemann, R. G. & Sweet, W. H (1965). Symptomatic occult hydrocephalus with 'normal' cerebrospinal fluid pressure: a treatable syndrome. *New Eng. J. Med.* **273**, 117.

Addison, T. (1855). *On the Constitutional and Local Effects of Disease of the Supra-renal Capsules.* London: Highley.

Adelson, L. (1972). The battering child. *J. Amer. med. Ass.* **222**, 159–161.

Adler A. (1924) *Individual Psychology.* London: Kegan Paul.

Adler, A. (1938). *Social Interest: a Challenge to Mankind.* London: Faber.

Adrian, E. D. & Yamagiwa, K. (1935). The origin of the Berger rhythm. *Brain,* **58**, 323.

Agras, S., Sylvester, D., & Oliveau, D. (1969) The epidemiology of common fears and phobias. *Compr. Psychiat.* **10**, 151–156.

Alanen, Y. O. (1958). The mothers of schizophrenic patients. *Acta psychiat. neurolog. Scand.* **33**, 124.

Alarcon, R. de., & Carney, M. W. P. (1969). Severe depressive mood changes following slow-release intramuscular fluphenazine injection. *Brit. med. J.* **3**, 564–587.

Alexander, E. R., Crow, T. J., & Hamilton, S. M. (1973). Water intoxication in relation to acute psychotic disorder. *Brit. med. J.* **1**, 89.

Alexander, F. (1929). The Psychoanalysis of the Total Personality. Nervous and Mental Disease Monograph Series, No. 52. Washington: Nervous and Mental Disease Publishing Coy.

Alexander, F. (1930). The neurotic character. *Int. J. Psycho-Anal.* **11**, 292.

Alexander, F. (1943). Fundamental concepts of psychosomatic research: psycho-genesis, conversion, specificity. *Psychosom. Med.* **5**, 205.

Alexander, F. (1952). *Psychoanalysis and Psychotherapy.* London: Allen & Unwin.

Alexander, F. & French, T. M. (1946). *Psychoanalytic Therapy.* New York: Ronald Press Coy.

Alexander, G. L. & Norman, R. M (1966). *The Sturge-Weber Syndrome.* Bristol: John Wright.

Allan, J. D., Cusworth, D. C., Dent, C. E. & Wilson, V. K. (1958). A disease probably hereditary, characterized by severe mental deficiency and a constant gross abnormality of aminoacid metabolism. *Lancet* i, 182.

Allen, C. (1962). *A Textbook of Psychosexual Disorders.* London: Oxford University Press.

Allen, F. H. (1942). *Psychotherapy with Children.* New York: Norton.

Allen, R. P., Faillace, L. A., & Reynolds, D. M. (1971). Recovery of memory functioning in alcoholics following prolonged alcohol intoxication. *J. nerv. ment. Dis.* **153**, 417–423.

Allison, A. C. & Paton, G. R. (1966). Chromosomal abnormalities in human diploid cells infected with mycoplasma and their possible relevance to the aetiology of Down's syndrome (Mongolism). *The Lancet,* 2, 1229–1230.

Allison, R. S. (1966*a*). Perseveration as a sign of diffuse and focal brain damage–I. *Brit. med. J.* 2, 1027.

Allison, R. S. (1966*b*). Perseveration as a sign of diffuse and focal brain damage–II. *Brit. med. J.* 2, 1095.

Allport, G. W. (1961). *Pattern and Growth in Personality.* New York: Holt, Rinehart & Winston.

Alvarez, W. C. (1929). Ways in which emotion can affect the digestive tract. *J. Amer. med. Ass.* **92**, 1231.

Alvord, E. C., Stevenson, L. D., Vogel, F. S. & Engle, R. L. (1950). Neuropathological findings in phenyl pyruvic oligophrenia (phenyl-ketonuria). *J. Neuropath.* **9**, 298.

Alzheimer, A. (1907). Über eine eigenartige Erkrankung der Hirnrinde. *Allg. Z. Psychiat.* **64**, *146.*

Amdur, M. J., & Harrow, M. (1972). Conscience and depressive disorders. *Brit. J. Psychiat.* **120**, 259–264.

Ames, F. (1955). The hyperventilation syndrome. *J. ment. Sci.* **101**, 466.

Anastasi, A. (1954). *Psychological Testing.* New York: Macmillan.

Anastasi, A. & Foley, J. (1948). A proposed reorientation in the heredity-environment controversy. *Psychol. Rev.* **55**, 239.

Anderson, E. W. (1933). A study of the sexual life in psychoses associated with childbirth. *J. ment. Sci.* **79**, 137.

Anderson, I. (1950). Alopecia areata: a clinical study. *Brit. med. J.* 2, 1250.

Anderson, J. (1968). Psychiatric Aspects of Primary Hyperparathyroidism. *Proc. roy. Soc. Med.* **61**, 1123–4.

Anderson, O. D. & Liddell, H. S. (1935). Observations on experimental neurosis in sheep. *Arch. Neurol. Psychiat.* **34**, 330.

Andreason, N. J. C., Noyes, R., & Hartford, C. E. (1973). Factors influencing adjustment of burn patient during hospitalization. *Psychosom. Med.* **34**, 517–525.

Andreasson, R. (1962). Alcohol and road traffic: an international survey of the discussions. In *Alcohol & Road Traffic.* Proceedings of Third International Conference. pp. 66–78. London: Brit Med. Assoc.

Andreski, S. (1972). *Social Sciences as Sorcery.* London: Deutsch.

Angst, J., Weis, P., Grof, P., Baastrup, P. C., & Schou, M. (1970). Lithium prophylexis in recurrent affective disorders. *Brit. J. Psychiat.* **116**, 604–614.

Ansell, G. B. & Dohmen, H. (1956). The depression of phospholipid turnover in brain tissue by chlorpromazine. *J. Neurochem.* **1**, 150.

Antebi, R. N. (1963). Seven principles to overcome resistance in hypnoanalysis. *Brit. J. med. Psychol.* **36**, 341.

Apley, J. (1959). Psychosomatic disorders in children. *Lancet,* i, 641.

Apley, J., Philips, M. & Westmacott, I. (1960). Psychogenic disorders in children; an experiment in management. *Brit. med. J.* 1960, 1, 190.

Appelby, B. P. (1960). A study of premenstrual tension in general practice. *Brit. med. J.* **1**, 391.

Argyll Robertson, D. (1869*a*). On an interesting series of eye-symptoms in a case of spinal disease with remarks on the action of belladonna on the iris, etc. *Edinb. med. J.* XIV, 696.

Argyll Robertson, D. (1869*b*). Four cases of spinal myosis; with remarks on the action of light on the pupil. *Edinb. med. J.* XV, 487.

Arieti, S. (1955). *Interpretation of Schizophrenia.* New York: Brunner.

Arieti, S. (1959*a*). Manic-depressive psychosis. In *American Handbook of Psychiatry,* ed. Arieti, S. New York: Basic Books.

Arieti, S. (1959*b*). Schizophrenia: the manifest symptomatology, the psychodynamic and formal mechanisms. In *American Handbook of Psychiatry,* ed. Arieti, S. New York: Basic Books.

Arieti, S. (1970). Cognition and feeling. In *Feelings and Emotions,* ed. Arnold, M. B. New York: Academic Press.

Armitage, G. H. & Sim, M. (1960). Barbiturate addiction and sensitivity. *Brit. J. med. Psychol.* 33, 149.

Arnold, M. B. (1970). Perennial problems in the field of emotion. In *Feelings and Emotions,* ed. Arnold, M. B. New York: Academic Press.

Asatoor, A. M., Levi, A. J. & Milne, M. D. (1963). Tranylcypromine and cheese. *Lancet,* ii. 733.

Asch, S. S. (1971). Wrist scratching as a symptom of anhedonia: a predepressive state. *Psychoanal. Quart.* **40**, 603–617.

Ashby, W. R. (1948). The homeostat. *Electron. Engng.* **20**, 379.

Ashby, W. R. (1950). Cybernetics. In *Recent Progress in Psychiatry,* pp. 94–110, ed. Fleming, G. W. T. H. London: Churchill.

Ashby, W. R. (1963). Induction, prediction and decision-making in cybernetic systems. In *Induction: some current issues.* Middletown, Connecticut: Wesleyan University Press.

Ashby, W. R. & Bassett, M. (1949). The effect of leucotomy on creative ability. *J. ment. Sci.* **95**, 418.

Ashcroft, G. W., Ecclestone, D. & Waddell, J. L. (1965). Recognition of amphetamine addicts. *Brit. med. J.* **1**, 57.

Asher, R. (1949). Myxoedematous madness. *Brit. med. J.* 2, 555.

Asher, R. (1951). Munchausen's syndrome. *Lancet,* i, 339.

Asher, R. (1954). The physical basis of mental illness. *Trans. med. Soc. Lond.* **70**, 93.

Asher, R. (1956). Arrangements for the mentally ill. *Lancet,* ii, 1265.

Aula, P., & Nichols, W. W. (1967). The cytogenetic effects of mycoplasma in human leukocyte cultures. *J. Cell Physiol.* **70**, 281–289.

Aungle, P. G. (1959). The care and treatment of psychopathic offenders in Norway, Sweden and Denmark. *J. ment. Sci.* **105**, 428.

Ayd, F. J. (1957). A critique of chlorpromazine and reserpine therapy. In *Tranquilizing Drugs,* ed. Himwich, H. E. Amer. Assoc. for the Advancement of Science Publ. No. 46. Washington. D.C.

Baastrup, P. C., Poulsen, J. C., Schou, M. & Thomsen, K. Prophylactic lithium: double blind discontinuation (1970) in manic-depression and recurrent depressive disorders. *Lancet,* ii, 326–330.

Baastrup, P. C. & Schou, M. (1967). Lithium as a prophylactic agent: its effect against recurrent depression and manic-depressive psychosis. *Arch. gen. Psychiat.* **16**, 162–172.

Babcock, H. (1930). An experiment in the measurement of mental deterioration. *Arch. Psychol.* **18**, 5.

Babinski, J. F. (1908). My conception of hysteria and hypnotism. *Alien. & Neurol.* **1**, 1.

Baer, R. L. & Sulzberger, M. B. (1952). Attempts at passive transfer of allergic eczematous sensitivity in man. *J. invest. Derm.* **18**, 53.

Bailey, P. & Gibbs, F. A. (1951). The surgical treatment of psychomotor epilepsy. *J. Amer. med. Ass.* **145**, 365.

Bailey, P., Green, J. R., Amador, L. & Gibbs, F. A. (1953). Treatment of psychomotor states by anterior temporal lobectomy. *Res. Publ. Ass. nerv. ment. Dis.* **31**, 341.

Bailey, P. & von Bonin, G. (1951). The isocortex of man. *Illinois Monogr. med. Sci.* **6**, 1 & 2.

Baillarger, J. (1854). *Essai de classification des maladies mentales. (Lecon faite a la Salpêtrière le 9 Avril,* 1854). Paris: V. Masson.

Bain, A. D., & Sutherland, G. R. (1973) Antenatal screening for Down's syndrome. *Lancet,* i, 423.

Baker, A. A. (1958). Breaking up the mental hospital. *Lancet,* ii, 253.

Baker, A. A. (1961). Pulling down the old mental hospital. *Lancet,* i, 656.

Bakwin, H. (1944). Psychogenic fever in infants. *Amer. J. Dis. Child.* **67**, 176.

Bale, R. N. (1973). Brain damage in diabetes mellitis. *Brit. J. Psychiat.* **122**, 337–341.

Balint, M. (1957). *The Doctor, His Patient and the Illness.* London: Pitman.

Bancroft, J. & Marks, I. (1968). Electric aversion therapy of sexual deviations. *Proc. roy. Soc. Med.* **61**, 796–799.

Bänder, A. (1950). Über zwei verschiedene chromoffine Zelltypen in Nebennierenmark und ihre Beziehung zum Adrenalin–und Arterenolgehalt. *Verh. anat. Ges. Jena.* **48**, 172.

Bannister, R. (1970). The place of isotope encephalography by the lumbar route in neurological diagnosis. *Proc. roy. Soc. Med.* **63**, 921–925.

Barber, T. X. (1962). Towards a theory of hypnosis: posthypnotic behaviour. *Arch. gen. Psychiat.* 7, 321.

Barger, G. & Dale, H. H. (1910). The presence in ergot and physiological activity of β-imidazolylethylamine. *J. Physiol.* **40,** 38 (Abstr.).

Barker, J. C. (1958). Electroplexy (E.C.T.) techniques in current use: a report of a questionnaire recently circulated to hospitals. *J. ment. Sci.* **104,** 1069.

Barker, J. C. & Baker, A. A. (1959). Deaths associated with electroplexy. *J. ment. Sci.* **105,** 339.

Barker, J. C. & May, A. (1959). Prolonged apnoea following E.C.T. modified by suxemethonium (Brevedil 'E'). *J ment. Sci.* **105,** 496.

Barker, J. C., Thorpe, J. G. Blakemore, C. B., Lavin, N. I. & Conway, C. G. (1961). Behaviour therapy in a case of transvestism. *Lancet,* i, 510.

Barker, M. G. (1968). Psychiatric illness after hysterectomy. *Brit. med. J.* 2, 91- 95.

Barnes, M. & Berke, J. (1971). Mary Barnes: *Two Accounts of a Journey Through Madness.* London: McGibbon & Kee.

Barnes, R. & Schottstaedt, W. W. (1960). The relation of emotional state to renal excretion of water and electrolytes in patients with congestive heart failure. *Amer. J. Med.* **29,** 217.

Baron, D. N., Dent, C. E. Harris, H., Hart, E. W. & Jepson, J. B. (1956). Hereditary pellagra-like skin rash with temporary cerebellar ataxia, constant renal amino-aciduria, and other bizarre biochemical features. *Lancet,* ii, 421.

Barraclough, B. M. & Shea, M. (1970). Suicide and Samaritan clients. *Lancet,* ii, 868–70.

Barraclough, M. A. & Sharpey-Schafer, E. P. (1963). Hypotension from absent circulatory reflexes: effects of alcohol, barbiturates, psychotherapeutic drugs, and other mechanisms. *Lancet,* i, 1121.

Bartlett, E. M. (1965). Exceptional children. In *Modern Perspectives in Child Psychiatry,* ed. Howells, J. G. Edinburgh: Oliver & Boyd.

Barton, R. (1965). Diabetes insipidus and obsessional neurosis: a syndrome. *Lancet,* i. 133.

Baruk, H. (1956). Un grave probleme de moral médicale. *Presse méd.* **64,** 371.

Batchelor, I. R. C. (1954). Alcoholism and attempted suicide. *J. ment. Sci.* **100,** 451.

Batchelor, I. R. C. & Napier, M. B. (1953). Attempted suicide in old age. *Brit. med. J.* 2, 1186.

Bayle, A. L. J. (1822). Recherches sur les maladies mentales. M.D. Thesis, Paris.

Beach, F. A. (1948). *Hormones and Behaviour: a Survey of Interrelationships between Endocrine Secretions in Patterns of Overt Response.* New York: Hoeber.

Bearcroft, J. S. & Donovan, M. D. (1965). Psychiatric referrals from courts and prisons. *Brit. med. J.* 2, 1519.

Beard, B. H. (1971). The quality of life before and after renal transplantation. *Dis. nerv. Syst.* 32, 24–31.

Beaumont, W. (1833). *Experiments and Observations on the Gastric Juice and the Physiology of Digestion,* ed. Combe, A. (1838). Edinburgh: Maclachlan & Stewart.

Beckenstein, N. & Gold, L. (1945). Problems of senile arteriosclerotic mental patients: a review of 200 cases. *Psychiat. Quart.* 19, 398.

Beech, H. R., Davies, B. M. & Morgenstern, F. S. (1961). Preliminary investigations of the effects of sernyl upon cognitive and sensory processes. *J. ment. Sci.* **107,** 509.

Behcet, H. (1937). Über regidivierende Apthöse, durch ein Virus verursachte; Geschwüre am Mund, am Auge und an den Genitalien. *Dermat. Wchschr.* **105,** 1152–1157.

Behrman, J. & Levy, R (1970). Neurophysiological studies on patients with hysterical disturbances of vision. *J Psychosom. Res.* 14, 187–194.

Behrman, S. (1972). Mutism induced by phenothiazines. *Brit. J. Psychiat.* 121, 599–604.

Bellak, L. (1948). *Dementia Praecox: the Past Decade's Work and Present Status: a Review and Evaluation.* New York: Grune.

Bellak, L. *et al.* (1952). *Manic-depressive Psychosis and Allied Conditions.* New York: Grune.

Belson, W. A. (1957). 'The Hurt Mind', An enquiry into some of the effects of the series of five television broadcasts about mental illness and its treatment. British Broadcasting Corporation. Audience Research Report.

Bemporad, J. F., Pfeifer, C. M., Gibbs, L., Cortner, R. H., & Bloom, W. (1971). Characteristics of encopretic patients and their families. *J. Amer. Acad. Child Psychiat.* **10,** 272–292.

Benchimol. A. B. & Schlesinger, P. (1953). Beriberi heart disease. *Amer. Heart J.* **46,** 245.

Benda, C. E. (1947). *Mongolism and Cretinism: a Study of the Clinical Manifestations and the General Pathology of Pituitary and Thyroid Deficiency.* London: Heinemann.

Benda, C. E. (1953). Research in congenital acromicria (mongolism) and its treatment. *Quart. Rev. Pediat.* **8,** 79.

Bender, L. (1938). A visual motor Gestalt test and its clinical use. *Amer. Orthopsychiat. Ass. Res. Monogr.* No. 3.
Bender, L. (1945). Infants reared in institutions permanently handicapped. *Child Welfare League of America Bull.* **14**, No. 7.
Bender, L. (1950). Postencephalitic behavior disorders. In *Anxiety,* ed. Hoch, P. H. & Zubin, J. New York: Grune & Stratton.
Bender, L. (1951). The psychological treatment of the brain-damaged child. *Quart. J. Child. Behav.* **3**, 123.
Bender, L. (1953). Childhood schizophrenia. *Psychiat. Quart.* **27**, 663.
Bender, L. (1956). *Psychopathology of Children with Organic Brain Disorders.* Springfield, Illinois: Thomas.
Bender, L. & Schilder, P. (1937). Suicidal pre-occupation and attempts in children. *Amer. J. Orthopsychiat.* **7**, 225.
Bengtsson, M., Holmberg, S. & Jansson, B. (1969). A psychiatric-psychological investigation of patients who had survived circulatory arrest. *Acta Psychiat. Scand.* **45**, 327–346.
Bennett, A. E. (1940). Preventing traumatic complications in convulsive shock therapy by curare. *J. Amer. med. Ass.* **114**, 322.
Bennett, D., Folkard, S. & Nicholson, A. K. (1961). Resettlement unit in a mental hospital. *Lancet* ii, 539.
Berg, C. (1948). *Clinical Psychology.* London: Allen & Unwin.
Berg, J. M. Brandon, M. W. & Kirman, B. H. (1959). Atropine in Mongolism. *Lancet,* ii, 441.
Berg, J.M. & Kirman, B. H. (1959). Some aetiological problems of mental deficiency. *Brit. med. J.* **2**, 848.
Berg, J. M., Smith, G. F., Ridler, M. A. C., Dutton, G., Green, E. A. & Richards, B. W. (1966). On the association of broad thumbs and first toes with other physical peculiarities and mental retardation. *J. Ment. Def. Res.* **10**, 204.
Berger, H. (1929). Über das Elektroenkephalogram des Menschen. *Arch. Psychiat. Nervenkr.* **87**, 527.
Bergler, E. (1946). Problems of suicide. *Psychiat. Quart.* Suppl., **20**, 261.
Bernard, C. (1865). *Introduction a l'étude de la médicine experimentale.* Paris: Baillière. Eng. trans. by Greene, H. C. (1927), *An Introduction to the Study of Experimental Medicine.* New York: Macmillan.
Bernfeld, S. (1928). Über Faszination. *Imago,* **14**, 76.
Bernhardson, G., & Gunne, L-M. (1972). Forty-six cases of psychosis in cannabis abusers. *Int. J. Addiction.* **7**, 9–16.
Bernstein, F. (1924). Ergebnisse einer biostatischen zusammenfassenden Betrachung über die erblichen Blutsrukturen des Menschen. *Klin. Wschr.* **3**, 1495.
Berry, C. & Orwin, A. (1966). 'No fixed abode': a survey of mental hospital admissions. *Brit. J. Psychiat.* **112**, 1019.
Berry, C. & Sim, M. (1968). Schizophrenia: a follow up of patients treated in a general hospital unit. (To be published).
Bethell, M. F. (1965). Toxic psychosis caused by inhalation of petrol fumes. *Brit. med. J.* **2**, 276.
Bethune, H. C. & Kidd, C. B. (1961). Psychophysiological mechanisms in skin diseases. *Lancet,* ii, 1419.
Bettelheim, B. (1969). *The Children of the Dream. Communal Child-Rearing and its Implications for Society.* London: Thames & Hudson.
Betts, T. A., Kalra, P. L. Cooper, R., & Jeavons, P. M. (1968). Epileptic fits as a probable side-effect of amitriptyline: report of seven cases. *Lancet,* i, 390–392.
Bibring, G. L. (1959). Some considerations of the psychological processes in pregnancy. *Psychoanal. study Child.* **14**, 113.
Bibring, G. L. *et al.* (1961). A study of the psychological processes in pregnancy and of the earliest mother-child relationship. *Psychoanal. Study Child,* **16**, 9–72.
Bickel, H. (1954). The effects of a phenylalanine-free and phenylalanine poor diet in phenylpyruvic oligophrenia. *Exp. Med. Surg.* **12**, 114.
Bickers, W. (1958). Premenstrual tension: a water-toxicity syndrome. *Virginia med. Mth.* **85**, 613.
Bickford, J. A. R. & Ellison, R M. (1953). The high incidence of Huntington's chorea in the Duchy of Cornwall. *J. ment. Sci.* **99**, 291.
Bickford, R. G. (1948). Electroencephalographic and clinical responses to light stimulation in normal subjects. *Electroenceph. clin. neurophysiol.* **1**, 126.
Bierer, J. (1951) *The Day Hospital.* London: Lewis.
Bierer, J. (1959). Theory and practice of psychiatric day hospitals. *Lancet,* ii 901.

Binet, A. & Simon, T. (1905). Méthodes nouvelles pour le diagnostic du niveau intellectual des anormaux. *Année psychol.* 11, 191.

Birtchnell, J. (1970). The relationship between attempted suicide, depression and parent death. *Brit. J. Psychiat.* 116, 307–313.

Birtchnell, J. (1970). Depression in relation to early and recent parent death. *Brit. J. Psychiat.* 116, 299–306.

Birtchnell, J. (1970). Recent parent death and mental illness. *Brit. J. Psychiat.* 116, 289–297.

Birtchnell, J. (1970). Early parent death and mental illness. *Brit. J. Psychiat.* 116, 281–288.

Blacher, R. S. (1972). The hidden psychosis of open-heart surgery: with a note on the sense of awe. *J. Amer. med. Ass.* 222, 305–308.

Blachly, P. H. (1973). Naloxone for diagnosis in methadone programs. *J. Amer. med. Ass.* 224, 334–335.

Blackwell, B. (1963). Hypertensive crisis due to monoamine-oxidase inhibitors. *Lancet,* ii, 849.

Blackwell, B. & Shepherd, M. (1968). Prophylactic lithium: another therapeutic myth? an examination of the evidence to date. *Lancet,* i, 968–971.

Blaschko, H. (1957). Formation of catecholamines in the animal body. *Brit. med. Bull.* 13, 162.

Blaschko, H. (1959). The development of current concepts of catecholamine formation. *Pharm. Rev.* 11, 307.

Blau, J. N. & Hinton, J. M. (1960). Hypopituitary coma and psychosis. *Lancet,* i, 408.

Bleuler, E. P. (1911). *Dementia Praecox or the Group of Schizophrenics.* Transl. by Ziskin. New York. 1950.

Bleuler, E. P. (1913). Autistic thinking. *Amer. J. Insan.* 69, 873.

Bleuler, E. P. (1924). *Textbook of Psychiatry.* Transl. by Brill A. A. New York: Macmillan.

Bleuler, M. (1951). Psychiatry of cerebral diseases. *Brit. med. J.* 2, 1233.

Bleuler, M. (1954). *Endokrinologische Psychiatrie.* Stuttgart: Thieme.

Blonstein, J. L. (1963). Neurological disease in boxers. *Lancet,* ii, 937.

Bloodstein, O. (1958). *Stuttering–A Symposium.* Ed. Eisenson, J. New York: Harper.

Boakes, A. J., Laurence, D. R. Teoh, P. C., Barar, F. S. K. Benedikter, L. T. Prichard, B. N. C. (1973). Interactions between sympathomimetic amines and antidepressant agents in man. *Brit. med. J.* 1, 311–315.

Board of Control (1947). Pre-frontal Leucotomy in 1000 Cases. London: H.M.S.O.

Boardman, R. H., Lomas, J. & Markowe, M. (1956). Insulin and chlorpromazine in schizophrenia: a comparative study in previously untreated cases. *Lancet,* ii, 487.

Bonhoff, G. & Lewrenz, H. (1954). *Über Weckamine.* Berlin: Springer.

Bonn, J. A. (1973). Progress in Anxiety States. *Proc. roy. Soc. Med.* 66 249–252.

Böök, J. A. & Reed, S.C. (1950). Empiric risk figures in mongolism. *J. Amer. Med. Ass.* 143, 730.

Borges Fortes, A. B. (1956). Tratamento da paralisia geral pela penicilina. *Arch. bras. Psychiat.* 51, 23.

Boslow, H. M. Rosenthal, D. & Gliedman, L. H. (1959). Psychiatric implications for the treatment of antisocial disorders under the law. *Brit. J. Delinq.* 10. 5.

Bossard, J. H. S. (1943). Family table talk: an area for sociological study. *Amer. Social Rev.* 8, 295.

Bostock, J. (1958). Exterior gestation, primitive sleep, enuresis and asthma: a study in aetiology, Part I & II. *Med. J. Aust.* 2, 149, 185.

Boswell, J. (1791). *The Life of Samuel Johnson, LL.D.* 6 vols. 1934–50. London: Oxford University Press.

Botterell, E. H., Callaghan, J. C. & Jousse, A. T. (1954). Pain in paraplegia: clinical management and surgical treatment. *Proc. roy. Soc. Med.* 47, 281.

Boulougouris, J. C. & Marks, I. M. (1969). Implosion (flooding)–a new treatment for phobias. *Brit. med. J.* 2, 721–723.

Bourne, H. (1953). The insulin myth. *Lancet,* ii, 964.

Bourne, H. (1955). Protophrenia: a study of perverted rearing and mental dwarfism. *Lancet,* ii, 1156.

Bourneville, D. (1880). Sclerose tuberouse de circumvolutions cerebrates: idiotie et épilepsie hémiplégique. *Arch. Neurol.* 1, 81.

Bovet, D., Longo, V. G. & Silvestrini, B. (1957). Les methodes d'investigations électrophysiologiques dans l'étude des médicaments tranquillisants. In *Psychotropic Drugs,* p. 193, ed. Garattini, S. and Ghetti, V. Amsterdam: Elsevier Publ. Co.

Bowen, M. (1960). A family concept of schizophrenia. In *The Etiology of Schizophrenia,* ed. Jackson, D. D. New York: Basic Books.

Bowlby, J. (1940). *Personality and Mental Illness.* London: Kegan Paul.
Bowlby, J. (1944). Forty-four juvenile thieves, their characters and home life. *Int. J. Psycho-Anal.* 25, 107.
Bowlby, J. (1951). Maternal care and mental health. *Wld. Hlth. Org. Monogr. Ser.* No. 2.
Bowlby, J. (1960). Grief and mourning in infancy and early childhood. In *The Psychoanalytic Study of the Child,* vol. 15. New York: International Universities Press.
Bowlby, J. (1969). *Attachment and Loss.* Vol. 1: Attachment. London: Hogarth Press.
Bowman, K. M. & Rose, M. (1951). A criticism of the terms 'psychosis', 'psychoneurosis' and 'neurosis'. *Amer. J. Psychiat.* **108**, 161.
Boyd, P., Layland, W. R. & Crickmay, J. R. (1971). Treatment and follow-up of adolescents addicted to heroin. *Brit. med. J.* 4, 604–605.
Bradley, P. B. (1957). Microelectrode approach to the neuropharmacology of the reticular formation. In *Psychotropic Drugs,* pp. 207, 209, ed. Garattini, S. and Ghetti, V. Amsterdam: Elsevier Publ. Co.
Bradley, P. B. & Wolstencroft, J. H. (1965). Actions of drugs on single neurones in the brain-stem. *Brit. med. Bull.* 21, 15.
Bradley, P. B., Wolstencroft, J. H., Hösli, L. & Avanzino, G. L. (1966). Neuronal basis for the central action of chlorpromazine. *Nature,* Lond. **212**, 1425.
Brain, W. R. (1962). *Diseases of the Nervous System,* 6th Ed. London: Oxford University Press.
Brain, W. R., Daniel, P. M. & Greenfield, J. G. (1951). Subacute cortical cerbellar degeneration and its relation to carcinoma. *J. Neurol. Neurosurg. Psychiat.* **14**, 59.
Brandon, S. (1970). Crisis theory and possibilities of therapeutic intervention. *Brit. J. Psychiat.* 117, 627–633.
Bratfos, O. (1970). Transition of neuroses and other minor mental disorders into psychoses. *Acta Psychiat. Scand.* 46, 35–49.
Breuer, J. & Freud S. (1895). *Studies in Hysteria.* New York: Nervous and Mental Disease Publishing Coy. 1936.
Brickner, R. M. (1936). *Intellectual Functions of the Frontal Lobes: a Study Based upon Observations of a Man after Partial Bilateral Frontal Lobectomy.* New York: Macmillan.
Bridenbaugh, R. H., Drake, F. R., & O'Regan, T. J. (1972). Multiple monitored electroconvulsive treatment of schizophrenia. *Compr. Psychiat.* 13, 9–17.
Brigden, W. & Robinson, J. (1964). Alcoholic heart disease. *Brit med. J.* 1, 450.
Brill, A. A. (1946). *Lectures on Psychoanalytic Psychiatry.* London: Garden City Books.
Brill, N. Q. & Storrow, H. A. (1963). Prognostic factors in psychotherapy. *J.A.M.A.* **183**, 913.
British Medical Journal (1955). Homosexuality and prostitution. B.M.A. memorandum of evidence for departmental committee. *Brit. med. J.* 2, 165, (Suppl.).
British Medical Journal (1958). Psychological medicine in general practice. *Brit. med. J.* 2, 585.
British Medical Journal (1959*a*). Monoamine oxidase inhibitors. *Brit. med. J.* 2, 1238.
British Medical Journal (1959*b*). Book review: *Class and Mental Illness. Brit. med. J.* 1, 154.
British Medical Journal (1960). Emotional stress and coronary thrombosis. *Brit. med. J.* 1, 866.
British Medical Journal (1961*a*). Sexual assaults on children. 1. Present procedure. *Brit. med. J.* 2, 1628.
British Medical Journal (1961*b*). Suicide Act. *Brit. med. J.* 2, 460.
British Medical Journal (1961*c*). Schizophrenic syndrome in childhood: Progress report (April 1961) of a working party. *Brit. med. J.* 2, 889.
British Medical Journal (1961*d*). Detention of criminals in mental hospitals. *Brit. med. J.* 2, 716.
British Medical Journal (1962*a*). Incurably of unsound mind. *Brit. med. J.* 2, 268.
British Medical Journal (1962*b*). Drugs for anxiety. *Brit. med. J.* 1, 38.
Britton, S. W. & Kline, R. F. (1939). Emotional hyperglycaemia and hyperthermia in tropical mammals and reptiles. *Amer. J. Physiol.* 125, 730.
Broadwin, I. T. (1932). Contribution to study of truancy. *Amer. J. Orthopsychiat.* 2, 253.
Brodie, B. B., Pletscher, A. & Shore, P. A. (1956). Evidence that serotonin has a role in brain function. *Science,* **122**, 968.
Brodie, H. K. H., Murphy, D. L., Goodwin, F. K., & Bunney, W. E. (1971). Catecholamines and mania: the effect of alpha-methyl-para-tyrosine on manic behaviour and catecholamine metabolism. *Clin. Pharmacol. Ther.* 12, 218–224.
Brooks, G. W. & Mueller, E. (1966). Serum urate concentrations among university professors. *J. Amer. med. Ass.* 195, 415.

Brown, D. G. & Bettley, F. R. (1971). Psychiatric treatment of eczema: a controlled trial. *Brit. med. J.* 2, 729–734
Brown, G. W., Birley, J. L. T., & Wing, J.K. (1972). Influence of family life on the course of schizophrenic disorders: a replication. *Brit. J. Psychiat.* **121**, 241–258.
Brown, G. W., Bone, M. Dalison, N. & Wing, J. K. (1968). *Schizophrenia and Social Care.* Maudsley Monographs No. 17.
Brown, G. W., Carstairs, G. M. & Topping, G. (1958). Post-hospital adjustment of chronic mental patients. *Lancet,* ii 685.
Brown, G. W., Monck, E. M., Carstairs, G. M., & Wing, J. K. (1962). Influence of family life on the course of schizophrenic illness. *Brit. J. prev. soc. Med.* 16, 55.
Brown, J. A. C. (1961). *Freud and the Post-Freudians.* Harmondsworth, Middlesex: Penguin Books Ltd.
Bruce, J. & Russell, G. F. M. (1962). Premenstrual tension: a study of weight changes and balances of water, sodium, and potassium. *Lancet,* ii, 267.
Bruch, H. (1940). Obesity in childhood. *Amer. J. Dis. Child.* **60**, 1082.
Bruch, H. (1941). Obesity in childhood and personality development. *Amer. J. Orthopsychiat.* 11, 467.
Bruch, H. (1957). *The Importance of Overweight.* New York: Norton & Co.
Bruch, H. (1966). Anorexia nervosa and its differential diagnosis. *J. nerv. ment. Dis.* **141**, 555.
Bruch, H. (1969). Hunger and instinct. *J. nerv. ment. Dis.* **149**, 91–114.
Bruner, J. S., Goodnow, J. S., & Austin, G. A. (1956). *A Study of Thinking.* New York: Wiley.
Bucy, P. C. & Klüver, H. (1955). An anatomical investigation of the temporal lobe in the monkey (macaca mulatta). *J. comp. Neurol.* **103**, 151.
Bumke, O. (1932). *Handbuch der geisteskrankheiten,* Bearb. von K. Beringer, *et al.* Hrsg. von Oswald Bumke, 11 vols 1928–32. Berlin: Springer.
Bumke, O. (1948). *Lehrbuch der geisteskrankheiten.* 7 Aufl. München: Bergmann.
Bunney, W. E., Davis, J. M., Weil-Malherbe, H. & Smith, E. R. B. (1967). Biochemical changes in psychotic depression: high norepinephrine levels in psychotic vs. neurotic depression. *Arch. gen. Psychiat.* **16**, 448–460.
Bunney, W. E., Goodwin, F. K., & Murphy, D. L. (1972). The 'switch process' in manic-depressive illness. III. Theoretical implications. *Arch. gen. Psychiat.* **27**, 312–317.
Bunney, W. E., Goodwin, F. K., Murphy, D. L., House, K. M. & Gordon, E. K. (1972). The 'switch process' in manic-depressive illness. II. Relationship to catecholamines, REM sleep, and drugs. *Arch. gen. Psychiat.* **27**, 303–309.
Bunney, W. E., Murphy, D. L., Goodwin, F. K., & Borge, G. F. (1972). The 'switch process' in manic depressive illness. I. A. systematic study of sequential behavioral changes. *Arch. gen. Psychiat.* **27**, 295–302.
Burgess, E. W. (1926). The family as a unity of interacting personalities. *The Family,* 7, 3.
Burns, B. H. & Howell, J. B. L. (1969). Disproportionately severe breathlessness in chronic bronchitis. *Quart J. Med.* **38**, 277–294.
Burns, C. L. C. (1941). Encopresis (incontinence of faeces) in children. *Brit. med. J.* 2, 767.
Burns, C. L. C. (1959). Truancy or School Phobia. National Association for Mental Health: proceedings of the 15th inter-clinic conference, p. 26. London.
Bursten, B. (1972). The manipulative personality. *Arch. gen. Psychiat.* **26**, 318–321.

Cade, J. F. J. (1972). Massive thiamine dosage in the treatment of acute alcoholic psychoses. *Aust. N.Z.J. Psychiat.* 6, 225–230.
Cade, J. F.S. (1949). Lithium salts in the treatment of psychotic excitement. *Med. J. Austral.* 2, 349.
Caffey, J. (1957). Some traumatic lesions in growing bones other than fractures and dislocations: clinical and radiological features. *Brit. J. Radiol.* **30**, 225–238.
Calderone, M. S. (ed.) (1958). *Abortion in the United States.* New York: Hoeber-Harper.
Calmeil, L. F. (1826). *De la paralysie considérée chez les aliénés.* Paris: Baillière.
Calne, D. B. (1973). The drug treatment of epilepsy. *Brit. J. Hosp. Med.* **9**, 171–175.
Cameron, N. (1938). Reasoning, regression and communication in schizophrenics. *Psychol. Monogr.* **50** (1).
Campbell, A. M. G., Evans M., Thomson, J. L. G., & Williams, M. J. (1971). Cerebral atrophy in young cannabis smokers. *Lancet,* ii, 1219–1224.
Campbell, C. M. (1943). Clinical studies in schizophrenia: a follow-up study of a small group of cases of deterioration with few special trends. (schizophrenic "surrender"). *Amer. J. Psychiat.* **99**, 475.

Campbell, D. R. (1971). The electroencephalogram in cannabis associated psychosis. *Canad. Psychiat. Ass. J.* **16**, 161–165.

Candy, J., Balfour, H. G., Cawley, R. H., Hildebrand, H. P., Malan, D. H., Marks, I. M., & Wilson, J. (1972). A feasability study for a controlled trial or formal psychotherapy. *Psychol. Med.* 2, 345–362.

Cannon, W. B. (1915). *Bodily Changes in Pain, Hunger, Fear and Rage.* New York: Appleton.

Cannon, W. B. (1939). *The Wisdom of the Body,* 2nd Ed. New York: Norton.

Canter, A. H. (1951). Direct and indirect measures of psychological deficit in multiple sclerosis. *J. gen. Psychol.* **44**, 3, 27.

Caplan, G. (1964). *Principles of Preventive Psychiatry.* New York: Basic Books.

Caplan, G. (1970). *The Theory and Practice of Mental Health Consultation.* New York: Basic Books.

Capstick, A. (1960). Recognition of emotional disturbance and the prevention of suicide. *Brit. med. J* 1, 1179.

Carlander, O. (1958) Pica och järnbrost. (Pica and iron deficiency.) *Svenska Läk.-Tidn.* **55**, 387.

Carlson, G. A. & Goodwin, F. K. (1973). The stages of mania: a longitudinal analysis of the manic episode. *Arch. gen. Psychiat.* **28**, 221–228.

Carothers, J. C. (1947). A study of mental derangement in Africans and an attempt to explain its peculiarities more especially in relation to the African attitude to life. *J. ment. Sci.* **93**, 548.

Carothers, J. C. (1953). The African mind in health and disease. A study in ethnopsychiatry. *Wld. Hlth. Org. Monogr. Ser.* No. 17.

Carse, J., Panton, N. E. & Watt, A. (1958). A district mental health service. *Lancet,* i, 39.

Carson, J. & Kitching, H. E. (1949). Psychiatric beds in a general ward. *Lancet,* i, 833.

Carstairs, G. M. (1956). Hinjra and Jiryan: two derivatives of Hindu attitudes to sexuality. *Brit. J. med. Psychol.* **29**, 128.

Carstairs, G. M. (1958). Some problems of psychiatry in patients from alien cultures. *Lancet,* i, 1217.

Carstairs, G. M. & Wing, J. K. (1958). Attitudes of the general public to mental illness. *Brit. med. J.* 2, 594.

Carter, C. O. & Evans, K. A. (1961). Risk of parents who have had one child with Down's syndrome (mongolism) having another child similarly affected. *Lancet,* ii, 785.

Cattell, J. McK. (1890). Mental tests and measurements. *Mind,* **15**, 373.

Cattell, R. B. (1937). *The Fight for Our National Intelligence.* London: King.

Cattell, R. B. (1946). *Description and measurement in Personality.* Yonkers, New York: World Books.

Cattell, R. B. (1957). *The Sixteen Personality Factor Questionnaire.* (Rev. Ed.) Champaign, Ill: IPAT.

Catterall, R. D. (1961). Collagen disease and the chronic biological false positive phenomenon. *Quart. J. Med.* **30**, 41.

Cawley, R. (1971). Evaluation of psychotherapy. *Psychol. Med.* 1, 101–103.

Cawley, R., Candy, J., Malan, D., & Marks, I. (1973). Dynamic psychotherapy: can it be evaluated? *Proc. roy. Soc. Med.* **66**, 943–945.

Celesia, G. G., & Barr, A. N. (1970). Psychosis and other psychiatric manifestations of levadopa therapy. *Arch. Neurol.* **23**, 193–200.

Cerletti, V. & Bini, L. (1938). L'Elettroshock. *Arch. Psicol neurol Psichiat.* **19**, 266.

Chambers, W. N. & Reiser, M. F. (1953). Emotional stress in the precipitation of congestive heart failure. *Psychosom. Med.* **15**, 38.

Chandler, J. H. (1955). Reserpine in the treatment of Huntington's chorea. *Univ. Mich. med. Bull.* **21**, 95.

Chapman, A. H. (1959). Psychogenic urinary retention in women: report of a case. *Psychosom. Med.* **21**, 119.

Chapman, W. P. (1958). Studies of the periamygdaloid area in relation to human behaviour. *Res. Publ. Ass. nerv. ment. Dis.* **36**, 258.

Charatan, F. B. & Brierley, J. B. (1956). Mental disorder associated with primary lung carcinoma. *Brit. med. J.* 1, 765.

Charcot, J.-M. (1877). *Diseases of the Nervous System.* London: New Sydenham Soc.

Chasin, R. M. (1967). Special clinical problems in day hospitalization. *Amer. J. Psychiat.* **123**, 779.

Chaudhary, N. A. & Truelove, S. C. (1962). The irritable colon syndrome: a study of the clinical features, predisposing causes and prognosis in 130 cases. *Quart. J. Med.* **31**, 307.

Cheney, C. O. (1934). *Outline for psychiatric Examinations.* Utica, New York: State Hospitals Press.
Chess, S. (1959). *An Introduction to Child Psychiatry.* New York: Grune & Stratton.
Chess, S. (1972). Neurological dysfunction and childhood behavioral pathology. *J. Autism Child. Schiz.* 2, 299–311.
Christodoresco, D., Collino, S., Zellingher, R., & Tăutu, C. (1970). Psychiatric disturbances in Turner's syndrome. *Psychiat. clin.* 3, 114–124.
Clark, D. H. (1958). Administrative therapy: its clinical importance in the mental hospital. *Lancet,* i, 805.
Clark, D. H. (1960). Principles of administrative therapy. *Amer. J. Psychiat.* 117, 506.
Clark, L. D., Hughes, R., & Nakishima, E. N. (1970). Behavioral effects of marihuana: experimental studies. *Arch. gen. Psychiat.* 23, 193–198.
Clark, R. E. (1949). Psychoses, income, and occupational prestige. *Amer. J. Sociol.* 54, 433.
Clarke, A. D. B. & Clarke, A. M. (1955). Pseudo-feeblemindedness—some implications. *Amer. J. ment. Defic.* 59, 507.
Clarke, A. M. & Clarke, A. D. B. (1958). *Mental Deficiency; the Changing Outlook.* London: Methuen.
Clarke, C. M., Edwards, J. H. & Smallpiece, V. (1961). Trisomy/normal mosaicism in an intelligent child with some mongoloid characters. *Lancet,* i, 1028–1030.
Cleckley, H. M. (1950). *The Mask of Sanity,* 2nd Ed. London: Kimpton.
Cleghorn, R. A. (1955). The hypothalamic-endocrine system. *Psychosom. Med.* 17, 367.
Clement, A. J. (1962). Atropine premedication for electric convulsion therapy. *Brit. med. J.* 1, 228.
Clouston, T. S. (1877). A case of general paralysis at the age of sixteen. *J. ment. Sci.* 23, 419.
Cobb, W. A. (1950). In *Electroencephalography,* ed. Hill. J. D. N. & Parr, G. London: McDonald.
Coe, R. M. (1970). *Sociology of Medicine.* New York: McGraw Hill.
Coekin, M. & Gairdner, D. (1960). Faecal incontinence in children: the physical factor. *Brit. med. J.* 2, 1175.
Cohen, B. H. Lilienfeld, A. M. & Sigler, A. T. (1963). Some epidemiologic aspects of mongolism: a review. *Amer. J. Pub. Health,* 53, 223.
Cohen, H. (Chairman) (1956). Report of the subcommittee on the medical care of epileptics. Central Health Services Council, Ministry of Health, Great Britain, H.M.S.O. London.
Cohen, H. (1958). Epilepsy as a social problem. *Brit. med. J.* 1, 672.
Cohen, I. M. & Archer, J. D. (1955). Liver function and hepatic complications in patients receiving chlorpromazine. *J. Amer. med. Ass.* 159, 99.
Collum, J. M. (1972). Identity diffusion and the borderline maneuver. *Compr. Psychiat.* 13, 179–184.
Colwell, C. & Post, F. (1959). Community needs of elderly psychiatric patients. *Brit. med. J.* 2, 214.
Committee of the Clinical Society of London (1888). Report on Myxoedema. *Trans. clin. Soc.* 21, 31, (Suppl.).
Conger, J. J. (1951). The effects of alcohol on conflict behavior in the albino rat. *Quart. J. Stud. Alcohol.* 12, 1.
Connell, P. H. (1958). *Amphetamine Psychosis.* Maudsley Monograph, No. 5, London: Chapman & Hall, for Inst. of Psychiatry.
Connell, P. H. (1965). Suicidal attempts in childhood and adolesence. In *Modern Perspectives in Child Psychiatry,* ed. Howells, J. G. Edinburgh: Oliver & Boyd.
Conroy, R. T. W. L., Hughes, B. D., & Mills, J. N. (1968). Circadian rhythm of plasma 11-hydroxycorticosteroids in psychiatric disorders. *Brit. med. J.* 2, 405–407.
Cooper, A. J. (1969). Clinical and therapeutic studies in premature ejaculation. *Compr. Psychiat.* 10, 285–295.
Cooper, A. J., Ismail, A. A. A., Phanjoo, A. L., & Love, D. L. (1972). Antiandrogen (cyproterone acetate) therapy in deviant hypersexuality. *Brit. J. Psychiat.* 120, 59–63.
Cooper, J. E., Kendell, R. E., Gurland, B. J., Sharpe, L., Copeland, J. R. M., & Simon, R. (1972). Psychiatric Diagnosis in New York and London. Maudsley Monograph No. 20. London: Oxford Univ. Press.
Copeland, J. R. M., Cooper, J. E., Kendell, R. E. & Gourlay, A. J. (1971). Differences in usage of diagnostic labels amongst psychiatrists in the British Isles. *Brit. J. Psychiat.* 118, 629–640.
Coppen, A., Brooksbank, B. W. L., Noguera, R. & Wilson, D. A. (1971). Cortisol in the cerebrospinal fluid of patients suffering from affective disorders. *J. Neurol. Neurosurg. Psychiat.* 34, 432–435.

Coppen, A. & Cowie, V. (1960). Maternal health and mongolism. *Brit. med. J.* 1, 1843.
Coppen, A. & Kessel, N. (1963). Menstruation and personality. *Brit. J. Psychiat.* **109, 711.**
Coppen, A., Shaw, D. M., Malleson, A. & Costain, R. (1966). Mineral metabolism in mania, *Brit. med. J.* 1, 71.
Coppen, A. J., (1959). Vomiting of early pregnancy: psychological factors and body build. *Lancet* i, 172.
Coppen, A. J. (1959). Body-build of male homosexuals. *Brit. med. J.* 2, 1443.
Coppen, A. J. & Shaw, D. M. (1963). Mineral metabolism in melancholia. *Brit. med. J.* 2, 1439.
Cormia, F. E. (1952). Experimental histamine pruritis: influence of physical and psychological factors on threshold reactivity. *J. invest. Derm.* 19, 21.
Corsellis, J. A. N. & Brieriey, J. B. (1954). An unusual type of pre-senile dementia. *Brain,* 77, 571.
Costain, R., Redfearn, J. W. T. & Lippold, O. C. J. (1964). A controlled trial of the therapeutic effects of polarization of the brain in depressive illness. *Brit. J. Psychiat.* **110**, 786.
Court Brown, W. M. (1962). Sex chromosomes and the law. *Lancet,* ii, 508.
Courvoisier, S., Fourncl, J., Ducrot, R., Kolsky, M. & Koetschet, P. (1953). Proprietes pharmacodynamiques du chlorhydrate de chloro-3 (diméthyl-amino-3 propyl)-10 phenothiazine. *Arch. int. Pharmacodyn.* 92, 305.
Cowie, E. (1971). Amniocentesis: a means of pre-natal diagnosis of conditions associated with severe mental sub-normality. *Brit. J. Psychiat.* **118**, 83–86.
Cowie, V. (1961). Children of psychotics: a controlled study. *Proc. roy. Soc. Med.* 54, 675.
Cox, J. (1965). A patient's view of psychotherapy. *Lancet,* ii, 103.
Craft, M. (1959). Psychiatric day hospitals. *Amer. J. Psychiat.* 116, 251.
Craft, M. (1969). The natural history of psychopathic disorder. *Brit. J Psychiat.* **115**, 39–44.
Crammer, J. L. (1959). Periodic psychoses. *Brit. med. J.* 1, 545.
Creak, M. (1959). Child health & child psychiatry: neighbours or colleagues? *Lancet,* i, 482.
Crichton Miller, H. (1931). The psychology of suicide. *Brit. med. J.* 2, 239.
Crichton-Miller, H. (1945). *Psychoanalysis and its Derivatives,* 2nd Ed. H.U.L. (Oxf.).
Critchley, M. (1929). The nature and significance of senile plaques. *J. Neurol. Psychopath.* **10**, 124.
Crichley, M. (1950). Migraine. *Brit. med. J.* 2, 996.
Critchley, M. (1953). *The Parietal Lobes.* London: Edward Arnold.
Critchley, M. (1962). Periodic hypersomnia and megaphagia in adolescent males. *Brain,* **85**, 627.
Critchley, M. & Earl, C. J. C. (1932). Tuberose sclerosis & allied conditions. *Brain,* 55, 311.
Crockett, R. W. (1960). Doctors, administrators and therapeutic communities. *Lancet,* ii, 359.
Cronin, D., Bodley, P., Potts, L., Mather, M. D., Gardner, R. & Tobin, J. C. (1970). Unilateral and bilateral ECT: a study of memory disturbance and relief from depression. *J. Neurol. Neurosurg. Psychiat.* 33, 705–713.
Crowley, R. M. (1939). Psychoanalytic literature on drug addiction and alcoholism. *Psychol. Rev.* 26, 39.
Crown, S. (1973). Psychotherapy. *Brit. J. Hosp. Med.* 9, 355–362.
Cruickshank, W. H. (1940). Psychoses associated with pregnancy and the puerperium. *Canad. med. Ass. J.* 43, 571.
Cruickshank, W. M. & Bice, H. V. (1955). In *Cerebral Palsy,* Chap. IV, ed. Cruickshank, W. M. and Raus, G. M. Syracuse, New York: Syracuse Univ. Press.
Culpan, R. H., Davies, B. M. & Oppenheim, A. N. (1960). Incidence of psychiatric illness among hospital out-patients. *Brit. Med. J.* 1, 855.
Culpin, M. (1929). Nervous illness in industry. *J. industr. Hyg.* 11, 114.
Cumming, G. (1961). *The Medical Management of Acute Poisoning.* London: Cassell.
Curran, D. & Garmany, G. (1961). Child psychiatry. *Lancet,* ii, 1249.
Curran, D. & Mallinson, P. (1944). Psychopathic personality. *J. ment. Sci.* 90, 266.
Curran, D. & Parr, D. (1957). Homosexuality: an analysis of 100 male cases seen in private practice. *Brit. med. J.* 1, 797.
Curran, F. J. (1944). Current views on neuropsychiatric effects of barbiturates and bromides. *J. nerv. ment. Dis.* **100**, 142.
Cust, G. (1958). The epidemiology of nocturnal enuresis. *Lancet,* ii, 1167.
Cutts, K. K. & Jasper, H. H. (1939). Effect of benzedrine sulfate and phenobarbital on behavior problem children with abnormal electroencephalograms. Arch. Neurol. *Psychiat.* 41, 1138.

Dagg, J. H., Goldberg, A., Lochhead, A. & Smith, J. A. (1965). The relationship of lead poisoning to acute intermittent porphyria. *Q. Jl. Med.* **34**, 163.
Dahlgren, K. G. (1945). *On Suicide and Attempted Suicide.* Universitiats Bokhandel, Lund.
Dallos, V. & Heathfield, K. (1969). Iatrogenic epilepsy due to anti-depressant drugs. *Brit. med. J.* **4**, 80–82.
Dally, P. J. & Sargant, W. (1960). A new treatment of anorexia nervosa. *Brit. med. J.* **1**, 1770.
Daly, D. D., & Mulder, D. W. (1957). Gelastic epilepsy. *Neurology.* **7**, 189.
Daly, R. F. (1969). Mental illness and patterns of behavior in IO XYY males. *J. nerv. ment. Dis.* **149**, 318–327.
Dancis J., Levitz, M. & Westall, R. G. (1960). Maple syrup urine disease: branched-chain keto-aciduria, *Pediatrics.* **25**, 72.
Dashe, A. M., Cramm, R. E., Crist, C. A., Habener, J. F. & Solomon, D. H. (1963). A water deprivation test for the differential diagnosis of polyuria. *J. Amer. med. Ass.* **185**, 699.
Davidson, S. (1961). School phobia as a manifestation of family disturbance: its structure and treatment. *J Child Psychol. Psychiat.* **1**, 270.
Davies, B. M. (1961). Oral sernyl in obsessive states. *J. ment. Sci.* **107**, 109.
Davies, B. M. & Beech, H. R. (1960). The effect of 1-arylcyclohexylanine (sernyl) on twelve normal volunteers. *J. ment. Sci.* **106**, 912.
Davies, B. M. & Morgenstern, F. S. (1960). A case of cysticercosis, temporal lobe epilepsy, and transvestism. *J. Neurol. Neurosurg. Psychiat.* **23**, 247.
Davies, D. L., Shepherd, M. & Myers, E. (1956). Two years' prognosis of 50 alcohol addicts after treatment in hospital. *Quart. J. Stud. Alcohol,* **17**, 485.
Davies, D. W. (1964). General medical problems in a psychiatric hospital. *Lancet,* i, 545.
Davies, F. L. (1960). Mental abnormalities following subdural haematoma. *Lancet,* i, 1369.
Davies, M. H. (1965). Mental changes following chest surgery. (Personal communication).
Davies, P. A. & Smallpiece, V. (1963). The single tranverse palmar crease in infants and children. *Develop, Med. Child Neurol.* **5**, 491.
Davis, H. V., Sears, R. R., Miller, H. C. & Brodbeck, A. J. (1948). Effects of cup, bottle and breast feeding on oral activities of newborn infants. *Pediatrics,* **2**, 549.
Davison, A. N. (1958). Physiological role of monoamine oxidase. *Physiol. Rev.* **38**, 729.
Dawson, E. B., Moore, T. D., & McGanity, W. J. (1972). Relationship of lithium metabolism to mental hospital admission and homicide. *Dis. Nerv. Syst.* **33**, 546–556.
Dax, E. C. (1970). Psychiatric aspects of poverty. *Med. J. Austral.* **2**, 815–817.
Day, G. (1946). Observations on the psychology of the tuberculous. *Lancet,* ii, 703.
Day, G. (1951). The psychosomatic approach to pulmonary tuberculosis. *Lancet,* i, 1025.
de Alarcon, R. & Carney, M. W. P. (1969). Severe depressive mood changes following slow-release intramuscular fluphenazine injection. *Brit. med. J.* **3**, 564–567.
Dean, S. R., & Thong, D. (1972). Shamanism versus psychiatry in Bali, 'Isle of the Gods': some modern implications. *Amer. J. Psychiat.* **129**, 59–62.
Delay, J. & Deniker, P. (1952). Utilization en therapeutique psychiatrique d'un phénothiazine d'action centrale élective (45–60 RP). *Année Med.-Psychol.* **110**, 112.
Delay, J., Pichot, P., Lemperière, T. & Nicolas-Charles, P. (1958). Effets psychophysiologiques de la psilocybine. *C.R. Acad. Sci.* **247**, 1235.
Dencker, S. J. (1960). Closed head injury in twins: Neurologic, psychometric, and psychiatric follow-up study of consecutive cases, using co-twins as controls. *Arch. gen. Psychiat.* **2**, 569.
Dencker, S. J. & Sandahl, A. (1961). Mental disease after operations for mitral stenosis. *Lancet,* i, 1230.
Denko, J. D. & Kaelbling, R. (1962). Psychiatric aspects of hypoparathyroidism. *Acta psychiat. Scand.* **38**, Suppl. 164.
Denny-Brown, D. (1943). Intellectual deterioration resulting from head injury. *Proc. Ass. Res. nerv. Dis.* **24**, 467. In Assoc. for Research in Nervous and Mental Disease *Trauma of the Central Nervous System.* Baltimore: Williams and Wilkins, 1945.
Denny-Brown, D. & Russell, W. R. (1941). Experimental cerebral concussion. *Brain,* **64**, 93.
De-Nour, A. K. (1969). Some notes on the psychological significance of urination. *J. nerv. ment. Dis.* **148**, 615–623
De-Nour, A. K., & Czaczkes, J. W. (1968). Emotional Problems and Reactions of the Medical Team in a Chronic Hemodialysis Unit. *Lancet,* ii, 987.
De-Nour, A. K., & Czaczkes, J. W. (1972). Personality factors in chronic hemodialysis patients causing noncompliance with medical regimen. *Psychosom. Med.* **34**, 333–344.
De-Nour, A. K., Shaltiel, J. & Czaczkes, J. W. (1968). Emotional reactions of patients on chronic hemodialysis. *Psychosom. Med.* **30**, 521–533.
Dent, C. E., (1957). The relation of the biochemical abnormality to the development of the mental defect in phenylketonuria. *Ross Pediatric Research Conferences,* **23**, 32.

Dent, J. Y. (1954). Dealing with the alcoholic at home. *Med. World Lond.* **81**, 245.
Dent, T., Edwards, J. H., & Delhanty, J. D. A. (1963). A partial mongol. *Lancet,* ii, 484–487.
Deri, S. K. (1949). *Introduction to the Szondi Test.* New York: Grune & Stratton.
De Ropp, R. S. (1958). *Drugs and the Mind.* London: Gollancz.
Despert, J. L. (1944). Emotional factors in some young children's colds. *Med. Clin. N. Amer.* **29**, 603.
Deutsch, H. (1946). *The Psychology of Women: a Psychoanalytic Interpretation,* Vol. 1, Girlhood. London: Research Books.
Devlin, L. (1964). The legal conception of guilt and punishment. *Lancet,* ii, 1130.
Dewhurst, K. (1969). The neurosyphilitic psychoses today: a survey of 91 cases. *Brit. J. Psychiat.* **115**, 31–38.
Dewhurst, K. E., El Kabir, D. J., Exley, D., Harris, G. W., & Mandelbrote, B. M. (1968). Blood-levels of thyrotrophic hormone, protein-bound iodine, and cortisol in schizophrenia and affective states. *Lancet,* **2**, 1160.
Dewhurst, W. G. (1969). Amines and abnormal mood. *Proc. roy. Soc. Med.* **62**, 1100–1107.
Dickinson, G. L. (1896). *The Greek View of Life,* p. 184. London: Methuen.
Dicks, H. V. (1963). Psychology of race prejudice. *Lancet,* i, 593.
Diethelm, O. (1955). *Etiology of Chronic Alcholism.* Springfield, Ill.: Thomas.
Dillon, H. & Leopold, R. L. (1961). Children and the post-concussion syndrome. *J. Amer. med. Ass.* **175**, 86.
Dimson, S. B. (1959). Toilet training and enuresis. *Brit. med. J.* **2**, 666.
Divry, P. (1927). Etude histo-chimique des plaques seniles. *J. belge Neurol. Psychiat.* **27**, 643.
Dixon, K. C. (1953). Cytochemical changes in necrotic grey matter of the brain. *J. Path. Bact.* **66**, 251.
Dixon, K. C. & Herbertson, B. M. (1950). Clusters of granules in human neurones. *J. Path. Bact.* **62**, 335.
Dixon, K. C. & Herbertson, B. M. (1951). Cytoplasmic glycolipids of brain. *J. Path. Bact.* **63**, 175.
Doll. E. A. (1941). The essentials of an inclusive concept of mental deficiency. *Amer. J. ment. Defic.* **46**, 214.
Donnelly, J. (1964). Aspects of the psychodynamics of the psychopath. *Amer. J. Psychiat.* **120**, 1149.
Donnelly, J. P. (1958). In *Abortion in the United States,* pp. 103, 104, ed. Calderone, M. S. New York: Hoeber-Harper.
Douglas, J. W. B. & Blomfield, J. M. (1958). *Children under Fire.* London: Allen & Unwin.
Draper, G. & Touraine, G. A. (1932). Man-environment unit and peptic ulcer. *Arch, intern. Med.* **49**, 616.
Drawneek, W., O'Brien, M. J., Goldsmith, H. J. & Bourdillon, R. E. (1964). Industrial methyl-bromide poisoning in fumigation: a case report and field investigation. *Lancet,* ii, 855.
Dreyfus, F. & Czaczkes, J. W. (1959). Blood cholesterol and uric acid of healthy medical students under the stress of an examination. *Arch. intern. Med.* **103**, 708.
Drillien, C. M. (1959). A longitudinal study of the growth and development of prematurely and maturely born children. *Arch. Dis. Childh.* **34**, 487.
Drummond, J. C. & Wilbraham, A. (1957). *The Englishman's Food.* London: Jonathan Cape.
Drury, A. N., Florey, H. & Florey, M. E. (1929). The vascular reactions of the colonic mucosa of the dog to fright. *J. Physiol.* **68**, 173.
Druss, R. G., O'Connor, J. F., & Stern, L. O. (1972). Changes in body image following ileostomy. *Psychoanal. Quart.*, **41**, 195–206.
Drye, J. C. & Schoen, A. M. (1958). Studies on the mechanisms of the activation of peptic ulcer after non-specific trauma. *Ann. Surg.* **147**, 738.
Dubois, P. (1949). *The Psychic Treatment of Mental Disorders,* 6th Ed. New York: Frank and Wognelle.
Dudley, D. L., Verhey, J. W., Masuda, M., Martin, C. J. & Holmes, T. H. (1969). Long term adjustment, prognosis and death in irreversible diffuse obstructive pulmonary syndromes. *Psyosom. Med.* **31**, 310–325.
Dudley, W. H.C., & Williams, J. G. (1972). Electroconvulsive therapy in delirium tremens. *Compr. Psychiat.* **13**, 357–360.
Dumont, M. P. (1972). The doctor and his changing community. *Modern Medicine,* Dec. 730–736.

Dunbar, F. (1943). *Psychosomatic Diagnosis.* New York: Hoeber.
Dunlap, C. B. (1927). Pathologic changes in Huntington's chorea. *Arch. Neurol. Psychiat.* **18**, 867.
Dunlap, H. F. & Moersch, F. P. (1935). Psychic manifestations associated with hyperthyroidism. *Amer. J. Psychiat.* **91**, 1215.
Dunlap, K. (1932). *Habits, Their Making and Unmaking.* New York: Liveright.
Dupont, A. & Clausen, J. (1968). The elfin-face syndrome. *The Lancet,* i, 209.
Dupont, R. L., & Grunebaum, H. (1968). Willing victims: the husbands of paranoid women. *Amer. J. Psychiat.* **125**, 151–159.
Durkheim, E. (1897). *Le Suicide.* Paris: Alcan.
Durton, J. H., & Milner, J. N. (1970). Relapsing encephalomyelitis. *Brain,* **93**, 715–730.
Duss, L. (1950). *La méthode des fables en psycho-analyse infantile.* Paris: L'Arche.
Dynes, J. B. & Poppen, J. L. (1949). Lobotomy for intractable pain. *J. Amer. med. Ass.* **140**, 15.

Eade, N. R. (1958). The storage and release of catecholamines. *Rev. Canad. Biol.* **17**, 299.
Earle, K. M. Baldwin, M. & Penfield, W. (1953). Incisural sclerosis and temporal lobe seizures produced by hippocampal herniation at birth. *Arch. Neurol. Psychiat.* **69**, 27.
Early, D. F. (1960). The industrial therapy organisation (Bristol); a development of work in hospital. *Lancet,* ii, 754.
Easson, W. M. (1966). Myxoedema with psychosis. *Arch. Gen. Psychiat.* **14**, 277.
East, W. N. (1942). *The Adolescent Criminal: a medico-sociological study of 4,000 male adolescents.* London: Churchill.
Eastwood, M. R. Mindham, R. H. S., & Tennent, T. G. (1970). The physical status of psychiatric emergencies. *Brit. J. Psychiat.* **116**, 545–550.
Eastwood, M. R. & Trevelyan, M. H. (1972). Relationship between physical and psychiatric disorder. *Psychol. Med.* **2**, 363–372.
Eaton, J. W. & Weil, R. J. (1955). The mental health of the Hutterites. In *Mental Health and Mental Disorder,* ed. Rose, A. M. New York: Norton.
Economo, C. von. (1917). Encephalitis lethargica. *Wien Klin. Wschr.* **30**, 581.
Edwards G., Hawker, A., Hensman, C. Peto, J., & Williamson V., (1973). Alcoholics known or unknown to agencies: epidemiological studies in a London suburb. *Brit. J. Psychiat.* **123**, 169–183.
Edwards H. (1970). The significance of brain damage in persistent oral dyskinesia. *Brit. J. Psychiat.* **116**, 271–275.
Efron, R. (1963). Temporal perception, aphasia and déjà vu. *Brain,* **86**, 403.
Egas Moniz, A. C. de A. F. (1936). *Tentatives opératoires dans le traitement de certaines psychoses.* Paris: Masson.
Egerton, N. & Kay, J. H. (1964). Psychologic disturbances associated with open heart surgery. *Brit. J. Psychiat.* **110**, 433.
Eisenberg, L. (1957). Psychiatric implications of brain damage in children. *Psychiat. Quart.* **31**, 72.
Eisler, R. M., & Polak, P. R. (1971). Social stress and psychiatric disorder. *J. nerv. ment. Dis.* **153**, 227–233.
Ekblad, M. (1955). Induced abortion on psychiatric grounds: a follow-up study of 479 women. *Acta psychiat. scand.* Suppl. 99.
Ekblad, M. (1961). The prognosis after sterilization on social-psychiatric grounds. *Acta Psychiat. Scand. Suppl.* **161**, Vol. 37.
Ekecrantz, L., & Rudhe, L. (1972). Transitional phenomena: frequency, forms and functions of specially loved objects. *Acta Psychiat. Scand.,* **48**, 261–273.
Elithorn, A., Glithero, E. & Slater, E. (1958). Leucotomy for pain. *J. Neurol. Neurosurg. Psychiat.* **21**, 249.
Elithorn, A., Piercy, M. F. & Crosskey, M.A. (1955). Prefrontal leucotomy and the anticipation of pain. *J. Neurol. Neurosurg. Psychiat.* **18**, 34.
Elkes, J., Elkes C. & Bradley, P. B. (1954). The effect of some drugs on electrical activity of the brain and on behaviour. *J. ment. Sci.* **100**, 125.
Ellenberger, H. (1953). Der Selbstmord im Lichte der Ethno-Psychiatrie. *Mschr. Psychiat. Neurol.* **125**, 347.
Ellery, R. S. (1927). Psychoses of the puerperium. *Med. J. Aust.* **1**, 287.
Ellinwood, E. H., (1971). Assault and homicide associated with amphetamine abuse. *Amer. J. Psychiat.* **127**, 1170–1175.
Ellis, H. (1902). Mescal, a study of a divine plant. *Pop. Sci. Mon.* **41**, 52.
Engel G. L. (1954*a*). Studies of ulcerative colitis. I. Clinical data bearing on the nature of the somatic process. *Psychosom. Med.* **16**, 496.

Engel, G. L. (1954*b*) Studies of ulcerative colitis. II. The nature of the somatic processes and the adquacy of psychosomatic hypotheses. *Amer. J. Med.* **16**, 416.
Engel, G. L. (1955). Studies of ulcerative colitis. III. The nature of the psychologic processes. *Amer. J. Med.* **19**, 231.
Engel. G. L. (1956). Studies of ulcerative colitis. IV. The significance of headaches. *Psychosom. Med.* **18**, 334.
Engel, G. L. (1958). Studies of ulcerative colitis. V. Psychological aspects and their implications for treatment. *Amer. J. digest. Dis. N.S.* **3**, 315.
Engel, G. L. (1962). *Psychological Development in Health and Disease.* Philadelphia: Saunders.
Engel, G. L. & Reichsman, F. (1956). Spontaneous and experimentally induced depressions in an infant with a gastric fistula: a contribution to the problem of depression. *J. Amer. Psychoanalyt. Ass.* **4**, 428.
Enoch, M. D. & Barker, J. C. (1965). Misuse of Section 29: fact or fiction. *Lancet,* i, 760.
Entwistle, C. & Sim, M. (1961). Tuberous sclerosis and fetishism. *Brit. med. J.* **2**, 1688.
Epstein, A. W. (1960). Fetishism: a study of its psychopathology with particular reference to a proposed disorder in brain mechanisms as an etiological factor. *J. nerv. ment. Dis.* **130**, 107.
Epstein, B. S., Epstein, J. A., & Postel, D. M. (1971). Tumors of spinal cord simulating psychiatric disorders. *Diis. nerv. Syst.* **32**, 741–743.
Epstein, R. S., Cummings, N. A., Sherwood, E. B. & Bergsma, D. R. (1970). Psychiatric aspects of Behcet's syndrome. *J. Psychosom. Res.* **14**, 161–172.
Eros, G. (1951). Observations on cerebral arterio-sclerosis. *J. Neuropath. exp. Neurol.* **10**, 257.
Esen, F. M. (1957). Congenital heart malformations in mongolism with special reference to ostium atrioventriculare commune. *Arch. Pediat.* **74**, 245.
Esmarch, F. & Jessen, W. (1857). Syphilis und Geistesstörung. *Allg. Z. Psychiat.* **14**, 20.
Esterson, A. (1970). *The Leaves of Spring.* London: Tavistock.
Esterson, A., Cooper, D. G. & Laing, R. D. (1965). Results of family-orientated therapy with hospitalized schizophrenics. *Brit. med. J.* **2**, 1462.
Estes, W. K. (1959). The statistical approach to learning theory. In *Study of a Science,* Vol. 2, ed. Koch, S. New York: McGraw-Hill.
Esquirol, J. E. D. (1838). *Des maladies mentales considérées sous les rapports médicals, hygiéneques, et médico-légals, Vols. 1 & 2.* Paris: Baillière.
Ettlinger, R. W. & Flordh, P. (1955). Attempted suicide: experience of 500 cases at a general hospital. *Acta psychiat. scand.* Suppl. 103.
Evans, C. R. (1966). The stuff of dreams. *The Listener.*
Evans, J. (1959). Psychosis and addiction to phenmetrazine (preludin). *Lancet,* ii, 152.
Evans, S. L., Reinhart, J. B. & Succop, R. A. (1972). Failure to thrive: a study of 45 children and their families. *J. Amer. Acad. Child Psychiat.* **11**, 440–457.
Evans, W. (1959). The electrocardiogram of alcoholic cardiomyopathy. *Brit. Heart J.* **21**, 445.
Eysenck, H. J. (1947). *Dimensions of Personality.* London: Routledge & Kegan Paul.
Eysenck, H. J. (1956). The questionnaire measurement of neuroticism and extroversion. *Riv. Psicol.* **50**, 113.
Eysenck, H. J. (1959). *Manual of the Maudsley Personality Inventory.* London: University of London Press.
Eysenck, H. J. (ed.) (1960). *Behaviour Therapy and the Nueroses.* London: Pergamon.
Eysenck, H. J. (1965). *Smoking, Health and Personality.* London: Weidenfeld and Nicholson.
Eysenck, H. J. & Rachman, S. J. (1965). The application of learning theory to child psychiatry. In *Modern Perspectives in Child Psychiatry,* ed. Howells, J. G. Edinburgh: Oliver & Boyd.

Fairhall, L. T. & Neal, P. A. (1943). Industrial manganese poisoning. *Nat. Inst. Hlth. Bull.* **182**.
Falconer, M. A., Hill, D., Meyer, A., Mitchell, W. & Pond, D. A. (1955). Treatment of temporal-lobe epilepsy by temporal lobectomy. *Lancet,* i, 827.
Falconer, M. A., Hill, D., Mayer, A. & Wilson, J. L. (1958). Clinical, radiological, and EEG correlations with pathological changes in temporal lobe epilepsy and their significance in surgical treatment. *Proc. Int. Colloq. on Temporal Lobe Epilepsy,* Bethesda, Maryland. Springfield, Ill.: Thomas.
Falconer, M. A. & Kennedy, W. A. (1961). Epilepsy due to small focal temporal lesions with bilateral independent spike-discharging foci. *J. Neurol. Neurosurg. Psychiat.* **24**, 205.

Falret, J. P. (1854). *Lecons cliniques de médecine mentale faites a l'hospice de la Salpêtrière*. Paris: Baillière. Quoted in *Some Historical Phases of the Manic-depressive Psychosis*, Vol. XI, Jeliffe, S. E. Baltimore: Williams & Wilkins. 1931.

Farberow, N. L. (1950). Personality patterns of suicidal mental hospital patients. *Genet. Psychol. Monogr.* 42, 3.

Farberow, N. L. & Shneidman, E. S. (1961). *The Cry for Help*. New York: McGraw Hill.

Faris, R. E. L. & Dunham, H. W. (1939). *Mental Disorders in Urban Area*, p. 134. Chicago: University of Chicago Press.

Farndale, J. (1961). *The Day Hospital Movement in Great Britain*. Oxford: Pergamon.

Feldman, R. G., Chandler, K. A., Levy, L. L. & Glaser, G. H. (1963). Familial Alzheimer's Disease. *Neurology*, 13, 811.

Feldstein, A., Hoagland, H. & Freeman, H. (1959). Monoamine oxidase, psychoenergizers and tranquillizers. *Science*, 130, 500.

Feldstein, A., Hoagland, H. & Freeman, H. (1959). Blood and urinary serotonin and 5-hydroxyindole acetic acid levels in schizophrenic patients and normal subjects. *J. nerv. ment. Dis.* 129, 62.

Fellman, J. H. (1958). Epinephrine metabolites and pigmentation in the central nervous system in a case of phenylpyruvic oligophrenia. *J. Neurol. Neurosurg. Psychiat.* 21, 58.

Fenichel, O. (1945). *The Psychoanalytic Theory of Neurosis*. New York: Norton.

Ferarro, A. (1959). Presenile psychoses. In *American Handbook of Psychiatry*, ed. Arieti, S. New York: Basic Books.

Ferenczi, S. (1926*a*). The further development of an active therapy in psychoanalysis. In *Further Contributions to the Theory and Technique of Psychoanalysis*. London: Hogarth Press.

Ferenczi, S. (1950). *Further Contributions to the Theory and Technique of Psychoanalysis*, 2nd Ed. London: Hogarth Press.

Ferenczi, S. & Rank, O. (1925). Developmental goals of psychoanalysis. In *The Development of Psychoanalysis*. New York: Nervous and Mental Diseases Publishing Coy.

Ferguson, R. S. (1961). Side-effects of community care. *Lancet*, i, 931.

Ferguson, J. K. W., Armstrong, J. D., Kerr, H. T. & Bell, R. G. (1956). A new drug for alcoholism treatment. *Canad. med. Ass. J.* 74, 793.

Fernando, S. J. M. (1967). Gilles de la Tourette's syndrome. *Brit. J. Psychiat.* 113, 607–617.

Fiamberti, A. M. (1950). *Acetylcholine in Physio-pathogenesis and Therapy in Schizophrenia*. Internat. Psychiat. Congress Report, 4, 79. Paris: Hermann et Cie.

Field, L. H. (1973). Benperidol in the treatment of sexual offenders. *Medicine, Science, and the Law*. 13, No. 3 July, 1973.

Fischer, K., & Dlin, B. M. (1972). Psychogenic determination of time of illness or death by anniversary reactions and emotional deadlines. *Psychosomatics*, 13. 170–173.

Fischer, M. Harvald, B., & Hague, M. (1969). A Danish twin study of schizophrenia. *Brit. J. Psychiat.* 115, 981-990.

Fischer-Williams, M. (1956). Treatment of chronic pain. *Brit. med. J.* 1, 533.

Flanagan, T. A., Goodwin, D. W., & Alderson, P. (1970). Psychiatric illness in a large family with familial hyperparathyroidism. *Brit. J. Psychiat.* 117, 693–698.

Flinn, R. H., Neal, P. A., Reinhart, W. H., Dallavalle, J. M., Fulton, W. B. & Dooley, A. E. (1940). *Chronic Manganese Poisoning in an Ore-crushing Mill*. U.S. Public Health Service Bulletin 247. Washington: Government Printing Office.

Florey, E. (1953). Naturwiss. *Arch. in Physiol.* 62, 33.

Fölling, A. (1934). Über Ausscheidung von Phenylbranztraubensäure in den Harn al Stoffwechselanomalie in Verbindung mit Imbezillität. *Z. phys. Chem.* 227, 169.

Forbes, A. & Morison, B. R. (1939). Cortical response to sensory stimulation under deep barbiturate narcosis. *J. Neurophysiol.* 2, 112.

Forssmann, H. & Hambert, G. (1963). Incidence of Klinefelter's syndrome among mental patients. *Lancet*, i, 274.

Forssmann, H., & Thuwe, I. (1966). One hundred and twenty children born after application for therapeutic abortion refused. *Acta Psychiat Scand.* 42, 71–88.

Foster, F. H. (1962). *Maori Patients in Mental Hospitals*. Department of Health, Wellington, New Zealand.

Foulkes, S. H. (1948). *Introduction to Group-analytic Psychotherapy*. London: Heinemann.

Foulkes, S. H. (1961). Psychotherapy 1961. *Brit. J. med. Psychol.* 34, 91.

Fox. C. A. (1949). Amygdalo-thalamic connections in Macaca mulatta. *Anat. Rec.* 103, 537.

Fox. T. F. (1951). Professional freedom. *Lancet*, ii, 115.

Frank, J. D., (1972). Common features of psychotherapy. *Aust. N.Z. J. Psychiat.* 6, 34–40.

Frank, R. T. (1931). The hormonal causes of premenstrual tension. *Arch. Neurol. Psychiat.* 26, 1053.
Fraser, H. F. & Grider, J. A. (1953). Symposium on drug addiction; treatment of drug addiction. *Amer. J. Med.* 14, 571.
Fraser, R. & Lewis, P. D. (1973). A case of abnormal thirst. *Brit. med. J.* 3, 214–219.
Frazer, J. G. (1911). *The Golden Bough.. Taboo and the Pride of the Soul,* 3rd Ed. London: Macmillan. 1955.
Freeman, H. L. (1960). Oldham and district psychiatric service. *Lancet* i, 218.
Freeman, H. L. & Kendrick, D. C. (1960). A case of cat phobia: treatment by a method derived from experimental psychology. *Brit. med. J.* 2, 497.
Freeman, T. & Gathercole, C. E. (1966). Perseveration: the clinical symptoms in chronic schizophrenia and organic dementia. *Brit. J. Psychiat* 112, 27.
Freeman, W. (1949). Transorbital leucotomy: the deep frontal cut. *Proc. roy. Soc. Med.* 42, 8 (Suppl.).
Freeman, W. (1953). Hazards of lobotomy: study of two thousand operations *J. Amer. med. Ass.* 152, 487.
Freeman, W. (1954). Changes in behaviour following lobotomy. The Malamud rating scale. *J. Neuropath. exp. Neurol.* 13, 90.
Freeman, W. (1959). Psychosurgery. In *American Handbook of Psychiatry,* Vol. 2, ed. Arieti, S. New York: Basic Books.
Freeman, W. (1971). Frontal lobotomy in early schizophrenia: long follow-up in 415 cases. *Brit. J. Psychiat.* 119, 621–624.
Freeman, W. & Watts, J. W. (1941). The frontal lobes and consciousness of the self. *Psychosom. Med.* 3, 111.
Freeman, W. & Watts, J. W. (1946). Pain of organic disease relieved by prefrontal lobotomy. *Lancet,* i, 953.
Freeman, W. & Watts, J. W. (1947). Retrograde degeneration of the thalamus following prefrontal leucotomy. *J. comp. Neurol.* 86, 65.
French, J. D., Hernandez-Peón, R. & Livingston, R. B. (1955). Projections from cortex to cephalic brain stem (reticular formation) in monkey. *J. Neurophysiol.* 18, 74.
French, J. D., Porter, R. W., Cavanaugh, E. & Longmire, R. L. (1954). Experimental observations on 'psychosomatic' mechanisms. I. Gastro-intestinal disturbances. *Arch. Neurol. Psychiat.* 72, 267.
French, J. D., Porter, R. W., Cavanaugh, E. B. & Longmire, R. L. (1957). Experimental gastroduodenal lesions induced by stimulation of the brain. *Psychosom. Med.* 19, 209.
French, T. M. & Alexander, F. (1941). Psychogenic factors in bronchial asthma. Psychosom. Med. Mongr. Suppl. IV, Vol. 1, No. 4; Vol. 2, Nos. 1 & 2. Washington, D.C.: National Research Council.
Freud, A. (1937). *The Ego and Mechanisms of Defence.* London: Hogarth.
Freud, A. (1946). *The Psycho-analytical Treatment of Children: Technical Lectures and Essays.* London: Imago.
Freud, S. (1895). Obsessions and phobias: their psychical mechanisms and their aetiology. In *Collected Papers I.* London: Hogarth Press,. 1924.
Freud, S. (1896). Further remarks on the defence neuro-psychoses. In *Collected Papers I.* London: Hogarth Press, 1924.
Freud, S. (1905). *Three Contributions to the Theory of Sex. (Drei abhandlungen zur Sexualtheorie).* Leipzig: Deuticke. New York: Nervous and Mental Disease Publishing Coy. 1910.
Freud, S. (1907). Obsessive acts and religious practices. In *Collected Papers II.* London: Hogarth Press. 1933.
Freud, S. (1908). Character and anal erotism. In *Collected Papers II,* p. 45. London: Hogarth Press. 1933.
Freud, S. (1909*a*) Analysis of a phobia in a five-year-old boy. In *Collected Papers III.* London: Hogarth Press. 1933.
Freud, S. (1909*b*). Notes upon a case of obsessional neurosis. In *Collected Papers II.* London: Hogarth Press. 1933.
Freud, S. (1910*a*). The future prospects of psychoanalytic therapy. In *Collected Papers II.* London: Hogarth Press. 1933.
Freud, S. (1910*b*). Observations on 'wild' psycho-analysis. In *Collected Papers II.* London: Hogarth Press. 1933.
Freud, S. (1911). Psycho-analytic notes upon an autobiographic account of a case of paranoia (dementia paranoides). In *Collected Papers III.* London: Hogarth Press. 1933.
Freud, S. (1912*a*). The employment of dream interpretation in psychoanalysis. In *Collected Papers II.* London: Hogarth Press. 1933.

Freud, S. (1912*b*). The dynamics of the transference. In *Collected Papers II.* London: Hogarth Press. 1933.

Freud, S. (1912*c*). Recommendations for physicians on the psychoanalytic method of treatment. In *Collected Papers II.* London: Hogarth Press. 1933.

Freud, S. (1913*a*). Fausse reconnaissance (déjà racouté) in psycho-analytic treatment. In *Collected Papers II.* London: Hogarth Press. 1933.

Freud, S. (1913*b*). Further recommendations in the technique of psychoanalysis on beginning the treatment: the question of the first communication: the dynamics of the cure. In *Collected Papers II.* London: Hogarth Press. 1933.

Freud, S. (1913*c*). Predisposition to obsessional neurosis. In *Collected Papers II.* London: Hogarth Press. 1933.

Freud, S. (1913*d*). *Totem and Taboo.* Trans. Strachey, J. (1950). London: Routledge & Kegan Paul.

Freud, S. (1914). Further recommendations in the technique of psychoanalysis: recollection, repetition and working through. In *Collected Papers II.* London: Hogarth Press. 1933.

Freud, S. (1915*a*). Further recommendations in the technique of psychoanalysis: observations on transference-love. In *Collected Papers II.* London: Hogarth Press. 1933.

Freud, S. (1915*b*). The unconscious. In *Collected Papers IV.* London: Hogarth Press. 1934.

Freud, S. (1917). Mourning and melancholia. In *Collected Papers IV.* London: Hogarth Press. 1934.

Freud, S. (1918). From the history of an infantile neurosis. In *Collected Papers III.* London: Hogarth Press. 1933.

Freud, S. (1919). Turnings in the ways of psychoanalytic therapy. In *Collected Papers II.* London: Hogarth Press. 1933.

Freud, S. (1922). *Group Psychology and the Analysis of the Ego.* Trans. Strachey, J. London: International Psycho-Analytic Press.

Freud, S. (1924*a*). Neurosis and psychosis. In *Collected Papers II.* London: Hogarth Press. 1933.

Freud, S. (1924*b*). The loss of reality in neurosis and psychosis. In *Collected Papers II.* London: Hogarth Press. 1933.

Freud, S. (1927). *The Ego and the Id.* London: Hogarth Press.

Friedhoff, A. J. & van Winkle, E. (1962). Isolation and characterization of a compound from the urine of schizophrenics. *Nature,* London. **194**, 897.

Friedman, M., Rosenman, R. H. & Carroll, V. (1958). Changes in the serum cholesterol and blood clotting time in men subjected to cyclic variations of occupational stress. *Circulation,* **17**, 852.

Friedman, M. & Rosenman, R. H. (1959). Association of specific overt behaviour pattern with blood and cardiovascular findings. *J. Amer. med. Ass.* **169**, 1286.

Friedman, P. (1959). The phobias. In *American Handbook of Psychiatry,* ed. Arieti, S. New York: Basic Books.

Froesch, E. R., Prader, A., Labhart, A., Stuber, H. W. & Wolf, H. P. (1957). Die hereditäre Fructoseintoleranz eine bisher nicht bekannte kongenitale Stoffwechselstörung. *Schweiz. med. Wschr.* **87**, 1168.

Frohlich, E. D. Dustan, H. P. & Page, I. H. (1966). Hyperdynamic beta-adrenergic circulatory state. *Arch. intern. Med.* **117**, 614.

Fromm, E. (1942). *The Fear of Freedom.* London: Paul.

Fromm, E. (1944). Individual and social origins of neurosis. *Amer. Sociol. Review,* **60**.

Fromm, E. (1949). *Man for Himself.* London: Paul.

Fry, W. J. (1956). Ultrasound in neurology. *Neurology,* **6**, 693.

Fullerton, D. T. & Munsat, T. L. (1966). Pseudo-myasthenia gravis: a conversion reaction. *J. nerv. ment. Dis.* **142**, 78.

Funkenstein, D. H., Greenblatt, M. & Solomon, H. C. (1950). A test which predicts the clinical effect of electroshock treatment on schizophrenic patients. *Amer. J. Psychiat.* **106**, 889.

Funkenstein, D. H. *et. al.* (1957). *Mastery of Stress.* Cambridge, Mass.: Harvard.

Gaddum, J. H. (1953). Antagonism between lysergic acid diethylamide and 5-hydroxytryptamine. *J. Physiol.* **121**, 15P.

Gaddum, J. H., Krivoy, W. A. & Laverty, G. (1958). The action of reserpine on the excretion of adrenaline and noradrenaline. *J. Neurochem.* **2**, 249.

Gahagan, L. H. (1962). Intravenous atropine premedication before electro-convulsion therapy. *Lancet,* i, 1305.

Gajdusek, D. C., & Gibbs, C. J: (1971). Transmission of two subacute spongiform encephalopathies of man (Kuru and Creutzfeldt-Jakob disease) to New World Monkeys. *Nature. Lond.* **230**, 588–591.

Gallagher, J. R., Gibbs, E. L. & Gibbs F. A. (1942). Relation between electrical activity of cortex and personality in adolescent boys. *Psychosom. Med.* **4**, 134.

Galton, F. (1869). *Hereditary Genius.* London: Macmillan.

Galton, F. (1875). The history of twins as a criterion of the relative powers of nature and nurture. *J. R. anthrop. Inst.* **5**, 391.

Galton, F. (1883). *Inquiries into Human Faculty and Development.* London: Macmillan.

Ganser, S. (1898). Über einen eigenartigen hysterischen Dämmerzustand. *Arch. Psychiat.* **30**, 633.

Gantt, W. H. (1944). Experimental basis for neurotic behaviour: origin and development for artificially produced disturbances of behaviour in dogs. *Psychosomat. Med. Monogr.* Suppl. 3, Nos. 3 & 4.

Ganz, V. H. Gurland, B. J., Deming, W. E., &. Fisher, B. (1972). The study of psychiatric symptoms of systemic lupus erythematosus: a biometric study. *Psychosom. Med.* **34**, 207–220.

Garratt, F. N., Lowe, C. R. & McKeown, T. (1958). Institutional care of the mentally ill. *Lancet,* i, 682.

Garron, D. C., Klawans, H. L., & Narin, F. (1972). Intellectual functioning of persons with idiopathic parkinsonism. *J. nerv. ment. Dis.* **154**, 445–452.

Gates, R. R. (1946). *Human Genetics* Vol. II, New York: Macmillan.

Gath, D., Tennent, G., & Pidduck, R. (1970). Psychiatric and social characteristics of bright delinquents. *Brit. J. Psychiat.* **116**, 151–160.

Geier, S. (1971). Minor seizures and behaviour. *Electroenceph. Clin. Neurophysiol.* **31**, 499–507.

Gelder, M. G., & Mathews, A. M. (1968). Forearm blood flow and phobic anxiety. *Brit. J. Psychiat.* **114**, 1371–1376.

Gelder, M. G. & Marks, I. M. (1966). Severe agoraphobia: a controlled prospective trial of behaviour therapy. *Brit. J. Psychiat.* **112**, 309.

Gelineau, J. B. E. (1880). De la narcolepsie. *Gaz. Hôp. Paris,* **53**, 626, 635.

Gellhorn, E., & Kiely, W. F. (1972). Mystical states of consciousness: neurophysiological and clinical aspects. *J. nerv. ment. Dis.* **154**, 399–405.

Gerstmann, J. (1940). Syndrome of finger agnosia, disorientation for right and left, agraphia and acalculia; local diagnostic values. *Arch. Neurol. Psychiat.* **44**, 398.

Gesell, A. *et al.* (1941). *The First Five Years of Life: a Guide to the Study of the Preschool Child.* London: Methuen.

Gibb. J. W. G. & MacMahon, J. F. (1955). Arrested mental development induced by lead poisoning. *Brit. med. J.* **1**, 320.

Gibbens, T. C. N. (1962). Shoplifting. *Med-leg. J.* **30**, 6.

Gibbens, T. C. N. (1966) Psychiatric research in delinquency behaviour. *Brit. med. J.* **2**, 695.

Gibbens T. C. N. & Prince, G. (1963). *Child Victims of Sex Offences.* London: Institute for the Study and Treatment of Delinquency.

Gibbens, T. C. N. & Silberman, M. (1960). The clients of prostitutes. *Brit. J. vener. Dis.* **36**, 113.

Gibbs, E. L. Gibbs F. A. & Fuster, B, (1948). Psychomotor epilepsy. *Arch. Neurol. Psychiat.* **60**, 331.

Gibbs, F. A. & Gibbs E. L. (1947). The electro-encephalogram in encephalitis. *Arch. Neurol, Psychiat.* **58**, 184.

Gibbs, F. A. & Gibbs, E. L. (1950). *Atlas of Electroencephalography.* Cambridge, Mass.: Addison-Wesley Press.

Gibbs, F. A., Gibbs, E. L. & Lennox, W. G. (1937). Epilepsy: a paroxysmal cerebral dysrhythmia. *Brain,* **60**, 377.

Gibbs, F. A., Gibbs, E. L. & Lennox, W. G. (1938). The likeness of the cortical dysrhythmias of schizophrenia and psychomotor epilepsy. *Amer. J. Psychiat.* **95**, 255.

Gilles de la Tourette, G. (1885). La maladie des tics convulsifs. *Sem. méd. Paris.* **19**, 153–156.

Gillespie, R. D. (1934). On alleged dangers of barbiturates. *Lancet,* i, 337.

Gillison, T. H. & Skinner, J. L. (1958). Treatment of nocturnal enuresis by the electric alarm. *Brit. med. J.* **2**, 1268.

Ginsberg, G. L. Frosch, W. A., & Shapiro, T. (1972). The new impotence. *Arch. gen. Psychiat.* **26**, 218–220.

Gitelson, M. (1951). Psychoanalysis and dynamic psychiatry. *Arch. Neurol. Psychiat.* **66** 280.
Gjessing, R. (1947). Biological investigation in endogenous psychoses. *Acta psychiat. Kbh.* Suppl. 47, 93.
Glass G. S., Heninger, G. R., Lansky, M., & Talan, K. (1971). Psychiatric emergency related to the menstrual cycle. *Amer. J. Psychiat.* 128, 705–711.
Glatt, M. M. (1959). An alcoholic unit in a mental hospital. *Lancet,* ii, 397.
Glatt, M. M. (1962). Suicide in alcoholics. *Brit. med. J.* **1**, *1079.*
Glatt, M. M. (1964). *Alcoholism in 'impaired' and drunken driving. Lancet,* i, 161.
Glover, E. (1949). *Psycho-analysis,* 2nd Ed. Chap. X, p. 145. London: Staples Press.
Goldberg, A., Rimmington, C. & Lochhead, A. C. (1967). Hereditary coprophyria. *Lancet,* i, 632.
Goldfarb, A. (1969). Predicting mortality in the institutionalized aged: a seven-year follow-up. *Arch. gen. Psychiat.* **21**, 172–176.
Goldfarb, W. (1943). Infant rearing and problem behavior. *Amer. J. Ortho-psychiat.* **13**, 249.
Goldfarb, W. (1961). Childhood schizophrenia. Commonwealth Fund. Cambridge, Mass.: Harvard University Press.
Goldstein, K. (1939). *The Organism: a Holistic Approach to Biology Derived from Pathological Data in Man.* New York: American Book Coy.
Goldstein, K. (1943). The significance of psychological research in schizophrenia. *J. nerv. ment. Dis.* 97, 261.
Gonen, J. Y. (1971). The use of psychodrama combined with videotape playback on an inpatient floor. *Psychiatry,* **34**, 198–213.
Goodman, L. S. & Gilman, A. (1955). *The Pharmacological Basis of Therapeutics.* New York: Macmillan.
Goodwin, D. W., Guze, S. B., & Robins, E. (1969). Follow-up studies in obsessional neurosis. *Arch. gen. Psychiat.* **20**, 182–187.
Goodwin, F. K. (1972). Behavioral effect of L-dopa in man. *Psychiatric Complications of Medical Drugs,* ed. Shader, R. I. New York: Raven Press.
Goodwin, F. K. Murphy, D. L. Dunner, D. L. & Bunney, W. E. (1972). Lithium response in unipolar versus bipolar depression. *Amer. J. Psychiat.* **129** 44–47.
Goody, W., Gautier-Smith, P. C. & Dunkley, E. W. (1960). Neurological practice in a mental observation unit. *Lancet,* ii, 1290.
Gordon, E. B. (1965). Carbon-monoxide encephalopathy. *Brit. med. J.* **1**, 1232.
Gordon, E. B. (1965) Mentally ill West Indian immigrants. *Brit. J. Psychiat.* **111**, 877.
Gordon, E. B. & Sim, M. (1967). The EEG in presenile dementia. *J. Neurol. Neurosurg. Psychiat.* **30**, 285.
Gordon, H. (1973) Abortion as a method of population regulation: the problems. *Brit. J. Hosp. Med.* 9, 303–306.
Goresky, V. B. (1948). Treatment of psychoneurosis in general practice. *Bull. Vancouver med. Ass.* **24**, 120.
Goresky, V. B. (1961). Pavlov or Freud. *Lancet,* i 721.
Goring, C. (1913). The English convict. London: H.M.S.O.
Gornall, A. G., Eglitis, B., Miller, A., Stokes, A. B. & Dewan, J. G. (1953). Long-term clinical and metabolic observations in periodic catatonia: an application of the kinetic method of research in three schizophrenic patients. *Amer. J. Psychiat.* **109**, 584.
Gottesman, I. I. & Shields, J. (1966). Schizophrenia in twins: sixteen years consecutive admissions to a psychiatric clinic. *Brit. J. Psychiat.* **112**, 809.
Gottesman, I. I., & Shields, J. (1973). Genetic theorizing and schizophrenia. *Brit. J. Psychiat.* **122**, 15–30.
Gottfries, C. G. (1971). Flupenthixol and trifluoperazine: a double-blind investigation in the treatment of schizophrenia. *Brit. J. Psychiat.* **119**, 547–548.
Gould, G. M. (1956). *Medical Dictionary,* 2nd Ed. New York: McGraw-Hill.
Gowdy, J. M. (1972). Stramonium intoxication: review of symptomatology in 212 cases. *J. Amer. Med. Ass.* 221, 585–587.
Grace, W. J., Wolf, S. & Wolff, H. G. (1951). *The Human Colon.* New York: Hoeber.
Graham, D. T. & Wolf, S. (1950). Pathogenesis of urticaria: experimental study of life situations, emotions and cutaneous vascular reactions. *J. Amer. med. Ass.* **143**, 1396.
Graham, G. S. (1957). Chlorpromazine jaundice in a general hospital. *Brit. med. J.* **2**, 1080.
Grant, E. C. (1965). The contribution of ethology to child psychiatry. In *Modern Perspectives in Child Psychiatry,* ed. Howells, J. G. Edinburgh: Oliver & Boyd.
Gray, S. J., Benson, J. A., Reifenstein, R. W. & Spiro, H. M. (1951). Chronic stress and peptic ulcer. *J. Amer. med. Ass.* **147**, 1529.

Green, J. R. (1965). The incidence of alcoholism in patients admitted to medical wards of a public hospital. *Med. J. Austral.* **i, 465.**

Green, J. R., Duisberg, R. E. H. & McGrath, W. B. (1951). Focal epilepsy of psychomotor type. *J. Neurosurg.* **8,** 157.

Green, M. A., Stevenson, L. D., Fonesca, J. E. & Wortis, C. B. (1952). Cerebral biopsy in patients with presenile dementia. *Dis. nerv. Syst.* **13,** 303.

Green, R. (1970). Persons seeking sex change: psychiatric management of special problems. *Amer. J. Psychiat.* **126,** 1596–1603.

Greenberg, S. I. (1955). Alopecia areata: a psychiatric study. *Arch. Derm. Syph. Chic.* **72,** 454.

Greene, E. B. (1941). *Measurement of Human Behaviour.* New York: Odyssey Press.

Greene, W. A., Goldstein, S. & Moss, A. J. (1972). Psychosocial aspects of sudden death. *Arch. Intern. Med.* **129,** 725–731.

Greenfield, J. G. (1934). Subacute spino-cerebellar degeneration occurring in elderly patients. *Brain,* **57,** 161.

Greenfield, J. G. & Bosanquet, F. D. (1953). The brain stem lesions in Parkinsonism. *J. Neurol. Neurosurg. Psychiat.* **16,** 213.

Greenland, C. (1961). Family care of mental patients. *Lancet,* ii, 605.

Greenson, R. R. (1958). Variations in classical psycho-analytic technique: an introduction. *Int. J. Psycho-Anal.* **39,** 200.

Greenson, R. R. (1959) The classic psycho-analytic approach. In *American Handbook of Psychiatry,* ed. Arieti, S. New York: Basic Books.

Greer, S. & Gunn, J. C. (1966). Attempted suicides from intact and broken parental homes. *Brit. med. J.* **2,** 1355.

Gregg, N. M. (1941). Congenital cataract following German measles in the mother. *Trans. ophthal. Soc. Aust.* **3,** 35.

Gregory, I. (1955). The role of nicotinic acid (niacin) in mental health and disease. *J. ment. Sci.* **101,** 85.

Gregory, I. (1960). Genetic factors in schizophrenia. *Amer. J. Psychiat.* **116,** 961.

Griffith, J. D., Cavanaugh, J., Held, J., & Oates, J. A. (1972). Dextroamphetamine: evaluation of psychomimetic properties in man. *Arch. gen. Psychiat.* **26,** 97–100.

Grinker, R. R., Korchin, S. J., Basowitz, H., Hamburg, D. A., Sabshin, M., Persky, H., Chevalier, J. A. & Board, F. A. (1957). A theoretical and experimental approach to problems of anxiety. In *Progress in Psychotherapy,* Vol. II, ed Masserman, J. H. & Moreno, J. L. New York: Grune.

Grinker, R. R. & Spiegel, J. P. (1945*a*). *Men under Stress.* Philadelphia: Blakiston.

Grinker, R. R. & Spiegel, J. P. (1945*b*). *War Neuroses.* Philadelphia: Blakiston.

Groddeck, G. W. (1928). *The Book of the It.* New York: Nervous and Mental Diseases Publishing Coy.

Groen, J. (1947). Psychogenesis and psychotherapy of ulcerative colitis. *Psychosom. Med.* **9,** 151.

Grossman, H. J. & Greenberg, N. H. (1957). Psychosomatic differentiation in infancy. 1. Autonomic activity in the newborn. *Psychosom. Med.* **19,** 293.

Grounds, D., Davies, B., & Mowbray, R. (1970). The contraceptive pill, side effects and personality: report of a controlled double blind trial. *Brit. J. Psychiat.* **116,** 169–172.

Grundfest, H. (1959). Synaptic and ephaptic transmission. In *Handbook of Physiology.* Amer. Physiol. Soc. Vol. 1, Section 1, 147.

Grünthal, E. (1926). Über die Alzheimersche Krankheit. Einè histopathologische, klinische Studie. *Z. ges. Neurol. Psychait.* **101,** 128.

Gull, W. W. (1874). Anorexia nervosa (apepsia hysterica, anorexia hysterica). *Trans. clin. Soc. Lond.* **7,** 22.

Gunn, J. & Fenton, G. (1971). Epilepsy, automatism and crime. *Lancet,* i, 1173–1176

Günther, H. (1912). Die Hämotoporphyrie. *Dtsch. Arch. klin. Med.* **105,** 89.

Gunzburg, H. C. (1958). Vocational and social rehabilitation of the feebleminded. In *Mental Deficiency; the Changing Outlook,* ed. Clarke & Clarke. London: Methuen.

Gupta, J. C., Deb, A. K. & Kahali, B. S. (1943). Preliminary observations on use of *Rauwolfia serpentina Benth* in treatment of mental disorders. *Indian M. Gaz.* **78,** 547.

Hackett, T. P., Cassem, N. H., & Wishnie, H. A. (1968). The coronary care unit: an appraisal of its psychological hazards. *New Eng. J. Med.* **279,** 1365–1370.

Hadfield, J. A. (1958). The cure of homosexuality. *Brit. med. J.* **1,** 1323.

Hahn, R. D. *et al.* (1959). Penicillin treatment of general paresis (dementia paralytica). *Arch Neurol. Psychiat.* **81,** 557.

Haider, I. & Oswald, I. (1970). Late brain recovery processes after drug overdose. *Brit. med. J.* **2,** 318–322.

Hakim, R. A. (1953). Indigenous drugs in the treatment of mental diseases. Sixth Gujurat and Saurashtra Provincial Medical Conference, Baroda, India.

Hald, J. & Jacobsen, E. (1948). A drug sensitizing the organism to ethyl alcohol. *Lancet,* ii, 1001.

Hall, C. S. (1938). The inheritance of emotionality. *Sigma Xi Quart.* **26,** 17.

Hallgren, B. (1959). Nocturnal enuresis; aetiologic aspects. *Acta paediat. Uppsala,* Suppl. **118,** 66.

Halliday, J. L. (1943). Concept of a psychosomatic affection. *Lancet,* ii, 692.

Hamerton, J. L., Briggs, S. M., Gianelli, F. & Carter, C. O. (1961). Chromosome studies in detection of parents with high risk of second child with Down's syndrome. *Lancet,* ii, 788.

Hamilton, M. (1960). A rating scale for depression. *J. Neurolog. Neurosurg. Psychiat,* **23,** 56–62.

Hamilton, M., & White, J. M. (1959). Clinical syndromes in depressive states. *J. ment. Sci.* **105,** 985–998.

Hanfmann, E. & Kasanin, J. (1942). Conceptual thinking in schizophrenia. *Nerv. ment. Dis. Monogr.* No. 67. New York: Nervous and Mental Disease Publishing Coy.

Harcourt, B. & Hopkins, D. (1972). Tapetoretinal degeneration in childhood presenting as a disturbance in behaviour. *Brit. med. J.* **1,** 202–205.

Hare, E. H., Dominian, J. & Sharpe, L. (1962). Phenelzine and dexamphetamine in depressive illness: a comparative trial. *Brit. med. J.* **1,** 9.

Hare, E. H. & Shaw, G. K. (1965). *Mental Health on a New Housing Estate: A Comparative Study of Health in Two Districts of Croydon.* Maudsley Monograph No. 12. London: Oxford University Press.

Hargreaves, M. A. (1962). Intravenous atropine premedication before electro-convulsive therapy. *Lancet,* i 243.

Harlow, H. F. (1959). Basic social capacity of primates. *Human Biology,* **31,** 40.

Harlow, J. M. (1869). *Recovery from the Passage of an Iron Bar through the Head.* Boston: Clapp.

Harper J. (1959). Out-patient adult psychiatric clinics. *Brit. med. J.* **1,** 357.

Harries, J. M. & Hughes, T. F. (1958). Enumeration of the 'cravings' of some pregnant women. *Brit. med. J.* **2,** 39.

Harrington, J. A. & Cross, K. W. (1959). Cases of attempted suicide admitted to a general hospital. *Brit. med. J.* **2,** 463.

Harris, A. (1957). Day hospitals and night hospitals in psychiatry. *Lancet,* i, 729.

Hartman, H. R. (1933). Neurogenic factors in peptic ulcer. *Med. Clin. N. Amer.* **16,** 1357.

Harvey, W. A. & Sherfey, M. J. (1954). Vomiting in pregnancy: a psychiatric study. *Psychosom. Med.* **16,** 1.

Haslam, J. (1798). *Observations on Madness and Melancholy: Including Practical Remarks on those Diseases; together with Cases; and an Account of the Morbid Appearances on Dissection,* 2nd Ed. (1809). London: Callow.

Hathaway, S. R. & McKinley, J. C. (1951). *Minnesota Multiphasic Personality Inventory: Manual* (revised). New York: Psychological Corporation.

Hatrick, J. A., & Dewhurst, K. (1970). Delayed psychosis due to L.S.D. *Lancet,* ii, 742–744.

Hauptmann, A. (1912). Luminal bei Epilepsie. *Münch. med. Wschr.* **59,** 1907.

Hawkings, J. R., Jones, K. S., Sim, M. & Tibbetts, R. W. (1956). Deliberate disability. *Brit. med. J.* **1,** 361.

Hawkings, J. R. & Tibbetts, R. W. (1956*a*). Carbon dioxide inhalation therapy in neurosis: a controlled clinical trial. *J. ment. Sci.* **102,** 52.

Hawkings, J. R. & Tibbetts, R. W. (1956*b*). Intravenous acetylcholine therapy in neurosis: a controlled clinical trial. *J. ment. Sci.* **102,** 43.

Hay, D., & Oken, D. (1972). The psychological stresses of intensive care unit nursing. *Psychosom. Med.* **34,** 109–118.

Hayek, F. A. (1970). 'Literarism' versus Scientism. *Times Lit. Suppl. No. 3560.* p.564.

Head, H. (1920). *Studies in Neurology.* London: Oxford Univ. Press.

Head, H. & Rivers, W. H. R. (1920). *Studies in Neurology,* 2 vols. London: Froude.

Healy, W. (1915). *The Individual Delinquent–a Textbook of Diagnosis and Prognosis.* Boston: Little Brown & Co.

Heath, R. G. & Norman, E. C. (1946). Electroshock therapy by stimulation of discrete cortical sites with small electrodes. *Proc. Soc. exp. Biol. N.Y.* **63,** 496.

Heine, B. (1970). Psychogenesis of hypertension. *Proc. roy. Soc. Med.* **63,** 1267–1270.

Heisel, J. S. (1972). Life changes as etiologic factors in juvenile rheumatoid arthritis, *J. Psychosom. Res.* **16,** 411–420.

Hemphill, R. E. (1952). Incidence and nature of puerperal psychiatric illness. *Brit. med. J.* 2, 1232.
Hemphill R. E. (1960). Psychiatric half-way hostel. *Lancet,* i 703.
Hemphill, R. E. (1962). Mental impairment in boxers. *Brit. med. J.* 2, 1962.
Hemphill, R. E., Leitch, A., Stuart J. R. (1958). A factual study of male homosexuality. *Brit. med. J.* 1, 1317.
Hemphill, R. E., Reiss, M. & Taylor, A. L. (1944). A study of the histology of the testis in schizophrenia and other mental disorders. *J. ment, Sci.* **90**, 681.
Henderson, D. (1956). Psychiatric evidence in court. *Brit. med. J.* 2, 1.
Henderson, D. K. (1939). *Psychopathic States.* New York: Norton.
Henderson, D. K. & Gillespie, R. D. (1950). *A Text-book of Psychiatry,* 7th Ed. Oxford Medical Publications.
Hendin, H. (1969). Black suicide. *Arch. gen. Psychiat.* **21**, 407–422.
Henriques, B. (1961). Sexual assaults on children. II. A magistrates' view. Brit. med. J. 2, 1629.
Henriques, F. (1962). *Prostitution and Society: a Survey. Vol. I. Primitive, Classical and Oriental.* London: MacGibbon & Kee.
Herridge, C. F. (1960). Physical disorders in psychiatric illness: a study of 209 consecutive admissions. *Lancet,* ii, 949.
Hersov, L. A. (1960*a*). Persistent non-attendance at school. *J. Child Psychol.* 1, 130.
Hersov, L. A. (1960*b*). Refusal to go to school. *J. Child Psychol.* 1, 137.
Herzberg, B. N., Draper, K. C., Johnson, A. L. & Nicol, G. C. (1971). Oral contraceptives, depression, and libido. *Brit. med. J.* 3, 495–500.
Heston, L. L., Lowther, D. L. W. & Leventhal, C. M. (1966). Alzheimer's disease: a family study. *Arch. Neurol.* (Chicago) **15**, 225.
Hiebel, G., Bonvallet, M. & Dell, P. (1954). Action de la chlorpromazine ('largactil' 45 60 RP). *Sem. Hôp. Paris,* **30**, 2346.
Hilgard, E. R. (1962). *Introduction to Psychology,* 3rd Ed. London: Methuen.
Hilgard, J. R., & Newman, M. F. (1959). Anniversaries in mental illness. *Psychiatry,* **22**, 113.
Hill, A. B. (1963). Medical ethics and controlled trials. *Brit. med. J.* 1 1043.
Hill, D. (1952). EEG in episodic psychotic and psychopathic behaviour: a classification of data. *Electroenceph. clin. Neurophysiol.* 4, 419.
Hill, D. (1957). Electroencephalogram in schizophrenia. In *Schizophrenic Somatic Aspects,* p. 33, ed. Richter, D. London: Pergamon.
Hill, D. (1958). Value of the E.E.G. in diagnosis of epilepsy. *Brit. med. J.* 1, 663.
Hill, D. (1968). Depression: disease, reaction or posture? *Amer. J. Psychiat.* **125**, 445–457.
Hill, D. & Sargant, W. (1943). A case of matricide. *Lancet,* i, 526.
Hill, D. & Watterson, D. (1942). Electro-encephalographic studies of psychopathic personalities. *J. Neurol. Psychiat.* 5, 47.
Hill, H. E. & Belleville, R. E. (1953). Effects of chronic barbiturate intoxication on motivation and muscular co-ordination. *Arch. Neurol. Psychiat.* **70**, 180.
Himmelhoch, J., Pincus J., Tucker, G. & Detre, T. (1970). Sub-acute encephalitis: behavioural and neurological aspects. *Brit. J. Psychiat.* **116**, 531–538.
Himwich, H. E. (1955). Prospects in psychopharmacology. *J. nerv. ment. Dis.* **122**, 413.
Himwich, H. E. (1956). Alcoholism and brain physiology. In *Alcoholism,* ed. Thompson, G. N. Springfield, Ill.: Thomas.
Himwich, H. E. (1957). Viewpoints obtained from basic and clinical symposia on tranquilizing drugs. In *Tranquilizing Drugs,* ed. Himwich, H. E. Amer. Assoc. for the Advancement of Science, Publ. No. 46. Washington, D.C.
Hinde, R. A. (1959). Some recent trends in ethology. In *Psychology, a Study of a Science,* Vol. 2, ed. Koch, S. New York: McGraw-Hill.
Hiroisi, S. & Lee, C. C. (1936). Origin of senile plaques. *Arch. Neurol. Psychiat.* **35**, 827.
Hirsch, S. R., Gaind, R., Rohde, P. D., Stevens, B. C. & Wing, J. K. (1973). Outpatient maintenance of chronic schizophrenic patients with long-acting fluphenazine: double-blind placebo trial. *Brit. med. J.* 1, 633–637.
Hjern, B. & Nylander, L. (1964). Acute head injuries in children. *Acta Paediat. Supp.* 152.
H.M.S.O. (1959). *Road Accidents,* 1959. H.M. Stationery Office.
Hobson, J. A. & Prescott, F. (1947). Use of *d*-tubocurarine chloride and thiopentone in electro-convulsion therapy. *Brit. med. J.* 1, 445.
Hoag, J. M., Norriss, N. G., Himeno, E. T., & Jacobs, J. (1971). The encopretic child and his family. *J. Amer. Acad. Child Psychiat.* **10**, 242–246.
Hoch, P. H. (1951). Experimentally produced psychoses. *Amer. J. Psychiat.* **107**, 607.
Hoch, P. H. (1955). Experimental psychiatry. *Amer. J. Psychiat.* **111**, 787.
Hoch, P. H., Cattell, J. P. & Pennes, H. H. (1952). Effects of mescaline and lysergic acid (δLSD-25). *Amer. J. Psychiat.* **108**, 579.

Hoch, P. H., Cattell, J. P., Strahl, M. O. & Pennes, H. H. (1962). The course and outcome of pseudoneurotic schizophrenia. *Amer. J. Psychiat.* **119,** 106.

Hoch, P. H. & Polatin, P. (1949). Pseudo-neurotic forms of schizophrenia. *Psychiat. Quart.* **23,** 248.

Hodgson, O. E. F. & Sim, M. (1959). Out-patient electroplexy: review of work of a general hospital clinic. *Lancet,* i, 1245.

Hoenig, J., Kenna, J., & Youd, A. (1970). Social and economic aspects of transsexualism. *Brit. J. Psychiat.* **117,** 163–172.

Hofmann, A., Heim, R., Brack, A. & Kobel, H. (1958). Psilocybin, ein psychotroper Wirkstoff aus dem mexikanischen Rauschpilz Psilocybe mexicana Heim. *Experimentia,* **14,** 107.

Hogben, L. (1931). *Genetic Principles in Medicine and Social Science.* London: Williams & Norgate.

Hogben, L. (1961). Whewell's Dilemma. An Essay on Some Taxonomical Concepts. A Farewell Address delivered in the Department of Zoology of the University of Birmingham.

Hogben, L. & Sim. M. (1953). The self-controlled and self-recorded clinical trial for low-grade morbidity. *Brit. J. prev. soc. Med.* **7,** 163.

Holland, J., Masling, J., & Copley, D. (1970). Mental illness in lower class normal, obese and hyperobese women. *Psychosom. Med.,* **32,** 351–357.

Hollingshead, A. B. & Redlich, F. C. (1958). *Social Class and Mental Illness.* New York: Wiley.

Hollister, L. E., & Gillespie, H. K. (1970). Marihuana, ethanol and dextroamphetamine: mood and mental function alterations. *Arch. gen. Psychiat.* **23,** 199–203.

Holmes, J. M. (1956). Cerebral manifestations of vitamin B_{12} deficiency. *Brit med. J.* **2,** 1394.

Holt, S. B. (1969). The genetics of dermal ridges. *Lancet,* i, 1969. 83.

Holtz, P. (1959). Role of L-dopa decarboxylase in the biosynthesis of catecholamines in nervous tissue and the adrenal medulla. *Pharm. Rev.* **11,** 317.

Holtz, P. & Heise, R. (1938). Fermentativer Abbau von 1-Dioxyphenylalanin durch Niere. *Arch. exp. Path. Pharmakol.* **191,** 87.

Horney, K. (1939). *New Ways in Psychoanalysis.* New York: Norton.

Horney, K. (1945). *Our Inner Conflicts: a Constructive Theory of Neurosis.* New York: Norton.

Horwitt, M. K. (1956). Fact and artifact in the biology of schizophrenia. *Science,* **124,** 429.

Horwitz, D., Lovenberg, W., Engelman, K. & Sjoerdsma, A. (1964). Monoamine oxidase inhibitors, tyramine and cheese. *J. Amer. med. Ass.* **188,** 1108.

Hourigan, K., Sherlock, S., George, P., & Mindel, S. (1971). Elective end-to-side portacaval shunt: Results in 64 cases. *Brit. med. J.* **4,** 473–477.

Housden, J. (1961). Neurotics nomine. *Lancet,* ii, 1453.

Hubble, D. V. (1953). Endocrine disorders. In *Diseases of Children,* Vol. 1, ed. Moncrieff A. & Evans, P. London: Arnold.

Hughes, P. H., Crawford, G. A., Barker, N. W., Schumann, S., & Jaffe, J. H. (1971). The social structure of a heroin copping community. *Amer. J. Psychiat.* **128,** 551–558.

Hughes, R. (1959). Some unusual cases of neurosyphilis. *J. Neurol. Psychiat.* **22,** 81.

Hughes, R. R. & Summers, V. K. (1956). Changes in the electroencephalogram associated with hypopituitarism due to post-partum necrosis. *Electroenceph. clin. Neurophysiol.* **8,** 87.

Hughes, W., Dodgson, M. C. H. & MacLennan, D. C. (1954). Chronic cerebral hypertensive disease. *Lancet,* ii, 770.

Hull, C. L. (1951). *Essentials of Behaviour.* New Haven, Conn: Yale University Press.

Hunt, J. McV. (1941). The effects of infant feeding frustration upon adult breeding in the albino rat. *J. abnorm. soc. Psychol.* **36,** 338.

Hunter, C. (1917). A rare disease in two brothers. *Proc. roy. soc. Med.* **10,** 104.

Hunter, H. (1947). Anxiety manifested by moderately elevated temperatures. *Rocky Mtn. med. J.* **44,** 908.

Hunter, R., Earl, C. J. & Thornicroft, S. (1964). An apparently irreversible syndrome of abnormal movements following phenothiazine medication. *Proc. roy. Soc. Med.* **57,** 758.

Hunter, R., Jones, M. & Mathews, D. M. (1967). Post-gastrectomy vitamin B_{12} deficiency in psychiatric practice. *Lancet,* i, 47.

Hunter, R. A. & Greenberg, P. H. (1954). Barbiturate addiction simulating spontaneous hyperinsulinism. *Lancet,* ii, 58.

Huntington, G. (1872). On chorea. *Med. Surg. Reptr.* **26,** 317.

Hurler, G. (1919). Über einen Typ multipler Abartungen, vorweigend am Skelettsystem. Z. *Kinderheilk.* **24,** 220.
Husler, J. (1931). Multiple Abartungen. In *Handbuch d. Kinderheilk,* ed. Pfaundler, M. von & Schlossmann, A. Berlin: Vogel.
Hutchinson, J. H., Stone, F. H. & Davidson, J. R. (1958). Photogenic epilepsy induced by the patient. *Lancet,* i, 243.
Huxley, A. (1954). *The Doors of Perception.* London: Chatto & Windus.

Ibor, J. L. (1952). Anxiety states and their treatment by intravenous acetyl choline. *Proc. roy. Soc. Med.* **45,** 511.
Illingworth, G. F. W., Scott, L. D. W. & Jamieson, R. A. (1944). Acute perforated peptic ulcer: frequency and incidence in the West of Scotland. *Brit. med. J.* **2,** 617.
Inciardi, J. A. & Chambers, C. D. (1971). Patterns of pentazocine abuse and addiction. *New York J. Med.* **71,** 1727–1733.
Ingalls, T. H. (1947). Etiology of mongolism: epidemiologic and teratologic implications. *Amer. J. Dis. Child.* **74,** 147.
Irwin, D. (1953). In *Emotional Factors in Skin Diseases.* Ed. Wittkower, E. & Russell, B. London: Cassell.
Isaacs, S. (1972). Neglect, cruelty, and battering. *Brit. med. J.* **3** 224–226.
Isbell, H. (1959). Comparison of the reactions induced by psilocybin and LSD 25 in man. *Psychopharmacologia,* **1,** 29.
Isbell, H., Altschul, S., Korentsky, C., Eisenman, A. J., Flanary, H. C. & Fraser, H. F. (1950). Chronic barbiturate intoxication: experimental study. *Arch. Neurol. Psychiat.* **64,** 1.
Isselbacher, K. J. & Greenberger, N. J. (1964). Metabolic effects of alcohol on the liver. *New Eng: J. Med.* **270,** 351, 402.
Itil, T. M., Polvan, N., & Holden, J. M. C. (1971). Clinical and electro-encephalengraphic effects of cinanserin in schizophrenic and manic patients. *Dis. nerv. Syst.* **32,** 193–200.

Jackson, J. H. (1894). The factors of insanities. In *Selected Writings,* Vol. 2, p. 411 (1932). London: Hodder & Stoughton.
Jacobs, H. & Russell, W. R. (1961). 'Functional' disorders: a follow-up study of out-patient diagnosis. *Brit. med. J.* **2,** 346.
Jacobs, P. A., Baikie, A. G., Court-Brown, W. M. & Strong, J. A. (1959). The somatic chromosomes in mongolism. *Lancet,* i, 710.
Jacobsen, C. F. (1936). Studies on cerebral function in primates. *Comp. Psychol. Mongr.* **13,** No. 3.
Jacobsson, L., & Ottosson, J.-O. (1971). Initial mental disorders in carcinoma of pancreas and stomach. *Acta Psychiat. Scand. Suppl.* **221,** 120–127.
Jacoby, M. G. (1958). Abuse of E.C.T. *Brit. med. J.* **1,** 282.
Jaffe, S. L. & Scherl, D. J. (1969). Acute psychosis precipitated by T-group experiences. *Arch. gen. Psychiat.* **21,** 443–448.
James, G. (1969). New dimensions in legal and ethical concepts for human research. N.Y. Acad. Sci. Conference on Human Research. *The Sciences,* **9,** (10). p.8.
James, W. (1890). *Principles of Psychology,* 2 vols. New York: Macmillan.
Janet, P. (1893). État mental des hysteriques. Les accidents mentaux. Paris: Rueff.
Jarvie, H. (1958). The frontal lobes and human behaviour. *Lancet,* ii, 365.
Jarvie, H. F. (1954). Frontal lobe wounds causing disinhibition: a study of six cases. *J. Neurol. Neurosurg. Psychiat.* **17,** 14.
Jasper, H. H. (1949*a*). Diffuse projection systems: the integrative action of the thalamic reticular system. *Electroenceph. clin. Neurophysiol.* **i,** 405.
Jasper, H. H. (1949*b*). Étude anatomo-physiologique des epilepsies. 2nd Int. E.E.G. Cong. Paris. *Rapp. Electroenceph. clin. Neurophysiol.* Suppl. 2, 99.
Jasper, H. H. & Rasmussen, T. (1958). Studies of clinical and electrical responses to deep temporal stimulation in man with some considerations of functional anatomy. *Res. Publ. Ass. nerv. ment. Dis.* **36,** 316.
Jaspers, K. (1946). *Allgemeine Psychopathologie,* 4 Aufl. Berlin: Springer.
Jaspers, K. (1963). *General Psychopathology.* Translated from the German 7th edition by Hoenig, J. & Hamilton, M. W. Manchester: The University Press.
Jefferson, G. (1944). The nature of concussion. *Brit. med. J.* **1,** 1.
Jefferson, J. W., (1972). Atypical manifestations of postural hypotension. *Arch. gen. Psychiat.* **27,** 250–251.
Jellinek, E. M. (1951). W.H.O. Expert Committee on Mental Health. Sub-committee on Alcoholism. Alcoholism. *Techn. Rep. Wld. Hlth. Org.* **42,** 20.

Jellinek, E. M. (1952). W.H.O. Expert Committee on Mental Health. Second report of the Alcoholic Sub-committee. *Tech. Rep. Wld. Hlth. Org.* No. 48,

Jellinek, E. M. (1960). Alcoholism, a genus and some of its species. *Canad. med. Ass. J.* **83**, 1341.

Jenkins, R. B., & Groh, R. H. (1970). Mental symptoms in parkinsonian patients treated with L-dopa. *Lancet,* ii, 177–180.

Jennett, W. B. (1962). Epilepsy After Blunt Head Injuries. London: Heinemann.

Jennings, R. (1962). Mental disorder and the Court of Protection. *Lancet,* i, 855.

Jeri, R. (1963). Las Manifestasciones Neurologicas del Carcinoma Broncogenica; Observasciones Clinico-Patologicas en una Series Constructiva de 383 Pacientes. Lima.

Jervis, G. A. (1948). Early senile dementia in mongoloid idiocy. *Amer. J. Psychiat.* **105**,102.

Johnson, A. M., Falstein, E. I., Szurek, S. & Svendsen, M. (1942). School Phobia. *Amer. J. Orthopsychiat.*11 702.

Jonas, S. (1969). The approach to heroin addiction. *Lancet,* ii, 383–384.

Jones, D. P. (1951). Recording of the basal electroencephalogram with sphenoidal needle electrodes. *Electroenceph. clin. Neurophysiol.* **3**, 100.

Jones, E. (1913). Hate and anal erotism in the obsessional neurosis. In *Papers on Psychoanalysis,* 3rd Ed. (1923). London: Baillière.

Jones, E. (1953–1957). *Sigmund Freud,* 3 vols. London: Hogarth Press.

Jones, K. (1955). *Lunacy, Law and Conscience. 1744–1845: the Social History of the Care of the Insane.* London: Routledge & Kegan Paul.

Jones, K. (1960). *Mental Health and Social Policy,* 1845–1959. London: Routledge & Kegan Paul.

Jones, K. S. & Tibbetts, R. W. (1959). Pituitary snuff, propantheline and placebos in the treatment of enuresis. *J. ment. Sci.* **105**, 371.

Jones, M. (1952). *Social Psychiatry, a Study of Therapeutic Communities.* London: Tavistock Publications.

Jones, M. (1956). Industrial rehabilitation of mental patients still in hospital. *Lancet,* ii, 985.

Jones, M. & Lewis, A. (1941). Effort syndrome. *Lancet,* i, 813.

Jones, W. L. (1971). Manifest dream content: an aid to communication during analysis. *Amer. J. Psychother.* **25**, 284- 292.

Joyce, C. R. B. (1959). Consistent differences in individual reactions to drugs and dummies. *Brit. J. Pharmacol.* **14**, 512.

Jung, C. G. (1906). *Über die Psychologie der Dementia praecox. Ein Versuch.* Halle: Marbold.

Jung, C. G. (1909). A lecture given at Clark University. In *Collected Works* London: Routledge.

Jung, C. G. (1910). The association method. *Amer. J. Psychol.* **21**, 219.

Juul-Jensen, P. (1964). Epilepsy: a clinical and social analysis of 1020 adult patients with epileptic seizures. *Acta neurol. Scand.* **40**, Suppl. 5, 126.

Kahlbaum, K. (1874). *Klinische Abhandlungen über psychische Krankheiten. Ht. I. Die Katatonie.* Berlin: Hirschwald.

Kahn, E. (1931). *Psychopathic Personalities.* New Haven: Yale University Press.

Kalinowsky, L. B. (1942). Convulsions in non-epileptic patients on withdrawal of barbiturates, alcohol and other drugs. *Arch. Neurol. Psychiat.* **48**, 946.

Kalinowsky, L. B. & Hoch, P. H. (1952). *Shock Treatment, Psychosurgery, and other Somatic Treatments in Psychiatry,* 2nd Ed. New York: Grune & Stratton.

Kallmann, F. J. (1952). Comparative twin study on the genetic aspects of male homosexuality. *J. nerv. ment. Dis.* **115**, 283.

Kallmann, F. J. (1953). *Heredity in Health and Mental Disorder.* New York: Norton.

Kanner, L. (1943). Autistic disturbances of affective contact. *Nerv. Child.* **2**, 217.

Kanner, L. (1957). *Child Psychiatry,* 3rd Ed. Springfield, Ill.: Thomas.

Kanner, L. (1960). *Textbook of Child Psychiatry.* Springfield, Ill.: Thomas.

Kanner, L., Rodriguez, A., & Ashenden, B. (1972). How far can autistic children go in matters of social adaptation? *J. Autism Childhd. Schizophrenia,* **2**, 9–33.

Kaplan, H. A. & Browder, J. (1954). Observations on the clinical and brain wave patterns of professional boxers. *J. Amer. med. Ass.* **156**, 1138.

Kardiner, A. (1939). *The Individual and His Society.* New York: Columbia University Press.

Karush, A. & Daniels, G. (1953). Ulcerative colitis: the psychoanalysis of two cases. *Psychosom. Med.* **15**, 140.

Katz, L. N. & Stamler, J. (1953). *Experimental Atherosclerosis.* Springfield, Ill.: Thomas.

Kay, D. W. K. (1953). Anorexia nervosa: a study in prognosis. *Proc. roy. Soc. Med.* **46**, 669.

Kay, D. W. K. (1972). Schizophrenia and schizophrenia–like states in the elderly. *Brit. J. Hosp. Med.* **8**, 369–376.

Kazamatsuri, H., Chien, C., & Cole, J. O. (1972*a*). Treatment of tardive dyskinesia. 1. Clinical efficacy of a dopamine-depleting agent, tetrabenazine. *Arch. gen. Psychiat.* **27**, 95–99.

Kazamatsuri, H., Chien, C., & Cole, J. O. (1972*b*). Treatment of tardive dyskinesia. 11. Short-term efficacy of dopamine-blocking agent, haloperidol and thiopropazate. *Arch. gen. Psychiat.* **27**, 100–103.

Kelly, D. Guirguis, W. Frommer, E., Mitchell-Heggs, N. Sargant, W. (1970). Treatment ot phobic states with antidepressants: a retrospective study of 246 patients. *Brit. J. Psychiat.* **116**, 387–398.

Kelly, D., Mitchell-Heggs, N., & Sherman, D. (1971). Anxiety and the effects of sodium lactate assessed clinically and physiologically. *Brit. J Psychiat.* **119**, 129–141.

Kelly, D. H. W. (1967). The technique of forearm plethysmography for assessing anxiety. *J. Psychosom. Res.* **10**, 373–382.

Kelly, G. A. (1955). *The Psychology of Personal Constructs.* New York: Norton.

Kelman, H. (1957). A unitary theory of anxiety. *Amer. J. Psychoan.* **17**, 127.

Kendell, R. E. (1968). *The Classification of Depressive Illnesses.* Maudsley Monogr., No. 18. London.

Kendrick, J. P. & Gibbs, F. A. (1957). Origin, Spread and neurosurgical treatment of the psychomotor type of seizure discharge. *J. Neurosurg.* **14**, 270.

Kennedy, P. F., Hershon, H. I. & McGuire, R. J. (1971). Extra-pyramidal disorders after prolonged phenothiazine therapy. *Brit. J. Psychiat.,* **118**, 509–518.

Kennedy, W. A. (1959). Clinical and electroencephalographic aspects of epileptogenic lesions of the medial surface and superior border of the cerebral hemisphere. *Brain,* **82**, 147.

Kennedy, W. A. & Hill, D. (1958). The surgical prognostic significance of the electroencephalographic prediction of Ammon's horn sclerosis in epileptics. *J. Neurol. Neurosurg. Psychiat.* **21**, 24.

Kennell, J. H., Slyter, H., & Klaus, M. H. (1970). The mourning response of parents to the death of a new-born infant. *New Eng. J. Med.,* **283**, 344–349.

Kenyon, F. E. (1965). Hypochondriasis: a survey of some historical, clinical and social aspects. *Brit. J. med. Psychol.* **38**, 117.

Kenyon, F. E. (1968). (a) Studies in female homosexuality. IV. social and psychiatric aspects. *Brit. J. Psychiat.* **114**, No. 516. 1337–1343.

Kenyon, F. E. (1968). (b) Studies in female homosexuality. V. sexual development, attitudes and experience. *Brit. J. Psychiat.* **114** No. 516. 1343–1350.

Kerridge, J. C. (1952) A technique of recording from the basal areas of the skull ('sphenoidal' electrodes). *Electroenceph. clin. Neurophysiol.* **4**, 254.

Kessel, N. (1965*a*). Self-poisoning. Part I. *Brit. med. J.* **2**, 1265.

Kessel, N. (1965*b*). Self-poisoning. Part II. *Brit. med. J.* **2**, 1336.

Kessel, N. & Grossman, G. (1961). Suicide in alcoholics. *Brit. med. J.* **2**, 1671.

Kety, S. S. (1959). Biochemical theories of schizophrenia. Parts 1 & 2. *Science,* **129**, 1528, 1590.

Keup, W. (1970). Psychotic symptoms due to cannabis abuse. *Dis. Nerv. Syst.* **31**, 119–126.

Khan, A. U. (1971). 'Mama's boy' syndrome. *Amer. J. Psychiat.* **128**, 712–717.

Kidd, H. B. (1961). A team system in a mental hospital. *Lancet,* ii, 703.

Kierkegaard, S. A. (1844). *The Concept of Dread.* London: Oxford University Press.

Kiev, A. (1972). *Transcultural Psychiatry.* New York: The Free Press.

Kiloh, L. G. & Garside, R. F. (1963). The independence of neurotic depression and endogenous depression. *Brit. J. Psychiat.* **109**, 451–463.

King, A. & Little, J. C. (1959). Thiopentone treatment of the phobic anxiety-depersonalization syndrome: a preliminary report. *Proc. roy. Soc. Med.* **52**, 595.

Kinsey, A. C., Pomeroy, W. B. & Martin, C. E. (1948). *Sexual Behavior in Human Male.* Philadelphia: Saunders.

Kinsey, A. C., Pomeroy, W. B., Martin, C. E. & Gebhart, P. H. (1953). *Sexual Behavior in the Human Female.* Philadelphia: Saunders.

Kirby, G. H. (1921). Some problems of the mental reaction types associated with organic brain disease. *St. Hosp. Quart. N.Y.* **6**, 467.

Kirman, B. H. (1951). Epilepsy in mongolism. *Arch. Dis. Childh.* **26**, 501.

Kishimoto, K. (1962). Preliminary theory about psychotherapy based on Oriental thought. *Acta psychotherap. et psychosom.* **10**, 428.

Kissen, D. M. (1958). *Emotional Factors in Pulmonary Tuberculosis.* London: Tavistock Publications.

Kissen, D. M. (1963). Personality characteristics in males conducive to lung cancer. *Brit. J. med. Psychol.* **36**, 27.
Kissen, D. M. (1964). Personality and lung cancer. *Lancet,* ii, 216.
Kissen, D. M. (1966). Psychological factors, personality and prevention in lung cancer. *Med. Offr.* **106**, 135.
Klaber, R. & Wittkower, E. D. (1939). The pathogenesis of rosacea: review with special reference to emotional factors. *Brit. J. Derm.* **51**, 501.
Klein, M. (1932). *The Psycho-analysis of Children.* London: Hogarth.
Klein, M. (1948). *Contributions to Psycho-analysis 1921–1945.* London: Hogarth.
Klein, R. & Mayer-Gross, W. (1957). *The Clinical Examination of Patients with Organic Cerebral Disease.* London: Cassel.
Kleist, K. (1926). *Episodische Dämmerzustände.* Leipzig: Thieme.
Kline, N. S. (1954). Use of Rauwolfia serpentini Bentham in neuropsychiatric conditions. *Ann. N.Y. Acad. Sci.* **59**, 107.
Klingler, J. & Gloor, P. (1960). The connections of the amygdala and of the anterior temporal cortex in the human brain. *J. comp. Neurol.* **115**, 333.
Klüver, H. & Bucy, P. C. (1938). An analysis of certain effects of bilateral temporal lobectomy in the Rhesus monkey. *J. Psychol.* **5**, 33.
Knapp, P. H. (1969). The asthmatic and his environment. *J. nerv. ment. Dis.* **149**, 133–151.
Knight, G. (1965). Stereotactic tractotomy in the surgical treatment of mental illness *J. Neurol. Neurosurg. Psychiat.* **28**, 304.
Knight, R. P. (1937). The psychodynamics of chronic alcoholism. *J. nerv. ment. Dis.* **86**, 538.
Knox, S. J. (1960). Psychogenic urinary retention after parturition resulting in hydronephrosis. *Brit. med. J.*2, 1422.
Knox, S. J. (1963). Psychiatric aspects of mitral valvotomy. *Brit. J. Psychiat.* **109**, 656.
Koelle, G. B. (1961). In *Regional Neurochemistry,* ed. Kety, S. S. & Elkes, J. Proc. IVth International Neurochemical Symposium, p. 312.
Kohs, S. C. (1923). *Intelligence Assessment: a Psychological and Statistical Study based upon the Block-design Test.* New York: Macmillan.
Kolansky, H. & Moore, W. T. (1971). Effects of marihuana on adolescents and young adults. *J. Amer. Med. Ass.* **216**, 486–492.
Kolb, L. (1925). Pleasure and deterioration from neurotic addiction. *Ment. Hyg. N.Y.* **9**, 699.
Kolb, L. C. (1954). *The Painful Phantom.* Psychology, Physiology and Treatment. Springfield, Ill.: Thomas.
Korsakoff, S. S. (1887). Ob alkoholnom paralichie. *Westnik Psychiatrii,* **4**.
Kozol, H. L. (1946). Pretraumatic personality and psychiatric sequelae of head injury. II. Correlation of multiple, specific factors in the pretraumatic personality and psychiatric reaction to head injury, based on analysis of one hundred and one cases. *Arch. Neurol. Psychiat.* **56**, 245.
Kraepelin, E. (1909–13). *Psychiatrie.ein Lehrbuch für Studierende und Artze,* 8 Auf. Leipzig: Barth.
Krafft-Ebing, R. (1894). *Psychopathia Sexualis, with Special Reference to Contrary Sexual Instinct: a Medico-Legal Study,* 7th Ed. Trans. Chaddock, C.G. Philadelphia: Davis.
Kraines, S. H. (1957). *Mental Depressions and Their Treatment.* New York: Macmillan.
Krapf, E. E. (1957). On the pathogenesis of epileptic and hysterical seizures. *Bull. Wld. Hlth. Org.* **16**, 749.
Krauss, S. (1961). Prognosis in schizophrenia. *Brit. med. J.* **1**, 1392.
Kreindler, A., Hornet, T. & Appel, E. (1959). Complex forms of cerebral senility. *Rum. med. Rev.* 3(2), 43.
Kreitman, N., Sainsbury, P. Pearce, K. & Costain, W. R. (1965). Hypochondriasis and depression in out-patients at a general hospital. *Brit. J. Psychiat.* **111**, 607.
Kreitman, N., Smith, P., & Tan, E. S. (1970). Attempted suicide as language: an empirical study. *Brit. J. Psychiat.* **116**, 465–473.
Kretschmer, E. (1925). *Korperbau und Charackter,* 4 Aufl. Berlin: Springer. Trans. Sprott, W. J. H. (1936). London: Kegan Paul.
Kretschmer, E. (1926). *Hysteria.* New York: Nervous and Mental Diseases Publishing Coy.
Kringlen, E. (1964). Discordance with respect to schizophrenia in monozygotic male twins: some genetic aspects. *J. nerv. ment. Dis.* **138**, 26.
Krynauw, R. A. (1950). Infantile hemiplegia treated by removal of one cerebral hemisphere. *S. Afric. Med. J* 24, 243–267.
Kubie, L. S. (1958). The investigation of the pharmacology of psychological processes: some methodologic considerations from the point of view of clinical psychoanalysis. In *Psychopharmacology: Pharmacologic Effects on Behavior,* ed. Pennes, H.H. New York: Hoeber.

Kubie, L. S., & Mackie, J. B. (1968). Critical issues raised by operations for gender transmutation. *J. nerv. ment. Dis.* **147**, 431–443.
Kühn, R. (1957). Uber die Behandlung depressiver Zustände mit einem Iminodibenzylderivat. (G22355). *Schweiz. med. Wschr.* **87**, 1135.
Kumar, K. & Wilkinson, J. C. M. (1971). Thought-stopping: a useful treatment in phobias of "internal stimuli". *Brit. J. Psychiat.* **119**, 305–307.
Kuno, Y. (1934). *The Physiology of Human Perspiration.* London: Churchill.
Kutner, S. J., & Brown, W. L. (1972). Types of oral contraceptives, depression and premenstrual symptoms. *J. nerv. ment. Dis.* **155**, 153–162.

Laborit, H., Huguenard, P. & Alluaume, R. (1952). Un nouveau stabilisateur végétatif (LE 4560 RP). *Presse Méd.* **60**, 206.
La Brosse, E. H., Axelrod, J. & Kety, S. S. (1958). O-methylation, the principal route of metabolism of epinephrine in man. *Science,* **128**, 593.
Lader, M., & Sartorius, N. (1968). Anxiety in patients with hysterical conversion symptoms. *J. Neurol. Neurosurg. Psychiat.* **31**, 490–495.
Lader, M. H. (1968). Prophylactic lithium? *Lancet,* ii, 103.
Laing, R. D. (1960). *The Divided Self: An Existential Study in Sanity and Madness.* London: Tavistock.
Laing, R. D. (1972). *The Politics of the Family and Other Essays.* London: Tavistock.
Laing, R. D., & Esterson, A. (1964). *Sanity, Madness and the Family.* Vol. 1. Families of Schizophrenics. London: Tavistock.
Laitinen, L. V. (1972). Stereotactic lesions of the knee of the corpus collosum in the treatment of emotional disorders. *Lancet,* i, 472–475.
Lambo, T. A. (1959). Mental health in Nigeria: research and its technical problems. *Wld. ment. Hlth.* **2**, 131.
Lambo, T. A. (1960). Further neuropsychiatric observations in Nigeria. *Brit. med. J.* **2**, 1696.
Lancet, (1949*a*). A psychiatrist looks at tuberculosis. *Lancet,* ii, 805.
Lancet, (1949*b*). Disabilities: 26. Enuresis. *Lancet,* i, 537.
Lancet (1949*c*). Disabilities No. 34. Homosexuality. *Lancet* ii, 128.
Lancet (1958). Book Review. *Social Class and Mental Illness. Lancet,* ii, 888.
Lancet (1960*a*). The mongol chromosome and some others. *Lancet,* ii, 1068.
Lancet (1960*b*). School phobia. *Lancet,* i, 270.
Lancet (1961) Compensation for cupidity. *Lancet,* i, 1099.
Lancet (1962). Attitude and prejudice: a UNESCO conference. *Lancet,* i, 154.
Landau, R., Harth, P., Othnay, N., & Sharfhertz, C. (1972). The influence of psychotic parents on their children's development. *Amer. J. Psychiat.* **129**, 38–43.
Landers, J. J., MacPhail, D. S. & Simpson, R. C. (1954). Group therapy in H.M. Prison, Wormwood Scrubs–the application of analytical psychology. *J. ment. Sci.* **100**, 953.
Landzkowsky, P. (1959). Investigation into the aetiology and treatment of pica. *Arch. Dis. Childh.* **34**, 140.
Langdon Down, J. L. H. (1866). Observations on an ethnic classification of idiots. *Clin. Lect. Rep. Lond. Hosp.* **3**, 259.
Langfeldt, G. (1937). Prognosis in schizophrenia and factors influencing course of disease. *Acta psychiat et neurol. Scand.* Suppl. 13.
Larson, J. W., Swenson, W. M., Utz, D. C. & Steinhilber, R. M. (1963). Psychogenic urinary retention in women. *J.A.M.A.* **184**, 697.
Larsson, T. & Sjögren, T. (1954). A methodological, psychiatric and statistical study of a large Swedish rural population. *Acta psychiat. scand.* Suppl. 89.
Lascelles, P. T., & Lewis P. D. (1972). Hypodipsia and hypernatraemia associated with hypothalamic and suprasellar lesions. *Brain,* **95**, 249–264.
Lawson, I. R., & McLeod, R. D. M. (1969). The use of imipramine ("Tofranil") and other psychotropic drugs in organic emotionalism. *Brit. J. Psychiat.* **115**, 281–285.
Layne, O. L., & Yudofsky, S. C. (1971). Postoperative psychosis in cardiotomy patients: the role of organic and psychiatric factors. *New Eng. J. Med.* **284**, 518–520.
Lazarte, J. A., Peterson, M. C., Baars, C. W. & Pearson, J. S. (1955). Huntington's chorea. Results of treatment with reserpine. *Proc. Staff Meet. Mayo Clinic,* **30**, 358.
Le Beau, J. (1954). *Psycho-chirurgie et fonctions mentales: techniques–résultats applications physiologiques.* Paris: Masson.
Leff, J. P., & Wing, J. K. (1971). Trial of maintenance therapy in schizophrenia. *Brit. med. J.* **3**, 599–604.
Lehmann, H. E. & Hanrahan, G. E. (1954). Chlorpromazine: new inhibiting agent for psychomotor excitement and manic states. *Arch. Neurol. Psychiat.* **71**, 227.

Leigh, D. (1952). Pellagra and the nutritional neuropathies: a neuropathological review. *J. ment. Sci.* **98**, 130.

Lejuene, J., Lafourcade, J., Berger, R. Vialatte, J., Boeswillwald, M., Seringe, P. & Turpin, R. (1963). Trois cas de délétion partielle du bras court d'un chromosome 5. *C.R. Acad. Sci. Paris,* **257**, 3098.

Lennard Jones, J. E. & Asher, R. (1959). Why do they do it? a study of pseudocide. *Lancet* i, 1138.

Lennox, B. (1961). Chromosomes for beginners. *Lancet,* i, 1046.

Lennox, W. G. (1943). Amnesia, real and feigned. *Amer. J. Psychiat.* **99**, 732.

Lennox, W. G. (1947*a*). The genetics of epilepsy. *Amer. J. Psychiat.* **103**, 457.

Lennox, W. G. (1947*b*). Sixty-six twin pairs affected by seizures. *Ass. Res. nerv. Dis. Proc.* **26**, 11.

Lennox, W. G., Gibbs, E. L. & Gibbs, F. A. (1939). The inheritance of epilepsy as revealed by the electro-encephalograph. *J. Amer. med. Ass.* **113**, 1002.

Lennox, W. G., Gibbs, E. L. & Gibbs, F. A. (1940). Inheritance of cerebral dysrhythmia and epilepsy. *Arch. Neurol. Psychiat.* **44**, 1155.

Leonhard, K. (1957). Aufteilung der endogenen Psychosen. Berlin: Akademie-Verlag.

Lesch, M. & Nyhan, W. L. (1964). A familial disorder of uric acid metabolism and central nervous system function. *Amer. J. med.* **36**, 561.

Levin, B., Fajerman, J., & Jacoby, N. M. (1972). Mucopolysaccharidosis. *Proc. roy. Soc. Med.* **65**, 339–341.

Levin, M. (1948). Bromide psychoses: four varieties. *Amer. J. Psychiat.* 104, 798.

Levin, M. (1959). Toxic psychoses. In *American Handbook of Psychiatry*, Vol. 2, ed. Arieti, S. New York: Basic Books.

Levin, S. (1971). The psychoanalysis of shame. *Int. J. Psycho-Anal.* **52**, 355–362.

Levine, M. (1942). *Psychotherapy in Medical Practice.* New York: Macmillan.

Levine, S. & Stephens, R. (1971). Games addicts play. *Psychiat. Quart.* **45**, 582–592.

Levy, D. M. (1934). Experiments on the sucking reflex and social behavior of dogs. *Amer. J. Orthopsychol.* **4**, 203.

Levy, D. M. (1943). *Maternal Over-protection.* New York: Columbia University Press.

Levy, D. M. (1950). On evaluating the 'specific event' as a source of anxiety. In *Anxiety,* p. 140, ed. Hoch, P. H. & Zubin, J. New York: Grune & Stratton.

Levy, R., & Meyer, V. (1971). Ritual prevention in obsessional patients. *Proc. roy. Soc. Med.* **64**, 1115–1118.

Levy, S. & Goodman, L. (1952). Juvenile familial amaurotic idiocy (Vogt-Spielmeyer disease). *Amer. J. ment. Defic.* **57**, 63.

Lewis, A. (1935). Problems of obsessional illness. *Proc. roy. Soc. Med.* **29**, 325.

Lewis, A. (1942). Discussion on differential diagnosis and treatment of postcontusional states. *Proc. roy. Soc. Med.* **35**, 607.

Lewis A. B. (1966). Effective utilization of the psychiatric hospital. *J.A.M.A.* **197**, 871.

Lewis, H. (1965). The psychiatric aspects of adoption. In *Modern Perspectives in Child Psychiatry,* ed. Howells, J.G. Edinburgh: Oliver & Boyd.

Lewison, E. (1965). An experiment in facial reconstructive surgery in a prison population. *Canad. med. Ass. J.* **92**, 251.

Leyberg, J. T. (1959). A district psychiatric service: the Bolton pattern. *Lancet,* ii, 282.

Liberson, W. T. (1947). Some technical observations concerning brief stimulus therapy. *Dig. Neurol. Psychiat.* **15**, 72.

Liberson, W. T. & Wilcox, P. H. (1945). Electric convulsive therapy: comparison of 'brief stimuli technique' with Freidman-Wilcox-Reiter technique. *Dig. Neurol. Psychiat.* **13**, 292.

Lidberg, L. (1971). Frequency of concussion and type of criminality: a preliminary report. *Acta Psychiat. Scand.* **47**, 452–461.

Lidz, R. W. & Lidz, T. (1949). The family environment of schizophrenic patients. *Amer. J. Psychiat.* **106**, 332.

Lidz, R. W. & Lidz, T. (1969). Homosexual tendencies in mothers of schizophrenic women. *J. nerv. ment. Dis.* **149**, 229–235.

Lidz, T. (1949). Emotional factors in the etiology of hyperthyroidism: the report of a preliminary survey. *Psychosom. Med.* **11**, 2.

Lidz, T., Cornelison, A. R., Fleck, S. & Terry, D. (1957). The interfamilial environment of schizophrenic patients, (2) marital schism and marital skew. *Amer. J. Psychiat.* **114**, 241.

Lieber, A. L., & Sherin, C. R. (1972). Homicides and the lunar cycle: toward a theory of lunar influence on human emotional disturbance. *Amer. J. Psychiat.* **129**, 69–74.

Lightbody, M. & Jacobson, S. (1965). A therapeutic community in an acute admission unit of a mental hospital. *Brit. med. J.*1, 47.
Liley, A. W. (1972). The foetus as a personality. *Aust. N.Z. J. Psychiat.* **6**, 99–105.
Lindberg, B. (1948). What does the abortion-seeking woman do when the psychiatrist refuses it? *Svenska Läk.–Tidn.* **45**, 1381.
Lindemann, E. (1945). Psychiatric problems in conservative treatment of ulcerative colisis. *Arch. Neurol. Psychiat.* **53**, 322.
Lindstrom, P. A. (1954). Prefrontal ultrasonic irradiation–a substitute for lobatomy. *Arch. Neurol. Psychiat.* **72**, 399.
Lipowski, Z. J. (1966). Psychopathology as a science: its scope and tasks. *Compr. Psychiat.* **7**, 175.
Lipowski, Z. J. (1974). Physical illness, the patient and his environment: psychosocial foundations of medicine. In *American Handbook of Psychiatry,* ed. Arieti, S. Vol 4. New York: Basic Books.
Lippold, O. C. J. & Redfearn, J. W. T. (1964). Mental changes resulting from the pasage of small direct currents through the brain. *Brit. J. Psychiat.* **110**, 768.
Lishman, W. A. (1968). Brain damage in relation to psychiatric disability after head injury. *Brit. J. Psychiat.* **114**, 373–410.
Lissauer, H. & Storch, E. (1901). Über einige Fälle atypischer progressiver Paralyse. Nach einem hinterlassenem. Manuscript Dr. H. Lissauers. *Mschr. Psychiat. Neurol.* **9**, 401.
Litman, R. E., & Swearingen, C. (1972). Bondage and suicide. *Arch. gen. Psychiat.* **27**, 80–85.
Little, J. C. (1969). The athlete's neurosis–a deprivation crisis. *Acta Psychiat. Scand.* **45**, 187–197.
Litvak, R., & Kaelbling, R. (1971). Agranulocytosis, leukopenia, and psychotropic drugs. *Arch. gen. Psychiat.* **24**, 265–267.
Locket, S. (1957). *Clinical Toxicology*. London: Kimpton.
Locock, C. (1857). Analysis of fifty-two cases of epilepsy observed by the author (contribution to the discussion). *Lancet,* i, 529.
Logan, F. A. (1959). The Hull-Spence approach. In *Psychology, a Study of a Science,* Vol. 2, ed. Koch, S. New York: McGraw-Hill.
Logue, V., Durward, M., Pratt, R. T. C., Piercy, M., & Nixon, W. L. B. (1968). The quality of survival after rupture of an anterior cerebral aneurysm. *Brit. J. Psychiat.* **114**, 137–159.
Loiseau, P., Cohadon, F., & Cohadon, S. (1971). Gelastic epilepsy: a review and report of five cases. *Epilepsia,* **12**, 312–323.
Lolli, G. (1956). Alcoholism as a disorder of the love disposition. *Quart. J. Stud. Alcohol.* **17**, 96.
Lorente De Nó, R. (1933). Vestibulo-ocular reflex arc. *Arch. Neurol. Psychiat.* **30**, 245.
Lorenz, K. (1937). The nature of instinct. In *Instinctive Behaviour.* Translated by Schiller, C.H. 1957. New York: International Universities Press.
Lorenz, M. (1953). Language behaviour in manic patients: a qualitative study. *Arch. Neurol. Psychiat.* **69**, 14.
Lorenz, M. & Cobb, S. (1952). Language behaviour in manic patients. *Arch. Neurol. Psychiat.* **67**, 763.
Lowenfeld, H., & Lowenfeld, Y. (1970). Our permissive society and the superego: some current thoughts about Freud's cultural concepts. *Psychoanal. Quart.* **39**, 590–608.
Lowenfeld, M. (1939). The world pictures of children: a method of recording and studying them. *Brit. J. med. Psychol.* **18**, 65.
Lowinger, P., & Dobie, S. (1969). What makes the placebo work? a study of placebo response rates. *Arch. gen. Psychiat.* **20**, 84–88.
Luby, E. D., Cohen, B. D., Rosenbaum, G., Gottlieb, J. S. & Kelley, R. (1959). Study of a new schizophrenomimetic drug–sernyl. *Arch. Neurol. Psychiat.* **81**, 363.
Lucas, R. N. & Falkowski, W. (1973). Ergotamine and methysergide abuse in patients with migraine. *Brit. J. Psychiat.* **122**, 199–203.
Ludwig, A. M. (1968). The influence of nonspecific healing techniques with chronic schizophrenics. *Amer. J. Psychother.* **22**, 382–404.
Luossenhop, A. J., de la Cruz, T. C., Fenichel, G. M. (1970). Surgical disconnection of the cerebral hemispheres for intractable seizures: results in infancy and childhood. *J. Amer. Med. Ass.* **213**, 1630–1636.
Luria, A. R. (1965). Two kinds of motor perseveration in massive injury of the frontal lobes. *Brain,* **88**, 1.
Lyon, M. F. (1961). Gene action in the X-chromosome of the mouse (Mus musculus L.). *Nature,* **190**, 372.

Lyon, R. L. (1962*a*). Huntington's chorea in the Moray Firth area. *Brit. med. J.* **1**, 1301.
Lyon, R. L. (1962*b*). Non-hereditary chronic adult chorea as a clinical entity. *Brit. med. J.* **1**, 1306.
Lyon, R. L. (1962*c*). Drug treatment of Huntington's chorea: a trial with thiopropazine. *Brit. med. J.* **1**, 1308.
Macalpine, I. (1958). Is alopecial areata psychosomatic? A psychiatric study. *Brit. J. Derm.* **70**, 117.
Macalpine, I. & Hunter, R. (1966). The 'insanity' of King George III: a classic case of porphyria. *Brit. med. J.* **1**, 65.
Macalpine, I. & Ross, J. P. (1956). Oedème bleu. *Lancet*, i, 78.
MacCarthy, D., Lindsay, M. & Morris, I. (1962). Children in hospital with mothers. *Lancet*, i, 603.
McCarthy, J. P. (1971). Some less familiar drugs of abuse. *Med. J. Austral.* **2**, 1078–1081.
McClary, A. R., Meyer, E. & Weitzman, E. L (1955). Observations on the role of the mechanism of depression in some patients with lupus erythematosus. *Psychosom. Med.* **17**, 311.
McCord, W., McCord, J. & Gudeman, J. (1959). Some current theories of alcoholism: a longitudinal evaluation. *Quart. J. Stud. Alcohol*, **20**, 724.
McCown, I. A. (1959). Boxing injuries. *Amer. J. Surg.* **98**, 509.
McCullagh, E. P. & Tupper, W. R. (1940). Anorexia nervosa. *Ann. intern. Med.* **14**, 817.
MacDougall, A. A. (1958). Regressive shock therapy. *Brit. med. J.* **1**, 1180.
McGee, T. F., Schuman, B. N., & Racusen, F. (1972). Termination in group psychotherapy. *Amer. J. Psychother.* **26**, 521–532.
MacGregor, R. (1964). *Multiple Impact Therapy with Families*. Maidenhead: McGraw-Hill.
McIlwain, H. & Greengard, O. (1957). Excitants and depressants of the central nervous system, on isolated electrically-stimulated cerebral tissues. *J. Neurochem.* **1**, 348.
Mackay, D. M. & McCullough, W. S. (1952). The limiting information capacity of a neuronal link. *Bull. math. Biophys.* **14**, 127.
McKegney, F. P., Gordon, R. O., & Levine, S. L. (1970). A psychosomatic comparison of patients with ulcerative colitis and Crohn's disease. *Psychosom. Med.* **32**, 153–166.
MacKenna, R. M. B. & Macalpine, I. (1951). Application of psychology to dermatology. *Lancet*, i, 66.
McKeown, T. (1958). The concept of a balanced hospital community. *Lancet*, i, 701.
McKinley, C. K., Ritchie, A. M., Griffin, D., & Bondurant, W. (1970). The upward mobile negro family in therapy. *Dis. nerv. Syst.* **31**, 710–715.
McKissock, W. (1943). The technique of prefrontal leucotomy. *J. ment. Sci.* **89**, 194.
McKissock, W. (1951). Rostral leucotomy. *Lancet*, ii, 91.
McLardy, T. (1950). Uraemic and trophic deaths following leucotomy: neuro-anatomical findings. *J. Neurol. Neurosurg. Psychiat.* **13**, 106.
McLardy, T. (1951). A case of Marchiafava's disease (primary degeneration of the corpus callosum). *Proc. roy. Soc. Med.* **44**, 685.
MacLean, P. D. (1949). Psychosomatic disease and the 'Visceral brain': recent developments bearing on the Papez theory of emotion. *Psychosom. Med.* **11**, 338.
MacLean, P. D. (1952). Some psychiatric implications of physiological studies on fronto-temporal portion of limbic system (visceral brain). *Electroenceph. clin. Neurophysiol.* **4**, 407.
MacLean, P. D. (1955). The limbic system (visceral brain) in relation to central gray and reticulum of the brain stem: evidence of interdependence in emotional processes. *Psychosom. Med.* **17**, 355.
McMenemey, W. H. (1940). Alzheimer's disease–a report of 6 cases. *J. Neurol. Psychiat.* **3**, 211.
McMichael, J. (1961). Reorientations in hypertensive disorders. *Brit. med. J.* **2**, 1239.
Macmillan, D. (1958). Community treatment of mental illness. *Lancet*, ii, 201.
Macmillan, D. (1960). Preventive geriatrics: opportunities of a community mental health service. *Lancet*, ii, 1439.
MacMillan, Lord, (1937). *Law and Other Things*. Cambridge University Press.
McMurray, W. C., Mohyuddin, F., Rossiter, R. J., Rathbun, J. C., Valentine, G. H., Koegler, S. J. & Zarfas, D. E. (1962). Citrullinuria: a new aminoaciduria associated with mental retardation. *Lancet*, i, 138.
Macht, L. B., & Mack, J. E. (1968). The firesetter syndrome. *Psychiatry*, **31**, 277–288.
Mackiewicz, J. & Reid, A. A. (1965). Clinical and neuropathological investigations of four cases of Huntington's chorea treated with high doses of reserpine. *Med. J. Austral.* i, 833.

Mackwood, J. C. (1949). The psychological treatment of offenders in prison. *Brit. J. Psychol.* (Gen. Section), **40**, 5.

Magoun, H. W. & Rhines, R. (1946). An inhibitory mechanism in the bulbar reticular formation. *J. Neurophysiol.* **9**, 165.

Maher-Loughnan, G. P., Macdonald, N. Mason, A. A. & Fry, L. (1962). Controlled trial of hypnosis in the symptomatic treatment of asthma. *Brit. med. J.* **2**, 371.

Mahl, G. F. (1949). Effect of chronic fear on the gastric secretion of HCl in dogs. *Psychosom. Med.* **11**, 30.

Mahl, G. F. (1950). Anxiety, HCl secretion and peptic ulcer aetiology. *Psychosom. Med.* **12**, 158.

Mahl, G. F. (1952). Relationship between acute and chronic fear and the gastric acidity and blood sugar levels in *Macaca mulatta* monkeys. *Psychosom. Med.* **14**, 182.

Maier, N. R. F. (1949). *Frustration: the Study of Behaviour without a Goal.* New York: McGraw-Hill.

Main, T. F. (1958). Mothers with children in a psychiatric hospital. *Lancet,* ii, 845.

Malamud, N. & Saver, G. (1954). Neuropathologic findings in disseminated lupus erythemotosus. *Arch. Neurol. Psychiat.* **71**, 723.

Malan, D. H. (1963) *A Study of Brief Psychotherapy.* London: Tavistock Publications.

Malinowski, B. K. (1929). *The Sexual Life of Savages in North-Western Melanesia.* London: Routledge.

Malmquist, C. P. (1971). Melancholic violence and cognitive dysfunction. *Brit. J. med. Psychol.* **44**, 267–276.

Malzberg, B. (1956). A statistical review of mental disorders in later life. In *Mental Disorders in Later Life,* 2nd Ed., ed. Kaplan, O.H. California: Stanford University Press.

Man, P. L. & Bolin, B. J. (1969). Further explanation of unilateral electroshock treatment. *Dis. nerv. Syst.* **30**, 547–551.

Mann P. J. G. & Quastel, J H. (1940). Benzedrine (β-phenyl*iso*propylamine) and brain metabolism. *Biochem. J* **34**, 414.

Mann, P. J. G., Tennenbaum, M. & Quastel, J. H. (1939) Acetylcholine metabolism in the central nervous system. *Biochem. J* **33**, 1506.

Marazzi, A. S. & Hart, E. P. (1955). Relationship of hallucinogens to adrenergic cerebral neurohumors *Science,* **121**, 365.

Marfan, B. J. A. (1896). Un cas de déformation congenitale des quatre membres plus prononcée aux extrémités. *Bull. Soc. méd. Hôp. Paris* **13**, 220.

Margolin, S. (1951). The behaviour of the stomach during psychoanalysis. *Psychoanal. Quart.* **20**, 349.

Margolis L. H. Simon, A. & Bowman, K. M. (1952). Selective utilization of unilateral lobotomy. *J. nerv. ment. Dis.* **116**, 392.

Marinacci, A. A. (1956). Electroencephalography in alcoholism. In *Alcoholism,* ed. Thompson, G.N. Springfield, Ill.: Thomas.

Marks, I., Boulougouris, J. & Marset, P. (1971). Flooding versus desensitization in the treatment of phobic patients: a crossover study. *Brit. J. Psychiat.* **119**, 353–375.

Marrack, D., Rose, F. C. & Marks, V. (1961). Glucagon and tolbutamide tests in the recognition of insulinomas. *Proc. roy. Soc. Med.* **54**, 749.

Martin, D. V. (1962). *Adventure in Psychiatry.* Oxford: Bruno Cassirer.

Martin, M. E. (1958). Puerperal mental illness: a follow-up study of 75 cases. *Brit. med. J.* **2**, 773.

Marshall, J. H. L., Davis, J. M. & Janowsky, D. S. (1970). Chlorpromazine dose regulated by plasma levels. *Arch. gen. Psychiat.* **22**, 289–296.

Martin, H. (1970). Antecedents of burns and scalds in children. *Brit. J. med. Psychol.* **43**, 39–47.

Martland, H. S. (1928). Punch drunk. *J. Amer. med. Ass.* **91**, 1103.

Masserman, J. H. (1943). *Behaviour and Neurosis. An Experimental Psychoanalytic Approach to Psychobiologic Principles.* Chicago: University of Chicago Press.

Masserman, J. H. (1955). *The Practice of Dynamic Psychiatry.* Philadelphia: Saunders.

Masserman, J. H., Jaques, M. G. & Nicholson, M. S. (1945). Alcohol as a preventive of experimental neuroses. *Quart. J. Stud. Alcohol.* **6**, 281.

Masserman, J. H. & Yum, K. S. (1946). An analysis of the influence of alcohol on experimental neuroses in cats. *Psychosom. Med.* **8**, 36.

Masters, W. H., & Johnson, V. E. (1970). *Human Sexual Inadequacy.* Boston: Little Brown.

Matarazzo, R. G., Bristow, D. & Reaume, R. (1963). Medical factors relevant to psychologic reactions in mitral valve disease. *J. nerv. ment. Dis.* **137**, 380.

Matthew, G. K. (1971). Measuring need and evaluating services. In *Psychiatric Hospital Care*, ed. McLochlan, G. London: Ballière, Tindall & Cassell.
Matthew, H. Proudfoot, A. T., Aitken, R. C. B., Raeburn, J. A., Wright, N. (1969). Nitrazepam–a safe hypnotic. *Brit. med. J.* 3, 23–25.
Matthew, H. Proudfoot, A. T. Brown, S. S., Smith, A. C. A. (1968). Mandrax poisoning: Conservative management of 116 patients. *Brit. med. J.* 2, 101–102.
Mattinson, J. (1970). *Marriage and Mental Handicap.* London: Duckworth.
Mattsson, A., & Agle, D. P. (1972). Group therapy with parents of hemophiliacs: therapeutic process and observations of parental adaptation to chronic illness in children. *J. Amer. Acad. Child Psychiat.* **11**, 558–571.
Mattsson, A., Gross, S., & Hall, T. W. (1971). Psychoendocrine study of adaptation in young hemophiliacs. *Psychosom. Med.* **33**, 215–225.
Maughs, S. (1941). Concept of psychopathy and psychopathic personality: its evolution and historical development. *J. crim. Psychopath.* 2, 329, 465.
Mautner H. (1959). *Mental Retardation: Its Care, Treatment and Physiological Base.* New York: Pergamon.
Mawson, A. B. (1970). Methohexitone–assisted desensitisation in treatment of phobias. *Lancet,* i, 1084–1086.
Mawdsley, C. & Ferguson, F. R. (1963). Neurological disease in boxers. *Lancet,* ii, 795.
Maxwell, J. D., & Williams, R. (1973). *Drug induced jaundice. Brit. J. Hosp. Med.* **9**, 193–200.
May, A. R. (1961). Prescribing community care for the mentally ill. *Lancet,* i, 760.
May, R. (1950). *The Meaning of Anxiety.* New York: Ronald.
May, R. (1959). The existential approach. In *American Handbook of Psychiatry.* ed. Arieti, S. New York: Basic Books.
Mayer-Gross, W. (1951). Experimental psychoses and other mental abnormalities produced by drugs. *Brit. med. J.* 2 317.
Mayer-Gross, W. & Guttmann, E. (1937). Scheme for the examination of organic cases. *J. ment. Sci.* **83**, 440.
Mayer-Gross, W., Slater, E. & Roth, M. (1960). Clinical Psychiatry. 2nd. Ed. London: Cassell
Mayerhofer, E. (1939) Die mongoloide Idiote in ihrer Beziehung zum Curettage-Abortus. *Ann. Pediat.* **154**, 57.
Mayor's Committee on Marihuana (1944). *The Marihuana Problem in the City of New York.* Philadelphia: Jaques Cattell.
Mead G. H. (1934). *Mind, Self and Society.* Chicago: University of Chicago Press.
Mead, M. (1928). *Enquiry into the Question of Cultural Stability in Polynesia.* New York: Columbia University Press.
Mead, M. (1931). *Growing up in New Guinea.* London: Routledge.
Mead, M. (1935). *Sex and Temperament in Three Primitive Societies.* London: Routledge.
Mead, M. (1936). *Coming of Age in Samoa.* 'Blue Ribbon'. Since published Harmondsworth: Penguin.
Mead, M. (1950). *Male and Female.* London: Gollancz.
Meares, A. (1960). *A System of Medical Hypnosis.* Philadelphia: Saunders.
Meares, A. (1962). What makes the patient better? Atavistic regression as a basic factor. *Lancet,* i, 151.
Meares, R. & Horvath, T. (1972). 'Acute' and 'chronic' hysteria. *Brit. J. Psychiat.* **121**, 653–657.
Mears, E. (1958). Dyspareunia. *Brit. med. J.* 2, 443.
Medical Research Council (1956). The genetic effects of radiation. In *Hazards to Man of Nuclear and Allied Radiations.* London: H.M.S.O.
Meduna, L. J. (1936). *Die Konvulsionstherapie der Schizophrenie.* Halle: Marhold.
Meduna, L. J. (1950). *Carbon Dioxide Therapy.* Springfield, Ill.: Thomas.
Mehlman, R. D. & Griesemer, R. D. (1968). Alopecia areata in the very young. *Amer. J. Psychiat.* **125**, 605–614.
Meigs, J. W. & Hughes, J. P. W. (1952). Acute carbon monoxide poisoning: an analysis of one hundred and five cases. *Arch. Industr. Hyg.* **6**, 344.
Mei-Tal, V. Meyerowitz, S. & Engel, G. L. (1970). The role of psychological process in a somatic disorder: multiple sclerosis: I. The emotional setting of illness onset and exacerbation. *Psychosom. Med.,* 32, 67–86.
Melby, J. C., Street, J. P. & Watson, C. J. (1956). Chlorpromazine in the treatment of porphyria. *J. Amer. med. Ass.* **162**, 174.
Mellins, R. B. & Jenkins, C. D. (1955) Epidemiological and psychological study of lead poisoning in children. *J. Amer. Med. Ass.* **158**, 15.

Mendel, G. (1865). Versuche uber Pfanzen-hybriden. *Verh. d. Naturf. Vereins in Brunn* 4, 3. Reprinted in German in Vol. 42 No. 1 of the *J. Hered.* Translation into English; published as an appendix to Bateson s *Mendel's Principles of Heredity*. Later published as a pamphlet by Harvard University Press.

Mendelson, J. H. & Mello, N. K. (1966). Experimental analysis of drinking behavior of chronic alcoholics. *Ann. N.Y. Acad. Sci.* 133, 828–845.

Mendelson, J. H., Ogata, M., & Mello, N. K. (1971). Adrenal function and alcoholism. I Serum cortisol. *Psychosom. Med.* 33, 145–157.

Mendlewicz, J., Schulman, C. C., De Schutter, B., & Wilmotte, J. (1971). Chronic prostatitis: psychosomatic incidence. *Psychother. Psychosom.* 19, 118–125.

Menninger, K. (1938). *Man against Himself.* New York: Harcourt.

Menninger, K. A. (1941). Recognizing and renaming 'psychopathic personalities . *Bull. Menninger Clin.* 5, 150.

Mental Health Research Fund (1962). Depression and Suicide. Pamphlet No. 2.

Merck, (1961). *The Merck Manual,* 10th Ed. New Jersey: Merck, Sharp & Dohme Research Laboratories.

Merritt, H. H. (1958). Medical treatment in epilepsy. *Brit. med. J.* 1, 666.

Merritt, H. H. & Putnam, T. J. (1938). Sodium diphenyl hydantoinate in the treatment of convulsive disorders. *J. Amer. med. Ass.* 111, 1068.

Merry, J (1966). The 'loss of control' myth. *Lancet,* i, 1257.

Merskey, H. & Spear, F. G. (1967). *Pain: psychological and psychiatric aspects.* London: Bailliere, Tindall & Cassell.

Mestitz, P. (1957). A series of 1817 patients seen in a casualty department. *Brit. med. J.* 2, 1108.

Métraux, R. W. (1950). Speech profiles of the pre-school child 18 to 54 months. *J. Speech Dis.* 15, 37.

Meyer, A. (1901). On parenchymatous systemic degenerations mainly in the central nervous system. *Brain,* 24, 47.

Meyer, A. (1906) Fundamental conceptions of dementia praecox. *Brit. med. J.* 2 757.

Meyer, A. (1929). 'Über eine der amyotrophischen Lateralsclerose nah stehende Erkrankung mit psychischen Störungen. Zugleich ein Beitrag zur Frage der spastischen Pseudo-sklerose (A. Jakob) . *Z. ges. Neurol. Psychiat.* 121, 107.

Meyer, A. (1950). Anatomical lessons from prefrontal leucotomy. In *Perspectives in Neuropsychiatry,* ed. Richter, D.

Meyer, A. (1952). *The Collected Papers of Adolf Meyer,* Vol. IV. Baltimore: Johns Hopkins Press.

Meyer, A. & Beck, E. (1954). *Prefrontal Leucotomy and Related Operations: Anatomical Aspects of Success and Failure.* Edinburgh: Oliver & Boyd.

Meyer, A., Falconer, M. A. & Beck, E. (1954). Pathological findings in temporal lobe epilepsy. *J. Neurol. Neurosurg. Psychiat.* 17, 276.

Meyer, A., Jeliffe, S. E. & Hoch, A. (1911). *Dementia Praecox: a Monograph.* Boston: Badger.

Meyer, H. J. (1939). Über chronischen Schlafmittelmissbrauch und Phanodormpsychosen. *Psychiat.-neurol. Wschr.* 41, 275.

Meyer, V. (1960). Effects of brain damage. In *Handbook of Abnormal Psychology,* ed. Eysenck, H. J. (1960). London: Pitman.

Michael, R. P. (1957). Treatment of a case of compulsive swearing. *Brit. med. J.* 1, 1506.

Michael, S. T. & Langner, T. S. (1963). Social mobility and psychiatric symptoms. *Dis. Nerv. System,* 24, 128.

Miller, F. J. W., Court, S. D. M., Walton, W. S. & Knox, E. G. (1960). *Growing up in Newcastle-on-Tyne: a Continuing Study of Health and Illness in Young Children within their Families.* London: Oxford University Press.

Miller, H. (1961*a*). Accident neurosis. *Brit. med. J.* 1, 919.

Miller, H. (1961*b*). Accident neurosis. *Brit. med. J.* 1, 992.

Miller, H., & Cartlidge, N. (1972). Simulation and malingering after injuries to the brain and spinal cord. *Lancet,* i, 580–585.

Miller, H. & Stern, G. (1965). The long-term prognosis of severe head injury. *Lancet,* i, 225.

Miller, N. E., & Banuazizi, A. (1968). Instrumental learning by curarized rats of a specific visceral response, intestinal or cardiac. *J. Compar. Physiol. Psychol.* 65, 1–7.

Milligan, W. L. (1951). Non-convulsive stimulation therapy: a new psychiatric treatment. *Lancet,* i, 938.

Milne, M. D. (1964). Disorders of amino-acid transport. *Brit. med. J.* 1, 327.

Mindham, R. H. S., (1970). Psychiatric symptoms in Parkinsonism. *J. Neurol. Neurosurg. Psychiat.* 33, 188–191.

Miskolczy, D. (1959). Histopathological characteristics of senile psychoses. *Rum. med. Rev.* 3(2), 62.
Mitchell, S. W. (1881). *Fat and Blood and How to Make Them,* 2nd Ed. London; Lippincott.
Mitchell, W. Falconer, M. A & Hill D. (1954). Epilepsy with fetishism relieved by temporal lobectomy. *Lancet,* ii, 626.
Mittelman, B. & Wolff, H. G. (1942). Emotions and gastroduodenal functions: experimental studies on patients with gastritis, duodenitis and peptic ulcer. *Psychosom. Med.* **4**, 5.
M.O.H. (1960). Drug addiction: interim report of the interdepartmental committee. London: H.M.S.O.
Moncrieff, A. A., Koumides, O. P., Clayton, B. E., Patrick, A. D., Renwich. A. G. C. & Roberts, G. E. (1964). Lead poisoning in children. *Arch. Dis. Childh.* **39**, 1.
Money, J. (1970). Behavior genetics: principles, methods and examples from XO, XXY & XYY syndromes. *Seminars Psychiat.* 2, 11–29.
Monroe, R. R. (1970). *Episodic Behavioral Disorders: A Psychodynamic and Neurophysiologic Analysis.* Cambridge: Harvard University Press.
Monroe, R. R. & Drell, H. J. (1947). Oral use of stimulants obtained from inhalers. *J. Amer. med. Ass.* **135**, 909.
Moore, M. T. & Book, M. H. (1970). Study of sudden death caused by phenothiazines. *Psychiat. Quart.* **44**, 389–402.
Morel, B. A. (1860). *Traités des maladies mentales.* Paris: Masson.
Moreno, J. L. (1958). Fundamental rules and techniques of psychodrama. In *Progress in Psychotherapy. vol. III. Techniques of psychotherapy,* ed. Masserman, J. H. & Moreno, J. L. New York: Grune & Stratton.
Moreno, J. L. (1959). Psychodrama. In *American Handbook of Psychiatry,* ed. Arieti, S. New York: Basic Books.
Morgan, D. H. (1966). The 'loss of control' myth. *Lancet,* ii, 54.
Morison, R. S., Dempsey, E. W. & Morison, B. R. (1941). Cortical responses from electrical stimulation of the brain stem. *Amer. J. Physiol.* **131**, 732.
Morison, R. S. & Dempsey, E. W. (1942). A study of thalamo-cortical relations. *Amer. J. Physiol.* **135**, 281.
Morley, J. (1952). Insulin tumours of the pancreas. *Brit. J. Surg.* **40**, 97.
Morphew, J. A. & Sim, M. (1969). Gilles de la Tourette's syndrome: a clinical and psychopathological study. *Brit. J. med. Psychol.* **42**, 293–301.
Morrison, J. R. (1973). Catatonia: retarded and excited states. *Arch. gen. Psychiat.* **28**, 39–41.
Morse, M. E. (1923). The pathological anatomy of the ductless glands in a series of dementia praecox cases. *J. Neurol. Psychopath.* **4**, 1.
Morton, L. T. (1956). Daniel McNaughton's signature. *Brit. med. J.* **1**, 107.
Moruzzi, G. & Magoun, H. W. (1949). Brain stem reticular formation and activation of the EEG. *Electroenceph. clin. Neurophysiol.* **1**, 455.
Mott, F. W. (1919). Normal and morbid conditions of the testes from birth to old age in one hundred asylum and hospital cases. *Brit. med. J.* **2**, 655.
Motto, J. A. (1970). Newspaper influence on suicide: a controlled study. *Arch. gen. Psychiat.* 23, 143–148.
Mowrer, O. H. & Mowrer, W. M. (1938). Enuresis—method for its study and treatment. *Amer. J. Orthopsychiat.* **8**, 436.
Moynihan, N. H. (1965). Alcohol-withdrawal syndrome. *Brit. med. J.* **1**, 450.
M.R.C. (1963). Treatment of phenylketonuria. *Brit. med. J.* **1**, 1691.
M.R.C. (1965). Clinical trial of the treatment of depressive illness: report to the Medical Research Council by its Clinical Psychiatry Committee. *Brit. med. J.* **1**, 881.
Muellner, S. R. (1960). Development of urinary control in children. *J. Amer. med. ass.* **172**, 1256.
Munthe, A. (1929). *The Story of San Michele.* London: Murray.
Murphy, G. (1928). *Historical Introduction to Modern Psychology,* 5th Ed. London: Routledge and Kegan Paul.
Murphy, G. (1947). *Personality, a Biosocial Approach.* New York: Harper.
Murphy, H. B. M. (1973). Current trends in transcultural psychiatry. *Proc. roy. Soc. Med.* **66**, 711–716.
Murphy, H. B. M., & Raman, A. C. (1971). The chronicity of schizophrenia in indigenous tropical peoples: results of a twelve year follow-up survey in Mauritius. *Brit. J. Psychiat.* **118**, 489–497.
Murray, H. A. (1943). *Thematic Apperception Test Manual.* Cambridge, Mass.: Harvard University Press.
Murray, R. M. Greene, J. G., & Adams, J. H. (1971). Analgesic abuse and dementia. *Lancet,* ii, 242–245.

Murray, R. M., Timbury, G. C., & Linton, A. L. (1970). Analgesic abuse in psychiatric patients. *Lancet,* i, 1303–1305.

Mushatt, C. (1954). Psychological aspects of non-specific ulcerative colitis. In *Recent Developments in Psychosomatic Medicine,* ed. Wittkower, E. D. & Cleghorn, R. A. London: Pitman.

Nadler, R. P. (1968). Approach to psychodynamics of obscene telephone calls. *New York J. Med.* 68, 521–526.

Navon, R., & Padeh, B. (1971). Pre-natal diagnosis of Tay-Sachs genotypes. *Brit. med. J.,* 4, 17–20.

Neff, K. E., Denney, D., & Blachly, P. H. (1972). Control of severe agitation with droperidol. *Dis. nerv. Syst.* 33, 594–597.

Nelson, R. A. & Mayer, M. M. (1949). Immobilization of Treponema pallidum *in vitro* by antibody produced in syphilitic infection. *J. exp. Med.* **89**. 369.

Nelson, W. E., Vaughan, V. C. & McKay, R. J. (1969). Eds. *Textbook of Pediatrics,* 9th. edn. Philadelphia: Saunders.

Nemiah, J. C. (1950). Anorexia nervosa: a clinical psychiatric study. *Medicine (Baltimore),* 29, 225.

Neubürger, K. T. (1930). Arteriosclerosis. In *Handbuch der Geisteskrankheiten,* ed. Bumke, O. Berlin: Springer.

Neuhaus, E. C. (1958). A personality study of asthmatic and cardiac children. *Psychosom. Med.* 20, 181.

Neumann, M. A. & Cohn, R. (1953). Incidence of Alzheimer's disease in a large mental hospital. *Arch. Neurol. Psychiat.* 69, 615.

Nevin, S., McMenemey, W. H., Behrman, S. & Jones, D. P. (1960). Subacute spongiform encephalopathy—a subacute form of encephalopathy attributable to vascular dysfunction (spongiform cerebral atrophy). *Brain,* **83, 519–564.**

Newman, L. E., & Stoller, R. J. (1971). The oedipal situation in male transsexualism. *Brit. J. med. Psychol.* 44, 295–303.

Newman, M. B., & San Martino, M. R. (1971). The child and the seriously disturbed parent: patterns of adaptation to parental psychosis. *J. Amer. Acad. Child Psychiat.* **10**, 358–374.

Nichols, L. A. (1956). Enuresis: its background and cure. *Lancet,* ii, 1336.

Nicolson, G. A., Greiner, A. C., McFarlane, W. J. G. & Baker, R. A. (1966). Effect of penicillamine on schizophrenic patients. *Lancet,* i, 344.

Nielson, J. (1971). Prevalence and a 2½ years incidence of chromosome abnormalities among all males in a forensic psychiatric clinic. *Brit. J. Psychiat.* **119**, 503–512.

Nielsen, J., Tsuboi, T., Stürup, G., & Romano, D. (1968). XYY chromosomal constitution in criminal psychopaths. *Lancet,* ii, 576.

Nishizono, M., (1969). Japanese characteristics of the doctor-patient relationship in psychotherapy. In *Proceedings of the 7th International Congress of Psychotherapy.* Vol. 1. 46–51, Basel: Karger.

Noble, J. & Mathews, H. (1969). Adult poisoning from tricyclic anti-depressants. *Clin. toxicol.* 2, 403–421.

Noble, P., Hart, T., & Nation, R. (1972). Correlates and outcome of illicit drug use by adolescent girls. *Brit. J. Psychiat.* **120, 497–5**0**4.**

Noguchi, H., & Moore, J. W. (1913). A demonstration of Treponema pallidum in the brain in cases of general paralysis. *J. exp. Med.* 17, 232.

Nolan, J. P. (1965). Alcohol as a factor in the illness of university service patients. *Amer. J. med. Sci.* 249, 135.

Norton, A. (1961). Mental hospital ins and outs. A survey of patients admitted to a mental hospital in the past 30 years. *Brit, med. J.* 1, 528.

Novak, J. Corke, P., & Fairley, N. (1971). 'Petit mal status' in adult. *Dis. nerv. Syst.* 32, 245–248.

Noyes, A. P. & Kolb, L. C. (1958). *Modern Clinical Psychiatry.* Philadelphia: Saunders.

Nunberg, H. (1931). The synthetic function of the ego. *Int. J. Psycho-Anal.* X11, 123.

O'Connor, J. F. (1957). Psychiatric manifestations in patients with lupus erythematosus. *Arch. Neurol. Psychiat.* 77, 166.

O'Connor, N. (1958). Learning and mental defect. In *Mental Deficiency: the Changing Outlook,* p. 175, ed. Clarke, A. M. & Clarke, A. D. B. London: Methuen.

O'Connor, W. A. (1948). Some notes on suicide. *Brit J. med. Psychol.* 21, 222.

Offord, D. R., Aponte, J. F. & Cross, L. A. (1969). Presenting symptomatology of adopted children. *Arch. gen. Psychiat.* **20**, 110–116.

Ogata, M., Mendelson, J. H., Mello, N. K., & Majchrowicz, E. (1971). Adrenal function and alcoholism. II. Catecholamines. *Psychosom. Med.* **33**, 159–180.
Ogden, D. A. (1959). Use of surgical rehabilitation in young delinquents. *Brit. med. J.* **1**, 432.
Ogilvie, C. M. (1955). The treatment of pulmonary tuberculosis with iproniazid (1-isonicotinyl 2-isopropyl hydrazine) and isoniazid (isonicotinyl hydrazine). *Quart. J. Med.* **24**, 175.
Olds, J., Killam, K. F. & Eiduson, S. (1957). Effects of tranquillizers on self-stimulation of the brain. In *Psychotropic Drugs*, p. 235, ed. Garattini, S. & Ghetti, V. Amsterdam: Elsevier Publishing Co.
Olds, J. & Milner, P. (1954). Positive reinforcement produced by electrical stimulation of septal area and other regions of rat brain. *J. Comp. Physiol. Psychol.* **47**, 419.
Oppenheim, H. (1890). Zur Pathologie der Grosshirngeschwülste. *Arch. Psychiat. Nervenkr.* **21**, 560, 705.
Oppenheim, H. (1891). Zur Pathologie der Grosshirngeschwülste. *Arch. Psychiat. Nervenkr.* **22**, 27.
Orton, S. T. (1937). *Reading, Writing and Speech Problems in Children.* New York: Norton.
Orwin, A. (1971). Respiratory relief: a new and rapid method for the treatment of phobic anxiety. *Brit. J. Psychiat.* **119**, 635–637.
Orwin, A. & Sim. M. (1965). The mental hospital: effects of an alternative psychiatric service. *Lancet*, i, 644.
Osmond, H. & Hoffer, A. (1959). Schizophrenia: a new approach. *J. ment. Sci.* **105**, 653.
Oswald, I. (1960). Falling asleep open-eyed during intense rhythmic stimulation. *Brit. med. J.* **1**, 1450.
Otenasek, F. J. (1948). Prefrontal lobotomy for the relief of intractable pain. *Bull. Johns Hopk. Hosp.* **83**, 229.

Palmer, H. A. (1939). Vertebral fractures complicating convulsion therapy. *Lancet*, ii, 181.
Palmer, H. A. (1945). Abreactive techniques—ether. *J. R. Army med. Cps.* **84**, 86.
Pampiglione, G. (1952). Induced fast activity in the EEG as an aid in the location of cerebral lesions. *Electroenceph. clin. Neurophysiol.* **4**, 79.
Papez, J. W. (1937). A proposed mechanism of emotion. *Arch. Neurol. Psychiat.* **38**, 725.
Pare, C. M. B., Rees L. & Sainsbury, M. J. (1962). Differentiation of two genetically specific types of depression by the response to anti-depressants. *Lancet*, ii, 1340.
Pargiter, R. A. & Hodgson, T. D. (1959). The mental welfare officer and the psychiatrist. *Lancet*, ii, 727.
Parkes, C. M. (1973). Factors determining the persistence of phantom pain in the amputee. *J. Psychosom. Res.* **17**, 97–108.
Parkes, C. M. Benjamin, B. & Fitzgerald, R. G. (1969). Broken heart: a statistical study of increased mortality among widowers. *Brit. med. J.* **1**, 740–743.
Parkin, D. & Stengel, E. (1965). Incidence of suicidal attempts in an urban community. *Brit. med. J.* **2**, 133.
Parnell, R. W. (1951). Mortality and prolonged illness among Oxford undergraduates. *Lancet*, i, 731
Parr, D. (1957). Alcoholism in general practice. *Brit. J. Addict.* **54**, 25.
Parr, D. & Swyer, G. I. M. (1960). Seminal analysis in 22 homosexuals. *Brit. med. J.* **2**, 1359.
Parrish, H. M. (1957), Epidemiology of suicide among college students. *Yale J. Biol. Med.* **29**, 585.
Partridge, G. E. (1930). Current conceptions of psychopathic personality. *Amer. J. Psychiat.* **10**, 53.
Partridge, M. (1950). *Pre-frontal leucotomy: a Survey of* 300 *Cases Personally Followed over* 1½–3 *Years.* Oxford: Blackwell.
Patch, I. C. L. (1970). Homeless men: London survey. *Proc. roy. Soc. Med.* **63**, 437–441.
Paterson, A. & Zangwill, O. L. (1944). Recovery of spatial orientation in the post-traumatic confusion state. *Brain*, **67**, 54.
Paton, W. D. M. (1973). Cannabis and its problems. *Proc. roy. Soc. Med.* **66**, 718–721.
Patten, J. P. (1968). Chlorpromazine and dystonic reactions. *Brit. med. J.*, **1**, 642–643.
Paul, N. L., Fitzgerald, M. A. & Greenblatt, M. (1956). Five-year follow-up of patients subjected to three different lobotomy procedures. *J. Amer. med. Ass.* **161**, 815.
Paulett, J. D. (1956). Neurotic ill-health: a study in general practice. *Lancet*, ii, 37.
Pavlov, I. P. (1921). *Lectures on Conditioned Reflexes, Vol.* 2. *Conditioned Reflexes and Psychiatry* (Trans. 1941). London: Lawrence & Wishart.
Pavlov, I. P. (1927). *Conditioned Reflexes.* London: Oxford University Press.
Pecknold, J. C., Ananth, J. V., Ban, T. A. & Lehmann, H. E. (1971). Lack of indication of use of antiparkinson medication: a follow-up study. *Dis. nerv. Syst.* **32**, 538–541.

Pemberton, J. (1949). Illness in general practice. *Brit, med. J.* **1**, 306.
Penfield, W. (1958). Pitfalls and success in surgical treatment of focal epilepsy. *Brit. med. J.* **1**, 669.
Penfield, W. (1968). Engrams in the human brain: mechanisms of memory. *Proc. roy. Soc. Med.* **61**, 831–840.
Penfield, W. & Jasper, H. (1954). *Epilepsy and the Functional Anatomy of the Human Brain.* London: Churchill.
Penrose, L. S. (1933). *Mental Defect.* London: Sidgwick & Jackson.
Penrose, L. S. (1949). *The Biology of Mental Defect* (Revised edition 1954). London: Sidgwick & Jackson.
Penrose, L. S. (1954). Observations on the aetiology of mongolism. *Lancet,* ii, 505.
Penrose, L. S. (1955). Memorandum prepared for the British Medical Association Committee on Homosexuality and Prostitution.
Penrose, L. S. (1959). *Outline of Human Genetics.* London: Heinemann.
Penrose, L. S. (1962). Paternal age in mongolism. *Lancet,* i, 1101.
Penrose, L. S., Ellis, J. R. & Delhanty, J. D. A. (1960). Chromosomal translocations in mongolism and in normal relatives. *Lancet,* ii, 409.
Penrose, L. S. & Marr, W. B. (1943). Results of shock therapy evaluated by estimating chances of patients remaining in hospital without such treatment *J. ment. Sci.* **89**, 374.
Penrose, R. J. J. (1972). Life events before subarachnoid haemorrhage. *J. Psychosom. Res.* **16**, 329–333.
Peters, R. S. (1958). *The Concept of Motivation.* London: Routledge & Kegan Paul.
Petersdorf, R. G. & Bennett, I. L. (1957). Factitious fever. *Ann. intern. Med.* **46**, 1039.
Peterson, F. (1912). Bull. Ont. Hosps. Insane, **5**, 107. Quoted by Greenland, C. (1961). *Lancet,* ii, 605.
Petit Dutaillis, D., Christophe, J., Pertuiset, B., Dreyfus-Brisac, C. & Blanc, C. (1954). Lobectomie temporale bilatérale pour épilepsie. Evolutions des perturbations fonctionelles postoperatoires. *Rev. neurol.* **91**, 129.
Pfalzner, P. M. (1970). Computers. *The Sciences,* **10**, No. 9, p. 4.
Phillips, R. M. & Hutchinson, J. T. (1954). Intravenous acetylcholine in treatment of neuroses. *Brit, med. J.* **1**, 1468.
Piaget, J. (1953). *The Origin of Intelligence in the Child.* Translated by Cook, M. London: Routledge & Kegan Paul.
Pick, A. (1892). Über die Beziehungen der senilen Hirnatrophie zur Aphasie. *Prag. med. Wschr.* **17**, 165.
Pilling, L. F., Barry, M. J. & Parkin, T. W. (1962). Electroshock therapy of a depressed patient with complete heart block. *Amer. J. Psychiat.* **119**, 788.
Pilowsky, I., & Sharp, J. (1971). Psychological Aspects of Pre-eclamptic Toxaemia: a Prospective Study. *J. Psychosom. Res.* **15**, 193–197.
Pincus, G. & Hoagland, H. (1950). Adrenal cortical responses to stress in normal man and in those with personality disorders. 1. Some stress responses in normal & psychotic subjects. 2. Analysis of the pituitary-adrenal mechanism in man. *Amer. J. Psychiat.* **106**, 641.
Pinkerton, P. (1958). Psychogenic megacolon in children: the implications of bowel negativism. *Arch. Dis. Childh.* **33**, 371.
Pinkerton, P. (1960). Faecal incontinence in children. *Brit. med. J.* **2**, 1451.
Pintner, R. & Paterson, D. G. (1917). *A Scale of Performance Tests.* New York: Appleton.
Pippard, J. (1955). Second leucotomies. *J. ment. Sci.* **101**, 788.
Pius XII, (1952). Les limites morales des méthodes de recherche et de traitement. *Osservatore romano.* **92**, 218. Quoted by Beecher, H. K. in *Experimentation in Man,* p. 66. Springfield, Ill.: Thomas.
Pletscher, A. (1959). Significance of monoamine oxidase inhibition for the pharmacological and clinical effects of hydrazine derivatives. *Ann. N.Y. Acad. Sci.* **80** 1039.
Poirier, L. J. (1952). Anatomical and experimental studies on the temporal pole of the macaque. *J. comp. Neurol.* **96**, 209.
Poirier, L. J. & Shulman, E. (1954). Anatomical basis for the influence of the temporal lobe on respiration and cardiovascular activity. *J. comp. Neurol.* **100**, 99.
Polani, P. E., Briggs, J. H., Ford, C. E., Clarke, C. M. & Berg, J. M. (1960). A mongol girl with 46 chromosomes. *Lancet,* i, 721–724.
Polatin, P., & Fieve, R. R. (1971). Patient rejection of lithium carbonate prophylaxis. *J. Amer. med. Ass.* **218**, 846–866.
Pollack, M. & Krieger, H. P. (1958). Oculo-motor and postural patterns in schizophrenic children. *Arch. Neurol. Psychiat.* **79** 720.
Pollitt, J. & Young, J. (1971). Anxiety state or masked depression?: a study based on the action of monoamine oxidase inhibitors. *Brit. J. Psychiat.* **119**, 143–149.

Pollitt, J. D. (1965). Suggestions for a physiological classification of depression. *Brit. J. Psychiat.* **111**, 489.

Pollock, H. M., Malzberg, B. & Fuller, R. G. (1939). *Hereditary and Environmental Factors in the Causation of Manic-depressive Psychoses and Dementia Praecox.* Utica, N.Y.: State Hospital Press.

Polonio, P. & Figueiredo, M. (1955). On structure of mental disorders associated with childbearing. *Mschr. Psychiat. Neurol.* **130**, 304.

Pond, D. A. (1961). Psychiatric aspects of epileptic and brain-damaged children. *Brit. med. J.* **2**, 1454.

Pool, A. (1959). Organisation of Community Care for Oldham and District. Paper read to the Northern and Midland Sections of the Royal Medico-Psychological Association.

Pool, J. L. (1949). Topectomy: a surgical procedure for the treatment of mental illness. *J. nerv. ment. Dis.* **110**, 164.

Poppen, J. L. (1948). Technic of prefrontal lobotomy. *J. Neurosurg.* **5**, 514.

Popper, H. (1965). Hepatic drug reactions simulating viral hepatitis. In *Therapeutic Agents and the Liver,* eds. McIntyre, N. and Sherlock, S. Oxford: Blackwell.

Posner, L. B., McCottry, C. M. & Posner, A. C. (1957). Pregnancy craving and pica. *Obstet. and Gynec.* **9**, 270.

Potter, H. W. (1933). Schizophrenia in children. *Amer. J. Psychiat.* **12**, 1254.

Poussaint, A. F. & Ditman, K. S. (1965). A controlled study of imipramine (Tofranil) in the treatment of childhood enuresis. *J. Pediat.* **67**, 283.

Powdermaker, F. (1948). The techniques of the initial interview and methods of teaching them. *Amer. J. Psychiat.* **104**, 642.

Powell, W. J. & Klatskin, G. (1968). Duration of survival in patients with Laennec's cirrhosis. *Amer. J. Med.* **44**, 406–420.

Pratt, R. T. C., Warrington, E. K. & Halliday, A. M. (1971). Unilateral E.C.T. as a test for cerebral dominance, with a strategy for treating left-handers. *Brit. J. Psychiat.* **119**, 79–83.

Preston, J. B. (1956). Effects of chlorpromazine on the central nervous system of the cat: a possible neural basis for action. *J. Pharmacol.* **118**, 100.

Pribram, K. H. & Fulton, J. F. (1954). An experimental critique of the effects of anterior cingulate ablations in monkey. *Brain,* **77**, 34.

Price, W. H. & Jacobs, P. A. (1970). The 47, XYY male with special reference to behavior. *Seminars Psychiat.* **2**, *30–39.*

Price, W. H. & Whatmore, P. B., (1967). Behaviour disorders and pattern of crime among XYY males identified at a maximum security hospital. *Brit. med. J.,* **1**, 533–536.

Prichard, J. C. (1835). *A Treatise on Insanity and other Disorders affecting the Mind.* London: Sherwood, Gilbert & Piper.

Prien, R. F., Caffey, E. M., & Klett, C. J. (1972). A comparison of lithium carbonate and chlorpromazine in the treatment of excited schizo-affectives: Report of the Veterans Administration and National Institute of Mental Health Collaborative Study Group. *Arch. gen. Psychiat.,* **27**, 182–189.

Priest, R. G. (1970). Homeless men: A U.S.A.–U.K. comparison. *Proc. roy. Soc. Med.* **63**, 437–441.

Prince, M. (1906). *The Dissociation of a Personality.* New York: Longmans.

Prince, R. (1960). Use of Rauwolfia for the treatment of psychoses by Nigerian native doctors. *Amer. J. Psychiat.* **117**, 147.

Prinzmetal, M. & Bloomberg, W. (1935). Use of benzedrine for treatment of narcolepsy. *J. Amer. med. Ass.* **105**, 2051.

Prugh, D. G. (1951). The influence of emotional factors on the clinical course of ulcerative colitis in children. *Gastroenterology,* **18**, 339.

Putnam, T. J. & Cushing, H. (1925). Chronic subdural hematoma, its pathology, its relation to pachymeningitis hemorrhagica and its surgical treatment. *Arch. Surg.* **11**, 329.

Querido, A. (1955). The Amsterdam psychiatric first-aid scheme and some proposals for new legislations. *Proc. roy. Soc. Med.* **48**, 741.

Rachman, S. & Teasdale, J. (1969). *Aversion Therapy and Behaviour Disorders. An analysis.* London: Routledge and Kegan Paul.

Rado, S. (1928). The problem of melancholia. *Int. J. Psycho-Anal.* **9**, 420.

Rado, S. (1933). Psychoanalysis of pharmacothymia. *Psychoanal. Quart.* **2**, 1.

Rado, S. (1959). Obsessive behaviour: so-called obsessive-compulsive neurosis. In *American Handbook of Psychiatry.* ed. Arieti, S. New York: Basic Books.

Raffle, P. A. B. (1959). Stress as a factor in disease. *Lancet,* ii 839.

Rahe, R. H. & Lind E. (1971). Psychosocial factors and sudden cardiac death: a pilot study. *J. Psychosom. Res.* 15, 19–24.

Rahe, R. H., & Paasikivi, J. (1971). Psychosocial factors and myocardial infarction. II. an out-patient study in Sweden. *J. Psychosom. Res.* 15, 33–39.

Ramer, B. S., Zaslove, M. O., & Langan, J. (1971). Is methadone enough? The use of ancillary treatment during methadone maintenance. *Amer. J. Psychiat.*, 127, 1040–1044.

Ramon y Cajal, S. (1909). Histologie du systeme nerveuse de l'homme et des vetébrés. Paris: Maloine.

Ramsey, T. A., Mendels, J., Stokes, J. W., & Fitzgerald, R. G. (1972). Lithium carbonate and kidney function: a failure in renal concentrating ability. *J. Amer. med. Ass.* 219, 1446–1449.

Rank, O. (1952*a*). *The Trauma of Birth.* New York: Brunner.

Rank, O. (1952*b*). *The Myth of the Birth of the Hero.* New York: Brunner.

Rapoport, A. (1959). Mathematics and cybernetics. In *American Handbook of Psychiatry*, ed. Arieti, S. New York: Basic Books.

Raskin, N. & Ehrenberg, R. (1956). Senescence, senility and Alzheimer's disease. *Amer. J. Psychiat.* 113, 133.

Rasmussen, T. B. & Jasper, H. H. (1957). Temporal lobe epilepsy: indications for operation and surgical technique. *Proc. 2nd Int. Colloq. on Temporal Lobe Epilepsy, Bethesda, Maryland.* Springfield, Ill.: Thomas.

Raven, J. C. (1951). *Controlled Projection for Children.* London: Lewis.

Rawnsley, K. (1968). Case self-selection and psychosomatic research. *Proc. roy. Soc. Med.* 61, 1126–1128.

Raymond, M. J. (1956). Case of fetishism treated by aversion therapy. *Brit. med. J.* 2, 854.

Raymond, M. J., Lucas, C. J., Beesley, M. L., O'Connell, B. A. & Roberts, J. A. F. (1957). A trial of five tranquillizing drugs in psychoneurosis. *Brit. med. J.* 2, 63.

Read, A. E., Laidlaw, J. & McCarthy, C. F. (1969). Effect of chlorpromazine in patients with hepatic disease. *Brit. med. J.* 3, 497–499.

Read, A. E., Laidlaw, J. & Sherlock, S. (1961). Neuropsychiatric complications of portacaval anastomosis. *Lancet*, i, 961.

Rechtschaffen, A., Wolpert, E. A., Dement, W. C., Mitchell, S. A. & Fisher, C. (1963). Nocturnal sleep of narcoleptics. *EEG & Clin. Neurophysiol.* 15, 599.

Rees, L. (1953). Psychological concomitants of cortisone and ACTH therapy. *J. ment. Sci.* 99, 497.

Rees, L. (1957). An aetiological study of chronic urticaria and angio-neurotic oedema. *J. psychosom. Res.* 2, 172.

Rees, L. (1963). The significance of parental attitudes in childhood asthma. *J. Psychosom. Res.* 7, 181.

Regestein, Q. R., Rose, L. I., & Williams, G. H. (1972). Psychopathology in Cushing's syndrome. *Arch. intern. Med.* 130, 114–117.

Reich, W. (1925). *Der Triebhafte Charakter.* Int. Psycho-Anal. Verlag. Wien.

Reich, W. (1933). *Charakteranalyse. Technik und Grundlagen für Studierende und Praktizierender Analytiker.* Wien. English trans. *Character-analysis,* 3rd Ed., trans. Wolfe, T. P. New York. 1949.

Reichard, S. & Tillman, C. (1950). Patterns of parent-child relationships in schizophrenia. *Psychiatry*, 13, 247.

Reik, T. (1968). The psychological meaning of silence. *Psychoanal. Rev.*, 55, 172–186.

Reimann, H. A. (1932). Habitual hyperthermia. *J. Amer. med. Ass.* 99, 1860.

Reimann, H. A. (1936). The problem of the long continued, low grade fever. *J. Amer. med. Ass.* 107, 1089.

Reinhold, M. (1960). Relationship of stress to the development of symptoms in alopecia areata and chronic urticaria. *Brit. med. J.* 1, 846.

Reiser, M. F., Weiner, H. & Thaler, M. (1957). Patterns of object relationships and cardiovascular responsiveness in healthy young adults and patients with peptic ulcer and hypertension. *Psychosom. Med.* 19, 498.

Reiss, M. (1955). Psychoendocrinology. *J. ment. Sci.* 101 683.

Reiter, P. J. (1969). On flupentixol, an anti-depressant of a new chemical group. *Brit. J. Psychiat.* 115, 1399–1402.

Report of the Royal Commission on the Law relating to Mental Illness and Mental Deficiency (1957). (Cmnd. 169.) London: H.M.S.O.

Resnik, H. L. P. (1972). Erotized repetitive hangings: a form of self-destructive behavior. *Amer. J. Psychother.* 26, 4–21.

Rey, J. H. & Coppen, A. J. (1959). Distribution of androgyny in mental patients. *Brit. med. J.* 2, 1445.

Reynolds, E. H., Preece, J. M., Bailey, J., & Coppen, A. Folate deficiency in depressive illness. *Brit. J. Psychiat.* 117, 287–292.

Rhoads, J. M., & Feather, B. W., (1972). Transference and resistance observed in behaviour therapy. *Brit. J. med. Psychol.* 45, 99–103.

Rich, D. G., & Greenfield, N. S., (1969). Psycho-physiological correlates of *La Belle Indifférence. Arch. gen. Psychiat.* 20, 239–245.

Rich, E., & Gendelman, S. (1973). Psychiatric aspects of normal pressure hydrocephalus. *J. Amer. med. Ass.* 223, 409–412.

Richter, C.P. (1957). On the phenomenon of sudden death in animals and man. *Psychosom. Med.* 19, 191.

Riesman, D. *et al.* (1950). *The Lonely Crowd.* New Haven, Conn.: Yale.

Ritchie, E. A. (1956). Toxic psychosis under cortisone and corticotrophin. *J. ment. Sci.* 102, 830.

Rivers, W. H. R. (1920). *Instinct and the Unconscious.* Cambridge: University Press.

Roberts, A. H. (1964). Housebound housewives: a follow-up study of a phobic anxiety state. *Brit. J. Psychiat.* 110, 191.

Roberts E., Frankel, S. & Harman, P. J. (1950). Amino-acids of nervous tissue. *Proc. Soc. exp. Biol.* 74, 383.

Roberts, G. F. (1953). *The Rhesus Factor*, 3rd Ed. London: Heinemann.

Robertson, G. G. (1946). Nausea and vomiting of pregnancy; a study in psychosomatic and social medicine. *Lancet*, ii, 336.

Robertson, J. (1958*a*). *Young Children in Hospital.* London: Tavistock Publications.

Robin, A. A., & Freeman-Browne, D. L. (1968). Drugs left at home by psychiatric in-patients. *Brit. med. J.* 2, 424–425.

Rodriguez, A., Rodriguez, M. & Eisenberg, L. (1959). The outcome of school phobia: a follow-up based on 41 cases. *Amer. J. Psychiat.* 116, 540.

Rogers, C. R. (1942). *Counselling and Psychotherapy; Newer Concepts in Practice.* Boston; Houghton.

Rogers, C. R. (1951). *Client-centered Therapy.* Boston: Houghton Mifflin.

Rogers, M. P., & Whybrow, P. C. (1971). Clinical hypothyroidism occurring during lithium treatment: two case histories and a review of thyroid function in 19 patients. *Amer. J. Psychiat.* 128, 158–163.

Rollin. H. R. (1963). Social and legal repercussions of the Mental Health Act, 1959. *Brit. med. J.* 1,786.

Rollin, H. R. (1965). Unprosecuted mentally abnormal offenders. *Brit. med. J.* 1, 831.

Rollin, H. R. (1966). Mental hospitals without bars, a contemporary paradox. *Proc. roy. Soc. Med.* 59, 701.

Rolph, C. H. (ed.) (1955). *Women of the Streets.* London: Secker & Warburg.

Rolph, C. H. (1972). Scientific explanations of social inaction. *Times Lit. Suppl.* No 3961. pp. 1455–1456.

Romano, J., Michael, M. & Merritt, H. H. (1940). Alcoholic cerebellar degeneration. *Arch. Neurol. Psychiat.* 44, 1230.

Rome, H. P. & Braceland, F. J. (1952). Psychological response to corticotrophin, cortisone and related steroid substances. *J. Amer. med. Ass.* 148, 27.

Rook, A. (1959). Student suicides. *Brit. med. J.* 1, 599.

Rorschach. H. (1921). *Psychodiagnostics: a Diagnostic Test based on Perception.* Trans. Lemkau, P. & Kronenberg, B. (1942). New York: Grune & Stratton.

Rosen, I. (1968). The basis of psychotherapeutic treatment of sexual deviation. *Proc. roy. Soc. Med.* 61, 793–796.

Rosen, J. N. (1953). *Direct Analysis.* New York: Grune & Stratton.

Rosenbaum, M. & Maltby, G. L. (1943). Relation of cerebral dysrhythmia to eclampsia. *Amer. J. Obstet. Gynec.* 45, 992.

Rosenblatt, G., Hartmann, E., & Zwilling, G. R. (1973). Cardiac irritability during sleep and dreaming. *J. Psychosom. Res.* 17, 129–134.

Rosenzweig, S., Fleming, E. E. & Clark, H. J. (1947). Revised scoring manual for the Rosenzweig picture-frustration study. *J. Psychol.* 24, 165.

Ross, T. A. (1936). *An Enquiry into Prognosis in the Neuroses.* Cambridge.

Ross, T. A. (1937). *The Common Neuroses: Their Treatment by Psychotherapy*, 2nd Ed. London: Arnold.

Ross, W. D., Browning, J. S. & Kaplan, S. M. (1961). *Emotional Aspects in the Medical Management of Rheumatoid Arthritis.* Basle: Geigy.

Roth, M. (1959). The phobic anxiety-depersonalization syndrome. *Proc. roy. Soc. Med.* 52, 587.

Roth, M. (1960). Problems of an ageing population. *Brit. med. J.* 1, 1226.

Roth, S. (1970). The seemingly ubiquitous depression following acute schizophrenic episodes: a neglected area of clinical discussion. *Amer. J. Psychiat.* **127**, 51–58.

Rothschild, D. (1941). The clinical differentiation of senile and arteriosclerotic psychoses. *Amer. J. Psychiat.* **98**, 324.

Rothschild, D. (1956). Senile psychoses and psychoses with cerebral arteriosclerosis. In *Mental Disorders in Later Life,* 2nd Ed., ed. Kaplan, O. J. California: Stanford University Press.

Rowbotham, G. F., MacIver, I. N., Dickson, J. & Bousfield, M. E. (1954). Analysis of 1400 cases of acute injury to the head. *Brit. med. J.* **1**, 726.

Rubenstein, J. H. & Taybi, H. (1963). Broad thumbs and toes and facial abnormalities: a possible mental retardation syndrome. *Amer. J. Dis. Child.* **105**, 588.

Rubin, B. (1972). Prediction of dangerousness in mentally ill criminals. *Arch. gen. Psychiat.* **27**, 397–407.

Rüdin, E. (1916). *Studien über Verberung und Entstehung geistiger Störungen. Vol.* 1. *Zur Verberung und Neuentstehung der Dementia Praecox.* Berlin: Springer.

Ruesch, J. (1951). Part and whole, the sociopsychological and psychosomatic approach to disease. *Dialectica,* **5**, 99.

Ruesch, J. (1966). Hospitalization and social disability. *J. nerv. ment. Dis.* **142**, 203.

Ruesch, J., Harris, R. E. & Bowman, K. M. (1943). Pre- and post-traumatic personality in head injuries. In *Trauma of the Central Nervous System.* Baltimore: Williams & Wilkins.

Rundle, A., Coppen, A. & Cowie, V. (1961). Steroid excretion in mothers of mongols. *Lancet,* ii, 846.

Russek, H. I. & Zohman, B. L. (1958). Relative significance of heredity, diet and occupational stress in coronary heart disease of young adults; based on an analysis of 100 patients between the ages of 25 and 40 years and a similar group of 100 normal control subjects. *Amer. J. med. Sci.* **235**, 266.

Russell, D. H., & Bender, E. H. (1970). Legal implications of the XYY syndrome. *Seminars Psychiat.* **2**, 40–42.

Russell, R. J., Page, L. G. M. & Jillett, R. L. (1953). Intensified electro-convulsant therapy: review of five years' experience. *Lancet,* ii, 1177.

Russell, W. R. & Esper, M. L. E. (1961). *Traumatic Aphasia, a Study of Aphasia in War Wounds of the Brain.* Oxford University Press.

Rutter, M. (Ed.) (1970). *Study Group on Infantile Autism,* arranged by the Institute for Research into Mental Retardation. London: Churchill.

Rutter, M. (1972). Maternal deprivation reconsidered. *J. Psychosom. Res.* **16**, 241–250.

Rylander, G. (1939). Personality changes after operations on the frontal lobes. *Acta psychiat. Kbh.* Suppl. **20**.

Rylander, G. (1972). Psychoses and the punding and choreiform syndromes in addiction to central stimulant drugs. *Psychiat. Neurol. Neurochir.* **75**, 203–212.

Ryle, A. & Lunghi, M. (1971). A therapist's prediction of a patient's Dyad Grid. *Brit. J. Psychiat.* **118**, 556–560.

Sachs, B. (1887). On arrested cerebral development, with special reference to its cortical pathology. *J. nerv. ment. Dis.* **14**, 541.

Sainsbury, P. (1955). *Suicide in London; an Ecological Study.* Maudsley Monograph, 1. London: Chapman & Hall.

Sainsbury, P. (1968). Suicide and Depression. A. Coppen and A. Walk. Eds. *Recent developments in affective disorders: a symposium.* Beir. J. Psychiat., Special Publication, No. 2. Hedley Bros., Ashford, Kent.

Sainsbury, P. (1973). Suicide: opinions and facts. *Proc. roy. Soc. Med.* **66**, 579–587.

Sainsbury, P. & Collins, J. (1966). Some factors relating to mental illness in a New Town. *J. Psychosom. Res.* **10**, 45.

Salzer, H. M. & Lurie, M. L. (1953). Anxiety and depressive states treated with isonicotinyl hydrazide (isoniazid). *Arch. Neurol. Psychiat.* **70**, 317.

Sandison, R. A. (1954). Psychological aspects of LSD treatment of the neuroses. *J. ment. Sci.* **100**, 508.

Sandison, R. A., Spencer, A. M. & Whitelaw, J. D. A. (1954). The therapeutic value of lysergic acid diethylamide in mental illness. *J. ment. Sci.* **100**, 491.

Sandler, B. (1968). Emotional stress and infertility. *J. Psychosom. Res.* **12**, 51–59.

Sargant, W. (1951). Leucotomy in psychosomatic disorders. *Lancet,* ii, 87.

Sargant, W. & Craske, N. (1941). Modified insulin therapy in war neuroses. *Lancet,* ii, 212.

Sargant, W. & Dally, P. (1962). Treatment of anxiety states by anti-depressant drugs. *Brit. med. J.* **1**, 6.

Sargant, W. & Slater, E. (1954). *An Introduction to Physical Methods of Treatment in Psychiatry*. Edinburgh: Livingstone.
Sarwer-Foner, G. J. (1972). Denial of death and the unconscious longing for indestructibility and immortality in the terminal phase of adolescence. *Canad. Psychiat. Ass. J.* 17, Suppl. 2, 551–557.
Sarwer-Foner, G. J. (1972). On human territoriality: a contribution to instinct theory. *Canad. Psychiat. Ass. J.* 17, Suppl. 2, SS-169–SS-183.
Saul, L. J. (1946). Relations to mother as seen in cases of allergy. *Nerv. Child.* 5, 332.
Schachter, S. (1970). Identity and peripheralist-centralist controversies. In *Feelings and Emotions,* ed. Arnold, M. B. New York: Academic Press.
Schachter, S., Goldman, R., & Gordon, A. (1968). Effects of fear, food deprivation and obesity on eating. *J. Personal & Soc. Psychol.* 10, 91–97.
Schaudin, F. R. (1905). Zur Kenntnis den Spirochaete pallida. *Dtsch. med. Wschr.* 31, 1065.
Schaffer, H. R. (1958). Objective observations of personality development in early infancy. *Brit. J. med. Psychol.* 31, 174.
Schayer, R. W., Wu, K. Y. T., Smiley, R. L. & Kobayashi, Y. (1954). Studies on monoamine oxidase in intact animals. *J. biol. Chem.* 210, 259.
Schilder, P. (1935). *The Image and Appearance of the Human Body. Studies in the Constructive Energies of the Psyche.* London: Kegan Paul.
Schildkraut, J. J. & Kety, S. S. (1967). Biogenic amines and emotion: pharmacological studies suggest a relationship between brain biogenic amines and affective state. *Science,* 156, 21–30.
Schmale, A. M. & Iker, H. P. (1966). The affect of hopelessness and the development of cancer. *Psychosomatic Medicine,* 28, 714.
Schmidt, W., Smart, R. G. & Popham, R. E. (1962). The role of alcoholism in motor vehicle accidents. In *Alcohol & Road Traffic.* Proceedings of Third International Conference. pp. 90–98. London: Brit. Med. Assoc.
Schneider, G. (1957). Les psychoses puerpérales. *Schweitz. med. Wschr.* 87, 1145.
Schneider, J. A., Plummer, A. J., Earl, A. E. & Gaunt, R. (1955). Neuropharmacological aspects of reserpine. *Ann. N.Y. Acad. Sci.* 61, 17.
Schneider, K. (1925). Wesen und Erfassung des Schizophrenen. *Z.ges. Neurol. Psychiat.* 99, 542–547.
Schneider, K. (1934). *Die psychopathischen Persönlichkeiten,* ed. 3. Leipzig: Deuticke.
Schofield, M. (1965). *The Sexual Behaviour of Young People.* London: Longmans.
Schottstaedt, W. W., Grace, W. J. & Wolff, H. G. (1956). Life situations, behaviour, attitudes, emotions and renal excretion of fluid and electrolytes. I, II, III, IV, *J. psychosom. Res.* 1, 75, 147, 203, 287.
Schou, M., Amdisen, A. & Baastrup, P. C. (1971). The practical management of lithium treatment. *Brit. J. Hosp. Med.* 6, 53–60.
Schou, M., Amdisen, A., Eskjaer Jensen, S. & Olsen, T. (1968). Occurrence of Goitre during Lithium Treatment. *Brit. med. J.* 6, 710–713.
Schou, M., Amdisen, A., & Steenstrup, O. R. (1973b). Lithium and Pregnancy. II. Hazards to Women given Lithium during pregnancy and delivery. *Brit. med. J.,* 2, 137–138.
Schou, M., Goldfield, M.D., Weinstein, M. R. & Villeneuve, A. (1973a). Lithium and Pregnancy, I. Report from the Register of Lithium Babies. *Brit. med. J.* 2, 135–136.
Schou, M., Juel-Nielsen, N., Strőngren, E., & Voldby, H. (1954). The treatment of manic psychoses by the administration of lithium salts. *J. Neurol. Neurosurg. Psychiat.* 17, 250–260.
Schreber, D. P. (1903). *Denkwürdigkeiten eines Nervenkranken.* Oswald Mutze, Leipzig. Trans. Macalpine, I. & Hunter, R. A. (1955). London: Dawson.
Schuckit, M., Robins, E., & Feighner, J. (1971). Tricyclic antidepressants and monoamine oxidase inhibitors: combination therapy in the treatment of depression. *Arch. gen. Psychiat.* 24, 509–514.
Schuckit, M. A. & Winokur, G. (1972). A short term follow-up of women alcoholics. *Dis. Nerv. Syst.* 33, 672–678.
Schüller, A. (1907). Infantilism. Über Infantilismus. *Wien. med. Wschr.* 57, 625.
Schulman, J. L. & Stern, S. (1959). Parents' estimate of the intelligence of retarded children. *Amer. J. ment. Defic.* 63, 696.
Schultz, L. G. (1968). The victim-offender relationship. *Crime Delinq.* 14, 135–141.
Schvarcz, J. R., Driollet, R., Rios, E., & Betti, O. (1972). Stereotactic hypothalamotomy for behaviour disorders. *J. Neurol. Neurosurg. Psychiat.* 35, 356–359.
Schwartz, M. S. & Scott, D. F. (1971). Isolated petit-mal status presenting *de novo* in middle age. *Lancet,* ii, 1399–1401.
Scott, J. (1778). An account of a remarkable imperfection of sight. *Phil. Trans.* 68, 611.

Scott, J. A. (1958). Problem families: a London survey. *Lancet,* i, 204.
Scott, M. (1970). Transitory psychotic behaviour following operation for tumors of the cerebello-pontine angle. *Psychiat. Neurol. Neurochir.* 73, 37–48.
Scott, P. D. (1960). The treatment of psychopaths. *Brit. med. J.* 1, 1641.
Scott, P. D. (1965). The Ganser syndrome. *Brit. J. Criminol.* 5, 127.
Scott, P. D. (1966). Medical aspects of delinquency. *Hosp. Med.* 1, 219, 259.
Scott, P. D. (1970). Punishment or treatment: prison or hospital. *Brit. med. J.* 2, 167–169.
Scoville, W. B. (1949). Selective critical undercutting as a means of modifying and studying frontal lobe function in man; preliminary report of 43 operative cases. *J. Neurosurg.* **6**, 65.
Scoville, W. B. & Milner, B. (1957). Loss of recent memory after bilateral hippocampal lesions. *J. Neurol. Neurosurg. . Psychiat.* **20**, 11.
Scully, C. (1973). Down's syndrome. *Brit. J. Hosp. Med.,* **10**, 89–98.
Seager, C. P. & Foster, A. R. (1958). Addiction to unrestricted drugs. *Brit. med. J.* **2**, 950.
Sedal, L., Korman, M. G., Williams, P. O., & Mushin, G. (1972). Overdosage of tricyclic antidepressants: a report of two deaths and a prospective study of 24 patients. *Med. J. Austral.* **2**, 74–79.
Sedvall, G., Jönsson, B., & Petterson, U., (1969). Evidence of an altered thyroid function in man during treatment with lithium carbonate. *Acta Psychiat. Scand. Suppl.* **207**, 59–67.
Seglow, J., Kellmer-Pringle, M., & Wedge, P. (1972). *Growing up Adopted.* National Foundation of Educational Research in England & Wales.
Seguin, É. (1866). *Idiocy, and its Treatment by the Physiological Methods* Teachers Coll. Columbia Univ. Bin. Publ. 1907. New York: Wood.
Segundo, J. P., Naquet, R. & Buser, P. (1955). Effects of cortical stimulation on electro-cortical activity in monkeys. *J. Neurophysiol.* **18**, 236.
Seitz, P. F. D. (1954). Psychological aspects of skin diseases. In *Recent Developments in Psychosomatic Medicine,* eds. Wittkower, E. D. & Cleghorn, R. A. p. 245. London: Pitman.
Seligman, R., Macmillan, B. G., & Carroll, S. S. (1971). The burned child: a neglected area of psychiatry. *Amer. J. Psychiat.* **128** 52–57.
Selye, H. (1950*a*). Stress and the general adaption syndrome. *Brit. med. J.* **1**, 1383.
Selye, H. (1950*b*). *The Physiology and Pathology of Exposure to Stress.* Montreal: Acta Inc.
Selye, H. (1956). *The Stress of Life.* New York: McGraw-Hill.
Seman, J. H. (1956). Premature ejaculation: a new approach. *J. Urology,* **49**, 533–537.
Semrad, E. V. & Arsenian, J. (1951). The use of group processes in teaching group dynamics. *Amer. J. Psychiat.* **108** 358.
Serry, M. (1969). Lithium retention and response. *Lancet,* i, 1267–1268.
Shagass, C. (1954). The sedation threshold: a method for estimating tension in psychiatric patients. *EEG & Clin. Neurophysiol.* **6**, 222.
Shapiro, A. K., Wilensky, H., & Struening, E. L. (1968). Study of the placebo effect with a placebo test. *Compr. Psychiat.* **9**, 118–137.
Sharpey-Schafer, E. P., Hayter, C. J. & Barlow, E. D. (1958). Mechanism of acute hypotension from fear or nausea. *Brit. med. J.* **2**, 878.
Shattock, F. M. (1950). The somatic manifestations of schizophrenia: a clinical study of their significance. *J. ment. Sci.* **96**, 32.
Shaw, C. H. & Wright, C. H. (1960). The married mental defective: a follow-up study. *Lancet,* i, 273.
Shaw, D. M. (1966). Mineral metabolism, mania and melancholia. *Brit. med. J.* **2**, 262.
Sheehan, H. L. & Summers, V. K. (1949). The syndrome of hypopituitarism. *Quart. J. Med.* **18**, 319.
Sheldon, J. H. (1960). Problems of an ageing population. *Brit. med. J.* **1**, 1224.
Sheldon, W. H. (1949). *Varieties of Delinquent Youth: an Introduction to Constitutional Psychiatry.* New York: Harper.
Sheldon, W. H., Stevens, S. S. & Tucker, W. B. (1940). *The Varieties of Human Physique: an Introduction to Constitutional Psychology.* New York: Harper.
Shepherd, M. (1957). *Studies of Major Psychoses in an English County.* London: Chapman & Hall.
Sheridan, M. D. (1956). The intelligence of 100 neglectful mothers. *Brit. med. J.* **1**, 91.
Sherlock, E. B. (1911). *The Feebleminded: a Guide to Study and Practice.* London: Macmillan.
Sherwood, S. L. (1952). Intraventricular medication in catatonic stupor. *Brain,* **75**, 68.
Shneidman, E. S. & Farberow, N. L. (ed.) (1957). *Clues to Suicide.* New York: McGraw-Hill.

Shochet, B. R., Lisansky, E., Schubart, A. E., Fiocco, V., Kurland, S., & Pope, M. (1969). A medical-psychiatric study of patients with rheumatoid arthritis. *Psychosomatics,* **10,** 271–279.

Shopsin, B., & Gershon, S., (1971). Plasma cortisol response to dexamethasone suppression in depressed and control patients. *Arch. gen. Psychiat.* **24,** 320–326.

Shorvon, H. J. (1947). Prefrontal leucotomy and the depersonalization syndrome. *Lancet,* ii, 714.

Shorvon, H. J., Hill, D. N., Burkitt, E. & Halstead, H. (1946). The depersonalization syndrome. *Proc. roy. Soc. Med.* **39,** 779.

Shorvon, H. J. & Richardson, J. S. (1949). Sudden obesity and psychological trauma. *Brit. med. J.* **2,** 951.

Shulman, R. (1967). Psychiatric aspects of pernicious anaemia: a prospective controlled investigation. *Brit. med. J.* **2,** 266.

Siegfried, S. (1951). Psychiatrische Untersuchungen über die Folgen der künstlichen schwangerschaftsunterbrechung. *Schweiz. Arch. Neurol. Psychiat,* **67,** 365.

Sieveking, E. H. (1857). Analysis of fifty-two cases of epilepsy observed by the author. *Lancet,* i, 528.

Sifneos, P. E. (1968). "The motivational process": a selection and prognostic criterion for psychotherapy of short duration. *Psychiat. Quart.* **42,** 271–279.

Silverman, D. (1943). Psychoses in prisoners: study of 500 psychotic prisoners. *J. crim. Psychopath.* **4,** 703.

Silverman, M. (1961). A comprehensive department of psychological medicine. *Brit. med. J.* **2,** 698.

Sim, M. (1945). The N.C.O. as a psychiatric casualty: a study of 627 cases admitted to a psychiatric hospital. *J. R. Army med. Cps.* **85,** 184.

Sim, M. (1946*a*). A comparative study of disease incidence in admissions to a base psychiatric hospital in the Middle East. *J. ment. Sci.* **92,** 118.

Sim, M. (1946*b*). Quantitative estimation in psychiatric diagnosis. *J. R. Army med. Cps.* **87,** 281.

Sim, M. (1947). Electronarcosis. *Lancet,* ii, 294.

Sim, M. (1956). Hannah, Mother of Samuel: a psychopathological contribution to Old Testament Criticism. *Bgham. med. Rev.* **19,** 121.

Sim, M. (1963*a*). Abortion and the psychiatrist. *Brit. med. J.* **2,** 1061.

Sim, M. (1963*b*). *Guide to Psychiatry* Edinburgh: Livingstone.

Sim, M. (1970). Childhood autism. *Brit. med. J.* **1,** 300.

Sim, M. (1972). Psychiatric aspects of abortion. *Prevent,* **3,** 25–28.

Sim, M. (1972). Imipramine and pregnancy. *Brit. med. J.* **2,** 45.

Sim, M., & Bale, R. N. (1973). Familial pre-senile dementia: the relevance of a histological diagnosis of Pick's disease. *Brit. J. Psychiat.* **122,** 671–673.

Sim, M. & Brooke, B. N. (1958). Ulcerative colitis; a test of psychosomatic hypotheses. *Lancet,* ii, 125.

Sim, M., Emens, J. M., & Jordan, J. A. (1973). Psychiatric aspects of female sterilization. *Brit. med. J.* **3,** 220–222.

Sim, M. & Houghton, H. (1966). Phobic anxiety and its treatment. *J. nerv. ment. Dis.* **143** 484.

Sim, M. & Smith, W. T. (1955). Alzheimer's disease confirmed by cerebral biopsy: a therapeutic trial with cortisone and ACTH. *J. ment. Sci.* **101,** 604.

Sim, M. & Sussman, I. (1962). Alzheimer's disease: its natural history and differential diagnosis. *J. nerv. ment. Dis.* **135,** 489.

Sim, M. & Tibbetts, R. W. (1958). Anorexia nervosa. *Brit. med. J.* **2,** 447.

Sim, M., Turner, E. & Smith, W. T. (1966). Cerebral biopsy in the investigation of pre-senile dementia. 1. clinical aspects. *Brit. J. Psychiat.* **112,** 119.

Simon, J. L. & Taube, H. (1946). A preliminary study on the use of methedrine in psychiatric diagnosis. *J. nerv. ment. Dis.* **104,** 593.

Simpson, S. L. (1957). Hormones and behaviour patterns. *Brit. med. J.* **2,** 839.

Sinclair, R. J. C., Kitchin, A. H. & Turner, R. W. D. (1960). The Marfan syndrome. *Quart. J. Med.* **29,** 19.

Sinclair-Gieben, A. H. C. (1960). Treatment of status asthmaticus by hypnosis. *Brit. med. J.* **2,** 1651.

Singer, K. (1962). Huntington's chorea in the Chinese. *Brit. med. J.* **1,** 1311.

Singer, K. & Cheng, M. N. (1971). Thiopropazate hydrochloride in persistent dyskinesia. *Brit. med. J.* **4,** 22–25.

Siomopoulos, V. (1971). Hysterical psychosis: psychopathological aspects. *Brit. J. med. Psychol.* **44,** 95–100.

Sjögren, T. (1950). Hereditary congenital spino-cerebellar ataxia accompanied by congenital cataract and oligophrenia; genetic and clinical investigation. *Confin. neurol.* **10**, 293.
Sjögren, T., Sjögren, H. & Lindgren, A. G. H. (1952). Morbus Alzheimer and morbus Pick: genetic, clinical and patho-anatomical study. *Acta psychiat. scand.* **Suppl. 82.**
Skinner, A. E. & Castle, R. L. (1969). *78 Battered Children.* London: National Society for Prevention of Cruelty to Children.
Skinner, B. F. (1938). *The Behavior of Organisms.* New York: Appleton-Century-Crofts.
Skinner, B. F., Solomon, H. C. & Lindsley, O. R. (1954). A new method for the experimental analysis of the behavior of psychotic patients. *J. nerv. ment. Dis.* **120,** 403.
Skottowe, I. (1942). Mental disorders in pregnancy and the puerperium. *Practitioner,* **148,** 157.
Slaney, G. & Brooke, B. N. (1959). Cancer in ulcerative colitis. *Lancet,* ii, 694.
Slater, E. (1943). The neurotic constitution: a statistical study of two thousand neurotic soldiers. *J. Neurol. Psychiat.* **6,** 1.
Slater, E. T. O. (1944). Genetics in psychiatry. *J. ment Sci.* **90,** 17.
Slater, E. (1953). Psychotic and neurotic illnesses in twins. *Spec. Rep. Ser. med. Res. Coun. Lond.* No. 278.
Slater, E. (1954). The McNaghten Rules and modern concepts of responsibility. *Brit. med. J.* 2, 713.
Slater, E. & Beard, A. W. (1963). The schizophrenia-like pyschoses of epilepsy. 1. psychiatric aspects. *Brit. J. Psychiat.* **109,** 95.
Slater, E., Beard, A. W. & Gilthero, E. (1963). The schizophrenia-like psychoses of epilepsy. *Brit. J. Psychiat.* **109,** 95.
Slater, E., & Roth, M. (1969) *Clinical Psychiatry,* pp. 322–323. London: Ballière, Tindall & Cassell.
Slater, P. (1969). Theory and Technique of the repertory grid: being a review of *The Evaluation of Personal Constructs* by D. Bannister and J. M. M. Mair. *Brit. J. Psychiat.* **115**, 1287–1296.
Slavson, S. R. (1950). *Analytic Group Psychotherapy with Children, Adolescents and Adults.* New Y ork: Columbia University Press.
Smith, A. D. M. (1960). Megaloblastic madness. *Brit. med. J.* 2, 1840.
Smith, M., Culpin, M. & Farmer, E. (1927). *A Study of Telegraphist's Cramp.* Industrial Fatigue Research Board. Report No. 43. London: H.M.S.O.
Smith, R. P., Wagman, A. I., Wagman, A. I., Pfeiffer, C. C. & Riopelle, A. J. (1957). Effects of some tranquillizing and depressant drugs on conditioned avoidance behaviour in monkeys. *J. Pharmacol.* **119,** 317.
Smith, S. (1961). Psychiatry in general hospitals: Manchester's integrated scheme. *Lancet,* i, 1158.
Smythies, J. R. (1958). Biochemical concepts of schizophrenia. *Lancet,* ii, 308.
Smythies, J. R. (1960). Recent advances in the biochemistry of psychoses. *Lancet,* i, 1287.
Snider, J. G., & Osgood, C. E. (1969). (eds.) *Semantic Differential Technique.* Chicago: Aldine.
Snyder, W. *et al.* (1947). *Casebook of Non-directive Counselling.* Boston: Houghton.
Soddy, K. (1947). Psychological aspects of accidents and accident prevention. *Brit. med. J.* 2, 623.
Soddy, K. (1954). Homosexuality. *Lancet,* ii, 541.
Solomons, B. (1931). Insanity and its relation to the parturient state. *J. ment Sci.* **77**, 701.
Sours, J. A. (1962). Akinetic mutism simulating catonic schizophrenia. *Amer. J. Psychiat.* **119**, 451.
Sourkes, T. L. (1965). The action of *a*-methyldopa in the brain. *Brit. med. Bull.* **21**, 66.
Sparrow, J. (1969). Without the death penalty: deterring criminals kindly. *The Times* (London), 31st December.
Sparrow, J. H. A. (1966). *Controversial Essays.* London: Faber.
Spearman, C. E. (1927). *The Abilities of Man.* London: Macmillan.
Speller, S. R. (1961). *The Mental Health Act, 1959.* The Institute of Hospital Administrators, 75 Portland Place, London W.1.
Sperling, M. (1946). Psychoanalytic study of ulcerative colitis in children. *Psychoanal. Quart.* **15**, 302.
Spicer, C. C., Stewart, D. N. & Winser, D. M. de R. (1944). Perforated peptic ulcer during the period of heavy air raids. *Lancet,* i, 14.
Spiegel, J. P. & Bell, N. W. (1959). The family of the psychiatric patient. In *American Handbook of Psychiatry,* ed. Arieti, S. New York: Basic Books.
Spillane, J. D. (1962). Five boxers. *Brit. med. j.* 2, 1206.

Spitz, R. A. (1946). Hospitalism, a follow-up report on investigation described in Vol. 1, 1945. *Psychoanal. Stud. Child.* 2, 113.
Stabenau, J. R., Creveling, C. R., & Daly, J. (1970). The 'pink spot', 3, 4–Dimethoxyphenylethylamine, common tea, and schizophrenia. *Amer. J. Psychiat.* 127, 611–616.
Stafford-Clark, D. & Taylor, F. H. (1949). Clinical and electro-encephalo-graphic studies of prisoners charged with murder. *J. Neurol. Neurosurg. Psychiat.* 12, 325.
Stallard, F. (1966). The therapeutic community. *Proc. roy. Soc. Med.* 59, 700.
Standing Medical Advisory Committee (1972). Medical memorandum on drug dependence. London: D.H.S.S.
Stanley-Jones, D. (1947). Sexual inversion: an ethical study. *Lancet,* i, 366.
Steel, R. (1960). G.P.I. in an observation ward. *Lancet,* i, 121.
Steinach, R. (1913). Feminierung von Männchen und Maskulierung von Weibchen. *Zbl. Physiol.* 27, 717.
Steinhilber, R. M., Pearson, J. S. & Rushton, J. G. (1960). Some psychologic considerations of histamine cephalgia. *Proc. Mayo Clin.* 35, 691.
Stengel, E. (1941). An aetiology of fugue states. *J. ment. Sci.* 87, 572.
Stengel, E. (1948). A study of the symptomatology and differential diagnosis of Alzheimer's disease and Pick's disease. *J. ment. Sci.* 89, 1.
Stengel, E. (1952). Enquiries into attempted suicide. *Proc. roy. Soc. Med.* 45, 613.
Stengel, E. (1961). Behaviour therapy and abnormal psychology. *Brit. med. J.* 2, 156.
Stengel, E. (1964). *Suicide and Attempted Suicide.* Harmondsworth: Penguin Books.
Stengel, E. & Cook, N. G. (1958). *Attempted Suicide.* Maudsley Monographs, No. 4. London: Chapman & Hall.
Stern, E. S. (1957). Operation sesame. *Lancet,* i, 577.
Stern, K. & Reed, G. E. (1945). Presenile dementia (Alzheimer's disease): its pathogenesis and classification with two case reports. *Amer. J. Psychiat.* 102 191.
Stevens, B. (1969). Impact of community-orientated psychiatry on marriage and fertility of psychotic women. *Brit-Med. J.* 4, 22-24.
Stevenson, G. H. & McCausland, A. (1953). Prefrontal leucotomy for the attempted prevention of recurring manic-depressive illness. *Amer. J. Psychiat.* 109, 662.
Stevenson, R. L. (1886). *The Strange Case of Dr. Jekyll and Mr. Hyde.* 1950. London: Macdonald.
Stokes, J. W., Mendels, J., Secunda, S. K. & Dyson, W. L. (1972). Lithium excretion and therapeutic response. *J. nerv. ment. Dis.* 154, 43–48.
Stoll, W. A. (1947). Lysergsäure-diathylamid, ein Phantastikum aus der Mutterkorngruppe. *Schweiz Arch. Neurol, Psychiat.* 60, 279.
Stoller, A. & Collmann, R. D. (1965). Incidence of infective hepatitis followed by Down's syndrome nine months later. *Lancet,* ii, 1221.
Stott, D. H. (1957). Physical and mental handicaps following a disturbed pregnancy. *Lancet,* i, 1006.
Strachan, R. W. & Henderson, J. G. (1965). Psychiatric syndromes due to avitaminosis B_{12} with normal blood and marrow. *Quart. J. Med.* 34, 303.
Strauss, A. A. & Kephart, N. C. (1955). *Psychopathology and Education of the Brain-injured Child. Vol. II. Progress in Theory and Clinic.* New York: Grune & Stratton.
Strauss, A. A. & Lehtinen, L. E. (1947). *Psychopathology and Education of the Brain-injured Child. Vol. I.* New York: Grune & Stratton.
Strecker, E. A. (1946). *Their Mothers' Sons. The Psychiatrist Examines an American Problem.* Philadelphia: Lippincott.
Strecker, E. A. & Ebaugh, F. G. (1940). *Practical Clinical Psychiatry,* 5th edition. Philadelphia: Blakiston.
Strich, S. J. (1956). Diffuse degeneration of the cerebral white matter in severe dementia following head injury. *J. Neurol. Neurosurg. Psychiat.* 19 163.
Strich, S. J. (1961). Shearing of nerve fibres as a cause of brain damage due to head injury: a pathological study of twenty cases. *Lancet,* ii, 443.
Strom-Olsen, R. (1950). Enuresis in adults and abnormality of sleep. *Lancet,* ii, 133.
Struve, F. A., Becka, D., & Klein, D. F. (1972). The B-Mitten E.E.G. pattern in process and reactive schizophrenia and affective states. *Clin. Electroenceph.* 3, 136–144.
Stunkard, A. (1972). New therapies for the eating disorders: behavior modification of obesity and anorexia nervosa. *Arch. gen. Psychiat.* 26, 391–398.
Stunkard, A. J., & Fox, S. (1971). The relationship of gastric motility and hunger: a summary of the evidence. *Psychosom. Med.,* 33, 123–134.
Stunkard, A. J., Grace, W. J. & Wolff, H. G. (1955). The night eating syndrome: a pattern of food intake among certain obese patients. *Amer. J. Med.* 19, 78.

Stürup, G. K. (1948). The management and treatment of psychopaths in a special institution in Denmark. *Proc. roy. Soc. Med.* **41**, 765.
Stürup, G. K. (1952). The treatment of criminal psychopaths in Herstedvester. *Brit. J. med. Psychol.* **25**, 31.
Stürup, G. K. (1964). The treatment of chronic criminals. *Bull. Menninger Clin.* **28**, 229.
Stürup, G. K. (1972). Treating 'untreatable' criminals. *Federal Probation,* **36**, 22–25.
Sullivan, A. J. (1936). Psychogenic factors in ulcerative colitis. *Amer. J. digest. Dis.* **2**, 651.
Sullivan, H. S. (1948). *Conceptions of Modern Psychiatry.* New York: Norton.
Sullivan, H. S. (1954). *The Psychiatric Interview.* New York: Norton.
Surridge, D. (1969). An investigation into some psychiatric aspects of multiple sclerosis. *Brit. J. Psychiat.* **115**, 749–764.
Surman, O. S., Gottlieb, S. K., Hackett, T. P., & Silverberg, E. L. (1973). Hypnosis in the treatment of warts. *Arch. gen. Psychiat.* **28**, 439–441.
Suttie, I. D. (1935). *The Origins of Love and Hate.* London: Kegan Paul.
Swan, C., Tostevin, A. L., Mayo, H. & Black, G. H. B. (1943). Congenital defects in infants following infectious diseases during pregnancy. *Med. J. Aust.* **2**, 201.
Swan, C., Tostevin, A. L., Mayo, H. & Black, G. H. B. (1944). Further observations on congenital defects in infants following infectious diseases during pregnancy, with especial reference to rubella. *Med. J. Aust.* **1**, 409.
Swanson, D. W. (1968). Adult sexual abuse of children (the man and circumstances). *Dis. Nerv. Syst.* **29**, 677–683.
Swanson, D. W., & Dinello, F. A. (1970). Follow-up of patients starved for obesity. *Psychosom. Med.* **32**, 209–214.
Sweeny, J. S. (1934). Menstrual edema. *Amer. J. med. Ass.* **103**, 234.
Symonds, C. (1960). Disease of mind and disorder of brain. *Brit. med. J.* **2**, 1.
Symonds, C. (1962). Concussion and its sequelae. *Lancet,* i, 1.
Szasz, T. S. (1949). Factors in the psychogenesis of peptic ulcer. *Psychosom. Med.* **11**, 300.
Szasz, T. S. (1951). Physiologic and psychodynamic mechanisms in constipation and diarrhoea. *Psychosom. Med.* **13**, 112.
Szasz, T. S. (1957). Psychiatric expert testimony: its covert meaning and social function. *Psychiatry,* **20**, 313.
Szasz, T. S. (1961). *The Myth of Mental Illness; foundations of a theory of personal conduct.* London: Secker & Warburg (1962).

Talbott, J. A., & Teague, J. W. (1969). Marihuana psychosis: acute toxic psychosis associated with the use of cannabis derivatives. *J. Amer. med. Ass.* **210**, 289–302.
Talland, G. A., Sweet, W. H., & Ballantine, H. T. (1967). Amnesic syndrome with anterior communicating artery aneurysm. *J. nerv. ment. Dis.* **145**, 179–192.
Tamerin, J. S., & Neumann, C. P. (1971). Prognostic factors in the evaluation of addicted individuals. *Int. Pharmacopsychiat.* **6**, 69–76.
Tanay, E. (1971). Psychiatric aspects of homicide prevention. *Amer. J. Psychiat.* **128**, 815–818.
Tappan, P. W. (1949). *Juvenile Delinquency.* New York: McGraw-Hill.
Tay, W. (1881). Symmetrical changes in the region of the yellow spot in each eye of an infant. *Trans. Ophthal. Soc. U.K.* **1**, 55.
Taylor, H. C. (1958). In *Abortion in the United States,* p. 164. ed. Calderone, M. S. New York: Hoeber-Harper.
Teicher, J. D. & Jacobs, J. (1966). Adolescents who attempt suicide—preliminary findings. *Amer. J. Psychiat.* **122**, 1248.
Temkin, O. (1945). *The Falling Sickness: a History of Epilepsy from the Greeks to the Beginnings of Modern Neurology.* Baltimore: Johns Hopkins.
Terman, L. M. (1916). *The Measurement of Intelligence.* Boston: Houghton Mifflin.
Terzian, H. & Dalle Ore, G. (1955). Syndrome of Klüver and Bucy reproduced in man by bilateral removal of the temporal lobes. *Neurology,* **5**, 373.
Tetlow, C. (1955). Psychoses of childbearing. *J. ment. Sci.* **101**, 629.
Theorell, T., & Rahe, R. H. (1971). Psychosocial factors and myocardial infarction—I. an in-patient study in Sweden. *J. Psychosom. Res.* **15**, 25–31.
Thigpen, C. H. & Cleckley, H. M. (1957). *The Three Faces of Eve.* New York: McGraw-Hill.
Thompson, G. N. (ed.) (1956). *Alcoholism.* Springfield, Ill.: Thomas.
Thomson, I. G., & Rathod, N. H. (1968). Aversion therapy for heroin dependence. *Lancet,* ii, 382–384.
Thurstone, L. L. (1935). *Vectors of Mind: Multiple-factor Analysis for the Isolation of Primary Traits.* Chicago: University of Chicago Press.
Tibbetts, R. W. (1949). Leucotomy and hypertension. *Brit. med. J.* **2**, 1452.

Tibbetts, R. W. & Hawkings, J. R. (1956). The placebo response. *J. ment. Sci.* **102**, 60.
Tienari, P. (1963). Psychiatric illnesses in identical twins *Acta psychiat. Scand. Suppl.* **171**, Vol. 39. Copenhagen: Munksgaard.
Tinbergen, N. (1951). *Study of Instinct.* London: Oxford University Press.
Titchener, J. L. & Golden, M. (1963). Prediction of therapeutic themes from observations of family interaction evoked by 'revealed differences' technic. *J. nerv. ment. Dis.* **136**, 464.
Tizard, J. & Grad, J. C. (1961). *The Mentally Handicapped and Their Families: A Social Survey.* Maudsley Monograph no. 7. London: Oxford University Press.
Tizard, J. P. M., Stapleton, T., Cox, P. J. N. & Davis, J. A. (1959). The role of the paediatrician in mental illness. *Lancet,* ii, 193.
Todd, J., Collins, A. D., Martin, F. R. R. & Dewhurst, K. E. (1962). Mental symptoms due to insulinomata: report on two cases. *Brit. med. J.* 2, 828.
Toolan, J. M. (1962). Suicide and suicidal attempts in children and adolescents. *Amer. J. Psychiat.* **118**, 719.
Tooth, G. C. & Brooke, E. M. (1961). Trends in the mental hospital population and their effect on future planning. *Lancet,* i, 710.
Tooth, G. C. & Newton, M. P. (1961). *Leucotomy in England & Wales, 1942–1954.* Rep. publ. Hlth. med. Subj. Lond. No. 104. H.M.S.O.
Tow. P.M. (1955). *Personality Changes Following Frontal Leucotomy.* London: Oxford University Press.
Tredgold, R. F. (1947). Manic states in the Far East. *Brit. med. J.* 2, 522.
Trethowan, W. H. & Cobb, S. (1952). Neuropsychiatric aspects of Cushing's syndrome. *Arch. Neurol. Psychiat.* **67**, 283.
Trousseau, A. (1873). *Clinique Médicale de l'Hôtel-Dieu de Paris.* 4th edn., p. 109. Paris: Ballière.
Tuke, D. H. (1882). *Chapters in the History of the Insane in the British Isles.* London: Kegan Paul.
Turek, I., Kurland, A. A., Hanlon, T. E., & Bohm, M. (1972). Tardive dyskinesia: its relation to neuroleptic and antiparkinson drugs. *Brit. J. Psychiat.* **121**, 605–612.
Turner, E. (1963). A new approach to unilateral and bilateral lobotomies for psychomotor epilepsy. *J. Neurol. Neurosurg. Psychiat.* **26**, 285.
Turner, E. A. (1954). Cerebral control of respiration. *Brain,* **77**, 448.
Turner, E. A. (1962). Personal communication.

Ulett, G. A., Akpinar, S., & Itil, T. M. (1972). Quantitative E.E.G. analysis during hypnosis. *Electroenceph. clin. Neurophysiol.,* 33, 361–368.

Valentine, G. H. (1969). *The Chromosome Disorders.* 2nd edn. London: Heinemann.
Van Wagenen, W. P., & Herren, R. Y. (1940). Surgical division of commissural pathways in corpus callosum: relation to spread of epileptic attack. *Arch. Neurol. Psychiat.* **44**, 740–759.
Venables, J. F. (1930). Anorexia nervosa. *Guy's Hosp. Rep.* **80**, 213.
Verplanck, W. S. (1955). The control of the content of conversation: reinforcement of statements of opinion. *J. Abnorm. Soc. Psychol.* **51**, 668–676.
Vickers, G. (1958). Congress on Stress and Mental Illness. *Lancet,* i, 205.
Vickers, G. (1965). *The Art of Judgment: a study of policy-making.* London: Chapman & Hall.
Victor, M., Adams, R. D. & Mancall, E. L. (1959). A restricted form of cerebellar cortical degeneration occurring in alcoholic patients. *Arch. Neurol.* **1**, 579.
Vining, C. W. (1952). Feeding disorders in children: their interpretation. *Lancet,* ii, 99.
Virchow, R. (1849). *Scientific Methods and Therapeutic Standpoints.* Quoted by R. M. Coe (1970). In *Sociology of Medicine.* New York: McGraw Hill.
Vogt, M. (1958). Pharmacology of tranquillizing drugs. *Brit. Med. J.* 2, 965.
von Bergmann, G. & Katsch, G. (1913). Über Darmbewegung und Darmform. Experimentelles und Klinisches. *Dtsch. med. Wschr.* **39**, 1294.
Von Domarus, E. (1944). The specific laws of logic in schizophrenia. In *Language and Thought in Schizophrenia,* p. 104, ed. Kasanin, J. S. Berkeley: University of California Press.

Wagner, von Jauregg, J. (1887). Über die Einwirkung fieberhafter Erkrankingen auf Psychosen. *Jb. Psychiat. Neurol.* 7, 94.
Walker, J. G., Emlyn-Williams, A., Craigie, A., Rosenoer, V. M., Agnew, J. & Sherlock, S. (1965). Treatment of chronic portal-systemic encephalopathy by surgical exclusion of the colon. *Lancet,* ii, 861.

Wall, P. D. & Davis, G. D. (1951). Three cerebral cortical systems affecting autonomic functions. *J. Neurophysiol.* **14**, 507.
Wallerstein, R. S. (1956). Comparative study of treatment methods for chronic alcoholism: the alcoholism research project at Winter VA hospital. *Amer. J. Psychiat.* **113**, 228.
Walshe, F. M. R. (1958*a*). The role of injury, of the law and of the doctor in the aetiology of the so-called traumatic neurosis. *Med. Press,* **239**, 493.
Walshe, F. M. R. (1958*b*). *Diseases of the Nervous System,* 9th Ed. Edinburgh: Livingstone.
Walshe, F. M. R. (1965). *Further Critical Studies in Neurology and other Essays and Addresses,* Edinburgh: Livingstone.
Walter, W. G. (1953). *The Living Brain.* London: Duckworth.
Walter, W. G., Dovey, V. J. & Shipton, H. (1946). Analysis of the electrical response of the human cortex to photic stimulation. *Nature, Lond.* **158**, 540.
Walton, J. N. Ellis, E. & Court, S. D. M. (1962). Clumsy children: developmental apraxia and agnosia. *Brain,* **85**, 603.
Waskowitz, C. H. (1959). The parents of retarded children speak for themselves. *J. Paediat.* **54**, 319.
Wassermann, A., Neisser, A. & Bruck, C. (1906). Eine serodiagnostische Reaktion bei Syphilis. *Dtsch. med. Wschr.* **32**, 745.
Watts, C. A. H. & Watts, B. M. (1952). *Psychiatry in General Practice.* London: Churchill.
Wayne, H. L., Shapiro, A. K., & Shapiro E. (1972). Gilles de la Tourette's syndrome: electroencephalographic investigation and clinical correlation. *Clin. Electroenceph.* **3**, 160–168.
Weatherall, M. (1962). Tranquillisers. *Brit. med. J.* **1**, 1220.
Wechsler, D. (1939). *The Measurement of Adult Intelligence.* Baltimore: Williams & Wilkins.
Weeks, H. A. (1958). *Youthful Offenders at Highfields: an Evaluation of the Effects of the Short-term Treatment of Delinquent Boys.* Ann Arbor: University of Michigan Press.
Wegmann, T. G. & Smith, D. W. (1963). Incidence of Klinefelter's syndrome among juvenile delinquents and felons. *Lancet,* i, 274.
Weidmann, H., Taeschler, M. & Konzlett, H. (1958). Zur Pharmakologie von Psilocybin, einem Wirkstoff aus Psilocybe mexicana Heim. *Experimentia,* **14**, 378.
Weiner, H., Thaler, M., Resier, M. F. & Mirsky, I. A. (1957). Etiology of duodenal ulcer. 1. Relation of specific psychological characteristics to rate of gastric secretion (serum pepsinogen). *Psychosom. Med.* **19**, 1.
Weinstein, M. R., & Fischer, A. (1971). Combined treatment with E. C.T. and antipsychotic drugs in schizophrenia. *Dis. nerv. Syst.* **32**, 801–808.
Weiskrantz, L. & Wilson, W. A. (1955). Effects of reserpine on emotional behaviour of normal and brain-operated monkeys. *Ann. N.Y. Acad. Sci.* **61**, 36.
Weisman, G., Feirstein, A., & Thomas, C. (1969). Three-day hospitalization–a model for intensive intervention. *Arch. gen. Psychiat.* **21**, 620–629.
Weiss, E. & English, O. S. (1943). *Psychosomatic Medicine: the Clinical Application of Psychopathology to General Medical Problems.* Philadelphia: Saunders.
Weiss, T., & Engel, B. T. (1971). Operant conditioning of heart rate in patients with premature ventricular contractions. *Psychosom. Med.* **33**, 301–321.
Weissenberg, S. (1926). Über Enkopresis. *Z. Kinderheilk,* **40**, 674.
Welford, A. T. (1962). On changes of performance with age. *Lancet,* i, 335.
Welt, L. (1887–88). Über Charakterveränderungen des Menschen infolge von Läsionen der Stirnhirns. *Dtsch. Arch. klin. Med.* **42**, 339.
Weppner, R. S., Stephens, R. C.,& Conrad, H. T. (1972). Methadone: some aspects of its legal and illegal use. *Amer. J. Psychiat.* **129**, 451–455.
Wernicke, C. (1881). *Lehrbuch der Gehirnkrankheiten,* Vol. 2. Berlin: Fischer and Kassel.
Wertham, F. & Wertham, F. (1934). *The Brain as an Organ: its Postmortem Study and Interpretation.* New York: Macmillan.
Westphal, C. (1872). Die Agoraphobie: eine neuropathische Erscheinung. *Archiv. Psychiatrie,* **3**, 138.
Westwood, G. (1960). *A Minority: a Report on the Life of the Male Homosexual in Great Britain.* London: Longmans.
Whipple. A. O. & Frantz, V. K. (1935). Adenoma of islet cells with hyper-insulinism. *Ann. Surg.* **101**, 1299.
White, H. C. (1961). Hypnosis in bronchial asthma. *J. psychosom. Res.* **5**, 272.
White, H. C. & Sim, M. (1959). Imipramine hydrochloride in the treatment of depression. *Bgham. med. Rev.* **20**, 480.
White, H. C. & Warburton, J. (1962). Personal communication on the use of psilocybin.
White, K. L. & Long, W. N. (1958). The incidence of 'psychogenic' fever in a university hospital, *J. chron. Dis.* **8**, 567.

White, M. A., Prout, C. T., Fixsen, C. & Foundeur, M. (1957). Obstetrician's role in post-partum mental illness. *J. Amer. med. Ass.* **165**, 138.

White, W. A. (1935). *Outline of Psychiatry,* 14th Ed. Washington: Nervous and Mental Disease Publishing Coy.

Whitehead, T. N. (1938). *The Industrial Worker: a Statistical Study of Human Relations in a Group of Manual Workers.* Cambridge, Mass.: Harvard University Press.

Whiteley, S., Briggs, D., & Turner, M. (1972). *Dealing with Deviants.* London: Hogarth Press.

Whitfield, A. G. W. (1955). Chlorpromazine jaundice. *Brit. med. J.* **1**, 784.

Whitlock, D. G. & Nauta, W. J. H. (1956). Subcortical projections from the temporal neocortex in macaca mulatta. *J. comp. Neurol.* **106**, 183.

Whitlock, F. A. (1961). Some psychiatric consequences of gastrectomy. *Brit. med. J.* **1**, 1560.

Whitlock, F. A. (1967). The Ganser syndrome. *Brit. J. Psychiat.* **113**, 19.

Whitlock, F. A. & Edwards, J. E. (1968). Pregnancy and attempted suicide. *Comp. Psychiat.* **9**, 1–12.

Whittaker, S. R. F. & Whitehead, T. P. (1956). Acute and latent porphyria. *Lancet,* i, 547.

WHO Expert Committee on Mental Health. Sub Committee on alcoholism (1951) *Alcoholism.* Tech. Rep. Wld. Hlth. Org. No. 42.

WHO Expert Committee on Mental Health (1952). Subcommittee on alcoholism. Second Report. Tech. Rep. Wld Hlth. Org. No. 48.

WHO Expert Committee on Mental Health (1955). *Alcohol and Alcoholism* Tech. Rep. Wld. Hlth. Org. No. 94.

WHO (1959). *Mental Health Problems of Ageing and the Aged.* Sixth report of the expert committee on mental health. Tech. rep. Wld. Hlth. Org. No. 171. Geneva.

WHO. (1969). *Expert Committee on Drug Dependence. Wld. Hlth. Org. tech. Rep.* Ser. 407. Reprint.

Whitten, C. F., Pettit, M. G., & Fischhoff, J. (1969). Evidence that growth failure from maternal deprivation is secondary to undereating. *J. Amer. med. Ass.* **209**,1675–1682.

Whybrow, P. C., Kane, F. J., & Lipton, M. A. (1968). Regional ileitis and psychiatric disorder. *Psychosom. Med.* **30**, 209–221.

Wickramasekera, I. (1972). Electromyographic feedback training and tension headache: preliminary observations. *Amer. J. Clin. Hypn.* **15**, 83–85.

Wiener, J. M., Delano, J. G. & Klass, D. W. (1966). An EEG study of delinquent and non-delinquent adolescents. *Arch. Gen. Psychiat.* **15**, 144.

Wiener, N. (1948). *Cybernetics: or Control and Communication in the Animal and the Machine.* New York: Wiley.

Wikler, A. (1951). Merchanisms of action of drugs that modify personality function. *Amer. J. Psychiat.* **108**, 590.

Wikler, A. (1952). A psychodynamic study of a patient during experimental self-regulated re-addiction to morphine. *Psychiat. Quart.* **26**, 270.

Wikler, A. (1952). Reactions of dogs without neo-cortex during cycles of addiction to morphine and methadone. *Arch. Neurol. Psychiat.* **67**, 672.

Wilcox, P. H. (1946). Brain facilitation not brain destruction, the aim in electroshock therapy. *Dis. nerv. Syst.* 7, 201.

Wilcox, P. H. (1948). Shock therapy. In *Progress in Neurology and Psychiatry,* Ed. Spiegel E. A. Vol. 3, p. 567. New York: Grune & Stratton.

Wilkinson, R. (1973). *The Broken Rebel. A Study in Culture, Politics, and Authoritarian Character.* London: Croom Helm.

Wilks, S. (1868). Lectures on diseases of the nervous system. General paralysis of the insane. *Med. Times Gaz.* 2, 470.

Willcox, W. (1934). The uses and dangers of hypnotic drugs other than alkaloids. *Brit. Med. J.* **1**, 415.

William, W. (1949). A society of Alcoholics Anonymous. *Amer. J. Psychiat.* **106**, 370.

Williams, D. (1941*a*). The electro-encephalogram in acute head injuries. *J. Neurol. Psychiat. Neurosurg.* **4**, 107.

Williams, D. (1941*b*). The electro-encephalogram in chronic post-traumatic states. *J. Neurol. Psychiat. Neurosurg.* **4**, 131.

Williams, D. (1950). New orientations in epilepsy. *Brit. med. J.* **1**, 685.

Williams, D. (1956). The structure of emotions reflected in epileptic experiences. *Brain,* **79**, 29.

Williams, D. (1958). Modern views on the classification of epilepsy. *Brit. med. J.* **1**, 661.

Williams, D. & Sweet, W. H. (1944). The constitutional factor in anaesthetic convulsions. *Lancet,* ii, 430.

Williams, E. (1958). Anorexia nervosa: a somatic disorder. *Brit. med. J.* **2**, 190.
Williams, G. E. & Johnston, A. M. (1956). Recurrent urinary retention due to emotional factors: report of a case. *Psychosom. Med.* **18**, 77.
Williams, G. P. & Glatt, M. M. (1965). Unrecognized drinking. *Lancet,* ii, 1294.
Williams, L. N., (1969). L.S.D. and manslaughter. *Lancet,* ii, 332.
Wilson, G. W. (1941). A study of structural and instinctual conflict in cases of hay fever. *Psychosom. Med.* **3**, 51.
Wilson, P. J. F. (1973). The surgical treatment of epilepsy. *Brit. J. Hosp. Med.* **9**, 161–168.
Wilson, S. A. K. (1955). *Neurology,* 2nd Ed. Vol. 3, ed. Bruce, A. N. London: Butterworth.
Wing, J. K. & Hailey, A. M. (Eds) (1972). *Evaluating a Community Psychiatric Service.* The Camberwell Register: 1964–71. London: Oxford Univ. Press.
Wing, L. (1964). Autistic Children. London: National Association for Mental Health.
Winnicott, D. W. (1951). Leucotomy in psychosomatic disorders. *Lancet,* ii, 314.
Winnicott, D. W. (1953). Transitional objects and transitional phenomena. *Int. J. Psychoanal.* **34**, 89–97.
Wiseman, F. (1961). Psychiatry and law: use and abuse of psychiatry in a murder case. *Amer. J. Psychiat.* **118**, 289.
Wishnie, H. A., Hackett, T. P., & Cassem, N. H. (1971). Psychological hazards of convalescence following myocardial infarction. *J. Amer. med. Ass.* **215**, 1292–1296.
Wittkower, E. (1938). Ulcerative colitis: personality studies. *Brit. med. J.* **2**, 1356.
Wittkower, E. (1949). *A Psychiatrist looks at Tuberculosis.* London: National Association for the Prevention of Tuberculosis.
Wittkower, E. & Wilson, A. T. M. (1940). Dysmenorrhoea and sterility: personality studies, *Brit. med. J.* **2**, 586.
Wittkower, E. D. (1970). Transcultural psychiatry in the Caribbean: past, present and future. *Amer. J. Psychiat.* **127**, 162–166.
Wittkower, E. D. & Lester, E. P. (1962). *Psychosomatic Aspects of Skin Disorders.* Basle: Geigy.
Wittkower, E. D. & Russell, B. (1953). *Emotional Factors in Skin Disease.* New York: Hoeber.
Wittkower, E. D. & White, K. L. (1959). Psychophysiologic aspects of respiratory disorders. In *American Handbook of Psychiatry,* Vol. 1, ed. Arieti, S. New York: Basic Books.
Wolf, A. & Cowen, D. (1952). Histopathology of schizophrenia and other psychoses of unknown origin. In Milbank Memorial Fund, *The Biology of Mental Health and Disease,* p. 469. New York: Hoeber.
Wolf, S. & Wolfe, H. G. (1947). *Human Gastric Function: an Experimental Study of a Man and His Stomach,* 2nd Ed. New York: Oxford University Press.
Wolfenden, J. (Chairman) (1957). *Report of the Departmental Committee on Homosexual Offences and Prostitution.* Home Office Committee on homosexual offences and prostitution. Cmd. 247. London: H.M.S.O.
Wolfers, H. (1970). Psychological aspects of vasectomy. *Brit. med. J.,* **4**, 297–300.
Wolff, H. G. (1948). Headache and Other Head Pain. New York: Oxford University Press.
Woloshin, A. A., & Pomp, H. C. (1969). *Implementation barriers to community mental health programs.* Vol. 2., pp. 6–15.
Wolpe, J. (1958) *Psychotherapy by Reciprocal Inhibition.* Stanford, California: Stanford University Press.
Woodruff, R. A., Pitts, F. N., & McClure, J. N. (1968). The drug modification of E.C.T. I. Methohexital, Thiopental and pre-oxygenation. *Arch. gen. Psychiat.* **18**, 605–611.
Woodruff, R. A., Robins, L. N. Winokur, G., & Reich, T. (1971). Manic-depressive illness and social achievement. *Acta Psychiat. Scand.* **47**, 237–249.
Woodward, M. (1965). Piaget's theory. In *Modern Perspectives in Child Psychiatry,* ed. Howells, J. G. Edinburgh: Oliver & Boyd.
Woolley, D. W. & Shaw, E. (1954). A biochemical and pharmacological suggestion about certain mental disorders. *Science,* **119**, 587.
Wootton, B. (1963). The law, the doctor and the deviant. *Brit. med. J.* **2**, 197.
Worster-Drought, C., Greenfield, J. G. & McMenemey, W. H. (1940). A form of familial presenile dementia with spastic paralysis (including the pathological examination of a case). *Brain,* **63**, 237.
Wortis, J. (1937). Note on body build of male homosexual. *Amer. J. Psychiat.* **93**, 1121.
Wortis, J. (1950). *Soviet Psychiatry.* Baltimore: Williams & Wilkins.
Wortis, S. B. & Pfeffer, A. Z. (1950). Management of alcoholism. Veterans *Adm. techn. Bull. T.B.* 10–67, pp. 1–23, Oct. 31.

Wright, J. T., & Das, A.K. (1973). Urinary excretion of homovanillic acid (HVA) and vanillylmandelic acid (VMA) in patients with diarrhoea of presumed nervous origin. *J. Psychosom. Res.* 17, 155–157.
Wycis, H. T. & Spiegel, E. A. (1956). Treatment of certain types of chorea, athetosis and tremor by stereoencephalotomy. *J. int. Coll. Surg.* 25, 202.

Yap, P. M. (1951). Mental diseases peculiar to certain cultures: a survey of comparative psychiatry. *J. ment. Sci.* 97, 313.
Yap, P. M. (1952). The Latah reaction: its pathodynamics and nosological position. *J. ment. Sci.* 98, 515.
Yudkin, J. (1956). Man's choice of food. *Lancet,* i, 645.

Zeller, E. A., Barsky, J., Berman, E. R. & Fouts, J. R. (1952). Action of isonicotinic acid hydrazide and related compounds on enzymes of brain and other tissues. *J. Lab. clin. Med.* **40**, 965.
Zeller, E. A., Barsky, J., Fouts, J. R. Kircheimer, W. F. & Van Orden, L. S. (1952). Influence of isonicotinic acid hydrazide (INH) and isonicotinyl-2-isopropyl hydrazide (IIH) on bacterial and mammalian enzyme. *Experimentia* (*Basel*), **8**, 349.
Zelman, S., & Guillan, R. (1970). Heat stroke in phenothiazine-treated patients: a report of three fatalities. *Amer. J. Psychiat.* **126**, 1787–1790.
Ziegler, F. J., Rodgers, D. A., & Prentiss, R. J. (1969). Psychosocial response to vasectomy. *Arch. Gen. Psychiat.* 21, 46–54.
Zilboorg, G. (1928). Post-partum schizophrenia. *J. nerv. ment. Dis.* **68**, 370.
Zilboorg, G. (1929). Dynamics of schizophrenic reactions related to pregnancy and childbirth. *Amer. J. Psychiat.* **8**, 733.
Zilboorg, G. (1931). Depressive reactions related to parenthood. *Amer. J. Psychiat.* **10**, 927.
Zilboorg, G. (1936*a*). Differential diagnostic types of suicide. *Arch. Neurol. Psychiat.* **35**, 270.
Zilboorg, G. (1936*b*). Suicide among civilized and primitive races. *Amer. J. Psychiat.* **92**, 1347.
Zwerling, I. & Rosenbaum, M. (1959). Alcoholic addiction and personality. In *American Handbook of Psychiatry,* ed. Arieti, S. New York: Basic Books.

Index